MW00668463

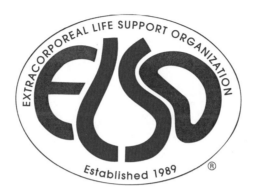

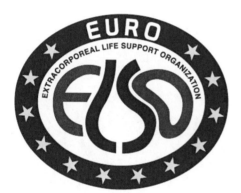

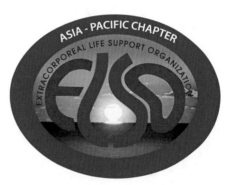

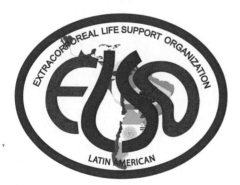

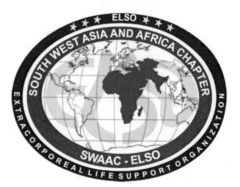

lostov

# Extracorporeal Life Support: The ELSO Red Book

# 6th Edition

Graeme MacLaren, MD, MSc
Daniel Brodie, MD
Roberto Lorusso, MD, PhD
Giles Peek, MD
Ravi Thiagarajan, MD, MPH
Leen Vercaemst, RN, ECCP

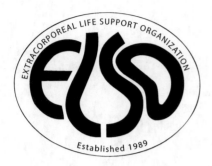

Extracorporeal Life Support: The ELSO Red Book

6th Edition

Editor-in-chief: Graeme MacLaren
Editors: Daniel Brodie, Roberto Lorusso, Giles Peek, Ravi Thiagarajan, Leen Vercaemst
Manuscript Editor: Cindy Cooke
Cover Design: Velia Antonini, Sudeep Chatterjee
Back Cover: ECMO team taking care of a patient during the COVID-19 pandemic. Clinica Las Condes, Santiago de Chile 2021. Photographer: Francisca Selman. Provided by: Rodrigo Diaz.
Layout: Peter Rycus, Christine Stead

©2022 Extracorporeal Life Support Organization, Ann Arbor, Michigan

Previous editions 1996, 2000, 2005, 2012, 2017

Printed in the United States of America

ISBN 978-0-9656756-8-0

v1.00

# Dedication

Toward the end of 2019, a hitherto unknown coronavirus triggered the most devastating pandemic in over 100 years, infecting hundreds of millions of people; causing millions of deaths; and crippling international travel, trade, and society.

Across the globe, healthcare professionals cared for unprecedented numbers of critically ill patients, regardless of the risks, and often at great personal cost.

This book is dedicated to them.

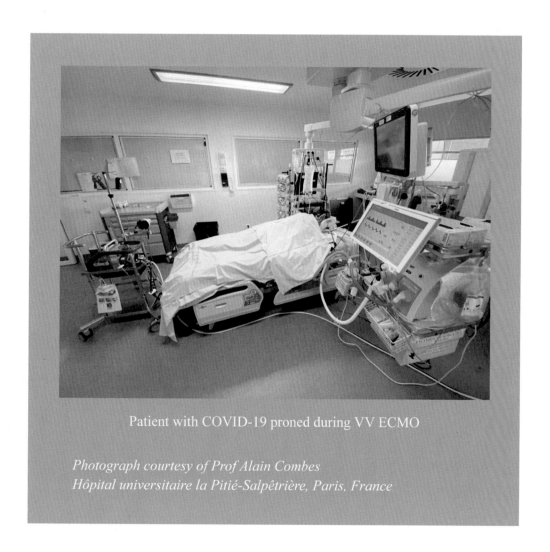

Patient with COVID-19 proned during VV ECMO

*Photograph courtesy of Prof Alain Combes*
*Hôpital universitaire la Pitié-Salpêtrière, Paris, France*

# Foreword

Göttingen, July 13th, 2022

When dealing with any medical problem which requires a conceptual, technical, and practical resolute intervention, three basic questions have to be answered: Why do it? How to do it? When to do it? ie, what are the indications for a given approach; how should the technique be applied; and the timing of application and withdrawal. The Sixth Edition of what is now simply called 'The Red Book' answers all these questions regarding extracorporeal life support (ECLS) through simple, clear, and essential concepts and language. It is emotional and an honor for me that I had the fortune to follow the development of extracorporeal support throughout five decades, to present this book, realizing in the meantime how ECLS has been disseminated throughout the world, adding a powerful therapeutic tool to our instruments to preserve life. This is a great credit to the Extracorporeal Life Support Organization (ELSO), whose membership has exponentially increased over time and provided education, data sharing, and supported several research initiatives. ELSO and 'The Red Book' are the fruit of a multinational collaboration of experts dedicated to the advancement in the field and education of new members and centers.

I cannot end this Foreword without mentioning Drs. Kolobow and Zapol, mentors and friends who recently left us. These giants, decades ago, had a dream that we now see realized.

Nobody knows the future, but I am pretty sure that the passion and enthusiasm which characterizes ECLS people, far more than other medical disciplines, will allow further dreams and advances. To these people, my Foreword is dedicated.

Luciano Gattinoni

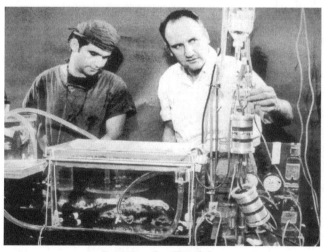

Drs. Zapol and Kolobow

# List of Contributors

Mohd Hafiz Abdul-Aziz, BPharm PhD
Research Fellow & Clinical Research Pharmacist
The University of Queensland, Brisbane, Australia
*Chapter 49*

Darryl Abrams, MD
Associate Director, Medical ECMO Program
Columbia University Medical Center, New York, USA
*Chapters 43, 57*

Cara Agerstrand, MD
Director of the Medical ECMO Program
Columbia University Medical Center, New York, USA
*Chapters 7, 24, 34, 46*

Ali Akil, MD
Thoracic surgeon, Leader of ECMO Divison
Thoracic Surgery and Lung Support, Ibbenbueren, Germany
*Chapter 51*

Peta M. A. Alexander, MBBS
Director of Cardiac ECMO
Boston Children's Hospital, Boston, Massachusetts, USA
*Chapters 20, 41, 58, 60*

Gail Mary Annich, MD MS FELSO
Director of Resuscitation/Mass Casualty HSC
The Hospital for Sick Children, Toronto, Canada
*Chapters 6, 14*

Marta Velia Antonini, CCP MS
Cardiovascular Perfusionist
Bufalini Hospital - AUSL della Romagna, Cesena, Italy
*Chapters 7, 53, 54*

Toshiyuki Aokage, MD PhD
Asst. Prof., Emergency & Critical Care Medicine
Okayama University Hospital, Okayama, Japan
*Chapter 55*

Jutta Arens, PhD
Chair of Engineering Organ Support Technologies
University of Twente, The Netherlands
*Chapter 3*

Erin August, RN MSN
Adult ECMO Coordinator
Memorial Regional Hospital, Florida, USA
*Chapter 46*

Jenelle H. Badulak, MD
Emergency Medicine & Intensive Care
University of Washington, Seattle, Washington, USA
*Chapter 2*

Ryan Pasquale Barbaro, MD MSc FELSO
Service Chief, Pediatric Critical Care
University of Michigan, Ann Arbor, Michigan, USA
*Chapters 13, 58, 60*

Kali Alyssa Barrett, MD MSc
Critical Care Physician
University Health Network, Toronto, Canada
*Chapter 56*

Nicholas A. Barrett, MBBS
Director of Critical Care
Guy's & St Thomas' NHS Trust, London, UK
*Chapter 26*

David J. Barron, MBBS MD
Division Head, Cardiovascular Surgery
Hospital for Sick Children, Toronto, Canada
*Chapter 18*

Robert H. Bartlett, MD FELSO
Professor of Surgery, Emeritus
University of Michigan, Ann Arbor, Michigan, USA
*Chapters 1, 5, 45*

Andriy Batchinsky, MD
Director, AREVA Innovation Institute
The Geneva Foundation, San Antonio, Texas, USA
*Chapter 6*

John Samuel Beca, MBChB
Director of Surgery and Intensive Care
Starship Children's Hospital, Auckland, New Zealand
*Chapter 53*

Thomas Bein, MD
Senior Professor, Faculty of Medicine
University of Regensburg, Germany
*Chapter 57*

Dorothy M Beke, MS RN CPNP-PC/AC
CICU Nurse Practice Specialist
Boston Children's Hospital, Boston, Massachusetts,
USA
*Chapter 18*

Jan Bělohlávek, MD PhD
Professor of Medicine
Deputy Head, Dept. of CV Medicine
General University Hospital, Prague, Czech Republic
*Chapter 32*

Melania M. Bembea, MD MPH PhD
Director, Johns Hopkins Pediatric ECMO Program
Johns Hopkins University, Baltimore, Maryland, USA
*Chapters 39, 55*

Christoph Benk, PhD
Chief Perfusionist
University Hospital Freiburg, Germany
*Chapter 42*

Christian Bermudez, MD
Director of Thoracic Transplantation
Hospital of the University of Pennsylvania, Phila-
delphia, Pennsylvania, USA
*Chapters 40, 53*

Mark S. Bleiweis, MD
Congenital Heart Center Director
University of Florida, Florida, USA
*Chapters 20, 31*

Adam Blumenberg, MD MA
Assistant Professor of Emergency Medicine
Columbia University Medical Center, New York, USA
*Chapter 37*

Benjamin Bongiorno, RN
Hôpital Pitié-Salpêtrière
Paris, France
*Chapter 28*

Matthew J. Brain, MBBS PhD
Intensive Care Staff Specialist
Launceston General Hospital, Launceston, Australia
*Chapter 5*

Susan L. Bratton, MD MPH
Emeritus Professor of Pediatrics
University of Utah, Utah, USA
*Chapter 16*

Nicolas Bréchot, MD PhD
Medical ICU
Pitié-Salpêtrière University Hospital, Paris, France
*Chapter 36*

Brian C. Bridges, MD
ECMO Medical Director
Vanderbilt University Medical Center, Nashville,
Tennessee, USA
*Chapter 42*

Daniel Brodie, MD FELSO
Director, Adult ECMO Program
Columbia University Medical Center, New York, USA
*Chapters 2, 23, 52, 57, 58*

Thomas Brogan, MD FELSO
Medical Director, Pediatric ECMO Program
Seattle Children's Hospital, Seattle, Washington, USA
*Chapter 13*

Lars Mikael Broman, MD PhD
Principal Investigator ECMO Centre Karolinska
Karolinska University Hospital, Stockholm, Sweden
*Chapter 2*

Katherine Louise Brown, MD MPH
Professor of Pediatric Cardiac Intensive Care
Great Ormond Street Hospital, London, UK
*Chapter 22*

Hergen Buscher, MD
Senior Specialist Intensive Care
St Vincent's Hospital, Sydney, UNSW, Australia
*Chapter 27*

Warwick Butt, MB BS FELSO
Consultant, Intensive Care
Royal Childrens Hospital, Melbourne, Australia
*Chapter 36*

Daniele Camboni, MD MHBA
Cardiac Surgeon
University Medical Center Regensburg, Germany
*Chapter 33*

Jeremy Cannon, MD, SM
Trauma Program Medical Director
University of Pennsylvania, Philadelphia, USA
*Chapter 35*

Rachel Chapman, MD
Medical Director, NICCU
Children's Hospital Los Angeles, California, USA
*Chapter 8*

Ivan J. Chavez, MD
Interventional Cardiology
Minneapolis Heart Institute, Minnesota, USA
*Chapter 4*

Ira M. Cheifetz, MD
Chief, Cardiology and Cardiac Critical Care
Rainbow Babies & Children's Hospital, Cleveland, Ohio, USA
*Chapter 14*

Yih-Sharng Chen, MD PhD
Director of Cardiovascular Center
National Taiwan University Hospital, Taiwan
*Chapters 32, 38*

Hwa Jin Cho, MD PhD
Associate Professor
Chonnam National University Hospital, Gwangju, S. Korea
*Chapter 18*

Sung-Min Cho, DO MHS
Director, Adult ECMO Research
Johns Hopkins Hospital, Baltimore, Maryland, USA
*Chapter 33*

Alain Combes, MD PhD FELSO
Head of ICU, Director of ECMO program
APHP Sorbonne Universite Paris, France
*Chapters 30, 44, 58*

Steven A. Conrad, MD PhD MCCM FELSO
Director, Extracorporeal Organ Support Program
Louisiana State University Health, Shreveport, Louisiana, USA
*Chapter 2*

Mackenzie R. Cook, MD
Assistant Professor of Surgery
Oregon Health & Science University, Portland, USA
*Chapter 46*

David S. Cooper, MD MPH
Medical Director, The Heart Institute
Cincinnati Children's Hospital Medical Center, Cincinnati, USA
*Chapters 17, 42*

Jessica B. Cornman, PT DPT PCS
Pediatric Physical Therapist, PhD Student
UF Health and the University of Florida, USA
*Chapter 47*

Matthew E. Cove, MBChB
Senior Consultant, Department of Medicine
National University Hospital, Singapore
*Chapter 43*

Susana Cruz Beltran, MD
Pediatric Cardiac Anesthesiologist
University of Florida, Florida, USA
*Chapter 50*

Marta Cucchi, MSc TND BSN
Senior Pediatric Cardiac Intensive Care Nurse
Maastricht University, The Netherlands
*Chapter 47*

Marcelo Cypel, MD MSc
Surgical Director Transplant Centre at UHN
University of Toronto, Toronto, Canada
*Chapters 40, 47*

Heidi Dalton, MD MCCM FELSO
Director of ECLS Research/ Program Development
INOVA Health System, Falls Church VA, USA
*Chapters 13, 58*

Mark Davidson, MBChB BSc
Director Cardiac & ECLS Service
Royal Hospital for Children Glasgow, UK
*Chapter 14*

Carl F. Davis, MB BCh BAO MCh
Consultant Paediatric & Neonatal Surgeon
Royal Hospital for Children, Glasgow, UK
*Chapter 8*

Filip De Somer, PhD ECCP
Chief perfusionist
University Hospital Ghent, Belgium
*Chapter 7*

Joseph Dearani, MD
Consultant
Mayo Clinic, Rochester, Minnesota, USA
*Chapter 31*

Erik DeSoucy, DO
Trauma and Critical Care Surgeon
Brooke Army Medical Center, Fort Sam Houston, Texas, USA
*Chapter 35*

Matteo Di Nardo, MD
Senior Consultant, Pediatric ICU
Children's Hospital Bambino Gesù, IRCCS, Italy
*Chapters 39, 60*

Janet Diaz, MD
World Health Organization
Geneva, Switzerland
*Chapter 59*

Rodrigo Diaz, MD MB FELSO
OR and ECMO Chief
Clinica Red Salud Santiago, Chile
*Chapters 53, 59*

Michele B. Domico, MD
Associate Director, Cardiovascular ICU
Children's Hospital of Orange County, California, USA
*Chapter 22*

Dirk W. Donker, MD PhD
Professor Cardiovascular Respiratory Physiology
University of Twente, Enschede, The Netherlands
*Chapters 28, 48*

Ghislaine Douflé, MD MME
Critical care physician
Toronto General Hospital, University of Toronto, Canada
*Chapter 48*

Yves d'Udekem, MD PhD
Division Chief of Cardiac Surgery
Children's National Hospital, Washington, DC, USA
*Chapter 41*

Amy L. Dzierba, PharmD
Critical Care Pharmacist
NewYork-Presbyterian Hospital, New York, USA
*Chapter 37*

Alyaa Elhazmi, MD
Member, MOH National ECMO Program
Ministry of Health (MOH), Saudi Arabia
*Chapter 52*

Eddy Fan, MD PhD
Medical Director, ECLS Program
University Health Network, Toronto, Canada
*Chapters 23, 48, 58*

Jeffrey J. Fanning, MD
Chief, Pediatric Medicine; Director, ECLS
Medical City Children's Hospital, Dallas, Texas, USA
*Chapter 60*

Gail Faulkner, RGN RSCN
ECMO Co-ordinator
University Hospitals of Leicester, UK
*Chapter 9*

Simon J. Finney, MBChB MSc PhD
Consultant in Intensive Care Medicine and ECMO
Barts Health NHS Trust, London, UK
*Chapter 52*

Stefan Fischer, MD MSc
Head of Thoracic Surgery and Lung Support
Ibbenbueren General Hospital, Germany
*Chapter 51*

Dale Fisher, MBBS
Infectious Disease Physician
National University Hospital, Singapore
*Chapter 59*

James D. Fortenberry, MD FELSO
Chief Medical Officer
Children's Healthcare of Atlanta, Georgia, USA
*Chapter 1*

John F. Fraser, MBChB PhD FELSO
Director Critical Care Research Group and ICU
Prince Charles Hospital & U Queensland, Brisbane, Australia
*Chapter 58*

Justin Fried, MD
Associate Director of Cardiac Care Unit
Columbia University Medical Center, New York, USA
*Chapter 27*

Janene H. Fuerch, MD
Clinical Assistant Professor
Stanford University School of Medicine, Palo Alto, California, USA
*Chapter 9*

David Furfaro, MD
Associate MICU Director
Beth Israel Deaconess Medical Center, Boston, USA
*Chapter 24*

Francis Fynn-Thompson, MD
Surgical Director, Advanced Cardiac Therapies
Boston Children's Hospital, Boston, USA
*Chapter 22*

Luciano Gattinoni, MD FELSO
Guest Professor
University of Medicine of Göttingen, Germany
*Foreword*

Katja M. Gist, DO MSc
Co-Director, Center for Acute Care Nephrology
Cincinnati Children's Hospital Medical Center, Ohio, USA
*Chapter 42*

Giacomo Grasselli, MD
Medical Director of Adult ICU
Policlinico Hospital, University of Milan, Italy
*Chapter 23*

Anne-Marie Guerguerian, MD PhD
Medical Director, SickKids ECLS Program
The Hospital for Sick Children, Toronto, Canada
*Chapter 21*

Yigit S. Guner, MD MS
Associate Professor of Surgery
UC Irvine, Children's Hospital of Orange County, California, USA
*Chapter 11*

Amy E. Hackmann, MD
Assoc Prof, Chief of ECMO and Temporary MCS
UT Southwestern Medical Center, Dallas, Texas, USA
*Chapters 4, 30, 40, 51*

Jonathan Haft, MD
Director, Extracorporeal Life Support
University of Michigan, Ann Arbor, Michigan, USA
*Chapter 41*

Jumana Yusuf Haji, MBBS MD
Consultant cardiac critical care ECMO director
Sir HN Reliance Hospital Mumbai, India
*Chapter 52*

Matthew T. Harting, MD MS
Medical Director, Pediatric ECLS
Children's Memorial Hermann Hospital, Houston, Texas, USA
*Chapter 11*

Chris Harvey, MB ChB
ECMO Director
University Hospitals of Leicester, UK
*Chapters 10, 25*

Ibrahim Fawzy Hassan, MD
ECMO Program Director
Hamad Medical Corporation, Qatar
*Chapter 53*

Jonathan Hastie, MD
Medical Director of Cardiothoracic ICU
New York Presbyterian/Columbia, New York, USA
*Chapter 50*

Micheal Heard, RN FELSO
Advanced Technologies Coordinator
Children's Healthcare of Atlanta, Georgia, USA
*Chapters 14, 60*

Daniel L Herr, MD MS
Director Critical Care
Hilton Head Hospital, Okatie, South Carolina, USA
*Chapters 24, 47*

Carol Hodgson, PhD PT MPhil
Specialist ICU Physiotherapist, Alfred Health
Monash University and Alfred Health, Australia
*Chapters 26, 47, 58*

Aparna Hoskote, MBBS MD
Clinical Lead Pediatric Cardiac Intensive Care
Great Ormond Street Hospital for Children, London, UK
*Chapter 12, 22*

Xiaotong Hou, MD PhD
Director of Center for Cardiac Intensive Care
Beijing Anzhen Hospital, Beijing, China
*Chapter 57*

Katarzyna Hryniewicz, MD
Medical Director VA ECMO Program
Allina Health Minneapolis Heart Institute, Minnesota, USA
*Chapter 27*

Maayke Hunfeld, MD PhD
Pediatric Neurologist
Erasmus Medical Center, The Netherlands
*Chapter 16*

Rob Hyslop, RN
ECMO Coordinator
Medical City Children's Hospital, Dallas, Texas, USA
*Chapter 60*

Shingo Ichiba, MD PhD
Professor of Intensive Care Medicine
Tokyo Women's Medical University, Tokyo, Japan
*Chapter 35*

Hanneke Ijsselstijn, MD PhD
Associate Professor
Erasmus MC, Sophia, Rotterdam, The Netherlands
*Chapter 12*

Jeffrey Phillip Jacobs, MD
Professor of Surgery and Pediatrics
University of Florida, Florida, USA
*Chapters 21, 31*

Ina Jochmans, MD PhD
Abdominal Transplant Surgeon
KU Leuven, University Hospitals Leuven, Belgium
*Chapter 45*

Timothy J. Jones, MD
Congenital Cardiac Surgeon
Birmingham Women's and Children's Hospital, UK
*Chapters 17, 54*

Jae Seung Jung, MD PhD
Director of ICU
Korea University Anam Hospital, South Korea
*Chapter 29*

Madelyn Kahana, MD
Director, PICU
Nemours Children's Hospital, Orlando, Florida, USA
*Chapter 50*

Christian Karagiannidis, MD
Head ARDS and ECMO Centre Cologne-Merheim
University Witten/Herdecke, Germany
*Chapter 43*

Javier Kattan, MD
Medical School & ECMO UC Program Director
Pontificia Universidad Católica de Chile
*Chapter 11*

Christa Jefferis Kirk, PharmD BCCP
Heart Center Clinical Pharmacy Specialist
Seattle Children's Hospital, Washington, USA
*Chapter 49*

Roxanne Kirsch, MD MBE
Interim Division Chief Cardiac Critical Care
The Hospital for Sick Children, Toronto, Canada
*Chapter 18*

Theo Kofidis, MD PhD
Head, Dept of Cardiothoracic and Vascular Surgery
National University Hospital, Singapore
*Chapter 51*

Mariusz Kowalewski, MD PhD
Assistant Professor, Cardiac Surgery Department
Central Clinical Hospital, Warsaw, Poland
*Chapter 38*

Ahmed Labib, MBBCh MSc
Senior Consultant MICU
Hamad General Hospital, Doha, Qatar
*Chapter 46*

Kevin P. Lally, MS MD
Chairman, Department of Pediatric Surgery
McGovern Medical School at UTHealth Houston,
Texas, USA
*Chapter 11*

Giovanni Landoni, MD
Full Professor
Vita-Salute San Raffaele University, Milan, Italy
*Chapter 38*

Peter C. Laussen, MBBS
Executive Vice President Health Affairs
Boston Children's Hospital, Boston, Massachusetts, USA
*Chapters 21, 55*

Robert Burnham Laverty, MD
General Surgery Resident
Brooke Army Medical Center, Fort Sam Houston,
Texas, USA
*Chapter 35*

Guillaume Lebreton, MD PhD
Director of Perfusion, ECMO and MCS programs
Pitié-Salpêtrière Hôpital, Sorbonne University, Paris,
France
*Chapter 29*

Laurance Lequier, MD
Medical Director PICU
Stollery Children's Hospital, Alberta, Canada
*Chapter 19*

Roberto Lorusso, MD PhD FELSO
Professor of Cardiac Surgery and ECLS
Deputy Director Cardio-Thoracic Surgery Dept.
Maastricht University Medical Centre, The Netherlands
*Chapters 1, 2, 4, 27, 38, 44*

Peter Simon Macdonald, MBBS PhD MD
Medical Director, Heart Transplant Unit
St Vincent's Hospital, Sydney, Australia
*Chapter 45*

Graeme MacLaren, MBBS MSc FELSO
Director of Cardiothoracic ICU
National University Hospital, Singapore
*Chapters 2, 6, 15, 24, 31, 36, 49, 52, 59*

Purnema Madahar, MD MS
Assistant Director of Medical ICU
Columbia University Medical Center, USA
*Chapter 23*

Brian E. Malley, MD
Clinical Instructor in Critical Care Medicine
University of Pittsburgh, Pennsylvania, USA
*Chapter 25*

Silvia Mariani, MD PhD Fellow
Cardiac Surgeon
Maastricht University, The Netherlands
*Chapter 27*

Gennaro Martucci, MD PhD
Attending for Anesthesia and Intensive Care
IRCCS-ISMETT, Palermo, Italy
*Chapter 6*

Eva Miranda Marwali, MD PhD
Pediatric Cardiac Intensivist
NCC Harapan Kita, Jakarta, Indonesia
*Chapter 52*

Phillip E. Mason, MD MS
ECMO Medical Director
Brooke Army Medical Center, Fort Sam Houston, Texas, USA
*Chapter 7*

Timothy M. Maul, CCP FPP PhD
Perfusionist and Senior Research Scientist
Nemours Children's Health, Orlando, Florida, USA
*Chapters 3, 44*

Tommaso Mauri, MD
Associate Professor of Critical Care
University of Milan, Milano, Italy
*Chapter 5*

Michael Mazzeffi, MD
Professor of Anesthesiology
University of Virginia Health
Charlottesville, Virginia, USA
*Chapter 33*

David Michael McMullan, MD
Chief, Cardiac Surgery
Seattle Children's Hospital, Seattle, Washington, USA
*Chapters 19, 51, 52*

Malaika M. Mendonca, MD
Senior Consultant, ECMO Program Director
Children`s University Hospital, Bern, Switzerland
*Chapter 22*

Elizabeth A. Moore, MBA RN BSN
Associate Director, Heart and Vascular Center
University of Iowa Hospitals and Clinics, Iowa, USA
*Chapters 52, 54*

Nicholas Moore, MBBS
Department of Anaesthesia & Heartlink
University of Leicester Hospitals, UK
*Chapter 50*

Gordon Morewood, MD MBA
Professor & Chair, Department of Anesthesiology
Temple University, Philadelphia, Pennsylvania, USA
*Chapter 56*

Tracy Morrison, RN FELSO
Miami Valley Hospital
Dayton, Ohio, USA
*Chapter 55*

Wynne Morrison, MD MBE
Professor, Critical Care & Palliative Care
Univ of Pennsylvania School of Medicine,
Philadelphia, Pennsylvania, USA
*Chapter 57*

Andrea Moscatelli, MD
Director Emergency Department and NICU-PICU
IRCCS Istituto Gainnina Gaslini, Genova, Italy
*Chapter 9*

Katie Moynihan, MBBS
Cardiac Intensivist
Boston Children's Hospital, Boston, Massachusetts, USA
*Chapter 57*

Thomas Müller, MD FELSO
Head of Medical Intensive Care Unit
University Hospital Regensburg, Germany
*Chapters 26, 42*

Dana A. Mullin, CCP MS
Chief Perfusionist, ECMO Services and Education
New York Presbyterian Hospital, New York, USA
*Chapter 54*

Priya Nair, MD
Director of Intensive Care
St Vincents Hospital, Sydney, Australia
*Chapter 34*

Vinodh Bhagyalakshmi Nanjayya, MD
Head of Cardiothoracic ICU
Alfred Hospital, Melbourne, Australia
*Chapter 29*

Emily Elizabeth Naoum, MD
Obstetric Anesthesiologist, Intensivist
Massachusetts General Hospital, Boston, Massachusetts, USA
*Chapter 34*

Viviane G. Nasr, MD MPH
Associate Professor
Boston Children's Hospital, Boston, Massachusetts, USA
*Chapter 50*

Mark T. Ogino, MD FELSO
Chief Partnership Officer
Nemours Children's Health, Delaware, USA
*Chapters 9, 52, 54*

Shinichiro Ohshimo, MD PhD
Associate Professor of ER/ICU
Hiroshima University, Hiroshima, Japan
*Chapter 38*

Neil Orford, MBBS PhD
Senior ICU Consultant
University Hospital Geelong, Geelong, Australia
*Chapter 52*

P. Pearl O'Rourke, MD FELSO
Harvard Medical School, Boston, Massachusetts, USA
*Chapter 1*

Matthew L. Paden, MD
Professor of Pediatric Critical Care
Children's Healthcare of Atlanta, Georgia, USA
*Chapters 42, 60*

Federico Pappalardo, MD
Director Cardiothoracic ICU
AO SS Antonio e Biagio, Alessandria, Italy
*Chapter 44*

David Paredes-Zapata, MD CETC UEMS
Consultant Transplant Coordination, Asst Prof
Hospital Clinic, University of Barcelona, Spain
*Chapter 45*

Bhavesh Patel, MD
Consultant, Critical Care Medicine
Mayo Clinic, Phoenix, Arizona, USA
*Chapter 28*

Giles J. Peek, MD FELSO
Professor of Surgery and Pediatrics
University of Florida, Florida, USA
*Chapters 4, 10, 31, 37, 51*

Vin Pellegrino, MBBS FELSO
Head of ECMO Clinical Services
Alfred Health, Melbourne, Australia
*Chapter 25*

Tanya Perry, DO
Cardiac ICU/Ventricular Assist Device Program
Cincinnati Children's Hospital Medical Center, Cincinnati, Ohio, USA
*Chapter 17*

Antonio Pesenti, MD FELSO
Director of Anesthesia, Critical Care and Emergency
Fondazione IRCCS Cà Granda Ospedale Maggiore
Policlinico, Milano, Italy
*Chapter 43*

Thomas Pranikoff, MD
Surgeon-in-Chief, Brenner Children's
Atrium Health Wake Forest Baptist, Winston-Salem,
North Carolina, USA
*Chapter 15*

Susanna Price, MD PhD
Clinical Lead Cardiogenic Shock Programme
Royal Brompton, Harefield Hospitals, London, UK
*Chapter 32*

Parthak Prodhan, MD MBA
Director of Pediatric Cardiothoracic ICU
Arkansas Children's Hospital, Arkansas, USA
*Chapter 16*

Ahmed Abdulhamid Rabie, MD
Director of ECMO Program, ICU Consultant
King Saud Medical City, Riyadh, Saudi Arabia
*Chapter 52*

Lakshmi Raman, MD
Medical Director of ECMO, Childrens Health
UT Southwestern Medical Center, Dallas, Texas, USA
*Chapter 16*

Raj Ramanan, MD
Medical Director, ECMO
University of Pittsburgh Medical Center, Pittsburgh,
Pennsylvania, USA
*Chapter 25*

Kollengode Ramanathan, MD
Senior Consultant, Cardiothoracic ICU
National University Hospital, Singapore
*Chapters 34, 54*

Hannah Rando, MD MPH
Postdoctoral Research Fellow
Johns Hopkins Hospital, Baltimore, Maryland, USA
*Chapter 33*

Jordi Riera, MD PhD
Intensivist. Director of adult ECMO Program
Hospital Universitari Vall d'Hebron, Barcelona,
Spain
*Chapter 47*

Natalie Rintoul, MD
Medical Director Neonatal Surgical Service/ECMO
Children's Hospital of Philadelphia, Pennsylvania, USA
*Chapter 8*

Jason A. Roberts, PhD BPharm BAppSc
Professor of Medicine & NHMRC Leadership Fellow
The University of Queensland, Brisbane, Australia
*Chapter 49*

Teryn R. Roberts, PhD
Principal Investigator
AREVA Research Program, San Antonio, Texas, USA
*Chapter 6*

Peter Paul Roeleveld, MD PhD
Medical Director of PICU
Leiden University Medical Center, The Netherlands
*Chapters 18, 51*

Alvaro Rojas-Pena, MD
Assistant Research Scientist of Surgery
University of Michigan, Ann Arbor, Michigan, USA
*Chapter 45*

Erika B. Rosenzweig, MD
Director, Pulmonary Hypertension Center
Columbia University, New York, USA
*Chapter 31*

Jose Alfonso Rubio Mateo-Sidron, MBBS
ICU Consultant
Hospital Universitario 12 de Octubre, Madrid, Spain
*Chapter 28*

Peter Rycus, MPH FELSO
Executive Director
Extracorporeal Life Support Organization (ELSO)
*Chapter 60*

Lindsay M. Ryerson, MD
Pediatric cardiac intensivist
Stollery Children's Hospital, Edmonton, Canada
*Chapter 6*

Pranya Sakiyalak, MD
Bangkok Heart Hospital
Bangkok, Thailand
*Chapter 56*

Leonardo Salazar, MD MSc
Director ECMO and VAD program
Fundacion Cardiovascular de Colombia, Colombia
*Chapter 30*

Bernadette Sanchez Elliott, BSN RN
Adult ECLS Transport Program Manager
Brooke Army Medical Center, Fort Sam Houston,
Texas, USA
*Chapter 46*

Anna Mara Scandroglio, MD
Director of Cardiothoracic ICU
San Raffaele Hospital, Milano, Italy
*Chapter 38*

Gregory Schears, MD
Professor of Anesthesiology
Mayo Clinic, Rochester, Minnesota, USA
*Chapter 31*

Peter Schellongowski, MD
Consultant of Medical Intensive Care
Dept. of Med. I, Medical University of Vienna, Austria
*Chapter 39*

Luregn J. Schlapbach, MD PhD
Head, Department of Intensive Care
University Children's Hospital Zurich, Zurich,
Switzerland
*Chapter 13*

Matthieu Schmidt, MD PhD
Professor of Intensive Care
Pitié-Salpêtrière Hôpital, Paris, France
*Chapters 5, 39, 47, 59*

Steven M. Schwartz, MD MS
Chief, Department of Critical Care Medicine
The Hospital for Sick Children, Toronto, Canada
*Chapters 18, 55*

Ayan Sen, MD MSc
Chair, Department of Critical Care Medicine
Mayo Clinic, Arizona, USA
*Chapter 28*

Omar M. Sharaf, BS
Research Fellow
University of Florida Health, Florida, USA
*Chapter 31*

Kiran Shekar, MBBS PhD
Senior Intensivist & Director of Research
The Prince Charles Hospital, Brisbane, Australia
*Chapters 29, 49*

Lara Shekerdemian, MBChB MD MHA
Pediatrician In-Chief, Professor of Pediatrics
Texas Children's Hospital, College of Medicine,
Houston, Texas, USA
*Chapters 19, 56*

Jayne Sheldrake, MSC BSc
ECLS Clinical Nurse Consultant
Alfred Health, Melbourne, Australia
*Chapter 24*

Riyan Sukumar Shetty, MBBS MD
Consultant, Pediatric Cardiac ICU & ECMO Director
Narayana Institute of Cardiac Sciences, Bengaluru,
Karnataka, India
*Chapter 56*

Billie Lou Short, MD FELSO
Chief, Division of Neonatology
Children's National Hospital, Washington DC, USA
*Chapters 1, 8*

Farah Siddiqui, MBChB DM
Consultant in Fetal and Maternal Medicine
University Hospitals of Leicester NHS Trust,
Leicester, UK
*Chapter 34*

Simon Sin Wai Ching, MBBS
Director of Critical Care Medicine Unit
LKS Faculty of Medicine University of Hong Kong,
Hong Kong
*Chapter 54*

Kai Singbartl, MD MPH
Intensivist & Hospital Medical Director
Mayo Clinic, Phoenix, Arizona, USA
*Chapter 28*

Jonathan Hayden Smith, MBChB
Paediatric Cardiothoracic Anaesthesia
Freeman Hospital, Newcastle upon Tyne, UK
*Chapter 41*

Elena Spinelli, MD
Intensivist
Ospedale Maggiore Policlinico, Milano, Italy
*Chapter 43*

Christine Stead, MHSA
Chief Executive Officer
Extracorporeal Life Support Organization (ELSO)
*Chapter 55*

R. Scott Stephens, MD
Director, Oncology/Bone Marrow Transplant ICU
Johns Hopkins University, Baltimore, Maryland, USA
*Chapter 39*

Yuriy Stukov, MD
Research Fellow
University of Florida, Florida, USA
*Chapter 4*

Erik Su, MD
Assistant Professor, ACHD ICU
Texas Children's Hospital, Houston, Texas, USA
*Chapter 48*

Alexander Supady, MD MPH
Attending Physician
Medical Center, University of Freiburg, Germany
*Chapters 42, 57*

Denise Suttner, MD
Director Neonatal Services, Director of ECMO
UC San Diego, Rady Childrens Hospital, San Diego,
California, USA
*Chapter 11*

Justyna Swol, MD PhD
Clinical Scientist
Paracelsus Medical University Nuremberg, Germany
*Chapters 35, 53*

Sarah Tabbutt, MD PhD
Professor of Pediatrics
University of California, San Francisco, California, USA
*Chapter 17*

Koji Takeda, MD
Director, Cardiac Transplant and ECMO
New York-Presbyterian/Columbia University, New
York, USA
*Chapter 38*

Ravi R. Thiagarajan, MBBS MPH FELSO
Professor of Pediatrics, Harvard University
Chief, Cardiac Critical Care
Boston Children's Hospital, Boston, Massachusetts,
USA
*Chapters 6, 17, 21, 44, 48, 60*

Pierre Tissieres, MD DSc
Director Pediatric ICU
AP-HP Paris Saclay University, Bicetre Hospital, Le
Kremlin-Bicêtre, France
*Chapter 13*

Joseph E. Tonna, MD MS
Section Head, Cardiothoracic Critical Care
University of Utah Health, Utah, USA
*Chapters 27, 60*

John M. Toomasian, MS CCP FELSO
Senior Research Scientist, ECLS Laboratory
University of Michigan, Ann Arbor, Michigan, USA
*Chapter 3*

Sebastian C. Tume, MD
Director of Cardiac Intensive Care Unit
Texas Children's Hospital, Houston, Texas, USA
*Chapter 20*

Eleonore Valencia, MD
CICU Staff Physician
Boston Children's Hospital, Boston, Massachusetts,
USA
*Chapters 37, 49*

Anne Marie Valente, MD
Director, Boston Adult Congenital Heart Program
Boston Children's Hospital, Harvard Medical School,
Boston, USA
*Chapter 31*

Arno van Heijst, MD PhD
Pediatrician-neonatologist
Sophia Childrens Hospital, Rotterdam, The Netherlands
*Chapter 12*

Krisa Van Meurs, MD
Lucile Packard Children's Hospital at Stanford, Palo
Alto, California, USA
*Chapter 9*

Christophe Vandenbriele, MD PhD
Consultant Cardiac Intensive Care
University Hospital Leuven, Belgium
*Chapter 6*

Leen Vercaemst, RN ECCP FELSO
Clinical Perfusionist, ECMO Coordinator
University Hospital Leuven, Belgium
*Chapters 3, 7, 42*

Alain Vuylsteke, BSc MD MA
Consultant in Anaesthesia and Intensive Care
Royal Papworth Hospital, Cambridge, UK
*Chapter 26*

Kevin M. Watt, MD PhD
Division Chief of Clinical Pharmacology
University of Utah, USA
*Chapter 49*

Chris L. Wells, PhD PT CCS ATC
EBP & Research Coordinator
University of Maryland Medical Center, USA
*Chapter 47*

Claire Anne Westrope, MBChB
Consultant PICU|ECMO
University Hospitals Leicester NHS Trust, UK
*Chapter 8*

Glenn J.R. Whitman, MD
Professor and Director, CVSICU
Johns Hopkins School of Medicine, Baltimore,
Maryland, USA
*Chapter 30*

Christopher Wilcox, DO MS
Assistant Professor
Johns Hopkins Hospital, Baltimore, Maryland, USA
*Chapter 30*

K. Taylor Wild, MD
Fellow Physician
Children's Hospital of Philadelphia, Pennsylvania, USA
*Chapter 8*

Demetris Yannopoulos, MD
Professor of Medicine
University of Minnesota, Minneapolis, USA
*Chapters 32, 46*

Jonathan C. Yeung, MD PhD
Assistant Professor
University of Toronto, Toronto, Canada
*Chapter 39*

Bishoy Zakhary, MD
Director of ECMO
Oregon Health & Science University, Oregon, USA
*Chapter 54*

David Zonies, MD MPH MBA
Associate Chief Medical Officer
Oregon Health & Science University, Oregon, USA
*Chapter 46*

# Preface to the 6<sup>th</sup> Edition

Much has changed in the world of extracorporeal life support (ECLS) since the Fifth Edition of the Extracorporeal Life Support Organization (ELSO) Red Book was published in 2017. An ever-increasing amount of research has been published, many centers have developed new programs, and ECLS has become better established as support for numerous conditions. However, none of these changes approach the impact of the emergence of Coronavirus disease 2019 (COVID-19) on the ECLS community, on the ICU community, and on healthcare professionals worldwide. The most devastating emerging infectious disease outbreak since the Influenza A(H1N1) pandemic of 1918, COVID-19 has caused several million deaths, catastrophic social disruption, unprecedented travel restrictions, and widespread economic hardship. The impact on healthcare professionals has been immense, leading to mass resignations in many regions. Throughout this time, the role of ECLS has been re-examined as life support therapy for patients with the most severe pulmonary or cardiac failure, capturing widespread medical and media attention.

ELSO has continued to evolve to meet the needs of the ECLS community. Seven hundred twenty-nine international centers were registered ELSO members at the beginning of 2022, representing a >50% increase since the last edition was published. ELSO has updated important clinical guidelines, established a comprehensive online training program and certification for adult ECLS practitioners, and published a number of pivotal studies in the field.

As with previous editions, and in the spirit of academic collaboration, any figure, table, or text not previously bound by copyright may be reproduced in scientific publications without further permission, conditional on the source being referenced. Common abbreviations can be found in the glossary. This edition of the ELSO Red Book will be available both as a hard copy and an electronic reference as we work toward developing a dedicated online platform fit for our times.

Throughout the book, the terms ECLS and ECMO (extracorporeal membrane oxygenation) are essentially used interchangeably. Those interested in learning the exact differences between the two are directed to Chapter 2 on Nomenclature. While many prefer the more accurate term ECLS, ECMO has fewer syllables, is easier to say in conversation, and has become so firmly established that it is hard to imagine it being laid aside.

Although the COVID-19 pandemic has adversely impacted so many lives, it has also shown the resilience of healthcare professionals in the face of overwhelming clinical demand, fostering many significant international collaborations, and demonstrated that the ECLS community can share protocols, data, and research in order to fulfill our fundamental mission of saving lives. We hope that the Sixth Edition of the ELSO Red Book will contribute to this mission. We would like to thank the many experts who gave freely of their time and energy to contribute to this book despite the ongoing pandemic; Peter Rycus, Cindy Cooke, and Christine Stead for their invaluable help in organization and editing; and Dr Robert H. Bartlett for setting all our feet upon the road.

Graeme MacLaren
Roberto Lorusso
Ravi Thiagarajan

Daniel Brodie
Giles Peek
Leen Vercaemst

**Thank you, Robert H. Bartlett, for 50 Years of ECLS**

2022 marks the 50-year anniversary of the first ever clinical report of ECLS. Dr Robert H. Bartlett was there taking care of patients from the beginning and yet continues to guide the evolution of ECLS and the organization that he founded, ELSO.

His deep commitment to advancing the art and science of critical care medicine has saved many thousands of lives and fostered a flourishing global ECLS community.

On behalf of ELSO and the wider community, we thank him for his unwavering dedication.

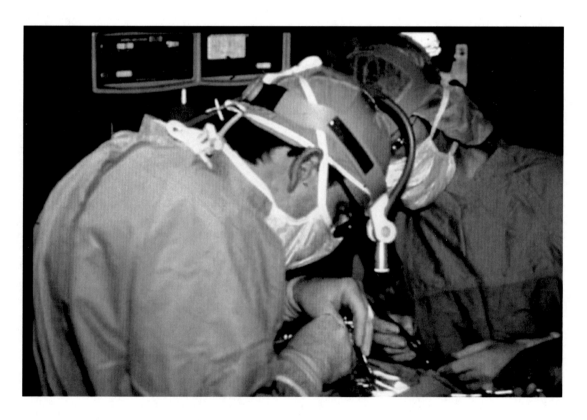

**Dr. Robert H. Bartlett - A Lifetime of Commitment**

# Table of Contents

## Section I. ECLS: General Principles

## Section II. Neonatal Respiratory Failure

## Section III. Pediatric Respiratory Failure

**Section IV. Neonatal and Pediatric Cardiac Failure**

## Section VII. Special Indications

# 1

## The History and Development of Extracorporeal Support

*James D. Fortenberry, Robert H. Bartlett, P. Pearl O'Rourke, Billie Lou Short, Roberto Lorusso*

### The History and Development of Extracorporeal Support

*"During that long night, helplessly watching the patient struggle for life as her blood became darker... the idea naturally occurred to me that if it were possible to remove continuously some of the blue blood...put oxygen into that blood... and then to inject continuously the now-red blood back into the patient's arteries, we might have saved her life."*

*-John Gibbon MD*

### Extracorporeal Support: Earliest Beginnings

Surgeon John Gibbon eloquently described the anguish and powerlessness he felt as a young research fellow in 1931 over the loss of a young patient to a pulmonary embolism.[1] The memory of that single patient was the impetus for Dr. Gibbon to embark on an effort dedicated to the proposition that mimicking or replacing normal human body cardiopulmonary functions during an acute illness could save lives. However, the remarkable story of the development of extracorporeal support can be traced as far back as 1693, when Jean Baptiste Denis performed experiments cross-transfusing the blood of a human with the "gentle humors of a lamb" to determine if living blood could be transmitted

between two species (Figure 1-1). Benjamin Ward Richardson MD, noted British physician and anesthetist, conducted experiments in the 1860s using injected oxygen and blood driven by a syringe to the right heart to generate artificial circulation in an animal model.

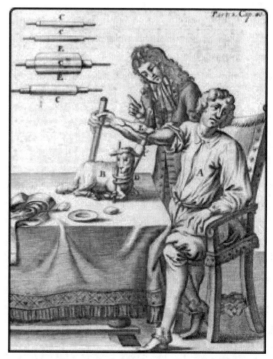

**Figure 1-1.** Woodcarving of experiments circa 1693 by Jean Baptiste Denis to drain human blood into a sheep (Source: Jefferson Medical Archives).

Results were promising, but limited by lack of anticoagulation, leading Richardson to note, "I infer that resuscitation [and artificial circulation]…is a possible process, and that it demands only the elements of time, experiment and patience for its development of a demonstrable fact of modern science."[2] In the 1920s Russian physician Sergei Brukhonenko and collaborators developed a total body perfusion system, called the 'autojector,' using excised donor animal lungs for blood oxygenation, and later a bubble oxygenator, to perform successful animal experiments with isolation of the heart.[3]

Dr. Gibbon began his journey to further advance the field of extracorporeal support in humans in the 1930s. Collaborating with his wife Mary at Jefferson Medical School in Philadelphia, Dr. Gibbon developed a freestanding roller pump device for extracorporeal support. The initial Gibbon heart-lung machine was the size of a spinet piano that created thin films of deoxygenated blood passing over a screen

exposed to oxygen.[1,4]  Twenty-two years would pass before Dr. Gibbon was able to use the device in the operating theater. On May 6, 1953, he performed the first successful extracorporeally assisted repair of an atrial septal defect in 18-year-old Cecilia Bavolek (Figure 1-2).

The esteemed cardiac surgeon C. Walton Lillehei, MD (Figure 1-3) further advanced extracorporeal circulation in the operating room in 1954 when he performed cardiac surgery via cross circulation and then progressed to using a bubble oxygenator which he had invented with Richard DeWall. The remarkable chronicles of early extracorporeal development were captured by Dr. Lillehei in the first edition of the ELSO Red Book.[4,5]

While use of extracorporeal support proved feasible in limited settings in the operating theater, more prolonged use past several hours outside of the OR remained problematic. Early attempts in the ICU for extracorporeal support were limited by the nature of available artificial lung devices and blood gas interfaces, which tended to induce blood component damage from the direct exposure to oxygen gas.[6,7]

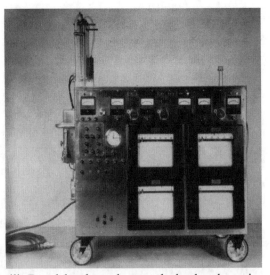

**Figure 1-2.** Left: John H. Gibbon MD and patient Cecilia Bavolek, who underwent the landmark repair in 1953 of an atrial septal defect utilizing an extracorporeal circuit. The two pose before the covered "lung" ten years after the procedure. Right: original device, approximately the size of a spinet piano (Source: Jefferson University Archives).

Bubble oxygenators did not create an interface between blood and gas, producing hemolysis within hours.

The next steps in the development of extracorporeal support were a testimony to the collaboration between biomedical engineers, physiologists, physicians, and surgeons to create devices that could provide support for more extended time periods inside and outside the OR without massive hemolysis and plasma leakage across any membrane or interface. Two basic innovations drove this breakthrough: the invention of silicone and the ability to allow prolonged circuit-blood exposure through controlled anticoagulation.[8] The development of synthesis of silicone rubber by Kammermeyer in 1957 revolutionized the artificial lung.[8,9] Silicone possessed the strength to withstand hydrostatic pressure and yet remain permeable to gas transfer. Collaborative innovators, including Drs. Theodor Kolobow, Al Gazzaniga, Phil Drinker, and Robert Bartlett pioneered

experiments in developing a silicone membrane lung that allowed prolonged circulation[1]. Kolff and Kolobow independently identified and advanced the use of silicone membranes for gas exchange, and Kolobow identified the enhanced gas exchange activity of a spiral-wrapped silicone membrane.[9,10] The use of this spiral-wrapped silicone 'membrane oxygenator' also led to the use of the term extracorporeal membrane oxygenation (ECMO). Bypass became feasible in animal models for days at a time.[11]

Bartlett and Drinker also recognized that the cardiac patient in the operating room needed "infinite" anticoagulation due to stagnation in open surgical repair, but with long-term circulating flow, significantly less heparin would be required.[7] They showed circuits could be used for days using minimal heparin without clot formation or hemorrhage.[11,12] Bartlett and Drinker also described and developed an approach to continuously titrate coagulation and

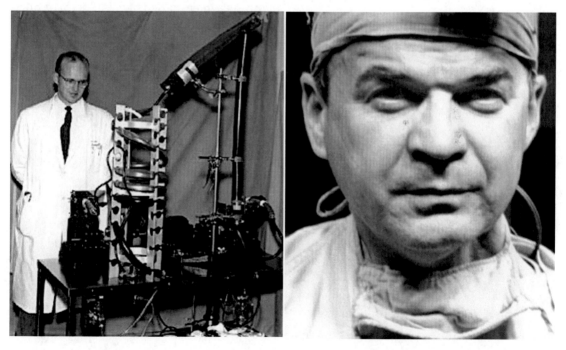

**Figure 1-3.** Bubble oxygenator first used in 1954. Left: Inventor Richard DeWall and device. Right: Dr. C. Walton Lillehei, cardiovascular surgeon and innovator in cardiopulmonary bypass.

heparin dosing via the activated clotting time, a time honored approach that has remained in place for over 40 years.[7]

The benefits of extracorporeal support with membrane oxygenators during a procedure and recovery postoperatively in children with congenital heart disease encouraged physicians to expand its operating room use. Baffes et al.[13] first reported the use of extracorporeal support for palliative neonatal cardiac surgery procedures, followed by experiences from other centers. In 1972, Bartlett, Gazzaniga, and associates first successfully used cardiac ECMO for 36 hours in a 2-year-old infant with cardiac failure following a Mustard procedure for correction of transposition of the great vessels; they subsequently reported a growing series of pediatric cardiac cases.[14] Indications in these patients related to low cardiac output due to ventricular failure or pulmonary vasospastic crisis following surgical repair of complex heart lesions.

With this improved technology, extracorporeal support was extended outside of the operating theater. Dr. J.D. Hill reported on the first successful cannulation and prolonged extracorporeal circuit use in a patient in an intensive care setting in 1972.[15] The patient was a 24 year old male with a ruptured aorta and posttraumatic acute respiratory distress syndrome following a motorcycle accident, who was supported with a membrane lung developed by Morrie Bramson. The patient received venoarterial support for 75 hours, with subsequent decannulation and survival. Adult ECMO support efforts continued, although survival rates were initially low.

Meanwhile, the use of ECLS in neonates also expanded. Dorsons and White reported experience with trials of extracorporeal support[16, 17] in moribund patient cases at the end of life, demonstrating the capability of the support system to provide adequate oxygenation.

Surgeon Dr. Robert Bartlett (Figure 1-4), who has been called the father of modern

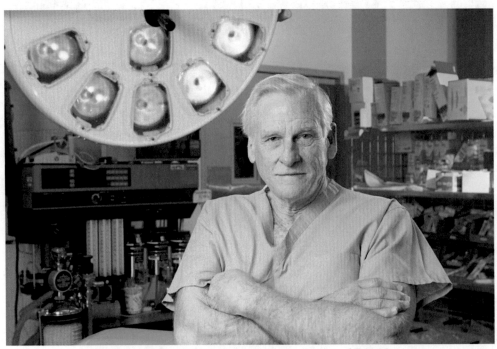

**Figure 1-4.** Dr. Robert H. Bartlett. The Father of ECMO.

extracorporeal support, made a therapeutic decision in 1975 that brought this burgeoning technology to neonates. Faced with a newborn infant dying from meconium aspiration pneumonia and resultant pulmonary hypertension, Bartlett and colleagues brought an ECMO oxygenator to the NICU bedside from the laboratory, and sought consent from the infant's mother, who had delivered her after crossing the Mexican border into Orange County, California. She signed the consent and then disappeared, leaving her baby behind. The nursing staff named the child Esperanza, Spanish for "hope."[18] She received ECMO support for 72 hours, and then was decannulated with recovery, and a subsequent life with children of her own (Figure 1-5).[19,20] Bartlett's success and further experience helped drive growing successful expansion of use in neonates around the world. From 3 survivors among 16 patients treated by Bartlett and colleagues, clinical outcomes consistently improved,[21-23] which promoted the interest and application in the surgical and intensive care communities. Published reports showed ongoing improvements in outcomes, increasing survival rates to 75% for neonatal diseases previously associated with only 10% survival.

Expansion of the use of ECMO in neonates ran counter to typical use of new medical and technologic interventions, which had typically advanced first in adults. With growing interest, the medical community sought randomized, controlled trial (RCT) evidence of the benefits of neonatal extracorporeal support over standard therapies. Dr. Bartlett and colleagues at the University of Michigan initiated an ECMO RCT with an intriguing statistical twist to give preference in the trial to a therapy which appeared superior. Their "randomized play the winner" approach began with randomization but gave increased preference based on the success or failure of the previous patient. During the study, the first patient receiving ECMO survived. The next patient, randomized to standard care, died. Increased preference went to ECMO, and the next ten patients, all receiving ECMO, survived. The study[24] was published in 1985 to significant controversy and discussion, including concern that control patients did not undergo informed consent. The findings, however, encouraged growing use of ECMO support in neonates.

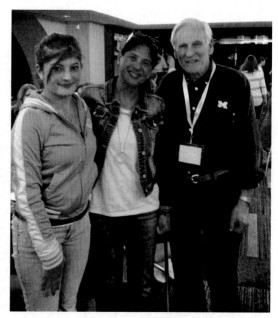

**Figure 1-5.** Left: Esperanza, the first infant successfully placed on ECMO for primary respiratory failure. Right: Esperanza and daughter with Dr. Bartlett at ELSO conference.

A second prospective trial effort took advantage of ECMO and traditional, non-ECMO therapy being provided in separate intensive care units. Dr. Pearl O'Rourke, a pediatric critical care physician at Boston Children's Hospital, led a two-phase RCT. The study design included a phase one approach with a traditional 50/50 randomization of patients until one arm had four deaths or there was a statistical difference between the two arms, followed by a phase two utilizing an adaptive design to favor the "winner" of the first phase. Overall, 19/20 (97%) of ECMO patients survived compared to 60% of standard control patients.[25] The study, published in 1989, engendered controversy in the medical community and in the media.[26,27] Ironically, an outcry arose from many medical professionals and the lay press that randomization to standard therapy without ECMO was unethical, implying a loss of equipoise and subtly demonstrating recognition that ECMO had become a standard of care.

The long-desired RCT evidence for outcome benefit in neonatal ECMO for persistent pulmonary hypertension was provided by a study performed in the United Kingdom from 1993 to 1995[28] that remains to date the largest randomized ECMO trial in children. The study, authored by Drs. David Field, Richard Firmin, and colleagues, enrolled 55 centers and took advantage of the country's regionalized medical/ECMO system, with randomization either to stay in the referral center for standard therapy or transfer to the regional ECMO center. A significant survival difference (60% in ECMO patients vs. 40% with standard therapy; number needed to treat: 3 to 4) supported the superiority of ECMO in severe neonatal respiratory failure and etched the value of ECMO in stone. Centers performing ECMO grew from only 18 worldwide in the 1980s to over 100 centers in the early 1990s. In great part due to technological advances, application of ECMO to neonatal and pediatric populations became a common practice.

**Global Spread of ECMO**

Even absent the elusive "perfect" trial, support for, and use of ECMO in neonates grew globally. Neonatal ECMO served as a role model for rapid propagation of medical technology for treatment of disease and served as a demonstration model in a National Institutes of Health workshop for diffusion of technology in 1990 (Figure 1-6), outlining the meteoric rise from concept to clinically accepted, if still controversial, therapy. The NIH workshop Chair, Dr. Anne Lennarson-Greer, noted, "The diffusion of an innovation is a highly social process. The spread of even a simple technology..is characterized by many interpersonal contacts and differentiated social roles."[29]

The concept of rapid technology diffusion as a social enterprise aptly described ECMO well before the days of social media. Dissemination of information for ECMO accelerated with the initiation of meetings and networks dedicated

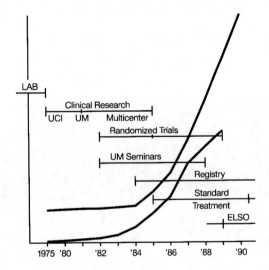

**Figure 1-6.** Graphic representation of development and propagation of ECMO, from NIH Report of the Workshop on Diffusion of ECMO Technology, 1993.

to ECMO issues. Multiple centers sprang up nationally and internationally, often with movement of physicians and staff to develop a new center, and always with collaboration from the experienced centers. For instance, in 1983, only three institutions regularly performing ECMO (Medical College of Virginia, University of Michigan, and University of Pittsburgh) were

| MEMBERS | LOCATION |
|---|---|
| Robert Bartlett | Ann Arbor, MI |
| William Kanto | Augusta, GA |
| Fred Ryckman | Cincinnati, OH |
| Larry Cook | Louisville, KY |
| Martin Keszler | Washington, DC |
| Billie Lou Short | Washington, DC |
| P. Pearl O'Rourke | Seattle, WA |
| J. Devn Cornish | San Diego, CA |
| Charles Stolar | New York, NY |
| Michael Klein | Detroit, MI |
| Phyllis McClelland | Ann Arbor, MI |
| Sandy Snedecor | Ann Arbor, M |

**Table 1-1:** ELSO's First Steering Committee

represented at one of the meetings. By 1986, nineteen institutions provided ECMO support to neonates.[30] A voluntary alliance of these active centers emerged. In 1989, a steering committee formed (Table 1-1 and Figure 1-7) and created the bylaws to form the Extracorporeal Life Support Organization (ELSO). The purpose of ELSO was to pool common data on ECMO use, compare outcomes, and exchange ideas for optimal use of ECMO support. ELSO meetings attracted representatives from the small number of institutions performing ECMO to present their experience. The growing interest in ECMO led to the development of a week-long meeting totally dedicated to ECMO directed by Dr. Billie Short and sponsored by DC Children's National Medical Center. Attendance was broadened by a growing international community experience. The community of international ECMO experience also grew with the first European symposium on extracorporeal lung support in Paris in 1991. This meeting was associated with the foundation of the European Extracorporeal Life Support Organization (EESO). In 1994, the

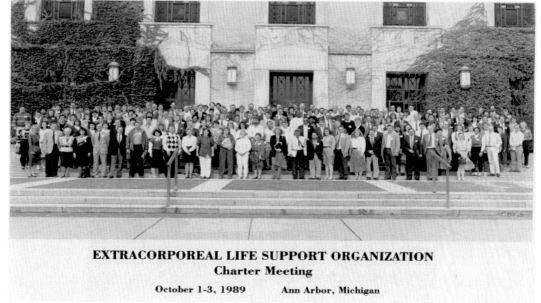

**EXTRACORPOREAL LIFE SUPPORT ORGANIZATION**
**Charter Meeting**
October 1-3, 1989      Ann Arbor, Michigan

**Figure 1-7.** Above: Attendees at Charter Meeting of the Extracorporeal Life Support Organization, October 1989.

international ECMO conference represented the first combined meeting of ELSO and EESO.

ELSO became the epicenter for the development of thought and definition of the operation of an ECMO center and guidelines which could be utilized by a growing number of centers. In addition, it became the steering organization for future randomized trial work. Awards for ELSO Centers of Excellence were developed to provide center recognition around ELSO recommendations. The Award of Excellence has received recognition by entities such as the annual *US News and World Report* survey as a marker of institutional quality.

Key efforts of ELSO included the publication of manuals and textbooks to help codify approaches to ECMO care. The need for a collated text of ECMO knowledge was recognized. Two members of the steering committee, Drs. Robert Arensman and Devn Cornish, edited the inaugural edition of this textbook, now known as the 'Red Book,' in 1992. The Red Book is now entering its 6th edition in 2022 as a collaboration of experts in the global ECMO community.

A critical element of propagation of ECMO technology was the development of a standardized international patient database to track results and provide evaluation of indications and outcomes in a large population, a huge improvement over traditional small case series experience. This early database, which transitioned into the ELSO Registry (Chapter 60),[31] allowed for participating institutions to collate and compare outcomes with national and international centers. International ELSO Registry involvement grew from 80 centers in 1990 to over 764 active centers in 2022, and well over 600 centers contributing data (Figure 1-8). From Registry inception to date in 2022, the Registry database has captured over 175,000 patients and provided data for hundreds of publications and countless queries for centers seeking experience around ECMO use in a specific condition. The Registry is the largest repository of extracorporeal support data in the world and is considered the gold standard for reporting US and international ECLS outcomes. Use of neonatal ECMO peaked in 1992 at around 1500 annual cases. The development

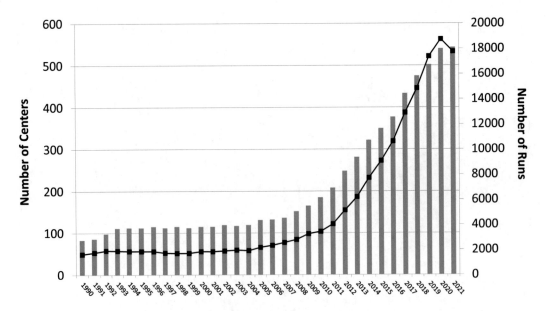

**Figure 1-8.** Growth of ELSO Centers 1989-2021 (ELSO Registry centers actively providing data annually to 2021) and total recorded ELSO Registry runs by year.

of additional new therapies such as inhaled nitric oxide as well as advances in mechanical ventilation likely contributed to a decline in the numbers of neonates requiring ECMO, to current levels half of those at the peak.

Efforts to use ECMO for pediatric cardiac and respiratory failure rose with the success of neonatal ECMO and its availability in growing numbers of centers. A variety of case series supported the efficacy of ECMO in pediatric respiratory failure.[32,33] However, the relatively low numbers of pediatric patients suitable for ECMO across the U.S. precluded a definitive trial. A multicenter RCT was attempted in the 1990s by Fackler and Heulitt, but was stopped due to enrollment difficulties, and lower than expected mortality in the study population.[34] In the absence of a pediatric RCT, the most significant case-control study[35] demonstrated improved outcomes associated with use of ECMO. To date, no new pediatric RCTs are on the horizon. Efforts in pediatrics became focused on delineating optimal timing and indications for support,[36] pushing the envelope for pediatric indications,[37,38] and determining relationships between center volumes and outcome.[39]

**Perseverance: Experience and Growing Indications in ECMO**

Since the initial efforts of Dr. Gibbon, clinicians sought to utilize the benefits of ECMO to allow recovery in adult cardiac and respiratory failure. However, the road to acceptance of the benefits of ECMO in adults was a slow one. The first attempt at an ECMO RCT was actually an NIH-supported adult trial directed by Zapol et al. comparing venoarterial (VA) ECMO to standard therapy for severe respiratory failure.[40] The study, while well intentioned, was hampered by a variety of factors, including the choice of moribund patients for study entry, participation of the majority of centers with no previous ECMO experience, and the utilization of VA cannulation patients potentially requiring only respiratory support. The trial utilized the relatively poor-performing technology available at the time, and lung protective strategies were not utilized in either arm. The study demonstrated very poor survival (approximately 10%) in both study arms. These findings, although clearly underlining the complexity of the clinical scenario (66% mortality in total population and 90% in severe ARDS patients), put a chill on subsequent extension of ECLS in adult respiratory failure.

In a later adult RCT in 1994,[41] patients with ARDS were randomized to receive either extracorporeal $CO_2$ removal with VA support or standard therapy utilizing a computerized protocol for ventilator management. The study again showed no difference in outcomes. Study design concerns included the lack of experience with extracorporeal use in some centers as well as extremely high blood loss in ECMO patients. Despite these disappointing study results, physicians such as Dr. Luciano Gattinoni[42] and Dr. Bartlett persevered in its use in adults, reporting significant survival improvement compared to historical controls.

Advances in ECMO experience, equipment, and expertise paved the way for a groundbreaking RCT in adult respiratory failure, the 2009 United Kingdom Conventional ventilatory support vs. Extracorporeal membrane oxygenation for Severe Adult Respiratory failure (CESAR) trial,[43] under the leadership of Dr. Giles Peek. The CESAR trial took advantage of the regionalized ECMO system which had allowed the success of the neonatal UK trial, with patients randomized to either remain at a standard treatment center or be transferred to a regional ECMO center. The study also utilized venovenous (VV) cannulation, with its inherent advantages. Patients receiving care at the ECMO center demonstrated significantly improved intact survival compared to standard center treatment (63% vs. 47%, RR 0.69). The study results, while controversial due to some methodological limitations, served to support the growing interest in adult therapeutic potential.

The timing of release of the CESAR results shortly preceded the 2009 worldwide Influenza A(H1N1) pandemic. The acute, severe, fulminant nature of respiratory failure with H1N1 led providers to seek ECMO as a therapeutic option, with encouraging findings supporting potential ECMO benefit.[44,45] The convergence helped supercharge international growth of ECMO use. Both ELSO Registry reports[31,46] and studies of independent national data registries[47] demonstrated a marked rise in adult cannulation in subsequent years, with a continued upward trajectory to the present day.

This rise in use of extracorporeal support was fuelled by several major advancements in equipment, including improvements in oxygenator components, ECLS circuit and configuration, and vascular access. Femoro-femoral cannulation with reduced cannula sizes, prevention of limb ischemia through selective distal perfusion, active drainage of limb venous flow, and attention paid to left ventricular unloading all played a critical role in enhanced ECLS management, reduced complication rates, and improved outcome. Vascular access techniques transitioned from surgical cutdown and insertion towards emphasis on peripheral access employing the Seldinger technique, with thin, small size, percutaneous cannulas, often characterized by nonthrombogenic surfaces. Cannula design (double lumen cannula for VV ECMO[48,49] or low profile cannulas for arterial access) and the routine application of distal limb perfusion in case of femoral artery cannulation for peripheral VA were additional breakthroughs for successful ECMO application, with significant reductions in postprocedural complications. These innovations increased use of VV cannulation, with transition from routine use of VA cannulation to a predominance of VV use for pediatric respiratory failure in 2012.[31]

Coating and heparin-bonded circuit surfaces,[50] together with the miniaturization and integration of pump systems, led to the development of more simplified, portable, and efficient ECLS systems. The most significant recent step was the development of the polymethyl pentene membrane oxygenator, with low priming volumes, low internal resistance, high oxygenation efficiency, and long-lasting membrane performance.[51] Preferential use of centrifugal pumps for pediatric and adult support also grew.

Several trends in management also altered ECMO care. In Europe, efforts to allow patients to remain awake and enhance mobility were popularized, particularly by the ECMO team at the Karolinska Institute,[52] allowing for longer runs, bridging for transplant, and the capacity for ambulatory ECMO.[53,54] Primary use of ECMO for extracorporeal carbon dioxide removal opened the door for potential support for a large number of adults with chronic obstructive pulmonary disease.[55] ECMO teams also pushed the envelope in expanding indications for extracorporeal support previously considered contraindications, with reports of improved outcomes in trauma, malignancy, and sepsis on ECMO.[56,57] The use of ECLS for acute extracorporeal support during cardiopulmonary resuscitation (ECPR) also became a burgeoning, if somewhat controversial indication for support, with growing use in both children and adults in emergency department and invasive cardiology settings.[58-60] One recent randomized trial demonstrated 43 percent healthy survival with ECPR compared to 7 percent with standard CPR in out of hospital cardiac arrest.[61]

Global growth of ECMO use has character-ized recent decades. ECLS use in Europe has been both longstanding and innovative. In particular, the enhanced use in adult respiratory and cardiac failure has been propagated in great part by experience and expertise in European centers. International center growth also resulted in the establishment of ELSO global chapters tied to every inhabited continent. EuroELSO was chartered in 2011 as a sequel to the previous European Extracorporeal Support Organization (Table 1-2). Asia Pacific ELSO (APELSO) soon followed, being chartered in 2013, and Latin American ELSO (LA-ELSO) and the South West Asia and Africa ELSO chapters (SWAAC) followed later in 2013, all with the support of then-ELSO chair Steve Conrad. These vibrant organizations allowed accelerated growth of international ECMO patient capture in the Registry, robust scientific

conferences, expanded training courses, and enhanced global networking among ECMO providers and centers. Individual membership in ELSO was also initiated in 2016 to draw in members from around the world, exclusive of a member's institutional ELSO center status.

As ECMO advanced, so ELSO continued its progress as the definitive organization for education and information regarding ECMO worldwide. Following its recognition as an independent nonprofit organization, ELSO administration transitioned from the University of Michigan in 2018. A separate governing board of directors now leads the organization in association with the longstanding ELSO steering committee. The growth of the organization led to the hiring of Christine Stead as ELSO's first chief executive officer. Under her wise and energetic guidance, ELSO continues to grow as a highly professional organization, headquartered in separate offices in Ann Arbor. (Figure 1-9)

Adult ECMO predominantly fueled the rapid growth of ECLS use from the period of 2010 to the present time (Figure 1-8).[62,63] While the CESAR trial had provided significant encouragement in adult use, investigators continued to seek evidence of the benefits of ECMO therapy itself exclusive of overall management at an ECMO center. To address some of these concerns, Combes and co-

| YEARS | CHAIR |
|---|---|
| **ELSO** | |
| 2020-2022 (Present) | Matthew Paden |
| 2018-2020 | Mark Ogino |
| 2016-2018 | Michael McMullan |
| 2014-2016 | James Fortenberry |
| 2012-2014 | William Lynch |
| 2010-2012 | Steve Conrad |
| 2007-2010 | Mike Hines |
| 2004-2007 | Heidi Dalton |
| 2002-2004 | Joseph Zwischenberger |
| 2000-2002 | Ronald Hirschl |
| 1997-2000 | Charles Stolar |
| 1994-1997 | Michael Klein |
| 1993-1994 | Billie Lou Short |
| 1989-1993 | Robert Bartlett |
| **Euro ELSO** | |
| 2022 - Present | Nicholas Barrett |
| 2019-2022 | Jan Belohlavek |
| 2017-2019 | Alain Combes |
| 2014-2017 | Roberto Lorusso |
| 2012-2014 | Giles Peek |
| **Asia Pacific ELSO** | |
| 2020-Present | John Fraser |
| 2017-2020 | YS Chen |
| 2013-2017 | Graeme MacLaren |
| **Latin American ELSO** | |
| 2022 - Present | Rene Gomez |
| 2017-2021 | Leonardo Salazar |
| 2015-2017 | Luiz Caneo |
| 2013-2015 | Rodrigo Diaz/Javier Kattan (Co-chairs) |
| **South and West Asia ELSO** | |
| 2022 (Present) | Poonam Malhotra |
| 2021 | Akram Abdalbary |
| 2020 | Yatin Mehta |
| 2019 | Ibrahim Fawzy Hassan |
| 2018 | Venkat Goyal |
| 2017 | Malaika Mendonca |
| 2014 -2016 | Suneel Poobani |

**Table 1-2:** ELSO Presidents and Chapter Chairs

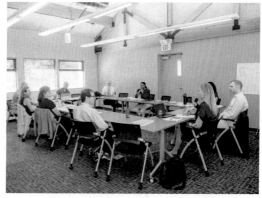

**Figure 1-9.** Meeting facilities at ELSO Headquarters, Ann Arbor, Michigan.

investigators designed and led the ambitious European Extracorporeal membrane Oxygenation to rescue Lung Injury in severe ARDS (EOLIA) multi-center trial,[64] comparing use of ECMO instituted as soon as patients met high risk criteria compared to continued conventional care. The findings were both provocative and encouraging. The study was stopped with overall survival not meeting statistical significance (65% randomized initially to ECMO vs. 54%; p = .07). However, when including crossover to ECMO (35 salvage patients), survival for all ECMO patients was indeed significant (65% compared to 42% with no ECMO; p = .001). The study brought robust conversation in the ICU and ECMO communities and further assessment by Bayesian methodology, which supported significant (88-99%) posterior probability of mortality benefit for ECMO in the trial.[65]

The COVID-19 pandemic, caused by multiple strains of a novel coronavirus, changed the world and further advanced ECMO into the forefront of care. Severe pneumonia impacted millions worldwide with severe morbidity and death, and ECMO was used in thousands of patients who were dying despite aggressive medical and ventilatory management. Worldwide, demand and use of ECMO exploded, with many ICUs managing as many as ten to twenty patients simultaneously. ELSO was directly involved in providing data, center referrals and guidelines for early use of ECMO. [66,67] Many new ECMO centers were established to deal with the pandemic, leading to need for rapid education and support from ELSO. Mainstream media also latched on to the provision of lifesaving COVID-19 care with ECMO, and shared the need, use and shortages of equipment. The ELSO Registry team created real time data capture and analytic capabilities to meet acute information needs. The ELSO Registry informed the most influential early report[68], demonstrating mortality of 39 percent (38 percent with VV ECMO), in line with other ARDS-related conditions receiving ECMO. ELSO investigators provided data for over 4800 ECMO patients in 2020[69]. They demonstrated evolving ECMO outcomes over time with decreasing survival during the pandemic, possibly due to patient selection, patient treatment differences, and experience with ECMO support for COVID-19. Cumulative meta-analysis supported benefits of ECMO for COVID-19 survival with refractory cases.[70] Reports of survival with SARS-CoV-2 infection after months on ECMO without any lung function led to reassessment of concepts of 'irreversible' lung disease. Successful lung transplantation was also reported in COVID-19 patients, establishing the feasibility of lung transplantation for acute infectious respiratory failure, many of whom were bridged to transplant on ECMO.[71]

| FELSO AWARD RECIPIENTS | |
|---|---|
| Inaugural Class – 2015 | Class – 2018 |
| Robert H. Bartlett MD | Alain Combes MD |
| Konrad Falke MD | James Fortenberry MD |
| Luciano Gattinoni MD | Roberto Lorusso MD |
| John Gibbon MD | Graeme MacLaren MD |
| Robert E. Gross MD | |
| J. Donald Hill MD | Class – 2019 |
| Theodor Ted Kolobow PhD | Daniel Brodie MD |
| Pearl O'Rourke MD | Tom Brogan MD |
| Billie Short MD | James Connelly, RRT |
| John Toomasian CCP | Don Granoski, RRT |
| | Thomas Mueller MD |
| Class – 2016 | Ravi Thiagarajan MD |
| Warwick Butt MD | |
| J. Devn Cornish MD | Class – 2020 |
| Robin Chapman RN | Gail Annich MD |
| Jean-Yves Chevalier MD | Venkat Goyal MD |
| Richard Firmin MD | Richard Martin |
| Masahiro Nagaya MD | Mark Ogino MD |
| Antonio Pesenti MD | |
| Giles Peek MD | Class – 2021 |
| Peter Rycus MPH | W. Cory Ellis |
| Charles Stolar MD | John Fraser MD |
| Jay Zwischenberger MD | |
| Warren Zapol MD | |
| | |
| Class – 2017 | |
| Steve Conrad MD | |
| Heidi Dalton MD | |
| Rodrigo Diaz MD | |
| Bjorn Frencker MD | |
| Barb Haney RN | |
| Phoebe Hankins | |
| Micheal Heard RN | |
| Tracy Morrison RN | |
| Andrezj (Andrew) Sosnowski MD | |
| Palle Palmer MD | |

**Table 1-3:** FELSO Recipients

The COVID-19 pandemic response illustrates well the evolution of the indications and evolving value of ECMO. The next chapter in the development of extracorporeal support remains to be written, but it was the authors of the preceding work who have penned its opening chapters. In 2015, ELSO established the Fellowship in the Extracorporeal Support Organization, an honorary designation to recognize these pioneering contributors to the ECMO story (Table 1-3). The ECMO story to date is an incredible combination of innovation, ingenuity, commitment, care, and community. It is also clear that much work remains to be done to improve ECMO technology, predict outcomes, fine tune best indications, and meet the next challenge.[47,63] As we seek to fulfill Dr. Gibbons' quest for lifesaving support, we should be encouraged by the inspiring words of Sir Winston Churchill, "The future is unknowable, but the past should give us hope."[72]

**Technology and Clinical Indications for ECMO: the Future is Bright**

Based on its expanding use, it is clear that ECMO will play a major role in several clinical scenarios. Enhanced knowledge, expertise, and technology will encourage the expansion of current indications as well as the identification of new ones. Improved and better engineered ECMO-related components such as new cannulas, pumps and oxygenators; clinical trials and investigations that shed light on the benefits of ECMO, and improved understanding of patient management, all support a bright future. (Figure 1-10). There is substantial investment in companies, engineers, research and development groups, and investigators who are actively exploring advances in mechanical support. Major breakthroughs can be expected and will hopefully lead to improved organ recovery and ultimately improved patient outcomes. Finally, the recent events related to the COVID-19 pandemic clearly emphasize the need for the health-care community to be prepared to support dedicated personnel, centers, and companies that can meet the need for ECMO in unprecedented conditions and numbers.

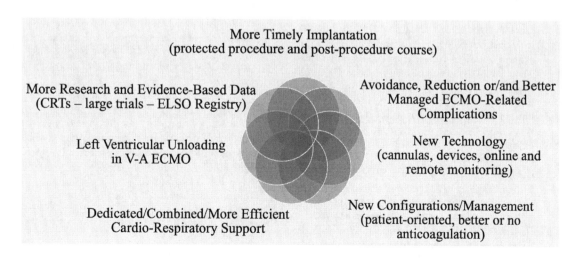

**Figure 1-10:** Improvements in ECMO-related components and care.

# References

1. Bartlett RH. Extracorporeal Life Support: Gibbon fulfilled. J Am Coll Surg 2014; 218:317-327.
2. Richardson BW. An inquiry into the possibility of restoring the life of warm blooded animals in certain cases where the respiration, circulation and the ordinary manifestations of organic motion are exhausted or have ceased. Proceedings of the Royal Sociey of London, 13:358-371, 1865.
3. Konstantinov I, Alexi-Meshkishvili V. Sergei S. Brukhonenko: the development of the first heart-lung machine for total body perfusion. Ann Thoracic Surg 2000; 69:962-6.
4. Lillehei CW. History of the development of extracorporeal circulation, in Arensman RM, Cornish JD, eds. Extracorporeal Life Support in Critical Care (1st edition), Boston: Blackwell Publications, 1993.
5. Kanto WP, Shapiro MB. The development of prolonged extracorporeal circulation, in Zwischenberger JB, Bartlett RH, eds. ECMO: Extracorporeal Cardiopulmonary Support in Critical Care, Ann Arbor, MI: ELSO, 1995.
6. Lee WH, Krumhaar D, Fonkalsrud EW, et al. Denaturation of plasma proteins as a cause of morbidity and death after intracardiac operations. Surgery. 1961; 50:29-39.
7. Custer JR. The evolution of patient selection criteria and indications for extracorporeal life support in pediatric cardiopulmonary failure: next time let's not eat the bones. Organogenesis. 2011;7(1):13-22.
8. Kammermeyer K. Silicone rubber as a selective barrier. Ind Eng Chem. 1957;49:1685.
9. Kolff WJ, Effler DB, Groves LK, Peereboom G, Moraca PP. (1956). Disposable membrane oxygenator (heart-lung machine) and its use in experimental surgery. Cleve Clin Q. 156;23(2):69-97.
10. Kolobow T, Zapol W, Pierce JE et al. Partial extracorporeal gas exchange in alert newborn lambs with a membrane artificial lung perfused via an AV shunt for periods up to 96 hours. Trans Am Soc Artif Intern Organs. 1968;14:238.
11. Bartlett RH, Isherwood J, Moss RA, Olszewski WL, Polet H, Drinker P. A toroidal flow membrane oxygenator: four day partial bypass in dogs. Surg Forum. 1969;20:152-3.
12. Kolobow T, Zapol WM, Sigmon RL, Pierce J. Partial cardiopulmonary bypass lasting up to seven days in alert lambs with membrane lung blood oxygenation. J Thorac Cardiovasc Surg. 1970;60(6):781-788.
13. Baffes TG, Fridman JL, Bicoff JP, Whitehill JL. Extracorporeal circulation for support of palliative cardiac surgery in infants. Ann Thorac Surg 1970;10(4):354-363.
14. Bartlett RH, Gazzaniga AB, Fong SW, Jefferies MR, Roohk HV, Haiduc N. Extracorporeal membrane oxygenator support for cardiopulmonary failure. Experience in 28 cases. J Thorac Cardiovc Surg. 1977;73(3):375-386.
15. Hill JD, O'Brien TG, Murray JJ et al. Prolonged extracorporeal oxygenation for acute post-traumatic respiratory failure (shock-lung syndrome): use of the Bramson Membrane Lung. N Engl J Med. 1972;286(12):629-634.
16. Dorson W Jr, Baker E, Cohen ML, et al. (1969). A perfusion system for infants. Trans Am Soc Artif Intern Organs. 1969;15:155-60.
17. White JJ, Andrews HG, Risemberg H, et al. (1969). Prolonged respiratory support in newborn infants with a membrane oxygenator. Surgery 1969;70(2):288-296.
18. Bartlett RH. Esperanza. Trans Am Soc Artif Intern Organs. 1985; 31:723-735.
19. Bartlett RH. Artificial organs: basic science meets critical care. J Am Coll Surg. 2003; 196(2):171-179.
20. Wolfson PJ. The development and use of extracorporeal membrane oxygenation in neonates. Ann Thorac Surg. 2003;76(6):S2224-2229.
21. Bartlett RH. Extracorporeal life support in the management of severe respiratory failure. Clin Chest Med. 2000;21(3):555-561.
22. Bartlett RH, Gazzaniga AB, Jefferies R, Huxtable RF, Haiduc RF, Fong SW. (1976). Extracorporeal membrane oxygenation (ECMO) cardiopulmonary support in infancy. Trans Am Soc Artif Organ. 1976;22:80-93.
23. Bartlett RH, Andrews AF, Toomasian JM, Haiduc NJ, Gazzaniga AB (1982). Extracorporeal membrane oxygenation for newborn respiratory failure : forty-five cases. Surgery. 1982;92(2):452-433.
24. Bartlett RH, Roloff DW, Cornell RG, Andrews AF, Dillon PW, Zwischenberger JB. Extracorporeal circulation in neonatal respiratory failure: a prospective randomized study. Pediatrics. 1985;76(4):479-487.
25. O'Rourke PP, Crone RK, Vacanti JP, et al. Extracorporeal membrane oxygenation and conventional medical therapy in neonates with persistent pulmonary hypertension of the newborn: a prospective randomized study. Pediatrics. 1989;8(6):957-963.
26. Knox RA. A Harvard study on newborns draws fire. Boston globe, August 7, 1989:25.
27. Marwick C. NIH Research Risks Office reprimands hospital institutional review board. JAMA. 1990;263:2420.
28. UK Collaborative ECMO Trial Group. UK collaborative randomized trial of neonatal

extracorporeal membrane oxygenation. Lancet. 1996;348(9020):75-82.

29. Wright L, Ed. Report of the Workshop on Diffusion of ECMO Technology; National Institutes of Health, 1993.

30. Custer JR, Bartlett RH. Recent research in extracorporeal life support for respiratory failure. ASAIO J. 1992;38(4):754-771.

31. Paden ML, Conrad SA, Rycus PT, Thiagarajan RR; ELSO Registry. Extracorporeal Life Support Organization Registry report 2012. ASAIO J. 2013;59(3):202-10.

32. Moler FW, Palmisano J, Custer JR. Extracorporeal life support for pediatric respiratory failure: predictors of survival from 220 patients. Crit Care Med. 1993;21(10):1604-1611.

33. Pettignano R, Fortenberry JD, Heard M, et al. Primary use of the venovenous approach for extracorporeal membrane oxygenation in pediatric acute respiratory failure. Pediatr Crit Care Med. 2003; 4(3):291-298.

34. Fackler J, Bohn D, Green T, et al. ECMO for ARDS; stopping a RCT. Am J Resp Crit Care Med. 1997;155:A504.

35. Green TP, Timmons OD, Fackler JC, Moler FW, Thompson AE, Sweeney MF. The impact of extracorporeal membrane oxygenation on survival in pediatric patients with acute respiratory failure. Pediatric Critical Care Study Group. Crit Care Med. 1996;24(2):323-329.

36. Zabrocki LA, Brogan TV, Statler KD, Poss WB, Rollins MD, Bratton SL. Extracorporeal membrane oxygenation for pediatric respiratory failure: survival and predictors of mortality. Crit Care Med. 2011;39(2):364-370.

37. Gow KW, Heiss K, Wulkan ML, et al. Extracorporeal life support for support of children with malignancy and respiratory or cardiac failure. The Extracorporeal Life Support Organization Experience. Crit Care Med. 2009: 37(4):1308-1316.

38. MacLaren G, Butt W, Best D, Donath S, Taylor A. Extracorporeal membrane oxygenation for refractory septic shock in children: one institution's experience. Pediatr Crit Care Med. 2007; 8(5):447-451.

39. Barbaro RP, Odetola FO, Kidwell, K, et al. Association of hospital-level volume of extracorporeal membrane oxygenation case and mortality. Analysis of the Extracorporeal Life Support Organization registry. Am J Respir Crit Care Med. 2015; 191(8):894-901.

40. Zapol WM, Snider MT, Hill JD et al. Extracorporeal membrane oxygenation in severe acute respiratory failure. A randomized prospective study. JAMA. 1979;242(20):2193-6.

41. Morris AH, Wallace CJ, Menlove RL, et al. Randomized clinical trial of pressure-controlled inverse ratio ventilation and extracorporeal CO2 removal for adult respiratory distress syndrome. Am J Resp Crit Care Med. 1994;149(2 Pt 1):295-305.

42. Gattinoni L, Pesenti A, Bombino M et al. Role of extracorporeal oxygenation in adult respiratory distress syndrome management. New Horiz. 1993;1(4):603-612.

43. Peek GJ, Mugford M, Tiruvoipati R et al. Efficacy and economic assessment of conventional ventilatory support versus extracorporeal membrane oxygenation for severe adult respiratory failure (CESAR): a multicentre randomised controlled trial. Lancet. 2009;374(9698):1351-1363.

44. Davies A, ANZIC ECMO Investigators et al. Extracorporeal membrane oxygenation for 2009 influenza A (H1N1) acute respiratory distress syndrome. JAMA. 2009: 304:1888-1895.

45. Noah MA, Peek G, Finney S, et al. Referral to an extracorporeal membrane oxygenation center and mortality among patients with severe 2009 influenza A (H1N1). JAMA. 2011;306(15):1659-68.

46. Thiagarajan RR, Barbaro RP, Rycus PT, et al. ELSO member centers. Extracorporeal Life Support Organization Registry International Report 2016. ASAIO J. 2017 Jan/Feb;63(1):60-67.

47. Karagiannisidis C, Brocie D, Strassman S, et al. ECMO: evolving epidemiology and mortality. Intensive Care Med. 2016; 42(5):889-96.

48. Wang D, Zhou X, Liu X, Sidor B, Lynch J, Zwischenberger JB (2008). Wang-Zische double lumen cannula. Toward percutaneous and ambulatory paracorporeal artificial lung. ASAIO J. 54(6):606-11.

49. Javidfar J, Wang D, Zwischenberger JB, et al. Insertion of bicaval dual lumen extracorporeal membrane oxygenation catheter with image guidance. ASAIO J. 2011;57(3):203-205.

50. Harig F, Feyrer R, Mahmoud FO, Blum U, von der Emde J. Reducing the post-pump syndrome by using heparin-coated circuits, steroids, or aprotinin. Thorac Cardiovasc Surg. 1999; 47(2):111-118.

51. Lim MW. The history of extracorporeal oxygenators. Anaesthesia. 2006;61(10):984-994.

52. Frenckner B, Palmer K, Linden V. Extracorporeal respiratory support and minimally invasive ventilation in severe ARDS. Minerva Anestesiologica 2002; 68:381.

53. Turner DA, Cheifetz IM, Rehder KJ, et al. Active rehabilitation and physical therapy during ECMO while awaiting lung transplantation: a practical approach. Crit Care Med. 2011; 39(12):2593-2598.

54. Agerstrand CL, Bacchetta MD, Brodie D. ECMO for adult respiratory failure: current use and evolving applications. ASAIO J. 2014; 60(3):255-262.

55. Abrams DC, Brenner K, Burkart KM, et al. Pilot study of extracorporeal carbon dioxide removal to facilitate extubation and ambulation in exacerbations

of chronic obstructive pulmonary disease. Ann Am Thoracic Soc. 2013; 10(4):307-14.

56. Gow KW, Heiss KF, Wulkan ML, et al. Extracorporeal life support for support of children with malignancy and respiratory or cardiac failure: the ELSO experience. Crit Care Med. 2009; 37(4):1308-1316.

57. MacLaren G, Butt W, Best D, Donath B. Central extracorporeal membrane oxygenation for refractory pediatric septic shock. Pediatr Crit Care Med. 2011; 12(2):133-136.

58. Thiagarajan RR, Laussen P, Rycus PT, Bartlett RH, Bratton SL. Extracorporeal membrane oxygenation to aid cardiopulmonary resuscitation in infants and children. Circulation. 2007;116(15):1693-1700.

59. Raymond TT, Cunnyngham CB, Thompson MT, Thomas JA, Dalton HJ, NAdkarni VM. Outcomes among neonates, infants, and children after extracorporeal cardiopulmonary resuscitation for refractory in hospital pediatric cardiac arrest: a report from the National Registry of Cardiopulmonary Resuscitation. Pediatr Crit Care Med. 2010; 11(3):362-371.

60. Sakamoto T, Morimura N, Nagao K et al. Extracorporeal cardiopulmonary resuscitation versus conventional cardiopulmonary resuscitation in adults with out-of-hospital cardiac arrest: a prospective observational study. Resuscitation. 2014;85(6): 762-8.

61. Yanapoulos D, Bartos J, Raveendran G et al. Advanced reperfusion strategies for patients with out-of-hospital cardiac arrest and refractory ventricular fibrillation (ARREST): a a phase 2, single centre, open-label, randomized controlled trial. Lancet. 2020; 396:1807.

62. Fan E, Gattinoni L, Combes A, et al. Venovenous extracorporeal membrane oxygenation for acute respiratory failure: a clinical review from an international group of experts. Intensive Care Med. 2016;42(5):712-724.

63. Brodie D, Stlustsky AS, Combes A. Extracorporeal life support for adults with respiratory failue and related indications: a review. JAMA. 2019; 322:557-568.

64. Combes A, Hajage D, Capellier G, et al; EOLIA Trial Group, REVA, and ECMONet: Extracorporeal membrane oxygenation for severe acute respiratory distress syndrome. N Engl J Med 2018; 378:1965–1975.

65. Goligher E, Tomlinson G, Hajage D et al. ECMO for severe acute respiratory distress syndrome and posterior probability of mortality benefit in a post hoc Bayesian analysis of a randomized clinical trial. JAMA. 2018; 320:2251-2259.

66. Bartlett RH, Ogino MT, Brodie D et al. Initial ELSO guidance document: ECMO for COVID-19 patients with severe cardiopulmonary failure. ASAIO J. 2020. 66:472-474.

67. Badulak J, Antonini M, Stead C et al. Extracorporeal Membrane Oxygenation for COVID-19: Updated 2021 guidelines from the Extracorporeal Life Support Organization. ASAIO J. 2021;67:485-495.

68. Barbaro RP, MacLaren G, Boonstra P et al. Extracorporeal membrane oxygenation in COVID-19: an international cohort study of the Extracorporeal Life Support Organization registry. Lancet. 2020; 396:1071-78.

69. Barbaro RP, MacLaren G, Boonstra A. Extracorporeal membrane oxygenation in COVID-19: evolving outcomes from the Extracorporeal Life Support Organization registry. Lancet. 2021: 398:1230-38.

70. Bertini P, Guarracino F, Falcone M. ECMO in COVID-19 patients: A systematic review and meta-analysis. J Cardiothorac Vasc Anesth. 2021. S1053-0770.

71. Roach A, Chikwe J, Catarino P et al. Lung transplantation for COVID-19-related respiratory failure in the United States. New Engl J Med. 2022; 386:1187-1188.

72. Churchill, W (1958), cited in Winston S, Langsworth RM. Churchill: In His Own Words, Ebury Press, 2008.

# 2

## Nomenclature

*Lars Mikael Broman, Jenelle H. Badulak, Daniel Brodie, Graeme MacLaren, Roberto Lorusso, Steven A. Conrad*

### Introduction

Nomenclature is a body or system of names and definitions, especially for use in specialty, and in particular, scientific fields. The creation and maintenance of a flexible nomenclature for ECLS is of the utmost importance, especially in times of rapid expansion to new providers, the development of the technology itself, along with evolving methods, modalities, and configurations of this advanced technology. However, the growing number of clinical approaches and devices in ECLS have led to ambiguity concerning the use of terms and abbreviations in the literature and other communication among peers, as well as reporting to registries and studies. Furthermore, indications have widened from bridge to recovery to alternate outcomes including bridge

to bridge, bridge to organ recovery, bridge to transplant, and bridge to destination.

The concept of extracorporeal organ support (ECOS) has emerged as a unifying description of all extracorporeal techniques used in the support of acute organ failure in the critically ill patient (Figure 2-1).[1] Support is grouped on the failing organ system, with extracorporeal life support targeting cardiopulmonary failure, the focus of this chapter. Other categories include renal, hepatic, and immunologic support, and this list is expected to grow in the future.

With expansion of ECLS around the world, the risks of miscommunication in clinical practice and research increased. For this reason, ELSO organized a task force of international experts representing specialties involved in ECLS to develop appropriate nomenclature. The product of the task force, the ELSO Maastricht

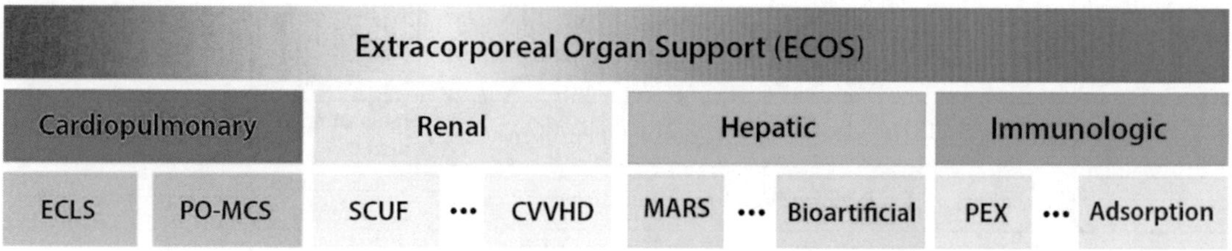

**Figure 2-1.** Chart showing the domains of extracorporeal organ support with some examples of support technologies. ECLS nomenclature is expanded in Figure 2-2.
Abbreviations: ECLS, extracorporeal life support; PO-MCS, pump-only mechanical circulatory support; SCUF, slow continuous ultrafiltration; CVVHD, continuous venovenous hemodialysis; MARS®, molecular absorbent recirculating system; PEX, plasma exchange

Treaty for Nomenclature in Extracorporeal Life Support was published in two parts. Part 1 of the ELSO Maastricht Treaty for Nomenclature in Extracorporeal Life Support provided the foundational nomenclature on terminology, abbreviations, definitions, and fundamental cannulation descriptions for ECLS to establish consistency for clinical application, documentation, followup, research, and quality assurance.[2] Part 1 also provides for standardization of units and measurements (Table 2-1). Part 2 of the Treaty expanded the nomenclature for cannulation configuration to provide a more thorough system for both clinical practice and research.[3] Both peripheral and central cannulation descriptors are included. The system has four hierarchies of increasing detail to manage complex cannulation configurations with precision and lack of ambiguity.

**Fundamental Nomenclature**

The term ECLS denotes extracorporeal support of cardiopulmonary function using an extracorporeal circuit incorporating (at a minimum) a pump and membrane lung. Systems applied for oxygenation and/or cardiac support are termed extracorporeal membrane oxygenation (ECMO), while extracorporeal carbon dioxide removal ($ECCO_2R$) is used to denote systems primarily targeted at $CO_2$ removal (Figure 2-2). Under each of these system categories are several support modes. A support mode describes an intended use such as venoarterial ECMO or venovenous $ECCO_2R$, in which venoarterial or venovenous describe the intended direction of flow and imply the condition supported. Modes (abbreviated without hyphens) describe intended support applications and are distinct from cannulation configurations. The latter, described in a separate section below, contain hyphens as part of the abbreviation convention.

| PHYSICAL CONCEPT | UNIT | DEFINITION | SPECIFICS | UNIT CONVERSION |
|---|---|---|---|---|
| Pressure | Millimeters of mercury (mmHg) | Preferred unit of pressure for ECLS, applied to absolute fluid pressures within the ECLS circuit and to partial pressures of gases in blood. | | 1 mmHg = 1/7.5 kPa; 1 mmHg = 1.36 $cmH_2O$ |
| Volumetric Flow | Liters per minute (L/min) | Preferred unit of volumetric flow for ECLS, applied to both blood flow and sweep gas flow. | | |
| Length | Centimeter (cm) | Preferred unit for cannula length, cannula insertion depth, and device dimension measurements. | | |
| | Meter (m) | Preferred unit for circuit tubing length and other lengths that exceed approximately 50 cm | | |
| | Inch (in) | Preferred unit for circuit tubing diameter. | Inner tubing diameter | 1 in = 25.4 mm |
| | French (Fr) | Preferred unit for cannula diameter. | Outer cannula diameter | 1 Fr = 1/3 mm |
| Area | Square meter ($m^2$) | Preferred unit for surface area, such as artificial membrane lung surface area. | | |
| Temperature | Degrees Centigrade (C°) | Preferred unit for temperature, including body temperature, blood temperature, and circuit component temperatures. | | |

**Table 2-1.** Physical units recommended for use in extracorporeal life support (ECLS).

Four support modes for ECMO are in common use and described in the nomenclature. Venoarterial (VA) describes venous drainage with systemic arterial return, venovenous (VV) describes venous drainage with venous return, and venopulmonary (VP) describes venous drainage with pulmonary artery return.[4] One hybrid mode, venovenoarterial (VVA), is in common use and describes venous drainage with simultaneous venous and systemic arterial return.[5] Other hybrid configurations have been used in selected circumstances. These are not included in the nomenclature due to infrequent use but described according to the underlying modes.

Conditions treated along with some common applications are also given in Figure 2-2. Cardiac ECMO refers to venoarterial ECMO for cardiac failure. Venoarterial support is also used for extracorporeal cardiopulmonary resuscitation (ECPR), the use of VA ECMO to initiate circulation when conventional CPR cannot achieve sustained return of spontaneous circulation (ROSC). ECPR is defined as VA ECMO support started when 20 minutes of ROSC cannot be achieved by conventional CPR. VA ECMO used to support low cardiac output following ROSC by conventional CPR is considered an application of cardiac ECMO and not ECPR. VA ECMO is also used for extracorporeal interval support for organ recovery (EISOR), in which ECMO is initiated following cardiac death to maintain organ blood flow in support of organ retrieval for transplantation (see Chapter 45).

Venovenous (VV) ECMO is used in the setting of hypoxemic respiratory failure (respiratory ECMO) when pulmonary function is insufficient to maintain adequate gas transfer. Venopulmonary (VP) ECMO is used in the support hypoxemic respiratory failure, most commonly when RV failure accompanies pulmonary dysfunction.

Extracorporeal $CO_2$ removal can be applied in venovenous or arteriovenous modes for management of hypercapnia, either in support

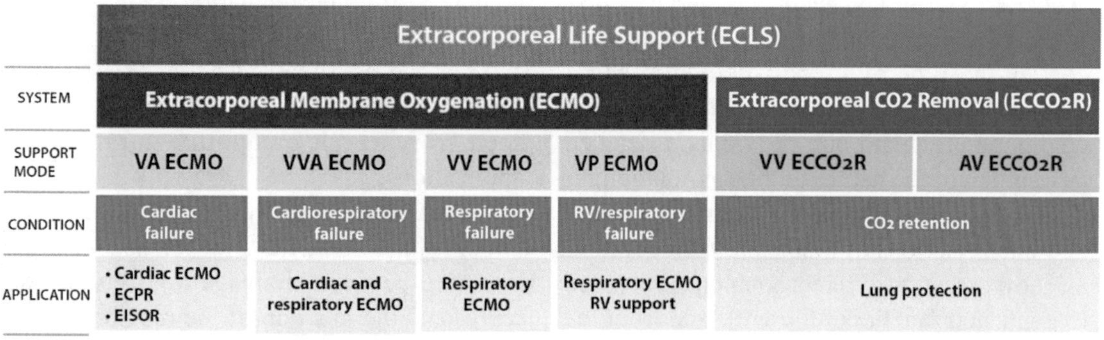

| Extracorporeal Life Support (ECLS) | | | | | | |
|---|---|---|---|---|---|---|
| SYSTEM | Extracorporeal Membrane Oxygenation (ECMO) | | | | Extracorporeal CO2 Removal (ECCO2R) | |
| SUPPORT MODE | VA ECMO | VVA ECMO | VV ECMO | VP ECMO | VV ECCO2R | AV ECCO2R |
| CONDITION | Cardiac failure | Cardiorespiratory failure | Respiratory failure | RV/respiratory failure | CO2 retention | |
| APPLICATION | • Cardiac ECMO<br>• ECPR<br>• EISOR | Cardiac and respiratory ECMO | Respiratory ECMO | Respiratory ECMO RV support | Lung protection | |

**Figure 2-2.** Chart showing nomenclature for extracorporeal life support in which a membrane lung is incorporated with a pump for cardiopulmonary support. ECMO and ECCO2R distinguish the use of ECLS for support of blood flow with oxygenation (ECMO) and carbon dioxide removal (ECCO2R). The support modes describe the general intent of support along with the major approaches to vascular access, as well as different applications to support targeted conditions.
Abbreviations: ECCO2R, extracorporeal carbon dioxide removal; ECLS, extracorporeal life support; ECMO, extracorporeal membrane oxygenation; ECPR, extracorporeal cardiopulmonary resuscitation; EISOR, extracorporeal interval support for organ recovery; AV, arteriovenous, VA, venoarterial, VV, venovenous, VVA, venovenoarterial.

of lung protective strategies during mechanical ventilation or as an alternative to mechanical ventilation. The arteriovenous mode is becoming less common with the development of dedicated venovenous $ECCO_2R$ systems that can be applied with dual-lumen cannulas similar in design to hemodialysis catheters (Chapter 43).[6]

**Abbreviations for Cannulation Configuration**

Increasing complexity of cannulation, partly driven by individualization of patient treatment, has also created a need of stratification. One key concept introduced by the Maastricht Treaty was a uniform nomenclature for cannulation configuration analogous to chemical formulae. The main properties of this nomenclature system were designed to allow for flexibility for adoption of future changes in management, device development, and other relevant changes. In July 2020, an ELSO Registry amendment created a fourth core category of ECMO, venopulmonary (VP) mode, to the already acknowledged modes venovenous (VV), venoarterial (VA), and venovenoarterial (VVA).

The emphasis of the nomenclature is to convey the type of support delivered and a blueprint of how the circuit and cannulation configuration is laid out, providing a detailed description of the nature of the cannulation for vascular access. Prior inconsistent descriptions and interpretations of mode and configuration, and how to refer to different components, has led to confusion that hopefully will fade from the two recent ELSO initiatives.[2,3] One spinoff after the release of the ELSO Maastricht Treaty Part 2 in 2019[3] was the development and publication of a free online tool to support ECLS providers to describe cannulation configurations uniformly (https://ecls.eurosets.com).

The nomenclature for cannulation configuration is hierarchical, initially starting at the highest level with one of the four modes. By adding additional levels, it describes increasing detail as the user or data recipient requires. The

abbreviation for a given configuration varies from simple to complex, covering the whole range from simple cannulation strategies to composites of different combinations of hybrid modes and hybrid methods. The ECLS provider may adopt and use the nomenclature according to their goals and the level of depth required for the task at hand, eg, quality assurance, research and development, communication with other clinicians, and so on. The goal at large is to offer consistency for clinical and research descriptions.

The four levels of the ECLS cannulation nomenclature are:

1. Basic configuration and flow direction,
2. Cannulation site,
3. Tip position,
4. Cannula dimension.

The rules for each level are provided in detail in the two publications describing the fundamental nomenclature for ECLS.[2,3] A summary of the Maastricht Treaty for nomenclature and cannulation configuration in ECLS follows. Emphasis is placed on Levels 1 and 2 as they are suitable for clinical use. Levels 3 and 4 are additional levels of detail typically seen in research or quality improvement applications.

Abbreviations are read in the direction of circuit blood flow, ie, from left to right. The interface between drainage and return sides represents the position of the membrane lung (ML) and is denoted as follows; one single ML "-", two MLs in parallel "=", two MLs in series "+", or no ML "x". The drainage side is to the left of the marker, and the return side is to the right. Levels two, three and four may be used in part and independently of the other ones. For easier understanding of abbreviated items in the following text, Table 2-2.

## Peripheral Cannulation Configuration

### *Basic Configuration (Level 1)*

The major cannulas are printed in uppercase letters. Consider two examples: V-V and V-A. In both cases, the uppercase letter to the left of the hyphen is one drainage cannula placed on the venous side (V) of the patient's circulation. In V-V, the V to the right of the hyphen represents a venous (V) return cannula. In the second example, the A indicates an arterial return cannula. In both examples, the drainage and return sides are separated by one ML (the hyphen) in the circuit. In a pumpless circuit (ie, driven by patient's blood pressure) for carbon dioxide removal, the drainage would be from an artery and the return to the venous side, designated as A-V.

*Multiple cannulas.* Additional cannulas are put to the outside of the original remaining cannula on the respective drainage or return side. Hence, a second venous drainage cannula is marked as a "V" placed to the left of the original "V". Thus, a dual-drainage VA mode configuration would be VV-A. If converting a VA patient into the hybrid mode VVA by adding an additional return cannula to the venous side,[5] the configuration would be V-AV placing the new cannula letter outside of the primary arterial return cannula. Thus, the configuration also provides inherent information of chronology. If the original mode was VV converted to VVA by adding an arterial return cannula, the configuration change would be from a V-V to a V-VA. If mode at implantation is VVA, the formula may be used to show priority of support, ie, if a cardiac problem is the primary reason for support, the abbreviation would be V-AV.

*Secondary cannulas.* To distinguish a smaller secondary (low-flow) cannula or catheter from a major high-flow cannula, the abbreviation representing this item is printed in lowercase letters. A common use for a secondary cannula is distal anterograde perfusion of the cannulated leg in VA ECMO with a femoral return cannula.[7] This smaller (5-8 Fr) cannula is denoted with a lowercase "d" (distal). The abbreviation "d" is placed directly after the cannula it is connected to, ie, V-Ad. Other examples are venting catheters, cephalad drainage catheters,[8-10] or use of distal venous drainage catheters.[11] The recent development of a femoral arterial cannula with an in-situ distal perfusion port, which obviously cannot be separated from the cannula, is abbreviated -Ad to mark this unique feature (Table 2-3).

| MODE | ABBREVIATION | SPECIFICS | COMMENT |
|---|---|---|---|
| Venovenous | VV | | Provides gas exchange of oxygen and carbon dioxide mainly via diffusion and the Haldane effect |
| Venoarterial | VA | | Provides circulatory support (ECLS/MCS), in combination with gas exchange if a membrane lung is connected into the circuit |
| Venopulmonary | VP | | Provides right ventricular support, and gas exchange if a membrane lung is applied to the circuit |
| Venovenoarterial | VVA | hybrid | Provides circulatory and gas exchange support via arterial and venous return |

**Table 2-2.** Support modes for ECLS, describing the intended organ support mode without designating the cannulation configuration.

***Use of prefixes***. A prefix expressed with lowercase letters within parentheses can be added to provide detail. For example, AV ECCO$_2$R in a pumpless circuit [18-19] can be indicated by placing "(pl)" directly before the drainage cannula, eg, (pl)A-V. Use of a dual-lumen cannula (DLC) is used in VV or VP ECLS is indicated by placing "(dl)" first "V", eg, (dl)V-V.[12] A VA ECMO configuration using both limbs of a DLC cannula for drainage with a separate arterial return cannula would be abbreviated (dl)VV-A. If a DLC is used for drainage and return in a VVA support mode, the cannulation configuration would be (dl)V-VA. If a secondary additional drainage cannula is added to a DLC VV support mode, it would be designated as (dl)Vcep-V.

### Cannulation Site (Level 2)

Level 2 describes which vessel is cannulated, in which a lowercase subscript directly follows the upper or lowercase letter marking the corresponding cannula. Left ("l") or right ("r") side follow directly upon vessel cannulation site as part of the subscript. Generic examples are Vx-Ay, (dl)Vx-V, Vxr-Ayl, with indexes for different cannulation sites presented in Table 2-3, and full description in the publication.[3]

Since dual lumen cannulas are placed in a single vessel, the subscripts described above are used and placed after first V. Using the side descriptor is not necessary since the site and side of cannulation are typically determined by the cannula design and thus need not be reported. The subscripts can be used, however, for atypical insertions, or with the introductions of new cannula designs if needed to avoid ambiguity.

New peripheral surgical approaches in ECLS include cannulation into a vascular chimney graft applied to the side of a vessel both in peripheral and central cannulation ECLS.[13] The use of a grafted cannulation is denoted with the descriptor "g" as exemplified by Vj-Asrg, describing a VA configuration with a jugular venous drainage, one ML, and arterial return via a chimney graft applied to the right subclavian artery.

### Additional Levels

Clinical application of the nomenclature is well suited by Levels 1 and 2. The two additional levels of detail serve to support situations where further detail is of importance, such as research publications and quality management.

Level 3 provides for description of cannula tip location. Descriptors can be applied to both major and minor cannulas immediately after the site and side descriptors. Table 2-3 lists descriptors for tip location such as "svc" for superior vena cava.

Level 4 gives the system for describing cannula diameter (in Fr) and length (in cm), and is intended to be used for major cannulas only. This descriptor consists of the diameter followed by the length and separated by a slash "/", eg, 23/15. The length is optional, and the diameter may be used alone without a trailing slash.

### Central Cannulation

Since site and tip position in most cases coincide, central cannulation terminology is more direct. Nevertheless, the rules and hierarchy apply in this case as well. All abbreviations for anatomical entities applicable to major cannulas are expressed as uppercase two-letter combinations, eg, PA for pulmonary artery and AO for the aorta (Table 2-3). The membrane lung and secondary cannulas are described according to the basic convention. Central cannulation approaches include a multitude of devices. Example: RA-PA is a central cannulation VP ECMO (supporting gas exchange and the right ventricle).

| Level 1 – Basic Cannulation Configuration ||||
|---|---|---|---|
| *Configuration* | *Abbrev* | *Specifics* | *Comment* |
| Cannula placed in an artery | A | | Return of oxygenated blood or drainage for pumpless CO2 removal |
| Cannula placed in a vein | V | | Drainage or return site |
| Cannula placed in pulmonary artery | P | | Drainage or return of oxygenated blood |
| One membrane lung | - | | |
| Two parallel membrane lungs | = | | |
| Two serial membrane lungs | + | | |
| Configuration | x | | |
| Combining central and peripheral cannulation | / | | Marks the separation of peripheral and central parts of a combined single circuit |
| Multiple independent circuits | \ | | Marks the separation of two independent configurations used in in parallel |
| Dual-lumen cannula (for V-V) | (dl)V-V | (ca) (bc) | (ca) for (dl) if cavo-atrial DLC (bc) for (dl) if bi-caval DLC |
| Dual-lumen cannula + arterial return | (dl)V-VA | (ca) (bc) | DLC with one arterial reinfusion cannula indexed accordingly (mode: VVA) |
| Dual-lumen cannula + arterial return | (dl)VV-A | (ca) (bc) | DLC with Y-piece using both limbs for venous drainage, and one arterial reinfusion cannula (mode: VA) |
| Dual-lumen cannula with return in the pulmonary artery | (dl)V-P | | Venopulmoarterial ECMO supporting the right ventricle. May be equivalent to percutaneous "oxyRVAD" |
| Dual-lumen cannula with return in the PA | (dl)VxP | | Venoarterial ECLS supporting the right ventricle. |
| Pumpless | (pl)A-V | | (pl) indicates pumpless driven circuit, A-V |

**Table 2-3.** Abbreviations used for describing cannulation configurations in ECLS. Level 1 shows abbreviations for major flow cannula and membrane lung configuration for peripheral and central cannulations. Level 2 shows abbreviations describing the actual vessels cannulated. Level 3 provides for describing the cannula tip position, while Level 4 allows description of the cannula size (length and diameter).

Abbreviations: DLC, dual-lumen cannula; ECLS, extracorporeal life support; ECMO, extracorporeal membrane oxygenation; MCS, mechanical cardiac support; ML, extracorporeal membrane lung

23

| Configuration | Abbrev | Specifics | Comment |
|---|---|---|---|
| Cephalad draining catheter | cep | | Drainage of venous blood from the jugular bulb, same side as "V" cannula on neck |
| Venting catheter | vnt | | Cardiac atrial or ventricular venting catheter |
| Distal cannula | d | | In V-A for perfusion of cannulated leg on same side as "A". In V-V or V-A for drainage of venous congestion of cannulated leg |
| Distal perfusion within the cannula | Ad | | Ad underlined indicates dual port femoral arterial cannula (designed with distal port) |
| **Level 1 - Central Cannulation** | | | |
| *Configuration* | *Abbrev* | *Specifics* | *Comment* |
| Cannula placed in RA | RA | | |
| Cannula placed in RV | RV | | |
| Cannula placed in PA | PA | | Direct cannulation |
| Cannula placed in LA | LA | | |
| Cannula placed in LV | LV | | |
| Cannula placed in aorta | AO | | Typically ascending aorta |
| Cannula placed in the innominate artery | IA | | Chimney graft may be used |
| Transvalvular left ventricular support | TVLS | | Transvalvular axial pump |
| Transvalvular right ventricular support | TVRS | | Transvalvular axial pump |
| Left ventricular assist device | LVAD | | If a membrane lung is put into the circuit: oxyLVAD |
| Right ventricular assist device | RVAD | | If a membrane lung is put into the circuit: oxyRVAD |

Table 2-3 Continued.

| Level 2 – Cannulated Vessel | | | |
|---|---|---|---|
| *Vessel* | *Simple approach* | *Extended approach* | *Comment* |
| Atrium | a | a<br><br>(al) | Right atrium if index for venous cannula (tip position mid to upper part), left atrium if index for venting catheter |
| Carotid artery | car | carl/carr | Left or right side |
| Femoral vessel | f | fl/fr<br><br>flg/frg | Artery or vein, left or right side<br><br>Chimney graft on left/right femoral artery |
| Jugular vein | j | jl/jr | Via left or right jugular vein |
| Subclavian vessel | s | sl/sr<br><br>slg/srg | Artery or vein, left or right side<br><br>Chimney graft on left/right subclavian artery |
| Level 3 – Cannula Tip Position | | | |
| *Position* | *Simple approach* | *Extended approach* | *Comment* |
| Iliacal vessel or low inferior vena cava | i | il/ir | Artery or ven, left or right side |
| Inferior vena cava | ivc | ivc | Venous cannula tip position at level of liver vein |
| Superior vena cava | svc | svc | Venous cannula tip position in superior vena cava |
| Distal perfusion | | dt | Perfusion of cannulated leg via femoral artery on same side |
| Distal perfusion | | dp | Perfusion via the dorsal foot or posterior tibial artery on same side |
| Level 4 – Cannula Size | | | |
| Diameter in French (Fr) | 25/…. | | 1 Fr = 1/3 mm (outer cannula diameter) |
| Length in centimeters | …/18 | | Do not print length alone |

Table 2-3 Continued.

## Combination of Central and Peripheral Applications

To provide clarity on the use of circuits combining central and peripheral cannulation, the configuration is still formulated in the direction of flow, but the junction between the two parts of the circuit is marker with a slash "/". An example of such a configuration is Vjra-/IAg, which is VA support with peripheral venous drainage from the right atrium via a cannula placed through the right jugular vein (peripheral component), one membrane lung, and return flow into a chimney graft (g) on the innominate artery (IA, central component). Such an approach is often used for bridging to lung transplant.

## Independent Circuits

If two independent extracorporeal circuits are used simultaneously, their respective configuration abbreviations are separated by a back slash "\". The nomenclature allows for combined use of both central and peripheral circuits.[14] An example is Vfl-Afrdt\Vja-Asg, where the first circuit (Vfl-Afrdt\) drains via the left femoral vein with return flow via one membrane lung into the right femoral artery with a distal perfusion cannula in the right groin. The second circuit (\Vja-Asg) drains via a jugular cannula with the tip in the (right) atrium and return flow via either subclavian artery where the cannula is put into a chimney graft.

## Commentary

Although comprehensive, the nomenclature is intended to describe widely adopted approaches, and special applications may not fit within this nomenclature. These special applications should be described accordingly. Once in more widespread use, the nomenclature can be adapted to include these new approaches.

Currently, cannula length of dual-lumen cannulas is not reported; however, with new devices emerging on the market, for example a dual-lumen cannula for femoral insertion, this may be a descriptor that will be added. The current nomenclature also does not provide information on cannula design, such as single-stage vs. multi-stage. Including such information would add unnecessary complexity without sufficient additional information to justify it.

The final tip position of drainage and return cannulas has an impact on patient support, in particular with respect to recirculation during VV ECMO, but also in VA ECMO using a femoral return cannula, where differential hypoxia (formerly known as North-South or Harlequin syndrome) can occur.[15-17] Blood flowing antegrade from native cardiac ejection and blood from the extracorporeal circuit flowing retrograde from the femoral artery cannula flow in opposing directions within the aorta. These competing flows meet at a mixing point (mixing zone, water-shedding zone), usually somewhere along the thoracic aorta. If respiratory failure is present, poorly oxygenated blood ejected from the left ventricle will perfuse the upper body, and well oxygenated blood will perfuse the lower body. The configuration solutions to the problem would be to consider conversion to VV or convert to VVA ECMO with an additional return cannula in the SVC.

Another rarely discussed issue related to the dual circulation with femoral VA ECMO is differential carbon dioxide tension (which can be found on the ELSO website www.elso.org for the Red Book). Upper body $PaCO_2$ is determined by lung ventilation and lower body $PaCO_2$ by circuit sweep gas flow. This phenomenon may easily pass undetected depending on where blood gases are sampled, and which regional blood stream supplies the respiratory center in the brainstem. Hypo or hypercarbia may develop in one or the other region depending on the interaction of the patient's own ventilation regulated by the respiratory center, degree of sedation and neuromuscular blockade, ventilator settings, cardiac output, and ECMO blood flow.

## Conclusion

The ELSO Maastricht Treaty for nomen-clature ECLS provides a uniform, informative, and flexible system to describe ECLS practice and cannulation configurations.[2,3] A free online tool for the peripheral cannulation segment is available (https://ecls.eurosets.com).

# References

1. Ranieri VM, Brodie D, Vincent JL: Extracorporeal organ support: From technological tool to clinical strategy supporting severe organ failure. JAMA 318 (12): 1105-1106, 2017.

2. Conrad SA, Broman LM, Taccone FS, et al: The Extracorporeal Life Support Organization Maastricht Treaty for nomenclature in extracorporeal life support. A position paper of the Extracorporeal Life Support Organization. Am J Respir Crit Care Med 198 (4): 447-451, 2018.

3. Broman LM, Taccone FS, Lorusso R, et al: The ELSO Maastricht Treaty for ECLS Nomenclature: abbreviations for cannulation configuration in extracorporeal life support - a position paper of the Extracorporeal Life Support Organization. Crit Care 23 (1): 36, 2019.

4. Aggarwal V, Einhorn BN, Cohen HA: Current status of percutaneous right ventricular assist devices: First-in-man use of a novel dual lumen cannula. Catheter Cardiovasc Interv 88 (3): 390-6, 2016.

5. Biscotti M, Lee A, Basner RC, et al: Hybrid configurations via percutaneous access for extracorporeal membrane oxygenation: a single-center experience. ASAIO J 60 (6): 635-42, 2014.

6. Taccone FS, Malfertheiner MV, Ferrari F, et al: Extracorporeal CO2 removal in critically ill patients: a systematic review. Minerva Anestesiol 83 (7): 762-772, 2017.

7. Madershahian N, Nagib R, Wippermann J, Strauch J, Wahlers T: A simple technique of distal limb perfusion during prolonged femoro-femoral cannulation. J Card Surg 21 (2): 168-9, 2006.

8. Avalli L, Maggioni E, Sangalli F, Favini G, Formica F, Fumagalli R: Percutaneous left-heart decompression during extracorporeal membrane oxygenation: an alternative to surgical and transeptal venting in adult patients. ASAIO J 57 (1): 38-40, 2011.

9. Kim HE, Jung JW, Shin YR, Park HK, Park YH, Shin HJ: Left Atrial Decompression by Percutaneous Left Atrial Venting Cannula Insertion during Venoarterial Extracorporeal Membrane Oxygenation Support. Korean J Thorac Cardiovasc Surg 49 (3): 203-6, 2016.

10. Skarsgard ED, Salt DR, Lee SK, Extracorporeal Life Support Organization R: Venovenous extracorporeal membrane oxygenation in neonatal respiratory failure: does routine, cephalad jugular drainage improve outcome? J Pediatr Surg 39 (5): 672-6, 2004.

11. Le Guyader A, Lacroix P, Ferrat P, Laskar M: Venous leg congestion treated with distal venous drainage during peripheral extracorporeal membrane oxygenation. Artif Organs 30 (8): 633-5, 2006.

12. Javidfar J, Brodie D, Wang D, et al: Use of bicaval dual-lumen catheter for adult venovenous extracorporeal membrane oxygenation. Ann Thorac Surg 91 (6): 1763-8; discussion 1769, 2011.

13. Chicotka S, Rosenzweig EB, Brodie D, Bacchetta M: The "Central Sport Model": Extracorporeal Membrane Oxygenation Using the Innominate Artery for Smaller Patients as Bridge to Lung Transplantation. ASAIO J 63 (4): e39-e44, 2017.

14. Porizka M, Rulisek J, Flaksa M, et al: Dual veno-arterial extra-corporeal membrane oxygenation support in a patient with refractory hyperdynamic septic shock: a case report. Perfusion 37 (3): 306-310, 2022.

15. Brodie D, Slutsky AS, Combes A: Extracorporeal life support for adults with respiratory failure and related indications: A review. JAMA 322 (6): 557-568, 2019.

16. Falk L, Sallisalmi M, Lindholm JA, et al: Differential hypoxemia during venoarterial extracorporeal membrane oxygenation. Perfusion 34 (1_suppl): 22-29, 2019.

17. Hou X, Yang X, Du Z, et al: Superior vena cava drainage improves upper body oxygenation during veno-arterial extracorporeal membrane oxygenation in sheep. Crit Care 19: 68, 2015.

# 3

## The Circuit

*Leen Vercaemst, Timothy M. Maul, Jutta Arens, John M. Toomasian*

### Introduction

The ECLS circuit is designed to support the function of a failing respiratory (sometimes referred to as extracorporeal lung assist, or ECLA) and/or cardiac system.[1] The circuit is comprised of one or more cannula(s), a blood pump, an artificial lung, connectors, tubing, circuit monitoring and temperature control devices. In rare instances, the circuit can be directly connected from an artery to a vein without the need for a blood pump (pumpless extracorporeal lung assist, or PECLA). Throughout this chapter, all combinations or modalities will be referred to as ECLS for simplicity.

Variations in circuitry depend on the individual component design and composition, and clinical needs of the patient. These issues require detailed attention and management. There is also a variety of hardware controlling these circuits with different monitoring and safety features. The same circuitry can be adapted for intra- and interhospital transport. Depending on the position of the drainage and return cannulas in the vascular system, ECLS can provide either respiratory and/or hemodynamic support. High blood flow rates may be required, depending on the degree of organ failure or metabolic needs of an individual patient. To ensure sufficient support, all components need to be correctly selected, sized, and carefully managed.

Historically, ECLS circuit components were adapted from cardiopulmonary bypass equipment used for cardiac surgery. Many of these devices are labelled for short-term use, typically less than six hours. These devices have been used for ECLS safely off-label for days, weeks, or months at a time.[2,3] Recently, some newer devices and cannulas have received regulatory clearance for extended use for periods up to 30 days. Existing devices may be reclassified as long-term use devices based on the interests of manufacturers, regulatory agencies, and country of use.

In this chapter, ECLS circuit components will be described, and their proper assembly and operation will be outlined.[4] This includes descriptions of disposable components, hardware, information provided by the device manufacturer, and some supporting tools to monitor circuit function. This chapter in previous editions of the Red Book provided specific commercial examples used in the ECLS circuit.[5] However, descriptions of industry products will not be provided here. For information on specific devices, the reader is referred to 'Instructions for Use' (IFU) provided by the manufacturer that describe the materials, indications for use, and operational parameters for clinical application.

## Circuit Components and Composition

The main components of the circuit are drainage cannula(s), pump, artificial lung with integrated heat exchanger, and return cannula(s). These are interconnected with PVC tubing with an inner diameter of 3/8" (inch) in adults, or 1/4" or 3/16" in children (Figure 3-1).

The extracorporeal volume and blood-to-polymer exposure impact patient blood composition, inflammatory processes, and coagulation (see Chapter 6). The volume to fill (prime) the circuit typically ranges from 100–250 mL in neonates to 500–700 mL in adults. The priming fluid composition depends on the relative blood dilution (circuit versus patient volume) and aims to maintain a physiological intravascular composition (especially the hemoglobin level needed for oxygen transport) despite the expansion of the patient's circulating volume.

The knowledge of basic physiology of flow and physics of laminar flow through tubing as described by the Hagen-Poiseuille Law equation (Equation 1), illustrating the relationship between flow and resistance in a tube.

$$Q = \frac{\Delta P \cdot \pi \cdot R^4}{8 \cdot L \cdot \mu}$$

Equation 1

The Hagen-Poiseuille Law states that volumetric flow (Q) is proportional to the 4th power of the tubing pathway's radius ($R^4$), pressure drop ($\Delta P$) across the pathway, and inversely proportional to the pathway length (L) and dynamic fluid viscosity ($\mu$). Resistance to flow ($pR^4/8L\mu$) within the ECLS circuit should be minimized. This provides important

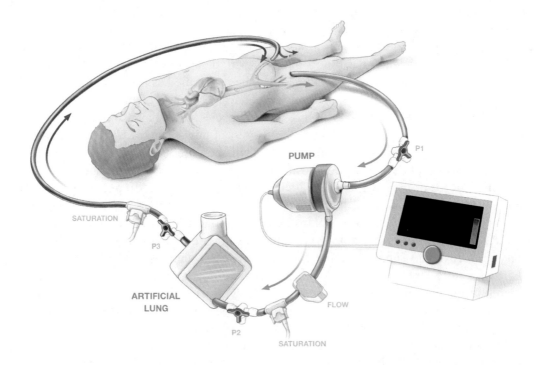

**Figure 3-1.** The ECLS circuit. (Illustration by Stephanie Philippaerts–copyright protected–Produced for UZ Leuven.)

guidance in the selection, composition, and management of the circuit. However, low resistance comes at the price of larger priming volume (Table 3-1). Therefore, both should be carefully balanced accounting for the individual patient needs.

### *Cannulas*

Cannulas (Figure 3-2) are integral parts of the circuit and provide the intravascular connections between the patient and circuit. They have a tremendous bearing on the ability of the circuit to provide sufficient flow and support and are often a limiting factor. Cannulas come in a variety of sizes, lengths, and designs. These features are important with respect to the desired flow. Cannulas are selected based on cannulation site, insertion method (percutaneous or surgical), intended purpose (blood drainage or return), desired flow rate (relative to patient size), and vessel condition.

The most important variable for flow is the diameter (radius x 2), which is expressed in millimeters (mm) or French (Fr) (1 Fr=3 mm) and refers to the outer diameter of the cannula. The inner diameter can vary between different manufacturers, depending on the wall thickness of the canula. However, it is the inner diameter that defines the resistance of the canula (Equation 1). Since 2021, the international standard on cannulas for extracorporeal circulation (ISO 18193:2021) requires manufacturers to provide the inner diameter of the cannula on packaging in addition to the outer diameter. The cannula length is a function of the size of the patient and the desired site for placement of blood drainage and return. Practitioners should keep in mind that cannula length linearly increases resistance to flow. Each specific cannula has its own flow/pressure curve, which can be found in the IFU to facilitate proper cannula selection. Generally, practitioners target working pressure drops <50 mmHg for drainage cannulas and <100 mmHg for return cannulas.

Information given by the manufacturers in the IFU typically includes the pressure drop (a surrogate for resistance) from cannula inlet to outlet that occurs at various flow rates. Historically, this information was based upon water as the test fluid (with a much lower viscosity compared to blood), and thus underestimated the true resistance of the cannula. The new standard ISO 18193, published in 2021, requires manufacturers to determine the resistance by using a blood analogue fluid with a viscosity matching that of blood. In approximately the next 5 years, there will be descriptive information on cannulas concerning the pressure drop based on both water and blood analogues.

Cannulas are typically manufactured using PVC or polyurethane polymers and can be surface coated to improve hemocompatibility. Wire reinforcement is typically integrated within the wall to avoid kinking and collapsing and for radiographic visualization. Some cannulas contain additional radiographic

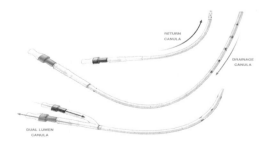

**Figure 3-2.** Cannulas. (Illustrations by Stephanie Philippaerts–copyright protected–Produced for UZ Leuven.)

| TUBING NOMINAL (inner) DIAMETER | | PRIMING VOLUME PER LENGTH | RESISTANCE PER LENGTH AT 1 L/min BLOOD FLOW* | SURFACE AREA PER LENGTH |
|---|---|---|---|---|
| 3/1" | (4.76 mm) | 17.8 mL/m | 35 mmHg/m/($L_{Blood}$/min) | 0.015 m²/m |
| 1/4" | (6.35 mm) | 31.7 mL/m | 11 mmHg/m/($L_{Blood}$/min) | 0.020 m²/m |
| 3/8" | (9.53 mm) | 71.3 mL/m | 2 mmHg/m/($L_{Blood}$/min) | 0.030 m²/m |
| 1/2" | (12.7 mm) | 126.7 mL/m | <1 mmHg/m/($L_{Blood}$/min) | 0.040 m²/m |
| *Calculated using Hagen-Poiseuille equation and blood viscosity of 0.0035 Ns/m² | | | | |

**Table 3-1.** Typical tubing diameters and their resulting priming volume and resistance as a function of length.

markers in the tip or along the body length to aide practitioners in assessing correct placement. Generally, a central hole is found at the tip as the main area for flow in or out of the cannula. Often, side holes are added as an alternative pathway through which the blood can drain or be returned to the patient. The position of the side holes can be near the tip or placed at intervals ("multistage") along the length of the cannula. The presence of these side holes in the drainage cannulas avoids suction of the cannula to the wall of the blood vessel by providing various flow paths. Side holes in return cannulas allow for a fountain effect to prevent jetting, or in the case of femoral arterial cannulas, competition with antegrade flow from the heart. Fluid dynamic studies have demonstrated that flow preferentially moves through side holes proximal to the source of flow, and that blood stasis at the distal side holes can occur if the blood flow is low enough.[6] Additionally, there are stent-like designs which can expand the cannula diameter in the vessel after placement.[7]

ECLS cannulas can be built as single-lumen, meaning that two separate cannulas are used for drainage and return of blood, or as dual-lumen, where a single cannula is internally divided to provide drainage and return flow. There are two general designs of dual-lumen cannulas: bicaval and unicaval.

The bicaval design is for placement reaching from the superior vena cava (SVC) into the inferior vena cava (IVC) and thus has the return opening as a side hole in the right atrium. The blood is drained from both the SVC (using side holes) and IVC (using side holes and the open tip). In this design, the return pathway within the cannula consists of a circle segment on one side of the lumen, leaving a crescent-shaped area for drainage. The return path is usually collapsible to allow the use of a dilator and guidewire for placement. The unicaval design aims for placement with drainage side holes in the SVC and a single point of return at the open tip either in the right atrium directed towards the tricuspid valve, or in the pulmonary artery.

Both general designs have their benefits and disadvantages. The bicaval design requires exact and precise placement. If the blood outlet port is not correctly positioned in the right atrium, recirculation can occur (oxygenated blood reentering the cannula rather than moving forward in the pulmonary circulation). On the other hand, because it drains blood from both superior and inferior vena cavae, recirculation can be reduced.[8] Careful monitoring with various imaging techniques is necessary to properly place the cannula and avoid perforation of the right ventricle or IVC. The unicaval design drains blood solely from the SVC, which can increase recirculation.[9] However, it is easier to place because the tip only needs to be advanced through the superior vena cava to the right atrium.

**Blood Pumps – Physics, Design, and Impact on Performance**

The blood pump is the heart of the circuit. Numerous pump designs have been used in clinical application, the majority being roller or centrifugal pumps. Both pump types have different operating characteristics. The roller pump is a volume displacement pump, while the centrifugal pump is categorized as a pressure generating pump. While the roller pump was the historical gold standard, there has been a steady shift over the years towards the use of a centrifugal pump.[2]

*Volume Displacement Pumps (Roller Pumps)*

Volume displacement pumps were first developed for cardiopulmonary bypass and found some success as mechanical circulatory assist devices or early ventricular assist devices. Volume displacement for these applications is generally accomplished via a pure mechanical-fluid interaction (eg, roller pump, Figure 3-3 left) or an intermediate gas (eg, pneumatic membrane pump). In essence, with each revolution or cycle of a mechanical actuator, a specific volume of blood is displaced. Volume displacement pumps typically displace the same amount of volume per revolution or cycle, enabling calculation of flow rate rather than requiring direct measurement. However, the use of a flow meter can corroborate the exact flow rate. Since blood is assumed to be an incompressible fluid, the prescribed blood volume is generated without regard to inlet or outlet pressures. Thus, high afterload can create an enormous strain on the pump, the associated peripheral tubing, and the cellular elements in the blood, which may lead to tubing rupture or hemolysis.[10] Conversely, a low preload or inlet obstruction may result in gaseous microemboli formation from dissolved gas, which is referred to as outgassing or cavitation. Therefore, additional monitoring and servo regulation of the volume displacement pump for both inlet and outlet pressure are necessary. Volume displacement pumps tend to be larger than centrifugal pumps that provide the same cardiac output. Although most volume displacement pumps produce small to moderate pulses with each stroke/compression of the tubing, the pulse wave is typically dampened in the membrane lung.

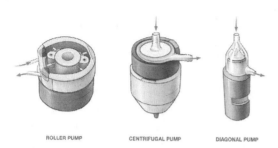

ROLLER PUMP   CENTRIFUGAL PUMP   DIAGONAL PUMP

**Figure 3-3**. Typical blood pumps utilized in ECLS. (Illustration by Stephanie Philippaerts–copyright protected–Produced for UZ Leuven.)

## Pressure Generating Pumps (Centrifugal Pumps)

A centrifugal pump, a pressure generating pump, is a newer type of ECLS blood pump. However, centrifugal pumps have been utilized previously in other clinical applications, including cardiopulmonary bypass. To make these devices suitable for blood contact, advanced mechanical design and fluid dynamics must be met to achieve hemocompatibility. Figure 3-3 also shows two general types of pressure generating pumps used for ECLS - centrifugal and diagonal. The flow path of the blood through the device generally determines its classification. Centrifugal pumps use centripetal motion to draw in fluid on one axis and exit the fluid on the other orthogonal axis. Diagonal pumps are essentially a hybrid of centrifugal and axial (fluid inlet and outlet along the same general axis) pumps and are also referred to as mixed flow pumps. Pressure generating pumps are mechanically complicated in terms of sensors, controllers, and general equipment, but more compact than their volume displacement counterparts. Pressure generating pumps are also more difficult to conceptually understand regarding their technical behaviour, physiologic interactions, and clinical use.

A pressure generating pump uses a moving series of blades attached to a central rotating mass, referred as an impeller. The impeller produces rotational velocity in a fluid. Many impeller designs exist. Some rest on a central bearing or bearings. Other designs are magnetically levitated by means of magnetic coupling. When rotating, impellers create a sub atmospheric pressure or suction at the central blood inlet, impart rotary motion to the fluid, and drive the fluid to the outlet port by centrifugal forces. The rotary motion or velocity creates a pressure gradient across the pump that drives fluid from high to low pressure. During normal operation, most pressure generating blood pumps run at a constant pump speed;

however, some pumps may also be run in a more pulsatile flow mode. This pulsatility is achieved by modulating the pump speed at a certain frequency and amplitude.

All pressure generating pump types require a certain circumferential speed as a function of impeller diameter to generate a given blood flow. The generated pressure gradient is dependent on the density and viscosity of the fluid and mechanical aspects of the pump (impeller diameter, blade dimensions, fluid gaps, etc.). These latter topics are beyond the scope of this chapter but are found in mechanical engineering and biomedical engineering textbooks.[11] Importantly for practitioners, the pump speed required for a given flow rate alone does not provide a measure of the pump's quality.

The many designs of pressure generating pumps have been referred to as centrifugal, kinetic, or constrained vortex, but are all nonocclusive pumps. These pumps produce flow if enough energy is applied to overcome the pressure gradient, which is the mathematical difference between upstream (inlet) and downstream (outlet) pressure. The physics of this design allows for reversed flow if downstream pressure/afterload is greater than the pump pressure gradient or if the pump is not running. These pumps are preload and afterload sensitive because the flow rate is dependent on the pump pressure gradient. External monitoring of total volumetric flow rate through ultrasonic or eddy current techniques is required because they do not produce the same amount of volumetric flow at the same pump speed due to this pre- and afterload dependency. Many practitioners and manufacturers utilize pressure monitoring at the pump inlet and outlet to guide clinical practice.

Table 3-2 highlights some of the key features of these pumps with respect to their operation and under various preload and afterload conditions.

When using a centrifugal pump, the achieved flow is related to the set pump speed (in revolutions per min, RPM); if increasing pump speed no longer results in higher flows, then the physical limits have been reached. Outlet tubing

| CHANGE IN FLOW RATE | PUMP SPEED | PUMP INLET PRESSURE | PUMP OUTLET PRESSURE | POST ARTIFICIAL LUNG PRESSURE | MAP* | CAUSE |
|---|---|---|---|---|---|---|
| Increased ↑ | Increased ↑ | Decreased ↓ | Increased ↑ | Increased ↑ | Increased or Same ↑ / → | **Pump speed increased** |
| Increased ↑ | Same → | Increased ↑ | Increased ↑ | Increased ↑ | Same or Increased → / ↑ | **Preload (CVP* or better cannula position) is increased** |
| Increased ↑ | Same → | Decreased ↓ | Decreased ↓ | Decreased ↓ | Decreased ↓ | **Afterload (patient MAP or cannula resistance) decreased** |
| Decreased ↓ | Decreased ↓ | Increased ↑ | Decreased ↓ | Decreased ↓ | Same or Increased → / ↑ | **Pump speed reduced** |
| Decreased ↓ | Same → | Decreased ↓ | Decreased ↓ | Decreased ↓ | Same or Increased → / ↑ | **Preload (CVP* usually or position of cannula) is decreased** |
| Decreased ↓ | Same → | Increased ↑ | Increased ↑ | Decreased ↓ | Same or Increased → / ↑ | **Resistance is building in artificial lung (eg, clots)** |
| Decreased ↓ | Same → | Increased ↑ | Increased ↑ | Increased ↑ | Increased ↑ | **Afterload (patient MAP or cannula resistance) is increased** |

*MAP: Mean arterial pressure; CVP: central venous pressure

**Table 3-2**. Key features of pressure generating pumps and their responses to changes.

can generally be safely clamped with pressure generating pumps because the maximum positive pressures are about 600 mmHg at the pump outlet under maximum pump speed. However, at the pump inlet, subatmospheric pressures down to -250 to -300 mmHg can be generated, risking cavitation. These micro-air bubbles cause additional shear stress to the blood cells, resulting in augmented hemolysis. When these implode in the positive pressure zone (pump exit), serious blood cell damage may occur. Undissolved micro-bubbles may pass the artificial lung, increasing the risk of clotting and gaseous embolism. In addition, high suction forces can result in blood vessel collapse around the cannula, causing the drainage tubing to rhythmically move in a process referred to as "chattering" or "chugging". This can lead to occluded cannula holes, reduced net drainage, damage to vessel intima, extreme negative pressures pulses (-600 to -650 mmHg), and hemolysis due to high shear rates at the canula tip.

Another factor that can affect the hemocompatibility is pump efficiency. Pump efficiency is determined by how much energy imparted to the spinning impeller goes towards creating forward flow in the blood. Pumps that are inefficient tend to generate vortices, internal recirculation, and heat, which can lead to blood coagulation and damage.[12] Pump efficiency is determined by the pump type, the size of the pump, the rotational speed, and the gaps between the rotating impeller and the housing of the pump. Blood pumps are typically tested by the manufacturers at maximum speed where the most significant blood cell damage is anticipated. However, there is some evidence that operating pumps at lower flow rates and below their efficiency points also increases blood cell damage.[13-15] Therefore, in 2022 the ISO 18242 standard will be updated with an amendment stating that the manufacturer must identify the worst-case scenario. These may include running the pump at flow rates that it was not designed for (eg, very low flow rates) and subsequently test for blood cell damage at these worst-case conditions. Additionally, clots either aspirated or generated internally on bearings, blades, etc. can also cause acute blood cell damage or cause the pump to acutely fail without warning. Unfortunately, there is no validated in vitro test method yet to test devices for flow-induced thrombogenicity.

### *Artificial Lung*

A principal requirement of any ECLS circuit is the ability to simulate lung function using an artificial lung. The device adds oxygen ($O_2$) and removes carbon dioxide ($CO_2$) from the blood. Often referred to as a gas exchange device, oxygenator, or membrane lung, the artificial lung's clinical gas exchange requirements for $O_2$ transfer must be at least 50 $mL_{O2}/L_{blood}$. This value typically supports the baseline metabolism of an adult. The artificial lung provides $O_2$ and $CO_2$ gas transfer by diffusion. Its capacity is expressed as rated blood flow, which is the maximum blood flow up to which the artificial lung can increase the inlet $O_2$ saturation from $65 \pm 5\%$ to 95% with a hemoglobin (Hb) of 12 g/dL. Adult artificial lungs have rated blood flow rates of up to 7 L/min. For lower flow applications or neonatal and pediatric purposes, smaller artificial lungs are available with rated blood flows of 800–2400 mL/min.

The development of artificial lungs has a long history and has been described in several articles.[16-18] Blood enters the artificial lung through tubing from the outlet of the blood pump and is distributed (manifolded) to a large gas exchange surface area before being collected and delivered back to the patient from the outlet port of the artificial lung. This gas exchange surface is the principal interface between the blood and gas phases. The larger the physical barrier of the gas exchange surface, the more resistance to diffusion, resulting in less total oxygen and $CO_2$ transfer. Reduction or elimination of the barrier was considered an early solution to lower resistance in many early artificial lungs including screen, bubble, and disc artificial lungs. However, these designs had significant challenges with hemocompatibility related to the direct air-blood interface. This interface caused proteins to denature, induced inflammation, and caused blood cell trauma. Next generation silicone membrane materials provided one of the first semi-permeable barriers to blood and air. This permitted sufficient diffusion for clinically applicable artificial lungs.

The production of silicone membrane materials was limited to thicknesses around 100 μm because of the mechanical strength and rupture potential. This created a finite membrane resistance that limited gas transfer and resulted in devices with large surface areas and high flow resistance.[19] A significant breakthrough to this limitation came with the advent of the microporous hollow fiber membrane materials. These fibers are composed of polymers, initially made from polypropylene (PP). They have an outer diameter of approximately 300 μm and a much smaller wall thickness of 50 μm. The key to PP fiber function is the fiber walls, which are porous with pore sizes of approximately 30 nm. Related to the hydrophobic nature of the PP fiber, the surface tension of the water in the plasma prevented fluid from entering the pore; thus, creating a stable, infinitely thin air-blood interface. This translated to the fact that hollow fiber artificial lungs were 2-times more efficient than their silicone membrane counterparts,[19] which permitted smaller artificial lungs to be created (both in surface area and subsequently priming volume).

Polypropylene hollow fiber membrane devices were not without problems that became apparent with long-term use. Over time, plasma proteins are deposited on the PP fiber surface. Since most proteins are amphiphilic (having both hydrophobic and hydrophilic portions), the protein buildup eventually breaks the surface

tension applied to the pores and plasma enters the inside of the fibers.[20-22] The presence of fatty acids, particularly lipids or cholesterol, may accelerate this surface tension degradation. Although the pores in these artificial lungs were too small for the cellular elements of blood to cross, plasma would cross into the gas phase and drastically reduce the efficiency of the artificial lung. This was related to the fact that gas had to diffuse through the liquid inside the membrane pores, eventually through the fluid where the red cells were situated. 'Plasma leakage' was clinical validation that this phenomenon was occurring, characterized by a large amount of yellow foam exiting from the gas vent outlet. Once gas exchange function was impaired, the artificial lung had to be replaced.

Preventing plasma leaks or plasma infiltration in long-term applications requires an asymmetric (narrowing) or blind (closing) design of the pores. Contemporary artificial lungs use a different material, commonly referred to as polymethylpentene (PMP).[19,21,23] Polymethylpentene hollow fibers are microporous on the gas side and have a dense outer layer (3–5 μm thick) which is resistant to plasma leakage. However, it is impermeable to anesthetic gases. The PMP hollow fiber membrane has an outer diameter of approximately 380 μm and a wall thickness of 90 μm. The efficiency of PMP is slightly less than the microporous PP,[24] but through creative fiber orientations and improved design, these artificial lungs meet the metabolic requirements of patients and allow for use up to 30 days compared to 6 hours for most PP devices.[21] PMP fiber artificial lungs provide gas exchange for a significantly longer duration; eg, one patient survived after 605 days of ECLS with only a few device changes being required.[65]

In the design of the membrane fiber bundles, the larger the thickness of the fluid layers in contact with the barrier, the greater resistance to diffusion. Creating artificial lungs with small gaps between membranes reduce the fluid component thickness but at the expense of increased resistance to flow. Therefore, most artificial lung manufacturers trade off resistance and gas exchange values through empirical or computational design. In addition to membrane gaps, blood pathways influence surface area and resistance.[20,25-28] Figure 3-4 depicts two common pathways–axial and transverse flow. Transverse flow designs have relatively low internal resistance and are more prone to low flow zones with stasis with a higher required surface area. Axial flow designs have a relatively higher internal resistance with relatively good blood washout and lower surface area required. Both designs meet manufacturing standards for mass transfer and principally differ on their resistance to flow and surface area for gas exchange. Each design features two blood ports (blood in and blood out) and two gas ports (gas inlet and gas exhaust). Many designs are manufactured with an integrated heat exchanger, which is connected to a separate heating device via inlet and outlet water ports, enabling maintenance of a desired blood temperature. Some designs may contain access ports for pressure monitoring, blood sampling, air evacuation or connection to peripheral support therapies (eg, renal replacement therapies).

During normal operation, both PMP and PP devices remove a significant amount of water.

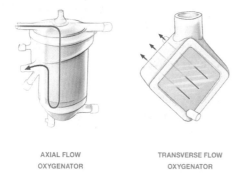

AXIAL FLOW
OXYGENATOR

TRANSVERSE FLOW
OXYGENATOR

**Figure 3-4.** Two general designs of artificial lungs. (Illustration by Stephanie Philippaerts–copyright protected–Produced for UZ Leuven.)

Water vapor loss from the gas outlet of the artificial lung can amount to over 1 L of water per day depending on the blood temperature, device fluid pressure inside the blood phase, and gas flow rate. Several mathematical relationships have been generated to describe the insensible losses through the artificial lung.[29,30] In addition, at lower gas flow rates, the water vapor condenses on the inside of the fibers related to cooler gas temperatures. This condensation can limit gas exchange in a similar fashion to plasma leakage in the PP devices, particularly because the $CO_2$ diffusional gradient is much lower than $O_2$. When this presents, a simple maneuver of temporarily raising the gas flow rate and purging the water droplets from the device ("sighing") can prevent changing out the artificial lung and is a tool that can be used to return the artificial lung to its prior gas exchange efficiency. Proper positioning of the artificial lung should be done in a manner that directs the gas flow from the top to the bottom of the artificial lung to optimize gravity in addition to the gas flow.

Ventilation gas (sweep gas) is delivered to the artificial lung via an air/$O_2$ blender. The gas composition is set depending on the desired $O_2$ transfer, whereas the sweep gas flow rate is set according to the desired $CO_2$ clearance. The sweep gas flow rate is generally established at equal to or half of the blood flow rate (depending on level of patient hypercapnia)[31] and then subsequently changed by Equation 2, which is based on one used by clinicians for ventilator tidal volume management.[32,33]

$$Sweep_{New} = Sweep_{Current} \frac{pCO_2}{desired\ pCO_2}$$

Equation 2

During support, clots might build up inside the artificial lung, which may impact the artificial lung's internal resistance. This is reflected by the pressure drop ($\Delta P$) over the artificial lung's blood pathway ($\Delta P = P_{inlet} - P_{outlet}$)

as a function of a given flow ($\Delta P/Q$). This gradient may gradually rise if the thrombus expands. Higher internal resistance will require higher pump speed to displace the same forward flow and might eventually prevent blood flow through the artificial lung in very extreme cases.

The artificial lung's performance may be checked by measuring the outlet blood gas on a regular basis. This should result in the blood being fully saturated or having a $PaO_2$ (mmHg) exceeding 2–5 times the set $FsO_2$ (%) ($FsO_2$).[1] For example, the $PaO_2$ should be $\geq 60$–150 mmHg if the $FsO_2$ is set to 30%. If the outlet blood gas value worsens, the post artificial lung blood gas may reflect a partially clotted surface and may investigated further by calculation of artificial lung gas transfer ($O_2$ content post artificial lung – $O_2$ content pre artificial lung). If gas transfer is no longer meeting specifications of the artificial lung's IFU, then the performance relative to the patient's metabolic oxygen requirement requires closer observation.

Over time, clots in the artificial lung may contribute to an altered hematological profile such as rising D-dimers, decreasing fibrinogen and increased clotting times despite low heparin concentrations. This may result in a consumptive coagulopathy. In cases where rising free hemoglobin and mechanically induced hemolysis is suspected, it is important to investigate the presence of nonphysiological circuit pressures, clots inside the pump housing, or if increased shear stress forces or diverts blood through a smaller effective area.

Any one or a combination of the three preceding situations (increased resistance, decreased performance, or consumptive coagulopathy/hemolysis) may prompt clinicians to consider changing the artificial lung. However, this decision is multifactorial, depending on the clinical condition of the patient, the prospect of weaning from ECLS, and available resources.

## Circuit Composition

### *Tubing + Connectors: Requirements, Physical Specifics*

The circuit's components are interconnected by tubing, creating an extracorporeal circuit with a relatively high extracorporeal volume, and allowing relative high blood flows. Tubing diameter should be large enough to accommodate the required flows at physiological pressures. Tubing diameter refers to the inner diameter and is expressed in inches (''). Adult sized pumps, artificial lungs, and cannulas are interconnected by 3/8'' tubing, pediatric circuits usually contain 1/4'' tubing. Because tubing length linearly adds to resistance, priming volume, and surface area (Table 3-1), it should be kept as short as possible to minimize these effects and still allow safe mobilization and transport of the patient. Sections of tubing may be joined by plastic (typically polycarbonate) connectors. These connectors often have one or more Luer lock ports to allow continuous pressure monitoring or provide access to the blood for sampling or fluid infusion. Connectors may also have a Y configuration to split or join flows from multiple cannulas. Because of physical limitations, each connector effectively presents a diameter change to the flowing blood, which results in turbulent flow zones, contributing to hemolysis and coagulation activation. Tubing connectors and cannulas should be secured by straps to prevent dislodgment from pressure or mechanical movement. Connectors should be limited on the drainage line because the blood is under negative pressure and may entrain air. Current best practices recommend that all infusion or sampling connectors be placed between the pump and artificial lung where they will experience positive pressure.

### Coatings

The concept of precoating or surface modification has been utilized early in the design of ECLS circuitry to control the adsorption of plasma proteins to the ECLS circuit. Surface coating materials have been developed, mimicking the vascular wall to reduce blood-surface reactions. Table 3-3 provides a general description of these coatings and their effects on thrombosis and inflammation. Published studies involving coatings are performed as in vitro short-term blood studies and/or as clinical studies in cardiopulmonary bypass settings. As a result, the clinical evidence for their efficacy is often conflicting, resulting in recommendations in favor of coatings.[34] Importantly, there is no evidence that coated circuits do any harm, and their true utility may be in those rare clinical cases where anticoagulation protocol deviation is necessary or other factors that are not controlled for may be influenced. In patients with heparin induced thrombocytopenia (HITT), a weakly heparin-bonded coating should be avoided. Table 3-3 describes some of the impact on coagulation and inflammation related to surface coatings.[35,36]

### Circuit Monitoring

Circuit monitoring is required to ensure the proper function of the ECLS circuit and to guide management. Common circuit monitoring techniques include flow, pressure, and saturation monitoring through integrated or external sensors (Figure 3-5). Because centrifugal pumps are commonly used, external flow monitoring is required because the operator can only set the pump speed, and the resulting flow is impacted by pre- and afterload. Modern flowmeters utilize ultrasound techniques, which with some manufacturers also provide detection of macro (>500 mm) air. Pressure monitoring is performed through inline (blood contacting) or noninvasive methods and can be performed in any of the three different pressure regions (prepump, postpump, and post artificial lung). Each region ideally contains one

| CLASSIFICATION | COATING | COAGULATION IMPACT | INFLAMMATION IMPACT | REFERENCES |
|---|---|---|---|---|
| Anticoagulation | Covalently bonded heparin | Reduced thrombosis and platelet adhesion | Reduced interleukin and white cell activation | 29-40,41 |
| Anticoagulation with Negative Charge/Reduced Surface Tension | Covalently bonded heparin, sulfate and sulfonate groups, polyethylene oxide | Reduced thrombosis, fibrinogen, and albumin adhesion | Reduced inflammatory markers | 42-44 |
| Passivation | Covalently bonded synthetic albumin | Reduced fibrinogen and platelets on the surface | Reduced complement activation | 45 |
| Reduced Surface Tension | Amphiphilic polymer coating | Reduced coagulation and platelet deposition | Reduced inflammatory markers | 45 |
| Passivation | Polyethylene oxide | Reduce fibrinogen and albumin adhesion | Reduced inflammatory markers | 42-44,46 |
| Passivation | poly2-methoxylacrylate | Reduced coagulation and platelet activation | Reduced leukocyte activation/adhesion, and complement activation | 47-49 |
| Passivation | Polycaprolactone-Polydimethylsiloxane-Polycaprolactone integrated into plastic | Reduced thrombin and platelet activation | Reduced complement generation, increased IL-10 (anti-inflammatory) | 50-52 |
| Passivation | Phosphorylcholine | Reduced fibrinogen and platelet binding | Increased T-cell activation through IL-8 | 53 |

**Table 3-3.** ECLS Coatings, classifications, and impact on the coagulation and inflammatory systems.

pressure sensor for direct or indirect continuous monitoring. Pressure monitoring may give useful information on the functionality of the circuit and/or the condition of the patient. The pump inlet pressure (often denoted P1) is mostly a negative pressure reflecting the availability of volume to the pump inlet and should not exceed -100 mmHg to avoid chattering of the drainage lines or collapsing the vessel. Postpump, or pre-artificial lung pressure (often denoted P2) is the highest pressure in the circuit and reflects the resistance at the entrance of the artificial lung through to the return cannula tip. Post-artificial lung pressure (often denoted P3) is lower than P2 due to pressure drop over the artificial lung and reflects the resistance along the tubing, cannula, and in the returning vessel. The difference in P2 and P3, is denoted as ΔP and reflects the internal resistance of the artificial lung.

Oxygen saturation of the drained blood $(S_{pre}O_2)$ and the blood leaving the artificial lung $(S_{post}O_2)$ is often monitored to indicate efficiency of ECLS support and artificial lung performance, respectively. $S_{pre}O_2$ reflects the $O_2$ saturation from blood leaving the venous cannulation site and should ideally be kept above 65–70%. Values can be higher in cases of decreased oxygen extraction or metabolism or contamination of the drainage blood with ECLS circuit blood (recirculation in V-V ECMO) or with arterial blood (left heart venting or atrial septal defects). $S_{post}O_2$ should be 100% to indicate blood is fully saturated by the artificial lung. Several instances can lead to low device outlet saturations $(S_{post}O_2)$. These include a low inlet saturation $(S_{pre}O_2)$ (eg, <60%) at or near the rated flow of the artificial lung, a $FsO_2$ below 60%, or a failing artificial lung. Monitoring the artificial lung can be done via integrated $O_2$ saturation sensors or separate inline (blood contacting) or clamp-on (nonblood contacting) continuous $O_2$ saturation monitoring devices.[62] These devices typically use absorbance at specific red wavelengths to indicate $O_2$ saturation and will also provide estimates of hematocrit. Saturation values are less significant if the hemoglobin concentration is not accounted for and managed appropriately.[63]

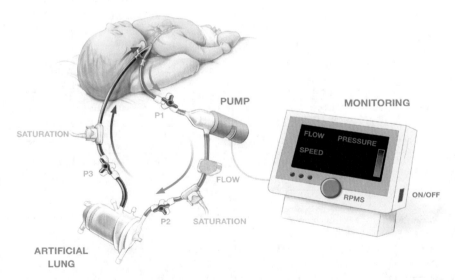

**Figure 3-5.** Circuit monitoring featuring flow, pressure prepump (P1), pressure pre artificial (P2) and post artificial (P3) lung, and O₂ saturation pre and post artificial lung. (Illustration by Stephanie Philippaerts–copyright protected–Produced for UZ Leuven.)

### *Pump Console or Hardware*

Most centrifugal pump systems are operated via manufacturer or device specific hardware, or consoles, all containing different operating, monitoring, and safety features. The main function of the hardware is to set pump speed and to measure and display the resulting flow. Some devices contain an integrated pressure regulator, allowing the operator to set a negative pressure limit, resulting in an automatic reduction in pump speed as soon this limit is reached. Alarm features vary, but most devices display a 'low flow', 'pressure limit', 'air bubble', and 'back flow' alarm. Modern consoles contain backup batteries in the event of central power supply loss or transport, and a motor backup (manual or electric) in case of motor failure.

Many factors are considered in choosing the pump console. Local experience and hardware complexity are often program specific. For intrahospital transport, the console must be easily and safely portable. For interhospital transport, the system must be safe and approved for transport via ambulance, helicopter, or fixed-wing aircraft. Using the same pump or system within a hospital network ensures safety and quality of care and facilitates interchanging or loaning devices or disposables between participating departments and hospitals. In each specific program, the nature of the program's cardiac, respiratory, or emergency support awaiting referral may have a different support duration. Extended support over days, weeks, or months might benefit from more advanced devices which may be more costly. This impacts on the economics approved term of usage, reimbursement, and other local budget considerations. Regardless of these factors, any system must ensure reliable technical support as well as manufacturer support for backup consoles that is available at all times, and fast delivery of circuits and other disposables. Team training with the relevant equipment to ensure efficient intervention in case of emergency is a key component of programmatic success (Chapters 7 and 54).

### *Temperature Regulation Devices*

During support, the blood is continuously exposed to the ambient temperature of the environment. The oxygen in the sweep gas comes from a cold liquid oxygen source and the subsequent evaporative vapor loss across the membrane dissipates heat, which may cool the patient. Therefore, nearly all patients, in particular infants and small children, may require direct blood warming to maintain normal body temperature. For this reason, blood path warming via a heat exchanger is integrated into most artificial lungs. This integrated heat exchanger is connected via tubing to a thermal regulation device that uses water as an energy transfer medium. In general, the temperature of the warming fluid is maintained between 36 to <38.5° C, which is related to the heat exchanger efficiency and thermal regulation device to achieve normothermia. The heat exchanger material is typically stainless steel, polyethylene terephthalate (PET), or polyurethane. These areas are glued (or potted) to separate the sterile blood path away from the nonsterile water path.

Warming the gas source or employing topical warming methods in small patients (ie, warm air blanket) may also prove effective. For larger patients, direct blood warming may be implemented, but is often not required and is discontinued if temperature autoregulation is maintained.

While thermal regulation devices are mainly used to maintain normothermia, mild hypothermia may be considered to decrease metabolic demands or for neuroprotection.

Several water-based thermal regulation units that have been used to maintain the circuit temperature, but various regulatory agencies have typically not granted full ECLS indications because these devices lack patient blood feedback regulatory mechanisms. Without such precautions, patient blood temperatures can be raised or lowered to dangerous levels without careful attention.

In 2014, infections related to the use of contaminated water-containing thermal recirculation devices were reported in patients on cardiopulmonary bypass. These infections were caused by *Mycobacterium chimaera*. It was hypothesized that the contaminated water was aerosolized by the device's cooling fan and that the *M. chimaera* resulted in infections in surgical patients. As a result, many manufacturers and institutional infection control teams have implemented strict cleaning and maintenance guidelines for any thermal regulation devices associated with cardiopulmonary bypass or ECLS.[64]

**Summary**

The development of ECLS circuit components has progressed from the early days of being handmade by practitioners towards an expanding variety of choices from multiple manufacturers. Because there can often be subtle but important differences between these components, it is incumbent upon practitioners at all levels of ECLS care to fully understand each of the specific circuit components used at their local institution. This will enhance the physiologic understanding of the ECLS system as a whole and aide in troubleshooting when situations invariably arise that deviate from the normal clinical picture, and will ultimately ensure that each patient receives the highest level of safe and effective care during the temporary period of ECLS support.

## References

1. Conrad SA, Broman LM, Taccone FS, et al. The Extracorporeal Life Support Organization Maastricht Treaty for Nomenclature in Extracorporeal Life Support. A Position Paper of the Extracorporeal Life Support Organization. Am J Respir Crit Care Med. 2018;198(4):447-451.

2. Hayes MM, Fallon BP, Barbaro RP, et al. Membrane Lung and Blood Pump Use During Prolonged Extracorporeal Membrane Oxygenation: Trends From 2002 to 2017. ASAIO J. 2021;67(9):1062-1070.

3. Philipp A, De Somer F, Foltan M, et al. Life span of different extracorporeal membrane systems for severe respiratory failure in the clinical practice. PLoS ONE. 2018;13(6):e0198392.

4. Gajkowski EF, Herrera G, Hatton L, Velia Antonini M, et al. ELSO Guidelines for Adult and Pediatric Extracorporeal Membrane Oxygenation Circuits. ASAIO J. 2022;68(2):133-152.

5. Toomasian JM, Vercaemst L, Bottrell S, et al. The Circuit. In: Brogan TV, Lequier L, Lorusso R, Maclaren G, Peek GJ, eds. Extracorporeal Life Support: The ELSO Red Book. 5th ed. Ann Arbor: ELSO; 2017:49-80.

6. Rauh P, Benk C, Beyersdorf F, et al. Determination of local flow ratios and velocities in a femoral venous cannula with computational fluid dynamics and 4D flow-sensitive magnetic resonance imaging: A method validation. Artif Organs. 2021;45(5):506-515.

7. Mueller XM, Tevaearai HT, Jegger D, et al. The Smart Cannula: A New Concept for Improved Venous Drainage with No Impact on Blood Cells Integrity. ASAIO J. 2002;48(2):132.

8. Palmer O, Palmer K, Hultman J, et al. Cannula Design and Recirculation During Venovenous Extracorporeal Membrane Oxygenation. ASAIO J. 2016;62(6):737-742.

9. Rasooli R, Jamil M, Rezaeimoghaddam M, et al. Hemodynamic performance limits of the neonatal Double-Lumen cannula. J Biomech. 2021;121:110382.

10. Xu Z, Yang M, Wang X, et al. The Influence of Different Operating Conditions on the Blood Damage of a Pulsatile Ventricular Assist Device. ASAIO J. 2015;61(6):656-663.

11. Smith PA, Wang Y, Gross-Hardt S, et al. Chapter 10 - Hydraulic design. In: Gregory SD, Stevens MC, Fraser JF, eds. Mechanical Circulatory and Respiratory Support. Academic Press; 2018:301-334.

12. Dasse KA, Gellman B, Kameneva MV, et al. Assessment of hydraulic performance and biocompatibility of a MagLev centrifugal pump system designed for pediatric cardiac or cardiopulmonary support. ASAIO J. 2007;53(6):771-777.

13. Gross-Hardt S, Hesselmann F, Arens J, et al. Low-flow assessment of current ECMO/ECCO2R rotary blood pumps and the potential effect on hemocompatibility. Crit Care. 2019;23(1):348.

14. Fiusco F, Broman LM, Prahl Wittberg L. Blood Pumps for Extracorporeal Membrane Oxygenation: Platelet Activation During Different Operating Conditions. ASAIO J. 2022;68(1):79-86.

15. Fuchs G, Berg N, Broman LM, et al. Flow-induced platelet activation in components of the extracorporeal membrane oxygenation circuit. Sci Rep. 2018;8(1):13985.

16. Lim MW. The history of extracorporeal oxygenators. Anaesthesia. 2006;61(10):984-995.

17. Stammers AH. Historical aspects of cardiopulmonary bypass: from antiquity to acceptance. J Cardiothorac Vasc Anesth. 1997;11(3):266-274.

18. DeWall RA. The evolution of the helical reservoir pump-oxygenator system at the University of Minnesota. Ann Thorac Surg. 2003;76(6):S2210-2215.

19. Federspiel W, Henchir K. Lung. Artificial: basic principles and current applications. In: Encyclopedia of Biomaterials and Biomedical Engineering: LZ. Informa Healthcare; 2004:910.

20. Wegner JA. Oxygenator anatomy and function. J Cardiothorac Vasc Anesth. 1997;11(3):275-281.

21. Toomasian JM, Schreiner RJ, Meyer DE, et al. A polymethylpentene fiber gas exchanger for long-term extracorporeal life support. ASAIO J. 2005;51(4):390-397.

22. Eash HJ, Jones HM, Hattler BG, et al. Evaluation of plasma resistant hollow fiber membranes for artificial lungs. ASAIO J. 2004;50(5):491-497.

23. Eya K, Tatsumi E, Taenaka Y, et al. Development of a membrane oxygenator for long-term respiratory support and its experimental evaluation in prolonged ECMO. ASAIO J. 1996;42(5):M832-836.

24. Osipov OA. Gas permeability of polymer films for use in membrane oxygenators. Biomed Eng (NY). 1973;7(1):19-21.

25. Schaadt J. Fiber manufacturing, membrane classification, and winding technologies associated with membrane oxygenators. J Extra Corpor Technol. 1998;30(1):30-34.

26. Hirschl RB. Devices. In: Zwischenberger JB, Bartlett RH, eds. ECMO: Extracoporeal Cadiopulmonary Support in Critical Care. Ann Arbor, MI: Extracoporeal Life Support Organization; 1995:159-190.

27. Galletti P, Colton C. Artificial Lungs and Blood-Gas Exchange Devices. In: Bronzino JD, ed. The Biomedical engineering handbook. Boca Raton: CRC Press : IEEE Press; 1995:1879-1897.

28. Mockros L, Cook K. Engineering Design of Thoracic Artificial Lungs. In: The Artificial Lung. Austin: Landes Biosciences Publishers; 2002:33–64.

29. Chang LL, Tam OY, Kwan MC, et al. Insensible water loss through adult extracorporeal membrane oxygenation circuit: an in vitro study. ASAIO J. 2014;60(5):508-512.

30. Lawson D, Holt D. Insensible water loss from the Jostra Quadrox D oxygenator: an in vitro study. Perfusion. 2007;22(6):407-410.

31. Romano TG, Mendes PV, Park M, et al. Extracorporeal respiratory support in adult patients. J Bras Pneumol. 2017;43(1):60-70.

32. Joyce CJ, Udy A, Weeden M, et al. What Determines the Arterial Partial Pressure of Carbon Dioxide on Venovenous Extracorporeal Membrane Oxygenation? ASAIO J. 2021.

33. Wexler HR, Lok P. A simple formula for adjusting arterial carbon dioxide tension. Canadian Anaesthetists' Society Journal. 1981;28(4):370-372.

34. Fleisher LA. Evidence-Based Practice of Anesthesiology. Philadelphia: Elsevier Health Sciences; 2013.

35. Willers A, Arens J, Mariani S, et al. New Trends, Advantages and Disadvantages in Anticoagulation and Coating Methods Used in Extracorporeal Life Support Devices. Membranes (Basel). 2021;11(8).

36. Maul TM, Massicotte MP, Wearden PD. ECMO Biocompatibility: Surface Coatings, Anticoagulation, and Coagulation Monitoring. In: Firstenberg M, ed. Extracorporeal Membrane Oxygenation - Advances in Therapy. Croatia: InTech; 2016.

37. Fukutomi M, Kobayashi S, Niwaya K, et al. Changes in platelet, granulocyte, and complement activation during cardiopulmonary bypass using heparin-coated equipment. Artif Organs. 1996;20(7):767-776.

38. Niimi Y, Ishiguro Y, Nakata Y, et al. Platelet adhesion to heparin coated oxygenator fibers under in vitro static conditions: impact of temperature. ASAIO J. 2001;47(4):361-364.

39. Mangoush O, Purkayastha S, Haj-Yahia S, et al. Heparin-bonded circuits versus nonheparin-bonded circuits: an evaluation of their effect on clinical outcomes. Eur J Cardiothorac Surg. 2007;31(6):1058-1069.

40. Wendel HP, Scheule AM, Eckstein FS, et al. Haemocompatibility of paediatric membrane oxygenators with heparin-coated surfaces. Perfusion. 1999;14(1):21-28.

41. Wendel HP, Ziemer G. Coating-techniques to improve the hemocompatibility of artificial devices used for extracorporeal circulation. Eur J Cardiothorac Surg. 1999;16(3):342-350.

42. Urlesberger B, Zobel G, Rodl S, et al. Activation of the clotting system: heparin-coated versus non coated systems for extracorporeal circulation. Int J Artif Organs. 1997;20(12):708-712.

43. Palatianos GM, Foroulis CN, Vassili MI, et al. A prospective, double-blind study on the efficacy of the bioline surface-heparinized extracorporeal perfusion circuit. Ann Thorac Surg. 2003;76(1):129-135.

44. Ashraf S, Tian Y, Cowan D, et al. Release of proinflammatory cytokines during pediatric cardiopulmonary bypass: heparin-bonded versus nonbonded oxygenators. Ann Thorac Surg. 1997;64(6):1790-1794.

45. Plotz FB, van Oeveren W, Bartlett RH, et al. Blood activation during neonatal extracorporeal life support. J Thorac Cardiovasc Surg. 1993;105(5):823-832.

46. Kopp R, Mottaghy K, Kirschfink M. Mechanism of complement activation during extracorporeal blood-biomaterial interaction: effects of heparin coated and uncoated surfaces. ASAIO J. 2002;48(6):598-605.

47. Ikuta T, Fujii H, Shibata T, et al. A new poly-2-methoxyethylacrylate-coated cardiopulmonary bypass circuit possesses superior platelet preservation and inflammatory suppression efficacy. Ann Thorac Surg. 2004;77(5):1678-1683.

48. Kagisaki K, Masai T, Kadoba K, et al. Biocompatibility of heparin-coated circuits in pediatric cardiopulmonary bypass. Artif Organs. 1997;21(7):836-840.

49. Johnson G, Curry B, Cahalan L, et al. Effects of surface-bound and intravenously administered heparin on cell-surface interactions: inflammation and coagulation. Perfusion. 2013;28(3):263-271.

50. Eynden FV, Carrier M, Ouellet S, et al. Avecor Trillium Oxygenator Versus Noncoated Monolyth Oxygenator: A Prospective Randomized Controlled Study. J Card Surg. 2008;23(4):288-293.

51. Marcoux J, Sohn N, McNair E, et al. Outcomes comparison of 5 coated cardiopulmonary bypass circuits versus an uncoated control group of patients undergoing cardiac surgery. Perfusion. 2009;24(5):307-315.

52. Sohn N, Marcoux J, Mycyk T, et al. The impact of different biocompatible coated cardiopulmonary bypass circuits on inflammatory response and oxidative stress. Perfusion. 2009;24(4):231-237.

53. Zimmermann AK, Weber N, Aebert H, et al. Effect of biopassive and bioactive surface-coatings on the hemocompatibility of membrane oxygenators. Journal of Biomedical Materials Research Part B: Applied Biomaterials. 2007;80B(2):433-439.

54. Chen H, Zhang Z, Chen Y, et al. Protein repellant silicone surfaces by covalent immobilization of poly(ethylene oxide). Biomaterials. 2005;26(15):2391-2399.

55. Tanaka M, Motomura T, Kawada M, et al. Blood compatible aspects of poly(2-methoxyethylacrylate) (PMEA)--relationship between protein adsorption

and platelet adhesion on PMEA surface. Biomaterials. 2000;21(14):1471-1481.

56. Ueyama K, Nishimura K, Nishina T, et al. PMEA coating of pump circuit and oxygenator may attenuate the early systemic inflammatory response in cardiopulmonary bypass surgery. ASAIO J. 2004;50(4):369-372.

57. Zimmermann AK, Aebert H, Reiz A, et al. Hemocompatibility of PMEA coated oxygenators used for extracorporeal circulation procedures. ASAIO J. 2004;50(3):193-199.

58. Gu YJ, Boonstra PW, Rijnsburger AA, et al. Cardiopulmonary bypass circuit treated with surface-modifying additives: a clinical evaluation of blood compatibility. Ann Thorac Surg. 1998;65(5):1342-1347.

59. Allen S, McBride WT, Young IS, et al. A clinical, renal and immunological assessment of Surface Modifying Additive Treated (SMART™) cardiopulmonary bypass circuits. Perfusion. 2005;20(5):255-262.

60. Rodriguez RA, Watson MI, Nathan HJ, et al. Do surface-modifying additive circuits reduce the rate of cerebral microemboli during cardiopulmonary bypass? J Extra Corpor Technol. 2006;38(3):216-219.

61. Campbell EJ, O'Byrne V, Stratford PW, et al. Biocompatible surfaces using methacryloylphosphorylcholine laurylmethacrylate copolymer. ASAIO J. 1994;40(3):M853-857.

62. Zakhary B, Vercaemst L, Mason P, et al. How I approach membrane lung dysfunction in patients receiving ECMO. Crit Care. 2020;24(1):671.

63. Bartlett RH. Physiology of Extracorporeal Gas Exchange. Compr Physiol. 2020;10(3):879-891.

64. Center for Disease Control. Non-tuberculous Mycobacterium (NTM) Infections and Heater-Cooler Devices Interim Practical Guidance. Updated October 27, 2015. January 26, 2022. https://www.cdc.gov/HAI/pdfs/outbreaks/CDC-Notice-Heater-Cooler-Units-final-clean.pdf.

65. Nelson-McMillan K, Vricella LA, Stewart FD, et al. Recovery from Total Acute Lung Failure After 20 Months of Extracorporeal Life Support. ASAIO J. 2020;66(1):e11-e14.

# 4

## Cannulation

*Giles Peek, Ivan Chavez, Amy E. Hackmann, Yuriy Stukov, Roberto Lorusso*

### Introduction

In this chapter we will systematically address cannulation of patients of all age groups for all forms of ECLS. Extracorporeal Life Support (ECLS) includes venoarterial (VA) and venovenous (VV) Extracorporeal Membrane Oxygenation (ECMO) as well as arteriovenous and venovenous Extracorporeal Carbon Dioxide Removal (ECCO$_2$R).

### Basic Principles

When cannulating a patient for ECLS, it is helpful to ask several questions in order to plan the best strategy:

- How much flow is required?
- Where should I drain and where should I return the blood?
- Which cannulation technique shall we use?
- How long will the patient require ECLS?
- How soon does the patient need ECLS?
- Who is the best person to cannulate?
- What is my anticoagulation strategy?
- How can a safe cannulation be carried out?

The **required extracorporeal flow rate** will determine the size of cannula(s) that are needed and thereby dictate the approach. For example, an adult whose jugular and femoral veins are 35 mm in diameter who needs a flow of 500-1000 ml/min for VV ECCO$_2$R can have a 23 Fr double lumen cannula inserted in either vessel. A 15 kg child with sepsis who requires 200 ml/kg/min of flow and who has a right jugular vein which is blocked from a previous PICU episode and a 4 mm femoral artery and a 5 mm femoral vein will likely need transthoracic cannulation. Cannula manufacturer's Instructions for Use (IFU) give expected flow rates at different pressure drops which can help guide cannulation decisions. ECMO cannula flow is governed by Poiseuille's Law, which states that the flow rate is directly proportional to the driving pressure multiplied by the fourth power of the radius, divided by the length. Thus, doubling the length of a cannula halves the flow rate at a given pressure, and doubling the diameter increases the flow rate by 16 times. Side hole profile is also important; flow in a venous cannula will be preferentially through the side holes furthest from the tip, closest to the pump, as these holes experience the largest pressure gradient.[1] Figures 4-19 and 4-20 (see end of this chapter) give recommendation for cannula sizes vs. patient size for peripheral and central cannulation. These recommendations should be refined locally with the aid of the cannula manufacturer's IFUs.

Patients who have a postoperative cardiac arrest after heart surgery and are cannulated through their sternotomy for ECPR are likely to only require ECMO for a week because they will either recover, succumb, or be converted to a durable ventricular assist device. Transthoracic cannulation with an open chest is sufficient for their needs, although recent studies have shown better outcomes with peripheral configurations.[2,3] A patient who is planned to have ECMO as a bridge to lung or heart transplantation, however, may need ECMO for several months and needs to have a cannulation approach which will allow them to mobilize. Similar techniques and may also be applied to paracorporeal VAD cannulation.

Our postoperative patient in cardiac arrest clearly needs ECMO flow starting within the next few minutes if ECPR has any chance of success, so the simplest approach of reopening the sternum is the best.

The best person to cannulate is determined by balancing the type of cannulation against the urgency. The necessity for post-cannulation definitive treatment should also be taken into account. A patient needing percutaneous coronary intervention (PCI) may well be best treated in the cardiac catheterization laboratory (cath lab) from the outset. Non surgeons (eg, Intensivists, Cardiologists, and Interventional Radiologists) may the best cannulators in many situations but should always form part of a multidisciplinary team to ensure timely surgical help is available if needed.

Most patients require a bolus of Heparin (75-100 u/kg) to a maximum of 5000u prior to cannulation, although some patients may be unable to receive heparin because of heparin induced thrombocytopenia, and some patients may already be anticoagulated. Patients at high risk of bleeding may be managed without any anticoagulation (eg, postcardiotomy, drowning or accidental hypothermia patients). In these cases, blood must not be left sitting stagnant in the cannulas, and flow should be started as soon as possible. During surgical cannulation,

heparin is given once the target vessels have been dissected, while during percutaneous cannulation it is given once the target vessels have been cannulated with the micropuncture sheath or small cannula, prior to passing the guidewire. If ECMO flow is delayed, the cannulas must be filled with heparinized saline to prevent clot formation.

The following discussion is subdivided as follows:

- Section 1: Percutaneous VA ECMO in all ages. Percutaneous distal perfusion cannulas and LV venting are included here.
- Section 2: Percutaneous Adult VV ECMO, which also applies to older children.
- Section 3: Percutaneous RVAD cannulation, including oxy-RVAD.
- Section 4: Adult Surgical V-A Cannulation. This section is also applicable to older children and surgical V-V cannulation. This includes chimney grafts, axillary artery cannulation, surgical distal perfusion cannulas, and seldom used vessels.
- Section 5: Transthoracic ECMO cannulation in all age groups, including non-sternotomy access.
- Section 6: Neck cannulation of babies and children for VA and VV ECMO, including the Semi-Seldinger technique.
- Section 7: How to make an airless connection.
- Section 8: Tables of cannula size vs. patient weight for peripheral and central cannulation (Figures 4-19 and 4-20).

We encourage cannulators to read the entire chapter rather than just the section they believe to be apposite to their needs.

## Section 1: Percutaneous VA ECMO Cannulation in Older Children and Adults

This section is written from the perspective of cannulation in the cath lab because this is the optimal venue for VA ECMO cannulation, due to the co-location of imaging technology, vascular access equipment, and a skilled team. When cannulating in more austere environments, thought should be given to duplicating the technology of the cath lab as closely as possible. Cannulation may be emergent, urgent (patient in shock, but not in cardiac arrest), or elective, and may be needed for periprocedural support (PCI or percutaneous valve procedure) or for primary support of cardiogenic shock. It is important, however, to balance the need for supported PCI with VA ECMO in patients with peripheral vascular disease who may experience an increased incidence of ECMO complications. Surgical arterial cannulation of the axillary artery (Section 4) can be considered because it is usually free of significant disease. Transcaval aortic access[4] (Figure 4-1) is another consideration in experienced hands to bypass significant iliofemoral disease. As patients

with peripheral vascular disease may have limited access, the return arterial canula can be entered with an access needle and sheath to provide access to the coronary arteries at one arterial site (Figure 4-2). Finally, developing pre or postclosure techniques for decannulation following complex supported PCI is essential, which are discussed in Chapter 29.

Preprocedural planning to ensure availability of appropriate equipment, disposables, and personnel is essential. Cannula sizes are given in Section 8.

The patient is prepped and draped in the usual sterile fashion. The appropriate level for vascular entry is estimated by positioning the tip of a hemostat fluoroscopically in the medial third of the femoral head (Figure 4-3), which approximates the position of the inguinal ligament. Vessel entry above the inguinal ligament risks retroperitoneal bleeding, which can be life threatening. The skin crease is an unreliable landmark, especially in obese patients and should not be used because it usually approximates the superficial femoral artery (after the origin of the profunda), which can be associated with bleeding, ischemia,

**A** **B** **C** **D**

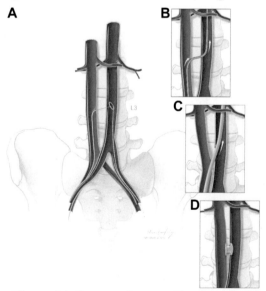

**Figure 4-1.** Transcaval access. The abdominal aorta is accessed via the inferior vena cava thereby bypassing any severe iliofemoral disease. A puncture is used to access the infrarenal abdominal aorta at its closest proximity by imaging. The guidewire is snared in the abdominal aorta and advanced to the appropriate position for cannulation. An Amplatz plug is then utilized following the procedure for closure of the aortotomy.

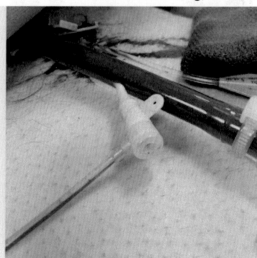

**Figure 4-2.** A sheath is placed in the soft part of the arterial return cannula to provide access for coronary angiography and PCI in emergency situations or where access is limited due to peripheral vascular disease.

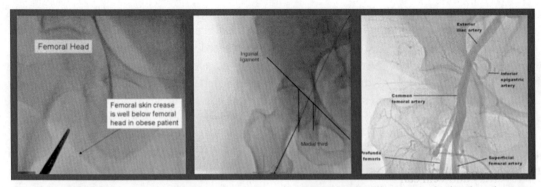

**Figure 4-3.** Fluoroscopic landmarks are useful for estimating the location of the common femoral artery above the bifurcation located in the medial third of the femoral head (center) as confirmed by angiography (right). The inguinal crease is an unreliable landmark especially in obese patients and should be avoided (left).

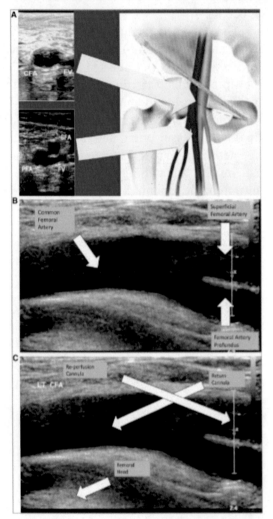

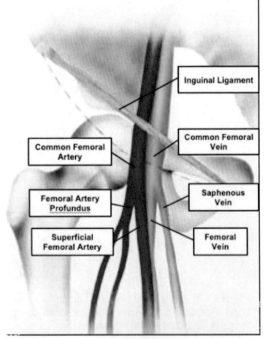

**Figure 4-4.** A) Vascular ultrasound in the transverse plane at the common femoral artery and vein and below the bifurcation of the common femoral artery and their anatomical correlation. Importantly, notice that the femoral vein courses below the superficial femoral artery below the bifurcation. B) Transverse ultrasound demonstrating common femoral artery and vein and bifurcation. C) Notice the relationship of the common femoral artery and the femoral head. Approximate placement of cannula and perfusion catheter are demonstrated.

pseudoaneurysm formation, and AV fistula. Fluoroscopic positioning cannot identify high common femoral artery bifurcations or the presence of atherosclerosis. Vascular ultrasound should therefore be used in all cases.[5]

Ultrasound-guided vessel entry may be performed in the transverse and longitudinal views. It is preferable to begin with the transverse view where the bifurcation of the common femoral artery and vein can be rapidly identified (Figure 4-4). The common femoral artery

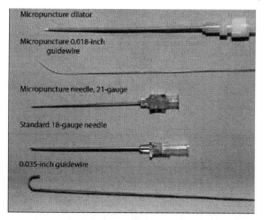

**Figure 4-5.** Comparison of the 21-gauge micropuncture needle, 0.018 guidewire and sheath with the standard 18-gauge needle and 0.035 guidewire.

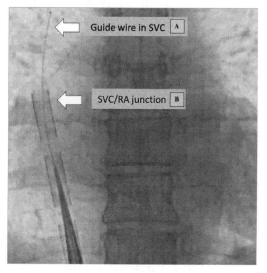

**Figure 4-6.** Guidewire position to the right of the spine confirms inferior vena cava position (A), SVC/RA Junction (B).

bifurcates into the superficial and deep femoral (profunda) arteries. The femoral vein is medial to the common femoral artery proximal to its bifurcation. Notice, however, that distal to the common femoral artery bifurcation, the femoral vein lies posterior to the superficial femoral artery (Figure 4-4A). This is an important relationship because vessel entry distal to the bifurcation of the common femoral artery risks inadvertent entry through the superficial femoral artery into the femoral vein which can be complicated by inappropriate venous cannulation and AV fistula formation. The transverse ultrasound view is less likely to facilitate the anterior vessel entry that is necessary for large bore cannulation (Figure 4-4B). Anterior vessel puncture is easier to visualize in the longitudinal view and can also confirm intraluminal placement of the guidewire. It is easier to visualize the femoral head (Figure 4-4C). It readily identifies the portion of the common femoral artery as it dives into the pelvis cephalad to the femoral head to avoid entry above the inguinal ligament. It also approximates the trajectory of the common femoral, facilitating vessel entry and cannula placement along the axis of the vasculature. Longitudinal ultrasound can be more challenging to perform compared to transverse ultrasound.

Ultrasound-guided vessel entry is performed using a micropuncture needle. The advantage of using a micropuncture technique is that the small needle can be removed if vessel entry is incorrect (Figure 4-5). The small size of the micropuncture sheath allows for angiographic evaluation of the entry site and vasculature. This sheath is small enough that it can also be removed if the entry site is unsatisfactory with easier hemostasis. Once satisfactory vessel entry and intraluminal wire placement is confirmed, an 0.038" guidewire is inserted via the micro puncture sheath under fluoroscopic control. Guidewire position to the left of the spine confirms an aortic position. Guidewire position to the right of the spine confirms inferior vena cava position (Figure 4-6). Note that this may not be true for patients with congenital heart disease.

If possible, femoral arterial and venous cannulation should be done contralaterally to avoid placing the cannulas in the same leg, with concomitant compromise of both arterial inflow and venous return (Figure 4-7). It is preferable that the venous drainage cannula be placed in the right femoral vein, giving a more direct route to the right atrium. The arterial cannula is then placed in the left common femoral artery. Limb ischemia can be avoided by placing an anterograde distal perfusion cannula or dedicated cannula with distal perfusion hole included (Figure 4-8). It is preferable to place this in advance if the patient's stability allows and limb ischemia is anticipated especially with larger 19 to 21 Fr arterial cannulas. If the cannulation is emergent, the distal perfusion cannula can be placed after the patient is stabilized on VA ECMO (Figure 4-9). Placing an anterograde distal perfusion catheter (DPC) after cannulation can be challenging. In both cases vascular ultrasound is used, and anterograde vessel entry is made with a micro puncture needle in the common or superficial femoral artery. The guidewire is then advanced fluoroscopically into the SFA. Beware the position of the femoral vein lying posterior to the SFA. If the wire is in the superficial femoral artery, wire advancement should be unimpeded because there are few side branches. If the profunda is accidently entered, wire advancement is difficult because the profunda has 5 perforating branches which may catch the tip of the wire. Angiography can also assist in delineating the anatomy. Once proper wire placement is confirmed, a short armored 6–8 Fr sheath is preferred because larger and longer sheaths can be associated with vascular trauma, bleeding, and spasm. More distal cannula insertion is also possible, always through an ultrasound-guided visualization of the superficial femoral artery. Once inserted, the side arm of the sheath can be connected to the side port of the arterial cannula (Figure 4-7A). If longer term use is planned or a cannula without a

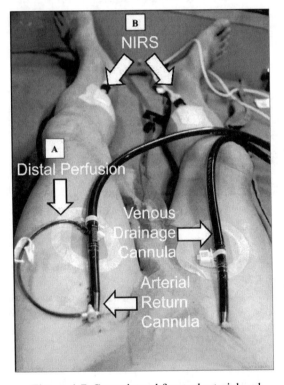

**Figure 4-7.** Contralateral femoral arterial and venous cannulation. A) Side arm of the sheath can be connected to the side port of the arterial cannula for distal limb perfusion. B) NIRS Assessment of the patient's lower extremities perfusion.

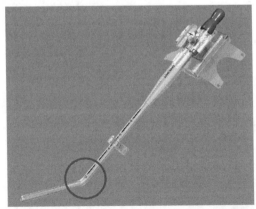

**Figure 4-8.** New cannula with the additional hole at the level of the elbow (circle) which guarantees distal limb perfusion. It remains to be seen how stable the cannula position is and whether mobilization will be possible.

side port is used, a 3/8" 3/8" ¼" Y can be placed in the arterial line, allowing a short segment of ¼" tubing with a 1/4-Perfusion connector to be used to connect to the stopcock on the sheath. This allows the use of a transonic flow meter on the ¼" tubing which gives confirmation of adequate flow. Assessment of perfusion of the patient's lower extremities should be continuously monitored by the use of Near-Infrared Spectroscopy (NIRS) (Figure 4-7B). NIRS probes can be placed on both legs prior to cannulation and can be used to assess perfusion and guide the decision to place a DPC. DPCs can sometimes be avoided when smaller 15 to 17 Fr arterial cannulas are used. If the NIRS is >50-60% bilaterally then a distal perfusion catheter is not necessary. For larger cannulas (19-21 Fr), DPCs are strongly recommended. If NIRS is <50-60% or the differential between the arterial cannulated leg vs. the venous cannulated leg exceeds 20%, then a DPC is indicated. The patient should not leave the lab until a definitive determination for the need of a distal perfusion catheter has been made. If an anterograde DPC is not possible, the retrograde technique should be used (see Section 4: Posterior Tibial Artery). Failure to adequately perfuse the leg has a large negative impact on patient survival.

Once ultrasound-guided vessel entry had been performed, appropriate intraluminal wire placement and anatomical wire relationships have been confirmed, cannulation can proceed (Figure 4-10). Beginning with the venous cannula, advance the 0.038 guidewire into the right atrium. Some operators prefer to stabilize the wire by passing it into the SVC or even the subclavian vein. Make a small skin incision (<1 cm) along the guide wire and dissect to the fascia using a small Kelly clamp. Next, serially dilate the tract and venotomy with supplied dilators to a size just below the size of the venous cannula. Ensure that the dilators move independently of the guidewire at all times and that the guidewire does not kink (Figure 4-11). Fluoroscopy is helpful to confirm the wire position (intrahepatic veins or in the contralateral leg) and show guidewire kinking

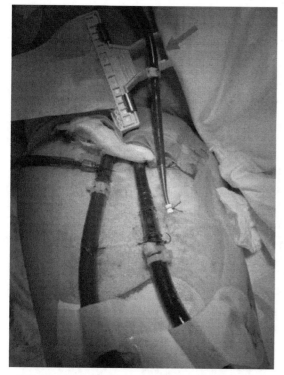

**Figure 4-9.** Distal superficial femoral artery percutaneous cannulation using a Seldinger neonatal ECMO cannula in case of impossible access at the groin to cannulate the proximal superficial femoral artery.

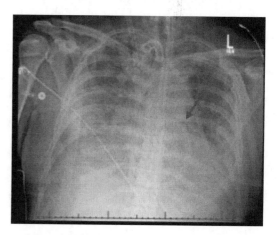

**Figure 4-10.** Chest x-ray demonstrating a 19 Fr single-lumen venous cannula in the main pulmonary artery.

in case of resistance. A 25 Fr multistage cannula should suffice in most adults. Next, advance the venous cannula under fluoroscopic guidance so that the tip is in the mid-right atrium or into the RA/SVC junction (Figure 4-6B). Remove the dilator and guidewire, de-air, and clamp. The venous cannula can be connected to the circuit at this point, which has the advantage of allowing transfusion via the cannula, which will displace the blood in the lumen and reduce clot formation and can also be helpful in the event of blood loss during a complicated arterial cannulation. Alternatively, both cannulas can be connected to the circuit at the end. The arterial cannula is inserted in the same manner. ECMO flow is commenced, and cannulas are secured to the skin using multiple sutures.

The use of appropriate ultrasound-guided vessel entry anteriorly and along the axis of the vasculature should facilitate uncomplicated cannulation in most cases. Challenging access, such as in patients that are obese or in patients under cardiac massage, need special consideration. In these cases, advancing cannulas may be difficult because anterior vessel entry is not always achieved and the tissue that needs to be dilated can be substantial. This can lead to cannula kinking, bleeding, and vascular trauma. This is especially important for arterial cannulation. In these situations, the

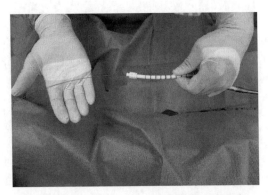

**Figure 4-11.** An assistant holds the cannula, allowing it to pass over the guidewire. Sometimes a twisting motion is necessary as the subcutaneous tissues are encountered.

use of extra support wires such as a superstiff wires, are essential. Once access is obtained, a small sheath is placed over a guidewire. Next, a 6 Fr JR4 or multipurpose coronary catheter is advanced over an 0.038 guide wire into the descending aorta under fluoroscopic guidance to the proximal descending thoracic aorta. Next, the standard guide wire is exchanged for the extra support guide wire under fluoroscopic guidance. The coronary catheter and arterial sheath are removed, and dissection and dilation of the tract and cannulation can proceed. A similar process may be used for venous cannulation.

Once VA ECMO has been initiated, potential complications are systematically eliminated. A right radial arterial catheter helps to confirm an adequate pulse pressure (>10 mmHg). A poorly ejecting left ventricle with echocardiographic evidence of poor left ventricular ejection and aortic valve opening mandates immediate intervention to avoid left ventricular stasis and thrombosis (see Chapter 28).

### Section 2: Percutaneous VV ECMO Cannulation in Older Children and Adults

Children over approximately 10 kg and adults who require VV support can usually be cannulated percutaneously using either a single double-lumen cannula, two or three single lumen cannulas, or a mixture. Ultrasound-guided target vein access using a micropuncture system should be used. Image guidance is mandatory for insertion of bicaval double lumen cannulas to allow positioning of the tip in the inferior vena cava and the return hole in front of the tricuspid valve. The consensus is that fluoroscopy is the ideal modality because it allows the entire guidewire to be seen in one image and reduces the chance of a transtricuspid RV guidewire loop forming, with potentially disastrous consequences. Some centers have reported good experience with TEE guidance, however. Fluoroscopic guidance is not mandatory for single lumen jugular or femoral cannula insertion; however, its use is encouraged.[6]

## Bicaval Double-lumen, Single Cannula

Originally described by Jay Zwischenberger and Dongfang Wang, drainage is achieved via two sites, at the superior and inferior vena cava levels, with the return exit port located at the level of the tricuspid valve. The separation of drainage and return flows results in very low levels of recirculation. Currently, two manufacturers market such a type of double-lumen cannula. Designed for right internal jugular insertion, they may also be inserted from the left jugular or the left subclavian if the target vessels and innominate vein are large enough. The left subclavian gives a particularly comfortable fixation and is popular for long-term support such as for bridge to lung transplantation. The smallest cannula which will provide adequate support should be chosen because there is a higher incidence of intracranial bleeding with the larger sizes, probably related to venous obstruction. Accurate insertion to the correct depth and radial orientation as shown below is essential for proper function.

The initial jugular vein puncture is made using ultrasound guidance and a micropuncture set. If possible, the needle path should be made anterior to the sternocleidomastoid muscle to facilitate dilatation of the track and reduce the possibility of hematoma formation. Heparin is usually given after the micropuncture sheath has been placed. A superstiff guidewire is easier to screen into the IVC and forms a better conduit for dilatation than the standard wire included in the dilator kit. Note that the pediatric size cannulas have ¼" connectors and are sized for a 0.025" wire, whereas the adult cannulas take an 0.038" wire. Prior to passing the dilator, a small skin incision is made large enough to pass the tapered tip of the dilator but smaller than the

cannula so that the skin will grip the cannula tightly and reduce the chances of cannula movement and cannulation site infection. It is usually possible to dilate to one size smaller than the cannula in a single pass if using the gently tapered dilators with a superstiff wire. Attention to not moving the wire in space and not kinking the wire as the dilator and cannula are passed is essential. Some operators find it useful to hold the wire in one hand and the cannula in the other to ensure they can feel if the wire starts dragging as it becomes kinked. If the track will not dilate easily, or if using the blunt tapered dilators then revert to serial dilations, increasing the diameter each time.

It is possible to place a double lumen cannula next to an in-situ internal jugular line if the patient is receiving inotropes down this line and it is the only access. If time allows, it might be better to place venous access elsewhere, double pump the inotropes, and then wire out the in-situ line. When doing so, screening the wire can make the procedure more reliable. If the in-situ line does not have a distal lumen of at least 18G, the 0.038 wire will not pass and a staged approach with a smaller wire must be taken. Make sure the wire is long enough to allow the exchange without losing instrumentation of the vein. A trick to obtain the correct size intermediate wire if cannulating in a peripheral hospital is to ask for an exact duplicate of the line the patient has in. A note of caution: when wiring out in-situ central lines, remember that the line may have been inserted through the accompanying artery even though the line appears to be in a perfect position in the vein. This is less common now that ultrasound guided insertion is the norm, but it has happened. It is heralded by a difficult insertion followed by massive hemorrhage and hemodynamic collapse.

The cannula is screened to the correct depth with the tip in the IVC and the return orifice in the right atrium pointing anteromedially towards the tricuspid valve. To achieve this, the return lumen is oriented as shown in Figure 4-12. Remove the dilator and connector covers, allow the lumens to fill with blood, clamp, connect, unclamp, and go on ECMO. Note the color differential between the arterial lumen and the drainage lumen. This indicates that the sweep gas is on and that the heart is propelling blood forwards. If the cardiac output decreases, the venous lumen will become red. This will also occur if the return orifice slips down into the IVC, allowing recirculation. Echocardiography can be used to confirm or fine tune the position. The cannula is fixed in place with multiple sutures. These should not be tied tight on the skin otherwise they will strangulate the tissue and erode through. Note the suture on the arterial lumen maintaining correct orientation. A film dressing with an adhesive chlorhexidine gel pad is very effective in both maintaining cannula position and preventing cannula site infection.

### Two Single-Lumen Cannulas

The configuration with a separate draining and perfusion cannula is still the most frequently used strategy for VV ECMO. Cannulation may be femoral-jugular, jugular-femoral, or femorofemoral. The most following factors should be considered:

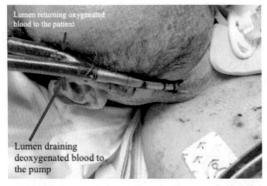

**Figure 4-12.** Bicaval Double-lumen, Single Cannula positioning: return lumen should be oriented anteromedially.

- Cannula access feasibility
- Cannula size
- Efficiency of the chosen VV mode
- Performance of the right ventricle or cardiac biventricular function
- Indications for VV ECMO
- Predicted duration of support.

Femorofemoral access has high recirculation, up to 60% in some cases, however it may be the only possible access, and, despite the recirculation, it seems to work in most circumstances. Jugular drainage-femoral reinfusion has more recirculation than the converse but can give more oxygen delivery if a larger jugular cannula is used allowing an increase in ECMO flow. This may be an important consideration in smaller children. Placing a smaller jugular reinfusion cannula and draining from the intrahepatic IVC with a 25Fr multistage cannula is a good solution in a patient at risk of intracranial hemorrhage in order to avoid a large cannula obstructing the jugular vein. Single-lumen cannulas should be inserted using ultrasound guidance for the initial puncture as described in Section 1. The guidewires should be screened, if possible, but it is not mandatory. This makes the two single-lumen cannula technique the best choice when cannulating for VV ECMO when screening is not available. If ultrasound guidance is also not available, the initial puncture can be made using the landmark technique and the venous position should be confirmed by pressure transduction or manometry prior to giving heparin and dilating the track.

### Three Single-Lumen Cannulas

This may be necessary if the patient remains hypoxic and needs higher ECMO flows. This can happen with either a large patient or if the cardiac output is high. An additional drainage cannula is inserted to complement the two-cannula configuration above. For example, draining from the jugular and iliac veins, returning to the contralateral femoral vein up to the right atrium. Alternatively, draining cannulas in both femoral veins (one from the iliac vein and the other from the intra-hepatic IVC) and returning to the jugular vein. The subclavian vein or the pulmonary artery as a return cannula is also possible. An additional femoral drainage cannula can also be inserted for a patient with a bicaval double lumen cannula in situ. A 25 Fr hybrid arterial/venous cannula with the tip in the low IVC will typically add 0.5-1.5 L/min to the ECMO flow of an adult (dl)V-V, flow becoming limited by the size of the return lumen as well as venous drainage.

## Section 3: Pulmonary Artery Cannulation, Percutaneous RVAD

Cannulation of the pulmonary artery (PA) has brought several new ECLS options. It can be drained for LV unloading, analogous to a pulmonary artery vent during open heart surgery, or for re-infusion. Cannulation can be surgical or percutaneous. Cannulas may be single-lumen or double-lumen. Flow from RA or RV to PA can provide direct right ventricular assist (RVAD) or include an oxygenator to support gas exchange (oxyRVAD).[7]

Currently, there are two double-lumen percutaneous PA cannulas commercially available. One type is placed from the right internal jugular vein, blood is drained from the RA. The cannula traverses the tricuspid and pulmonic valves and returns blood to the pulmonary arteries. A single-center study demonstrated improved outcomes from severe ARDS using this strategy versus traditional VV ECMO.[8] The second design drains from the RA and RV and returns to the PA, clinical experience is still limited with this newer model.

The 2-cannula approach utilizes a multistage drainage cannula placed in the SVC, IVC, or RA from the desired access vessel. The PA is cannulated fluoroscopically using a balloon tipped 7 Fr Berman wedge catheter. The balloon is then inflated in a wedged position to maintain distal catheter location while a stiff 180 cm wire is advanced into the distal PA. The 19 Fr wire-wound single-stage venous cannula is then advanced into the PA. Attention must be paid to keep the guidewire distally in the branch PAs during insertion because the stiffness of the cannula will tend to pull the wire back into the right ventricle. Figure 4-10 shows a patient supported with a 25 Fr multistage venous cannula from the right internal jugular vein into the IVC and a 19 Fr left subclavian single stage venous cannula with its radiolucent 5 cm multihole tip in the main pulmonary artery. Overall, the larger lumens of the two cannulas allow for higher flow rates compared to the double lumen approach.

## Section 4: Surgical Cannulation for VA (VV) ECMO in Older Children and Adults

This section covers the extrathoracic noncervical vessels which are useful for ECMO cannulation and details surgical approaches to these vessels. It also includes a surgical technique for placing a retrograde distal perfusion cannula in the posterior tibial artery. Of course, the techniques may also be used to insert a venous cannula in the event of V-V ECMO being needed. Surgical cannulation may be needed if percutaneous cannulation has failed, or if percutaneous cannulation is not possible for anatomic or logistical reasons. It may only be necessary to insert the arterial cannula surgically because of venous cannulas being already in-situ in a patient on V-V ECMO or a decision to place the venous cannula percutaneously at another site to the artery. This approach has great merit because it allows less extensive dissection and preserves the vein more effectively.

## Femoral

The femoral vessels can be used from 15-20 kg upwards. Experienced operators may use the femoral vein in even smaller patients, but venous congestion usually occurs (see Section 6). The patient is positioned supine with a roll under the buttock (or buttocks) if time allows. The feet are moved to the edge of the bed to open the femoral triangle. The position of the femoral artery is confirmed by palpation, ultrasound, or by identifying the midpoint of the inguinal ligament between the anterior-superior iliac spine and the pubic tubercule depending on the scenario. The femoral vessels can be exposed via several incisions. A vertical incision has the advantage of speed and allowing the abdominal wall and inguinal ligament to be identified as a known point of anatomy. Its disadvantage is that it makes tunneling the lines through the skin flap more difficult. An oblique

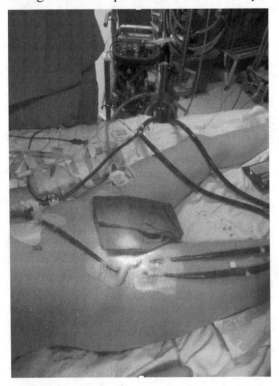

**Figure 4-13.** Hockey stick incision: open right femoral artery and vein cannulation with DPC.

skin crease incision gives good position of the skin flaps but can be more difficult to expose sufficient distal vessel without a large extension. A hockey stick extension down the course of the saphenous vein solves this problem and is the preferred approach (Figure 4-13).

Dissection with electrocautery is deepened through superficial fascia (fat) until the deep fascia is reached. Remember the saphenous vein is in this layer. If you find it, follow it up to the saphenofemoral junction. A large self-retaining retractor is helpful here. Divide the deep fascia in line with the vessels. Divide the circumflex arterial and venous branches if necessary, an automatic Ligaclip applicator can speed up this process. Dissect up and down the artery until you can identify the bifurcation of the common femoral artery into superficial and deep branches (profunda). Go around each of them with a right-angle instrument and place a vessel loop. Give the heparin, tunnel the arterial cannula through the skin flap and cannulate the vessel using one of the three techniques discussed below (see Vessel Cannulation Techniques). Connect to the circuit. Cannulate the vein percutaneously on the opposite side if possible. If using the femoral vein on the same side, it can be dissected out as for the artery, but a potentially better approach is to avoid dissecting the vein and use the stump of the saphenous vein to pass a guidewire up into the femoral vein. Alternatively, perform a direct puncture of the vein through the skin flap and then use a Semi-Seldinger technique (see Section 6). When decannulating, the artery is decannulated first, the wound is closed, and then the cannula can be withdrawn as for a percutaneous cannula or left in place if the patient is being converted from VVA to VV. Once on ECMO, place an anterograde distal perfusion cannula in either the distal CFA or the proximal SFA using either a 6 Fr armored sheath, as described in Section 1, or 8-12 Fr neonatal arterial ECMO cannula depending on the size of the artery. This is tunneled through the superior skin flap. The DPC is secured either with a purse string or by ligation. Connection as described in Section 1, and shown in Figure 4-14, to allow a flow meter to be used. Apply some fibrin glue if desired and close the wound over the cannulae.

**Right Axillary/Subclavian Artery**

Assuming a left aortic arch with a normal branching pattern, the right axillary artery has several advantages and disadvantages. First, the upper limb is less prone to ischemia due to the collateral circulation. Second, it moves the mixing point into the ascending aorta thereby ameliorating any differential hypoxemia. Finally, it is comfortable for the patient and is well suited for mobilization and bridge to transplantation. Disadvantages include the risk of hyperperfusion and/or thromboembolism of the cannulated arm. The cannulation usually follows an open approach, although, as experience with percutaneous intraaortic balloon pump insertion increases, it will not be long before percutaneous insertion becomes

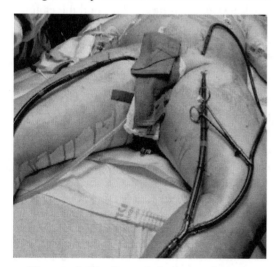

**Figure 4-14.** Open left femoral artery cannulation with DPC, percutaneous right femoral vein cannulation for ECPR, partial clamp of DPC limb to balance DPC and arterial cannula flow pending application of Transonic flowmeter.

routine. The artery is exposed via a subclavicular incision which is deepened through pectoralis major and minor to expose the subclavian vein. The branches on the superior aspect are divided, the vein is encircled with a vessel loop and retracted inferiorly. This exposes the artery which is similarly controlled. The cords of the brachial plexus surround the artery more distally and should be avoided, for a distal approach it is not necessary to mobilize the vein as much. Cannulation is by the purse string or chimney technique (Figure 4-15). Usually, the cannula is tunneled. The muscles are repaired during wound closure.

*Please see www.elso.org for Subclavian Cannulation video.*

### Left Subclavian Vein

This vessel is useful if the right jugular vein is unavailable, for instance the skin is infected, burnt, absent, or blocked. The presence of a normal innominate vein should be checked if a double-lumen cannula is to be inserted. A smaller return cannula should work perfectly well in a patient without an innominate vein who has a persistent left SVC to coronary sinus. Of course, the subclavian vein can be accessed percutaneously, however many centers have had bad experiences with a bleeding subclavian on

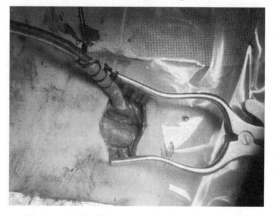

**Figure 4-15.** Chimney technique for arterial cannulation.

ECMO and try to avoid using them. One way to reduce the risk of bleeding is to cut down on the cephalic vein in the deltopectoral groove and follow it up to the clavi-pectoral triangle just before it drains into the axillary vein. A guidewire can be inserted through the cephalic vein into the right atrium or left SVC under fluoroscopy, allowing dilatation and insertion of a tunneled ECMO cannula. It is not necessary to dissect the axillary vein. The wound is closed over the cannula. Decannulation is comparable to a percutaneous cannula.

### *Iliac Vessels, Abdominal Aorta and IVC*

The *McEverdy extraperitoneal approach* can be used to access these vessels. The iliacs follow a line from the umbilicus to the mid-point of the inguinal ligament. A transverse incision half-way along this line is deepened through the external and internal obliques, exposing transversus abdominus, which is then divided parallel with the fibers, exposing the peritoneum. The peritoneum is displaced medially without opening it until the iliac vessels are reached. They are then cannulated using the Purse String or Chimney techniques.

### *Vessel Cannulation Techniques*

### Ligation

This is the technique outlined in Section 6 used to cannulate the carotid and jugular in newborns. It can only be used in arteries with an adequate collateral circulation or if a distal perfusion cannula is inserted. As such, it can be helpful in the femoral artery. Note that ligating the subclavian artery distal to the thyrocervical and thoraco-acromial trunks will result in arm ischemia.

### Purse String

This can be useful if inserting a cannula significantly smaller than the target vessel. A purse-string suture of appropriate size is placed, and the cannula is then inserted through purse string. The vessel can be opened with a knife and the cannula passed with a blunt introducer as would be the normal approach during cannulation for CPB. If using a Seldinger type cannula, the vessel can be opened in the same way, but with an incision only large enough to admit the tip of the introducer. This is inserted into the arteriotomy/venotomy, and the preloaded guidewire is then advanced through the introducer into the vessel. The cannula can then be pushed safely forwards. Seldinger type cannulas can also be inserted using the semi-Seldinger technique outlined in Section 6, the puncture being made through the purse string. The purse string can be secured with a tourniquet or tied as discussed in Section 5. If cannulating a vein which is contralateral to the artery and is possibly suitable for percutaneous decannulation, the purse string should be tied on the vein only and not tied around the cannula.

### Chimney

A vascular graft, typically a preclotted woven polyethylene terephthalate type, is anastomosed to the target vessel and then used as a conduit to insert the cannula. This preserves the vessel from ligation. The graft is tunneled to just under the skin entry/exit point of the cannula. This allows for decannulation without dissecting out the vessel again. The cannula can be removed, and the graft oversewn or clipped. The cannula is inserted through the graft with the guidewire loaded as above. The artery is controlled by pinching the graft closed around the cannula and the wire is advanced by feel, the cannula is then pushed over it. It is better to have the cannula sitting in the vessel past the anastomoses, otherwise the anastomosis is subject to high pressure which can result in hemorrhage. It also predisposes to the graft twisting like a "Tootsie-roll" (DM McMullan, personal communication). The graft is sized according to the vessel and cannula to be inserted. When using this technique for intraoperative cannulation during CPB, the cannula is often omitted and a ¼" connector ligated directly into an 8 mm conduit. This technique has also been used during ECMO but does not feel as secure. When tying the graft around the cannula it is recommended to use at least two heavy silk ties, one just around the conduit and another tied around the conduit and then tied again around the cannula. In addition, a purse string suture in the distal conduit is tied and then tied around the cannula. The graft is sized so that it can be buried beneath the skin to reduce the infection risk. An interesting variation of the chimney technique on the axillary artery using a y-graft allows concomitant implantation of ECLS return as well as an Impella device through the same prosthetic graft (Figure 4-16).[9]

### Posterior Tibial Artery

This is a good solution to insert a retrograde distal perfusion cannula following percutaneous femoral artery cannulation if an anterograde

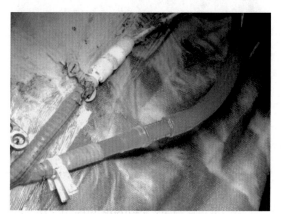

**Figure 4-16.** Single arterial access using an y-graft for concomitant implantation of ECLS return and Impella device (ECMELLA).

DPC cannot be inserted. The posterior tibial artery is exposed by a longitudinal incision posterior to the medial malleolus. It lies deep to the fascia and is surrounded by venae comitantes much like the radial artery. Having exposed the top of the vessel it is best not to go around it or to dissect the veins off the artery. Using a micropuncture needle passed through the skin flap, insert the small guidewire into the artery and then the 5 Fr sheath. The sheath itself can be used as the cannula, or it can be exchanged for a 14G Jelco IV cannula or a wire wound 5 Fr cardiology sheath. The micropuncture sheath has the best performance because it is thin and a straight though connection, rather than a right angle. The sheath is easiest to secure because it has a right-angle connection, but this detracts from its hemodynamic performance. Connect to the circuit using a ¼"/Male-Luer connector. Use a flow meter as described in Section 1. Flow will usually be over 100 ml/min and can be increased by means of a Hoffman partial occlusion clamp on the arterial line distal to the DPC-Y connector, although it may be necessary to increase RPM if doing this. Adequacy of limb flow is confirmed by examination and NIRS (Section 1).

### Section 5: Transthoracic ECMO Cannulation in All Age Groups, Including Nonsternotomy Access

Central cannulation is used for post-cardiotomy patients, particularly intraoperatively when unable to wean from CPB, or from post-CPB impaired uni or biventricular function. This approach is also preferred in the intensive care unit for postoperative ECPR or refractory shock, providing more efficient heart drainage, central perfusion avoiding coronary artery and supra-aortic vessel hypoxemia, or to provide higher flows due to the more efficient right heart drainage.

Central cannulation, based on the above-mentioned features, may also be considered in case of high-flow ECLS-related settings (eg, septic shock), but also as an alternative to femoral/axillary artery cannulation in case of an absence of or complicated vascular access, particularly in cases of limb ischemia; in case of the requirement for other devices; or after occurrence of vascular injury following cannulation.

The arterial cannula may be the CPB cannula, or the chimney technique can be used. The latter may be fashioned to enter the mediastinum via a dedicated small incision laterally at the jugular level (Figure 4-17). This technique may allow decannulation without the need to reopen the sternum.[10] Closing the sternum, if possible, reduces the risks of infection and bleeding. If using Paracorporeal VAD cannulas which are designed for a substernal path, they should be routed to avoid compression of the right atrium and ventricle, which can cause tamponade and prevent weaning. When not using these cannulas, exiting the neck or through an intercostal space may be preferable to the epigastrium.

Partial central cannulation may be used with femoral vein drainage and aortic arterial return. Other possibilities for central cannulation include Right Atrium-Left Atrium or Right Atrium-Pulmonary Artery or Pulmonary Artery-Left Atrium. While in the first two configurations, the RV is bypassed thereby providing RV support. In the last mode, this is effectively 'central VV ECMO' since the RV is not bypassed and supported. The first two configurations might be useful in patients awaiting lung transplant and requiring prolonged extracorporeal gas exchange and RV support in the presence of high pulmonary vascular resistance.

Central cannulation may be performed leaving the sternum opened in case the right ventricle remains dilated despite ECMO-based drainage, or to allow quick access to the mediastinum in the event of bleeding. Cannulas may exit the mediastinal cavity either through a subxiphoid, jugular (Figure 4-18), or intercostal route. Postcardiotomy-based issues related to

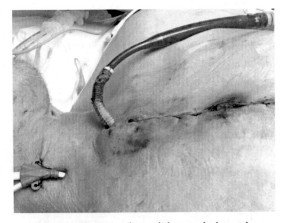

**Figure 4-17.** Central arterial cannulation using a chimney graft to the ascending aorta and brought outside the jugulum for a subsequent minimally invasive cannula removal without reopening the chest. The chimney graft may also be tunneled to the neck and cut shorter so that it sits just under the skin.

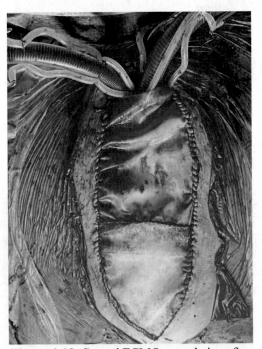

**Figure 4-18.** Central ECMO cannulation after cardiac surgery with the cannula exit point at the jugular level, with bovine pericardium closure of the skin leaving the sternum open. The snares may also be secured inside the chest to reduce contamination.

cannulation can also be found in the ELSO Monograph on this topic.

### *Right Atrium via Subcostal Approach or Anterior Mediastinotomy*

The right atrium can be cannulated via a right 4th intercostal anterior mediastinotomy. It can also be approached via a subcostal incision. These can be helpful in patients with previous healed sternotomy, especially if the SVC is blocked, absent, or connected to the pulmonary artery (Bi-directional Glenn).

### *Left Ventricle via Apex*

A small thoracotomy over the apex of the left ventricle can be used to insert an LV vent (Chapter 51).

### *Left Atrium*

An LA vent can be inserted via the right superior pulmonary vein through a median sternotomy, or via the left atrial appendage through a small left thoracotomy. Often the vent can be advanced across the mitral valve.

### **Sternotomy for Cannulation Disaster**

In the event of a failure to cannulate via the neck or groin accompanied by vessel disruption and hemodynamic collapse, the prognosis is dire. Immediate median sternotomy accompanied by trans-thoracic V-A cannulation and cooling (or using CPB and cooling) may possibly allow salvage. The neck vessels can be approached by joining the transverse incision to the sternotomy and then dissecting the innominate vein, aortic arch, innominate artery and then following the vessels up into the neck until the breach is reached and controlled. Right atrial or right ventricular injury can be repaired directly. Injury in the abdomen can be accessed by extending the sternotomy downwards. If necessary, the diaphragm can be divided to expose the supra-hepatic IVC and facilitate liver mobilization.

### *Hybrid Configurations (V-AV, V-VA, VV-AV, and others)*

For a detailed description of the nomenclature and definitions of hybrid configurations, please see Chapter 2.

Hybrid configurations include the presence of return perfusion towards both the venous and arterial systems. This usually means arterial return cannulas in the femoral artery and the right internal jugular vein. However, pulmonary artery cannulation as discussed above is also covered by this definition. Hybrid configurations may be used to treat or prevent differential hypoxia (formerly known as Harlequin Syndrome or North/South Syndrome) occurring during femoral VA ECMO. The hypoxic blood in the ascending aorta arch and branches (especially the coronary arteries and brachiocephalic vessels) is heralded by reduced $PaO_2$ in the right radial artery. Hybrid reconfiguration provides adequate oxygenated blood flow to the left ventricle and coronary arteries, promoting recovery and weaning. Additional benefits include prevention of cerebral hypoxia-ischemia.

During hybrid configurations, flow will preferentially go to the low resistance venous return line leaning to systemic arterial hypoperfusion. This must be controlled by increasing resistance on the venous return line by application of a Hoffman partial occlusion clamp, which is adjusted to give the desired partition between arterial and venous return lines. At least two flow meters are needed to measure the total flow and flow in at least one line. It may be necessary to increase RPM to achieve the desired balance of venous and arterial flows.

## Section 6: Babies and Children

Babies and children needing ECLS may range from around 2 kg to 150 kg. Obesity in children is challenging because the patient often has much smaller blood vessels than their size alone would suggest. Ultrasound imaging of target vessels is therefore essential. V-A ECMO cannulation in babies and small children is done by surgical cutdown on the right neck vessels. The risks of carotid ligation increase with age and is therefore best avoided in adolescents and older children. Femoral arterial cannulation, with suitable distal perfusion, is possible in children from around the age of 5, but reconstruction is challenging, and most centers avoid the femoral artery until patients are well over 20 kg. Postoperative cardiac surgery patients are almost always cannulated through the chest using the fresh sternotomy (see above). In this section we will discuss V-A cannulation via the neck, V-V cannulation in babies, and V-V cannulation in children.

### V-A Cannulation via the Neck

The patient is positioned supine with a shoulder roll, the head turned 45 degrees to the left. The ventilator tubing is arranged so that it is on the bed and not crossing the chest or neck. The endotracheal tube is supported with rolled towels in such a way that it can be reached in the event that hand ventilation is required. A large bore extension line is flushed and connected to the intravenous access, ensure that it is not planned to remove this access during cannulation, as may be the case for an in-situ right jugular vein line. This line should be positioned so that the anesthesiologist or intensivist can reach it when the patient is draped. The earth plate for electrocautery is applied according to the manufacturer's instructions. The right side of the neck is prepped and draped. Remember that alcohol-based skin prep, oxygen, and electrocautery is an explosive mixture which can easily be avoided. A transverse incision is made in the skin crease one third of the way up the neck. The platysma is divided exposing the sternocleidomastoid muscle. Dissection is extended along its anterior border and the muscle is retracted laterally, exposing the posterior belly of the omohyoid muscle, which is divided. The carotid sheath is thereby exposed, the jugular vein and carotid artery are dissected free, preserving the vagus nerve. Each vessel is encircled with two #1 silk ligatures. Heparin 50-100 u/kg is administered and allowed to circulate. The cephalad ligature on the carotid is tied and the ends of the ligature are clipped to the drapes to anchor the vessel. A vascular clamp is applied caudally, and the carotid is opened using an arrowhead or transverse incision using an 11-blade placed through the vessel from the side with the blade pointed anteriorly and then cutting upwards. This method allows for a rapid arteriotomy with less risk of vessel transection. All of the arterial layers are then grasped on each side with fine DeBakey forceps, and the tip of the cannula is introduced, the clamp is then released, and the cannula is advanced with a circumferential twisting motion, to a depth of 2-3 cm in a newborn. The cannula is then secured by tying the caudal ligature around the carotid caudal to the arteriotomy. Further security is then provided by tying the ends of the cephalad ligature around the cannula. The ends of both ligatures are then clipped to the drapes on the medial side of the wound, thereby retracting the carotid cannula away from the jugular vein. The introducer is removed, the cannula is allowed to fill with blood, and a line clamp is then applied to the cannula above the wire reinforcement, but below the surface of the blood. The cannula is then connected to the arterial limb of the ECMO circuit which should be identified by tracing the line from the oxygenator, rather than trusting the color of the tape. Airless connection techniques are discussed in Section 7. The jugular vein is cannulated in the same fashion as the artery, with the caveat that it is more fragile and the cannula should be inserted 6-8 cm, placing the tip in the mid right atrium. It is better for the venous cannula to be slightly too high than too low. A low cannula can suck into the tricuspid valve, coronary sinus, or atrial wall, obstructing venous drainage. The clamps are removed, and flow is initiated.

Speed of ECMO initiation should be balanced between clinical need and the biochemistry of the prime. At one extreme, ECPR, will go immediately to full flow. At the other, a patient who is relatively stable will have ECMO started at around 25-50 ml/kg/min and will only increase to full flow after the prime and patient blood are fully mixed after 2-5 minutes. As ECMO flow builds up, the patient may become hypertensive, allowing pressors to be weaned rapidly. Conversely, if the prime is acidotic, hyperkalemic, and hypocalcemic, the patient may become hypotensive, which can be rectified by administration of calcium, bicarbonate (not concurrently in the same line) and rapid weaning of airway pressure to improve venous return.

Sweep gas should be started with an initial $FsO_2$ between 50-100%. It is important not to blow off too much $CO_2$ too quickly so sweep:blood flow ratio should not exceed 1:1 unless $CO_2$ is being bled into the sweep gas.

The cannulas are secured to the skin cephalad to the cannulation incision with two silk sutures to each. Care must be taken not to cause skin necrosis whilst tying these sutures. A technique of knotting the suture so it is loose on the skin and then passing the ends around the cannula where they are tied tightly is used. When tying around the cannula it is possible to tie so tightly that the spiral wire reinforcement is dislocated. This can cause cannula obstruction and should be avoided. A small amount of fibrillar hemostatic agent can be placed in the wound if desired. The incision is then closed around the cannulas with non-adsorbable sutures. Some surgeons like to insert a small

piece of silastic vessel loop under the ligature to protect the vessel and make decannulation easier. If this is done, ensure that the ligature is sufficiently tight by performing a tug-test on the cannula once secure; the vessel should move with the cannula without any slipping. In patients where several weeks of support are contemplated, the cannulas can be tunneled through the superior skin flap, allowing the wound to be closed. This requires a relatively stable patient and a good assistant.

**Potential Pitfalls**

If the neck is flexed to the left at the same time as the head is turned to the left, this can open up the subclavian origins with respect to the arteriotomy and venotomy and result in the cannula either impacting on the bifurcation or actually entering the subclavian artery or vein. This is usually obvious from the resistance and, in the case of the venous cannula, an inability to advance. It is usually possible to adjust the head position slightly and advance the cannula into the correct position by using a slight twisting motion to get past the subclavian orifice.

Placing the arterial cannula too deeply can result in impingement on the aortic valve. This is a potentially life-threatening complication if the valve is injured because the resultant aortic incompetence makes it impossible to maintain support. It is best avoided by limiting insertion depth to 2-3 centimeters. Echocardiography can be used to confirm cannula position and aortic valve function.

If the right jugular vein is very small (<10 Fr), it is important to check that you have the correct vessel, inside the carotid sheath, next to the carotid artery and vagus nerve. If this is the case, one should suspect the presence of a left SVC to coronary sinus, in which case the right jugular may be small. Echocardiography will demonstrate a large coronary sinus. It may also occur in situs inversus with dextrocardia so this should be suspected from the chest x-ray prior to cannulation. While an 8 Fr venous cannula is available, it does not usually provide adequate venous drainage for babies bigger than 2.5 kg. It may be possible in a situation where the vein is around 9 Fr to stretch it by using the semi-Seldinger technique (discussed in the next subsection) to insert a 10 Fr Seldinger venous cannula. If the cannula will not pass it can be guidewire-exchanged for the 8 Fr. These cannulas can be very useful when a right jugular central line is in-situ because the central line can be guidewire-exchanged for the cannula through the superior skin flap, removing the need to dissect the jugular vein around the in-situ line. If the central line puncture is too low to make this possible, then the vein must be dissected without disturbing the line, and then place the ligatures above and below the line. Removing the line prior to cannulation makes the dissection more difficult as the venotomy tends to start bleeding as soon as soon as the vein is exposed.

If only the 8 Fr venous cannula can be inserted, and venous drainage is inadequate, additional venous drainage can be obtained by inserting an 8 Fr arterial cannula to drain the superior portion of the right jugular vein. This cephalad cannula or 'brain-drain' is used routinely in some centers, which is probably not necessary but is a useful technique in this specific instance.

A technique of replacing the silk ligatures with silastic vessel loops has been described. The author has witnessed this technique result in inadequate fixation of the cannula, causing accidental decannulation, and is therefore unable to recommend the approach for anything other than short term use in the operating room. Another inadvisable approach is to use purse strings secured with tourniquets on the vessels. The tourniquets are left hanging out of the neck where they become an infection hazard and may become loose if the clamp springs open. Some surgeons try and reduce the infection risk by securing the tourniquet with vascular clips

and burying them in the neck wound. This is a good technique for transthoracic cannulation but tends to cause necrosis in the neck if the ECMO duration is prolonged beyond 1-2 weeks. Purse strings can be used successfully but are best tied around the cannula. Compared to the security of ligating the vessel around the cannula, this is a poor second.

The low approach where the vessels are dissected between the heads of sterno-cleidomastoid can also be used but it is more difficult, especially to do rapidly. In addition, this technique can result in the subclavian vessels being misidentified as the carotid and jugular and cannulated instead. This is not necessarily a disaster as these vessels have been used electively for cannulation.

### *Venovenous ECMO in Babies, the Semi-Seldinger Technique*

Right atrial double lumen venovenous cannulas for neonatal ECMO are best inserted using the semi-Seldinger technique via the right jugular vein. Older patients can be cannulated using a pure percutaneous technique as described above. The semi-Seldinger approach is often described as the "exposure-assisted" technique. The technique is the same as the V-A technique described above, but dissection stops once the anterior surface of the vein has been liberated. It is better to leave the remaining connective tissue intact and to avoid going around the vessel because this tissue can help to support the vein and reduce the risk of the vein tearing. A small stab incision is made in the superior skin flap. The vein is held with forceps and a micropuncture needle is introduced through the incision in the skin flap into the vein. The guidewire is passed and then the needle is exchanged for the 5 Fr micropuncture sheath. Heparin is then administered and allowed to circulate. The .025" guidewire for the cannula is then inserted to a depth of 10-12 cm, until ectopics are seen on the monitor, or resistance is felt. In both these later eventualities the wire should be withdrawn slightly. The sheath is withdrawn, and the wire is controlled in the vein with the left index finger; do not place a gauze swab in the wound. The left thumb traps the wire against the side of the baby's head. This will prevent excessive bleeding and give immediate warning if the wire moves. The cannula is positioned with the arterial limb anteriorly. Dilator and cannula are then advanced. Once the tip of the dilator is in the right atrium, the cannula is advanced off the dilator. The tip of the cannula should be in the mid-right atrium, at a depth of 6-8 cm. Imaging with echocardiography or fluoroscopy can be used to guide cannula placement, but it is not mandatory, unlike a bicaval double lumen cannula. The wire and dilator are removed, and the cannula is held by the assistant whilst the connections with the circuit are made and ECMO flow is initiated. The cannula is then secured to the skin with silk sutures as described for V-A cannulation. The wound is then closed, using a braided poly-glycolic acid suture to bring the sternomastoid over the vein, and a monofilament poliglecaprone 25 subcuticular suture to close the skin. Because the vein is not secured to the cannula it can be treated in the same way as a percutaneous cannula henceforth.

### Potential Pitfalls

If the vein is too small for the 13 Fr cannula, it is easy to convert to V-A. In fact, if you do not ask for the cannula until you see the vein it hardly counts as a "conversion," merely an adaptation of strategy. If the vein appears marginal and a decision is made to proceed with V-V cannulation in the hope that it might stretch and accept the cannula, there is always the possibility that the vein will tear, partially or completely, and even invert into the chest. This can be prevented by watching and feeling the vein very carefully during insertion. If it is not dilating do not push! Maintain the guidewire

tip in the right atrium, remove the cannula, control the vein with a finger, and insert a 12 Fr or 10 Fr Seldinger venous cannula over the wire. This will fill the hole in the vein and stop the bleeding. If the vein tore completely and retracted into the chest it may well come out with the cannula. Keep the wire in the atrium and try and grab the end of the vein as it comes out, then put the Next-Gen over the wire. It is very rare for a transected jugular vein to cause intra-pericardial or intrapleural bleeding, and it is only rarely necessary to open the chest to deal with this problem. Once the vein is cannulated, connected to the circuit, and secured to the skin, it can be retracted laterally, and the carotid dissected for V-A cannulation. Alternatively, it may be elected to use the two cannula V-V technique (see next section).

If guidewire instrumentation has been lost, the first step is to pack the wound and hold pressure for a few minutes. This allows the anesthetic team time to replace blood loss and prepare for more. It may be possible to dissect down the carotid sheath and grab the end of the vein because it will usually retract and may stop bleeding (until you grab it). Gently deliver it superiorly and put a vascular clamp on it. Having got distal control, try and find the proximal end of the transected vein and put a titanium vascular occlusion clip on it. It is usually best to now cannulate the carotid artery. Having done this, a 6-0 polypropylene purse string suture is placed in the ragged end of the jugular stump and snared. This serves two purposes; it prevents further retraction and can be used for initial hemostasis. The venous cannula can then be inserted, and the purse string tightened. It may be possible to place a silk ligature around the vein stump and cannula and tie them together in the normal way, or to place a 5-0 polypropylene on a 17 mm half-circle round-bodied needle around the vessel instead. In both cases after the ligature is tied, the ends should be looped around the cannula and tied again. The purse string can also be tied for further security.

## Ligation Technique

Some surgeons prefer to ligate the vein around the double lumen cannula as they feel nostalgic for the V-A cannulation technique. If using this approach, use the blind ended introducer in the cannula rather than the Seldinger introducer. The disadvantage of this approach is that cannula adjustment and decannulation require formal surgical re-exploration, and the vein is ligated.

### Two Cannula VV ECMO in babies

The classic approach to ECMO in nonambulatory patients has been that the femoral vessels are too small to cannulate and should be avoided. Two groups in Melbourne, Australia, and London, UK, did not get the memo and have been using a two-cannula technique with success in newborns.[11,12] A 10-12 Fr drainage cannula is placed in the jugular vein and a 6-8 Fr reinfusion cannula is placed in the femoral vein. There is significant venous congestion of the leg, but it is reportedly well tolerated. Knowing that this strategy is possible is very useful, even if the technique is not used routinely in most centers. It is likely that design of specific percutaneous neonatal femoral venous cannulas could make this a more attractive option.

### Single Cannula, Single Lumen VV ECMO in Babies and Fetuses

Tidal flow VV ECMO using a non-occlusive roller-pump has a long history in France. It will likely be the cannulation of choice for artificial placenta use.

## Section 7: Airless Connection Techniques

### The Bump

This is the best method because it is fast, does not require another person, and maintains an unbroken meniscus, thereby forming fewer bubbles. The primer sets zero RPM on the centrifugal pump, places a clamp on the venous line (and bridge if present), and removes the clamp on the arterial line. The cannulator removes their clamp on the arterial line, which is now open to the primer. The introducer is withdrawn from the arterial cannula which is occluded at the connector with a thumb. It is then clamped above the wire reinforcement and held upwards at an angle of 45 degrees to the floor, with the back of the connector inside the arterial line, which is held at a reciprocal angle. Touching the knuckles together gives a good reference to the operator and facilitates the correct rolling motion for connection. The primer then injects balanced electrolyte solution through a pigtail anywhere upstream of the venous line clamp. The fluid fills the connector, which is then rolled together as the primer continues to inject. The connection is examined for bubbles prior to pushing the connector fully home. Once the connection is made the primer closes the stopcock on the pigtail and places a clamp upstream of the pigtail in preparation for bumping the venous line. This is done in exactly the same manner and, with the pump at zero rpm and the bridge clamped, can be done from the same pigtail.

### The Fill

This method requires a skilled assistant. The connectors are held in the same attitude as the bump, but the assistant releases the clamp on the cannula very, very, very slightly to fill the connection. Overzealous unclamping results in a deluge of blood and lots of bubbles.

### The Drip

This technique has been the ECMO standard for many years. Fluid is drizzled into the connection from above using a syringe whilst the connectors are rolled together. Its advantage is that it is easy to understand. The disadvantage is that a nervous drizzler can create intractable bubbles, especially in ¼" tubing. A modification of this technique which can reduce bubble formation is where a 14G IV cannula (the soft part, not the pointy needle) is attached to the syringe, using a no touch technique if in the hands of an assistant who is not scrubbed, and then the cannula is inserted into the tubing and connector, ideally below the surface, and fluid is injected gently until the meniscus is at the end. The catheter is then withdrawn and used to accurately drip fluid into the connection, thereby avoiding the deluge.

### The Stop-Cock Fill

This is the technique used to insert a pigtail and can be used for cannulas with a Luer-lock connector which can accept a stopcock. The connection is made without trying to expel the air. The connection is then held higher than the patient, the patient clamp is removed, and air is aspirated from the stopcock with a syringe. It is preferable to replace the stopcock with a blind cap once this has been done to reduce clot formation in the connector.

### The Automatic Fill

This is an advanced technique for the single-handed operator. The connection is filled from the patient by placing the clamp so that it almost, but not quite, occludes the cannula which then slowly fills. It is difficult to achieve exactly the correct clamp position, especially on the arterial cannula. The connection is then made as for the bump/fill.

### The Squeeze

This is an advanced technique for the single-handed operator, it can be used if there is no drizzler available, for instance during an emergency circuit change when you are alone. The connector and cut end of the tubing are held parallel in the nondominant hand facing the ceiling. Using a syringe with 14G cannula as discussed in "the drip," both sides are filled until the meniscus is at the end. The syringe is then put down and the tubing is taken in the dominant hand, the index finger and thumb are used to hold the end of the tubing and the remaining three fingers are used to squeeze the tubing and advance the fluid as the connection is made simultaneously, expelling the air. Once the connection is made, do not release the squeeze otherwise cavitation will occur. Release the clamp on the patient side and then release the squeeze and examine the connection for bubbles.

### Section 8: Cannula Size Tables

These show a guide to cannula size choice against patient body weight (Figures 4-19 and 4-20). They should be used in conjunction with the manufacturers IFU. Vessels should be sized by imaging or direct inspection. They will usually stretch slightly, especially the vein, but this must be done gently. If resistance to cannula insertion is excessive, drop down a size. Always take a size above and below the expected size. These cannulas will usually provide 100 ml/kg/min for V-A flow and 80 ml/kg/min for (dl)V-V. If aiming for 200 ml/kg/min in univentricular or septic shock, then upsize to a venous cannula for double the bodyweight (or put two in) and upsize the arterial to 1.5 x the bodyweight and accept a higher line pressure. This may mean using transthoracic cannulation if the peripheral vessels will not accept such large cannulas.

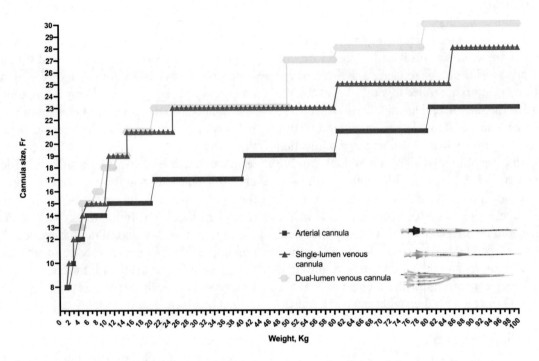

**Figure 4-19.** ECMO peripheral cannulation: relation of patient weight to cannula size.

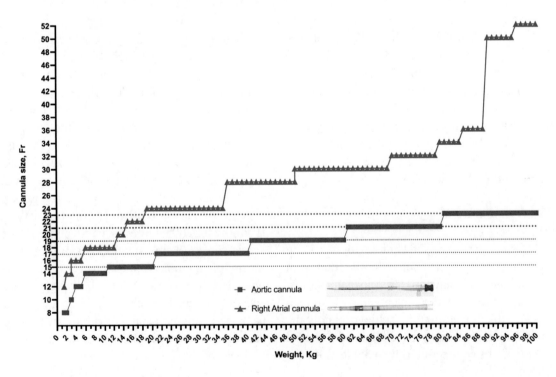

**Figure 4-20.** ECMO central cannulation: relation of patient weight to cannula size.

# References

1. Lindholm JA. Cannulation for veno-venous extracorporeal membrane oxygenation. J Thorac Dis. 2018 Mar;10(Suppl 5):S606-S612.
2. Kowalewski M, Zieliński K, Brodie D, et al. Venoarterial Extracorporeal Membrane Oxygenation for Postcardiotomy Shock-Analysis of the Extracorporeal Life Support Organization Registry. Crit Care Med. 2021 Jul 1;49(7):1107-1117.
3. Mariscalco G, Salsano A, Fiore A, et al. Peripheral versus central extracorporeal membrane oxygenation for postcardiotomy shock: Multicenter registry, systematic review, and meta-analysis. J Thorac Cardiovasc Surg. 2020 Nov;160(5):1207-1216.
4. Greenbaum AB, Babaliaros VC, Chen MY, et al. Transcaval Access and Closure for Transcatheter Aortic Valve Replacement: A Prospective Investigation. J Am Coll Cardiol. 2017 Feb 7;69(5):511-521.
5. Lorusso R, Shekar K, MacLaren G, et al. ELSO Interim Guidelines for Venoarterial Extracorporeal Membrane Oxygenation in Adult Cardiac Patients. ASAIO J. 2021 Aug 1;67(8):827-844.
6. Chacon MM, Shillcutt SK. Intraoperative Transesophageal Echocardiography-Guided Placement of Bicaval Dual-Lumen Extracorporeal Membrane Oxygenation Cannula. CASE (Phila). 2017;1(3):116-118. Published 2017 Jun 26.
7. Lorusso R, Raffa GM, Heuts S, et al. Pulmonary artery cannulation to enhance extracorporeal membrane oxygenation management in acute cardiac failure. Interact Cardiovasc Thorac Surg. 2020 Feb 1;30(2):215-222.
8. Cain MT, Smith NJ, Barash M, et al. Extracorporeal Membrane Oxygenation with Right Ventricular Assist Device for COVID-19 ARDS. J Surg Res. 2021 Aug;264:81-89.
9. Montagner M, Nersesian G, Eulert-Grehn JJ, et al. Single arterial access ECMELLA: A new concept and step-by-step procedure. Multimed Man Cardiothorac Surg. 2021 Apr 21;2021.
10. Lorusso R, Whitman G, Milojevic M, et al. 2020 EACTS/ELSO/STS/AATS expert consensus on post-cardiotomy extracorporeal life support in adult patients. Eur J Cardiothorac Surg. 2021 Jan 4;59(1):12-53.
11. Lillie J, Pienaar A, Budd J, et al: Multisite Veno-Venous Cannulation for Neonates and Nonambulatory Children. Pediatr Crit Care Med 2021; 22:692–700.
12. MacLaren G, Barbaro R, Peek G, Expanding Extracorporeal Membrane Oxygenation Cannulation Strategies in Neonatal Respiratory Failure, Pediatr Crit Care Med 2021; 22:756-758.

# 5

## The Physiology of Extracorporeal Life Support

*Robert H. Bartlett, Matthieu Schmidt, Matthew Brain, Tomasso Mauri*

ECLS (or ECMO) is the use of mechanical devices to support heart and/or lung function in severe heart or lung failure, unresponsive to optimal conventional care. With circulation and respiration supported by ECLS, damaging heart and lung treatment can be stopped (eg, vasopressors, high ventilator settings) while the failing organs are treated, recover, or can be replaced. Managing patients with ECLS actively differs from conventional care and requires a thorough understanding of cardiopulmonary physiology, pathophysiology, and ECLS physiology. This chapter includes a brief review of normal and abnormal cardiopulmonary physiology, and the physiology related to mechanical replacement of circulation and respiration.

### Cardiopulmonary Physiology

Figure 5-1 summarizes the essentials of normal cardiopulmonary physiology. All tissues of the body function by combining substrates (food) with oxygen, producing heat, energy, $CO_2$, and water in the process called metabolism. Metabolism is related most closely to oxygen consumption and is determined by measuring the amount of oxygen consumed per minute, which is called $VO_2$. The rate of metabolism for adults at rest is approximately 3 cc/kg/min or 120 cc/min/m$^2$ for a typical adult (children

4 cc/kg/min, infants 5 cc/kg/min). Metabolism is controlled by a center in the brain and increases or decreases depending on activity and other factors.

Metabolic rate increases with activity, fever, drugs, and hormones, and decreases with sleep, paralysis, and cooling. Metabolic rate increases as much as five times in extreme exercise. When the metabolic rate changes, the delivery of substrate and oxygen changes in proportion, accomplished by a change in cardiac output. The amount of oxygen available in the bloodstream for metabolism is normally five times the amount actually used by the tissues. A complex system of reflexes and hormones keeps this in balance, referred to as homeostasis.

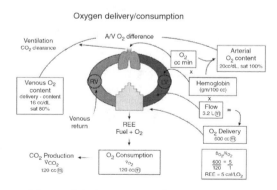

**Figure 5-1.** A summary of oxygen consumption, delivery, and metabolism. REE = resting energy expenditure.

Oxygen gets into the blood through the lungs and arrives in tissues via perfusion of the capillaries. About 20-25% of the oxygen is removed for metabolism (although the oxygen extraction ratio varies from organ to organ) so 75-80% of the oxygen is still in the venous blood on the way back to the heart and lungs. Carbon dioxide is produced during metabolism, the amount ($VCO_2$) of which is essentially the same as the amount of oxygen consumed (3 cc/kg/min). $CO_2$ comes out of the blood in the lungs and into the exhaled air. The amount of oxygen consumed and $CO_2$ produced is different for each organ but the average for all organs is measured by $O_2$ and $CO_2$ exchange in the lungs (Figure 5-2). These principles apply to all ages and sizes, and size-specific parameters are normalized to weight or BSA. Typical adult values are used in the examples in this chapter.

### Oxygen in Blood

The oxygen content is the amount of oxygen bound to hemoglobin plus the amount dissolved in plasma related to $PO_2$:

$$CO_2 (cc/dl) =$$
$$Hb\ (gm/dl) \times SO_2 \times 1.34\ (cc/gm) +$$
$$PO_2\ (mmHg) \times .003\ (cc/dl/mmHg)$$

Oxygen content is difficult to measure directly so it is typically calculated and reported by blood gas analyzers. It is the most important (and as a single value, perhaps the only important) measurement of oxygen in blood. In clinical practice, the amount of dissolved oxygen is less than 1% of the content, so the second half of the equation involving $PO_2$ is usually ignored. Figure 5-3 shows the relation among these measurements. Notice that there is twice as much oxygen in arterial blood at a normal hemoglobin (content 20 ml/dl) than in anemic blood (content 10 ml/dl), even though the oxygen saturation and $PO_2$ are the same in both samples.

The amount of oxygen delivered to metabolizing tissue is the oxygen content in arterial blood times the blood flow (cardiac output), called the oxygen delivery ($DO_2$).

$$DO_2\ (cc/min) =$$
$$CO_2\ (cc/dl) \times CO\ (1/min) \times 10\ (dl/l)$$

For an adult the normal $DO_2$ is 600 cc/min/m² (20 cc/dl × 3 l/min/m² x 10).

The normal amount of oxygen consumed by tissues at rest is 120 cc/min/m², abbreviated

### O₂ Content vs. PO₂ and SAT

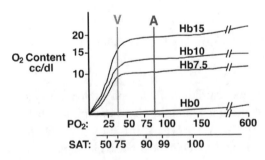

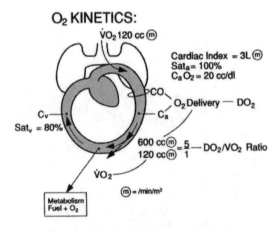

**Figure 5-2.** Oxygen delivery/consumption ($DO_2$/VO₂). Typical adult values are shown.

**Figure 5-3.** Oxygen in blood is measured as PO₂, oxyhemoglobin saturation, and oxygen content. Oxygen content is the only measurement of the amount of oxygen in blood, hence the most important measurement.

as $VO_2$. Figure 5-4 displays the relationship between these concepts. The $DO_2$ is controlled by homeostatic mechanisms to be 5 times $VO_2$, so in a resting adult 20% of the available oxygen is used for metabolism, leaving 80% in the venous blood. Therefore, the normal arterial oxygen values of a patient breathing air are $PO_2$ 90 mmHg, saturation 100%, $O_2$ content 20 cc/dl. Normal venous oxygen values are $PO_2$ 40 mmHg, saturation 80%, content 16 cc/dl. The $VO_2$ increases with exercise, catecholamine release or administration, and sepsis. The $DO_2$ adjusts to $VO_2$, maintaining the ratio at 5:1. $DO_2$ is limited primarily by cardiac output. If $VO_2$ increases relative to $DO_2$ (or if $DO_2$ is impaired), a higher fraction of the arterial oxygen content is removed by the tissues, so the content in the venous blood decreases from the normal 16 cc/dl to lower levels. This is well tolerated until the $DO_2/VO_2$ ratio is below 2:1 (50% extraction). At that point there is not enough oxygen available to maintain oxygen-dependent (aerobic) metabolism, and metabolism switches

to anaerobic processes which causes exhaustion and lactic acidosis. The $VO_2$ below this level then becomes dependent on the supply of $O_2$. Anaerobic metabolism is tolerated for a few hours at most, leading to cardiovascular and metabolic collapse if it persists.

## Cardiopulmonary Pathophysiology

The relationship between $DO_2$ and $VO_2$ can be affected by disease states, primarily those that affect oxygenation and cardiac output. If the $DO_2$ is decreased compared to $VO_2$ (eg, in low cardiac output states, anemia, or hypoxemia), $VO_2$ continues at the same rate, thus more oxygen is extracted per dl of blood, leaving less oxygen in venous blood. Normal aerobic metabolism continues in this setting. However, when the $DO_2$ is less than twice the $VO_2$, oxygen supply is inadequate to maintain aerobic metabolism and anaerobic metabolism ensues, producing lactic acid rather than $CO_2$. A $DO_2$:$VO_2$ ratio less than 2:1 leads to supply-

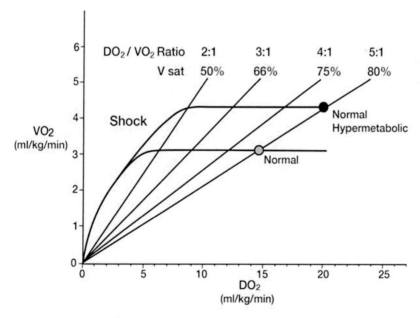

**Figure 5-4.** DO₂/VO₂ relationships during normal and elevated metabolic rate. DO₂ adjusts to changes in VO₂ over a wide range, maintaining DO₂ 5 times VO₂. If DO₂ drops below 5:1, normal aerobic metabolism continues, but if DO₂/VO₂ is less than 2:1, anaerobic metabolism and shock occurs.

dependency hypoxia and systemic acidosis, with resultant organ failure (Figure 5-4). A goal of managing any critically ill patient is to maintain $DO_2$:$VO_2$ close to normal (5:1), or at least more than the critical 2:1. So it is important to know the $VO_2$ and $DO_2$ when planning management.

**Cardiopulmonary Pathophysiology during ECLS**

ECLS is used when heart or lung failure is so severe that $DO_2$:$VO_2$ is less than 2:1, or when the interventions needed to keep $DO_2$ twice $VO_2$ are inherently damaging (eg, high airway pressure, high $FiO_2$, or vasoactive drugs at high doses). In its simplest form (venoarterial), ECLS maintains normal $DO_2$:$VO_2$ by draining most of the venous blood, pumping it through a membrane lung, and into the systemic circulation. Most of the blood bypasses the heart and lungs and the artificial organs replace the function of the diseased heart and lungs. This is shown in Figure 5-5, in a neonate, as an example. On ECLS, safe $DO_2$:$VO_2$ is restored, and the damaging ventilator settings and drugs are discontinued. This provides time for the organ dysfunction to be diagnosed and treated, leading to organ recovery in most cases.

**The ECLS Circuit**

**Cannulation.** Blood flow through the extracorporeal circuit is limited primarily by the size of the venous drainage catheter.

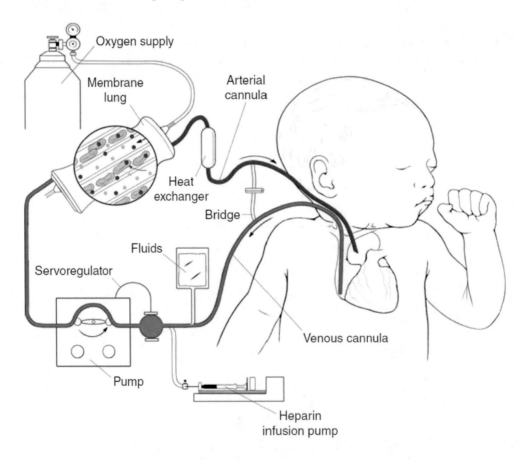

**Figure 5-5.** A simple diagram of VA ECMO, shown in a newborn.

Resistance to blood flow varies directly with the length of the catheter and inversely with the fourth power of the radius of the catheter. Consequently, the shortest and largest internal diameter catheter that can be placed in the right atrium via the access vein will allow the highest rate of extracorporeal blood flow. Blood drains through the venous tubing to a pump that directs the blood through the membrane lung and back into the patient.

**Blood Pumps.** Blood pumps are designed to direct the venous drainage through the membrane lung, then return it into the patient. Pumps can be centrifugal, servo-modified roller, or peristaltic. Centrifugal pumps modified for long-term use are the most commonly used. Rupture of the circuit can occur when the post pump pressure exceeds 300 mmHg, so pumps are modified to prevent overpressure.

Centrifugal pumps create suction which can lead to hemolysis when the suction pressure is high, so centrifugal pumps are operated under conditions to avoid high suction pressures. Generally, pressures no more negative than about -100 mmHg are targeted.

**Membrane Lung (Oxygenator).** Modern membrane lungs achieve gas exchange by perfusing venous blood through a network of thousands of small hollow fibers. The tubes are filled with continuously flowing gas (the "sweep gas"), either 100% oxygen or an air/oxygen mix, while blood flows exterior to the fibers. The hollow fibers are made of a material that allows gases to diffuse across the membrane wall but prevent liquids from passing through. Oxygen and $CO_2$ diffuse between the gas and the blood as a function of the gradient between the partial pressures on each side. When the gas is 100% oxygen, the gradient driving gas transfer is from 600 to 40 mmHg (venous blood) for $O_2$, and 45 to 0 (venous blood) for $CO_2$. Even though the gradient is much larger for oxygen, the solubility and diffusivity of $CO_2$ is much greater, so the amount of $O_2$ and $CO_2$ exchanged is roughly equal when to ratio of blood flow to gas flow is 1:1.

**Oxygen Transfer in Membrane Lungs.** The maximal $O_2$ transfer capacity of any membrane lung is determined by the gas exchange surface area and the amount of disruption of laminar flow as blood passes through the device. Laminar flow allows equilibration of blood of lower $PO_2$ at the membrane interface, reducing the gradient for diffusion. Laminar flow is disrupted by small secondary flows as the blood moves through the irregular blood flow path, mixing fully saturated red cells with deoxygenated red cells and maintaining the gradient. The amount of mixing by secondary flows is one of the most important factors in determining the maximal oxygenating capacity. All these factors are summarized in the concept of 'rated flow.' When venous blood is perfused at a low flow through a membrane lung there is sufficient time for equilibration and the hemoglobin saturation of the outlet blood is 100% saturated. As flow increases, a point is reached when the blood passes through so fast that not all the red cells are oxygenated, and the outlet saturation drops below 100% saturation. The flow of venous blood which exits the membrane lung at 95% saturation is defined as the 'rated flow' (standard venous blood is defined as Hb 12 gm/dl, and saturation 70%, Figure 5-6). Oxygenators for ECLS are chosen based on the rated flow for oxygenation. The size of the oxygenator is matched to the oxygen requirements of the patient.

As long as a membrane lung is perfused at a rate below rated flow, the amount of oxygen supplied by the membrane lung is the outlet minus inlet $O_2$ content difference (DO-I) times the flow. Normal DO-I difference is 5 cc/dl. Figure 5-7 shows the amount of oxygen supplied related to blood flow for different DO-I.

**$CO_2$ Transfer.** The amount of $CO_2$ cleared by any membrane lung is the inlet minus outlet $CO_2$ content difference (DI-O $CO_2$). At 1:1 gas to blood flow ratio, this will be about the same as oxygen. But when the sweep to blood flow ratio is increased to as high as 8:1, a much larger DO-I can be achieved and much more $CO_2$ can be removed. Therefore, when a membrane lung is used primarily for $CO_2$ removal, high gas:blood ratios are used, and $CO_2$ clearance can be achieved at a much lower blood flow than when the goal is oxygenation. The sweep gas flow rate is set by the operator based on the desired $PaCO_2$. These phenomena are demonstrated in Figure 5-8.

**Other Components**. The cannulas, pump, and membrane lung are connected by conduit tubing. It might seem desirable to have the circuit as close to the patient as possible, but usually the connection lines between the patient and the circuit are about 6 feet long because it is easiest to care for both the patient and the circuit when they are separated. One reason is because the pump and lung are mounted on a bulky cart which also carries the pump motor, a

large battery, a water bath for circulating warm water through the heat exchanger, an oxygen tank and gas regulator for travelling, and the monitors and displays. Monitors and alarms can include venous and arterial blood gases, pre and postpump pressure and flow, and blood temperature. There are access sites for infusion and blood sampling.

**ECLS Circuit Physiology**. The circuit blood and gas flow are set by the operator to match the needs of the patient. The amount of $O_2$ and $CO_2$ transfer is calculated based on all the information above, then adjusted to achieve the physiologic goals. Usually the circuit is set to totally support the circulation and respiration initially, then decreased as physiologic goals are met.

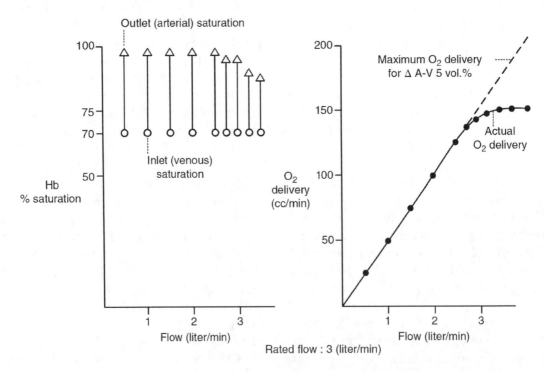

**Figure 5-6.** The concept of 'rated flow.' Venous blood perfused through a membrane lung exits at 100% saturation until a limitation is reached and blood exits at less than 100% saturation. The capacity of membrane lungs is described as 'rated flow.'

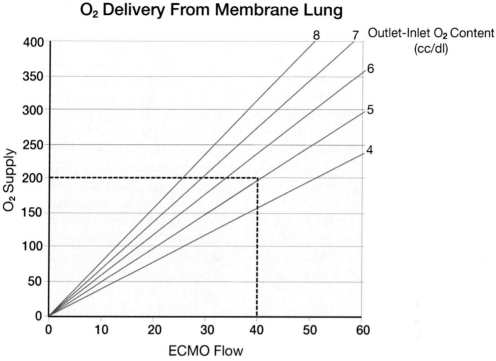

**Figure 5-7.** The amount of oxygen supplied by a membrane lung is the flow times the out-in $O_2$ content difference. Blood flow is in deciliters.

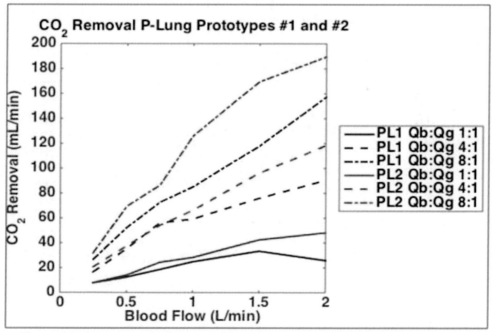

**Figure 5-8.** $CO_2$ removed when gas to blood flow is 1:1, 4:1, and 8:1. Data for two membrane lungs is shown (PL1 and PL2).

**Modes of Vascular Access and Perfusion**

*Venoarterial ECMO*

In venoarterial bypass (VA), the functions of both heart and lungs are replaced by artificial organs, either totally or partially. During partial VA bypass, perfusate blood mixes in the aorta with left ventricular blood which has traversed the lungs. Hence, the content of oxygen and $CO_2$ in the patient's arterial blood represents a combination of blood from these two sources, and the total systemic blood flow is the sum of the extracorporeal flow plus the amount of blood passing through the heart and lungs.

Hemodynamics of VA access are demonstrated in Figure 5-9. As venous blood is drained from the right atrium and perfused into the aorta, the total blood flow remains constant,

but the pulse contour decreases since there is less blood ejected from the left ventricle. When the extracorporeal flow is 100% of the venous return, the systemic pulse contour is flat. This is the situation in VA access for heart surgery (CPB). In CPB, the superior and inferior vena cavae are occluded proximal to the drainage cannulas, so that all the venous return (except the coronary sinus) goes through the circuit. In VA ECMO, the flow is maintained at about 80% of venous return, so 20% passes through the heart and lungs. The reason is to avoid stagnant flow and clotting in the pulmonary vessels and chambers of the heart (which can occur, even with systemic anticoagulation). Even in severe heart failure, the heart can usually pump a small amount of blood when 80% of the circulation is provided by the ECMO circuit. In practice, this proportion of extracorporeal to cardiac

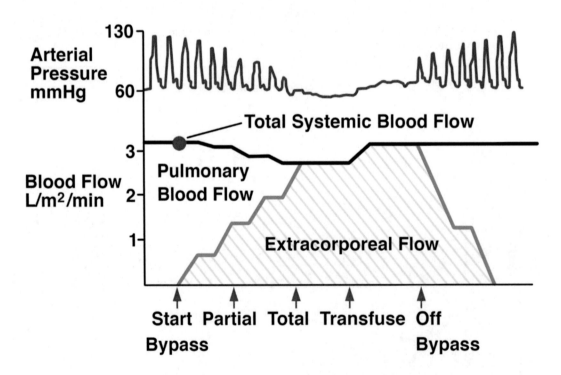

**Figure 5-9.** Physiology of VA perfusion. As extracorporeal flow increases, pulmonary flow decreases, and pulse pressure decreases until total extracorporeal flow is reached. During VA ECMO extracorporeal flow is ideally at 80% of total flow, so the pulse pressure is about 10 mmHg.

flow is represented by a pulse contour of about 10 mmHg. The best way to assess heart function in VA ECMO is by echocardiography.

If the heart is completely nonfunctional, all the venous return drains into the extracorporeal circuit and there is no arterial pulse contour. The patient is on total CPB (as during cardiac surgery). This is tolerated for a few hours (enough time to operate on the heart, then restore circulation), but in ECLS this leads to two problems. First, the left side of the heart gradually fills with blood from bronchial and Thebesian venous flow. This causes increased pressure in the left ventricle, atrium, and pulmonary circulation. When that pressure reaches 20-25 mmHg, pulmonary edema occurs and the LV becomes overdistended. This must be treated by draining blood from the left side of the circulation into the circuit. This is done by creating an atrial septal defect, or by placing a drainage cannula in the LA (or pulmonary artery)(see Chapters 4 and 51). The second problem is that blood in the cardiac chambers and pulmonary circulation will clot, even with systemic anticoagulation. This is treated by using higher levels of systemic anticoagulation and adding urgency to going from ECMO to a VAD and restoring the pulmonary circulation.

**VA ECMO Compared to CPB.** While the principles of gas exchange and blood flow are the same, there are several important differences between the conduct of ECLS and operating room bypass. Table 5-1 summarizes some of

| CPB vs. ECMO* | | |
|---|---|---|
| **Major Differences** | **OR CPB** | **ECMO** |
| Open Reservoir | Yes | No |
| Heparin (ACT) | >600 | 180 |
| Autotransfusion | Yes | No |
| Arterial Filter | Yes | NO |
| Patient | Asleep | Awake |
| Environment | OR, Hours | ICU, Days |
| *Venoarterial bypass, same devices, physiology | | |

**Table 5-1.** Comparison of CPB in the operating room and VA ECMO in the ICU.

the more important differences. Because the purpose of operating room CPB is to permit operations on the heart, total venoarterial bypass is always used, with airtight occlusion of the venous drainage catheters and arterial access, usually directly into the aorta. Because there is total stagnation of blood in the pulmonary circulation and some chambers of the heart, total anticoagulation is required, achieved by giving a huge dose of heparin to make the whole blood clotting time infinitely long. This anticoagulation, and uncontrolled blood flow into the operative field from the coronary sinus, bronchial veins, and Thebesian veins, results in continuous bleeding which is managed by aspiration and filtration of the shed blood with return to the venous reservoir (so called cardiotomy suction or autotransfusion). To minimize this bleeding into the field, and to minimize any risks associated with high blood flow, it is common practice to manage systemic perfusion at abnormally low levels of blood flow (2-2.4 $L/m^2/min$) and abnormally low hematocrit (typically 20%). This combination of low blood flow and low hematocrit leads to very low systemic oxygen delivery, which could result in oxygen debt and metabolic acidosis, except that total body hypothermia is usually implemented, maintaining the ratio of delivery to consumption in the normal range of 5:1. Therefore, a very efficient heat exchanger and a large water bath are required for cardiopulmonary bypass for heart surgery.

Aside from these differences in perfusion technology, the entire approach to management of extracorporeal circulation differs markedly comparing CBP to ECLS. Cardiopulmonary bypass is conducted in the operating room with the sole intention of operating upon the heart. There is an appropriate sense of urgency to minimize the time on bypass. Complications, including myocardial damage, renal failure, liver failure, hemolysis, and abnormal bleeding increase proportionate to the amount of time on bypass. Unlimited amounts of bleeding in the operating field are tolerated and managed by autotransfusion, with the realization that the effect of heparin will be reversed by protamine at the end of the procedure. An hour or two of rewarming and attempts to come off bypass is considered an exceedingly long and tedious interval. Sometimes huge doses of catecholamines are given to encourage a sluggish heart simply in order to come off bypass. If the patient cannot be weaned off bypass in a few hours, a mechanical support system (ECMO or VAD) must be instituted. The patient is anesthetized and paralyzed rendering neurologic evaluation impossible. Everyone caring for the patient measures success or failure in hours of CPB.

In contrast, ECLS is managed in the ICU by a team expecting days or weeks of continuous care. The patient is maintained awake or awakened at regular intervals to evaluate neurologic function. Feeding, ventilation, antibiotic management, renal function are all-important aspects of ECLS care. The use of inotropic drugs and high ventilator settings is minimal and weaning from bypass may proceed over a period of hours or days. The patient commonly lacks heart, lung, or renal function for days, and futility is conceded only after many days of vital organ failure.

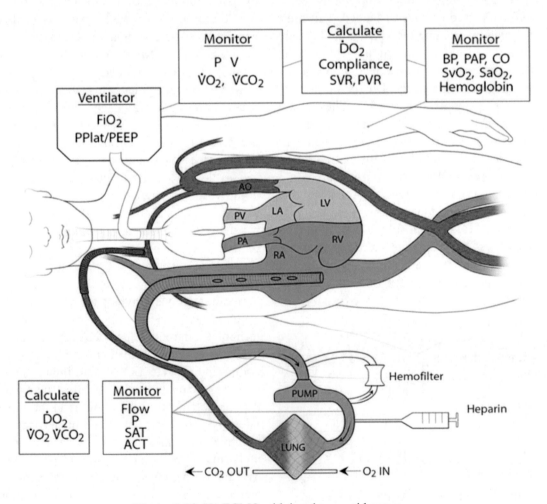

**Figure 5-10.** VA ECMO with jugular-carotid access.

**Gas Exchange in VA Access**. During VA ECMO, fully saturated blood from the circuit is perfused into the aorta and mixes with blood from the left ventricle. If the lungs are functioning well, the mixed blood is well oxygenated and has normal $PCO_2$. The patient can be weaned from the ventilator and managed awake and extubated. If the lungs are functioning poorly or not at all, the systemic blood gases will reflect the mixture of the cardiac and extracorporeal flows, resulting in lower oxygenation proximal to the site of mixing. If the mixing is in the proximal aorta, blood to the brain and coronary circulation is well oxygenated (as in neonatal VA ECMO with

carotid access). This is demonstrated in Figure 5-10. In femoral artery access, the mixing takes place in the mid aorta, so the upper body is perfused by the blood from the left ventricle. This can result in differential circulation with the lower body perfused by fully saturated red blood while the upper body is perfused with desaturated blue blood. This is referred to as differential hypoxemia (formerly known as the Harlequin or red feet blue head syndrome). This is demonstrated in Figure 5-11. The management of the differential hypoxemia is to perfuse some of the post oxygenator blood into the right atrium (combining VA with VV perfusion, or VVA). This is accomplished by

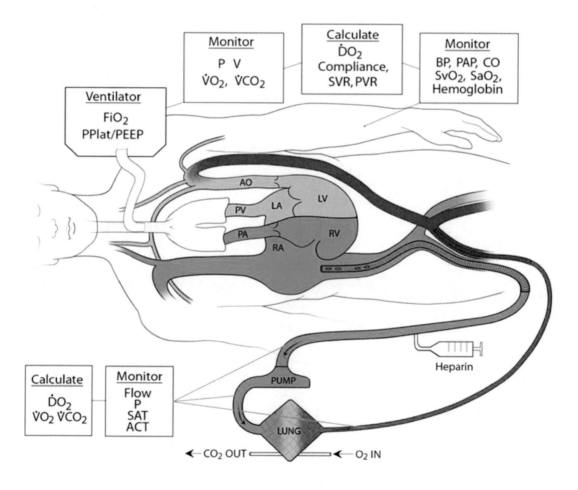

**Figure 5-11.** VA ECMO with femoral-femoral access.

inserting an infusion cannula via the jugular vein, or by perfusion of a second lumen in the drainage line as shown in Figure 5-12. The sweep gas is usually 100% oxygen (during VA access with no cardiac function, the oxygenator outlet will be the systemic $PO_2$, so the $FdO_2$ can be reduced if the operator wishes arterial $PO_2$ in the 100-200 range).

### *Hemodynamic Effects of VA ECMO*

By reinfusing blood directly into the arterial system, VA ECMO augments or replaces the cardiac output provided by the native heart. Since the heart and lungs are bypassed, native cardiac output decreases as extracorporeal flow increases, shifting systemic blood flow from pulsatile to nonpulsatile flow. VA ECMO thus provides systemic oxygen delivery and maintains systemic blood pressure. If the heart is not beating, all the systemic flow and oxygen delivery is provided by the ECMO circuit. In that case the left atrium and ventricle will gradually fill with pulmonary venous blood (from bronchial flow) and the left ventricle will become over distended and pressure >25 mmHg in the pulmonary circulation will cause pulmonary edema. If the left ventricle is not ejecting during VA ECMO it is necessary to decompress the left sided circulation as discussed previously.

VA ECMO flow determines arterial blood pressure (systemic vascular resistance). By controlling flow, we can maintain normal systemic perfusion by maintaining arterial pressure at 60-70 mmHg without vasoconstrictor

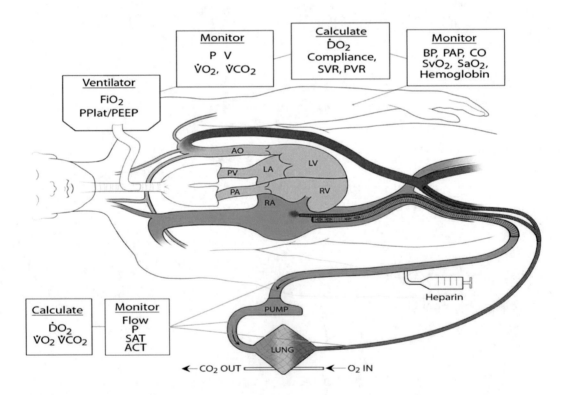

**Figure 5-12.** VA ECMO with some arterialized returned to the right atrium (VVA) to treat the differential circulation syndrome when lung function is compromised. Arterial blood is "Y'd" off the infusion line, through a second lumen in the drainage cannula.

drugs. Mixing of cardiac and retrograde ECLS flow does not add significantly to arterial pressure or systemic resistance. VA ECMO does not increase left ventricular afterload above normal. In fact, it decreases afterload by maintaining non pulsatile perfusion. When the heart is recovering and is regaining pulsatile flow, heart work can be minimized by unloading pressure during systole with an intraaortic balloon pump or using synchronized pulsatile ECMO flow.

**Managing VA ECMO Based on These Principles**. In VA access, the parameters described in Figures 5-9, 5-10-12 are monitored, and $VO_2$ and $DO_2$ are calculated from these measurements. That information informs the adjusting of ECMO variables and patient variables to maintain $DO_2:VO_2$ at 3:1 or higher.

1. Plan the circuit based on the best estimation of the metabolic rate (adults, 3-4 cc/kg/min for both $O_2$ and $CO_2$) and the drainage flow which can be achieved from the largest drainage cannula which can be placed. Plan for total support, realizing that there may be some native lung function and total support may not be necessary. For a septic 80 kg adult, you will need 5 L/min flow, and an oxygenator with rated flow over 5 L/min to supply 300 cc $O_2$/min.

2. On ECLS go to the highest flow to determine the maximum drainage capacity, following the pulse contour. If the drainage cannula is large enough, total bypass (nonpulsatile flow) will result. Then decrease the flow until the pulse contour is 10-15 mmHg. Vasoactive drugs should be decreased to low or absent levels. Use ECLS flow to control arterial pressure at 60-70 mmHg. If there is no LV function establish left atrial drainage.

3. When the patient is stable (usually 6-12 hours), determine the variables of $O_2$ kinetics, using the formulas described above. If oxygen supply is adequate ($DO_2:VO_2$ over 3) no changes are necessary.

If oxygen supply is inadequate ($DO_2:VO_2$ under 3) and the patient is anemic, transfuse to a higher hemoglobin (12-14 gm%). This will result in arterial saturation around 95% and venous saturation around 65% ($DO_2/VO_2$=3-4).

4. Manage the patient based on continuous venous and arterial saturation monitoring. Plot the position on Figure 5-4 frequently. Calculate the variables if oxygen supply seems excessive or inadequate.

5. When the native heart begins to recover (pulse contour increases when flow is decreased), turn down the flow, keeping the venous saturation >70%. When the native heart function is adequate, conduct a trial off bypass. When heart function is satisfactory, decannulate the patient.

### Venovenous ECMO

In VV ECMO, the perfusate blood is returned to the venous circulation and mixes with venous blood coming from the systemic organs, raising the oxygen content and lowering $CO_2$ content in the right atrial blood. This mixed blood, now higher in oxygen content with normal $PCO_2$ passes into the right ventricle, the lungs, and into the systemic circulation. Normal oxygen and $CO_2$ content in the pulmonary arterial blood can ameliorate vasoconstriction caused by hypoxemia, hypercarbia, or acidosis. Venovenous access is achieved by draining venous blood from the IVC via the femoral vein and reinfusing into the RA via the jugular (Figure 5-13), or by draining from the IVC and SVC and reinfusing into the RA via a separate lumen in a double lumen cannula (Figure 5-14).

Hemodynamics during venovenous access are not affected by the circuit. Since the volume of blood removed is exactly equal to the volume of blood reinfused, there is no net effect on central venous volume or pressure, right or left ventricle filling, or hemodynamics. The content of oxygen and $CO_2$ in the patient's arterial

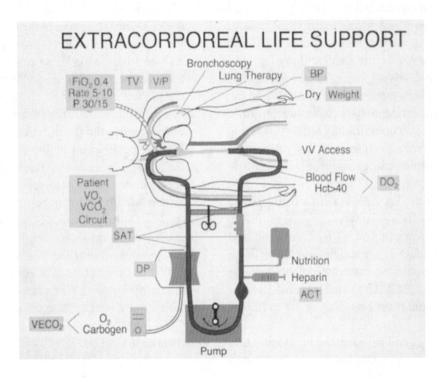

**Figure 5-13.** VV ECMO for respiratory support. 2-cannula access.

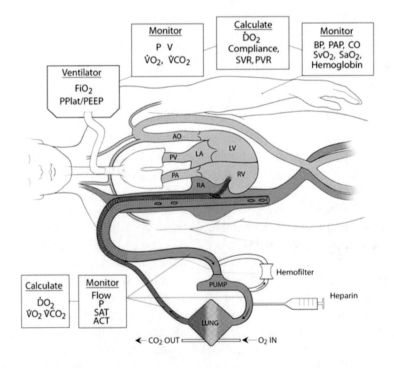

**Figure 5-14.** VV ECMO with a double lumen cannula.

blood represents that of mixed right ventricle blood modified by any pulmonary function that might exist. The systemic blood flow is the native cardiac output and is unrelated to the extracorporeal flow.

**Gas Exchange in VV ECMO.** In VV ECMO, some of the systemic venous return is drained into the ECLS system, oxygenated, and returned to the right atrium. Some of the systemic venous return goes directly to the right atrium where it mixes with the ECMO perfusate blood. The mixed blood passes through the right ventricle, native lungs, left heart, and into the systemic circulation. In severe respiratory failure, the native lungs contribute little or none to gas exchange, so the arterial oxygen and $CO_2$ levels are the result of mixing the oxygenated ECMO blood with the deoxygenated native venous blood. As a result, the arterial saturation ranges from 60% to 90%, depending on the relative amount of ECMO flow, native venous flow, lung function, and cardiac output. The desaturated arterial blood results in normal systemic oxygen delivery as long as the cardiac output and hemoglobin concentration (oxygen content) are adequate. These relationships are often confusing to ICU staff because the usual goal of management is to keep the arterial saturation over 90%.

In contrast, hypoxia in the setting of VV ECMO should be approached with reference to adequacy of oxygen delivery to the tissues ($DO_2:VO_2$) rather than a reference to a defined arterial $PaO_2$. Operating at $PaO_2$ 50-60 may be quite acceptable when considered within the context of the VV ECMO patient. A convenient single measurement goal is to keep the native venous saturation (the drainage sat) above 60%.

The major variable affecting systemic hemoglobin saturation in VV ECMO is the proportion of deoxygenated venous return that is routed through the oxygenator (ECMO flow) compared to native venous return which goes directly into the right ventricle. Attempts to reduce cardiac output to decrease the proportion of native (desaturated) venous return will not improve oxygen delivery. It may increase $SaO_2$ but decreases systemic oxygen delivery.

**Oxygenation.** To illustrate the principles, the discussion begins with the assumption that there is no native lung gas exchange (which is often the case in ECLS patients). In a membrane lung (as in the native lung), oxygenation is a much greater problem than $CO_2$ removal, so the initial focus is on oxygenation. The circuit and blood flow are planned for total oxygen supply ($VO_2$) at rest or during moderate exercise. For adults, this is 120 cc/min/m$^2$ (3 cc/kg/min) at rest or 250-300 cc of oxygen/min/m$^2$ with activity for average adults. The membrane lung must be large enough to transfer this amount of oxygen. All devices currently on the market can achieve this (see 'rated flow', above). The oxygen supply from the membrane lung is dependent on the blood flow, the hemoglobin concentration, and the difference between the outlet minus inlet $O_2$ content. Because the outlet blood is typically 100% saturated and $PO_2$ is over 500 mmHg, the dissolved oxygen can be as much as 10% of the oxygen content.

Blood flow is limited by the resistance to flow in the drainage cannula, the suction produced by the pump or siphon, and the geometry of the cannulated vessel (usually the vena cava or right atrium). Typical maximum flow at 100 cm/H$_2$O suction for common sizes of venous cannulas is 4-5 liters per minute.

**Relation of Extracorporeal Oxygenation to Systemic Oxygen Delivery**. Assuming that there is no native lung function, the systemic arterial content, saturation, and $PO_2$ will result from mixing the flow of oxygenated blood from the membrane lung with the flow of venous blood which passes into the right ventricle, not into the ECLS drainage cannula, (hereafter referred to as the native venous flow). The amount of oxygen in systemic arterial blood is the result of the mixture of these two flows (Figure 5-15).

**Calculations Related to Mixing Two Flows**. When two blood flows of different oxygen contents mix, the resultant oxygen content is the average of the amount of oxygen in each of the two flows (not the average of the partial pressures). The amount of oxygen contributed by each flow is the oxygen content (in cc/dL) in the blood times the flow rate (in dL/min). The equation summarizing these events is in Figure 5-16. The same calculation can be done using saturation rather than oxygen content. This calculation using saturation is done for simplicity and is not an exact representation of the amount of oxygen content but is useful at the bedside (Figure 5-17). The combinations of flow and oxygen (expressed as saturation) variations are shown in Figure 5-18. Of the variables in the equation, all are known

except the flow of venous blood which does not go through the extracorporeal circuit (the native venous flow). The native venous flow can be back calculated from the systemic arterial oxygen content or saturation. The total venous return (cardiac output) is the sum of the native venous and circuit flow.

**Systemic Arterial $PO_2$ Saturation, and Content During VV ECMO.** Use of these equations in venovenous patient physiology are shown in Figure 5-18. In these examples, one variable is changed while others are held constant to illustrate the principles. Clinically, all these variables may change simultaneously and at different rates. For simplicity of the examples, we assume no native lung function, and approximate the points on the graphs. We do not account for dissolved oxygen in calculation

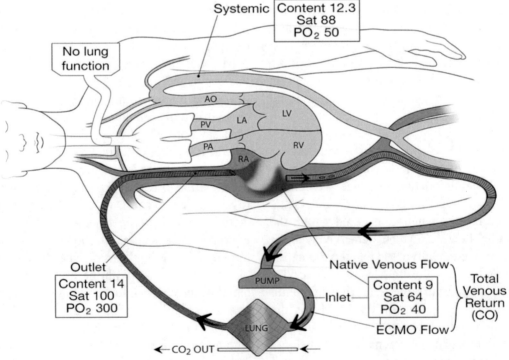

**Figure 5-15.** Mixing of perfusate with native venous flow during VV ECMO.

of $O_2$ content, although it can be significant when the $PO_2$ is over 300.

**Example 1: Typical VV physiology.** Suppose the extracorporeal flow for a 70 kg adult with no lung function is 4 L/min and the systemic $PO_2$ is 50 mmHg, saturation 88%, $O_2$ content 12.3 cc/dl. The Hb is 10.5 gm/dl and the venous blood saturation is 64%. The patient's oxygen consumption is 200 cc/min. The oxygen

**Mixing 2 Blood Flows of Different O2 Content (C1 and C2)**

*The resultant O2 content (C3) is the sum of each content x flow divided by total flow*

$$\frac{C_1 \times Flow_1}{Total\ Flow} + \frac{C_2 \times Flow_2}{Total\ Flow} = C_3$$

In VV ECMO, assuming no native lung function:
C1 and F2 are extracorporeal content and flow
C2 and F2 are the venous content and the native venous flow
The equation can be solved for cardiac output and native venous flow

$$Total\ Flow = Flow_1 \frac{(C_1 - C_2)}{C_3 - C_2} = Cardiac\ Output$$

$$Flow_2 = Total\ Flow - Flow_1 = Native\ Venous\ Flow$$

**Figure 5-16.** The relationships among flow and O₂ content are shown in the equation. During ECMO all the variables are known except native venous flow (F2) and total flow (cardiac output). Native venous flow can be calculated. Cardiac output is F2 plus F1. This assumes no lung function and no recirculation.

**Mixing 2 Blood Flows in VV ECMO: Example 1**

*Using $O_2$ Content:*

$$\frac{14 \times 4}{4 + F2} + \frac{9 \times F_2}{4 \times F_2} = 12.3\ cc/dL$$

Cardiac Output = $\frac{4(14-9)}{(12.3-9)}$ = 6 L/min

Native Venous Flow = 6 − 4 = 2 L/min

*Using $O_2$ Saturation:*

$$\frac{100 \times 4}{4 + F2} + \frac{64 \times F_2}{4 \times F_2} = 90\%$$

Cardiac Output = $\frac{4(100-64)}{(90-64)}$ = 6 L/min

Native Venous Flow = 6 − 4 = 2 L/min

**Figure 5-17.** The relationships among flow and O₂ content using the data in Example 1. The same calculations are shown using saturation rather than content.

content of blood leaving the membrane lung is determined primarily by the concentration of hemoglobin. At hemoglobin concentration of 10.5 gm/dl and 64% saturation, the drainage (inlet) $O_2$ content is 9 cc/dl and the outlet content at 100% saturation is 14 cc/dl. The amount of oxygen supplied to the patient is the outlet minus inlet content (which is 5 cc/dl), times the flow (40 dl/min), which equals 200 cc oxygen supplied per minute. The native venous flow is calculated at 2 L/min (as per the equation in Figure 5-17) so the cardiac output is 6 L/min (native plus circuit venous flow). Systemic $DO_2$ is the arterial content (12.3 cc/dl) x 60 dl/min = 738 cc/$O_2$/min. $DO_2/VO_2$ ratio is 3.64. The $O_2$ content of native venous blood is the same as the drainage content (9 cc/dl). The final complete equation is 40 dl/min x 14 c/dl divided by 60 dl/min, plus 20 dl/min x 9 dl divided by 60 dl/min=12.3 cc/$O_2$/dl (corresponding to a $PO_2$ of approximately 50 mm/Hg). The calculation using saturation is 4 L/min x 100% + 2 L/min x 70% ÷ 6 L/min which yields a systemic arterial saturation of 88% (Point A, Figure 5-18).

**Example 2: Increased cardiac output at fixed ECLS flow.** If, in the same patient, the cardiac output (venous return) increases to 8 L/min and the circuit flow is fixed at 4 L/min, there will be native venous return at 64% saturation mixing with the fully saturated ECLS flow. The systemic arterial content will decrease to 11.5 and the saturation will decrease to 84% corresponding to $PO_2$ of 45 mmHg. The total amount of oxygen going to the patient is the same (200 cc/min), but the systemic saturation and $PO_2$ is lower. The systemic oxygen delivery is 920 cc/min. The $DO_2/VO_2$ is 4.6. There has been a gain in systemic oxygen delivery because of the higher cardiac output, despite a decrease in arterial saturation and content. If the patient's systemic oxygen consumption is 200 cc/min, systemic oxygen delivery is perfectly adequate and full aerobic metabolism is supported, even though the arterial $PO_2$ is 45 mmHg and arterial saturation is 84%. No changes are required but the ICU staff need to understand that the hypoxemia does not require intervention. Understanding this concept can be difficult when the plan is to keep the arterial saturation over 90%. (Point B, Figure 5-18)

**Example 3: Anemia.** The patient in Example 1 is moderately anemic (Hb 10, 5 gm%) but stable. Suppose the hemoglobin suddenly drops to 8 gm%. The venous drainage is fixed at 4 L/min by the resistance of the drainage cannula, and cardiac output is 6 L/min. The outlet content at 100% sat is 10.7. The amount of oxygen supplied by the membrane lung is 10.7 minus 9 which is 1.7 cc/dl, so the membrane lung is supplying only 68 cc/min. The native venous flow is 20 dl/min and content is 9 cc/dl. The arterial content has gone from 11.5 to 9.8, the arterial sat to 80%, and the $DO_2$ has gone from 738 cc/min to 588. This results in a $DO_2/VO_2$ ratio of 2.9 (assuming no difference

in metabolic rate). However, since only 68 cc of oxygen is being added per minute, and the oxygen consumption is 200 cc/min, venous (inlet) content and saturation decrease quickly. When the inlet content falls to 5.7 (saturation 50%), the membrane lung O-I difference is 5 cc/dl and the oxygen supplied is 200 cc/min. The mixture of the fully saturated blood at 40 dl/min and the 50% saturated native venous flow results in arterial saturation of 75% and arterial content 9 cc/dl. The systemic oxygen delivery is 540 cc/min and the $VO_2/DO_2$ ratio is 2.7. The patient can remain in steady state with arterial saturation 75% and venous saturation 50%, but any further decrease in hemoglobin or increase in metabolic rate will result in supply dependency and lactic acidosis (Point C, Figure 5-18).

**Example 4: Increased metabolic rate.** Suppose the patient in Example 1 becomes hypermetabolic ($VO_2$=250 cc/min). The size

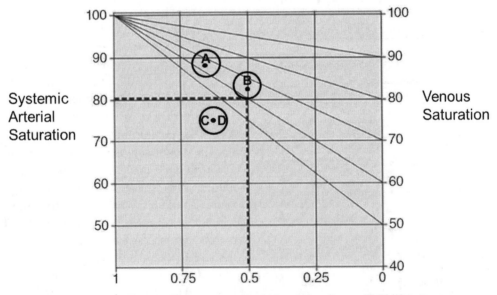

Arterial saturation and venous saturation at ratios of ECMO flow to native venous flow. (Assumes that ECMO flow is 100% saturated.)

**Figure 5-18.** Mixing of flows in VV ECMO. Data from examples 1 - 4 are shown.

of the venous cannula determines that the circuit flow is at maximum at 4 L/min, so the circuit oxygen delivery is limited to 200 cc/min. The cardiac output is 6 L/min. Going through the same arithmetic, the patient will fall behind at the rate of 50 cc of oxygen per minute and venous content and saturation will steadily decrease (eg. 70% to 45%). As venous saturation and content decrease, the oxygenator will still increase the outlet saturation to 100% and oxygen content to 14 cc/dl, so the circuit outlet minus inlet oxygen difference (oxygen supply) will go up as the venous saturation goes down (eg. from 5 to 6). Systemic saturation will decrease because the saturation and content of the native venous blood going through the heart and lungs will decrease. At venous content 7.5, the O-I content difference is 6.5 and the oxygen supplied is 260 cc/min. Steady state is reached with arterial saturation at about 75% and $PaO_2$ 35 mmHg. The $DO_2/VO_2$ is 2.1 and any increase in activity will lead to anaerobic metabolism which will produce lactate rather than $CO_2$, and lactic acidosis results. In time, this will lead to multiple organ failure and death (Point D, Figure 5-18).

How can systemic oxygen delivery be increased in Examples 3 and 4? Turning up the ventilator $FiO_2$ or airway pressure will not help. Furthermore, the whole objective is to avoid increasing $FiO_2$ and pressure from the mechanical ventilator. There are four alternatives. The first is to increase the hemoglobin concentration to normal. When hemoglobin goes from 10.5 to 15, systemic oxygen delivery goes to 930 cc/min, arterial saturation returns to 95%, venous saturation goes to 80%, and the patient is stable and well supported. The $DO_2/VO_2$ is 4.6. The second alternative is to increase the suction or add another cannula and increase the circuit flow from 4 to 5 L/min (maintaining Hb 10.5). The $DO_2$ increases to 792 cc/min, and the $DO_2/VO_2$ is 3.9. The third alternative is to paralyze and cool the patient, decreasing the $VO_2$ back to 200

cc/min. A fourth consideration is to add another membrane lung to increase the gas exchange surface, but $O_2$ supply is still limited by the blood flow, so this will not help.

The tradeoff between extracorporeal flow and hemoglobin is demonstrated in Figure 5-19. This example shows an 80 kg man with oxygen requirement of 240 cc/min, but the relationships remain the same for any size patient. Under most circumstances, the risks of increasing extracorporeal flow are greater than the risks of transfusion.

**Oxygenation in VV ECMO.** The combination of venous access cannula, membrane lung size, and hemoglobin concentration should be planned to match or exceed resting $VO_2$ (120 cc/m²/min for adults). The membrane lung will supply the most oxygen at a normal hemoglobin (15 gm/dl). All the important variables related to blood flow and oxygenation can be measured or calculated. It is essential to know the patient's oxygen consumption and systemic oxygen delivery to decide the best way to manage the extracorporeal circuit. Hypoxemia ($PaO_2$ 40-60, $SaO_2$ 70-90%) always occurs with venovenous support and is adequate to maintain normal oxygen delivery. If systemic oxygen delivery falls to a critical level (near twice consumption), circuit oxygen supply must be increased by: 1) transfusing to a higher hemoglobin or 2) adding additional venous drainage access to increase the flow. There is a tradeoff of risk between transfusion and increasing circuit flow which favors transfusion of RBCs. Membrane lungs function optimally at a normal hematocrit.

**Recirculation during VV ECMO.** Since VV ECMO reinfuses blood drained from the vena cavae or right atrium back into the central venous system, the potential exists for some of the returned blood to be drained by the circuit before it mixes with the native venous flow. Recirculation reduces the effective extracorporeal flow by the recirculated amount. For example, if total circuit flow is 5 L/min and recirculation is 20% (1 L/min), then only 4 L/min of oxygenated blood is available to the patient.

Determinants of recirculation include the type and placement of cannulas, and the extracorporeal flow in relation to cardiac output and vena caval native blood flow. Two-site single lumen cannulation is always associated with some recirculation, since the vena caval flow is less than the circuit drainage, necessitating blood from the atrium containing oxygenated blood from the circuit being drained as well. Three-site single lumen cannulation, in which both vena cavae are drained, reduces recirculation. Similarly, the dual lumen bicaval cannula provides drainage from both vena cavae and is associated with low recirculation.

Recirculation fraction is also related to overall circuit flow relative to cardiac output. As cardiac output decreases, the fraction increases, and becomes markedly elevated when cardiac output drops below extracorporeal flow. Increases in recirculation during extracorporeal support can result from dislodgement of cannulas, such as closer approximation of single-lumen cannulas from inadvertent advancement, or accidental withdrawal or advancement of a dual lumen cannula, in which the distal drainage port moves into the right atrium, or the reinfusion port advances into the inferior vena cava, respectively.

**Hemodynamics during VV ECMO**
Unlike venoarterial support, VV ECMO does not provide any direct hemodynamic support since there is no reinfusion of blood into the

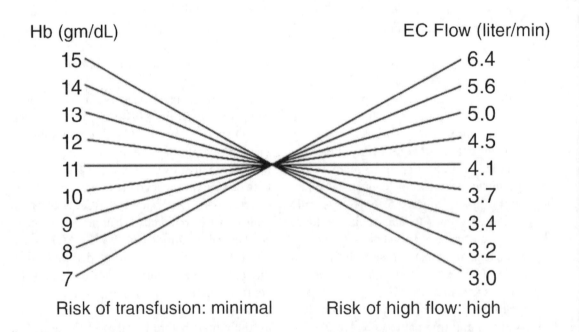

## Hb and flow in ECLS
## Typical 80 kg adult: total $O_2$ support

| Hb (gm/dL) | EC Flow (liter/min) |
|---|---|
| 15 | 6.4 |
| 14 | 5.6 |
| 13 | 5.0 |
| 12 | 4.5 |
| 11 | 4.1 |
| 10 | 3.7 |
| 9 | 3.4 |
| 8 | 3.2 |
| 7 | 3.0 |

Risk of transfusion: minimal    Risk of high flow: high

**Figure 5-19.** The tradeoff between hemoglobin and flow. The relationships to deliver 240cc $O_2$ per minute are shown, but the same calculations can be done for any oxygen supply.

arterial system. Venous return and pulsatility are unaffected since drainage and reinfusion are in equilibrium.

Despite the lack of direct support, however, myocardial function and cardiac output typically improve during VV support. Reduction in mechanical ventilatory support that is allowed from improved gas exchange reduces right ventricular afterload and improves RV function. Improved oxygenation of the pulmonary vascular bed can mitigate hypoxic vasoconstriction. Higher oxygen saturation of left ventricular blood results in improved myocardial oxygenation and reversal of hypoxia-induced myocardial depression. Reduction in acidosis from correction of hypercarbia and reversal of anaerobic metabolism also contribute to improved myocardial function.

This indirect support is usually sufficient to reduce or eliminate requirements for cardiovascular pharmacologic agents. Improved organ perfusion can help reverse renal, hepatic, and other organ failure.

## $CO_2$ Removal

$CO_2$ production is equal to $O_2$ consumption (when the Respiratory Quotient is 1), so the amount of $CO_2$ exchanged per minute is essentially the same as the amount of oxygen ($120$ cc/min/m$^2$ for adults). Because $CO_2$ is much more soluble and diffusible in blood than $O_2$, $CO_2$ clearance will exceed oxygenation in any circumstance, so all the circuit management is based on oxygenation. The sweep gas is always 100% oxygen in VV ECMO. Sweep gas flow rate is unrelated to oxygenation; it is only related to $CO_2$ clearance. If $CO_2$ clearance is the only or the major goal, much lower blood flow can be used, and hemoglobin concentration is not important. The amount of $CO_2$ elimination is a function of the membrane lung surface area and the gradient between the inlet $PCO_2$ (typically 50 mmHg) and the sweep gas (0). The systemic $PCO_2$ is the result of mixing circuit outlet blood ($PCO_2$ typically 30 mmHg) with native flow (typically 45 mmHg). Like oxygenation, the actual amount of $CO_2$ removed by the membrane lung is the inlet $CO_2$ content minus the outlet content times the flow. However, $CO_2$ content is difficult to measure or calculate, so actual $CO_2$ removal is measured as the % $CO_2$ in the exhaust gas times the gas flow. Unlike oxygenation, measuring or calculating the actual amount of $CO_2$ exchanged by the circuit is not critical; the sweep gas is simply adjusted to maintain the desired systemic $PCO_2$ (typically 40 mmHg).

One phenomenon unique to ECLS is the effect of water accumulation on the gas side of the membrane lung. This is the only circumstance in which $CO_2$ clearance is less than oxygenation. Understanding the reason is a good exercise in understanding how membrane lungs work.

## *Arteriovenous $CO_2$ Removal*

Arteriovenous (AV) extracorporeal circulation is commonly used for hemodialysis but not for cardiac or pulmonary support. The AV route can be used for gas exchange provided the arterial blood is desaturated, and the cardiovascular system can tolerate the arteriovenous fistula with a large enough flow to achieve adequate gas exchange. This is, after all, the mechanism of gas exchange in the placenta and fetus. Because of the blood flow requirements for gas exchange support, the arteriovenous route is not a reasonable approach to total extracorporeal respiratory support, except when the patient can tolerate a large arteriovenous shunt and an increase in cardiac output (such as a premature infant). However, AV flow through a membrane lung can provide significant $CO_2$ removal, decreasing the need for mechanical ventilation.

**ECLS Management when the Native Lung is Recovering**

All the preceding discussion describes a situation when there is no native lung function. As the native lung begins to recover, some oxygen and $CO_2$ exchange will occur. The effect will be to improve systemic arterial oxygenation and $PaCO_2$ with no change in the extracorporeal flow rate and hemoglobin. It is tempting to increase ventilator settings and $FiO_2$ in order to take advantage of this recovery, but this may add to lung injury and delay lung recovery. ECLS is continued during rest ventilator settings, and when arterial $PCO_2$ drops below 40 the sweep gas to the membrane lung can be proportionally decreased. When the systemic arterial saturation exceeds 95%, the extracorporeal flow can be gradually decreased (changing the ratio of circuit to native venous flow). When the extracorporeal support has decreased from total support to approximately 50%, extracorporeal support can be briefly discontinued (at moderate ventilator settings) to test native lung function. When native lung function is sufficient for total patient support, ECLS can be discontinued. Because reestablishing vascular access in ECLS can be difficult, it is wise to continue ECLS support for a day or two beyond this point to allow more lung recovery, unless there is a pressing reason to take the patient off ECLS (systemic bleeding or CNS complications).

***Managing VV ECMO Based on These Principles***

In venovenous access, the parameters described in Figures 5-13, 5-14, and 5-15 are monitored and $VO_2$, $DO_2$ are calculated from these measurements. That information is used to adjust the ECLS variables and the patient variables to maintain $DO_2/VO_2$ at 3:1 or higher.

1.  As in VA access, plan the circuit based on the best estimation of the metabolic rate (adults, 3-4 cc/kg/min for both $O_2$ and $CO_2$) and the drainage flow which can be achieved from the largest drainage cannula (or cannulas) which can be placed. Plan for total support, realizing that there may be some native lung function and total support may not be necessary. For a septic 80kg adult, you will need 5 L/min flow and an oxygenator with rated flow over 5 L/min to supply 300 cc $O_2$/min.

2.  On ECLS, go to the highest flow to determine the maximum drainage capacity, then turn down the ventilator to rest settings ($FiO_2$ 0.3, CPAP 10-15 cm $H_2O$) and wean off the vasoactive drugs. The hypermetabolism will decrease to baseline. The lungs may go to total consolidation. Adjust the sweep gas to keep the $PaCO_2$ 40 mm Hg.

3.  When the patient is stable (usually 6-12 hours), determine the variables of $O_2$ kinetics, using the formulas described above. If oxygen supply is adequate ($DO_2:VO_2$ over 3), no changes are necessary. If oxygen supply is inadequate ($DO_2:VO_2$ under 3) and the patient is anemic, transfuse to a higher hemoglobin (12-14 gm/dl). If $DO_2$ is still inadequate, change the drainage cannula to a larger size and increase flow.

4.  Manage the patient based on continuous venous and arterial saturation monitoring. Plot the position on Figure 5-4 frequently. Calculate the variables if oxygen supply seems excessive or inadequate.

5.  When the native lung begins to recover (the arterial saturation is >95%) turn down the flow, keeping the venous saturation >70%, and the sweep flow, keeping the $PaCO_2$ at 40. When native lung function is adequate, trial off ECLS then decannulate.

**Summary**

Managing a patient on ECLS requires a thorough understanding of normal and abnormal cardiopulmonary physiology, and a thorough understanding of the ECLS circuit. Based on this understanding, the ECLS system is used to replace part or all of heart and lung function, maintaining normal systemic physiology while the damaged organs can recover or be replaced.

# 6

## Adverse Effects of Extracorporeal Life Support

*Lindsay M. Ryerson, Gail Annich, Andriy Batchinsky, Gennaro Martucci, Teryn R. Roberts, Ravi R. Thiagarajan, Christophe Vandenbriele, Graeme MacLaren*

The use of ECLS can have a number of adverse consequences. These are primarily hematological in nature and relate to the biological conflict that occurs during extracorporeal exposure of blood to polymer circuitry components, in particular bleeding, thrombosis, and hemolysis. Nosocomial infections can also occur in all patient populations, increase in incidence with longer ECLS duration, and are arguably the principal reason why conventional VA ECMO can only be used as short-term support. The clinical significance of these adverse consequences varies. Thrombotic complications can be particularly problematic in small infants while nosocomial infections are more prevalent in older populations. This chapter will discuss the underlying pathophysiology and importance of the adverse consequences of ECLS, even when the circuit is otherwise functioning normally. Adverse events secondary to ECLS circuit malfunction, such as air emboli or pump failure, are described in Chapter 7. Complications which may be ascribed to either critical care or critical illness in ECLS patients are discussed in chapters focusing on specific populations (see Chapters 12, 16, 22, 26, and 33).

Several important factors contribute to the blood-polymer interaction (Figure 6-1). These interactions involve all the different

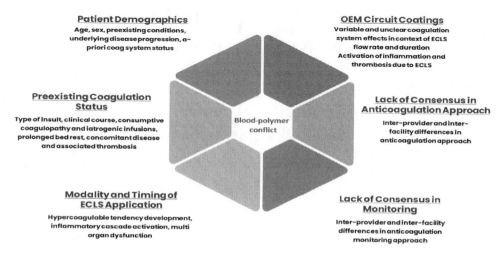

**Figure 6-1.** Patient dependent and ECLS dependent contributors to coagulation system management challenges.

blood components (platelets, leukocytes, red blood cells) as well as the endothelium and coagulation and inflammatory responses. The blood-polymer interface is a critical area of current research.

## Pathophysiology of Blood/Biomaterial Surface Interaction

Contact with synthetic, nonendothelial cell surfaces, shear stress, turbulent flow, cavitation, and osmotic forces may directly damage blood.[1] Plasma proteins and lipoproteins are progressively denatured during ECLS, increasing plasma viscosity and protein solubility, producing macromolecules, and increasing protein reactive side groups. Plasma IgG, IgA, IgM and albumin decrease more than expected from hemodilution. Red blood cells (RBCs) develop reversible echinocytic changes, but some are hemolyzed by shear forces and activated complement.[2,3] Platelets and white blood cells (WBCs) are also injured during perfusion; these impacts are described below. In addition, the effects of shear stress on platelets and other components of coagulation are also critically important. The higher the shear rate, the more platelet deposition and activation of FX by augmentation of the TF:VIIa complex, whereas at lower shear rates, less platelet deposition, but more fibrin deposition occurs.

Multiple blood cells and plasma protein systems are activated as part of a series of cellular and enzymatic reactions that occur during initiation and maintenance of ECLS. The response involves the contact and complement systems, coagulation, fibrinolysis and activation of most cell lines including platelets, neutrophils, monocytes, lymphocytes and endothelial cells.[4]

### *Platelets*

Platelets are the mainstay for hemostasis and together with endothelial cells preserve vascular wall integrity. Platelets respond to minimal stimulation and become activated when they encounter a thrombogenic stimulus such as injured endothelium, subendothelium, or artificial surfaces. Collagen exposure and von Willebrand Factor (vWF) released by the damaged blood vessel results in platelet adhesion. In high shear stress conditions (arteries and microvessels), high molecular weight vWF mediates platelet adhesion by binding to collagen and the nonactivated platelet through the platelet receptor glycoprotein (GP) Ib-IX-V. The adherence of platelets via GPIb to adsorbed vWF depends upon shear stress, which provides the conformational change in VWF needed to allow binding.[5] Fibrinogen binds to activated platelets through the receptor GPIIb-IIIa and acts as a bridge between platelets resulting in aggregation. Resting platelets with inactive GPIIb-IIIa have a low affinity for binding adsorbed fibrinogen. Once activated, conformational shape change of the platelet occur, and the high-affinity binding site of GPIIb-IIIa is exposed, binding soluble fibrinogen, which in turn leads to platelet aggregation and platelet leukocyte aggregates by the crosslinking of two GPIIb-IIIa receptors or by the crosslinking of GPIIb-IIIa with Mac-1 on the leukocyte.

Platelet activation and adhesion, as described above, occur during both CPB and ECLS, as well as with vascular access catheters and grafts. Both adherent platelets and platelet microparticles are procoagulant in nature, and therefore provide a continual, ongoing stimulus for the above-described physiologic platelet responses. During ECLS, platelet adhesion and aggregate formation reduce the circulating platelet count; however, high consumption and formation of microemboli, rather than occlusive thrombi, can occur even in the event of minimal adhesion to the circuitry surface. The circulating platelet pool during ECLS consists of decreased numbers of morphologically normal platelets, increased numbers of platelets at various stages of activation (eg, pseudopod formation, degranulation and membrane receptor loss), and immature platelets released from the bone marrow.

### Leukocytes

Neutrophils, monocytes, and lymphocytes are the main groups of cells involved in the inflammatory responses during ECLS. Exposure of patient blood to the extracorporeal circuit results in activation of innate immunity. Circulating leukocytes, including peripheral blood mononuclear cells (PBMCs), are stimulated in part by tissue factor activation,[6] complement[7] and endotoxin,[8] releasing numerous circulating proinflammatory cytokines (eg, TNF-$\alpha$, IL-1$\beta$) that activate circulating neutrophils facilitating their adhesion to the vascular surfaces of numerous organs. Leukocyte activation also releases an array of potent oxygen metabolites and proteolytic enzymes. The material characteristics of artificial surfaces modulate the absorption of proteins to the surface and therefore the level of activation.

Neutrophil counts decrease immediately after ECLS initiation because of dilution and recover slowly thereafter. The principal agonists for activating neutrophils during ECLS include kallikrein and C5a.[9] Both CPB and ECLS cause accumulation of activated neutrophils in pulmonary perivascular and interstitial tissue. This accumulation produces increased capillary permeability, interstitial edema, and large alveolar-arterial oxygen differences during and after perfusion.[10] During open heart surgery, monocytes are activated to express TF, in both the wound and extracorporeal circuit, but activation in the circuit is delayed for several hours.[11] Extracorporeal perfusion decreases the total number of lymphocytes and specific subsets of lymphocytes, particularly B lymphocytes, natural killer cells, helper T-cells, and T-suppressor lymphocytes.[12] Lymphocyte counts usually recover within 5

days of weaning from ECLS; slower recovery is associated with a poor prognosis.[13]

This proinflammatory response has been thought to be responsible for the physiologic derangements observed early after blood contacts the extracorporeal circuit. A compensatory, antiinflammatory response syndrome (CARS) also exists that is aimed at countering the proinflammation.[14] While CARS is a necessary response, an exaggerated or dysregulated CARS response can impair immunity thus rendering a host susceptible to infection and infectious sequelae such as sepsis and multiple organ dysfunction syndrome (MODS).[15]

### Endothelial Cells

Endothelial cells maintain the fluidity of blood and the integrity of the vascular system. Endothelial cells produce prostacyclin, heparin sulfate, tPA, and TFPI, which help regulate the coagulation pathway (Figure 6-2). Endothelial cells produce protein S, a necessary cofactor for normal protein C function; protein C is a natural anticoagulant. Endothelial cells also produce vasoactive substances and cytokines such as nitric oxide (NO), prostacyclin, endothelin-1, IL-1, IL-6, and platelet activating factor (PAF) as well as inactive substances such as histamine, norepinephrine, and bradykinin.[16]

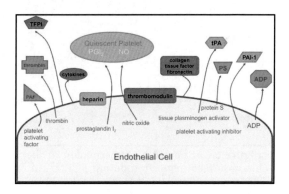

**Figure 6-2.** The endothelium maintains a delicate balance between thrombosis and anticoagulation during normal hemostasis.

## Complement

The alternative complement pathway, as opposed to the classic complement pathway, is primarily activated by foreign surfaces of microbial organisms or elements, particles, or biomaterial surfaces as part of this procoagulant activation and inflammation.[17] The alternative pathway does not require antibody or immune complexes for activation. Complement activation via the alternative pathway occurs spontaneously at a low rate, but as hydrolyzed C3 is formed, factor B becomes activated and then initiates the cleavage of C3 to form C3a and C3b. During ECLS or CPB, with a biomaterial surface to bind C3b covalently to its hydroxyl or amine groups, factor B and D binding occurs, and the alternative C3 convertase (C3bBb) is formed, creating a positive amplification loop.

## Initiation of ECLS: Coagulation Pathway Activation and Inflammatory Response

Exposure of blood to the nonbiologic surfaces of an extracorporeal circuit initiates a complex inflammatory response involving both the coagulation and the inflammatory response pathways (Figure 6-3).[7] This response leads

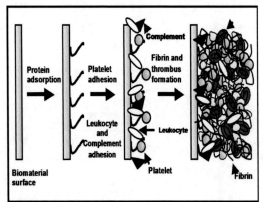

**Figure 6-3.** Simplistic representation of the blood-surface interaction during ECLS. This shows the components relevant to thrombosis; even though complement and leukocytes are considered to be involved with inflammation, they are also very relevant participants in thrombosis formation.

to capillary leak which can cause temporary dysfunction of every organ. In fact, the response to extracorporeal circulation is remarkably similar, clinically and biochemically, to that seen in the systemic inflammatory response syndrome (SIRS) and ARDS.[18]

## Activation of the Coagulation System during ECLS

Plasma proteins are adsorbed onto the biomaterial surface of the extracorporeal circuit to form a monolayer of bound proteins within seconds of contact.[19] Adsorbed FXII, FXI and fibrinogen undergo conformational changes, triggering activation of the contact system. The contact system consists of four primary plasma proteins: FXII, prekallikrein, high molecular weight kininogen (HMWK), and C-1 inhibitor. FXIIa, HMWK, FXI, FIX and FVIIIa work together to produce the tenase complex. The tenase complex binds FX to produce FXa. Activation of coagulation occurs through TF expression on activated cells (monocytes, macrophages, neutrophils, activated endothelial cells, smooth muscle cells, apoptotic cells), or cellular components (platelet microparticles or circulating vesicles). TF is a cell-bound glycoprotein expressed in the vascular subendothelium, and many other cells including activated monocytes.[20] TF complexes with FVII in conjunction with a phospholipid surface forming the TF:VIIa complex which in turn activates FX to FXa. FXa facilitates the conversion of prothrombin to thrombin, and fibrinogen to fibrin

Platelets adhere to the circuit surfaces and become activated, which leads to platelet aggregation and further activation of the coagulation system. Platelet activation and consumption occurs upon ECLS initiation causing decreases in platelet number and function within the first hour of ECLS.[21] With platelet activation, neutrophils also become activated producing cytokines and further contributing to the inflammatory response to extracorporeal circulation.[22]

The fibrinolytic system has the important role of limiting the extent of clot formation and eventually dissolving it. The presence of circulating thrombin stimulates endothelial cells to produce tPA, which participates in the cleavage of plasminogen to plasmin.[23] Plasmin lyses fibrin to dissolve clot and inhibits fibrinogen and factors V, VII, IX, and XI. The cleavage reaction to form plasmin produces D-dimers, which have been shown to be elevated during the course of neonatal ECLS as a marker of ongoing fibrinolysis.[24] Such significant activation of the coagulation system results in a pattern of consumptive coagulopathy, with half of infants and children in one study demonstrating deficiencies in both platelets and coagulation factors soon after the initiation of ECLS, even with the use of fresh frozen plasma (FFP) in the circuit priming volume.[25]

Despite the activity of plasmin and the fibrinolytic system described above, the use of an extracorporeal circuit results in continued activation of the coagulation system and generation of thrombin. Endogenous antithrombotic activity becomes overwhelmed and this necessitates the use of an exogenous anticoagulant to maintain the integrity of the extracorporeal circuit.

### Activation of the Innate Immune System and Resultant Immune Dysregulation

Activation of the coagulation system and thrombin generation does not occur in isolation, but in conjunction with the activation of the innate immune system. The initial activation of the innate immune system by the ECLS circuit cumulatively contributes to the SIRS response that can clinically manifest as hemodynamic instability and capillary leak. Thus, depending on the degree of the innate immune response, a slight increase in hemodynamic support may be necessary following the first few hours after initiation of ECLS. The initial SIRS response is counterbalanced by CARS to reestablish homeostasis and reset the innate immune system. However, a prolonged CARS response may lead to an acquired immunosuppressed state, placing the patient at risk for nosocomial infections.

### Blood-Compatible and Bioinspired Materials for ECLS

To improve the blood compatibility of ECLS devices, numerous material modification strategies are in development to make the foreign polymer surfaces that comprise the ECLS device potentially as safe for the blood as the vascular endothelium. The vascular endothelium is exceptionally intricate, however, and serves as more than a passive barrier that separates blood from foreign sources of activation. The endothelium actively regulates local blood fluidity and hemostasis by continuously modifying surface chemistry, excreted factors, flow distribution and permeability.[26,27] Further, the surface chemistry and functional characteristics of the endothelium are extremely heterogenous throughout the body, varied to support tissue-specific needs, local blood flow conditions and fluctuating metabolic demands.[28]

Design of "bioinspired" surface modifications for medical applications should involve consideration of the following characteristics observed in the natural blood vessel lining: 1) comprehensive and multifaceted—the surface should incorporate multiple complementary features to minimize thrombus deposition and cellular procoagulant and proinflammatory stimulation; 2) regionally specific—the surface features at specific locations within the medical device should be designed to address the regional flow dynamics and shear conditions, just as the vasculature surface in major arteries is substantially different than in veins and capillaries[29]; 3) responsive and adaptable—the vascular endothelium can act in both sensory and effective capacities to regulate hemostatic balance under varying physiological conditions and disease states; 4) durable—blood vessels are designed to maintain regional hemostasis indefinitely, and serious disease pathologies result from endothelial dysfunction and degradation.

### Clinically Available Biomaterials in ECLS

Clinically available biomaterial coatings for extracorporeal organ support devices currently do not incorporate these robust features of the vascular endothelium, and plausibly have failed to provide an efficacious solution to bleeding and thrombotic complications. Material modifications to improve blood compatibility typically involve application of a surface coating along the blood contact surface of the plastic, or incorporation of bioactive substances into the polymer matrix. These modifications can affect the physical properties and functionality of the materials, however, so care must be taken that the coatings do not alter device performance, such as impeding permeability of the fibers that compose a membrane lung.

The most commonly utilized antithrombogenic material modification for ECLS is immobilized heparin surface coating. Clinical studies comparing heparin-coated to uncoated circuitry for CPB and ECLS have shown that heparin coating may reduce inflammatory and complement activation,[30-32] reduce transfusion requirements,[30,33] and potentially reduce ICU length of stay[31,33]; however, most reported benefits are observed during short-term (~4-6 hours) use with tandem administration of systemic anticoagulation, leaving the long-term efficacy of this approach in lieu of systemic anticoagulation unestablished.[34,35]

Other clinically available blood-compatible materials have shown similar modest short-term benefits in CPB and ECLS, including surface passivation with albumin to competitively inhibit adsorption of procoagulant proteins such as fibrinogen and application of zwitterionic phosphorylcholine coatings that modify surface charge and hydrophilicity in a manner resembling endothelial cells. However, like immobilized heparin, there is no evidence to support the long-term safety and efficacy of these coatings, particularly in lieu of systemic anticoagulation.

### Investigational Biomaterials for ECLS

A number of investigational surface coatings have been identified as promising candidates for ECLS, many of which are inspired by features of the vascular endothelium. For example, NO-releasing materials that incorporate NO donor species such as diazeniumdiolated dibutylhexanediamine (DBHD/N2O2) and S-nitroso-N-acetylpenacillamine (SNAP) into a polymer surface or matrix can elute NO at a similar flux as occurs in the healthy endothelium, eliciting platelet quiescence and promoting an antithrombogenic environment as described earlier. One concern with NO-releasing materials is that only a finite store of NO donor species can be incorporated into the material, meaning NO flux can diminish over time. To address this, NO-catalyzing coatings have been developed that can generate NO from bioavailable donors in the patient's blood, such as S-nitrosothiols (RSNOs).[36-38] Other promising biomaterial approaches involve incorporation of bioactive substances that provide localized anticoagulation at the biomaterial interface, such as immobilization of direct thrombin inhibitors[39] and application of corn trypsin inhibitor as a selective fXIIa inhibitor.[40,41] Additional approaches target protein adsorption and thrombus deposition via passive barriers including slippery liquid infused surfaces,[42-44] fabrication of glycosaminoglycan polymer brushes,[45,46] and microstructured surfaces that reduce protein adsorption and platelet adhesion.[47] In order to replicate the multifaceted approach to hemostasis that is achieved in the endothelium, combination approaches that incorporate numerous aspects of the abovementioned surface modifications, such as dual nitric oxide release and slippery non-adhesive boundary layer coatings[48] or immobilized thrombin inhibitors combined with nitric oxide elution[49-51] are in development as well.

While the above-mentioned surface coatings have shown promise in various in vitro and in vivo models, the surface modifications are typically applied to the ECLS connective tubing and cannulas only; however, the blood pump and membrane oxygenators are critical functional components that could benefit from improved hemocompatibility. The membrane oxygenator presents key challenges to surface coating application, as the thin, strongly hydrophobic gas permeable fibers are sensitive to damage by common solvents and chemicals utilized in the coating process, and are not receptive to swelling of substances into the polymer matrix. Attempts have been made to seed endothelial cells onto the PMP fibers utilized in membrane oxygenators; however, the cells could not adhere to the hydrophobic material surface without addition of a titanium dioxide intermediary layer.[52] An alternative approach to membrane surface coating application is to apply NO gas into the sweep gas of the membrane oxygenator, enabling diffusion of NO into the blood to minimize platelet activation and thrombus deposition in the same manner as NO-releasing and NO-catalyzing surface coatings. This approach has been shown to potentially attenuate the inflammatory response during CPB in swine models,[53,54] was shown to reduce platelet loss in a neonatal ovine model of ECLS,[55] and was utilized in combination with NO-releasing circuit tubing in a pumpless venovenous ECLS model in sheep.[56] Early clinical evidence also suggests the safety and potential efficacy of NO gas administration via membrane oxygenator sweep gas during CPB and ECLS in children.[57-59] Additional information on current investigational coatings for ECLS is summarized in recent reviews.[60,61]

## Other Adverse Effects of ECLS

### Hemolysis

Hemolysis is characterized by mechanical damage to red blood cells and subsequent release of free hemoglobin in plasma, due to supraphysiologic shear stress that occurs during circulation of blood through extracorporeal circuits. Hemolysis leads to increased plasma levels of hemoglobin degradation products, including plasma free hemoglobin (PFHb) and heme, bilirubin as well as lactate dehydrogenase (LDH). High levels of PFHb and heme overwhelm normal neutralization by haptoglobin and hemopexin proteins, deplete endogenous nitric oxide, and thus promote vasoconstriction and platelet aggregation. Hemolysis is often associated, particularly in the pediatric population, with serious complications such as pump thrombosis, acute tubular necrosis, coagulopathy, and multiorgan dysfunction. Hemolysis associated with ECLS ranges between 5% and 18%.[62]

Normal shear stress in the circulatory system is between 1-10 Pa, but this is largely exceeded during extracorporeal circulation. Consequently, hemolysis occurs when there is turbulence, as in cases of high flow velocity due to small cannulas, or extremely negative circuit pressures in the setting of low preload, leading to cavitation. When blood flow becomes turbulent, the erythrocytes first deform to an ellipsoidal shape and finally progress to cell wall destruction, with consequences impacting blood flow through the microcirculation.

When hemoglobin is released outside of erythrocytes, it may result in deleterious effects on cells and tissues. PFHb and its components, heme and free iron, are capable of inducing potent free radical generation, which is widely known to disrupt cell membranes, damage proteins, DNA and lipids, induce SIRS, and thus lead to tissue and organ damage.[63] Furthermore, PFHb depletes endothelial-derived nitric oxide, one of the major regulators of microcirculation, leading to vasoconstriction and additional procoagulant state secondary to abnormal coagulation and platelet activation.[64]

Hemolysis screening is not standardized, and currently relies on plasma biomarkers. PFHb is the principal biomarker, and is considered an independent predictor of mortality and adverse clinical events during ECLS.[65-67] The cutoff for hemolysis for PFHb varies across studies. A value of >30 mg/dL is diagnostic of hemolysis, though the most commonly reported level is >50 mg/dL. Levels above 100 mg/dL are considered severe and should prompt immediate action.[66] Other biomarkers include LDH, bilirubin and aspartate transaminases, and have been found to show a relevant correlation with PFHb. These can be adopted if PFHb is not available.[68] The principal action to prevent or limit hemolysis is to avoid thrombosis in the circuit, change components or the entire circuit when thrombosis occurs, and avoid high pump speeds with inadequate proload and/or increased afterload.

## *Bleeding*

Bleeding occurs frequently in patients receiving ECLS and is associated with increased mortality.[69] Anticoagulation, dual antiplatelet therapy (DAPT) in patients with acute coronary syndrome (ACS) and/or PCI, platelet and clotting factor consumption, as well as the frequent development of acquired von Willebrand syndrome (AVWS), all increase the risk of bleeding in ECLS-supported patients (Figure 6-4).[70] The last of these may be caused by high shear and continuous flow in ECLS, leading to proteolysis of high-molecular-weight von Willebrand factor. This results in reduced platelet-binding affinity and the development of AVWS in the majority of patients within 24 hours of starting ECLS, but

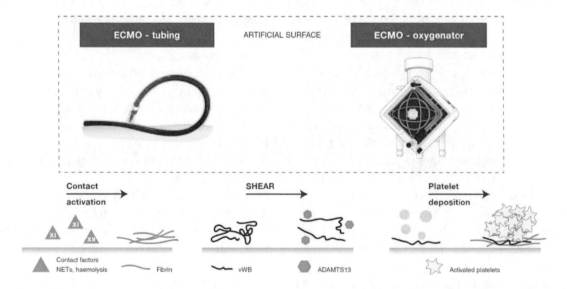

**Figure 6-4.** During ECMO, blood is continuously exposed to foreign body material (plastic surfaces in tubing and especially in the oxygenator); this causes a complex process of thrombus formation and consumptive coagulopathy due to contact activation resulting in fibrin deposition, high shear stress and von Willebrand deposition and platelet deposition/activation. (*vWB=von Willebrand molecule, NET=neutrophil-extracellular-traps, ADAMTS13=a disintegrin and metalloproteinase with a thrombospondin type 1 motif, member 13; after Vandenbriele[70]*)

which resolves rapidly after discontinuation.[71] The only treatment for ECLS-induced AVWS is decannulation, although novel techniques (eg, ADAMTS13 blocking agents) are under investigation.[72,73]

Bleeding is more common with nonpulsatile, continuous flow devices than with pulsatile assist devices, and greater at lower flow rates.[74] Most data pertaining to the frequency of bleeding and thrombotic complications come from retrospective analyses of large national databases. Among ACS patients with cardiogenic shock, bleeding complications occur in 40-70% of those treated with ECLS.[75,76] A metaanalysis of 20 studies including 1,866 adult patients treated with ECLS revealed lower extremity ischemia in 16.9%, stroke in 5.9% and major or significant bleeding in 40.8% of patients.[75] Bleeding is associated with an increased risk of death and with prolonged inotropic and ventilatory requirements.[77] Risk factors associated with major vascular complications in patients on ECLS are obesity, concomitant use of ECLS with other forms of mechanical circulatory support (MCS), SOFA-score at 24h post-ECLS and hematological disorders.[78]

Most ECLS-related bleeding are access site related, due to the need for large-bore access as well as continuous anticoagulation.[79,80] Meticulous cannulation techniques and the use of doppler ultrasound are required for percutaneous cannulation. Local source control is the best way to control access site-related bleeding. Oozing at the access site can be controlled by local tranexamic acid- or adrenalin-soaked gauze in conjunction with pressure. Ear-nose-throat (ENT) bleeds are common in patients on ECLS, and bleeding prevention and source control are key to success (eg, orogastric instead of nasogastric tubes, avoiding nasoendotracheal intubation in small children, mouth packing with tranexamic acid-soaked gauze, ENT-interventions, intranasal balloon compression). Only when no proper

hemostasis is obtained after optimal source control, lowering the UFH-target (and thus increasing the thrombotic risk) could be a next reasonable step. Cessation of UFH-treatment in combination with surgical or endovascular source control should only be considered for severe bleeding events, eg, retroperitoneal or intracerebral bleedings, and should be kept as short as possible to prevent pump thrombosis and/or systemic embolism.

### *Thrombosis*

Circuit thrombosis occurs following initiation of coagulation systems, platelet activation, and inflammatory and complement cascades after exposure to ECLS circuit materials as previously described. Circuit clots are more common on the venous side of the circuit due to areas of both stasis and turbulence. Thrombotic complications often have inconsistent definitions in the ECLS literature, making comparison between published reports difficult.[81-87] Standard definitions for thrombotic complications are necessary to determine clinically relevant outcomes and allow comparison between centers and publications. The ELSO Registry defines a circuit thrombotic complication as requiring either a change in the entire circuit or a circuit component, including tubing, connectors, cannulas or oxygenator. In the October 2021 ELSO International Registry report across all ages and indications, circuit change was reported in 2-17 % of all ECLS runs and thrombosis related to ECLS equipment components in 4–34% of all ECLS runs (Table 6-1).

Central nervous system infarction is the commonly measured parameter to assess thromboembolic complications in patients supported with ECLS. The ELSO Registry only includes patient thrombotic complications diagnosed by US, CT or MRI. The rates of stroke in ECLS patients varies by age and indication and ranges from 1–8% (Table 6-1). The total burden of patient thromboembolic events is likely underestimated due to difficulties in imaging critically ill patients on ECLS. Autopsy studies reveal higher rates of systemic thromboembolic complications, suggesting a significant burden of clinically unrecognized thromboembolic events.[88,89]

A recent systematic review of 34 studies described 201 individual adult patients treated with anticoagulation-free ECLS for a median of 4.75 days.[87] The overall incidence of thrombosis (patient or circuit requiring exchange) was 22.9%, which is comparable to thrombotic complications described in the literature of patients receiving systemic anticoagulation.[87] Conclusions must be interpreted in the context of retrospective data, inconsistent reporting of outcomes, and differences in circuit components and patient management.

The risk of circuit thrombosis and subsequent thromboembolic complications varies between adult and pediatric patients. Differences in cannulation strategies, smaller cannula sizes and circuitry, and lower flow rates all may contribute to the increased thrombotic complications in pediatric patients.

### Nosocomial Infection

Nosocomial infections are one of the most common adverse effects associated with ECLS, particularly in adult patients and in those receiving VA ECMO. The incidence is approximately 10-30 infections/1,000 ECLS days, but >100 infections/1,000 ECLS days have been described in some circumstances.[90,91] Differences across patient populations and inconsistently applied definitions explain at least some of this variation.[92] The preferred definitions are those of the Centers for Disease Control and Prevention National Healthcare Safety Network. The risk factors for infection during ECLS are shown in Table 6-2. One of the most important risk factors is the duration of ECLS, which represents both a risk and a consequence of nosocomial infection. Although many single-center studies of adult patients have not shown an association between infectious complications and mortality, large multicenter studies have consistently demonstrated this across all age groups.[90,91]

ECLS itself makes the diagnosis of infection more difficult because it can elicit a systemic inflammatory response which can be confused

| ECMO INDICATION | NEONATE | PEDIATRIC | ADULT |
|---|---|---|---|
| Respiratory ECMO Total Runs | 780 | 590 | 7917 |
| ECMO Equipment Thrombosis | 33.8% | 23% | 6.4% |
| Clots and Air Emboli | 1.2% | 0.7% | 0.2% |
| ECMO Circuit change | 16% | 17.1% | 10.6% |
| CNS infarction | 2.7% | 3.7% | 1.4% |
| Cardiac ECMO Total Runs | 531 | 1064 | 5146 |
| ECMO Equipment Thrombosis | 19.8% | 18.2% | 5.3% |
| Clots and Air Emboli | 0.3% | 0.3% | 0.1% |
| ECMO Circuit change | 9.9% | 9% | 2.8% |
| CNS infarction | 3.3% | 5.2% | 3.3% |
| ECPR ECMO Total Runs | 152 | 521 | 1559 |
| ECMO Equipment Thrombosis | 18.8% | 10.9% | 4.4% |
| Clots and Air Emboli | 0.1% | 0% | 0.2% |
| ECMO Circuit change | 7.2% | 5.9% | 1.8% |
| CNS infarction | 4% | 8% | 4.3% |

**Table 6-1.** Thrombotic complications reported to the ELSO Registry during 2016–2020: Data from the ECLS Registry Report: International Summary, October 2021.

with infection and because the heater-cooler masks any underlying fever. Current biomarkers such as C-reactive protein and procalcitonin are sensitive but not specific for infection and are not recommended for diagnostic purposes.[91] The most common types of infections are bloodstream infections, ventilator-associated pneumonia, and surgical site infections.

The organisms causing nosocomial infection are generally similar to those in critically ill, non-ECLS patients, such as *Staphylococcus* species, *Pseudomonas aeruginosa*, and Enterobacterales. Fungal infections such as *Candida* spp. are commonly seen in some patient populations, eg, neonates or those repeatedly exposed to broad-spectrum antibiotics. Rarely, unusual organisms may cause infection when they contaminate the heater-cooler, such as *Ralstonia picketii* and nontuberculous mycobacteria.[91] Some of these infections may be missed unless they are specifically looked for because they cannot be identified on routine microscopy and culture.

Treatment should be guided by local antibiograms, culture results, and directed at the probable site of infection. The pharmacokinetics and dynamics of many antibiotics are not well characterized on ECLS and therapeutic drug monitoring should be used when available, especially when prescribing drugs with narrow therapeutic indices (see Chapter 49). Conventional durations of antibiotic therapy may not be applicable in ECLS patients because source control is often impossible until the patient is decannulated, particularly with bloodstream infections.

Nosocomial infection mandates reassessment of the patient's clinical state because it may worsen other organ function and increase metabolic demand. This may require adjustments to the ECLS circuit, such as increasing circuit blood flow, or changes to the cannulation strategy to address evolving problems caused by worsening organ function, eg, differential hypoxemia.

More details on diagnosis and treatment can be found in chapters on specific patient populations.

| | RISK FACTOR | COMMENT |
|---|---|---|
| Patient Factors | Age | Adult patients at greater risk |
| | Severity of illness | Higher Sequential Organ Failure Assessment (SOFA) scores prior to cannulation are associated with greater risk |
| | Co-morbidities | eg, immunosuppression |
| | Hemorrhage | |
| ECLS Factors | ECLS duration | |
| | Cannulation strategy | Venoarterial ECMO is associated with increased risk than venovenous ECMO. Central ECMO is associated with greater risk than peripheral ECMO. Open cannulation is associated with greater risk than percutaneous cannulation. |
| | Surgery during ECLS | |
| | Mechanical complications | eg, pump failure |

**Table 6-2.** Important risk factors for nosocomial infection during ECLS.[90,91]

# References

1. Leverett LB, Hellums JD, Alfrey CP, et al. Red blood cell damage by shear stress. Biophys J. 1972;12:257-273.

2. Woodman RC, Harker LA. Bleeding complications associated with cardiopulmonary bypass. Blood. 1990;76:1680-1697.

3. Salama A, Hugo F, Heinrich D, et al. Deposition of terminal C5b-9 complement complexes on erythrocytes and leukocytes during cardiopulmonary bypass. N Eng J Med. 1988;318:408-414.

4. Bowen FW, Edmunds HL Jr. Coagulation, anticoagulation and the interaction of blood and artificial surfaces. In: Zwischenberger JB, Steinhorn RH, Bartlett, RH, eds. ECMO: Extracorporeal cardiopulmonary support in critical care. 2nd Ed. Ann Arbor, MI: ELSO; 2000:67-96.

5. Gorbet MB, Sefton MV. Biomaterial-associated thrombosis: roles of coagulation factors complement, platelets and leukocytes. Biomaterials. 2004;25:5681-5703.

6. Shibamiya A, Tabuchi N, Chung J, et al. Formation of tissue factor-bearing leukocytes during and after cardiopulmonary bypass. Thromb Haemost. 2004;92:124-131.

7. Wan S, LeClerc JL, Vincent JL. Inflammatory response to cardiopulmonary bypass: mechanisms involved and possible therapeutic strategies. Chest. 1997;112:676-692.

8. Tsunooka N, Maeyama K, Hamada Y, et al. Bacterial translocation secondary to small intestinal mucosal ischemia during cardiopulmonary bypass. Measurement by diamine oxidase and peptidoglycan. Eur J Cardiothorac Surg. 2004;25:275-280.

9. El Habbal MH, Carter H, Smith L, et al. Neutrophil activation in paediatric extracorporeal circuits: effect of circulation and temperature variation. Cardiovascular Research. 1995;29:102-107.

10. Ratliff NB, Young WG Jr, Hackel D, et al. Pulmonary injury secondary to extracorporeal circulation. An ultrastructural study. J Thorac Cardiovasc Surg. 1973;65:425-432.

11. Barstad RM, Ovrum E, Ringdal MA, et al. Induction of monocyte tissue factor procoagulant activity during coronary artery bypass surgery is reduced with heparin-coated extracorporeal circuit. Br J Haematol. 1996; 94:517-525.

12. DePalma L, Yu M, McIntosh CL, et al. Changes in lymphocyte subpopulations as a result of cardiopulmonary bypass. The effect of blood transfusion. J Thorac Cardiovasc Surg. 1991;101:240-244.

13. Kawahito K, Kobayashi E, Misawa Y, et al. Recovery from lymphocytopenia and prognosis after adult extracorporeal membrane oxygenation. Arch Surg. 1998;133:216-217.

14. Zimmerman JJ. Congenital heart disease, cardiopulmonary bypass, systemic inflammatory response syndrome, compensatory anti-inflammatory response syndrome, and outcome: evolving understanding of critical care inflammation immunology. Crit Care Med. 2002;30:1178-1179.

15. Mokart D, Capo C, Blache JL, et al. Early postoperative compensatory anti-inflammatory response syndrome is associated with septic complications after major surgical trauma in patients with cancer. Br J Surg. 2002; 89:1450-1456.

16. Vane JR, Anggard EE, Botting RM. Regulatory functions of the vascular endothelium. N Engl J Med. 1990;323:27-36.

17. Valhonart H, Swinford RD, Ingelfinger JR, et al. Rapid activation of the alternative pathway of complement by extracorporeal membrane oxygenation. ASAIO J. 1999;45:113-114.

18. Peek GJ, Firmin RK. The inflammatory and coagulative response to prolonged extracorporeal membrane oxygenation. ASAIO J. 1999;45:250-263.

19. Horbett TA. Principles underlying the role of adsorbed plasma proteins in blood interactions with foreign materials. Cardiovasc Pathol. 1993;2:137S.

20. Edgington TS, Mackman N, Brand K, et al. The structural biology of expression and function of tissue factor. Thromb Haemost. 1991;66:67-79.

21. Robinson TM, Kickler TS, Walker LK, et al. Effect of extracorporeal membrane oxygenation on platelets in newborns. Crit Care Med. 1993;21:1029-1034.

22. Fortenberry JD, Bhardwaj V, Niemer P, et al. Neutrophil and cytokine activation with neonatal extracorporeal membrane oxygenation. J Pediatr. 1996;128:670-678.

23. Levin EG, Marzec U, Anderson J, et al. Thrombin stimulates tissue plasminogen activator from cultured human endothelial cells. J Clin Invest. 1984;74:1988-1995.

24. Urlesberger B, Zobel G, Zenz W, et al. Activation of the clotting system during extracorporeal membrane oxygenation in term newborn infants. J Pediatr. 1996;129:264-268.

25. McManus ML, Kevy SV, Bower LK, et al. Coagulation factor deficiencies during initiation of extracorporeal membrane oxygenation. J Pediatr. 1995;126:900-904.

26. van Hinsbergh VWM. Endothelium—role in regulation of coagulation and inflammation. Seminars in Immunopathology. 2012;34:93-106.

27. Gimbrone MA, Jr. Vascular endothelium: nature's blood-compatible container. Ann N Y Acad Sci. 1987;516:5-11.

28. Aird William C. Phenotypic Heterogeneity of the Endothelium. Circulation Research. 2007;100:158-173.

29. dela Paz NG, D'Amore PA. Arterial versus venous endothelial cells. Cell Tissue Res. 2009;335:5-16.

30. Mahmood S, Bilal H, Zaman M, Tang A. Is a fully heparin-bonded cardiopulmonary bypass circuit superior to a standard cardiopulmonary bypass circuit? Interact Cardiovasc Thorac Surg. 2012;14:406-414.

31. Svenmarker S, Haggmark S, Jansson E, et al. Use of heparin-bonded circuits in cardiopulmonary bypass improves clinical outcome. Scandinavian cardiovascular journal : SCJ. 2002;36:241-246.

32. Wendel HP, Ziemer G. Coating-techniques to improve the hemocompatibility of artificial devices used for extracorporeal circulation. Eur J Cardiothorac Surg. 1999;16:342-350.

33. Mangoush O, Purkayastha S, Haj-Yahia S, et al. Heparin-bonded circuits versus nonheparin-bonded circuits: an evaluation of their effect on clinical outcomes. Eur J Cardiothorac Surg. 2007;31:1058-1069.

34. Silvetti S, Koster A, Pappalardo F. Do we need heparin coating for extracorporeal membrane oxygenation? New concepts and controversial positions about coating surfaces of extracorporeal circuits. Artif Organs. 2015;39:176-179.

35. Maul TM, Massicotte MP, Wearden PD. ECMO biocompatibility: surface coatings, anticoagulation, and coagulation monitoring. Extracorporeal Membrane Oxygenation-Advances in Therapy: InTechOpen; 2016.

36. Major TC, Brant DO, Burney CP, et al. The hemocompatibility of a nitric oxide generating polymer that catalyzes S-nitrosothiol decomposition in an extracorporeal circulation model. Biomaterials. 2011;32:5957-5969.

37. Roberts TR, Neufeld MJ, Meledeo MA, et al. A metal organic framework reduces thrombus formation and platelet aggregation ex vivo. J Trauma Acute Care Surg. 2018;85:572-579.

38. Neufeld MJ, Lutzke A, Jones WM, et al. Nitric oxide generation from endogenous substrates using metal-organic rrameworks: inclusion within poly(vinyl alcohol) membranes to investigate reactivity and therapeutic potential. ACS Appl Mater Interfaces. 2017;9:35628-35641.

39. Yu J, Brisbois E, Handa H, et al. The immobilization of a direct thrombin inhibitor to a polyurethane as a nonthrombogenic surface coating for extracorporeal circulation. J Mater Chem B. 2016;4:2264-2272.

40. Yau JW, Stafford AR, Liao P, et al. Corn trypsin inhibitor coating attenuates the prothrombotic properties of catheters in vitro and in vivo. Acta Biomaterialia. 2012;8:4092-4100.

41. Alibeik S, Zhu S, Yau JW, et al. Modification of polyurethane with polyethylene glycol–corn trypsin inhibitor for inhibition of Factor XIIa in blood contact. Journal of biomaterials science Polymer edition. 2012;23:1981-1993.

42. Roberts TR, Choi JH, Wendorff DS, et al. Tethered liquid perfluorocarbon coating for 72 hour heparin-free extracorporeal life support. ASAIO J. 2021;67:798-808.

43. Leslie DC, Waterhouse A, Berthet JB, et al. A bioinspired omniphobic surface coating on medical devices prevents thrombosis and biofouling. Nat Biotechnol. 2014;32:1134-1140.

44. Roberts TR, Harea GT, Singha P, et al. Heparin-free extracorporeal life support using tethered liquid perfluorocarbon: a feasibility and efficacy study. ASAIO J. 2020;66:809-817.

45. Hedayati M, Kipper MJ. Atomic force microscopy of adsorbed proteoglycan mimetic nanoparticles: Toward new glycocalyx-mimetic model surfaces. Carbohydrate Polymers. 2018;190:346-355.

46. Hedayati M, Reynolds MM, Krapf D, et al. Nanostructured surfaces that mimic the vascular endothelial glycocalyx reduce blood protein adsorption and prevent fibrin network formation. ACS Applied Materials & Interfaces. 2018;10:31892-31902.

47. Pham TT, Wiedemeier S, Maenz S, et al. Hemodynamic aspects of reduced platelet adhesion on bioinspired microstructured surfaces. Colloids and Surfaces B: Biointerfaces. 2016;145:502-509.

48. Goudie MJ, Pant J, Handa H. Liquid-infused nitric oxide-releasing (LINORel) silicone for decreased fouling, thrombosis, and infection of medical devices. Sci Rep. 2017;7:13623.

49. Devine R, Goudie MJ, Singha P, et al. Mimicking the endothelium: dual action heparinized nitric oxide releasing surface. ACS applied materials & interfaces. 2020;12:20158-20171.

50. Major TC, Brisbois EJ, Jones AM, et al. The effect of a polyurethane coating incorporating both a thrombin inhibitor and nitric oxide on hemocompatibility in extracorporeal circulation. Biomaterials. 2014;35:7271-7285.

51. Bellomo TR, Jeakle MA, Meyerhoff ME, et al. The effects of the combined argatroban/nitric oxide-releasing polymer on platelet microparticle-induced thrombogenicity in coated extracorporeal circuits. ASAIO J. 2020;67:573-582.

52. Pflaum M, Kühn-Kauffeldt M, Schmeckebier S, et al. Endothelialization and characterization of titanium dioxide-coated gas-exchange membranes for application in the bioartificial lung. Acta Biomaterialia. 2017;50:510-521.

53. Toomasian JM, Jeakle MMP, Langley M, et al. Nitric oxide attenuates the inflammatory effects of air during extracorporeal circulation. ASAIO J. 2020;66:818-824.

54. Qin Y, Zajda J, Brisbois EJ, et al. Portable nitric oxide (NO) generator based on electrochemical reduction of nitrite for potential applications in inhaled NO therapy and cardiopulmonary bypass surgery. Molecular Pharmaceutics. 2017;14:3762-3771.

55. Rossidis AC, Lawrence KM, Mejaddam AY, et al. The effects of nitric oxide in oxygenator sweep gas during extracorporeal circulation in a neonatal ovine model. ASAIO J. 2020;66:671-676.

56. Fallon BP, Lautner-Csorba O, Thompson AJ, et al. A pumpless artificial lung without systemic anticoagulation: the nitric oxide surface anticoagulation system. J Pediatr Surg. 2022;57:26-33.

57. Chiletti R, Horton S, Bednarz A, et al. Safety of nitric oxide added to the ECMO circuit: a pilot study in children. Perfusion. 2018;33:74-76.

58. Bennett M, Thuys C, Augustin S,et al. The safe addition of nitric oxide into the sweep gas of the extracorporeal circuit during cardiopulmonary bypass and extracorporeal life support. J Extra Corpor Technol. 2018;50:260-264.

59. James C, Millar J, Horton S, Brizard C, et al. Nitric oxide administration during paediatric cardiopulmonary bypass: a randomised controlled trial. Intensive Care Med. 2016;42:1744-1752.

60. Ontaneda A, Annich GM. Novel surfaces in extracorporeal membrane oxygenation circuits. Front Medicine. 2018;5:321.

61. Roberts TR, Garren MRS, Handa H, et al. Toward an artificial endothelium: Development of blood-compatible surfaces for extracorporeal life support. J Trauma Acute Care Surg. 2020;89:S59-S68.

62. Zangrillo A, Landoni G, Biondi-Zoccai G, et al. A meta-analysis of complications and mortality of extracorporeal membrane oxygenation. Crit Care Resusc. 2013;15:172-178.

63. Lin T, Kwak YH, Sammy F, et al. Synergistic inflammation is induced by blood degradation products with microbial Toll-like receptor agonists and is blocked by hemopexin. J Infect Dis. 2010;202:624-632.

64. Dufour N, Radjou A, Thuong M. Hemolysis and plasma free hemoglobin during extracorporeal oxygenation support: from clinical implications to laboratory details. ASAIO J. 2020;66:239-246.

65. Omar HR, Mirsaeidi M, Socias S, et al. Plasma free hemoglobin is an independent Predictor of mortality among patients on extracorporeal membrane oxygenation support. PLoS ONE. 2015;10:e0124034.

66. Lou S, MacLaren G, Best D, et al. Hemolysis in pediatric patients receiving centrifugal-pump extracorporeal membrane oxygenation: prevalence, risk factors, and outcomes. Crit Care Med. 2014;42: 1213–1220.

67. Okochi S, Cheung EW, Barton S, et al. An analysis of risk factors for hemolysis in children on extracorporeal membrane oxygenation. Pediatr Crit Care Med. 2018;19:1059–1066.

68. Ghaleb S, Reagor JA, Tarango C, et al. Correlation among hemolysis biomarkers in pediatric patients undergoing extracorporeal membrane oxygenation. J Extra Corpor Technol. 2021;53:125–129.

69. Chieffo A, Ancona MB, Burzotta F, et al. Observational multicentre registry of patients treated with IMPella mechanical circulatory support device in ITaly: the IMP-IT registry. Euro Intervention. 2020;15:e1343-e1350.

70. Vandenbriele C, Vanassche T, Price S. Why we need safer anticoagulant strategies for patients on short-term percutaneous mechanical circulatory support. Intensive Care Med. 2020;46:771-774.

71. Vandenbriele C, Balthazar T, Engelen M, et al. Acquired von Willebrand Syndrome in left Impella supported cardiogenic shock patients. Eur Heart J. 2020;41:1538.

72. Bartoli CR, Kang J, Restle DJ, et al. Inhibition of ADAMTS-13 by doxycycline reduces von Willebrand factor degradation during supraphysiological shear stress: therapeutic implications for left ventricular assist device-associated bleeding. JACC Heart Fail. 2015;3:860-869.

73. Deconinck SJ, Nix C, Bennek-Schopping E, et al. Inhibition of adamts13: a novel therapy to treat mechanical circulatory support-induced acquired von Willebrand syndrome. Eur Heart J. 2020;41:3836.

74. Ki KK, Passmore MR, Chan CHH, et al. Low flow rate alters haemostatic parameters in an ex-vivo extracorporeal membrane oxygenation circuit. Intensive Care Med Exp. 2019;7:51.

75. Cheng R, Hachamovitch R, Kittleson M, et al. Complications of extracorporeal membrane oxygenation for treatment of cardiogenic shock and cardiac arrest: a meta-analysis of 1,866 adult patients. Ann Thorac Surg. 2014;97:610-616.

76. Mazzeffi M, Greenwood J, Tanaka K, et al. Bleeding, transfusion, and mortality on extracorporeal life support: ECLS working group on thrombosis and hemostasis. Ann Thorac Surg. 2016;101:682-689.

77. Freund A, Jobs A, Lurz P, et al. Frequency and impact of bleeding on outcome in patients with cardiogenic shock. JACC Cardiovasc Interv. 2020;13:1182-1193.

78. Yang F, Hou D, Wang J, et al. Vascular complications in adult postcardiotomy cardiogenic shock patients receiving venoarterial extracorporeal membrane oxygenation. Ann Intensive Care. 2018;8:72.

79. Iannaccone M, Albani S, Giannini F, et al. Short term outcomes of Impella in cardiogenic shock: a review and meta-analysis of observational studies. Int J Cardiol. 2021;324:44-51.

80. Schrage B, Ibrahim K, Loehn T, et al. Impella support for acute myocardial infarction complicated by cardiogenic shock. Circulation. 2019;139:1249-1258.

81. Dalton HJ, Reeder R, Garcia-Filion P, et al. Factors associated with bleeding and thrombosis in children receiving extracorporeal membrane oxygenation. Am J Respir Crit Care Med. 2017;196:762–771.

82. Dalton HJ, Garcia-Filion P, Holubkov R, et al. Association of bleeding and thrombosis with outcome in extracorporeal life support. Pediatr Crit Care Med. 2015; 16:167–174.

83. Werho DK, Pasquali SK, Yu S, et al. Hemorrhagic complications in pediatric cardiac patients on extracorporeal membrane oxygenation: an analysis of the Extracorporeal Life Support Organization Registry. Pediatr Crit Care Med. 2015;16:276–288.

84. Thomas J, Kostousov V, Teruya J. Bleeding and thrombotic complications in the use of extracorporeal membrane oxygenation. Semin Thromb Hemost. 2018;44:20–29.

85. Yu JS, Barbaro RP, Granoski DA, et al. Prospective side by side comparison of outcomes and complications with a simple versus intensive anticoagulation monitoring strategy in pediatric extracorporeal life support patients. Pediatr Crit Care Med. 2017;18:1055–1062.

86. Barton R, Ignjatovic V, Monagle P. Anticoagulation during ECMO in neonatal and paediatric patients. Thromb Res. 2019;173:172–177.

87. Olson SR, Murphree CR, Zonies D, et al. Thrombosis and bleeding in extracorporeal membrane oxygenation (ECMO) without anticoagulation: a systematic review. ASAIO J. 2021;67:290-296.

88. Reed RC, Rutledge JC. Laboratory and clinical predictors of thrombosis and hemorrhage in 29 pediatric extracorporeal membrane oxygenation nonsurvivors. Pediatr Dev Pathol. 2010;13:385–392.

89. Rastan AJ, Lachmann N, Walther T, et al. Autopsy findings in patients on post-cardiotomy extracorporeal membrane oxygenation (ECMO). Int J Artif Organs. 2006; 29:1121-1131.

90. Bizzarro MJ, Conrad SA, Kaufman DA, et al. Extracorporeal life support organization task force on infections, extracorporeal membrane oxygenation: infections acquired during extracorporeal membrane oxygenation in neonates, children, and adults. Pediatr Crit Care Med. 2011;12:277-281.

91. MacLaren G, Schlapbach LJ, Aiken A. Nosocomial infections during extracorporeal membrane oxygenation in neonatal, pediatric, and adult patients: a comprehensive narrative review. Pediatr Crit Care Med. 2020;21:283-290.

92. Abrams D, Grasselli G, Schmidt M, et al. ECLS-associated infections in adults: what we know and what we don't yet know. Intensive Care Med. 2020;46:182-191.

# 7

## Circuit Malfunction and Crisis Management

*Phillip E. Mason, Marta Velia Antonini, Cara L. Agerstrand, M. Filip De Somer, Leen Vercaemst*

### Introduction

Patients supported with ECLS are at risk of a variety of complications that cause significant morbidity. Some complications, such as bleeding, venous thrombosis, and infection, are also common in non-ECLS patients, whereas other complications are particular to ECLS. For example, vessel perforation and lower extremity ischemia can occur because of cannulation problems (Chapter 4), while hemolysis and platelet dysfunction may result from the blood-polymer interaction (Chapter 6). Although modern ECLS circuits employing centrifugal pumps and polymethylpentene oxygenators provide a degree of safety not available in older equipment, circuit malfunctions do still occur. This chapter will focus on potentially catastrophic complications that require immediate intervention, including circuit air, pump failure, loss of circuit integrity, and inadvertent decannulation (Figure 7-1).

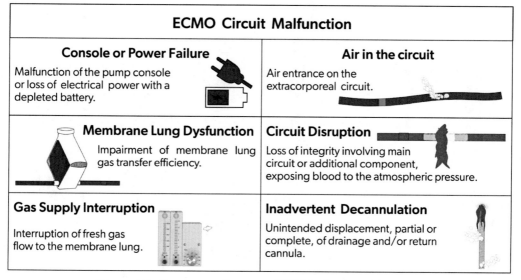

**Figure 7-1.** Summary of common ECMO circuit malfunctions.

**Prevention**

Rather than focus exclusively on managing circuit complications, ECLS program leaders should develop policies and procedures focused on preventing them in the first place.

A simplified circuit is generally considered a safer circuit. Any integration of access points into the ECLS circuit requires a considered risk:benefit assessment. For example, connecting continuous renal replacement therapy (CRRT) systems and intravenous infusion pumps directly to the ECLS circuit limits the need for additional vascular access and its associated complications, but also increases the risk of circuit malfunction. The additional connectors and access points required for these integrations are a nidus for clot formation and, when on the negative pressure side of the circuit, conduits for air entrainment into the circuit. External circuit monitoring devices provide valuable information and may allow early diagnosis of impending catastrophe. However, they are not without their own risk, again associated with the additional circuit access points they require. A careful assessment of risk and benefit should

be undertaken for each patient and program before integrating additional devices into the ECLS circuit, and the number of access points should be limited to the absolute minimum. Many successful programs avoid integration of additional devices completely, while others do so routinely.

Inadvertent decannulation is among the most uncommon but most dangerous ECLS related emergencies and it warrants exceptional efforts to avoid. Securing sutures should be placed at the time of cannulation and positioned to prevent both migration of the cannula and bowing of the cannula away from the skin between the skin entry site and the securing sutures. Sutures can break or loosen over time and should be inspected regularly and be replaced as needed. Additional adhesive devices can be used to secure tubing to the patient. Whatever the approach to cannula securement, it should be standardized. Depth of insertion and integrity of sutures and other securing devices should be noted and recorded at regular intervals (Figure 7-2).[1,2]

When central venous catheters lie in proximity to the drainage cannula there is a

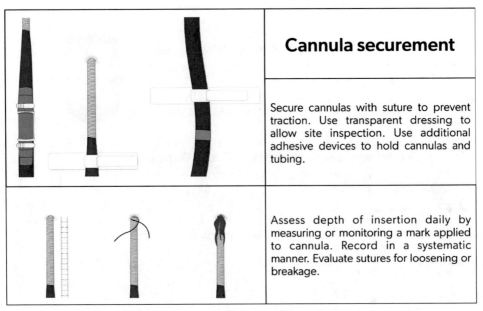

| | **Cannula securement** |
|---|---|
| | Secure cannulas with suture to prevent traction. Use transparent dressing to allow site inspection. Use additional adhesive devices to hold cannulas and tubing. |
| | Assess depth of insertion daily by measuring or monitoring a mark applied to cannula. Record in a systematic manner. Evaluate sutures for loosening or breakage. |

**Figure 7-2.** Cannula securement practices.

chance of air entrainment through the central line due to the negative drainage pressure. Personnel who administer medications or draw blood through central lines should take precautions to prevent exposing the line to air. The person responsible for managing the ECLS pump should be aware and in the immediate area when central lines are being placed.

Circuit thrombosis can cause sudden and catastrophic cessation of ECLS. Diligent attention to circuit monitoring may alert the team to impending failure and avoid the need for an emergent intervention.

Many centers use plastic ties ("zip ties") on all circuit connections to prevent accidental separation.

## Training

Despite the best efforts at prevention, circuit emergencies will occur. A team prepared by regular training on emergency procedures will provide an appropriate and timely response to mitigate the impact of such events.

Training on a primed circuit, termed "water drills," has long been the standard ECLS training activity. While water drills are an effective way of teaching the fundamentals of ECLS troubleshooting, high fidelity simulation is a more effective approach.[3-5] Elective circuit and component exchanges provide an opportunity for junior team members to practice a valuable emergency skill under supervision. The extent and frequency of training may vary depending on programmatic factors such as ECLS volume, program structure, and number of trained personnel. ELSO recommends training sessions of 4-8 hours occurring every six months as a starting point. At a minimum, each session should cover circuit ruptures and disruptions, component exchanges, air entrainment (venous/arterial), power or console failure, and inadvertent decannulation (see Chapter 54).[6]

## Preparation

A primed backup circuit should be readily available when managing a patient on ECLS. If patients are treated in multiple areas of the hospital, it is preferable to have a backup circuit for each geographic area, although equipment limitations may preclude this. Circuits primed with crystalloid in a sterile fashion can be safely maintained for 30 days or longer without loss of function or microbial contamination.[7-10] Each pump in use should have a back-up system (hand crank or second console) in the room and positioned for immediate use. A supply cart containing all supplies and equipment required to resolve circuit emergencies should be maintained on each unit where patients are treated on ECLS (Figure 7-3). Checklists and protocols covering all circuit related emergencies should be maintained and regularly reviewed with team members. A key component of these procedures is defining individual roles to avoid confusion during an emergency. The personnel responsible for troubleshooting the ECLS circuit should not simultaneously be responsible for patient management. Some circuit emergencies may result in massive and rapid blood loss. The historical practice of having blood products available in the room is excessive and unnecessary. However, all patients should have crossmatched blood available in the blood bank and the hospital should have a massive transfusion protocol that makes at least four units of uncrossmatched packed red blood cells available for immediate use.

## Specific Emergencies

### *Console or Power Failure*

A catastrophic malfunction of the ECLS pump console or loss of electrical power in combination with a depleted battery will cause an immediate loss of flow. Many ECLS systems employ a hand crank to operate the pump while some require a second console or motor as the backup system. When a console failure is suspected, a flow probe malfunction must first be excluded as this can mimic the appearance of console failure. As soon as it is determined that the pump is not functioning, the circuit should be clamped to prevent retrograde blood flow. After confirming the impeller is not spinning, the pump head should be removed and transferred to the hand crank or backup console. This will restore flow and support the patient until the problem can be fully resolved. Loss of power and console failure are the only indications to employ the hand crank. If the pump motor is still functioning, then transitioning to the hand crank will only cause delays and distract from other troubleshooting.

### *Circuit Air*

The impact of air entering the ECLS circuit can vary widely depending on the ECLS configuration, quantity of air, and location of air entry. A large amount of air may result in cessation of blood flow and have catastrophic consequences if it reaches the patient. Before discussing the response to air in the circuit, it should be noted that this complication is nearly always avoidable. Limiting access points on the negative pressure side of the circuit, exercising caution with central lines, and maintaining meticulous technique when operating stopcocks are all vital preventative strategies.

All modern ECLS systems have at least one integrated bubble detector which may be the first indicator of air in the ECLS circuit. Some

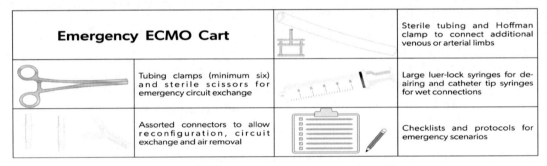

**Figure 7-3.** Basic content of an emergency ECMO cart.

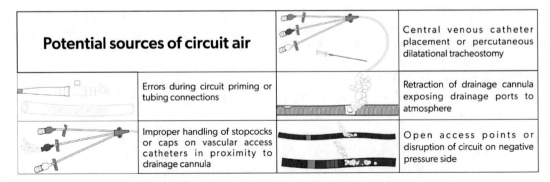

**Figure 7-4.** Potential sources of air in extracorporeal circuit.

ECLS systems allow the user to place the sensor in any location while in others it is fixed. In a user-configurable system, placing the bubble sensor before the membrane lung (ML) will alert the user earlier and may allow more time to intervene. Placing it after the ML will alert the user as the air is about to enter the patient but eliminates some alarms for inconsequential amounts of air that would remain in the ML and not pose an immediate risk to the patient. Most ECLS systems can be configured to stop the pump if air is detected or to alarm but provide no intervention. In some cases, such as centrally cannulated VA ECMO, even a small amount of air entering the patient can have adverse consequences and an automated pump stoppage in response to air detection may be warranted. While air entering a patient should never be considered acceptable, patients on VV ECMO may tolerate small amounts of air better than pump stoppage, which may cause rapid desaturation and cardiac arrest. A sensor placed before the ML and configured to stop the pump in response to bubble detection may create a dangerous situation in response to a small amount of air that would likely have been trapped in the ML. The decision to implement an automated intervention for air deserves thoughtful consideration and each program must weigh risks and benefits before settling on a standardized approach.

The operator should call for help as soon as air is detected within the circuit. The next immediate action is to determine if a significant amount of air will enter the patient, in which case the circuit should be clamped on the return limb as close to the patient as possible. In the absence of substantial air entry, it is generally preferable to maintain circuit flow while the problem is resolved as many patients will not tolerate complete cessation of blood flow. If blood flow is maintained, it is advisable to decrease flow to the lowest level tolerated to reduce air movement toward the patient. One person should be assigned to continuously monitor the arterial limb of the circuit and be prepared to clamp immediately if air moves toward the patient, while other team members troubleshoot the origin of the problem.

Determining the exact location of air in the circuit is critical. A circuit check should be conducted starting at one end of the circuit and proceeding methodically along its entire length with close inspection of each component. In addition to localizing the air, this will help diagnose its source, a critical step to ensure the problem does not recur (Figure 7-4). Air located between the ML and the patient is termed "arterial air" while air that lies before the ML is termed "venous air."

Once the location of the air is determined there are several techniques for removal. Air within the ML will usually rise to the highest point and may be aspirated through a pigtail or stopcock attached for this purpose. Some MLs have deairing ports that will allow air to exit passively. Users should be aware that these passive deairing ports often stop functioning after the membrane has been in use for an extended period. If air is visible in the tubing an attempt to move it to the ML using gravity is warranted, as the ML is the preferred location to remove air. Alternatively, a large quantity of air in the tubing can be isolated between two clamps and removed by cutting into the circuit, then reconnecting using a straight connector and wet connection technique. If air is located in the pump head, it may be necessary to remove the pump head from the motor assembly and position it so gravity will allow the air to exit and then be removed by one of the above techniques. Pump speed should be reduced to zero before removal from the motor, and the return limb of the circuit should always be clamped before proceeding.

In some cases of massive air entrainment, removal in a timely manner may be difficult or impossible. If the problem cannot be resolved rapidly and the patient is deteriorating, an immediate circuit change should be undertaken.

### Inadvertent Decannulation

Inadvertent decannulation occurs when a cannula is displaced from the vessel, either partially or completely. If the return cannula is involved there will be rapid exsanguination while displacement of the drainage cannula may result in air embolism or loss of flow as blood in the pump head is replaced by air. Either scenario will result in blood loss from the cannula site. The immediate reaction should be to call for help and immediately clamp the circuit near the patient. Life support interventions, such as increased ventilator support, blood product transfusion, vasopressor and inotropic agent administration, should be initiated immediately by a team distinct from the one troubleshooting the ECLS circuit. If the cannula is only partially removed and the patient is fully dependent on ECLS, reinsertion of the cannula may be attempted. This is a high-risk intervention that should only be undertaken by experienced personnel as a heroic effort to prevent death. If the cannula has been completely removed, pressure should be applied to the site to control bleeding.

### Loss of Circuit Integrity

Loss of circuit integrity refers to any breach that exposes a portion of the circuit to atmospheric pressure. Rupture of the main tubing is unusual with centrifugal pumps, although it is an ever-present risk with using roller pumps that can generate extremely high pressures and expose a section of tubing to continuous deformation by the pump head. However, there are ample ways in which circuit integrity can

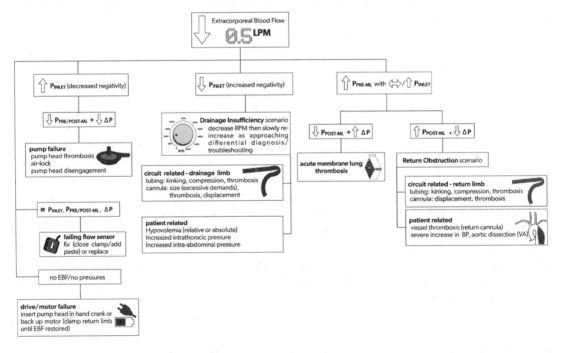

**Figure 7-5.** Algorithmic approach to a decrease in extracorporeal blood flow. LPM: liters per minute; $P_{INLET}$: drainage pressure, measure before centrifugal pump; $P_{PRE-ML}$: premembrane lung pressure, measured at membrane lung entrance; $P_{POST-ML}$: postmembrane lung pressure, measured at membrane lung exit, $\Delta P$: pressure drop between membrane lung entrance and exit, calculated as $\Delta P = P_{PRE-ML} - P_{POST-ML}$; EBF: extracorporeal blood flow; RPM: revolutions per minute; BP: blood pressure; VA: venoarterial configuration.

be compromised, even in centrifugal pump systems. Although unusual, any connection in the circuit tubing can become disconnected. Careless application of tubing clamps can cause a defect in the circuit tubing. Most commonly, circuit integrity is compromised when a stopcock or pigtail becomes disconnected or develops a defect. Typically, when a circuit breach occurs on the negative pressure side of the circuit, air entrainment is the primary risk, while blood loss is the primary concern on the positive pressure side.

A massive circuit breach will result in pump stoppage, although most events are less severe. Once identified, the location of the breach should be isolated between two clamps and the culprit component replaced. This will require a brief interruption of ECLS flow so arrangements must be made to support the patient during this time.

### Circuit Thrombosis or Occlusion

Sudden blood flow reduction with constant pump speed is often caused by decreased blood return to the pump, referred to as access insufficiency. Blood flow may also be reduced on VA ECMO if mean arterial pressure rises causing increased pump afterload. If these are excluded, the remaining causes of decreased pump flow relate to increased resistance to blood flow, usually from clot formation in the circuit, aspiration of clot from the venous system, or kinking of the ECLS circuit (Figure 7-5). When reduced flow is detected, circuit pressures should be noted if they are being monitored. Drainage pressures becoming more negative than baseline indicates obstruction between the drainage cannula and the pump inlet. If pre- and postmembrane pressures increase by similar amounts, obstruction between the ML and the return cannula should be suspected. Finally, if pre- and postmembrane differential increases, there is likely an obstruction to blood flow within the ML. After noting circuit pressures,

a methodical, end-to-end circuit check should be conducted to exclude kinks in the circuit, obvious clots in the oxygenator, or other easily correctable obstructions to blood flow. In the absence of a correctable cause, an emergency circuit exchange is usually indicated. Rarely, the problem will persist after circuit exchange if a clot has become lodged in the cannula. Aspirating the cannula with a large syringe may or may not resolve the problem.

Gradual accumulation of clot within the circuit leading to inefficient gas exchange, hematologic abnormalities or progressive resistance to blood flow is common and will be covered below.

### Gas Supply Interruption

Abrupt deterioration of an ECLS-supported patient requires an immediate assessment of the color differential between the pre- and post-ML blood. If both are dark red, it can be assumed that no gas exchange is occurring in the membrane. Since a decline in ML gas exchange efficiency usually occurs over a period of hours to days, abrupt changes suggest an interruption of fresh gas flow to the ML. A thorough assessment of the gas supply line starting at the ML and proceeding to the wall or tank will usually identify the problem. If the gas supply is from the wall, it should be moved to an alternative source to exclude a problem of the hospital gas supply. More often, the source will be a compressed oxygen cylinder that has been exhausted. One common scenario is a patient returning from an intrahospital transport using compressed gas where the operator fails to return the gas line to the wall source. The bottle will last a variable amount of time before causing gas supply failure and abrupt patient deterioration, a situation that can be avoided by using a checklist upon return from any venture outside the room.

## Pump Head Failure

The most common causes of ECLS flow cessation have been covered above: pump thrombosis, massive air entrainment, console, or power failure. Rarely, a stoppage can occur due to failure of the pump head itself or loss of the magnetic coupling between the pump head and drive motor.[11] These events may be accompanied by abnormal pump noise, sudden reduction in RPM, visible abnormalities, or vibrations. These scenarios usually represent a catastrophic failure that cannot be resolved. If pump head failure is suspected, help should be summoned immediately. If there is complete loss of flow, the circuit should be clamped. An emergency circuit exchange will usually be required to restore flow.

## Membrane Lung Dysfunction

Until now, the focus has been on abrupt or catastrophic ECLS related complications and malfunctions. However, gradual, more subtle derangements are far more common. Practitioners should monitor the ECLS circuit for obstruction to blood flow and impaired gas transfer from clot accumulation in the ML, and circuit related hematologic abnormalities (Figure 7-6). Monitoring resistance to blood flow detects obstruction due to clot formation in the ML or aspiration of a clot from the venous system into the circuit. If pre- and post-ML pressures are monitored, an increase in delta P at constant pump flow indicates increasing resistance. If pressures are not measured, increased resistance can be inferred when increased pump speed is required to maintain

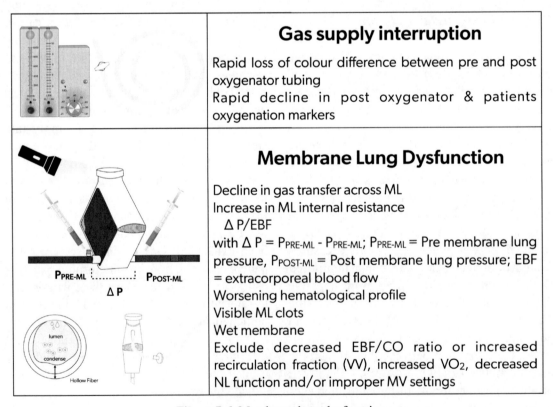

| | **Gas supply interruption** <br> Rapid loss of colour difference between pre and post oxygenator tubing <br> Rapid decline in post oxygenator & patients oxygenation markers |
|---|---|
| $P_{PRE-ML}$ ......... $P_{POST-ML}$ <br> $\Delta P$ <br> lumen <br> condense <br> Hollow Fiber | **Membrane Lung Dysfunction** <br> Decline in gas transfer across ML <br> Increase in ML internal resistance <br> $\Delta P/EBF$ <br> with $\Delta P = P_{PRE-ML} - P_{PRE-ML}$; $P_{PRE-ML}$ = Pre membrane lung pressure, $P_{POST-ML}$ = Post membrane lung pressure; EBF = extracorporeal blood flow <br> Worsening hematological profile <br> Visible ML clots <br> Wet membrane <br> Exclude decreased EBF/CO ratio or increased recirculation fraction (VV), increased $VO_2$, decreased NL function and/or improper MV settings |

**Figure 7-6.** Membrane lung dysfunction.

the same flow. Membrane lung efficiency is determined by calculating oxygen transfer. When oxygen transfer is below 150 ml/min, ML exchange should be considered.[12] Excessive clot formation in the ML can manifest as consumptive coagulopathy. Hemolysis may occur as a result clot formation in the ML or a clot in the pump head. The approach to monitoring for hematologic abnormalities will vary by program and may include measurements of plasma free hemoglobin, lactate dehydrogenase, D-dimer, and fibrinogen in addition to standard hematology and coagulation tests.[11]

Vigilant monitoring for ML dysfunction will detect abnormalities early and allow for elective replacement. The urgency of replacement should be based on the patient's condition and the rapidity of onset of ML dysfunction. Slowly progressive loss of gas transfer efficiency in a stable patient may warrant a period of observation rather than immediate replacement. Rapidly increasing resistance to blood flow may indicate impending circuit stoppage and should prompt immediate replacement. The decision to replace the entire circuit or only the ML is program dependent. However, it is often simpler to replace the entire circuit.

**Emergency Circuit Exchange**

Sudden circuit malfunctions with cessation of blood flow that cannot be resolved rapidly require an emergency circuit exchange (Figure 7-7). While a single skilled practitioner can accomplish a circuit change very rapidly, two equally skilled operators will accomplish

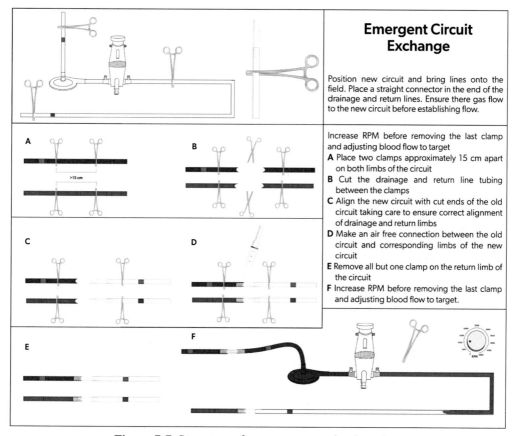

**Emergent Circuit Exchange**

Position new circuit and bring lines onto the field. Place a straight connector in the end of the drainage and return lines. Ensure there gas flow to the new circuit before establishing flow.

Increase RPM before removing the last clamp and adjusting blood flow to target
A Place two clamps approximately 15 cm apart on both limbs of the circuit
B Cut the drainage and return line tubing between the clamps
C Align the new circuit with cut ends of the old circuit taking care to ensure correct alignment of drainage and return limbs
D Make an air free connection between the old circuit and corresponding limbs of the new circuit
E Remove all but one clamp on the return limb of the circuit
F Increase RPM before removing the last clamp and adjusting blood flow to target.

**Figure 7-7.** Steps to perform emergency circuit exchange.

the same procedure in half the time. Emergency circuit changes call for two skilled personnel whenever possible, one for each limb of the circuit. Two additional personnel should be utilized to assist the primary operators with the wet connection. Necessary supplies should be preidentified and readily available. Sterile preparation should be rapid and can be limited to the portion of the ECLS tubing that will be cut to accomplish the change. The new circuit should be brought onto the field and straight connectors inserted into the cut ends of the tubing. Once the new circuit is laid out, a brief pause should occur to identify the drainage and return limbs of the existing and new circuits, and ensure the planned connections are correct. The existing circuit should be clamped in two locations per limb, about 15 cm apart and then cut between the clamps. The prepositioned ends of the new circuit are then connected, and flow resumed. A circuit check should follow and the previous ECLS settings established on the new circuit.

# References

1.  Bull T, Corley A, Lye I, Spooner AJ, et al. Cannula and circuit management in peripheral extracorporeal membrane oxygenation: An international survey of 45 countries. PLoS One. 2019;14(12):e0227248.

2.  Lucchini A, Elli S, Piovera D, et al. Management of vascular access for extracorporeal life support: A cohort study. J Vasc Access. 2021:11297298211056755.

3.  Zakhary BM, Kam LM, Kaufman BS, et al. The Utility of High-Fidelity Simulation for Training Critical Care Fellows in the Management of Extracorporeal Membrane Oxygenation Emergencies: A Randomized Controlled Trial. Crit Care Med. 2017;45(8):1367-1373.

4.  Brum R, Rajani R, Gelandt E, et al. Simulation training for extracorporeal membrane oxygenation. Ann Card Anaesth. 2015;18(2):185-190.

5.  Sakamoto S. Simulation-based training for handling extracorporeal membrane oxygenation emergencies. J Thorac Dis. 2017;9(10):3649-3651.

6.  ELSO Guidelines for Training and Continuing Education of ECMO Specialists. https://www.elso.org/ecmo-resources/elso-ecmo-guidelines.aspx. Accessed February 23, 2022.

7.  Deptula J, McGrath C, Preston T, et al. Sterility and performance of open and closed extracorporeal circuits after long-term dry-wet setups. Perfusion. 2021;36(2):130-137.

8.  Weinberg A, Miko B, Beck J, et al. Is it safe to leave an ECMO circuit primed? Perfusion. 2015;30(1):47-49.

9.  Tan VE, Evangelista AT, Carella DM, et al. Sterility Duration of Preprimed Extracorporeal Membrane Oxygenation Circuits. J Pediatr Pharmacol Ther. 2018;23(4):311-314.

10. Naso F, Gandaglia A, Balboni P, et al. Wet-priming extracorporeal membrane oxygenation device maintains sterility for up to 35 days of follow-up. Perfusion. 2013;28(3):208-213.

11. Lubnow M, Philipp A, Foltan M, et al. Technical complications during veno-venous extracorporeal membrane oxygenation and their relevance predicting a system-exchange--retrospective analysis of 265 cases. PLoS One. 2014;9(12):e112316.

12. Zakhary B, Vercaemst L, Mason P, et al. How I approach membrane lung dysfunction in patients receiving ECMO. Crit Care. 2020;24(1):671.

# 8

## Initiating Extracorporeal Life Support for Neonatal Respiratory Failure

*K. Taylor Wild, Rachel L. Chapman, Carl F. Davis, Natalie E. Rintoul, Claire Anne Westrope, Billie Lou Short*

### Introduction

Neonates with severe respiratory and/or cardiac failure refractory to maximal medical management, with a high likelihood of mortality and a potentially reversible etiology, are possible ECLS candidates. In the 2021 ELSO Registry report, most cases of neonatal ECLS had a primary respiratory diagnosis (74%), with the remainder having a primary cardiac cause.[1] Neonates continue to have the best survival across all groups and ECLS is now the standard of care in cases of oxygenation failure, severe hypoxic respiratory failure, and severe pulmonary hypertension with evidence of right ventricular dysfunction and/or left ventricular dysfunction refractory to less invasive management.[1] Management of these conditions generally involves mechanical ventilation and treatment of associated pulmonary hypertension with agents such as iNO.[2,3] Treatment commonly includes use of vasopressors and/or inotropes to support blood pressure, as well as consideration of stress hydrocortisone for pressor resistant hypotension. Preductal saturations between 88-95% are a good measure of oxygenation, while postductal $PaO_2$ levels are accepted down to 50 mmHg (6.7 kPa). Neonatal respiratory diseases that may require ECLS include: congenital diaphragmatic hernia (CDH), meconium aspiration syndrome (MAS), persistent pulmonary hypertension of the newborn (PPHN), hypoxic ischemic encephalopathy (HIE) accompanied by PPHN, neonatal pneumonia, sepsis with respiratory compromise, hyaline membrane disease accompanied by PPHN, and other congenital lung disorders.

### Neonatal Respiratory Diseases Predisposing to ECLS

In the 2021 ELSO Registry report, 4,036 infants required ECLS for a primary respiratory indication between 2016 and 2020, with 82% ECLS survival and 69% survival to discharge or transfer (Table 8-1).[1] Over the last 20 years, there has been a shift away from MAS to CDH as the most common diagnosis. CDH is covered in detail in Chapter 11. Congenital heart disease, myocarditis, cardiomyopathy, intractable arrhythmias with hemodynamic compromise, pulmonary hypertension, and univentricular circulation can all be indications for neonatal ECLS. Cardiac diagnoses are discussed in Chapter 17.

## Common Primary Etiologies for Neonatal ECLS

### *PPHN (Persistent Pulmonary Hypertension of the Newborn)*

PPHN occurs in 2/1000 live births when normal postnatal cardiopulmonary transition fails. There are 3 types: 1) vasoconstricted, but normally formed pulmonary vasculature (MAS, respiratory distress syndrome (RDS); 2) remodeled pulmonary vasculature with normal lung parenchyma (idiopathic PPHN, premature closure of the ductus, maternal medications ie, selective serotonin reuptake inhibitors, aspirin, indomethacin); and 3) hypoplastic pulmonary vasculature with hypoplastic lungs (CDH, oligohydramnios). Lethal forms of PPHN are found in several genetic disorders, including alveolar capillary dysplasia (ACD) and surfactant B deficiency, and should be considered in infants who cannot be weaned from ECLS.[4] Diagnosis may be made with genetic sequencing, lung biopsy, or at autopsy. In patients with a suspected form of lethal pulmonary hypertension, expedited exome sequencing should be considered.

### *Meconium Aspiration Syndrome (MAS)*

Meconium can reduce the antibacterial activity of amniotic fluid, increasing the risk of perinatal infection. Aspiration can also induce hypoxia secondary to airway obstruction, surfactant dysfunction, chemical pneumonitis, and pulmonary hypertension. VV ECMO is preferred.

### *Respiratory Distress Syndrome (RDS)/ Surfactant Deficiency*

While surfactant deficiency is more common in preterm infants due to insufficient alveolar production, full-term infants can also suffer from surfactant deficiency due to inactivation of surfactant from meconium or epithelial protein leak from lung injury. Although early surfactant replacement can reduce ECLS use, in some cases surfactant causes desaturation and worsening of ventilation, precipitating ECLS need.[5] Therefore, surfactant use in term infants is only recommended if $FiO_2$ is <50% or OI <25.

### *Neonatal Sepsis/Pneumonia*

Neonatal pneumonia and/or sepsis can be devastating conditions causing severe hypoxemic respiratory failure with or without shock and coagulopathy. Group B beta hemolytic streptococcus (GBS) and gram-negative organisms are the most common bacterial organisms.[6,7] Viral pneumonia is less common in neonates. The most common neonatal viruses are respiratory syncytial virus (RSV), herpes simplex virus (HSV), cytomegalovirus (CMV), and adenovirus. Infants infected with

| DIAGNOSIS | TOTAL RUN | % TOTAL RUNS | AVERAGE RUN TIME (Hrs) | SURVIVED | % SURVIVED |
|---|---|---|---|---|---|
| CDH | 1,301 | 32.6% | 325 | 730 | 56% |
| MAS | 611 | 15.3% | 151 | 559 | 91% |
| PPHN | 393 | 9.8% | 167 | 288 | 73% |
| RDS | 26 | 0.7% | 179 | 21 | 80% |
| Sepsis | 97 | 2.4% | 157 | 51 | 52% |
| Pneumonia | 17 | 0.4% | 387 | 7 | 41% |
| Air Leak Syndrome | 3 | 0.1% | 199 | 2 | 66% |
| Other | 1,543 | 38.7% | 184 | 1,120 | 72% |

**Table 8-1**. Neonatal respiratory ECLS by diagnosis from 2016-2020.[1]

HSV and adenovirus have a significantly lower survival rate when compared to infants with other viruses.[8,9] While ECLS has been used for pertussis infections in this age group, outcomes are generally poor.[10]

### *PPHN Associated with Hypoxic Ischemic Encephalopathy (HIE)*

Infants with HIE are at risk for abnormal pulmonary vasorelaxation and pulmonary hypertension and 4-9% will require ECLS.[11,12] Up to 30% of infants with HIE develop PPHN that may be due to in-utero and perinatal hypoxia and acidosis, ventricular dysfunction, and lung pathology such as MAS and pulmonary hemorrhage.[11,12] Despite improved neurologic outcomes with therapeutic hypothermia, morbidity and mortality from HIE remain high and the long-term effects are unclear.[13]

### Less Common Primary Etiologies for Neonatal ECLS

### *Tracheal Anomalies and Extrinsic Tracheobronchial Compression*

Infants with severe congenital tracheal anomalies such as tracheal stenosis and atresia, complete tracheal rings, and cartilaginous sleeve trachea are at risk for significant morbidity and mortality. Pulmonary artery anomalies and, occasionally, vascular stenting may also compress the tracheobronchial tree. While recent surgical advances have improved outcomes in these infants, many will not survive beyond the first few hours of life without aggressive cardiopulmonary support and/or emergent airway surgery. Perioperative ECLS can serve as a bridge to definitive tracheal reconstruction.[14-16]

### *Trisomy 21*

Neonates with trisomy 21 (T21) deserve special mention, as they are overrepresented in cases of severe pulmonary hypertension and the need for ECLS. 2.3% of neonates with T21 admitted to children's hospitals receive ECLS, and this is especially common in those with concomitant cardiac diagnoses.[17]

### *Gastrointestinal Diagnoses*

Patients with omphalocele and gastroschisis (less commonly) can develop PPHN related to lung hypoplasia and/or an aspiration pneumonitis/sepsis in the infants with gastroschsis.[18]

### *Congenital Anomalies of the Kidney and Urinary Tract*

Urinary obstruction (eg, posterior urethral valves) and renal dysplasia (eg, polycystic kidney disease, multicystic dysplastic kidneys) may be associated with oligohydramnios leading to pulmonary hypoplasia and pulmonary hypertension. In this population, ECLS is sometimes indicated to manage the associated pulmonary hypertension, not the pulmonary hypoplasia. While survival is overall low at 42%, survival is significantly better for obstructive urogenital lesions at 71% compared to primary intrinsic lesions at 16.6% (p=0.004).[19]

### *ECPR*

ECPR is the initiation of ECLS, including cannula placement, during ongoing CPR, so that the ECLS flow itself becomes part of the resuscitation. By necessity, patients are placed on V-A ECMO. This occurs more commonly in cardiac and pediatric patients.

## EXIT to ECLS

EXIT (ex-utero intrapartum treatment) may be performed for prenatally diagnosed cases of possible upper or main airway compression (neck or thoracic masses) with immediate placement of cannula and initiation of ECLS support before the cord is clamped and the infant is separated from placental bypass. The conceptual advantage is avoidance of clinical instability, hypoxia, and acidosis that occur and may worsen pulmonary hypertension. This has not been shown to increase survival in infants with CDH.[20,21]

### Pulmonary Lymphangiectasia

Congenital pulmonary lymphangiectasia is a rare developmental disorder of the lung characterized by subpleural, interlobar, perivascular, and peribronchial lymphatic dilatation. While mortality is very high, ECLS can sometimes serve as a bridge to diagnosis in the neonatal period.[22]

## Indications and Contraindications for ECLS in Neonates with Respiratory Failure

### Indications

In the early clinical trials that proved the safety and efficacy of ECLS, criteria included extreme abnormalities in Oxygenation Index (OI), alveolar-arterial oxygen difference (A-aDO), and hypoxemia.[23,24] OI can be determined using the calculation: OI = Mean Airway Pressure x $FiO_2$ x 100 divided by Postductal $PaO_2$. Better understanding of the role of pulmonary hypertension in these conditions and medical advances such as surfactant, iNO, and high frequency ventilation, have made historic treatments such as hyperventilation, hyperoxia, and alkalinization obsolete. These changes in practice, and a general acceptance that ventilation techniques should be lung protective, make the severity-of-illness measures difficult to translate from one era to another. Furthermore, predictors of mortality and morbidity can be institution dependent. For these reasons, universal acceptance of any one criterion for ECLS initiation is limited. With improved technology and a better understanding of its risks and benefits, the rationale to cannulate is based on decreasing morbidity as well as preventing death. Tools that predict morbidity are lacking and therefore many simply use the failure to respond to other therapies as the indication for ECLS. Beyond this, the most commonly used quantifier of disease severity for neonatal hypoxic respiratory failure remains the OI. The initial trials used an OI >40 as an enrollment criterion. At present, many centers still use an OI range of 40-45 as the primary indication for ECLS, though a figure of >25 may be more realistic in the present era of lung protective ventilation and iNO. Generally accepted indications for ECLS therapy include[25]:

1. Inadequate tissue oxygen delivery despite maximal therapy (eg, rising lactate, worsening metabolic acidosis, signs of end organ dysfunction)
2. Severe hypoxic respiratory failure with acute decompensation ($PaO_2$ <40 mmHg; 5.3 kPa)
3. Oxygenation Index with sustained elevation and no improvement
4. Severe pulmonary hypertension with evidence of right and/or left ventricular dysfunction.

Therapeutic options including surfactant and iNO have decreased ECLS use in neonates with respiratory failure.[1,26,27] Nonetheless, more than 4,000 neonates received ECLS between 2016-2020 because of failure of other therapies.[1] While infants should have the opportunity to respond to less invasive therapies, delaying ECLS cannulation may lead to worse outcomes.

The UK Collaborative ECMO trial was a large randomized controlled trial that demonstrated reduced morbidity and mortality in infants who received ECLS compared to conventional therapy.[28,29] Schumacher et al. documented that infants who received ECLS when the OI was >25 but <40 had shorter and less costly hospital stays with a trend toward improved outcomes. This study contained a small number of patients but indicates that earlier cannulation may reduce the morbidity associated with treatments for respiratory failure.[30] Radhakrishnan et al. compared the morbidity of patients with MAS to that in patients with all other respiratory conditions treated with ECLS. Overall, MAS patients had a significantly higher survival rate and significantly fewer complications per patient in each category compared to other patients, supporting the consideration of unique, relaxed ECLS entry criteria for infants with MAS.[31] Grist el al. reviewed neonatal patients to determine whether cannulation timing correlated to increased mortality. Elevated $CO_2$ gradient, anion gap, and Viability Index ($AGc+p(v-a)$ $CO_2$) were associated with higher mortality ($p<0.05$). The authors concluded that starting ECLS too late may cause reperfusion injury that reduces survival.[32] Thus, it is recommended that any neonate with respiratory failure and an OI of >25 be cared for in an ECLS center where timely initiation can occur if necessary. When oxygenation does not improve consistently by 6 hours of mechanical ventilation, infants should be referred to an ECLS center, as a high percentage will continue to worsen and require ECLS.[33,34] Regional ECLS centers should work with their referral centers to establish standard transfer protocols to prevent delays.

### Contraindications

Certain patients with complicating pathologies should not be considered for ECLS, regardless of the degree of respiratory failure. Even with technical progress, ECLS remains a high risk and resource intense intervention, thus it should only be utilized in patients with a high likelihood of survival. Pre-ECLS review of the history and physical examination are critical prior to cannulation to determine if there are contraindications for ECLS. Specific concerns regarding candidacy for ECLS should be discussed with the relevant medical subspecialists prior to cannulation, addressing the risks (including possible resource limitations) versus the potential benefits. As ECLS technology improves and medical therapies advance, candidacy becomes fluid and more neonates should be considered candidates. Some historical absolute contraindications are now considered relative contraindications. Generally accepted contraindications for neonatal respiratory ECLS are shown in Table 8-2.

| CONTRAINDICATIONS | RELATIVE CONTRAINDICATIONS |
|---|---|
| Lethal chromosomal disorder (includes trisomy 13, 18, but not 21) or other lethal anomaly | Irreversible organ damage (unless considered for organ transplant) |
| Severe brain damage | <2 kg |
| Uncontrollable bleeding | <34 weeks post-menstrual age |
| Significant intraventricular hemorrhage (generally >Grade III) | |
| Vessel size too small for cannulation | |

**Table 8-2.** Contraindications to Neonatal ECLS.

### Weight <2 kg and/or Gestational Age <34 weeks

For the past few decades, weight <2 kilograms (kg) and/or gestational age (GA) <34 weeks have been relative contraindications to ECLS. Intracranial hemorrhage (ICH) is a known complication of both ECLS and prematurity that may be related to physiologic instability of the germinal matrix during the first few days of life. The risk of ICH is thought to be higher for preterm neonates requiring ECLS given the need for continuous anticoagulation.[35] While weight <2 kilograms and <34 weeks postmenstrual were historically considered contraindications, newer studies have shown that although the rates of survival and cerebral infarction are worse at 29-33 weeks gestational age, the differences are modest and clinically acceptable.[35-40]

Early studies found an unacceptable risk of mortality and morbidities such as ICH among preterm and low birthweight (BW) neonates, leading to widely accepted ECLS inclusion criteria of gestational age GA ≥34 weeks and BW >2 kg.[35-37] However, modern practice has evolved since these early landmark studies.

In 2005, Chapman et al. performed a cross-sectional study that found that the lowest birth weight and gestational age at which respondents would consider placing a neonate on ECLS were frequently below recommended thresholds. Wide variability was also found in respondents' willingness to place neonates on ECLS in the presence of conditions such as ICH and HIE.[41] This variability is likely explained by more experience with ECLS, and the increasing complexity of the patient population.

While more recent studies have suggested decreased but still acceptable survival for neonates <34 weeks GA and BW <2 kg, these neonates are still at higher risk of mortality and morbidity compared to full-term infants.[35-37] Using the ELSO Registry from 1976 to 2008, Church et al. studied 752 neonates at 29-34 weeks GA. When compared to a survival rate of 58% for neonates born at 34 weeks GA, survival was statistically lower at 48% for neonates born between 29-33 weeks GA (p=0.05). While there was not a significant difference in ICH (17% vs. 21%, respectively, p=0.195), there was a significant difference in the incidence of cerebral infarction between groups (16% for 34 weeks vs. 22% for 29-33 weeks; p=0.03). Although survival was lower in the 29-33 weeks GA group, the difference was relatively modest, leading these authors to conclude that GA <34 weeks may not be an absolute contraindication to ECLS.[37] However, one important limitation of this study is that the postnatal age was not documented. It is possible that some of the neonates born at 29-33 weeks GA may have been several days to months old when cannulated onto ECLS. That being said, in a case series of three neonates born preterm with CDH and BW <2 kg from 2010 to 2015, all 3 survived with only mild developmental delay. The three patients were 31 4/7 weeks GA and 1.8 kg, 31 5/7 weeks GA and 1.5 kg, and 36 3/7 weeks GA and 1.64 kg.[38] These non-traditional ECLS candidates illustrate that ECLS can be performed with success and without complications in selected patients <34 weeks GA and <2 kg BW.

In 2011, Ramachandrappa et al. divided 21,218 neonates in the ELSO Registry into three groups: late preterm (34 0/7 to 36 6/7), early term (37 0/7 to 38 6/7), and full term (39 0/7 to 42 6/7). Survival was lowest in the late preterm neonates at 74% compared to 82% in the early term neonates, and 88.8% in the full-term neonates.[39] In 2004, Rozmiarek et al. divided all neonates (14,305) less than 30 days in the ELSO Registry from 1991 to 2002 into 2 groups, neonates with BW >2 kg (13,642) and neonates with BW ≤2 kg (663). They found a survival rate of 53% in the low BW neonates compared to 77% in the higher BW neonates (p<.0001) with no significant difference year to year over the course of the study. Using a regression analysis to determine the lowest BW at which a 40% survival probability could be achieved, they found a threshold weight of 1.6 kg.[40]

Another important group where ECLS may be considered is former preterm infants with bronchopulmonary dysplasia +/- pulmonary hypertension who develop respiratory failure, most often secondary to a viral respiratory infection. While there are limited data in this population, survival appears to be comparable to most other ECLS populations. However, there are high rates of severe pulmonary and neurodevelopmental sequelae among this already vulnerable population.[42-44] These more recent publications reporting improved survival and decreased ICH in infants at 32-34 weeks GA suggest high-volume centers should consider ECLS on a case-by-case basis. Careful neurodevelopmental followup will be essential to better inform practices changes on this select population. In the end, each patient must be evaluated individually and the decision based solely on what is in the patient's best interest.

Effective treatment of respiratory failure in preterm infants remains an unsolved problem. Despite significant advances, the increased rates of morbidity and mortality in the more preterm population suggests that alterations in traditional ECLS may still be necessary before acceptance of ECLS for patients <34 weeks gestation is widespread. Evolving technology such as an artificial placenta or pumpless ECLS without anticoagulation may facilitate continuing reevaluation of the boundaries of neonatal ECLS.[45,46]

### Cannula Size

Vessel size is the greatest limiting factor in the use of venovenous (V-V) ECMO in preterm neonates since the smallest V-V double lumen cannula currently available is 13 Fr (4.3 mm external diameter). In V-A ECMO, the carotid artery must be able to accommodate an 8 Fr (2.67 mm external diameter) arterial cannula to achieve adequate flow. While a 6 Fr cannula exists, it is not recommended due to the increased risk of hemolysis. Therefore, one must carefully consider the risks of VA ECMO, especially in this high-risk patient population (see Chapter 4).

### Intracranial Hemorrhage

Grade III or IV ICH, which can be detected by head ultrasound, is generally associated with an increased risk of poor neurodevelopmental outcomes.[47] Additional expansion of the hemorrhage, further compromising neurologic prognosis, is likely with the anticoagulation required for ECLS. Thus, all infants who are being considered for ECLS should have a pre-ECLS head ultrasound and infants with Grade III or IV ICH should not be offered ECLS. Infants with pre-ECLS grade I or II ICH have been successfully managed on ECLS without extension of hemorrhage. Even in this less severe situation, diligent monitoring of hemodynamics, clotting factors, platelets, bleeding times, anticoagulation, and imaging is required.

### Irreversible Organ Damage

Although infants with irreversible organ damage should not be offered ECLS unless they are eligible for transplantation, determination of irreversibility of organ function can be difficult. With advances in therapeutic capabilities, determining irreversible organ damage and eligibility for transplantation requires appropriate testing and input from organ subspecialists. In infants with HIE, it can be challenging to determine the degree of neurologic insult. Despite improved outcomes with therapeutic hypothermia, morbidity and mortality from HIE remain high. Centers must decide whether the degree of perinatal injury is suggestive of a poor neurologic outcome that would otherwise preclude ECLS. Given the acute illness, pre-ECLS neurologic evaluation can be especially challenging. With the exception of grade III or IV ICH, no clear set of measures defines how severe neurologic injury must be in order to exclude an infant from ECLS. In cases where there is strong evidence of hypoxic injury on brain imaging, abnormal EEG findings, significant metabolic acidosis, and low Apgar scores, it may be better to withhold ECLS.

Often pre-ECLS evaluations to determine irreversibility of organ damage are not always available or adequately predictive. In this setting, ECLS support can be offered expectantly. In these circumstances, reevaluation and discussions with consultants and parents should occur shortly after cannulation. If ECLS support is subsequently shown not to be in the infant's best interest, it should be discontinued.

### Chromosome Abnormalities

Patients with physical findings suggestive of trisomy 13 or trisomy 18 should have a pre-ECLS dysmorphology evaluation and ECLS is generally not offered or recommended (see Chapter 11). However, it has been rarely utilized in specific circumstances such as postcardiac surgery and based on individual phenotype.[48]

Guidance is less clear regarding other genetic syndromes. When possible, infants should have a genetic evaluation and testing prior to ECLS cannulation as donor blood in the ECLS prime can complicate testing after cannulation. While genetic results may not be available prior to initiating ECLS, rapid comprehensive genetic testing with either exome or genome sequencing can often provide results within a week and may guide future management. The increased availability of genetic testing may also present unique ethical challenges in cases of uncertain genetic results or syndromes with variable phenotypes. ECLS is no longer controversial in infants with trisomy 21.

### Pre-ECLS Ventilation Days

Evaluation for the appropriateness of ECLS should consider pre-ECLS ventilation days. While the number of days of ventilation required prior to ECLS has been shown to significantly decrease survival, Zabrocki et al. reviewed over 3,000 pediatric ECLS patients from 1993-2007 and found no association between pre-ECLS ventilation under 14 days and survival.[49] However, there is no doubt that long-term respiratory morbidity is likely to be reduced with earlier ECLS deployment to protect the lungs.

### ECLS Cannulation for Neonates with Respiratory Failure

#### Setup

The environment leading up to and during ECLS cannulation is usually stressful. Safe and efficient cannulation requires a number of teams (neonatal medical and nursing, surgical, operating room, perfusion, echocardiography, blood bank, laboratory) to function as one. Immediately prior to cannulation, the team should discuss the patient details and plan for cannulation to ensure that all personnel and equipment are present (or readily available) and that everyone understands their role and the sequence of events planned for successful cannulation. Starting ECLS flow rates (sweep gas and blood), blood products, resuscitation drugs, and the proposed loading dose of heparin are confirmed. Likely problems are anticipated and vocalized so all team members can prepare. Typical circuit design results in the need for blood prime to keep the hemoglobin stable, but circuit modifications can be considered to reduce this need. Each institution should have appropriate checklists to cover all these issues.

## Cannulation Strategy

There is ongoing debate in the ECLS community about the merits of VA vs. VV ECMO in the neonatal population. Renal complications and inotrope use are common in VV, whereas neurologic complications, including seizures and central nervous system infarcts, occur more frequently in VA.[50]

In neonates, V-V is almost always via a 13 Fr double lumen cannula (dl). Although (dl) V-V ECMO does not provide direct cardiac support, the delivery of well oxygenated blood to the right atrium invariably improves cardiac output, even in unstable neonates requiring high dose inotropic support.[51-53] In cases where (dl)V-V support proves inadequate, it can be converted to V-A. (dl)V-V ECMO is generally preferred for respiratory support because it avoids using a major artery, avoids potential systemic embolism, and provides oxygenated blood directly to the pulmonary circulation.

In contrast, VA ECMO provides both cardiac and respiratory support via an arterial cannula and a venous cannula. VA ECMO is often indicated in infants with low cardiac output as a result of sepsis, a cardiac anomaly, or in many infants with CDH (see Chapters 11 and 17). Arterial cannulas are sized down to 8 Fr, thus VA ECMO is also often required for smaller infants (<2.5 kg) where the right internal jugular vein is unlikely to accommodate the smallest double lumen venous cannula.

## Choice of Cannula and Vessel

Prior to cannulation, it is advisable to have a selection of cannulas immediately available, so alternative sizes can be chosen once the vessels have been visualized. Based on weight and required flow, each center should have a chart that helps with cannula selection based on known cannula pressure/flow characteristics. Cannulation is discussed in detail in Chapter 4.

## Pump Selection

There is variation amongst centers regarding the use of roller vs. centrifugal pumps for neonates. Pump selection is described in more detail in Chapter 3.

# References

1. Extracorporeal Life Support Organization (ELSO) Registry Report. International Summary. October, 2021.
2. Steinhorn RH. Neonatal pulmonary hypertension. Pediatr Crit Care Med. 2010 March; 11(2 Suppl): S79–S84.
3. The Neonatal Inhaled Nitric Oxide Study Group. Inhaled nitric oxide in full-term and nearly full-term infants with hypoxic respiratory failure. N Engl J Med. 1997; 336:597-604.
4. Tibballs J, Chow CW. Incidence of alveolar capillary dysplasia in severe idiopathic persistent pulmonary hypertension of the newborn. J. Paediatr. Child Health. 2002; 38:397–400.
5. Lotze A, Whitsett JA, Kammerman LA, et al. Surfactant protein A concentrations in tracheal aspirate fluid from infants requiring extracorporeal membrane oxygenation. Journal of Pediatrics. 1990; 116:435-440.
6. Mukhopadhyay S, Puopolo KM, Neonatal Early-Onset Sepsis: Epidemiology and Risk Assessment. NeoReviews. 2015; 16 (4): 221e-228.
7. Webber SI, Wilkinson AR, Lindsell D, et al. Neonatal pneumonia; Arch Dis Child. 1990 Feb;65(2):207-11.
8. Meyer TA, Warner BW. Extracorporeal life support for the treatment of viral pneumonia: collective experience from the ELSO registry. Extracorporeal Life Support Organization. J Pediatr Surg. 1997;32(2):232-236.
9. Ronchi A, Doern C, Brock E, et al. Neonatal adenoviral infection: a seventeen year experience and review of the literature. The Journal of Pediatrics. 2014;164(3):529-535.e4.
10. Pooboni S, Roberts N, Westrope C, et al. Extracorporeal life support in pertussis. Pediatr Pulmonol. 2003;36(4):310-315.
11. Agarwal P, Altinok D, Desai J, et al. In-hospital outcomes of neonates with hypoxic-ischemic encephalopathy receiving extracorporeal membrane oxygenation. J Perinatol. 2019;39(5):661–665.
12. Shankaran S, Pappas A, Laptook AR, et al. Outcomes of safety and effectiveness in a multicenter randomized, controlled trial of whole-body hypothermia for neonatal hypoxic-ischemic encephalopathy. Pediatrics. 2008;122:e791–8.
13. Field D. Neonatal ECMO study of temperature (Nest): a randomized controlled trial. Pediatrics. 2013;132(5):e1247-e1256.
14. Kunisaki SM, Fauza DO, Craig N, et al. Extracorporeal membrane oxygenation as a bridge to definitive tracheal reconstruction in neonates. Journal of Pediatric Surgery. 2008;43(5):800-804.
15. Alkhasov A, Razumovsky A, Gusev A, et al. Surgical treatment of patients with full tracheal rings: our experience. Journal of Laparoendoscopic & Advanced Surgical Techniques. Published online November 29, 2021:lap.2021.0337.
16. McMahon CJ, Ayoubi K, Mehanna R, et al. Outcome of congenital tracheal stenosis in children over two decades in a national cardiothoracic surgical unit. Cardiol Young. 2020;30(1):34-38.
17. Southgate WM, Annibale DJ, Hulsey TC, et al. International experience with trisomy 21 infants placed on extracorporeal membrane oxygenation. Pediatrics. 2001;107(3):549–52.
18. Baerg JE, Thirumoorthi A, Hopper AO, et al. The use of ECMO for gastroschisis and omphalocele: Two decades of experience. J Pediatr Surg. 2017 Jun;52(6):984-988.
19. Bagdure D, Torres N, Walker L, et al. Extracorporeal membrane oxygenation for neonates with congenital renal and urological anomalies and pulmonary hypoplasia: a case report and review of the extracorporeal life support organization registry. J Pediatr Intensive Care. 2017;06(03):188-193.
20. Kunisaki SM, Barnewolt CE, Estroff JA, et al. Ex utero intrapartum treatment with extracorporeal membrane oxygenation for severe congenital diaphragmatic hernia. J Pediatr Surg. 2007;42(1):98-104.
21. Stoffan AP, Wilson JM, Jennings RW, et al. Does the ex utero intrapartum treatment to extracorporeal membrane oxygenation procedure change outcomes for high-risk patients with congenital diaphragmatic hernia? Journal of Pediatric Surgery. 2012;47(6):1053-1057.
22. Mettauer N, Agrawal S, Pierce C, et al. Outcome of children with pulmonary lymphangiectasis: Pulmonary Lymphangiectasis. Pediatr Pulmonol. 2009;44(4):351-357.
23. Short BL, Miller MK, Anderson KD. Extracorporeal membrane oxygenation in the management of respiratory failure in the newborn. Clin Perinatol. 1987;14(3):737- 748.
24. Bartlett RH, Andrews AF, Toomasian JM, et al. Extracorporeal membrane oxygenation (ECMO) in neonatal respiratory failure: forty five cases. Surgery. 1982;92(2):425- 433.
25. Wild KT, Rintoul N, Kattan J, et al. Extracorporeal Life Support Organization (ELSO): Guidelines for Neonatal Respiratory Failure. ASAIO J. 2020;66(5):463-470.
26. Hintz SR, Suttner DM, et al. Decreased use of neonatal extracorporeal membrane oxygenation (ECMO): how new treatment modalities have affected ECMO utilization Pediatrics. 2000;106(6):1339-1343.
27. Rehder KJ, Turner DA, Bonadonna D, et al. Technological advances in extracorporeal membrane

oxygenation for respiratory failure. Expert Rev Respir Med. 2012;6(4):377-84.

28. McNally H, Bennett CC, Elbourne D, et al, for the UK Collaborative ECMO Trial Group. United kingdom collaborative randomized trial of neonatal extracorporeal membrane oxygenation: follow-up to age 7 years. Pediatrics. 2006;117(5):e845-e854.

29. Macrae DJ, Field DJ. Our study 20 years on: UK collaborative randomised trial of neonatal extracorporeal membrane oxygenation. Intensive Care Med. 2016;42(5):841-843.

30. Schumacher RE. Extracorporeal membrane oxygenation. Will this therapy continue to be as efficacious in the future? Pediatr Clin N Amer. 1993;40(5):1005-1022.

31. Radhakrishnan RS, Lally PA, Lally KP, et al. ECMO for meconium aspiration syndrome: support for relaxed entry criteria. ASAIO J. 2007;53(4):489-491.

32. Grist G, Whittaker C, Merrigan K, et al. Defining the late implementation of extracorporeal membrane oxygenation (ECMO) by identifying increased risk using specific physiologic cut-points in neonatal and pediatric respiratory patients. J Extra Corpor Technol. 2008; 41(4):213-219.

33. Paranka MS, Clark RH, Yoder BA, et al. Predictors of failure of high-frequency oscillatory ventilation in term infants with severe respiratory failure. Pediatr. 1995; 95(3):400-404.

34. Singh BS, Clark RH, Powers RJ, et al. Meconium aspiration syndrome remains a significant problem in the NICU: outcomes and treatment patterns in term neonates admitted for intensive care during a ten-year period. J Perinatol. 2009; 29(7):497-503.

35. Revenis ME, Glass P, Short BL: Mortality and morbidity rates among lower birth weight infants (2000 to 2500 grams) treated with extracorporeal membrane oxygenation. J Pediatr 1992, 121(3):452–458.

36. Cilley RE, Zwischenberger JB, Andrews AF, et al. Intracranial hemorrhage during extracorporeal membrane oxygenation in neonates. Pediatrics. 1986;78(4):699-704.

37. Chapman RL, Perterec SM, Bizzarro MJ, et al. Patient selection for neonatal extracorporeal membrane oxygenation: beyond severity of illness. J Perinatol. 2009;29(9):606-611.

38. Cuevas Guamán M, Akinkuotu AC, et al. Extracorporeal membrane oxygenation in premature infants with congenital diaphragmatic hernia. ASAIO Journal 2018;64(5):e126–9.

39. Ramachandrappa A, Rosenberg ES, Wagoner S, Jain L. Morbidity and mortality in late preterm infants with severe hypoxic respiratory failure on extra-corporeal membrane oxygenation. J Pediatr. 2011;159(2):192-8.e3.

40. Rozmiarek AJ, Qureshi FG, Cassidy L, et al. How low can you go? Effectiveness and safety of extracorporeal membrane oxygenation in low-birth-weight neonates. J Pediatr Surg. 2004;39(6):845-7.

41. Church JT, Kim AC, Erickson KM, et al. Pushing the boundaries of ECLS: Outcomes in <34 week EGA neonates. J Pediatr Surg. 2017;52(11):1810–1815.

42. Hibbs A, Evans JR, Gerdes M, et al. Outcome of infants with bronchopulmonary dysplasia who receive extracorporeal membrane oxygenation therapy. Journal of Pediatric Surgery. 2001;36(10):1479-1484.

43. Pena Hernandez A, Carr NR, McCurnin D, et al. Extracorporeal life support in pediatric patients with bronchopulmonary dysplasia and associated pulmonary hypertension. ASAIO Journal. 2020;66(9):1063-1067.

44. Kornhauser MS, Baumgart S, Desai SA, et al. Adverse neurodevelopmental outcome after extracorporeal membrane oxygenation among neonates with bronchopulmonary dysplasia. J Pediatr. 1998;132(2):307-311.

45. Partridge EA, Davey MG, Hornick MA, et al. An EXTrauterine environment for neonatal development: EXTENDING fetal physiology beyond the womb. Semin Fetal Neonatal Med. 2017;22(6):404-409.

46. Church JT, Coughlin MA, Perkins EM, et al. The artificial placenta: Continued lung development during extracorporeal support in a preterm lamb model. J Pediatr Surg. 2018;53(10):1896-1903.

47. Bolisetty A, Dhawan A, Abdel-Latif M, et al; New South Wales and Australian Capital Territory Neonatal Intensive Care Units' Data Collection. Intraventricular hemorrhage and neurodevelopmental outcomes in extreme preterm infants. Pediatrics. 2014;133(1):55-62. Pediatrics. 2019;144(3):e20192079.

48. Cleary JP, Janvier A, Farlow B, et al. Cardiac interventions for patients with trisomy 13 and trisomy 18: experience, ethical issues, communication, and the case for individualized family-centered care. World J Pediatr Congenit Heart Surg. 2022;13(1):72-76.

49. Zabrocki LA, Brogan TV, Statler KD, et al. Extracorporeal Membrane Oxygenation for Pediatric Respiratory Failure: Predictors of Mortality. Crit Care Med. 2011;39:364-370.

50. Rais-Bahrami K, Van Meurs K. Venoarterial versus venovenous ECMO for neonatal respiratory failure. Semin Perinatol. 2014 Mar;38(2):71-77.

51. Roberts N, Westrope C, Pooboni SK et al. Venovenous extracorporeal membrane oxygenation for respiratory failure in inotrope dependent neonates. ASAIO Journal 2003;49(5):558-571.

52. Bamat NA, Tharakan SJ, Connelly JT, et al. Venoarterial extracorporeal life support for neonatal respiratory failure: indications and impact on mortality. ASAIO Journal. 2017;63(4):490-495.

53. Sewell EK, Piazza AJ, Davis J, et al. Inotrope needs in neonates requiring extracorporeal membrane oxygenation for respiratory failure. J Pediatr. 2019;214:128-133.

# 9

## Management of Neonatal Patients with Respiratory Failure

*Janene H. Fuerch, Andrea Moscatelli, Gail Faulkner, Mark T. Ogino, Krisa Van Meurs*

### Introduction

ECLS for neonatal respiratory failure is utilized for a variety of diagnoses, including meconium aspiration syndrome (MAS), congenital diaphragmatic hernia (CDH), persistent pulmonary hypertension of the neonate (PPHN), respiratory distress syndrome (RDS), sepsis including viral or bacterial pneumonia, and air leak syndrome (Figure 9-1). The number of neonatal respiratory failure cases peaked in 1992 at approximately 1500 cases, falling steadily with the introduction of inhaled nitric oxide (iNO), surfactant, and high frequency ventilation.[1-3] The implementation of universal screening and intrapartum antimicrobial prophylaxis for women colonized with Group B Streptococcus (GBS) has also impacted the number of infants requiring ECLS for sepsis. Currently, annual neonatal respiratory failure cases remain steady at around 800 cases per year (Figure 9-2).[3] Reports describing the Neonatal ELSO Registry by Roy et al. and Mahmood et al. have demonstrated that while there has been little variation in the demographics such as mean gestational age, gender, or chronologic age at time of ECLS cannulation, there has been a dramatic change in the proportion

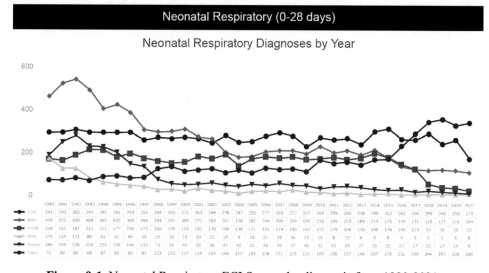

**Figure 9-1.** Neonatal Respiratory ECLS cases by diagnosis from 1990-2021.

of patients with specific diagnoses.[4,5] CDH (covered in Chapter 11) increased from 18% of the neonatal respiratory population in 1988 to 33% in 2020 and is now the second most common indication for neonatal ECLS, while RDS, MAS, pneumonia, and sepsis are now much less common indications for ECLS.[3]

The "other" diagnostic category which represents a collection of complex clinical conditions has been increasingly reported since 2000. A sharp rise has been seen in recent years and in 2020 the "other" category represented 44% of neonatal respiratory ECLS cases. The "other" category has been reported by Sharma et al. to include pulmonary hypoplasia, hypoxic ischemic encephalopathy (HIE), cardiopulmonary arrest, congenital anomalies, myocarditis, and inborn errors of metabolism, as well as patients with primary diagnoses "not otherwise specified" (NOS).[6] The authors speculated that these patients were not offered ECLS support in earlier eras due to a variety of reasons including poor prognosis, belief that the disease process was thought to be irreversible, or inability to survive until ECLS could be offered. Although neonatal ECLS cases have

decreased overall, currently ECLS runs are longer and survival rates are lower, suggesting that more challenging and critically ill patients are being managed with ECLS (Figure 9-3).[3]

The focus of this chapter is to describe the optimal management of the neonatal respiratory failure patient covering systems-based management, circuit considerations specific to the neonatal patient, and family support essential to the well-being of the family unit.

**Respiratory**

*Ventilation Strategies*

While on ECLS, the lungs are allowed to rest and recover from the underlying lung disease and from barotrauma often caused by pre-ECLS management. Rest settings on VV are usually higher than those used in VA. Typical VA settings are PIP (cmH$_2$0) 15-20, PEEP 5-10, Rate 12-20, iTime 0.5-1 second, and FiO$_2$ 0.21-0.3, while typical VV settings are PIP 15-25, PEEP 5-10, Rate 20-30, and FiO2 0.30-0.50.[7,8] A retrospective cohort analysis

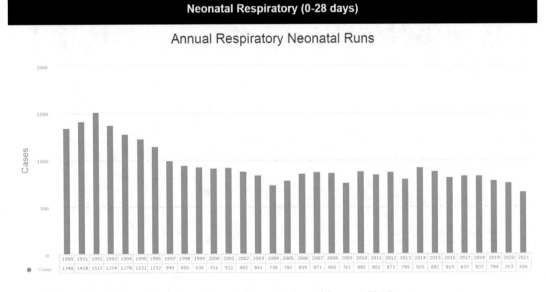

**Figure 9-2.** Decreasing cases of annual neonatal respiratory ECMO runs.

from the ELSO Registry from 2008–2013 revealed that while wide practice variation remains, an increasing number of centers (65%) are routinely using PEEP >6 cmH$_2$O and only 12% use HFOV during ECLS for lung rest.[9] Some centers advocate for higher PEEP to prevent alveolar collapse without compromising venous return. A multicenter study by Keszler et al. that found that PEEP of 12-14 cmH$_2$0 versus PEEP of 3-5 cmH$_2$0 was associated with more rapid lung recovery, shortened ECLS runs, improved lung compliance, and increased expansion on chest radiographs.[10]

The use of surfactant for neonatal respiratory failure prior to ECLS or while on ECLS has demonstrated significant benefit with decreased duration of ECLS, improved pulmonary mechanics, and reduced complications when compared with a placebo group.[11] Routine pulmonary clearance is essential while on ECLS. Gentle endotracheal tube (ETT) suctioning is recommended every 4-6 hours, avoiding deep suctioning. Suction catheters for nasal suction should be avoided to prevent trauma to soft tissues and bleeding.

Pulmonary hemorrhage was reported in 4% of neonatal patients undergoing ECLS from 2016-2020.[3] Treatment of pulmonary hemorrhage varies with the severity of the event and includes limiting suctioning, increasing PEEP, decreasing anticoagulation parameters, increasing platelet count target, and instillation of dilute epinephrine or recombinant factor VIIa through the ETT.[12,13] Surfactant can be useful as a therapy for significant pulmonary hemorrhage because hemorrhage results in surfactant inactivation and decreased lung compliance.[14]

Patient arterial blood gases, along with circuit pre and postoxygenator blood gases, are obtained every 6-12 hours. The usual practice is to obtain daily chest radiographs to confirm line, catheter, and tube position; assess lung volume changes following significant atelectasis or collapse; and to evaluate for free air. Endotracheal tube fixation should also be regularly monitored to avoid unplanned extubation.

Air leaks can be managed with lower ventilator settings, including low CPAP settings via an endotracheal tube, decreasing PEEP until no further air leaks are present, followed

| Overall Outcomes | | | | |
| --- | --- | --- | --- | --- |
| | Total Runs | Survived ECLS | | Survived to DC or Transfer |
| Neonatal | | | | |
| Pulmonary | 34,151 | 29,899 | 87% | 24,949 | 73% |
| Cardiac | 10,127 | 7,000 | 69% | 4,487 | 44% |
| ECPR | 2,420 | 1,685 | 69% | 1,031 | 42% |

| Overall Outcomes from 2017 to 2021 | | | | |
| --- | --- | --- | --- | --- |
| | Total Runs | Survived ECLS | | Survived to DC or Transfer |
| Neonatal | | | | |
| Pulmonary | 3,887 | 3,215 | 82% | 2,768 | 71% |
| Cardiac | 2,745 | 1,945 | 70% | 1,439 | 52% |
| ECPR | 822 | 534 | 64% | 368 | 44% |

**Figure 9-3.** Neonatal specific ECMO runs categorized by Pulmonary, Cardiac or ECPR indications with ECLS survival and survival to discharge or transfer. The highest rates of survival are for neonatal pulmonary indications.

by gentle and slow reexpansion of the lungs. A large or tension pneumothorax requires the careful placement of a chest tube by an experienced clinician. Daily chest radiographs, tidal volume measurements, and patient blood gases assist in formulating a weaning plan.

### Prone Positioning

While prone positioning requires significant coordination and can result in bleeding at the cannula site, it is well tolerated for neonatal and pediatric ECLS patients without decannulation or unplanned extubations (Figure 9-4).[15] Guérin et at. demonstrated that neonates with severe ARDS and severe hypoxemia can benefit from prone treatment.[16] When used in combination with VV ECMO, 18 hours of prone positioning improved both oxygenation and respiratory system compliance.[17]

### Extubation on ECLS

Extubation while on ECLS or 'awake ECLS' has been utilized in the adult population bridging to lung transplantation, and some pediatric centers have also reported successful extubation in patients with cardiogenic shock.[18] Most recently, a case series described the elective extubation of eight neonatal ECLS patients, with the greatest benefit in patients with a significant air leak. Three of the eight infants had resolution of the air leak and lung recruitment was achieved by spontaneous breathing. This led to successful weaning and decannulation.[19]

### Bronchoscopy

Multiple studies in the pediatric population on ECLS have illustrated the usefulness of bronchoscopy in patients with persistent atelectasis including removal of secretions,

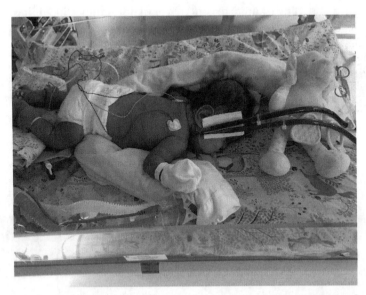

**Figure 9-4.** Proning Protocol: Head must be turned towards the right, to enable clear vision of the cannulas. The head of the bed should be raised to evenly distribute pressure across the shoulders, neck and head and avoid pressure injuries. Elevation of the arm in front of the face (as seen above) can also relieve pressure on the shoulder and neck. Care should be taken that the neonate does not move downwards which could force tension on the ECMO cannulas and lead to inadvertent decannulation. Optimal sedation is essential for successful prone positioning. [Guidelines available by contacting: gail.faulkner@uhl-tr.nhs.uk].

improvement in aeration, and identifying infectious etiology.[20,21] In an analysis of neonatal patients with CDH, 8 out of 17 patients received a therapeutic bronchoscopy on ECLS, of which a majority demonstrated radiologic improvement following bronchoscopy.[1] Overall, the procedure is well tolerated with only minor complications in the form of bleeding in 6% of the bronchoscopies performed.[21]

**Cardiovascular**

*Hemodynamic Support*

Neonates with respiratory failure being considered for ECLS often require pressors for hemodynamic support due to compromised cardiac function and hemodynamic instability. Once on bypass, ECLS blood flow should be gradually increased to 120 ml/kg/min (range 80-150 ml/kg/min) to provide adequate tissue perfusion and oxygenation. Following ECLS initiation, inotropic drugs are typically weaned, but this depends on the underlying pathology and mode of ECLS support. Per the 2021 ELSO Registry, 14.1% of neonates on ECLS received inotropes.[3] Several studies have found that use of inotropes has substantially decreased both in patients on VV and VA.[22,23] With VA support, hemodynamics are dependent on cardiac output (pump flow and native cardiac output) and vascular resistance. With signs of inadequate systemic perfusion pressure, therapeutic options include increasing pump flow, transfusion of blood products, or continued inotropic support. Patients with hypotension and decreased cardiac function may still be considered for VV ECMO. Strieper et al. evaluated cardiac function in 15 infants on VV ECMO and found borderline or normal cardiac indices prior to ECLS, with normalization of function on ECLS.[24] The authors concluded that VV ECMO did not worsen cardiac function, potentially due to avoidance of an increase in LV afterload as seen

with VA ECMO, as well as increased oxygen content provided to coronary arteries.

Systemic perfusion is best measured by mixed venous saturation, with normal values greater than 65% in neonates on VA ECMO. Other measures of systemic perfusion and oxygen delivery include lactate levels and near infrared spectroscopy (NIRS) of regional tissue beds, particularly the brain and kidneys. Mixed venous saturation is not accurate in a neonate on VV ECMO due to recirculation, where newly oxygenated blood delivered to the right atrium returns into the drainage lumen. Cannula adjustment, increasing intravascular volume, patient repositioning, or decreasing ECLS flow are potential treatments to reduce recirculation and improve oxygen delivery.

*Cardiac Stun and Cardiac Dysfunction*

Cardiac stun is a phenomenon seen uniquely in VA ECMO patients. It is diagnosed when the pulse pressure is <10 mmHg and is influenced by increased afterload produced with high ECMO flow, leading to increased left ventricular volumes and reduced left ventricular function.[25] Cardiac stun can also be caused by positioning of the arterial catheter tip too close to the coronary arteries, impacting filling. Cardiac stun in neonates with respiratory failure is usually transient, rarely if ever requires intervention, and is seen early after cannulation in more critically ill infants.[26]

*Hypertension*

Hypertension remains a complication while on ECLS, most commonly in neonates supported with VA; however, the incidence has decreased significantly from 12% in the 2015 ELSO Registry to 3.8% in the 2021 ELSO Registry report for unclear reasons.[3] Lowering pump flow or the use of anihypertensive medications are effective treatment strategies.

## Use of Echocardiography

Echocardiography and point-of-care ultrasound (POCUS) are being used more frequently in the NICU and have a variety of uses in ECLS patients. In the pre-ECLS patient, echocardiography is essential to rule out congenital heart disease, and once on bypass it is helpful in determining both arterial and venous cannula position as well as identifying changes in cardiac function and heart filling. In pediatric ECLS patients, echocardiography was superior to chest radiography for determination of cannula placement.[27] POCUS has also been useful in the identification of pericardial effusions and hemoperitoneums on ECLS.[28] Moscatelli et al. reported that ductal shunt and echocardiographic evidence of pulmonary hypertension such as septal morphology and systolic pulmonary arterial pressure estimated by tricuspid regurgitation are useful in monitoring the effect of lung recruitment on PVR in CDH.[29]

## Fluids, Electrolytes and Nutrition

The initial daily fluid intake is generally limited to 60-100 ml/kg/day because the usual neonatal ECLS patient is edematous due to substantial fluid overload as a result of pre-ECLS management. Transient renal dysfunction with oliguria is common and usually spontaneously resolves over the first 48-72 hours. A natural diuresis phase occurs as cardiac output improves, capillary leak resolves, and fluid mobilization takes place.

Acute kidney injury (AKI) and fluid overload are associated with increased morbidity and mortality, and duration of ECLS.[30-32] Early initiation of CRRT is associated with improved outcomes, including improved fluid balance and decreased duration of ECLS.[33-35] A dedicated CRRT machine connected to the circuit is currently the preferred modality, being more precise in fluid and solute management.[36,37]

Continuous venovenous hemodiafiltration (CVVHDF) may provide the maximum flexibility and effectiveness in terms of solute and fluid removal.[38]

Malnutrition is common in critically ill neonates and children, and adequate macronutrient delivery has been shown to improve outcome.[39-41] Early enteral nutrition is associated with less sepsis-related morbidity and cost, improved gastrointestinal immunologic function, and nitrogen balance than parenteral nutrition (PN).[42-44] Historically, neonates on ECLS were not fed enterally due to concerns regarding intestinal perfusion before ECLS, intestinal ischemia, and the risk of necrotizing enterocolitis, gut barrier function impairment, and obstructive intestinal distension. Several studies have documented enteral nutrition to be safe in neonatal and pediatric ECLS patients.[45] The American Society for Parenteral and Enteral Nutrition (ASPEN) published clinical guidelines for nutritional support in ECLS neonates in 2010.[46] These guidelines recommend that enteral feedings be initiated once the newborn has clinically stabilized. A reasonable approach is to optimize caloric intake through PN with a concomitant early and slow advancement of EN.[47]

In the ECLS neonate, dextrose and lipid emulsions are administered with proteins within 24 hours of cannulation to target caloric goals (80-120 kcal/kg/d), respecting the following recommended intakes: carbohydrates 5-10 mg/kg/min, lipids 3-4 g/kg/d, and proteins 3 mg/kg/d.[8] Intake should be adapted according to the phase of critical illness.[48,49] Excess calories are not helpful as they do not decrease protein catabolism, but can increase carbon dioxide production.[46] A small study supports the administration of lipids via a separate line whenever possible due to concerns of layering, agglutination, and clotting in low flow areas in the circuit.[50] Gastric ulcer prophylaxis is widely used in neonates on ECLS.[45,51,52]

## Hematologic

### *Inherent and ECLS-related Coagulation Abnormalities*

Normal neonatal hemostatic equilibrium involves procoagulant and anticoagulant factors that evolve from fetal to adult life.[53] In healthy term newborns, platelet count is normal or elevated and bleeding times are shortened, normalizing through the first month of life.[54] Due to minimal Vitamin K stores in neonates, a supplemental dose is given at birth to ensure the hepatic synthesis of Gla-proteins which contain four coagulation factors. Higher levels of Von Willebrand factor (VWF) balances inherent platelet hyperreactivity and thus normal hemostasis is maintained. In critically ill neonates, hemostatic equilibrium is disrupted due to lack of reserve capacity, immaturity of the coagulation system, and inflammatory responses, which ultimately result in a hemostatic imbalance. Furthermore, ECLS itself contributes to endothelial dysfunction and exacerbates the inflammatory response.[55] An increased incidence of hemolysis has been reported in neonates due to sheer stress of flow through smaller cannulas, fetal red cells which are more susceptible to mechanical stress, and higher hemoglobin concentration in neonates with increased blood viscosity.[56] Additionally, many newborns requiring ECLS exhibit coagulation derangements secondary to sepsis or hypoxia.

### *Anticoagulation*

Systemic anticoagulation is required for neonatal ECLS and is achieved with unfractionated heparin (UFH) or a direct thrombin inhibitor (DTI).[57,58] UFH is the most commonly used anticoagulant and works by directly binding antithrombin (AT) which then inhibits thrombin and factors Xa/XIIa/IXa. Appropriate UFH dosing varies

significantly in neonates because they maintain "lower concentrations of AT, large volume[s] of distribution, and increased rate[s] of clearance," with a ½ life of ~35 minutes.[59] DTIs (eg, bivalirudin, argatroban) instead bind directly to thrombin. The overall experience with DTIs remains limited in the neonatal population.[59] Currently, there is no consensus or recommendation for which anticoagulant is ideal for neonates.[8]

### *Unfractionated Heparin*

ELSO provides general guidelines for the management of UFH anticoagulation while on ECLS. Infants are anticoagulated with 50-100 units/kg body weight at the time of cannulation, before the neck vessels are entered, and the ECLS circuit is anticoagulated pre-ECLS with 50-100 units UFH/unit of packed red blood cells. After ECLS initiation, a UFH drip is started and titrated to keep the ACT or anti-Xa level in the desired range. A typical initial heparin infusion rate is 25-30 units/kg/hr.[8] Monitoring of coagulation factors, hematocrit, and platelet count are performed with the target values and frequency as noted (Table 9-1). Heparin-induced thrombocytopenia (HIT) is extremely rare in neonates.

| TEST | FREQUENCY | GOAL |
|---|---|---|
| Hematocrit | q 6-12 | >35-40% |
| Platelet count | q 6-12 | >50,000-100,000/μL |
| Fibrinogen | q 12-24 | >100 mg/dL or >150 mg/dL if bleeding or surgery planned |
| Antithrombin | daily | >50-80% (>0.5-0.8 u/mL) Consider use if on maximum dose of UFH and anti-Xa level is out of range |
| Anti-Xa | q6-12 | 0.3-0.7 u/mL |

**Table 9-1.** Recommended hematologic lab frequency while on ECLS.

### Activated Clotting Time (ACT) and Heparin Activity Level (anti-Xa)

The activated clotting time (ACT) has long been the standard for titrating heparin dosing; however, some centers are shifting away from this test. ACT is a global test of anticoagulation and is affected by platelet count, coagulation factor deficiency, hypofibrinogenemia, hemodilution, and hypothermia. Importantly, the ACT range varies by machine and cannot be used interchangably.[59]

Heparin activity level (anti-Xa) is an assay that quantifies the heparin effect by measuring how much exogenous factor Xa is inhibited by the patient's plasma. Anti-Xa assay differs from the ACT and aPTT because it is not influenced by coagulopathy, thrombocytopenia, or hemodilution and may be a better test to monitor the adequacy of heparinization. Khaja et al. compared aPTT and ACT values with heparin activity level of neonates on ECLS and found poor correlation.[60]

### Antithrombin

Antithrombin is an endogenous anticoagulant and inhibits coagulation through inactivation of factors IXa and Xa. Replacement of antithrombin is performed in ECLS patients to treat AT deficiency associated with bypass, to increase anti-Xa levels, and to potentially reduce UFH infusion rates. ELSO guidelines suggest that replacement for serum levels of 50-100% may be useful. Studies have recently raised the question of the utility of AT replacement in heparinized ECLS patients, particularly in light of the high cost and limited safety and efficacy data.[59]

### Direct Thrombin Inhibitors

A new generation of anticoagulants, DTIs have been FDA approved since 2000 for patients greater than 3 years of age, and have been used in adult patients with HIT and children with thrombosis. Activated partial thrombin time (aPTT) levels are the standard of care for monitoring DTIs. Buck et al. reviewed the literature on the use of bivalirudin in infants and children and found no difference in reported bleeding or clotting complications and less use of FFP and antithrombin.[50] Preoperative use of bivalirudin for 42 neonatal CDH patients on ECLS enabled rapid achievement of anticoagulation without bleeding complications; however, there was no relationship between the dose of bivalirudin administered and aPTT nor thromboelastography reaction time (TEG) levels.[61] DTIs have become increasingly used in the adult and pediatric ECLS populations and will likely increase in neonatal patients as new evidence and monitoring techniques (ie, plasma dilute thrombin time, ecarin chromogenic assay) become available.[59]

### Infection

Infection can be an indication for ECLS or can be acquired during the ECLS run. Sepsis now represents only 2% of neonatal cases in the ELSO Registry, likely due to the implementation of universal screening and intrapartum antibiotic prophylaxis for GBS-colonized women. In an analysis of ELSO data, Polito et al. reported that neonates with sepsis were at higher risk of neurologic injury (33%) when compared to other diagnostic categories.[62] The authors speculated that this increased risk was related to the disease process rather than to ECLS. Earlier use of ECLS may reduce morbidity and mortality. The American College of Critical Care Medicine recommends ECLS for refractory septic shock in neonates when medical management has failed.[63,64] Sepsis and ECLS are discussed further in Chapter 36.

Nosocomial sepsis on ECLS occurs in 2% of neonatal ECLS cases with an incidence of 10.1 infections per 1,000 ECLS days.[65] This rate is lower than for pediatric and adult

ECLS patients. The prevalence was highest in neonates supported with VA and increased with duration of ECLS. Neonates on ECLS for cardiac indications and ECPR had higher rates than those with neonatal respiratory failure. Coagulase negative staphylococci were the most common organisms, followed by Candida spp.[65,66] These species are found in association with support apparatus (eg, central lines, endotracheal tubes, and urinary catheters). The importance of reducing infection while on ECLS is highlighted by the findings demonstrating an increase in days on ECLS and lower survival rate in those neonates with documented nosocomial infections.[65,66] Two surveys of ELSO centers demonstrated a varying use of antibiotic prophylaxis while on ECLS, reflecting the uncertainty in the benefit of prophylactic antibiotics.[67,68] A review of the literature of studies regarding antibiotic prophylaxis while on ECLS found no significant difference in infection rate regardless of prophylactic antibiotic usage.[69]

## Neurologic System

Newborns have the highest rate of neurologic complications of any age group reported to the ELSO Registry and these complications are associated with higher mortality and adverse neurodevelopmental outcomes.[62] Neurologic injury can be attributed to the underlying disease process leading to ECLS as well as to accompanying hypoxia, hypotension, and hypocarbia. An analysis of brain injury in neonatal ECLS patients found that patients who developed neuroradiographic evidence of cerebral ischemia had higher relative increase in pH in the first 24 hours of bypass and larger $PaCO_2$ fluctuations while on ECLS. This finding underscores the importance of $PaCO_2$ monitoring in neonatal ECLS patients.[70] With cannulation there are further alterations in cerebral blood flow related to ligation of the right jugular vein and the right carotid artery,

potentially resulting in cerebral ischemia and reperfusion injury. Anticoagulation with bleeding complications and thrombosis with embolic phenomenon are competing risks which need careful management to avoid cerebral injury. Loss of cerebral autoregulation is an additional risk factor for neurologic injury, and severe impairment in autoregulation is reported in children who experience neurologic injury.[71] Risk factors for neurologic injury identified in a ELSO Registry study include lower birth weight and gestational age, need for cardiopulmonary resuscitation prior to ECLS, and use of VA ECMO.[62] For these reasons, ongoing assessment of the neurologic exam, head ultrasound, and consideration of newer neurodiagnostic modalities are warranted. Patient selection, earlier use of ECLS, and improved management practices on ECLS have the potential to improve survival and neurologic outcome. Prompt recognition and intervention for potentially treatable conditions are essential.

### Neuromonitoring

Current techniques for neuromonitoring of the neonatal ECLS patient include neurologic exam, head ultrasound, transcranial doppler, EEG, amplitude integrated EEG (aEEG), and NIRS. Close and frequent monitoring of the neurologic exam is warranted; however, multiple authors report that patients with neurologic injury had no clinical evidence of neurologic deficits at the time of injury detection.[72,73] A recent survey of neuromonitoring during ECLS by the EuroELSO Neurologic Monitoring and Outcome Working Group found that the majority of centers (79%) performed neuromonitoring in addition to neurologic examination.[72] The modalities used were NIRS (66%), intermittent EEG (35%), transcranial Doppler (29%), and brain biomarkers (25%).

Head ultrasound (HUS) is frequently performed prior to ECLS to identify preexisting intracranial hemorrhage or significant ischemic lesions because these may impact the decision to proceed with cannulation. Ongoing daily head ultrasounds are performed often for 5-7 days when the risk of hemorrhage is the highest and then less frequently, depending on the assessment of risk or new clinical findings, including seizures or drop in hematocrit.[74,75] Head ultrasound has a limited field of view and is unable to detect small hemorrhages or ischemic areas and the study has a poor correlation with later neuroimaging and neurodevelopmental outcomes.[73,76-79] Since HUS and clinical assessments are poor predictors of neurodevelopmental abnormalities, a brain MRI following ECLS is essential to identify injury and plan for neurodevelopmental interventional therapies.[8,73]

EEG and aEEG identify electrographic seizure activity as well as providing information about background brain activity and organization. Background activity on either EEG or aEEG is well correlated with neurodevelopmental outcome in neonates with hypoxic ischemic encephalopathy and neonates on ECLS.[80-83] Pappas et al. performed serial aEEG recordings and reported that aEEG predicted death or moderate-to-severe intracranial injury with a sensitivity of 1.0 and specificity of 0.75.[84]

EEG is the gold standard for seizure detection whereas aEEG is best used for screening for seizures and determining the background pattern. A single center study by Lin et al. reported electrographic seizure activity in 9% of neonatal respiratory failure patients (n=35), while ELSO Registry data in 2021 reported 5% with electrographic seizures and 2.4% with clinical seizures.[85] In the Lin study, seizures were subclinical in 83% and patients with seizures had higher mortality and unfavorable outcomes.

NIRS has emerged as a continuous, non-invasive technique which allows real-time measurement of regional oxygenation of cerebral and somatic tissue such as the kidney, providing useful information about hemodynamic status and identifies those at highest risk of adverse developmental outcomes with poor cerebral oxygen delivery and risk for cerebral injury. In the Cvetkovic study of neuromonitoring on ECLS, NIRS was used in 66% of those performing neuromonitoring.[89] Near-infrared light is emitted from a light source on a sensor, passes through the infant's underlying skin and tissue, and is partially absorbed by oxygenated and deoxygenated hemoglobin before being reflected back to a detector. A tissue saturation level (rSO2) is then calculated, reflecting a ratio of arterial and venous blood (approximately 25%:75%) and the regional balance between oxygen supply and demand of the underlying tissue. Tsou et al. reported on the use of NIRS monitoring in 153 neonatal and pediatric patients.[86] A decline in cerebral saturation, defined as any rSO2 $\leq$50% and any values >20% from baseline, was associated with abnormal short-term neurologic outcome, abnormal neuroimaging, and mortality.

### Therapeutic Hypothermia

Neonatal ECLS programs should be prepared to provide therapeutic hypothermia on ECLS for newborns who meet institutional criteria for therapeutic hypothermia. Cooling on ECLS is easily performed using the ECLS heater/cooling device to maintain a core patient temperature of 33-34 degrees $^\circ$C.[87] Due to the potential for a higher risk of bleeding with cooling on ECLS, an analysis of ELSO Registry data was performed.[88] No differences in complications or mortality were found between neonates with HIE who received (n=78) and who did not receive cooling on ECLS (n=109).

The Neonatal ECLS Study of Temperature (NEST) was a randomized controlled trial performed to determine if mild hypothermia to 34$^\circ$C would improve the outcome at 2 years of age in newborns receiving ECLS when compared to normothermia.[89] The use of mild hypothermia for newborns requiring ECLS without evidence of moderate or severe HIE did not result in an improved outcome.

### Sedation and Analgesia

Infants with severe respiratory failure frequently receive analgesia, sedation, and paralytics prior to cannulation. On ECLS, paralysis is usually discontinued; however, sedation and analgesia are continued due to the risks of agitation and concern for catheter security and decreased venous return. Excessive sedation limits the ability to interpret the neurologic exam. Opioids and benzodiazepines have unknown neurodevelopmental effects and prolonged use has been associated with tolerance, physical dependency, and subsequent withdrawal; therefore, the goal is always minimal sedation.[90] Routine pain level scoring should be implemented and appropriate responses evaluated throughout the ECLS course. Strategies to decrease cumulative doses and duration also merit consideration.[90] Commonly used drugs for analgesia and sedation include fentanyl, morphine, midazolam, and demedetomidine. Soothing music and a quiet environment should be considered to optimize nonpharmacologic management as well. No clinical guidelines have been published for sedation and analgesia for neonates on ECLS and this is an area that deserves further study.

## ECLS Circuit Considerations in the Neonate

### Configuration and Cannulas

VA ECMO is the most commonly used mode for respiratory support in newborns and provides direct hemodynamic support. VV ECMO has been used less frequently because one major brand of double-lumen VV catheter was recalled from the market in 2018, and there were several reports of cardiac perforations and cannula-related complications with bicaval double-lumen (BCDL) catheters.[91] (Figure 9-5).

A new double lumen mid-atrial cannula was FDA-approved in 2021 and is currently being used in neonates in the U.S. It can be placed either via open cutdown or percutaneously. Preliminary results are promising, and if confirmed by larger studies, this configuration might overcome the limitations of BCDL and multisite cannulation.[92] Others have described the feasibility of multisite jugular-femoral venvenous cannulation in newborns.[93] The access cannula is placed at the SVC (superior vena cava)/RA (right atrium junction) and return occurs in the common femoral vein (CFV). Detailed discussion regarding cannulation techniques are discussed in Chapter 4.

### Pump Selection

A retrospective analysis of the ELSO registry from 2002 to 2017 showed a progressive shift from roller heads to centrifugal pumps. In recent years, the proportion of roller pumps became negligible in the pediatric population while they still account for at least more than one-third of the neonatal runs.[94]

Hemolysis is a known problem with centrifugal pumps due to the shearing force on blood components created by the vortex in the pump head, resulting in elevated plasma-free hemoglobin (pfHb). Despite design improvements, there are recent reports of patients supported on centrifugal pumps exhibiting hemolysis.[95] According to a retrospective analysis of the ECLS registry from 2002 to 2017 (65,000 patients), hemolysis significantly increased in neonates with an overall incidence of 10.3% and an annual increase of 5.1%. A recent retrospective propensity-matched cohort study of the ELSO Registry showed increased mortality, hemolysis, and ECLS complications (cardiovascular, mechanical, renal, metabolic, neurologic, pulmonary, infectious, limb) in ECLS patients less than 10 kg supported with centrifugal pumps. Hemolysis was identified as a potential mediator of the relationship between centrifugal pump use and mortality.[96] In a metaanalysis of four studies, O'Halloran et al. found that roller pumps were associated with improved survival to discharge, fewer episodes of hemolysis, mechanical complications, cardiac complications, renal complications, and less inotropic support.[96,97] The studies mentioned above are retrospective and cannot demonstrate a causal relationship between centrifugal pumps use and mortality. As pump technology evolves, prospective data collection and comparative effectiveness research are essential to direct future clinical practice.[97,98]

## Tubing

The typical neonatal ECLS circuit comprises 1/4" polyvinylchloride (PVC) tubing, directly matching the cannula connectors. Reducing the tubing surface area is also essential to limit the inflammatory response and coagulation activation due to blood exposure to foreign plastic surface circuitry.[99] Although different kinds of coating (eg, heparin, phosphorylcholine) may help, clotting remains a significant problem in the neonate due to its intrinsic procoagulant state. Circuit clots are reported more commonly in neonates (25.8%) when compared to pediatric patients (20.4%) and adults (13.0%).[94]

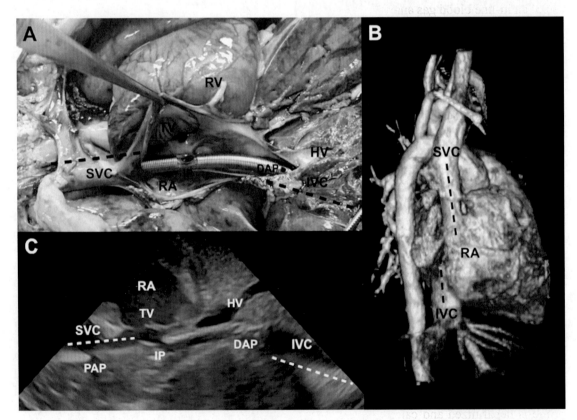

**Figure 9-5.** Picture showing anatomic (A) and radiologic correlates (CT scan reconstruction of the heart and great vessels [B], ultrasound long axis bicaval view [C]). The superior and inferior vena cava (IVC) lie on different planes (dashed lines). When the cannula is correctly positioned, the tip with the distal aspiration ports (DAPs) sits in the IVC, whereas the infusion port (IP) faces the tricuspid valve (TV) and the proximal aspiration ones are located in the superior vena cava (SVC) (A, C). HV = hepatic vein, PAP = proximal aspiration port, RA = right atrium, RV = right ventricle.

### Oxygenators and Gas Flow

The new generation of polymethylpentene (PMP) hollow fiber oxygenators are highly efficient in terms of ease of priming, reduced hemodynamic resistance, and less impairment of the coagulation cascade compared with the silicon membrane oxygenators.

Sweep gas flow is initiated at a 1:1 ratio of gas to blood flow and targeted to an arterial $pCO_2$ of 40-45 mmHg. When initiating ECLS support, it is critical to correct hypercapnia slowly and thus some centers now initiate a lower sweep gas to blood flow by protocol. Rapid changes in blood carbon dioxide levels may increase the incidence of neonatal brain injury.[100] The use of an in-line blood gas analyzing system is an important adjunct to monitor circuit carbon dioxide and blood pH levels.

### Circuit Prime

Priming practices are variable between centers. To prevent hemodilution and hemodynamic instability, the neonatal ECLS circuit is primed with packed red blood cells (PRBCs) and fresh frozen plasma (FFP) or 5% albumin to a hematocrit of 35-45%. Washing of PRBCs is not recommended because it damages the cells. FFP is preferred to albumin in many centers because of a lower tendency to foam during the priming process. PRBCs stored for less than seven days should be used to minimize the risk of hyperkalemia. Critically ill neonates are relatively immune-deficient and more prone to graft versus host disease and leukotropic virus transmission from the white blood cells contained in PRBCs. Use of leukodepleted PRBCs for priming is advisable.[101,102] The blood prime is heparinized and calcium is added to correct the hypocalcemia caused by citrate anticoagulation. Acidosis is corrected with bicarbonate. Priming is recirculated with the sweep gas set at minimal flow with 0.21 $FdO_2$.

The blood prime is warmed to 37° C unless the infant is undergoing hypothermia therapy.[58]

### Pump Flow

After cannulation, once ECLS is initiated, pump flow should be increased over several minutes. When going on VV bypass this is most important because prime blood may have elevated potassium levels that can cause myocardial dysfunction and even asystole if it is not introduced slowly into the systemic circulation. On VA bypass, flow is adequate if the venous saturation is greater than 70% and the patient is not acidotic or hypotensive after pressors have been weaned off, and the ventilator support is decreased to rest settings. On VV ECMO, support is adequate if arterial saturation is in an acceptable range on resting ventilator settings and the patient is not hypotensive or acidotic. Pump flow can range from 80-150 ml/kg/min. Flows in the higher limits are generally needed on VV ECMO to compensate for recirculation.

If the infant on VV bypass remains hypotensive or hypoxic, pressors can be continued, and ventilator pressures and $FiO_2$ increased to supplement ECLS support until the underlying barrier to delivering adequate oxygen through the circuit is corrected. These interventions can include: increasing ECLS pump flow, improving venous drainage, decreasing recirculation, PRBC transfusion. VV to VA conversion is sometimes necessary.

### Cephalad Jugular Drainage

Cephalad jugular drainage has been used to augment venous drainage if the primary cannula position is in an optimal position and venous drainage is inadequate to meet the oxygen demands of the patient. With VV ECMO, a cephalad drainage has several theoretical advantages including augmented venous return, reduced recirculation, and cerebral venous decompression. One study found a lower incidence of intracranial hemorrhage in VA and VV newborns managed with a cephalad drain compared to a historical cohort.[103] A single-center study of use of DLVV with cephalic drain reported that this approach supported 85% of their neonatal respiratory failure cases with a higher survival (89%) and lower rates of complications than reported by the ELSO Registry.[104] Challenges to cephalad cannula use include cannula placement, securing the cannula, and avoiding cannula clotting by monitoring with a flow probe.

**Nursing Management**

Neonatal patients on ECLS have special nursing requirements and practices should be reviewed and aligned to meet the needs of this unique group of patients. Together, the ECLS team must develop, verbalize, and implement patient management goals, which include review and assessment of daily patient and circuit parameters including hemodynamic monitoring, medications, anticoagulation management, and sedation guidelines. Joint rounding at the bedside is important in achieving this goal. Eye, bowel, and skin care are very important but easily overlooked by busy teams. Communication with all members of the multidisciplinary team must be clear, concise, and consistent to enable all team members to have a clear understanding of patient management. In summary, the nursing management of a neonate on ECLS must be individualized, goal directed, and holistic.[105]

**Family Support**

Interventions when caring for a neonate on ECLS must focus on family-centered care beginning with the referral process. Maternal transport to allow a mother to follow her baby to the ECLS center is often helpful. Families commonly are in crisis, finding it extremely difficult to process information.

Nursing interventions should promote positive psychosocial care to decrease these feelings of stress, anxiety, and loss of control. NICU nursing care now emphasizes parental involvement and positive touch as essential, and parents should be shown how they can touch, care for, and interact with their newborn on ECLS. Some ECLS centers report encouraging patient holding for bonding time with parents, and this is not only in the event of palliation, but rather as a routine daily practice. Parents should be empowered to develop a relationship with their baby despite the complexity of care. The ECLS team has to cope with parental distress and feelings of powerlessness. If parents require interpreters, the team members must access this support so the parents can ask questions and feel fully informed, thereby reducing their stress and anxiety. In the event of patient deterioration, hope of recovery must be balanced with the prospect of a negative outcome. This allows families to develop coping strategies. When faced with futility, the parents must never be made to feel that the decision to transition to comfort care from intensive care depends only on them.[106] Providing some control in the situation can be helpful (eg, creating a memory box, photographs, handprints and footprints, or saving locks of hair).

Other healthcare professionals with skills in end-of-life care include pastoral care, social workers, psychologists, and liaison nurses. These teams provide invaluable resources to aid the multidisciplinary team, parents, and other family members throughout this traumatic experience. The ECLS team should inquire about specific care needs, be aware of religious practices and beliefs, and ensure parents take regular breaks in order to eat, sleep, and take care of their personal needs.

One way of improving communication and complementing face-to-face communication is by encouraging parents to keep a diary of events. It acts as a tool for memory, not only for the parents, but for the child later in life. The diary allows the parents to write down notes, questions, or concerns, and assists in keeping other family members updated. Improving the quality and quantity of communication benefits the patient, family, and team while improving overall family wellbeing and satisfaction. By providing emotional support, clear and honest information, and communicating effectively, parents are enabled to feel safe, involved, and confident during this difficult time.

## Summary

It has been over 45 years since ECLS was first successfully used to treat Esperanza, a newborn with respiratory failure in 1975. As of January 2022, the ELSO Registry includes over 34,000 neonates with respiratory failure with an overall survival of 73%. The data gathered through the ELSO Registry, randomized controlled trials, and smaller clinical studies continue to demonstrate the success of ECLS in the neonatal population, especially when compared to other age and diagnostic groups. Therapies such as iNO, surfactant, intrapartum antibiotic prophylaxis, and HFOV have led to a decrease in the utilization of ECLS for certain neonatal disease states. This trend has resulted in fewer patients receiving ECLS treatment, and those that do have longer, more complicated runs with lower survival rates. More research is needed to understanding the growing "other" category so we can better manage this diverse and complex group of patients. Patient and circuit related complications continue to be a source of morbidity and mortality, with bleeding and clotting being the most common. The future challenge for neonatal ECLS centers lies in developing strategies to limit complications and improve survival, while treating fewer and more complex patients.

# References

1. Hintz SR, Suttner DM, Sheehan AM, et al. Decreased use of neonatal extracorporeal membrane oxygenation (ECMO): how new treatment modalities have affected ECMO utilization. Pediatrics. Dec 2000;106(6):1339-43.
2. Qureshi FG, Jackson HT, Brown J, et al. The changing population of the United States and use of extracorporeal membrane oxygenation. J Surg Res. Sep 2013;184(1):572-6.
3. Extracorporeal Life Support Organization (ELSO): ECMO registry of extracorporeal life support organization. http://www.elsoweb.net/registry.
4. Roy BJ, Rycus P, Conrad SA, et al. The changing demographics of neonatal extracorporeal membrane oxygenation patients reported to the Extracorporeal Life Support Organization (ELSO) Registry. Pediatrics. Dec 2000;106(6):1334-8.
5. Mahmood B, Newton D, Pallotto EK. Current trends in neonatal ECMO. Semin Perinatol. Mar 2018;42(2):80-88.
6. Sharma J, Sherman A, Rimal A, et al. Neonatal respiratory extracorporeal membrane oxygenation and primary diagnosis: trends between two decades. J Perinatol. Feb 2020;40(2):269-274.
7. Rais-Bahrami K, Van Meurs KP. Venoarterial versus venovenous ECMO for neonatal respiratory failure. Semin Perinatol. Mar 2014;38(2):71-7.
8. Wild KT, Rintoul N, Kattan J, Gray B. Extracorporeal Life Support Organization (ELSO): Guidelines for Neonatal Respiratory Failure. Asaio j. May 2020;66(5):463-470.
9. Alapati D, Aghai ZH, Hossain MJ, et al. Lung Rest During Extracorporeal Membrane Oxygenation for Neonatal Respiratory Failure-Practice Variations and Outcomes. Pediatr Crit Care Med. Jul 2017;18(7):667-674.
10. Keszler M, Ryckman FC, McDonald JV Jr, et al. A prospective, multicenter, randomized study of high versus low positive end-expiratory pressure during extracorporeal membrane oxygenation. J Pediatr. Jan 1992;120(1):107-13.
11. Lotze A, Knight GR, Martin GR, et al. Improved pulmonary outcome after exogenous surfactant therapy for respiratory failure in term infants requiring extracorporeal membrane oxygenation. J Pediatr. Feb 1993;122(2):261-8.
12. Welde MA, Sanford CB, Mangum M, et al. Pulmonary Hemorrhage in the Neonate. Neonatal Netw. Aug 1 2021;40(5):295-304.
13. Olomu N, Kulkarni R, Manco-Johnson M. Treatment of severe pulmonary hemorrhage with activated recombinant factor VII (rFVIIa) in very low birth weight infants. J Perinatol. Dec 2002;22(8):672-4.
14. Pandit PB, Dunn MS, Kelly EN, et al. Surfactant replacement in neonates with early chronic lung disease. Pediatrics. Jun 1995;95(6):851-4.
15. Haefner SM, Bratton SL, Annich GM,et al. Complications of intermittent prone positioning in pediatric patients receiving extracorporeal membrane oxygenation for respiratory failure. Chest. May 2003;123(5):1589-94.
16. Guérin C, Reignier J, Richard JC, et al. Prone positioning in severe acute respiratory distress syndrome. N Engl J Med. Jun 6 2013;368(23):2159-68.
17. Kimmoun A, Roche S, Bridey C, et al. Prolonged prone positioning under VV-ECMO is safe and improves oxygenation and respiratory compliance. Ann Intensive Care. Dec 2015;5(1):35.
18. Schmidt F, Jack T, Sasse M, et al. "Awake Veno-arterial Extracorporeal Membrane Oxygenation" in Pediatric Cardiogenic Shock: A Single-Center Experience. Pediatr Cardiol. Dec 2015;36(8):1647-56.
19. Costa J, Dirnberger DR, Froehlich CD, et al. Awake Neonatal Extracorporeal Membrane Oxygenation. Asaio j. May 2020;66(5):e70-e73.
20. Kamat PP, Popler J, Davis J, et al. Use of flexible bronchoscopy in pediatric patients receiving extracorporeal membrane oxygenation (ECMO) support. Pediatr Pulmonol. Nov 2011;46(11):1108-13.
21. Prentice E, Mastropietro CW. Flexible bronchoscopy for children on extracorporeal membrane oxygenation for cardiac failure. Pediatr Crit Care Med. Jul 2011;12(4):422-5.
22. Roberts N, Westrope C, Pooboni SK, et al. Venovenous extracorporeal membrane oxygenation for respiratory failure in inotrope dependent neonates. Asaio j. Sep-Oct 2003;49(5):568-71.
23. Knight GR, Dudell GG, Evans ML, et al. A comparison of venovenous and venoarterial extracorporeal membrane oxygenation in the treatment of neonatal respiratory failure. Crit Care Med. Oct 1996;24(10):1678-83.
24. Strieper MJ, Sharma S, Dooley KJ, et al. Effects of venovenous extracorporeal membrane oxygenation on cardiac performance as determined by echocardiographic measurements. J Pediatr. Jun 1993;122(6):950-5.
25. Schiller P, Vikholm P, Hellgren L. Experimental Venoarterial Extracorporeal Membrane Oxygenation Induces Left Ventricular Dysfunction. Asaio j. Sep-Oct 2016;62(5):518-24.
26. Martin GR, Short BL, Abbott C, O'Brien AM. Cardiac stun in infants undergoing extracorporeal membrane oxygenation. J Thorac Cardiovasc Surg. Apr 1991;101(4):607-11.
27. Thomas TH, Price R, Ramaciotti C, et al. Echocardiography, not chest radiography, for evaluation of cannula placement during pediatric

extracorporeal membrane oxygenation. Pediatr Crit Care Med. Jan 2009;10(1):56-9.

28. Noh CYK VK, Danzer E, Chock VY. Near-Infared Spectroscopy as a Hemodynamic Monitoring Tool during Neonatal Extracorporeal Life Support: A Case Series. The Journal of ExtraCorporeal Technology. 2021;54:61-6.

29. Moscatelli A, Pezzato S, Lista G, et al. Venovenous ECMO for Congenital Diaphragmatic Hernia: Role of Ductal Patency and Lung Recruitment. Pediatrics. Nov 2016;138(5).

30. Fleming GM, Sahay R, Zappitelli M, et al. The Incidence of Acute Kidney Injury and Its Effect on Neonatal and Pediatric Extracorporeal Membrane Oxygenation Outcomes: A Multicenter Report From the Kidney Intervention During Extracorporeal Membrane Oxygenation Study Group. Pediatr Crit Care Med. Dec 2016;17(12):1157-1169.

31. Selewski DT, Askenazi DJ, Bridges BC, et al. The Impact of Fluid Overload on Outcomes in Children Treated With Extracorporeal Membrane Oxygenation: A Multicenter Retrospective Cohort Study. Pediatr Crit Care Med. Dec 2017;18(12):1126-1135.

32. Gorga SM, Sahay RD, Askenazi DJ, et al. Fluid overload and fluid removal in pediatric patients on extracorporeal membrane oxygenation requiring continuous renal replacement therapy: a multicenter retrospective cohort study. Pediatr Nephrol. May 2020;35(5):871-882.

33. Blijdorp K, Cransberg K, Wildschut ED, et al. Haemofiltration in newborns treated with extracorporeal membrane oxygenation: a case-comparison study. Crit Care. 2009;13(2):R48.

34. Murphy HJ, Eklund MJ, Hill J, et al. Early continuous renal replacement therapy during infant extracorporeal life support is associated with decreased lung opacification. J Artif Organs. Dec 2019;22(4):286-293.

35. Murphy HJ, Cahill JB, Twombley KE, et al. Early Continuous Renal Replacement Therapy Improves Nutrition Delivery in Neonates During Extracorporeal Life Support. J Ren Nutr. Jan 2018;28(1):64-70.

36. Gorga SM, Lima L, Askenazi DJ, et al. Fluid Balance Management Informs Renal Replacement Therapy Use During Pediatric Extracorporeal Membrane Oxygenation: A Survey Report From the Kidney Intervention During Extracorporeal Membrane Oxygenation Group. Asaio j. May 10 2021.

37. Symons JM, McMahon MW, Karamlou T, et al. Continuous renal replacement therapy with an automated monitor is superior to a free-flow system during extracorporeal life support. Pediatr Crit Care Med. Nov 2013;14(9):e404-8.

38. Spector BL, Misurac JM. Renal Replacement Therapy in Neonates. Neoreviews. Dec 2019;20(12):e697-e710.

39. Heyland DK, Dhaliwal R, Drover JW, et al. Canadian clinical practice guidelines for nutrition support in mechanically ventilated, critically ill adult patients. JPEN J Parenter Enteral Nutr. Sep-Oct 2003;27(5):355-73.

40. Mehta NM, Bechard LJ, Cahill N, et al. Nutritional practices and their relationship to clinical outcomes in critically ill children--an international multicenter cohort study*. Crit Care Med. Jul 2012;40(7):2204-11.

41. Farr BJ, Rice-Townsend SE, et al. Nutrition Support During Pediatric Extracorporeal Membrane Oxygenation. Nutr Clin Pract. Dec 2018;33(6):747-753.

42. Mehta NM, Skillman HE, Irving SY, et al. Guidelines for the Provision and Assessment of Nutrition Support Therapy in the Pediatric Critically Ill Patient: Society of Critical Care Medicine and American Society for Parenteral and Enteral Nutrition. JPEN J Parenter Enteral Nutr. Jul 2017;41(5):706-742.

43. Kreymann KG, Berger MM, Deutz NE, et al. ESPEN Guidelines on Enteral Nutrition: Intensive care. Clin Nutr. Apr 2006;25(2):210-23.

44. Dellinger RP, Carlet JM, Masur H, et al. Surviving Sepsis Campaign guidelines for management of severe sepsis and septic shock. Crit Care Med. Mar 2004;32(3):858-73.

45. Ohman K, Zhu H, Maizlin I, et al. A Multicenter Study of Nutritional Adequacy in Neonatal and Pediatric Extracorporeal Life Support. J Surg Res. May 2020;249:67-73.

46. Jaksic T, Hull MA, Modi BP, et al. A.S.P.E.N. Clinical guidelines: nutrition support of neonates supported with extracorporeal membrane oxygenation. JPEN J Parenter Enteral Nutr. May-Jun 2010;34(3):247-53.

47. Jimenez L, Mehta NM, Duggan CP. Timing of the initiation of parenteral nutrition in critically ill children. Curr Opin Clin Nutr Metab Care. May 2017;20(3):227-231.

48. Mihatsch WA, Braegger C, Bronsky J, et al. ESPGHAN/ESPEN/ESPR/CSPEN guidelines on pediatric parenteral nutrition. Clin Nutr. Dec 2018;37(6 Pt B):2303-2305.

49. Moltu SJ, Bronsky J, Embleton N, et al. Nutritional Management of the Critically Ill Neonate: A Position Paper of the ESPGHAN Committee on Nutrition. J Pediatr Gastroenterol Nutr. Aug 1 2021;73(2):274-289.

50. Buck ML, Wooldridge P, Ksenich RA. Comparison of methods for intravenous infusion of fat emulsion during extracorporeal membrane oxygenation. Pharmacotherapy. Nov 2005;25(11):1536-40.

51. Kuusela AL, Ruuska T, Karikoski R, et al. A randomized, controlled study of prophylactic ranitidine in preventing stress-induced gastric

mucosal lesions in neonatal intensive care unit patients. Crit Care Med. Feb 1997;25(2):346-51.

52. Green DS, Abdel-Latif ME, Jones LJ, et al. Pharmacological interventions for prevention and treatment of upper gastrointestinal bleeding in newborn infants. Cochrane Database Syst Rev. Jul 2 2019;7(7):Cd011785.

53. Toulon P. Developmental hemostasis: laboratory and clinical implications. Int J Lab Hematol. May 2016;38 Suppl 1:66-77.

54. Strauss T, Sidlik-Muskatel R, Kenet G. Developmental hemostasis: primary hemostasis and evaluation of platelet function in neonates. Semin Fetal Neonatal Med. Dec 2011;16(6):301-4.

55. Graulich J, Walzog B, Marcinkowski M, et al. Leukocyte and endothelial activation in a laboratory model of extracorporeal membrane oxygenation (ECMO). Pediatr Res. Nov 2000;48(5):679-84.

56. Lou S, MacLaren G, Best D, Delzoppo C, Butt W. Hemolysis in pediatric patients receiving centrifugal-pump extracorporeal membrane oxygenation: prevalence, risk factors, and outcomes. Crit Care Med. May 2014;42(5):1213-20.

57. Fallon BP, Gadepalli SK, Hirschl RB. Pediatric and neonatal extracorporeal life support: current state and continuing evolution. Pediatr Surg Int. Jan 2021;37(1):17-35.

58. Connelly J, Blinman T. Special equipment considerations for neonatal ECMO. Semin Perinatol. Mar 2018;42(2):89-95.

59. McMichael ABV, Ryerson LM, Ratano D, Fan E, Faraoni D, Annich GM. 2021 ELSO Adult and Pediatric Anticoagulation Guidelines. Asaio J. Jan 19 2022.

60. Khaja WA, Bilen O, Lukner RB, et al. Evaluation of heparin assay for coagulation management in newborns undergoing ECMO. Am J Clin Pathol. Dec 2010;134(6):950-4.

61. Snyder CW, Goldenberg NA, Nguyen ATH, et al. A perioperative bivalirudin anticoagulation protocol for neonates with congenital diaphragmatic hernia on extracorporeal membrane oxygenation. Thromb Res. Sep 2020;193:198-203.

62. Polito A, Barrett CS, Wypij D, et al. Neurologic complications in neonates supported with extracorporeal membrane oxygenation. An analysis of ELSO registry data. Intensive Care Med. Sep 2013;39(9):1594-601.

63. Davis AL, Carcillo JA, Aneja RK, et al. American College of Critical Care Medicine Clinical Practice Parameters for Hemodynamic Support of Pediatric and Neonatal Septic Shock. Crit Care Med. Jun 2017;45(6):1061-1093.

64. Ramanathan K, Yeo N, Alexander P, et al. Role of extracorporeal membrane oxygenation in children

with sepsis: a systematic review and meta-analysis. Crit Care. Dec 7 2020;24(1):684.

65. Bizzarro MJ, Conrad SA, Kaufman DA, et al. Infections acquired during extracorporeal membrane oxygenation in neonates, children, and adults. Pediatr Crit Care Med. May 2011;12(3):277-81.

66. MacLaren G, Schlapbach LJ, Aiken AM. Nosocomial Infections During Extracorporeal Membrane Oxygenation in Neonatal, Pediatric, and Adult Patients: A Comprehensive Narrative Review. Pediatr Crit Care Med. Mar 2020;21(3):283-290.

67. Kao LS, Fleming GM, Escamilla RJ, et al. Antimicrobial prophylaxis and infection surveillance in extracorporeal membrane oxygenation patients: a multi-institutional survey of practice patterns. Asaio j. May-Jun 2011;57(3):231-8.

68. Glater-Welt LB, Schneider JB, Zinger MM, et al. Nosocomial Bloodstream Infections in Patients Receiving Extracorporeal Life Support: Variability in Prevention Practices: A Survey of the Extracorporeal Life Support Organization Members. J Intensive Care Med. Dec 2016;31(10):654-669.

69. O'Horo JC, Cawcutt KA, De Moraes AG, et al. The Evidence Base for Prophylactic Antibiotics in Patients Receiving Extracorporeal Membrane Oxygenation. Asaio j. Jan-Feb 2016;62(1):6-10.

70. Farhat A, Li X, Huet B, et al. Routine Neuroimaging: Understanding Brain Injury in Pediatric Extracorporeal Membrane Oxygenation. Crit Care Med. Mar 1 2022;50(3):480-490.

71. Joram N, Beqiri E, Pezzato S, et al. Continuous Monitoring of Cerebral Autoregulation in Children Supported by Extracorporeal Membrane Oxygenation: A Pilot Study. Neurocrit Care. Jun 2021;34(3):935-945.

72. Cvetkovic M, Chiarini G, Belliato M, et al. International survey of neuromonitoring and neurodevelopmental outcome in children and adults supported on extracorporeal membrane oxygenation in Europe. Perfusion. Sep 22 2021:2676591211042563.

73. Farhat A, Li X, Huet B, et al. Routine Neuroimaging: Understanding Brain Injury in Pediatric Extracorporeal Membrane Oxygenation. Crit Care Med. 2022 Mar 1;50(3):480-490.

74. Khan AM, Shabarek FM, Zwischenberger JB, et al. Utility of daily head ultrasonography for infants on extracorporeal membrane oxygenation. J Pediatr Surg. Aug 1998;33(8):1229-32.

75. Biehl DA, Stewart DL, Forti NH, et al. Timing of intracranial hemorrhage during extracorporeal life support. Asaio j. Nov-Dec 1996;42(6):938-41.

76. Cowan F, Mercuri E, Groenendaal F, et al. Does cranial ultrasound imaging identify arterial cerebral infarction in term neonates? Arch Dis Child Fetal Neonatal Ed. May 2005;90(3):F252-6.

77. Rollins MD, Yoder BA, Moore KR, et al. Utility of neuroradiographic imaging in predicting outcomes after neonatal extracorporeal membrane oxygenation. J Pediatr Surg. Jan 2012;47(1):76-80.

78. Lazar EL, Abramson SJ, Weinstein S, et al. Neuroimaging of brain injury in neonates treated with extracorporeal membrane oxygenation: lessons learned from serial examinations. J Pediatr Surg. Feb 1994;29(2):186-90; discussion 190-1.

79. Glass P, Bulas DI, Wagner AE, et al. Severity of brain injury following neonatal extracorporeal membrane oxygenation and outcome at age 5 years. Dev Med Child Neurol. Jul 1997;39(7):441-8.

80. Murray DM, Boylan GB, Ryan CA, et al. Early EEG findings in hypoxic-ischemic encephalopathy predict outcomes at 2 years. Pediatrics. Sep 2009;124(3):e459-67.

81. Del Río R, Ochoa C, Alarcon A, et al. Amplitude Integrated Electroencephalogram as a Prognostic Tool in Neonates with Hypoxic-Ischemic Encephalopathy: A Systematic Review. PLoS One. 2016;11(11):e0165744.

82. Chandrasekaran M, Chaban B, Montaldo P, et al. Predictive value of amplitude-integrated EEG (aEEG) after rescue hypothermic neuroprotection for hypoxic ischemic encephalopathy: a meta-analysis. J Perinatol. Jun 2017;37(6):684-689.

83. Hahn JS, Vaucher Y, Bejar R, Coen RW. Electroencephalographic and neuroimaging findings in neonates undergoing extracorporeal membrane oxygenation. Neuropediatrics. Feb 1993;24(1):19-24.

84. Pappas A, Shankaran S, Stockmann PT, Bara R. Changes in amplitude-integrated electroencephalography in neonates treated with extracorporeal membrane oxygenation: a pilot study. J Pediatr. Jan 2006;148(1):125-7.

85. Lin JJ, Banwell BL, Berg RA, et al. Electrographic Seizures in Children and Neonates Undergoing Extracorporeal Membrane Oxygenation. Pediatr Crit Care Med. Mar 2017;18(3):249-257.

86. Tsou PY, Garcia AV, Yiu A, et al. Association of Cerebral Oximetry with Outcomes after Extracorporeal Membrane Oxygenation. Neurocrit Care. Oct 2020;33(2):429-437.

87. Massaro A, Rais-Bahrami K, Chang T, et al. Therapeutic hypothermia for neonatal encephalopathy and extracorporeal membrane oxygenation. J Pediatr. Sep 2010;157(3):499-501, 501.e1.

88. Cuevas Guaman M, Lucke AM, Hagan JL, et al. Bleeding Complications and Mortality in Neonates Receiving Therapeutic Hypothermia and Extracorporeal Membrane Oxygenation. Am J Perinatol. Feb 2018;35(3):271-276.

89. Field D, Juszczak E, Linsell L, et al. Neonatal ECMO study of temperature (NEST): a randomized controlled trial. Pediatrics. Nov 2013;132(5):e1247-56.

90. Wildschut ED, Hanekamp MN, Vet NJ, et al. Feasibility of sedation and analgesia interruption following cannulation in neonates on extracorporeal membrane oxygenation. Intensive Care Med. Sep 2010;36(9):1587-91.

91. Lillie J, Boot L, Speggiorin S, et al. Factors Behind Decline of Venovenous Extracorporeal Membrane Oxygenation to Support Neonatal Respiratory Failure. Pediatr Crit Care Med. Aug 2020;21(8):e502-e504.

92. Gray BW CN, Chapman R, Chi A, et al. Early use experience of the novel Crescent RA Neonatal VV-ECMO Cannula among CHNC ECMO Focus Group members. February 13, 2022:

93. Lillie J, Pienaar A, Budd J, et al. Multisite Veno-Venous Cannulation for Neonates and Nonambulatory Children. Pediatr Crit Care Med. Aug 1 2021;22(8):692-700.

94. Hayes MM, Fallon BP, Barbaro RP, et al. Membrane Lung and Blood Pump Use During Prolonged Extracorporeal Membrane Oxygenation: Trends From 2002 to 2017. Asaio j. Sep 1 2021;67(9):1062-1070.

95. Neal JR, Quintana E, Pike RB, et al. Using Daily Plasma-Free Hemoglobin Levels for Diagnosis of Critical Pump Thrombus in Patients Undergoing ECMO or VAD Support. J Extra Corpor Technol. Jun 2015;47(2):103-8.

96. O'Halloran CP, Thiagarajan RR, Yarlagadda VV, et al. Outcomes of Infants Supported With Extracorporeal Membrane Oxygenation Using Centrifugal Versus Roller Pumps: An Analysis From the Extracorporeal Life Support Organization Registry. Pediatr Crit Care Med. Dec 2019;20(12):1177-1184.

97. Papadimas E, Leow L, Tan YK, et al. Centrifugal and Roller Pumps in Neonatal and Pediatric Extracorporeal Membrane Oxygenation: A Systematic Review and Meta-Analysis of Clinical Outcomes. ASAIO J. 2022 Mar 1;68(3):311-317.

98. Dalton HJ, Hoskote A. There and Back Again: Roller Pumps Versus Centrifugal Technology in Infants on Extracorporeal Membrane Oxygenation. Pediatr Crit Care Med. Dec 2019;20(12):1195-1196.

99. Gorbet MB, Sefton MV. Biomaterial-associated thrombosis: roles of coagulation factors, complement, platelets and leukocytes. Biomaterials. Nov 2004;25(26):5681-703.

100. Zhou W, Liu W. Hypercapnia and hypocapnia in neonates. World J Pediatr. Aug 2008;4(3):192-6.

101. Simancas-Racines D, Arevalo-Rodriguez I, Urrutia G, et al. Leukodepleted Packed Red Blood Cells Transfusion in Patients Undergoing Major Cardiovascular Surgical Procedure: Systematic

Review and Meta-Analysis. Cardiol Res Pract. 2019;2019:7543917.

102. Girelli G, Antoncecchi S, Casadei AM, et al. Recommendations for transfusion therapy in neonatology. Blood Transfus. Jul 2015;13(3):484-97.

103. O'Connor TA, Haney BM, Grist GE, et al. Decreased incidence of intracranial hemorrhage using cephalic jugular venous drainage during neonatal extracorporeal membrane oxygenation. J Pediatr Surg. Oct 1993;28(10):1332-5.

104. Roberts J, Keene S, Heard M, et al. Successful primary use of VVDL+V ECMO with cephalic drain in neonatal respiratory failure. J Perinatol. Feb 2016;36(2):126-31.

105. ECMO Specialist Training Manual - 4th Edition. Extracorporeal Life Support Organization. 2018.

106. Curley MA, Meyer EC. Parental experience of highly technical therapy: survivors and nonsurvivors of extracorporeal membrane oxygenation support. Pediatr Crit Care Med. Apr 2003;4(2):214-9.

# 10

## Weaning and Decannulation in Neonatal Respiratory Failure

*Giles J. Peek and Chris Harvey*

The guiding principle of this phase of patient care is that, in most cases, patients should not be decannulated if adequate gas exchange using lung protective ventilation cannot be achieved.

Newborns who require ECLS for respiratory failure usually have persistent pulmonary hypertension of the newborn (PPHN) as their dominant pathophysiology. As such, as soon as the pulmonary artery pressures become subsystemic, right to left shunting reverses and the patients improve dramatically. However, this by itself is insufficient. It is also essential to check that the lung compliance and chest x-ray appearance has returned to more normal levels and to estimate the pulmonary artery pressure using echocardiography to ensure that it has fallen to around half systemic. If this is the case, then the patient may be ready to wean from ECLS. Conducting a Cilley Study can give an indication of recovery. To do this the $FiO_2$ is turned to 100% and the patient's peripheral saturation is observed. If it rapidly climbs to 100% then pulmonary gas exchange has returned.

There is much confusing terminology employed to describe what happens next; however, the following definitions will be used throughout this chapter:

*Weaning* is the process where ECLS flow is reduced to determine if the patient is ready to trial-off ECLS.

*Trialing-Off* is the process where ECLS support is completely withdrawn allowing the patient's gas exchange and respiratory mechanics to be assessed to determine if the patient is ready to be decannulated.

*Decannulation* is the process of removing the ECLS cannulas.

### Weaning

The weaning process will be identical for patients who are on both VV and VA ECMO. The aim is to reduce the amount of ECMO support and begin the assessment of native gas exchange. The ability of the lungs to oxygenate blood usually returns before lung compliance will allow adequate ventilation for $CO_2$ removal because it is a function of the resolution of PPHN. Leaving the ventilator on rest settings of PC 20/10, SIMV 10, PS 10, Ti 1 sec, the $FiO_2$ is turned up to 60% and the flow is turned down from full flow of 100-120 ml/kg/min to around half flow. The sweep flow is left unchanged as oxygenation alone is being assessed. If the peripheral oxygen saturation is maintained, an arterial blood gas is drawn after around 20 minutes. If the $PaO_2$ is greater than 100 mmHg, then the ventilation can be partially normalized to PC 25/6, SIMV 15, PS 15, Ti 0.7, while the sweep is reduced to half its previous amount or $CO_2$ bleed in ($FsCO_2$) is doubled.

The lung mechanics are assessed, ventilation is optimized, and an arterial blood gas is repeated after 20 minutes. If the $PaCO_2$ is 35-45 mmHg it is likely that the patient can proceed with a trial-off. If a tidal volume of 6 ml/kg cannot be obtained with a PIP of 25, if the $PaCO_2$ is elevated, if the $PaO_2$ drops, or if there is any kind of hemodynamic instability, then the patient is not ready to be weaned. They should be placed back onto rest settings and the ECLS flow and sweep returned to preweaning settings. It may also be possible to reduce ECLS flow and sweep gas flow and $FsO_2$; however, these protocols tend to be used instead of trialing the patient off. They can be used as a prelude to a trial-off if desired. It is important to maintain circuit flow above 200 ml/min for a neonatal circuit (ie, one with a neonatal sized oxygenator and pump). If patient flow needs to be set lower than this, a bridge can be inserted and a Hoffman partial occlusion clamp (gate clamp) can be used to set the desired patient flow whilst circuit flow is maintained. Two Doppler flow meters (eg, Transonic Flow Monitors) should be used to calibrate this arrangement. Patients who are more likely to need gradual reduction or a prolonged weaning period include marginal congenital diaphragmatic hernia patients who may require 24-48 hours of gradual adjustment of ventilation and weaning of flow and sweep. It is important to remember that VA ECMO should not be run without sweep gas as this can result in fatal hypoxia.

**Trialing-Off**

This process will be different for VV and VA ECMO.

**VV ECMO Trial-Off**

Ventilation is increased, and the sweep gas is disconnected. Membrane $CO_2$ transport ceases immediately. Extracorporeal oxygenation slowly reduces until the venous drainage and return lines are the same color as the circuit becomes fully mixed with the patient's blood. Full mixing usually takes 20 minutes. If the flow has been previously weaned it should be turned back up to full flow to speed up the mixing. An arterial blood gas is taken every 20-30 minutes and ventilation is adjusted accordingly. The aim should be to have normal blood gases with $FiO_2$ <60% and PIP <28 cmH$_2$O. If more pressure is required or a higher $FiO_2$ then the patient is not ready to decannulate. An echocardiogram performed during the trial-off should demonstrate a PA pressure lower than 2/3$^{rd}$ systemic. If the PAP is higher that this the patient is not ready for decannulation. One of the advantages of VV ECMO is that the circuit blood flow continues to circulate and therefore is at no increased risk of clotting. Anticoagulation is left unchanged and any infusions running into the circuit are undisturbed. This is also true of Continuous Renal Replacement therapy (CRRT) connected to the circuit, which can be continued without alteration during the trial-off. Some patients are marginal during the usual 2-hour trial-off procedure, but the team may feel that ventilation or PA pressure may become acceptable with time for pulmonary toilet, adjustment of ventilation, sedation, and gentle lung recruitment. In this case, the trial-off can be extended until acceptable blood gases and PA pressures are obtained on lung protective ventilator settings. It is unusual to extend a VV trial-off beyond 24 hours because in most patients a decision to decannulate or go back onto ECMO can be made before 24 hours of trial-off. If performing a prolonged VV trial-off, blood gas frequency is reduced stepwise down to 6 hourly as the trial progresses.

**VA ECMO Trial-Off**

*Classic VA Trial-Off*

Often known as a "Clamp-Trial" or "Clamping-Off". Although this is considered the standard procedure, it is a laborious, labor intensive, and potentially dangerous technique. It can only run for 1-2 hours because the risk of cannula and circuit clot formation gradually increases as time goes on. The first step is to ensure all infusions are running into the baby rather than the circuit. This needs to be done several hours in advance to prevent swings in drug delivery caused when the circuit is clamped off. Next, the anticoagulation must be split between the circuit and the baby with a separate infusion for each. The dose of each infusion should be half of the total previous dose, each increased by approximately 10%. Use a bigger increase if the circuit has a significant clot burden. Now insert the bridge between the arterial and venous lines of the ECMO circuit. Then increase the ventilation to normal levels, clamp the patient off ECMO, recirculate around the bridge, and turn the sweep off. At 9 minutes draw an arterial blood gas and ACT sample from the patient and an ACT sample from the circuit. This will require 4 hands and two ACT machines. At 10 minutes clamp the bridge, open the venous and arterial lines, and allow flow to the baby for 20 seconds. This is called "flashing the cannulas." Ignore the massive swing in arterial pressure, it will occur in both directions as the bridge, venous and arterial lines are clamped and unclamped not entirely simultaneously. It only requires action if recovery to baseline is not prompt. Clamp off again and open the bridge. The ACTs should read in the next 2-4 minutes, adjust the anticoagulation on the baby and the circuit, including boluses if necessary. The blood gas should have read by now, adjust the ventilation as required. If no adjustments were made, repeat the ABG and ACTs again at 19 minutes. At 20 minutes and every 10 minutes thereafter flash the cannulas again. Repeat ABGs and ACTs just before the flash when needed. Once reasonable gas exchange is assured, measure the pulmonary artery pressure using echocardiography as described for VV

ECMO above. After 1 hour, make a tentative decision about decannulation. Decannulate or cap the cannulas before two hours. If the trial-off is deemed to have failed, restart the sweep and go back on ECMO, reset the ventilator to rest settings, put the anticoagulant infusion back to a single access point, and reset the dose. Make sure a backup circuit is readily available in case the circuit stops functioning. If the Pump Controlled Retrograde Trial-Off (PCRTO) technique (below) is adopted, it is very rare that this classic technique is needed.

### *Pump Controlled Retrograde Trial-Off (PCRTO)*

The pump controlled retrograde trial-off offers the advantage of permitting continued blood flow through the VA ECMO circuit and therefore eliminates the need for additional anticoagulation and significantly reduces the risk of circuit thrombosis.[1,2] The pump RPM is reduced until the patient's systemic pressure exceeds that generated by the ECMO pump and blood begins to flow in the reverse direction through the arterial cannula, around the ECMO circuit, before returning to the patient via the venous cannula. Depending on the pump manufacturer, it may be necessary to reverse the flow probe in order to measure the amount of retrograde flow. The pump now acts like a brake with increased RPM reducing the flow. A retrograde flow of around 100-150 mls/min is targeted because this is sufficient to maintain cannula patency without adverse effects on systemic blood flow and pressure. If retrograde flow is insufficient, then a 10 ml/kg bolus of fluid or a low dose epinephrine infusion (<0.1 µg/kg/min) may be all that is required to generate a sufficient driving pressure. With the sweep gas disconnected, the ventilation can then be adjusted as per arterial blood gas analysis. The bedside specialist needs to be aware that changes in the patient's arterial blood pressure lead to changes in flow and pump RPM may need adjusting throughout the trial-off. By utilizing this technique, it is possible to trial respiratory neonates cannulated for VA ECMO support for longer periods than with the classic technique. Trial-offs for up to 8 hours have been possible without circuit complications in neonates whose respiratory function remains marginal. As with a VV trial-off, the retrograde technique permits all drugs and CRRT running on the circuit to remain in place throughout the procedure with the need for additional intravenous access only once suitability for decannulation is established.

Occasionally, if a small 8 Fr arterial cannula is in situ and the clot burden in the oxygenator is such that the transmembrane gradient is higher than usual then this technique may fail, necessitating a return to the classic bridge technique.

### Leaving Cannulas in Place

Occasionally it is necessary to leave ECMO cannulas in place for a short period of time.[3,4] This eventuality may arise because of uncertainty regarding a patient's readiness to separate from ECMO, or for logistical reasons regarding OR and surgeon availability for decannulation. Finally, some patients on VV ECMO and CRRT may have difficult access for continued CRRT. In this situation the (dl)V-V or V-V single lumen cannulas can be used for continued hemofiltration. When electing to leave V-A neck cannulae in situ, the anticoagulation to the patient is continued and the cannula is flushed with heparinized saline 10 u/ml. This is achieved by cutting the tubing around 5 cm from the connector and inserting a blind ended ¼" ¼" leur connector with a pigtail. The blood is expelled from the cannula with the heparinized flush until the cannula is mostly clear of blood. An infusion of the same solution is then administered via the cannula at a rate of 1-5 ml/hr depending on institutional protocol. It is not recommended to use this technique to keep cannulas in for extended periods, but it

appears to be safe when used for a few hours or even overnight.

### Decannulation

The decision to decannulate is based on balancing several factors. These include resolution of the underlying disease process (eg, PPHN), development of complications such as intracranial hemorrhage, success margin of the trial-off, difficulty of recannulation, and finally the number and circumstances of previous trials off. This decision should be made by the multidisciplinary ECLS team, but the final casting vote must go to the person who will be tasked with recannulation in the event it is necessary. If recannulation is not to be offered in the event of subsequent deterioration this should be explicitly discussed with the parents prior to decannulation).[5,6] Informed consent should be obtained from the parents and documented according to institutional protocols. The procedure is different for the semi-Seldinger V-V cannulation, and for the V-V with ligation and V-A cannulation, which require formal surgical decannulation.

### *Semi-Seldinger V-V Decannulation*

The cannulation site is prepared and draped in the usual sterile fashion. The patient is placed 30 degrees head down, sedation is administered. Ketamine 1-2 mg/kg is often used. Paralysis is not essential but reduces the risk of air embolism, the risk of which is small in a patient receiving PEEP and in the Trendelenburg position. It is important to establish whether paralysis will lead to significant decreases in minute ventilation beforehand. For example, some patients may have satisfactory gas exchange when spontaneously triggering the ventilator but become hypercarbic when paralyzed. It is best to use a relatively short acting agent such as atracurium and adjusting mechanical ventilation to compensate for the loss of spontaneous effort. A horizontal mattress suture (u-stitch) is placed in the skin around the cannula using 2-0 silk (or equivalent). The patient is clamped off ECMO. As the cannula is removed by an assistant, the suture is tied. It is not usually necessary to hold pressure on the vein because there is rarely any bleeding. In fact, holding pressure is detrimental to underlying vein patency which is usually preserved by this technique. Apply a breathable dressing and reposition the patient. The suture can be removed after a week.

### *Formal Surgical Decannulation*

When the cannulas are ligated into the vessels, a formal surgical operation is required. Ensure that cross-matched blood is available at the patient's bedside. The patient is positioned as for cannulation, general anesthesia is administered, and the cannulation site is prepped and draped in the usual sterile fashion. The patient is clamped off and the circuit is recirculated around the bridge. The sutures which were used to close the cannulation wound are removed and the tip of the suction is used to remove blood clot, Surgicel, and exudate from around the vessels. If the cannulas have been in for more than 2 weeks, there may be healing around the vessels and dissection with electrocautery may be required. Gentle manipulation of the cannula in the vessel may aid in this, but beware if the cannula is loose in the vessel, or if the wound is obviously infected because vessel integrity may be compromised. It is best to approach one vessel at a time, with the artery being done first. The reason for this is that the arterial tissue is more robust than the vein and is less likely to disintegrate. Having the artery controlled gives different options for control of the vein. Place a right-angle instrument such as a Dennis-Brown around the carotid arterial cannula and use it to pull either a silastic vessel loop or a heavy silk tie around the artery. Clip each end of this separately on either side so that the loop will not interfere with the access. Dissect upwards and downwards so that the artery above and below the two ligation points is exposed. Put a vascular clamp on the artery caudal to the caudal ligature, only fasten it to one click. This serves to hold the cannula in. Using a 15 or 15c blade, cut the fixation sutures on the skin. Cut the cephalad ligature on the cannula, this leaves the cephalad ligation of the artery intact. Double check that the patient is clamped off ECMO. Hold the knot of the caudal ligature with DeBakey forceps. With a fresh blade, incrementally cut the caudal ligature near the knot using a stroking motion. It is usually possible to cut the ligature without damaging the artery. Hold the artery with DeBakey forceps behind the cannula, if the artery is transected hold the free edge of the arteriotomy instead. With the other hand hold the vascular clamp, ensure that you have an unobstructed view of the arteriotomy. Also ensure that your eyes are not directly in line with the vessel so that you are not blinded by the jet of blood. Release the clamp but keep it poised. Ask the assistant to remove the cannula on the command, apply the clamp. If reconstruction is planned, proceed (see below). If not, apply two titanium vascular clips to secure the artery, ensure that they are all the way across the vessel with no tissue in the clip apart from the artery. Apply one clip cephalad to the remaining ligature, remove the remaining ligature. Now remove the venous cannula in the same manner. Remember to warn the assistant that there is 6-8 cm in the patient and that there are multiple side holes. A natural reaction of inexperienced and insufficiently briefed assistants is to stop moving when they see blood. Of course, as soon as the first side hole of the cannula comes out of the vein it will bleed copiously, the remainder should be removed smartly. Only one vascular clip is needed on each end of the vein.

Irrigate the wound with antibiotic saline and obtain hemostasis as needed. If the wound appears relatively clean, a central venous catheter can be tunneled through the superior skin flap and inserted into the stump of the jugular vein.[7] The easiest technique is to use a micropuncture needle passed through the skin flap, holding the caudal stump in forceps in one hand and then advancing the needle in line with the vein whilst sucking on the syringe until blood is obtained. Usually this will be within 1 cm, care must be taken not to pass the needle into the chest. Having aspirated dark blood, pass the Seldinger wire then the micropuncture sheath, ensure it still aspirates freely, then exchange it for the line of choice. This line can then be removed as if it were percutaneously placed. The wound is closed by a single figure of eight Vicryl suture to bring the sternomastoid over the vessels. The skin is closed with either clips or interrupted monofilament sutures because it is usually quite inflamed.

If control of the artery is lost, it is often possible to grab it with DeBakey forceps and then either reapply the clamp or occlude it with a second pair of forceps. It can then be either secured with Ligaclips or oversewn with 5-0 Prolene. If the end cannot be grasped, digital pressure is applied which will usually achieve hemostasis. Once lost blood volume has been replenished and the hemodynamics have stabilized, the finger can be removed and the retracted end of the carotid can usually be found and grabbed in the few seconds before it starts bleeding again. Remember that the venous line is still in and can be used as a transfusion asset if required.

Once the arterial cannula is out and the artery secured or reconstructed, attention is turned to the venous cannula. If control of the vein is lost, and the steps described above for the artery are ineffective because the vein has disintegrated, it is possible to achieve hemostasis by the following method. The wound is rapidly closed with an over and over suture of the skin. The vein will bleed dramatically during this time and transfusion needs to keep pace. The wound is then compressed over the vein using a gauze swab which should achieve rapid hemostasis and restore stability. Pressure should be held without looking for 20 minutes. If bleeding recurs pressure should be reapplied for a further 20 minutes. This may need to be repeated until the anticoagulation has either worn off or been reversed. Using these two techniques it is almost never necessary to perform a median sternotomy to regain control.

Occasionally, the venous cannula may have been inserted by guidewire exchange of an in situ jugular central venous line. As such, the vein may not have been dissected during cannulation. In this case the artery can be decannulated as described above, the wound can then be closed, and the venous line can be removed using the V-V semi-Seldinger technique with a u-stitch in the skin. If the venous cannula and vein are seen during arterial decannulation, they should be decannulated surgically as described above.

**Vascular Reconstruction**

There is much institutional variation and discussion regarding whether the neck vessels should be reconstructed.[8-11] Against reconstruction is the risk of aneurysm formation,[12] risk of embolization, and long-term outcome of the reconstructed vessels. For reconstruction is the maintenance of four artery cerebral perfusion and the preservation of the vessels for future cannulation. Vessel reconstruction should not be attempted if the wound appears to be infected or severely inflamed, as is often the case after several weeks on ECLS. Neither should vessels be repaired if the anastomosis would be under tension. The two techniques in common use are direct closure of the arteriotomy and resection of the cannulation site with end-to-end anastomosis. Prior to reconstruction the artery and vein are bled from each end to ensure patency and that there is not clot present. Standard vascular surgical technique is used with magnification. Continuous 6-0 or 7-0 Prolene sutures are used. If the vein is fragile an interrupted technique with 8-0 Prolene can be used; however, reconstruction of small fragile veins is questionable in terms of long-term patency. Post reconstruction low dose anticoagulation such as heparin 10 u/kg/h or bivalirudin 0.05 mg/kg/h is continued until three doses of aspirin (1-5 mg/kg/day) have been given.

**Conclusion**

Coherent decision making, accompanied by smooth weaning, trialing-off and decannulation is essential in the delivery of high quality neonatal ECLS support. Clear communication with the parents is especially important during this phase of care. Particular attention should be directed to discussion regarding whether a second period of ECLS support is to be offered in the event of a recrudescence of primary illness.

# References

1. Westrope C, Harvey C, Robinson S, et al. Pump controlled retrograde trial off from VA-ECMO. ASAIO Journal. 2013;59(5).

2. Mattke CA, Haisz E, Pandya N, et al. Creating a controlled arterio-venous shunt by reversing the extracorporeal membrane oxygenation blood flow: A strategy for weaning patients off veno-arterial extracorporeal membrane oxygenation. Pediatric Critical Care Medicine. 2017 Oct 1;18(10):973–6.

3. Bobillo-Perez S, Cuaresma A, Girona-Alarcon M, et al. Weaning from neonatal and pediatric ECMO with stand-by cannula. Journal of Artificial Organs. 2021 Dec 1;24(4):507–10.

4. Thompson JL, Griffeth E, Rappa N, et al. Delaying Decannulation After Extracorporeal Membrane Oxygenation Is Safe and Advantageous. World journal for pediatric & congenital heart surgery. 2019 Jan 1;10(1):98–100.

5. Cooper DS, Thiagarajan R, Henry BM, et al. Outcomes of Multiple Runs of Extracorporeal Membrane Oxygenation: An analysis of the Extracorporeal Life Support Registry. Journal of Intensive Care Medicine. 2022 Feb 1;37(2):195–201.

6. Meehan JJ, Haney BM, Snyder CL, et al. Outcome after recannulation and a second course of extracorporeal membrane oxygenation. Journal of Pediatric Surgery. 2002;37(6):845–50.

7. Rauth TP, Scott BP, Thomason CK, et al. Central venous catheter placement at the time of extracorporeal membrane oxygenation decannulation: is it safe? Journal of Pediatric Surgery. 2008 Jan;43(1):53–8.

8. Sarioglu A, McGahren ED, Rodgers BM. Effects of carotid artery repair following neonatal extracorporeal membrane oxygenation. Pediatr Surg Int. 2000;16(1-2):15-8.

9. Duggan EM, Maitre N, Zhai A, Krishnamoorthi H, et al. Neonatal carotid repair at ECMO decannulation: Patency rates and early neurologic outcomes. Journal of Pediatric Surgery. 2015;50(1):64–8.

10. Spector ML, Wiznitzer M, Walsh-Sukys MC, et al. Carotid Reconstruction in the Neonate Following ECMO. Vol. 26, Journal of Pediatric Surgery. 1991.

11. Baumgart S, Streletz LJ, Needleman L, et al. Right common carotid artery reconstruction after extracorporeal membrane oxygenation: Vascular imaging, cerebral circulation, electroencephalographic, and neurodevelopmental correlates to recovery. The Journal of Pediatrics. 1994;125(2):295–304.

12. Jacobs JP, Goldman AP, Cullen S, Rocco D, Samanli U, Macrae DJ, Elliott MJ. Carotid artery pseudoaneurysm as a complication of ECMO. Ann Vasc Surg. 1997 Nov;11(6):630-3.

# 11

## Congenital Comorbidities and Extracorporeal Life Support for Respiratory Failure

*Kevin P. Lally, Javier Kattan, Yigit S. Guner, Matthew T. Harting, Denise M. Suttner*

Overall, use of ECLS in the newborn peaked in the early 1990s. Availability of nitric oxide, high frequency ventilation, and surfactant have resulted in a significant decline in several indications. Today, congenital diaphragmatic hernia (CDH) is the most common indication for ECLS in the newborn. The category "other" is the second most common (see Chapter 8). In this chapter, we discuss CDH as well as the other congenital comorbidities that may be faced both in determining indications as well as contraindications for initiation of ECLS.

### Congenital Diaphragmatic Hernia

As reported by the ELSO Registry, CDH is now the most common indication for neonatal respiratory ECLS. ECLS allows neonates with CDH the opportunity to recover from pulmonary hypertension and pulmonary hypertensive crisis, acute respiratory deterioration, and/or cardiac dysfunction. Approximately 30% of all CDH patients will receive ECLS and roughly half of infants undergoing ECLS for CDH do not survive. Although randomized clinical trials (RCT) have shown ECLS to be an effective intervention in neonatal respiratory failure, RCT-level evidence specific to CDH are lacking. In an effort to rectify this, Jancelewicz, using the CDH Study Group (CDHSG) data, showed that ECLS treatment results in improved survival, particularly among high-risk patients, compared to children treated with maximal medical management alone.[1] This study also highlighted the importance of high quality ECLS and the value of center CDH volume, showing that centers managing over 10 patients annually had significantly improved outcomes for high-risk patients with increased ECLS use. In light of this evidence, ECLS should be considered an important component in a multidimensional approach to CDH management. This section will highlight key recommendations and principles of ECLS for CDH. Recent ELSO guidelines include additional details specific to CDH.[2]

### Early Postnatal, Pre-ECLS Management

The primary goal of initial management after birth is to appropriately address the known, overarching pathophysiologic derangements, such as pulmonary hypertension, pulmonary hypoplasia, and cardiac dysfunction, mitigating progressive respiratory failure and cardiopulmonary decompensation. Many institutions have developed management guidelines such that the vast majority of infants with CDH after birth are managed with endotracheal intubation and mechanical ventilation.[3] Care should be taken to avoid ventilator associated trauma by keeping peak pressures below 26 mmHg, even with the initial intubation. Gastric decompression, arterial and venous access, and a controlled, calm environment are cornerstones of early management. Blood pH and gas exchange including preductal pulse oximetry, should be assessed, and monitored.[2,3] Chest radiography (Figure 11-1), echocardiography, and head ultrasonography provide critical information prior to ECLS initiation.

### Prenatal Diagnosis

Prenatal imaging can enhance the ability to predict severity of lung hypoplasia and subsequent outcome in CDH patients.[4-5] The most widely used and validated measure of prenatal CDH severity is the observed/expected lung-to-head ratio (o/e LHR), measured using ultrasound.[6] A second important marker of severity is the location of the liver or presence of liver herniation into the thorax ("liver up"). Magnetic resonance imaging (MRI)-based total fetal lung volume (TFLV) measurements have been shown to accurately predict the need

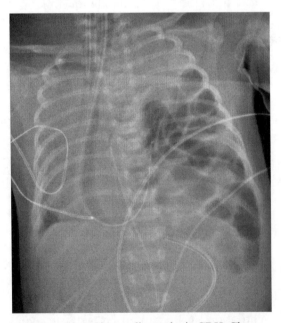

**Figure 11-1.** Chest radiography in CDH. Chest radiograph of a left CDH at diagnosis.

for ECLS in patients with CDH.[4] Syndromic presentation, abnormal genetic testing, and other significant anomalies including structural cardiac disease are important considerations for ECLS support. Major structural defects seen on fetal echocardiography require special consideration when determining ECLS candidacy.[7] In summary, a high risk of mortality and likelihood of ECLS may be expected with the following prenatal assessments[8,9]:

- LHR: <1 (less accurate outside gestational age 24-26 weeks),
- o/e LHR: <25%,
- Liver herniation: >20%,
- Observed/expected TFLV (o/e TFLV): <25%.

### Postnatal Risk Assessment

Between 20 and 40% of infants born with CDH are not detected prenatally. Multiple strategies for postnatal risk assessment exist.[10] The Brindle CDH mortality risk model is the updated version of the CDHSG equation and uses an integer score comprising low birth weight, low or missing Apgar scores, severe pulmonary hypertension by echocardiography, major cardiac anomaly, and chromosomal anomaly.[11] The probability of ECLS use in CDH patients can also be estimated using early postnatal blood gases and Apgar scores.[12] CDH-specific ECLS mortality risk models have also been developed and can be useful for risk assessment of both survivors and nonsurvivors.[13]

### Indications for ECLS

The degree of respiratory failure and overall magnitude of clinical illness in CDH depends on the severity of the existing pulmonary hypertension, pulmonary hypoplasia, and ventricular dysfunction. Therefore, most neonates with CDH who fail maximal management are candidates for ECLS, assuming there are no exclusion criteria. It is important to note that infants with CDH differ from other neonates with respiratory failure, such as meconium aspiration, given the anatomic changes in the thorax/vasculature, decreased lung volumes/degree of pulmonary hypoplasia, pulmonary hypertension secondary to pulmonary vasculopathy, and cardiac involvement.[14] Limits to medical management are different for CDH to avoid the cycle of hypoxemia, hypercarbia, acidosis, and barotrauma and volutrauma. When incorporated with a strategy of pressure-limited (gentle) ventilation and permissive hypercapnea, early use of ECLS may help minimize ventilator induced lung injury (VILI).[2] Many centers use a specific limit on ventilator parameters to avoid VILI and transition to ECLS support when a patient does not meet prespecified criteria.

Exceeding peak inspiratory pressure ($\leq$26 cm $H_2O$), HFOV to a MAP of 14-15 cm $H_2O$, and inability to maintain pH >7.2 (usually $PaCO_2$ <70 mmHg) are criteria commonly used as indications for ECLS.[2] General indications for ECLS in CDH are listed in Table 11-1.[15]

### Contraindications for ECLS

The most common contraindications to ECLS support in CDH are shown in Table 11-2.[13,16] ECLS support for neonates <34 weeks and <2 kg has been studied using the ELSO Registry.[17] Mortality rate was 71% for the BW <2 kg group, and 56.3% for the GA <34 weeks group. Low BW CDH infants had 2-fold increased odds of mortality compared to infants weighing >2 kg at birth.[17] For infants born with GA <34 weeks, there was a greater risk of severe

| ECMO INDICATION | RECOMMENDATIONS |
|---|---|
| Oxygenation & Ventilation Failure | 1. PIP >26-28 or MAP >15-18 to achieve preductal $O_2$ sats >85%. 2. Inability to achieve or maintain preductal $SpO_2$ >85% 3. Persistent severe respiratory acidosis ($pCO_2$ >70-80 mmHg) with pH <7.20 |
| Cardiovascular Failure | 1. Inadequate systemic oxygen delivery with metabolic acidosis 2. Severe refractory systemic hypotension 3. Severe left and/or right ventricular dysfunction |
| Acute Clinical Deterioration | 1. Preductal desaturation with inability to recover 2. Rapid cardiovascular deterioration 3. Escalating lactic acidosis |

**Table 11-1.** Indications for ECLS in patients with CDH.

| RELATIVE CONTRAINDICATIONS |
|---|
| Significant congenital anomalies (specific major cardiac or neurologic anomalies) |
| Lethal chromosomal abnormalities (Trisomy 18) or other lethal malformations |
| Grade III/IV intracranial hemorrhage |
| Weight <1.8 kg |
| Gestational age <32-34 weeks |
| Prolonged mechanical ventilation receiving prolonged high pressure (MAP >15-18 x 7 days) |

**Table 11-2.** Relative contraindications to initiating ECLS support in the CDH patient.

neurological events. This report showed that survival below 34 weeks of gestational age and 2 kg weight limit is possible, albeit with higher complications, consistent with other indications for ECLS.

Short-term survival is possible in patients with both CDH and congenital heart disease treated with ECLS.[18] Superimposed pulmonary hypoplasia/hypertension, with abnormal cardiopulmonary physiology, present difficult challenges when the goal is long-term survival, particularly congenital heart defects with single ventricle physiology. Paradoxically, high pulmonary vascular resistance (PVR) may delay increases in pulmonary blood flow, allowing time for interdisciplinary discussion. Use of ECLS in the setting of concomitant congenital heart disease and CDH should be done on a case-by-case basis and at centers with such experience.

### Mode and Pump Type for CDH

Infants with CDH often require more hemodynamic support compared to other conditions that require neonatal ECLS such as meconium aspiration. Traditionally, VA ECMO (used in more than 80% of CDH cannulations)-as opposed to VV ECMO (<20%)-is more commonly used.[19] Despite this, multiple studies have shown that patients with CDH can be effectively treated with both VA and VV ECMO modes. The most recent ELSO analysis did not identify any differences in mortality or rates of severe neurologic events when comparing VA and VV.[20] It is important to note that VV cannulation is not always anatomically possible due to venous vascular or mediastinal anatomic anomalies. Mediastinal shift is common and may make accurate cannula placement (with either VA or VV) difficult (Figures 11-2, 11-3). VV may not be possible in cases of extremely poor cardiac function such as significant biventricular dysfunction or in the rare setting of extracorporeal cardiopulmonary resuscitation (ECPR). Lastly, type of ECLS pump has also been specifically studied in a range of indications using ELSO data and, for patients <10 kg, roller pumps offered a survival advantage and centrifugal pumps were more likely to be associated with hemolysis.[21,22]

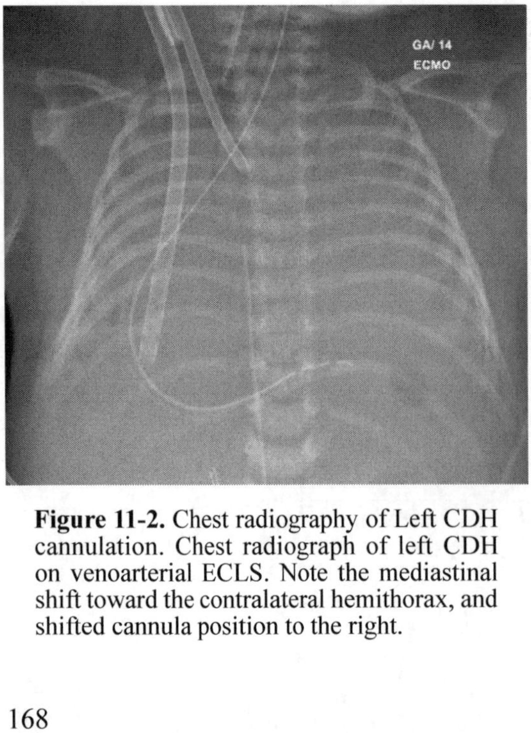

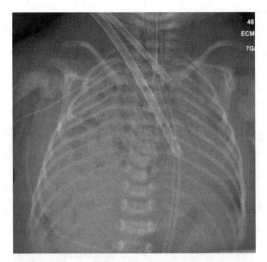

**Figure 11-2.** Chest radiography of Left CDH cannulation. Chest radiograph of left CDH on venoarterial ECLS. Note the mediastinal shift toward the contralateral hemithorax, and shifted cannula position to the right.

**Figure 11-3.** Chest radiography of Right CDH cannulation. Chest radiograph of right CDH on venoarterial ECLS. Note the mediastinal shift toward the contralateral hemithorax, and shifted cannula position to the left.

### Diaphragm Repair Relative to ECLS

Strategies for repair of the diaphragmatic defect in the setting of ECLS support include early repair (within 24-72 hours after cannulation), late repair prior to decannulation, or repair after decannulation (if able to discontinue ECLS). The challenges of surgery on ECLS include shifts in fluid status and increased risk of hemorrhage while anticoagulated. The potential advantages of surgery while on ECLS include avoidance of nonrepair (which has a 100% mortality), and the relief of intrathoracic compression early, allowing optimal pulmonary parenchymal expansion with pulmonary perfusion and restoration of normal anatomy.

Some evidence suggests that repair after decannulation is associated with optimal survival. A recent ELSO study evaluating 2224 patients with propensity matching showed that on-ECLS repair was associated with a greater than 3-fold higher odds of mortality compared with repair after ECLS.[23] Unfortunately, selection bias affects these studies, along with the inability to accurately risk stratify or predict successful weaning from ECLS. Also, there is an inability to account for the group of infants who died on ECLS prior to repair. In contrast, repair on ECLS may offer the best chance for survival. The most recent investigation from the CDH study group evaluated 1581 patients with CDH who received ECLS and performed two comparisons: 1) repair on ECLS to repair after ECLS, and 2) repair early on ECLS to repair later on ECLS. These groups were matched based on propensity scores and, importantly, the study accounted for nonrepaired patients. A center strategy of CDH repair on ECLS resulted in a 46% reduction in mortality rate compared to a strategy of repair after ECLS, while early repair on ECLS was associated with a 49% reduction in mortality rate compared to late repair on ECLS.[24] A risk-based strategy and an institution-based algorithm may be a hybrid approach which optimizes the strengths and minimizes the weaknesses regarding timing of diaphragmatic repair relative to ECLS, in that the highest risk infants who are unlikely to be weaned from ECLS may benefit from early repair at centers who do this routinely. Repair after ECLS is also a potentially valid option for specific infants with an optimized routine and with acknowledgment of the limitations of risk stratification, along with the potential for missing the repair window which optimizes survival.

The abdominal approach to repair is optimal for mitigating hemorrhage risk while allowing diaphragmatic defect repair (usually with a patch). Minimal dissection of the posterior rim of diaphragm is recommended, as this is an area of high risk for postoperative hemorrhage. Utilization of electrocautery and argon beam coagulation minimizes raw surface hemorrhage risk. A temporary abdominal closure (Gore-Tex® patch or temporary Silastic® sheet/silo) may be necessary and routine tube thoracostomy both allow the opportunity to expeditiously identify and correct hemorrhagic complications.[25] Surgicel®, Floseal®, or other hemostatic agents are used for coagulopathic hemorrhage. These measures collectively minimize bleeding risk and maximize the opportunity to identify and manage post-operative hemorrhage early.

Optimal management of anticoagulation prior to, during, and after the procedure must occur to limit bleeding complications. There is a dearth of evidence for optimal strategies in this area, so most institutional practices are based on anecdotal experience. Operating on ECLS includes the use of aminocaproic acid, decreasing anticoagulation parameters (such as ACT and/or Anti-Xa) to minimally acceptable levels, and optimizing platelet counts. Notably, there are a range of acceptable practices that vary based on surgeon and institutional experience and nuance.

### Length of Support and Weaning Strategies

According to ELSO data, CDH is the most common cause of neonatal ECLS runs >3 weeks.[26] Although prolonged ECLS support and second courses are associated with worse outcomes and increased risk of complications, more severe disease may require longer runs, and survival is possible after durations in excess of 4 weeks (Figure 11-4).[27] Data suggest that prolonged ECLS runs beyond 4-6 weeks may be of limited benefit, although universally accepted limits on length of treatment have not been established. Survival to discharge, related to length of ECLS treatment in CDH, has been shown to be approximately 50-60% after 2 weeks of ECLS, 40-50% at 3 weeks, and 20-40% at 4 weeks. After 5 weeks of ECLS, survival dropped to 15%, and after 40 days of ECLS support there were rare survivors.[27,28] Thus, arbitrary cutoffs for short duration of ECLS for CDH patients on ECLS may not be ideal. A prolonged run may be of benefit in selected patients.

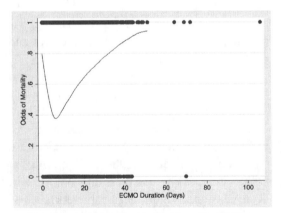

**Figure 11-4.** Survival over time in CDH patients receiving ECLS. Scatterplot of CDH patients in the ELSO database receiving ECLS (2000-2019, n= 5408 total patients) showing duration of ECLS management by mortality. Each dot represents an individual patient, with survivors on the 0 and deaths on the 1. Locally weighted scatterplot smoothing (LOWESS) curve demonstrates the association between ECLS duration and risk of mortality.

The ability to wean ECLS in the CDH patient is dependent upon recovery of ventricular function and improvement of pulmonary hypertension. Indicators of readiness to begin weaning include improvement in pulmonary hypertension, low ventilator settings, ventilator $FiO_2$ <0.4-0.5, adequate heart rate, minimal to no requirement for vasoactive support, and stable mixed venous oxygen saturation. Most CDH patients who receive ECLS demonstrate suprasystemic RV pressures on echocardiography, so a decrease in these pressures to subsystemic levels prior to decannulation is ideal, though not always achievable. In some cases, pulmonary hypertensive pharmacotherapy may be needed to improve cardiopulmonary function to either reach readiness for a trial off or facilitating a successful trial off. Options may include the use of sildenafil, bosentan, epoprostenol, and/or iNO. Their use may depend on institutional availability and practice patterns.

Protocols for trialing-off of ECLS vary by institution and by mode of support (see Chapters 10 and 19). If lung function is adequate at acceptable ventilator settings for a prolonged period of time, decannulation can be considered. The goal is to have a reasonable amount of latitude for worsening clinical condition such that increased need for ventilatory support and oxygenation can still be maintained. However, no specific guidance on ideal ventilator type or settings to optimize decannulation exist.

### Long-term Outcomes of CDH

CDH overall, and particularly those who receive ECLS, is associated with significant long-term morbidity. Overall, the reported incidence of chronic lung disease (CLD) in survivors of CDH is 33-52%, with ECLS utilization associated with a 9-fold increase in this complication. Many survivors require long-term treatment of pulmonary hypertension.[29] CDH survivors receiving ECLS also have an increased risk of growth failure. Up to 50-80% of CDH infants are diagnosed with clinical gastroesophageal reflux disease, with the highest risk seen in those requiring ECLS and/or a patch repair.[30] The potential for neurologic sequelae in CDH survivors is high, especially for those requiring ECLS hence, close neurodevelopment followup is warranted (see Chapter 12).

## Congenital Comorbidities and Neonatal ECLS

With the evolution of intensive care and ECLS, more complex and severe cases are selected to receive ECLS. Consequently, neonatal ECLS has seen an increase in mortality. Special attention to neonatal comorbidities during ECLS will help clinicians anticipate complications and perhaps impact outcome. Comorbidities related to ECLS for neonatal hypoxic respiratory failure (HRF) can be congenital or acquired. Congenital comorbidities are the primary focus of this section. Acquired conditions are discussed in Chapter 8.

### *Genetic*

ECLS has been used in children with genetic syndromes with good results, including high survival and few complications. Uppu conducted a retrospective review of children with congenital heart disease (CHD) and genetic syndromes who received ECLS and showed that ECLS duration, hospital LOS, and mortality were similar to patients without genetic abnormalities. In patients with genetic conditions, defined as chromosomal or syndromic abnormalities confirmed by a geneticist, renal insufficiency and need for dialysis were associated with mortality.[31]

### Trisomy 21

Cashen reported on 30 years of data from the ELSO Registry, including 623 patients with Down Syndrome (DS). During this period, there was no significant difference in survival between patients with or without DS.[32] Despite differences in indications for ECLS, by itself, the diagnosis of DS should not be considered a risk factor for ECLS.

### *Trisomy 13 and Trisomy 18*

In the 2013 ELSO Neonatal Respiratory Failure Supplement to the ELSO General Guidelines, both Trisomy 13 and 18 are listed as "lethal chromosome disorders" and contraindications to ECLS. In a 2016 article, Nelson reviewed the survival and surgical interventions for these diagnoses and found that, while most died in the first year of life, the 10-year survival was higher than previously reported.[33] A survey of ELSO Neonatal ECMO centers reported some would consider ECLS support for this population of patients.[34] In a recent review of the ELSO Registry, Alore found that while complications are frequent, the survival rate in 28 patients with Trisomy 13 and 18 was close to 45%. They concluded that these syndromes alone should not be viewed as absolute contraindications to ECLS, but rather considered during the evaluation of a patient's potential candidacy.[35]

### *Del22q11*

Prodhan compared institutional outcomes in patients with CHD on ECLS with and without del22q11 (DiGeorge) syndrome. Del22q11 syndrome did not confer a significant mortality or morbidity risk, including infectious complications or duration of ECLS.[36]

### *Pulmonary*

Disease categories for pulmonary congenital comorbidities can be grouped as: surfactant protein deficiencies, alveolar capillary dysplasia (ACD), anomalies of airways and lung parenchyma, thoracic dystrophies, and disorders of the diaphragm.

Neonates with an irreversible pulmonary dysplasia such as ACD, surfactant protein deficiency, and pulmonary lymphangiectasis may have a deteriorating clinical course requiring ECLS. These neonates are often difficult to distinguish from those with PPHN (Figure 11-5). However, an irreversible pulmonary dysplasia should be considered when ECLS is initiated on day of life ≥5 and/or the duration of ECLS ≥10 days.[37] In patients with an unusual presentation or ECLS course, further workup should be considered, including genetic testing and possible lung biopsy.

### *Gastrointestinal*

Congenital abdominal wall defects, especially omphalocele, may be associated with significant alterations in lung development. Although some patients may develop HRF, the use of ECLS to support these patients seems rare, likely due to the associated, irreversible pulmonary hypoplasia.[38]

### *Renal*

Newborns with congenital renal disease (CRD) may develop HRF from pulmonary hypoplasia, delayed lung maturation, or pulmonary hypertension.[39] Historically, the prognosis was poor, although successful support with ECLS in neonates with CRD has been reported.[39] Factors associated with successful

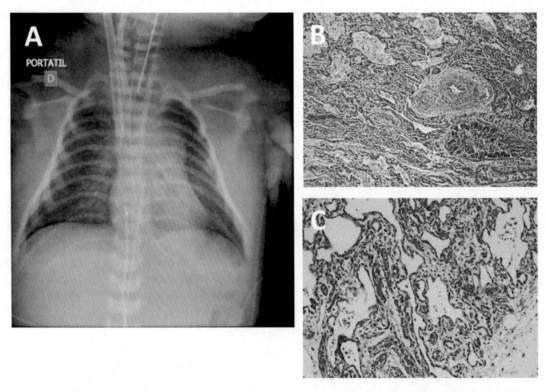

**Figure 11-5.** V-A ECLS in a newborn with PPHN, finally diagnosed as an alveolar capillary dysplasia by a biopsy. A: x-ray on ECLS; B & C: histology showing vascular and capillary misalignment.

long-term outcome include renal disease amenable to surgical correction, aggressive nutritional support, and a reliable social support system. Wightman utilized the ELSO Registry to investigate the prevalence and survival to discharge of neonates with underlying kidney disease who received ECLS from 1989 to 2012. The survival was much lower in neonates with kidney disease, 49% vs. 82% (pulmonary indication without congenital diaphragmatic hernia), 25% vs. 51% (pulmonary indication with congenital diaphragmatic hernia), and 21% vs. 41% (cardiac indication), suggesting that kidney disease be considered when evaluating ECLS candidacy.[40] Pre-ECLS evaluation should include serum creatinine and consideration for renal ultrasound if clinically warranted.

### Hematologic

A family history of blood dyscrasia should alert the clinician to possible hemostatic problems. Diagnostic confirmation in the neonatal period often proves difficult due to the dynamic nature of coagulation factors associated with gestational age and the impact of illness on neonatal levels. ECLS may mask congenital disorders due to consumption and replacement of coagulation factors. Suspicion of a congenital hematologic disorder may require workup after decannulation and disease recovery.

### Malignancies

The peak cancer incidence in children is the first year of life, and 13% of these cases are diagnosed in the neonatal period. The most common neonatal malignancies include neuroblastoma, leukemia, renal tumors, and sarcoma.[41] Some genetic conditions, such as Trisomy 21, are associated with neoplasms. Survival rates generally are lower for malignancies presenting in the neonatal period; however, newer drug therapies and interventions have resulted in a wide variation in survival rates and detailed evaluation of the malignancy is required for prognostication and will need to be considered to determine a neonate's candidacy for ECLS.

### Neurologic

### Hypoxic Ischemic Encephalopathy

Hypoxic Ischemic Encephalopathy (HIE) is associated with a poor prognosis.[42] Therapeutic hypothermia has become the standard treatment in neonates with moderate to severe HIE, with several trials showing improved long-term neurodevelopmental outcome.[43] Some patients with HIE will also have severe HRF and will meet criteria for ECLS.[44] With improved outcomes due to cooling, the decision regarding ECLS support in this high-risk population has become more complex. Currently, there are no clear set of measures that define how severe the damage must be to exclude an infant from ECLS. Additionally, the need to make a rapid decision in combination with medications such as narcotics, sedatives, and antiepileptic medications make performing a thorough neurologic evaluation to determine ECLS candidacy challenging. The decision to offer ECLS in this population has increased. Weems reported on a survey conducted in 2016. Compared to a similar survey in 2008, the number of providers who would never offer ECLS to a neonate with severe HIE decreased to 27% from 48%.[4]

### Vascular Variants

Common origin of the carotid arteries (COCA) is a normal anatomic variant reported in approximately 11% to 15% of the general population. Comparing institutional outcomes, Lamers found no difference in neurologic outcome or sequelae in neonates with and without COCA receiving VA ECMO. Despite concerns for vascular obstruction by the arterial cannula in this variant, COCA does not appear to increase the risk of neurologic injury.[46]

**Arteriovenous Fistula**

ECLS can support severely ill neonates with high-output heart failure secondary to intracranial arteriovenous fistula (AVF). Burry described the first successful novel approach to the management of high-output heart failure secondary to an intracranial AVF, performing an embolization in conjunction with ECLS. This was also the first report in which an ECLS cannula was used for intraarterial access for cerebral angiography.[47]

**Inborn Errors of Metabolism**

Acute signs of an inborn error of metabolism leading to clinical decompensation can present in a newborn as severe metabolic acidosis, cardiovascular failure and respiratory failure. Organic aciduria, urea cycle disorders, maple syrup urine disease, and fatty acid oxidation disorders can present with life threatening conditions. In addition to cardiac and respiratory support, ECLS in combination with hemodialysis can provide an efficient method to address hyperammonemia.[48]

**Conclusions**

Many neonates who meet ECLS criteria have comorbidities that may or may not impact outcome. The exclusion criteria for neonatal ECLS continues to evolve due to advances in care. Recent outcomes of ECLS in neonates reflect a more complex population. When time allows, thorough multiorgan evaluation and review of current guidelines remain important in determining ECLS candidacy.

# References

1. Jancelewicz T LM, Brindle ME, Stiles ZE, et al. Survival Benefit Associated With the Use of Extracorporeal Life Support for Neonates With Congenital Diaphragmatic Hernia. Ann Surg 2022;275:e256-e263.
2. Guner Y, Jancelewicz T, Di Nardo M, et al. Management of Congenital Diaphragmatic Hernia Treated With Extracorporeal Life Support: Interim Guidelines Consensus Statement From the Extracorporeal Life Support Organization. ASAIO J 2021;67:113-120.
3. Reiss I, Schaible T, van den Hout L, et al. Standardized postnatal management of infants with congenital diaphragmatic hernia in Europe: the CDH EURO Consortium consensus. Neonatology 2010;98:354-364.
4. Jani J, Cannie M, Sonigo P, et al. Value of prenatal magnetic resonance imaging in the prediction of postnatal outcome in fetuses with diaphragmatic hernia. Ultrasound Obstet Gynecol 2008;32:793-799.
5. Schaible T, Busing KA, Felix JF, et al. Prediction of chronic lung disease, survival and need for ECMO therapy in infants with congenital diaphragmatic hernia: additional value of fetal MRI measurements? Eur J Radiol 2012;81:1076-1082.
6. Snoek KG, Peters NCJ, van Rosmalen J, et al. The validity of the observed-to-expected lung-to-head ratio in congenital diaphragmatic hernia in an era of standardized neonatal treatment; a multicenter study. Prenat Diagn 2017;37:658-665.
7. Style CC, Olutoye OO, Verla MA, et al. Fetal echocardiography (ECHO) in assessment of structural heart defects in congenital diaphragmatic hernia patients: Is early postnatal ECHO necessary for ECMO candidacy? J Pediatr Surg 2019;54:920-924.
8. Oluyomi-Obi T, Kuret V, Puligandla P, et al. Antenatal predictors of outcome in prenatally diagnosed congenital diaphragmatic hernia (CDH). J Pediatr Surg 2017;52:881-888.
9. Kastenholz KE, Weis M, Hagelstein C, et al. Correlation of Observed-to-Expected MRI Fetal Lung Volume and Ultrasound Lung-to-Head Ratio at Different Gestational Times in Fetuses With Congenital Diaphragmatic Hernia. AJR Am J Roentgenol 2016;206:856-866.
10. Jancelewicz T, Brindle ME. Prediction tools in congenital diaphragmatic hernia. Semin Perinatol 2020;44:151-165.
11. Brindle ME, Cook EF, Tibboel D, et al. A clinical prediction rule for the severity of congenital diaphragmatic hernias in newborns. Pediatrics 2014;134:e413-419.
12. Jancelewicz T, Brindle ME, Harting MT, et al. Extracorporeal Membrane Oxygenation (ECMO) Risk Stratification in Newborns with Congenital Diaphragmatic Hernia (CDH). J Pediatr Surg 2018;53:1890-1895.
13. Guner YS, Nguyen DV, Zhang L, et al. Development and Validation of Extracorporeal Membrane Oxygenation Mortality-Risk Models for Congenital Diaphragmatic Hernia. ASAIO J 2018;64:785-794.
14. Harting MT. Congenital diaphragmatic hernia-associated pulmonary hypertension. Semin Pediatr Surg 2017;26:147-153.
15. Snoek KG, Reiss IK, Greenough A, et al. Standardized Postnatal Management of Infants with Congenital Diaphragmatic Hernia in Europe: The CDH EURO Consortium Consensus - 2015 Update. Neonatology 2016;110:66-74.
16. Barbaro RP, Bartlett RH, Chapman RL, et al. Development and Validation of the Neonatal Risk Estimate Score for Children Using Extracorporeal Respiratory Support. J Pediatr 2016;173:56-61.
17. Delaplain PT, Zhang L, Chen Y, et al. Cannulating the contraindicated: effect of low birth weight on mortality in neonates with congenital diaphragmatic hernia on extracorporeal membrane oxygenation. J Pediatr Surg. 2017;52:2018-2025.
18. Dyamenahalli U, Morris M, Rycus P, et al. Short-term outcome of neonates with congenital heart disease and diaphragmatic hernia treated with extracorporeal membrane oxygenation. Ann Thorac Surg 2013;95:1373-1376.
19. Guner YS, Khemani RG, Qureshi FG, et al. Outcome analysis of neonates with congenital diaphragmatic hernia treated with venovenous vs venoarterial extracorporeal membrane oxygenation. J Pediatr Surg 2009;44:1691-1701.
20. Guner YS, Harting MT, Fairbairn K, et al. Outcomes of infants with congenital diaphragmatic hernia treated with venovenous versus venoarterial extracorporeal membrane oxygenation: A propensity score approach. J Pediatr Surg 2018;53:2092-2099.
21. O'Halloran CP, Thiagarajan RR, Yarlagadda VV, et al. Outcomes of Infants Supported With Extracorporeal Membrane Oxygenation Using Centrifugal Versus Roller Pumps: An Analysis From the Extracorporeal Life Support Organization Registry. Pediatr Crit Care Med 2019;20:1177-1184.
22. Delaplain PT, Zhang L, Nguyen DV, et al. Effect of pump type on outcomes in neonates with congenital diaphragmatic hernia requiring ECMO. Perfusion 2018;33:71-79.
23. Delaplain PT, Harting MT, Jancelewicz T, et al. Potential survival benefit with repair of congenital diaphragmatic hernia (CDH) after extracorporeal membrane oxygenation (ECMO) in select patients: Study by ELSO CDH Interest Group. J Pediatr Surg 2019; 54:1132-1137.

24. Dao DT, Burgos CM, Harting MT, et al. Surgical Repair of Congenital Diaphragmatic Hernia After Extracorporeal Membrane Oxygenation Cannulation: Early Repair Improves Survival. Ann Surg 2021; 274:186-194.

25. Laje P, Hedrick HL, Flake AW et al. Delayed abdominal closure after congenital diaphragmatic hernia repair. J Pediatr Surg 2016;51:240-243.

26. Prodhan P, Stroud M, El-Hassan N, et al. Prolonged extracorporeal membrane oxygenator support among neonates with acute respiratory failure: a review of the Extracorporeal Life Support Organization registry. ASAIO J 2014;60:63-69.

27. Delaplain PT, Yu PT, Ehwerhemuepha L, et al. Predictors of long ECMO runs for congenital diaphragmatic hernia. J Pediatr Surg 2020;55:993-997.

28. Kays DW, Islam S, Richards DS, et al. Extracorporeal life support in patients with congenital diaphragmatic hernia: how long should we treat? J Am Coll Surg. 2014;218:808-817.

29. Wynn J, Krishnan U, Aspelund G, et al. Outcomes of congenital diaphragmatic hernia in the modern era of management. J Pediatr 2013;163:114-119.

30. Cortes RA, Keller RL, Townsend T, et al. Survival of severe congenital diaphragmatic hernia has morbid consequences. J Pediatr Surg. 2005;40:36-45.

31. Uppu SC, Goyal S, Gossett JM, et al. Extracorporeal membrane oxygenation in children with heart disease and genetic syndromes. Asaio J. 2013;59:52-56.

32. Cashen K, Thiagarajan RR, Collins JW Jr, et al. Extracorporeal membrane oxygenation in pediatric trisomy 21: 30 years of experience from the Extracorporeal Life Support Organization Registry. J Pediatr. 2015;167:403-408.

33. Nelson KE, Rosella LC, Mahant S, et al. Survival and surgical interventions for children with trisomy 13 and 18. JAMA. 2016;316:420-428.

34. Chapman RL, Peterec SM, Bizzarro MJ, et al. Patient selection for neonatal extracorporeal membrane oxygenation: beyond severity of illness. J Perinatol. 2009;29:606-611.

35. Alore EA, Fallon SC, Thomas JA, et al. Outcomes after extracorporeal life support cannulation in pediatric patients with trisomy 13 and trisomy 18. J Surg Res. 2021;257:260-266.

36. Prodhan P, Gossett JM, Rycus PT, et al. Extracorporeal membrane oxygenation in children with heart disease and del22q11 syndrome: a review of the Extracorporeal Life Support Organization Registry. Perfusion. 2015;30:660-665.

37. Lazar DA, Olutoye OO, Cass DL, et al. Outcomes of neonates requiring extracorporeal membrane oxygenation for irreversible pulmonary dysplasia: the Extracorporeal Life Support Registry experience. Pediatr Crit Care Med. 2012;13:188-190.

38. Baerg JE, Thirumoorthi A, Hopper AO, et al. The use of ECMO for gastroschisis and omphalocele: Two decades of experience. J Pediatr Surg. 2017;52:984-988.

39. Caesar RE, Packer MG, Kaplan GW, et al. Extracorporeal membrane oxygenation in the neonate with congenital renal disease and pulmonary hypoplasia. J Pediatr Surg. 1995;30:1560-1563.

40. Wightman A, Bradford MC, Symons J, et al. Impact of kidney disease on survival in neonatal extracorporeal life support. Pediatr Crit Care Med. 2015;16:576-582.

41. Linabery AM, Ross JA. Trends in childhood cancer incidence in the U.S. (1992-2004). Cancer. 2008;112:416-432.

42. Lee-Kelland R, Jary S, Tonk J, et al. School-age outcomes of children without cerebral palsy cooled for neonatal hypoxic-ischaemic encephalopathy in 2008-2010. Arch Dis Child Fetal Neonatal Ed. 2020;105:8–13.

43. Tagin MA, Woolcott CG, Vince MJ, et al. Hypothermia for neonatal hypoxic ischemic encephalopathy: an updated systematic review and meta-analysis. Arch Pediatr Adolesc Med. 2012;166:558–566.

44. Lakshminrusimha S, Shankaran S, Laptook A, et al. Pulmonary Hypertension Associated with Hypoxic-Ischemic Encephalopathy-Antecedent Characteristics and Comorbidities. J Pediatr. 2018;196:45-51.e3.

45. Weems MF, Upadhyay K, Sandhu HS. Survey of ECMO practices for infants with hypoxic ischemic encephalopathy. J. Perinatol 2018;38:1197–1204.

46. Lamers LJ, Rowland DG, Seguin JH. The effect of common origin of the carotid arteries in neurologic outcome after neonatal ECMO. J Pediatr Surg. 2004;39:532-536.

47. Burry M, Reig AS, Beierle EA, et al. Extracorporeal membrane oxygenation combined with endovascular embolization for management of neonatal high-output cardiac failure secondary to intracranial arteriovenous fistula. Case report. J Neurosurg. 2004;100:197-200.

48. Summar M, Pietsch J, Deshpande J, et al. Effective hemodialysis and hemofiltration driven by an extracorporeal membrane oxygenation pump in infants with hyperammonemia. J Pediatr. 1996;128:379-382.

# 12

## Complications, Followup, and Outcomes of Neonates with Respiratory Failure

*Hanneke IJsselstijn, Arno van Heijst, Aparna Hoskote*

## Introduction

The use of ECLS for life-threatening, reversible cardiorespiratory failure has transformed neonatal intensive care management, resulting in excellent survival outcomes over the years.[1-6] To date, almost 34.000 neonates have been treated with ECLS for neonatal respiratory failure, with an overall survival to discharge or transfer of 72% as reported to the ELSO Registry.[7] With such improved survival outcomes for neonatal ECLS, there is a growing population of childhood survivors. However, the long-term medical and neurodevelopmental outcomes remain of concern, particularly in certain diagnostic groups such as congenital diaphragmatic hernia (CDH).[4,5,8-11] If not appropriately identified and promptly managed, these may evolve over time into significant long-term neuropsychological sequelae with wide ranging implications for the health, education, and societal integration as these children grow into adulthood.[12]

In this chapter, we will review complications and survival outcomes and focus particularly on recently published data on long-term medical and neurodevelopmental outcomes after ECLS for severe respiratory failure in neonates. Outcomes in neonates with cardiac disease and those supported after extracorporeal cardiopulmonary resuscitation are covered in Chapter 22. We will discuss outcomes in neonates with CDH supported on ECLS separately because this subgroup is different with respect to survival rates and associated morbidities. Moreover, supported by the current literature, we will provide a structured framework and recommendations for multidisciplinary, longitudinal followup and discuss the recently published ELSO guidelines for followup.[13]

## Early Survival Outcomes and Complications

The survival outcome of neonates supported on ECLS for acute hypoxemic respiratory failure varies with the primary diagnosis, ranging from 97% in those supported for meconium aspiration syndrome (MAS) to as low as 50% in those supported for CDH.[1,14-18] The percentage survival to hospital discharge for different diagnostic categories is available on the ELSO Registry website.[7]

Due to the critical illness leading to ECLS and the complex nature of this therapy, neonates on ECLS are at risk of developing complications, some of which have significant impact on the outcome. The ELSO Registry reports an extensive list of complications within different categories in their biannual international summary.[19] In general, neonates who develop complications during ECLS have lower survival rates (Table 12-1).[19] We focus on some of the major complications that have an impact on survival and long-term outcome.

### *Bleeding, Thrombosis, and Hemolysis*

Complications related to bleeding, thrombosis, and hemolysis are relatively high and significantly add to the complexities of ECLS management in neonates. In a prospective observational study conducted in 8 hospitals (BATE study), Dalton et al. reported a high incidence of bleeding events (60%), thrombotic events (44%) and hemolysis (40%) in neonates on respiratory ECMO support. Circuit related thrombosis was reported in 40%, including entire circuit thrombosis in 28%, and bleeding related to cannula site (26%) and surgical

site bleeding (25%) was seen in a quarter of patients.[20] Surgical procedures such as repair of CDH on ECLS can also lead to substantial blood loss, requiring multiple blood transfusions.[21,22]

The management of anticoagulation on ECLS is often described as walking a tight rope balancing the risks of bleeding versus clotting. Factors unique to the neonatal population include developmental hemostasis coupled with hemostatic alterations that occur during ECLS.[23] Furthermore, mechanical factors such as small size of vessels, relatively large circuit volume to total blood volume, lower flows, and hemolysis from centrifugal pumps have been identified as important features that influence hematologic complications. In an ELSO Registry based propensity matched cohort study, O'Halloran et al. reported that hemolysis in centrifugal

| COMPLICATION | INCIDENCE | SURVIVAL |
|---|---|---|
| **Mechanical** | | |
| Thrombosis/clots in circuit | 33.6% | 53% |
| Cannula problems | 14.5% | 58% |
| Oxygenator failure | 5.4% | 51% |
| Pump failure | 0.6% | 48% |
| **Hemorrhagic** | | |
| Hemolysis (Hgb > 50 mg/dl) | 13.2% | 52% |
| Surgical site bleeding | 6.7% | 64% |
| Cannulation site bleeding | 6.3% | 64% |
| **Neurologic** | | |
| CNS hemorrhage (US/CT) | 7.3% | 41% |
| CNS infarction (US/CT/MRI) | 2.7% | 37% |
| Seizures | 2.4% | 51% |
| Other CNS hemorrhage | 4.0% | 37% |
| **Renal** | | |
| Renal replacement therapy required | 24.9% | 48% |
| **Cardiovascular** | | |
| Inotropes on ECLS | 14.1% | 58% |
| Cardiac arrhythmia | 4.3% | 53% |
| Hypertension(vasodilators) | 3.8% | 60% |
| **Pulmonary** | | |
| Pulmonary hemorrhage | 4% | 38% |
| **Infectious** | | |
| Culture proven infection | 2% | 37% |
| **Metabolic** | | |
| Hyperbilirubinemia | 9.7% | 48% |

**Table 12-1.** Important ECMO complications and outcome.[11]

pumps was associated with increased mortality in those weighing <10 kg, whereas Dalton et al. did not find any association of hemolysis and mortality. This issue continues to generate debate and discussion.[20,23,24]

### Neurological Complications

While mechanical complications related to thrombosis and clots in the circuit are most commonly reported (33.6%) in the ELSO Registry, neurological complications are the most worrying, with serious potential for mortality and significant neurologic morbidity in later life.[4,12,18,19,25-27] The prevalence of intracranial abnormalities in ECLS-treated neonates varies from 10 to 59%.[28] In an ELSO Registry study of 7190 neonates, Polito et al. reported that 20% of neonates developed neurologic complications, with significantly higher mortality than those without neurologic complications (62% vs. 36%).[29]

Based on severity and impact on outcomes, intracranial hemorrhage is a catastrophic complication.[30] It is also the most common patient-level complication that has shown to potentially add a further contribution of 28% to mortality.[18]

The BATE study identified relatively higher incidence of intracranial bleeding (22.5%) as compared to intracranial infarction (3%) in neonates on respiratory ECMO.[20] However, cerebral infarction from microthrombi may be altogether missed, undetected due to challenges in identification and thus underreported, leading to silent neurological injury that may potentially contribute to later neurologic morbidity.[19,30] Seizures during ECLS can result from hemorrhagic and/or ischemic lesions. The ELSO Registry reports an incidence of 2.4% and 5% (clinically evident and EEG confirmed, respectively), and they are associated with increased mortality and have a negative impact on neurodevelopmental outcomes.[29,31]

Risk factors for cerebral complications consist of individual risk factors and factors related to ECLS itself.[32] The pre-ECLS individual factors that have been identified to increase the risk of cerebral complications include lower gestational age at birth, birth weight < 3 kg, acidosis, pre-ECLS bicarbonate use, sepsis as the primary diagnosis, coagulopathy, age at initiation of ECLS, need for cardiopulmonary resuscitation prior to ECLS, prior ECLS exposure, fibrinogen concentration, VA ECMO, and use of therapeutic hypothermia.[32-34] Important risk factors related to ECLS therapy that are implicated in cerebral injury include disturbed autoregulation, alterations in cerebral blood flow, vascular cannulation, venous congestion, loss of arterial pulsatility, rapid shifts in carbon dioxide levels, blood pressure at initiation of ECLS, bloodstream contact with plasticizers, inflammatory response to ECLS, VA-bridge, bladder box alarms, and high intravascular volume administration.[32,35-38]

In a single-center study, Anton-Martin et al. showed that the traditional coagulation parameters were not different between the ones who developed neurological complications (intracranial hemorrhage and infarct) and the controls without neurological complications.[39,40] While it is important to meticulously monitor anticoagulation and maintain within therapeutic targets, it is crucial to remember that there may be a complex interplay of other interdependent and/or independent factors contributing towards cerebral injury.

There has been recent renewed interest in the concept of impaired cerebral autoregulation on ECLS.[37,38] Animal studies in the 1990s showed that both prolonged hypoxia, vascular ligation, and the initiation of ECLS can disturb cerebral autoregulation.[41,42] This has been postulated to be due to altered endothelial function as described in this animal model.[43] Disturbed autoregulation leads to ischemic lesions due to hypoperfusion or hemorrhagic complications due to hyperperfusion and can thus cause cerebral damage.[44]

In neonates with hypoxic ischemic encephalopathy, Cashen et al. reported that use of therapeutic hypothermia was independently associated with intracranial hemorrhage during the first 7 days of ECLS.[33] This is in contrast with an ELSO Registry study which found no differences in complications or mortality with hypoxic ischemic encephalopathy between those neonates who did and did not receive therapeutic hypothermia.[45]

### Renal Complications

In neonates on ECLS, acute kidney injury (AKI) is a commonly seen important complication and up to 25% of neonates may need renal replacement therapy.[19,46-49] Pre-ECLS factors such as lower pre-ECLS pH, need for cardiorespiratory resuscitation, inotropic drugs, the use of VA ECMO, and high lactate levels predominate as predisposing risk factors.[30,49] Zwiers et al. in their study of 242 neonates on ECLS, reported AKI in 64%: 30% qualified as at risk, 23% as injury and 11% as failure.[48] Dalton et al. reported that the presence of hemolysis (daily plasma free hemoglobin) was independently associated with development of renal failure during ECLS but not mortality. Furthermore, use of in-line renal replacement therapies may in turn increase hemolysis.[50] Neonatal nonsurvivors experienced more AKI than survivors (OR 3.2; p<0.001) and underwent more often renal replacement therapy (OR 2.5; p<0.001).[46] Liao et al. also found increased mortality in neonates with AKI.[49] Neonates with renal complications tend to have a longer ECLS run time.[47] Development of AKI and need for renal replacement therapy mandates appropriate dose adjustment of renally eliminated drugs and avoidance of nephrotoxic drugs.[51] Long-term followup of children with previous AKI on ECLS is described below.

### Infection

Critically ill neonates on ECLS are at increased risk of developing nosocomial infections and the incidence ranges from 2% in the ELSO Registry to 4.6% in other literature, depending on definitions used.[52] Bizzaro et al. reported an incidence of culture proven infection of 10.1/1000 ECLS days in neonates. The longer the ECMO run, use of VA ECMO, and a greater number of procedures for ECMO cannula placement have been reported as risk factors for acquired infection during ECMO.[53,54] The most common organisms include coagulase negative staphylococci and candida spp, and hence close surveillance and prompt treatment is important. Infections are associated with higher mortality rates and longer durations of hospital stay.[19,52] There is no current evidence to support use of prophylactic antibiotics for the prevention of nosocomial infections.[52]

### Key Factors Influencing Outcome

The key factors that influence outcome are patient selection, pre-ECLS status, the primary diagnosis and ECLS indication, timing of initiation of ECLS, associated morbidities, the ECLS run itself (type of cannulation, duration of ECLS, complications on ECLS), and post-ECLS morbidity and course.[1,15,55] It is notable that the use of VA ECMO has emerged as an important risk factor for complications. Over time, VA ECMO has become the most frequently used mode for neonatal respiratory failure, reflecting in part the preselection of sicker patients with hemodynamic instability for advanced life support, and to a lesser extent the nonavailability of appropriate VV cannulas. This change in the landscape of critically ill neonates requiring ECLS has led to longer ECLS run times, higher mortality rates, and increased long-term sequelae in survivors. Decreasing ECLS-related complications and ensuring long-term followup is essential in optimizing outcomes from this technically complex life-saving therapy for a specific subset of critically ill neonates.

It is important to recognize that not only complications arising during ECLS runs influence short-term outcome (survival) and long-term outcome (neurodevelopment). Very few of these risk factors are modifiable. A multicenter, randomized controlled trial conducted in the UK to study the benefit of systemic hypothermia in neonates supported on ECLS showed no benefit of hypothermia versus normothermia, but did highlight that up to 50% of neonates at 2 years had some form of neurodevelopmental issues as assessed by formal testing with Bayley Scales of Infant Development.[56]

Table 12-2 outlines the potential determinants of impaired outcome following neonatal ECLS.

## Late Survival Outcomes

Few studies describe long-term survival after neonatal ECLS. There is attrition over the years, influenced mainly by the presence of comorbidities related to the primary diagnosis and sequelae from complications. Iguchi et al. showed in a single-center retrospective study of 741 children (neonates and pediatric respiratory ECMO) that late death was related to comorbidities. Infants who were alive at 90 days had five-year survival estimates that were highest for MAS 97.9% (95% CI, 92.0-99.5%) and lowest for CDH 73.6% (52.3-86.5%).[14]

| OUTCOME PARAMETER | RISK FACTOR |
|---|---|
| Lung function/airflow obstruction | Diagnosis of RDS, diagnosis of CDH, prolonged duration ECMO, chronic lung disease |
| Exercise capacity | No significant determinants reported |
| Physical growth | Diagnosis of CDH |
| Sensorineural hearing loss | Diagnosis of CDH, prolonged duration ventilation,* prolonged duration ECMO, sepsis/bacterial meningitis,* administration of aminoglycosides,* severe birth asphyxia,* intracranial abnormalities,* clinical seizures before ECMO |
| Motor function development | Chronic lung disease, intracranial abnormalities, low feelings of social competence, reduced sport participation, diagnosis of CDH, duration of hospitalization |
| Intelligence | Low maternal education level, diagnosis of CDH, duration of hospitalization |
| Neuropsychological outcome | Highest mean airway pressure before ECMO, structural brain abnormalities, maximum vaso-inotropic score, chromosomal abnormality, acute neurologic event on ECMO, time to lactate clearance |
| Behavior | Need for extra help at school |
| *not specific for ECMO-treatment but for neonatal intensive care treatment; CDH=congenital diaphragmatic hernia; ECMO=extracorporeal membrane oxygenation; RDS=respiratory distress syndrome | |

**Table 12-2.** Potential determinants of impaired outcome following neonatal ECMO.[7]

## Long-term Medical Outcomes in Children without CDH

### *Lung Function*

Despite the fact that severe respiratory failure is the most common indication for ECLS in the neonatal period, lung function at followup usually reveals only mildly reduced forced expiratory flows. In survivors of the only randomized controlled neonatal ECLS trial recruited between 1993 and 1995, Beardsmore et al. showed slightly better lung function at 1-year followup in ECLS-treated children than in children receiving conventional treatment.[57] Lung function results of these UK ECMO Trial survivors did not significantly differ from those of a cohort of ECMO-treated infants born several years later.[58] In neonatal ECLS survivors, airflow obstruction is usually mild at school and adolescent age[11] and it remains stable over time in those without CDH.[12,59] Unfortunately, data on lung morphology after neonatal ECLS treatment is currently not available. Risk factors reported in the literature for persistent airflow obstruction after neonatal ECLS are: diagnosis of respiratory distress syndrome, CDH, prolonged duration of ECLS support, and having chronic lung disease (CLD).[12]

### *Exercise Tolerance*

Maximal exercise capacity at school age in ECLS survivors has been reported to be normal after ECLS for meconium aspiration syndrome or decreased in comparison to healthy peers in larger series that also included children who needed neonatal ECLS for other diagnoses.[12,60]

In a longitudinal study of 120 neonatal ECLS survivors aged 5 to 12 years, maximal exercise tolerance deteriorated significantly over time, irrespective of the underlying diagnosis.[61] Maximal exercise tolerance did not have any significant relationships with: time on ECLS, duration of ventilatory support prior to ECLS, total duration of ventilatory support, prevalence of CLD, physical growth parameters, spirometry results, and sports participation. Interestingly, the levels of exercise capacity estimated by the parents correlated positively with the measured maximal exercise tolerance scores.[61]

### *Renal Function*

Neonates with acute kidney injury (AKI) during critical illness and ECLS are at risk of developing chronic kidney disease (CKD) in childhood.[46,48,62] In a group of 169 neonatal ECLS survivors both with and without AKI, at least one sign of chronic kidney disease (proteinuria or eGFR <90 ml/min per 1.73 m$^2$) and/or hypertension was observed in 54 (32%) of children at a mean age of 8 years.[62] There is underappreciation and more often no long-term monitoring and screening for CKD in neonatal ECLS survivors.

### *Somatic Growth*

Physical growth is usually normal in children who required neonatal ECLS for diagnoses other than CDH.[12,63]

### *Vision*

Visual impairment is uncommon in children who underwent neonatal ECLS. At the 7-year followup of survivors recruited in the UK ECMO trial, seven (12.5%) children had mild to severe visual impairment, with only one having severe impairment, in comparison to 5.9% of controls with any kind of visual impairment.[5] Madderom et al. reported normal vision in 93.2% of five-year-old neonatal ECLS survivors, with only one child who had severe visual impairment.[25]

## Sensorineural Hearing Loss (SNHL)

Bilateral sensorineural hearing loss (SNHL) has been reported with a prevalence ranging from 3%-26% in early studies on neonates who received ECLS in the 1980s and 1990s.[64-66] A more recent Dutch study in 136 five-year-old neonatal ECLS survivors born between 1992 and 2005 reported a much lower prevalence at 3.7%.[67] Risk factors identified relate to the pre-ECLS clinical condition (seizures, $PaCO_2$ <30 mmHg, pH >7.5, use of furosemide) and neonatal intensive care therapies such as the use of aminoglycosides, neuromuscular blocking agents, and loop diuretics rather than ECLS-treatment itself.[8,12,66,68] This is attested by the finding that the proportion of SNHL was same (12%) in both the ECLS-treated and the conventionally treated neonates in the UK ECMO trial.[8] New studies are needed to establish whether innovations in intensive care treatment modalities have reduced the incidence of SNHL in neonatal ECLS survivors.

However, late presentation and identification of SNHL has been described despite normal initial clinical auditory brainstem responses before neonatal ICU discharge, which highlights the need for early, routine, audiologic evaluations throughout childhood for all ECLS survivors.[69] Early detection of hearing loss also provides a significant advantage for language and communication skills which is supported by the fact that in the Dutch study, language development was favorable.[67]

## Long-term Neurodevelopmental Outcomes

Neurodevelopmental sequelae are commonly described in several ECLS followup studies.[35,70,71] We describe the different neurodevelopmental and neuropsychological outcomes.

## Neuropsychological Development

The mental development scores of neonatal ECLS survivors when tested at the preschool age are generally favorable, with several reporting normal development, both with respect to overall cognition, and speech and language development.[4,67,72] In the UK ECMO trial, severe disability (defined as developmental quotient <70 on the Griffiths Mental Developmental Scales) was found in only 4% of ECMO-treated infants at 1 year and 17% at 4 years of age.[4,8] Interestingly, one third (33%) of the survivors experienced hyperactivity or behavioral difficulties when tested at 4 years.[8]

A recent study of neonatal ECLS survivors (n=24) reported developmental delay in nine children on assessment at 36 months with the Ages and Stages Questionnaire (parent administered questionnaire), with two-thirds showing abnormalities (ischemic changes, hemorrhage, or white matter changes) on magnetic resonance imaging (MRI) brain scan. In contrast, MRI abnormalities were noted less frequently in children without developmental delay.[73] In another study of 56 neonates who underwent neuroimaging (MRI or CT) post ECLS, 59% had ischemic and/or hemorrhagic abnormalities that correlated significantly with survival and pediatric cerebral performance score evaluated 3-4 years post ECLS discharge.[74]

Studies of children, when assessed at 5 years of age, have reported normal range of intelligence with one reporting language development even above average population norms.[25,75-77] However, at this age, new problems such as difficulties with visual-spatial and memory tasks may become apparent, which are often associated with concomitant behavioral problems such as hyperactivity, somatic complaints, and reported impaired health.[8,25,75]

Few studies have reported on neuro-developmental outcomes after the age of five years. In those tested, normal range intelligence scores at school age were not an unusual finding.[9,76] In the UK ECMO Trial, the cognitive outcome classification at 7 years of age was normal in 68% of the ECMO survivors and 70% in the conventionally treated group.[5] However, in the UK trial, 39% of children needed either special support at regular education or special educational needs. In a nationwide Dutch cohort, this was noted even in 48% of ECLS survivors.[5,9] Both studies reported problems with visual and spatial information-processing, hyperactivity, and attention or concentration problems (low working-speed).[5,9] These sometimes subtle neurodevelopmental deficits that preschool and school age children experience can put them at higher risk for school failure when compared to healthy children.[75,78] More profound neuropsychological assessments at 8 years in a cohort of children who survived neonatal critical illness revealed that intelligence was average, but children had problems with sustained attention and both immediate and delayed verbal memory as well as visuospatial memory.[26] The maximum dose of vasoactive medication was negatively associated with verbal and visuospatial memory, leading to the speculation that early cerebral hypoperfusion may have contributed. That similar findings were observed in children with CDH—also the group who did not need ECLS support—suggests that the severity of neonatal critical illness rather than treatment with ECLS determines these long-term neurodevelopmental problems.[26] A recent review of studies that used advanced neuroimaging techniques support this assumption.[79]

Parents reported more somatic problems for their 8-year-old children when compared to healthy peers.[9] On a positive note, these children seem to possess well-developed self-confidence and self-esteem.[9]

Thus far, only one study reported on neurodevelopmental assessments after school age. Adolescents treated with neonatal ECLS showed problems with short-term and long-term verbal memory, visual-spatial memory, and working memory. They reported more withdrawn or depressed behavior, somatic complaints, and social problems. However, they also reported positive feelings of self-esteem and an average health status.[27]

A recent U.S. study of adults who underwent ECLS for neonatal respiratory failure confirmed these positive feelings and less use of health care services in the past 12 months compared to national cohorts.[80] Interestingly, this study cohort had more education than national cohorts but learning problems were reported by 29.5%, along with significant limitations of physical, mental, and developmental domains. The results of this study may be biased by the low response rate of 8.9% of eligible candidates.[80]

Neonatal ECLS survivors without severe neurologic impairment usually have a neuropsychological profile that is characterized by an average intelligence; however, with significantly lower scores on attention or concentration (linked to working-speed and information processing speed) and memory tasks. Selective memory loss in late childhood has been identified in neonatal ECLS survivors without overt neurological impairment; however, a significant proportion did have reduced bilateral hippocampal volumes on brain MRI scans.[81,82] These problems highlight a significant concern because they put the children at risk of encountering difficulties as they get older when more demanding tasks require information to be processed faster, attention or concentration needs to be held longer, and more information must be stored in the (working) memory. These more subtle learning deficits can be classified as 'executive functioning skills'; skills needed to develop academic, behavioral, and social functioning. As these neuropsychological functions start to develop in early childhood but continue into young adulthood, these children are at risk for 'growing into deficits'.[83] Evaluation of intelligence is insufficient to detect neuropsychological deficits in an adequate and timely manner. When intervention is not provided at a young age, the neuropsychological deficits may put the child in a downward spiral, leading to academic failure and in consequence to emotional and behavioral problems. Children with visuospatial memory deficits may benefit from Cogmed Working Memory Training and timely guidance by local educational services should be advocated.[84]

### Motor Function Development

At preschool age, the motor function development scores of neonatal ECLS survivors are usually favorable, too.[12,72] In the UK ECMO Trial, significant motor function delay (scores <-2 SD) at 1 year of age was observed in 9% of ECMO-treated neonates and in 8% of those who had been treated conventionally.[4] However, when motor function tasks become more complex at older age, neonatal ECLS survivors here also seem to grow into their deficits: while 84% were reported normal at 1 year, only 43% reported normal at 5 years.[4,5] In the longitudinal nationwide Dutch study of neonatal ECLS survivors in the Netherlands, motor function performance was evaluated at 5, 8, and 12 years. Motor function was normal in 74, 75, and 41%, respectively.[85] Most problems were encountered with gross motor function, ie, ball skills and balance skills.[85] Interestingly, their actual motor function was worse than self-perceived motor function. In the same nationwide Dutch cohort, Toussaint and coworkers showed that in 135 eight-year-olds, standard deviation scores of perceived motor competence, social competence, and self-worth were all significantly higher than in healthy children: 0.18(0.94); 0.35(1.03); and 0.32(1.08), respectively. Self-reported feelings of social competence did correlate weakly but significantly with actual motor performance, but perceived motor competence and feelings of self-worth did not. The same cohort reported that their overall quality of life was impaired.[86]

This suggests that neonatal ECLS survivors may 'overrate' their actual motor performance and that monitoring of actual motor performance and education provision are important to enable timely and successful intervention. Further studies are needed to determine whether their parents are able to estimate adequately the motor performance.

## Outcomes Following ECLS in Congenital Diaphragmatic Hernia

### Medical Outcomes

**Lung Function.** Not surprisingly, CDH patients who need ECLS treatment are those with the most hypoplastic lungs and the most severe critical illness, needing prolonged ventilation and intensive care treatment. A longitudinal study on infant lung function testing in CDH patients at 6 and 12 months showed evidence of hyperinflation and abnormal airway patency indicative of impaired lung growth. Hyperinflation was most prominent in ECLS-treated infants who developed CLD.[59] The first studies in ECLS-treated CDH patients showed that lung function deteriorated over time: mean (SD) z-score $FEV_1$ decreased from -0.71 (0.40) at 5 years to -2.73 (0.61) at 12 years.[87,88] Later studies in children with CDH at school age—also the ones who did not need neonatal ECLS—revealed persistent airflow obstruction and reduced diffusion capacity which was more severe in children who had been treated with neonatal ECLS. Deterioration of airflow obstruction between 8 and 12 years was observed in all CDH patients, irrespective of ECLS treatment.[89] Worsening of airflow obstruction over time was recently confirmed; diaphragmatic defect size and need for oxygen at discharge but not ECLS-treatment had been reported as independent risk factors.[90] Ventilation-perfusion mismatch as a result of perfusion deficits on the ipsilateral side seem to deteriorate over time as well, especially in those with large diaphragmatic defects and need for oxygen at discharge.[91] Longitudinal MRI lung perfusion measurements have shown significantly reduced perfusion MRI values at 2 years in those who needed ECLS.[92] At 10 years, similar reduction of ipsilateral lung perfusion values was observed, with significantly lower pulmonary blood flows in those who needed neonatal ECLS. The ipsilateral pulmonary blood flow correlated positively with spirometric $FEV_1$.[93]

A significant deterioration of $FEV_1$ but to a much lesser extent has also been described in a longitudinal study of conventionally ventilated young adult CDH patients with mean (SD) z-score $FEV_1$ decreasing from -0.8 (1.2) to -1.3 (1.4) between 12 and 26 years of age.[88] Evaluations of lung function in young adults born with CDH who underwent neonatal ECLS treatment are currently being performed.

To date, only one study on long-term development of lung morphology using hyperpolarized $^3$He MRI in CDH patients is available, showing microstructural changes with significant differences in the ipsilateral and contralateral lungs.[94] In a case-control study of school-aged children with CDH, CT scans showed significantly more frequent subpleural triangles, architectural distortion, and linear opacities in CDH that in healthy controls.[95] In this single center cohort, the use of ECLS was not reported.

**Exercise Tolerance.** Although maximal exercise tolerance in ECLS-treated CDH patients tended to be worse than in other neonatal ECLS survivors, this difference was not statistically significant.[61] Maximal exercise capacity longitudinally evaluated in children with CDH at 5, 8, and 12 years has shown that the exercise capacity was below normal in all and deteriorated over time, with significantly lower values in those who underwent neonatal ECLS. It was negatively associated with duration on initial hospital stay and positively with diffusion capacity of the lungs.[96]

**SNHL.** Recently published data on SNHL in CDH patients show contradictory results, with the prevalence of significant SNHL ranging from 2.5% to 32%.[67,97-99] Differences may be partly explained from age at followup and selection bias. Illness severity (eg, need for prolonged ventilation or ECLS) is a predictor of SNHL in this population.

### Neuropsychological Development

A recent study of fetuses with CDH has identified small cerebellum and reduced middle cerebral artery flows on prenatal ultrasound examinations. However, the clinical significance for neurodevelopment is subject to future studies.[100] From the currently available data on neurodevelopmental outcome, it seems that the pathway of neuropsychological development in ECLS-treated CDH survivors is comparable to that of neonates treated with ECLS due to other underlying diseases. However, the CDH survivors are the ones that seem to experience the greatest deficits. Still, most studies reporting on neurodevelopment in children born with CDH within the first years of life do not provide separate data for the ECLS patients. Overall, the cognitive and language development scores at preschool age are normal to mildly delayed and the need for ECLS—amongst other factors indicating disease severity—is reported as an independent predictor of impaired mental development.[101,102]

At school age, intelligence is found in the average range but at eight years the mean (SD) IQ score was 84 (12) and 100 (20) in ECLS-treated and non-ECLS treated CDH patients, respectively.[26,103,104] Mean intelligence in ECLS-treated CDH children was 10 points lower than those who underwent ECLS for other underlying diagnoses in the neonatal period.[26] Eight-year-olds—both ECLS-treated and non-ECLS treated CDH patients—also experience concentration and attention problems, and have impaired verbal and visuospatial memory problems.[26,103] ECLS-treated CDH patients have significantly lower scores on visual motor integration compared with other neonatal ECLS patients; however, these scores are in the average range.[9] Verbal and visuospatial memory problems in children with CDH were not significantly worse than in children who needed ECLS for other causes of neonatal respiratory failure.[26] The children report that their perception of general health is reduced when compared to the reference norm, positively, they also report to have a well-developed feeling of self-confidence.[86,103]

*Motor Function*

Preschool motor development scores in CDH patients are usually reported to be normal or below the norm and seem to improve between 1 and 3 years of age.[101,102,105] In a study of 47 children with CDH where 26% were treated with ECLS, mild to severe motor function delay was reported in 45% and 19% at 1 and 3 years, respectively. At 5 years, 47% of ECLS-treated CDH children had normal motor function, the remaining 53% had motor delays, mainly in the gross motor function domains.[104]

Longitudinal evaluation of motor performance through the years (5-8-12 years), revealed that children born with CDH who needed ECLS experience motor problems at all ages.[85,104] A recent longitudinal study in children with CDH showed that motor performance was below normal at 5 years irrespective of ECLS treatment. However, at 8 and 12 years, the estimated mean z-scores for motor function in non-ECLS treated participants were not significantly lower than the norm scores, whereas the scores of ECLS-treated children with CDH were.[106] Irrespective of ECLS treatment, the length of initial hospital stay was significantly negatively associated with motor performance.[106]

**Recommendations for Long-term Followup**

All neonatal ECLS survivors should have general and specialist followup regardless of whether they have suffered neurological complications on ECLS.[13] Long-term followup should be offered as a standard of care in a structured and standardized approach.

There are multiple risk factors (eg, significant hypoxemia, severe acidosis, hemodynamic compromise, cardiac arrest, or acute neurological events on ECLS) that may categorize some neonates at increased risk for neurodevelopmental difficulties (see Appendix, p.773). It is important to identify and recognize these risk factors from the start of ECLS therapy and institute a structured, longitudinal followup for all neonates from discharge to adolescence tailored to the needs of the child and family.[13]

Most single-center published studies that have incorporated followup have used standardized assessments. However, substantial heterogeneity occurs with different instruments used for assessments at variable followup intervals after ECLS. The assessment tools recommended for use in any followup program have to be guided by culturally appropriate and locally available tests with age-appropriate references. As of now, there is no universal reporting of long-term outcome in the ELSO Registry. Restricting focus exclusively to hospital discharge offers an incomplete understanding of the relationship between therapy and disease, and their combined effects on health in later life.[107]

Routine standardized followup programs are offered by very few ECLS programs. A recent European survey of neurological followup reported marked variability in neurodevelopmental followup as well as in neuromonitoring practices during ECLS.[108] Longitudinal studies from the Netherlands have unequivocally demonstrated the value and benefits of early identification and intervention to the children and their families.[9,25,84,85] Other

ECLS programs have conducted followup assessments with a view to understanding the prevalence of the problem or as part of research trials, but few have long-term followup by a multidisciplinary team of specialists.[4,5,8,10,56,72,75,109-111] However, patients in followup studies are subject to an inherent selection bias because there is a higher mortality in those with neurologic complications on ECLS.[19] In addition, children who survive with severe neurodevelopmental disabilities might either refuse to join followup programs or, when they participate, be unable to perform the standardized tests. These children usually show lifelong morbidity related to cerebral damage and profound mental and motor disability. Since predictability of outcome increases when the outcome at young age is more severe, followup of these patients should focus on providing optimal management of their disabilities and preventing further complications.[112] In addition, honest evaluation of the costs and benefits of ECLS treatment for this group of children is desirable because insight into this matter, apart from 4- and 7-year evaluation of the UK neonatal ECMO trial, is largely lacking.[113,114]

Neonatal ECLS survivors without 'overt' neurologic complications usually have favorable outcomes in the first years of life, but they are at risk for academic, behavioral, and motor function problems at later age for which they need to be monitored. For this group, more subtle insults to the brain might have led to minor lesions, which may interfere with normal brain maturation. Moreover, they are at risk for reduced maximal exercise capacity, chronic kidney disease, and, in the case of CDH, for deterioration of lung function. Their long-term followup should focus on early recognition and offering timely interventions.

Neonates with an identified risk factor or who have developed a neurological complication on ECLS will benefit from more targeted followup. The ideal algorithm would incorporate followup, neuroimaging, and sequential age-appropriate neuropsychological testing up to adolescence in a risk stratified process depending on clinical neurological signs and MRI findings[73,74,115]

The recently published ELSO guideline for followup after neonatal and pediatric ECLS outlines recommendations for medical and specialist followup from hospital discharge until adolescence, individualized depending on clinical status and neurodevelopmental morbidities (see Appendix, p.773).[13] As it is now becoming increasingly clear that exclusive assessment of intelligence does not capture the full range of learning deficits that underlie academic and behavioral problems, structured assessment of specific domains of neurodevelopmental skills at different ages seems essential. Internationally agreed recommendations, made in conjunction with all ECLS centers, are crucial to reduce variability, inform, integrate, and improve followup care with the aim of engaging families, community health, and educational psychology services. With different followup protocols, including neuroimaging and neuropsychological testing, reflecting the degree of variability in the followup data that are acquired, a longitudinal followup pathway integrating neurological assessment starting from the time of referral of the child for ECLS right up to adolescence should be planned by the individual ECLS program with the guidelines set out in the ELSO guidelines.[13] An example of a followup schedule is shown in the Appendix (p.773).

Having a structured followup plan in place early facilitates family engagement and helps them understand the importance of followup. Involving parents right from the start is crucial to the success of the followup program. Furthermore, standardized followup pathways provide information and knowledge for local pediatricians and neonatologists who may or may not be aware of the later neurocognitive issues and neuropsychological sequelae and thus ensures evaluation and support for the child's ongoing developmental needs.[116] Finally, if this information was collated and analyzed, it could lead to greater understanding and identification of risk factors for specific patterns of brain injury and neurological deficits in neonatal ECLS survivors.

## Conclusions

- Pre-ECLS and on-ECLS risk factors need to be taken into account during post discharge followup programs. Neurological injury may be 'silent' in neonates.
- Locally available standardized assessment tools should be used in these programs. It is important to bear in mind that IQ alone is insufficient to track neurodevelopmental problems.
- ECLS survivors may 'grow into their deficits,' ie, early, subtle brain injuries may become more evident later in life when higher cognitive functioning is needed. Therefore, followup should be continued into adolescence
- ECLS healthcare professionals should inform parents about potential sequelae and recommend seeking advice in case of growth failure; reduced exercise tolerance; or neurodevelopmental problems, such as clumsiness, poor academic performance, or problems in behavior, concentration, or memory.
- Early recognition of morbidities and timely intervention is important to optimize participation in society.

# References

1. Karimova A, Brown K, Ridout D, et al. Neonatal extracorporeal membrane oxygenation: practice patterns and predictors of outcome in the UK. Archives of Disease in Childhood-Fetal and Neonatal Edition. 2009;94(2):F129-F132.

2. Mugdorf M ED, Field D. Extracorporeal membrane oxygenation for severe respiratory failure in newborn infants. Cochrane review. Cochrane Database Syst Rev. 2008 Jul 16;(3):CD001340.

3. Paden ML, Rycus PT, Thiagarajan RR. Update and outcomes in extracorporeal life support. Seminars in perinatology. 2014;38:65-70.

4. The collaborative UK ECMO (Extracorporeal Membrane Oxygenation) trial: follow-up to 1 year of age. Pediatrics. 1998 Apr;101(4):E1.

5. McNally H, Bennett CC, Elbourne D, et al. United Kingdom collaborative randomized trial of neonatal extracorporeal membrane oxygenation: follow-up to age 7 years. Pediatrics. 2006;117(5):e845-e854.

6. Jancelewicz T, Langham MR, Jr., Brindle ME, et al. Survival Benefit Associated With the Use of Extracorporeal Life Support for Neonates With Congenital Diaphragmatic Hernia. Ann Surg. Jan 1 2022;275(1):e256-e263.

7. ELSO. https://www.elso.org/Registry/ELSOLiveRegistryDashboard.aspx.

8. Bennett CC, Johnson A, Field DJ, et al. UK collaborative randomised trial of neonatal extracorporeal membrane oxygenation: follow-up to age 4 years. The Lancet. 2001;357(9262):1094-1096.

9. Madderom MJ, Reuser JJCM, Utens EMWJ, et al. Neurodevelopmental, educational and behavioral outcome at 8 years after neonatal ECMO: a nationwide multicenter study. Intensive care medicine. 2013;39(9):1584-1593.

10. Nield TA, Langenbacher D, Poulsen MK, et al. Neurodevelopmental outcome at 3.5 years of age in children treated with extracorporeal life support: relationship to primary diagnosis. The Journal of pediatrics. 2000;136(3):338-344.

11. Benjamin JR, Gustafson KE, Smith PB, et al. Perinatal factors associated with poor neurocognitive outcome in early school age congenital diaphragmatic hernia survivors. Journal of pediatric surgery. 2013;48(4):730-737.

12. Ijsselstijn H, van Heijst AFJ. Long-term outcome of children treated with neonatal extracorporeal membrane oxygenation: Increasing problems with increasing age. Elsevier; 2014:114-121.

13. Ijsselstijn H, Schiller RM, Holder C, et al. Extracorporeal Life Support Organization (ELSO) Guidelines for Follow-up After Neonatal and Pediatric Extracorporeal Membrane Oxygenation. Asaio j. Sep 1 2021;67(9):955-963.

14. Iguchi A, Ridout DA, Galan S, et al. Long-term survival outcomes and causes of late death in neonates, infants, and children treated with extracorporeal life support*. Pediatric Critical Care Medicine. 2013;14(6):580-586.

15. Lazar DA, Cass DL, Olutoye OO, et al. The use of ECMO for persistent pulmonary hypertension of the newborn: a decade of experience. journal of surgical research. 2012;177(2):263-267.

16. Kays DW. ECMO in CDH: Is there a role? Semin Pediatr Surg. Jun 2017;26(3):166-170. doi:10.1053/j.sempedsurg. 2017.04.006.

17. Guner YS, Delaplain PT, Zhang L, et al. Trends in Mortality and Risk Characteristics of Congenital Diaphragmatic Hernia Treated With Extracorporeal Membrane Oxygenation. Asaio j. Jul 2019;65(5):509-515.

18. Barbaro RP, Paden ML, Guner YS, et al. Pediatric Extracorporeal Life Support Organization Registry International Report 2016. Asaio j. Jul/Aug 2017;63(4):456-463.

19. ELSO. https://www.elso.org/Registry/InternationalSummary.aspx.

20. Dalton HJ, Reeder R, Garcia-Filion P, et al. Factors Associated with Bleeding and Thrombosis in Children Receiving Extracorporeal Membrane Oxygenation. Am J Respir Crit Care Med. Sep 15 2017;196(6):762-771.

21. Dalton HJ, Garcia-Filion P, Holubkov R, et al. Association of bleeding and thrombosis with outcome in extracorporeal life support. Pediatr Crit Care Med. Feb 2015;16(2):167-74.

22. Fallon SC, Cass DL, Olutoye OO, et al. Repair of congenital diaphragmatic hernias on Extracorporeal Membrane Oxygenation (ECMO): does early repair improve patient survival? J Pediatr Surg. Jun 2013;48(6):1172-6.

23. Barton R, Ignjatovic V, Monagle P. Anticoagulation during ECMO in neonatal and paediatric patients. Thromb Res. Jan 2019;173:172-177.

24. Dalton HJ, Hoskote A. There and Back Again: Roller Pumps Versus Centrifugal Technology in Infants on Extracorporeal Membrane Oxygenation. Pediatr Crit Care Med. Dec 2019;20(12):1195-1196.

25. Madderom MJ, Gischler SJ, Duivenvoorden H, et al. Neonatal extracorporeal membrane oxygenation: impaired health at 5 years of age. Pediatric Critical Care Medicine. 2013;14(2):183-193.

26. Leeuwen L, Schiller RM, Rietman AB, et al. Risk Factors of Impaired Neuropsychologic Outcome in School-Aged Survivors of Neonatal Critical Illness. Crit Care Med. Mar 2018;46(3):401-410.

27. Madderom MJ, Schiller RM, Gischler SJ, et al. Growing Up After Critical Illness: Verbal, Visual-Spatial, and Working Memory Problems in Neonatal Extracorporeal Membrane Oxygenation Survivors. Crit Care Med. Jun 2016;44(6):1182-90.

28. van Heijst AFJ, Amerik C, Ijsselstijn H. ECMO in neonates: Neuroimaging findings and outcome. Elsevier; 2014:104-113.

29. Polito A BC, Wypij D, Rycus PT, et al. Neurologic complications in neonatessupported with extracorporeal membrane oxygenation. An analysis of ELSO registry data. Intensive Care Med 2013;39(9):1594-1601.

30. Fletcher K, Chapman R, Keene S. An overview of medical ECMO for neonates. Semin Perinatol. Mar 2018;42(2):68-79.

31. Parish AP, Bunyapen C, Cohen MJ, et al. Seizures as a predictor of long-term neurodevelopmental outcome in survivors of neonatal extracorporeal membrane oxygenation (ECMO). J Child Neurol. Dec 2004;19(12):930-4.

32. de Mol AC, Liem KD, van Heijst AF. Cerebral aspects of neonatal extracorporeal membrane oxygenation: a review. Neonatology. 2013;104(2):95-103.

33. Cashen K, Reeder RW, Shanti C, et al. Is therapeutic hypothermia during neonatal extracorporeal membrane oxygenation associated with intracranial hemorrhage? Perfusion. Jul 2018;33(5):354-362.

34. Smith KM, McMullan DM, Bratton SL, et al. Is age at initiation of extracorporeal life support associated with mortality and intraventricular hemorrhage in neonates with respiratory failure? J Perinatol. May 2014;34(5):386-91.

35. Short BL. The effect of extracorporeal life support on the brain: a focus on ECMO. Semin Perinatol. Feb 2005;29(1):45-50.

36. Kazmi SO, Sivakumar S, Karakitsos D, et al. Cerebral Pathophysiology in Extracorporeal Membrane Oxygenation: Pitfalls in Daily Clinical Management. Crit Care Res Pract. 2018;2018:3237810.

37. Joram N, Beqiri E, Pezzato S, et al. Continuous Monitoring of Cerebral Autoregulation in Children Supported by Extracorporeal Membrane Oxygenation: A Pilot Study. Neurocrit Care. Jun 2021;34(3):935-945.

38. Joram N, Beqiri E, Pezzato S, et al. Impact of Arterial Carbon Dioxide and Oxygen Content on Cerebral Autoregulation Monitoring Among Children Supported by ECMO. Neurocrit Care. Oct 2021;35(2):480-490.

39. Anton-Martin P, Journeycake J, Modem V, et al. Coagulation Profile Is Not a Predictor of Acute Cerebrovascular Events in Pediatric Extracorporeal Membrane Oxygenation Patients. ASAIO J. Nov/Dec 2017;63(6):793-801.

40. Anton-Martin P, Raman L, Thatte N, et al. Pre-ECMO coagulopathy does not increase the occurrence of hemorrhage during extracorporeal support. Int J Artif Organs. May 29 2017;40(5):250-255.

41. Walker LK, Short BL, Traystman RJ. Impairment of cerebral autoregulation during venovenous extracorporeal membrane oxygenation in the newborn lamb. Crit Care Med. Dec 1996;24(12):2001-6.

42. Short BL, Walker LK, Bender KS, et al. Impairment of cerebral autoregulation during extracorporeal membrane oxygenation in newborn lambs. Pediatr Res. Mar 1993;33(3):289-94.

43. Ingyinn M, Rais-Bahrami K, Viswanathan M, et al. Altered cerebrovascular responses after exposure to venoarterial extracorporeal membrane oxygenation: role of the nitric oxide pathway. Pediatr Crit Care Med. Jul 2006;7(4):368-73.

44. Rhee CJ, da Costa CS, Austin T, et al. Neonatal cerebrovascular autoregulation. Pediatr Res. Nov 2018;84(5):602-610.

45. Cuevas Guaman M, Lucke AM, Hagan JL, et al. Bleeding Complications and Mortality in Neonates Receiving Therapeutic Hypothermia and Extracorporeal Membrane Oxygenation. Am J Perinatol. Feb 2018;35(3):271-276.

46. Askenazi DJ, Ambalavanan N, Hamilton K, et al. Acute kidney injury and renal replacement therapy independently predict mortality in neonatal and pediatric noncardiac patients on extracorporeal membrane oxygenation. Pediatric Critical Care Medicine. 2011;12(1):e1-e6.

47. Fleming GM, Sahay R, Zappitelli M, et al. The Incidence of Acute Kidney Injury and Its Effect on Neonatal and Pediatric Extracorporeal Membrane Oxygenation Outcomes: A Multicenter Report From the Kidney Intervention During Extracorporeal Membrane Oxygenation Study Group. Pediatr Crit Care Med. Dec 2016;17(12):1157-1169.

48. Zwiers AJ, de Wildt SN, Hop WC, et al. Acute kidney injury is a frequent complication in critically ill neonates receiving extracorporeal membrane oxygenation: a 14-year cohort study. Crit Care. 2013;17(4):R151.

49. Liao X, Cheng Z, Wang L, Li B. Analysis of the risk factors of acute kidney injury in patients receiving extracorporeal membrane oxygenation. Clin Nephrol. Oct 2018;90(4):270-275.

50. Dalton HJ, Cashen K, Reeder RW, et al. Hemolysis During Pediatric Extracorporeal Membrane Oxygenation: Associations With Circuitry, Complications, and Mortality. Pediatr Crit Care Med. Nov 2018;19(11):1067-1076.

51. Shah AG, Peahota M, Thoma BN, et al. Medication Complications in Extracorporeal Membrane Oxygenation. Crit Care Clin. Oct 2017;33(4):897-920.

52. MacLaren G, Schlapbach LJ, Aiken AM. Nosocomial Infections During Extracorporeal Membrane Oxygenation in Neonatal, Pediatric, and Adult Patients: A Comprehensive Narrative Review. Pediatr Crit Care Med. Mar 2020;21(3):283-290.

53. Bizzarro MJ, Conrad SA, Kaufman DA, et al. Infections acquired during extracorporeal membrane oxygenation in neonates, children, and adults. Pediatr Crit Care Med. May 2011;12(3):277-81.

54. Cashen K, Reeder R, Dalton HJ, et al. Acquired infection during neonatal and pediatric extracorporeal membrane oxygenation. Perfusion. Sep 2018;33(6):472-482.

55. Kugelman A, Gangitano E, Pincros J, et al. Venovenous versus venoarterial extracorporeal membrane oxygenation in congenital diaphragmatic hernia. Journal of pediatric surgery. 2003;38(8):1131-1136.

56. Field D. Neonatal ECMO Study of Temperature (NEST): a randomized controlled trial. Pediatrics. 2013;132(5):e1247-e1256.

57. Beardsmore C, Dundas I, Poole K, et al. Respiratory function in survivors of the United Kingdom extracorporeal membrane oxygenation trial. American journal of respiratory and critical care medicine. 2000;161(4):1129-1135.

58. Beardsmore CS, Westaway J, Killer H, et al. How does the changing profile of infants who are referred for extracorporeal membrane oxygenation affect their overall respiratory outcome? Pediatrics. 2007;120(4):e762-e768.

59. Spoel M, van den Hout L, Gischler SJ, et al. Prospective longitudinal evaluation of lung function during the first year of life after repair of congenital diaphragmatic hernia. Pediatric Critical Care Medicine. 2012;13(3):e133-e139.

60. Boykin AR, Quivers ES, Wagenhoffer KL, et al. Cardiopulmonary outcome of neonatal extracorporeal membrane oxygenation at ages 10–15 years. Critical care medicine. 2003;31(9):2380-2384.

61. van der Cammen-van Zijp MHM, Gischler SJ, Hop WCJ, et al. Deterioration of exercise capacity after neonatal extracorporeal membrane oxygenation. European Respiratory Journal. 2011;38(5):1098-1104.

62. Zwiers AJM, Ijsselstijn H, van Rosmalen J, et al. CKD and hypertension during long-term follow-up in children and adolescents previously treated with extracorporeal membrane oxygenation. Clinical Journal of the American Society of Nephrology. 2014;CJN. 02890314.

63. Majaesic CM, Jones R, Dinu IA, Montgomery MD, et al. Clinical correlations and pulmonary function at 8 years of age after severe neonatal respiratory failure. Pediatric pulmonology. 2007;42(9):829-837.

64. Cheung P-Y, Robertson CMT. Sensorineural hearing loss in survivors of neonatal extracorporeal membrane oxygenation. Developmental Neurorehabilitation. 1997;1(2):127-130.

65. Graziani LJ, Baumgart S, Desai S, et al. Clinical antecedents of neurologic and audiologic abnormalities in survivors of neonatal extracorporeal membrane oxygenation. Journal of child neurology. 1997;12(7):415-422.

66. Fligor BJ, Neault MW, Mullen CH, et al. Factors associated with sensorineural hearing loss among survivors of extracorporeal membrane oxygenation therapy. Pediatrics. 2005;115(6):1519-1528.

67. van den Hondel D, Madderom MJ, Goedegebure A, et al. Sensorineural hearing loss and language development following neonatal extracorporeal membrane oxygenation. Pediatric Critical Care Medicine. 2013;14(1):62-69.

68. Murray M, Nield T, Larson-Tuttle C, et al. Sensorineural hearing loss at 9–13 years of age in children with a history of neonatal extracorporeal membrane oxygenation. Archives of Disease in Childhood-Fetal and Neonatal Edition. 2010;96:F128-132.

69. Robertson CM, Tyebkhan JM, Hagler ME, et al. Late-onset, progressive sensorineural hearing loss after severe neonatal respiratory failure. Otol Neurotol. May 2002;23(3):353-6.

70. Bulas D, Glass P. Neonatal ECMO: neuroimaging and neurodevelopmental outcome. Elsevier; 2005:58-65.

71. Amigoni A, Pettenazzo A, Biban P, et al. Neurologic outcome in children after extracorporeal membrane oxygenation: prognostic value of diagnostic tests. Pediatric neurology. 2005;32(3):173-179.

72. Khambekar K, Nichani S, Luyt DK, et al. Developmental outcome in newborn infants treated for acute respiratory failure with extracorporeal membrane oxygenation: present experience. Archives of Disease in Childhood-Fetal and Neonatal Edition. 2006;91(1):F21-F25.

73. Dhar AV, Scott S, Anton-Martin P, et al. Neurodevelopmental Outcomes in Extracorporeal Membrane Oxygenation Patients: A Pilot Study. Asaio j. Apr 2020;66(4):447-453.

74. Farhat A, Li X, Huet B, et al. Routine Neuroimaging: Understanding Brain Injury in Pediatric Extracorporeal Membrane Oxygenation. Crit Care Med. Sep 22 2021.

75. Rais-Bahrami K, Wagner AE, Coffman C, et al. Neurodevelopmental outcome in ECMO vs near-miss ECMO patients at 5 years of age. Clinical pediatrics. 2000;39(3):145-152.

76. Goodman M, Gringlas M, Baumgart S, et al. Neonatal electroencephalogram does not predict cognitive and academic achievement scores at early school age in survivors of neonatal extracorporeal

membrane oxygenation. Journal of child neurology. 2001;16(10):745-750.

77. Hanekamp MN, Mazer P, van der Cammen-van MHM, et al. Follow-up of newborns treated with extracorporeal membrane oxygenation: a nationwide evaluation at 5 years of age. Critical Care. 2006;10(5):R127.

78. Schiller RM, Madderom MJ, Reuser JJ, et al. Neuropsychological Follow-up After Neonatal ECMO. Pediatrics. Nov 2016;138(5)doi:10.1542/peds.2016-1313.

79. IJsselstijn H, Hunfeld M, Schiller RM, et al. Improving Long-Term Outcomes After Extracorporeal Membrane Oxygenation: From Observational Follow-Up Programs Toward Risk Stratification. Front Pediatr. 2018;6:177.

80. Engle WA, West KW, Hocutt GA, et al. Adult Outcomes After Newborn Respiratory Failure Treated With Extracorporeal Membrane Oxygenation. Pediatr Crit Care Med. Jan 2017;18(1):73-79.

81. Cooper JM, Gadian DG, Jentschke S, et al. Neonatal hypoxia, hippocampal atrophy, and memory impairment: evidence of a causal sequence. Cerebral cortex. 2015;25(6):1469-1476.

82. Schiller RM, van den Bosch GE, Muetzel RL, et al. Neonatal critical illness and development: white matter and hippocampus alterations in school-age neonatal extracorporeal membrane oxygenation survivors. Dev Med Child Neurol. Mar 2017;59(3):304-310.

83. Davidson MC, Amso D, Anderson LC, et al. Development of cognitive control and executive functions from 4 to 13 years: Evidence from manipulations of memory, inhibition, and task switching. Neuropsychologia. 2006;44(11):2037-2078.

84. Schiller RM, Madderom MJ, van Rosmalen J, et al. Working Memory Training Following Neonatal Critical Illness: A Randomized Controlled Trial. Crit Care Med. Jul 2018;46(7):1158-1166.

85. van der Cammen-van MHM, Janssen AJWM, Raets MMA, et al. Motor Performance After Neonatal Extracorporeal Membrane Oxygenation: A Longitudinal Evaluation. Pediatrics. 2014;134(2):e427-e435.

86. Toussaint LC, van der Cammen-van Zijp MH, Janssen AJ, et al. Perceived Motor Competence Differs From Actual Performance in 8-Year-Old Neonatal ECMO Survivors. Pediatrics. Mar 2016;137(3):e20152724.

87. Spoel M, Laas R, Gischler SJ, et al. Diagnosis-related deterioration of lung function after extracorporeal membrane oxygenation. European Respiratory Journal. 2012;40(6):1531-1537.

88. Spoel M, van der Cammen-van Zijp M, Hop WCJ, et al. Lung function in young adults with congenital diaphragmatic hernia; a longitudinal evaluation. Pediatric pulmonology. 2013;48(2):130-137.

89. Toussaint-Duyster LCC, van der Cammen-van Zijp MHM, Spoel M, et al. Lung function in school-aged congenital diaphragmatic hernia patients; a longitudinal evaluation. Pediatr Pulmonol. Aug 2019;54(8):1257-1266.

90. Dao DT, Hayden LP, Buchmiller TL, et al. Longitudinal Analysis of Pulmonary Function in Survivors of Congenital Diaphragmatic Hernia. J Pediatr. Jan 2020;216:158-164.e2.

91. Dao DT, Kamran A, Wilson JM, et al. Longitudinal Analysis of Ventilation Perfusion Mismatch in Congenital Diaphragmatic Hernia Survivors. J Pediatr. Apr 2020;219:160-166.e2.

92. Weis M, Zoellner FG, Hagelstein C, et al. Lung Perfusion MRI After Congenital Diaphragmatic Hernia Repair in 2-Year-Old Children With and Without Extracorporeal Membrane Oxygenation Therapy. AJR Am J Roentgenol. Jun 2016;206(6):1315-20.

93. Groß V, Zahn K, Maurer K, et al. MR lung perfusion measurements in adolescents after congenital diaphragmatic hernia: correlation with spirometric lung function tests. Eur Radiol. Nov 6 2021.

94. Spoel M, Marshall H, H IJ, et al. Pulmonary ventilation and micro-structural findings in congenital diaphragmatic hernia. Pediatr Pulmonol. May 2016;51(5):517-24.

95. Tan JK, Banton G, Minutillo C, et al. Long-term medical and psychosocial outcomes in congenital diaphragmatic hernia survivors. Arch Dis Child. Aug 2019;104(8):761-767.

96. Toussaint-Duyster LCC, van der Cammen-van Zijp MHM, de Jongste JC, et al. Congenital diaphragmatic hernia and exercise capacity, a longitudinal evaluation. Pediatr Pulmonol. May 2019;54(5):628-636.

97. Wilson MG, Riley P, Hurteau A-M, et al. Hearing loss in congenital diaphragmatic hernia (CDH) survivors: Is it as prevalent as we think? Journal of pediatric surgery. 2013;48(5):942-945.

98. Morando C, Midrio P, Gamba P, Filippone M, et al. Hearing assessment in high-risk congenital diaphragmatic hernia survivors. International journal of pediatric otorhinolaryngology. 2010;74(10):1176-1179.

99. Amoils M, Janik MC, Lustig LR. Patterns and Predictors of Sensorineural Hearing Loss in Children With Congenital Diaphragmatic Hernia. JAMA Otolaryngol Head Neck Surg. 2015 Oct;141(10):923-926.

100. Van der Veeken L, Russo FM, Litwinska E, et al. Prenatal cerebellar growth is altered in congenital diaphragmatic hernia on ultrasound. Prenat Diagn. 2022 Mar;42(3):330-337.

101. Wynn J, Aspelund G, Zygmunt A, et al. Developmental outcomes of children with congenital diaphragmatic hernia: a multicenter prospective study. J Pediatr Surg. Oct 2013;48(10):1995-2004.

102. Danzer E, Gerdes M, D'Agostino JA, et al. Preschool neurological assessment in congenital diaphragmatic hernia survivors: outcome and perinatal factors associated with neurodevelopmental impairment. Early human development. 2013;89(6):393-400.

103. Madderom MJ, Toussaint L, van der Cammen-van MHM, et al. Congenital diaphragmatic hernia with (out) ECMO: impaired development at 8 years. Archives of Disease in Childhood-Fetal and Neonatal Edition. 2012:fetalneonatal-2012-303020.

104. Nijhuis-van der Sanden MW, Van Der Cammen-van Zijp MH, Janssen AJ, et al. Motor performance in five-year-old extracorporeal membrane oxygenation survivors: a population-based study. Crit Care. 2009;13(2):R47.

105. Danzer E, Gerdes M, D'Agostino JA, et al. Longitudinal neurodevelopmental and neuromotor outcome in congenital diaphragmatic hernia patients in the first 3 years of life. J Perinatol. Nov 2013;33(11):893-8.

106. de Munck S, van der Cammen-van Zijp MHM, Zanen-van den Adel TPL, et al. Persisting Motor Function Problems in School-Aged Survivors of Congenital Diaphragmatic Hernia. Front Pediatr. 2021;9:729054.

107. MacLaren G. Long-term outcomes after extracorporeal life support: what happens to the survivors? Pediatr Crit Care Med 2013; 14:646-647.

108. Cvetkovic M, Chiarini G, Belliato M, et al. International survey of neuromonitoring and neurodevelopmental outcome in children and adults supported on extracorporeal membrane oxygenation in Europe. Perfusion. Sep 22 2021:2676591211042563.

109. Jaillard S, Pierrat V, Truffert P, et al. Two years' follow-up of newborn infants after extracorporeal membrane oxygenation (ECMO). European journal of cardio-thoracic surgery. 2000;18(3):328-333.

110. Langenbacher D, Nield T, Poulsen MK. Neurodevelopmental Outcome of ECMO Survivors at Five Years of Age The Potential for Academic and Motor Difficulties. The Journal of Special Education. 2001;35(3):156-160.

111. Taylor AK, Cousins R, Butt WW. The long-term outcome of children managed with extracorporeal life support: an institutional experience. Crit Care Resusc. Jun 2007;9(2):172-7.

112. Marlow N, Wolke D, Bracewell MA, et al. Neurologic and developmental disability at six years of age after extremely preterm birth. New England Journal of Medicine. 2005;352(1):9-19.

113. Petrou S, Edwards L. Cost effectiveness analysis of neonatal extracorporeal membrane oxygenation based on four year results from the UK Collaborative ECMO Trial. Arch Dis Child Fetal Neonatal Ed. May 2004;89(3):F263-8.

114. Petrou S, Bischof M, Bennett C, et al. Cost-effectiveness of neonatal extracorporeal membrane oxygenation based on 7-year results from the United Kingdom Collaborative ECMO Trial. Pediatrics. May 2006;117(5):1640-9.

115. Bembea MM, Felling RJ, Caprarola SD, et al. Neurologic Outcomes in a Two-Center Cohort of Neonatal and Pediatric Patients Supported on Extracorporeal Membrane Oxygenation. Asaio j. Jan 2020;66(1):79-88.

116. Barbaro RP, Brodie D, MacLaren G. Bridging the Gap Between Intensivists and Primary Care Clinicians in Extracorporeal Membrane Oxygenation for Respiratory Failure in Children: A Review. JAMA Pediatr. May 1 2021;175(5):510-517.

# 13

## Initiating Extracorporeal Life Support for Pediatric Respiratory Failure

*Thomas V. Brogan, Ryan P. Barbaro, Pierre Tissieres, Luregn J. Schlapbach, Heidi Dalton*

Careful management of patients with moderate to severe lung disease (eg, pediatric acute respiratory distress syndrome [PARDS]) may obviate the need for ECLS or increase the likelihood of success once a patient is cannulated for ECLS. Unfortunately, strong evidence for the management of children with severe hypoxemic respiratory failure is sparse.

ECLS provides a means of patient support when mechanical ventilation proves inadequate or injurious. Decades of research have demonstrated that acute lung disease can be exacerbated by mechanical ventilation and even by enthusiastic spontaneous breathing. ECLS provides excellent gas exchange while permitting the clinician to minimize hazardous mechanical ventilation.

### Therapeutic Conditions that May Harm the Lung

Ventilator induced lung injury (VILI) results from the additive effects of conventional mechanical ventilation load (tidal volume, driving pressure, positive end expiratory pressure [PEEP], I:E ratio, flow and respiratory rate), considered as the "mechanical power" to injured lung parenchyma.[1] At the bedside, evaluation of mechanical power is made through analysis of three components: respiratory system elastance (overdistension/

recruitment), airway resistance, and PEEP. Practically, high mechanical power was shown to be associated in children with ARDS with fewer 28-day ventilator free days.[1] The effect of high mechanical power may prove to be particularly relevant in young children (<2 years of age), where higher chest wall compliance and increased energy transmission to the lung rather than the chest wall may predispose to increased VILI if treated with lower PEEP and high driving pressure.[1]

The pivotal studies of Amato et al. found that, among 3562 adults, driving pressure ($\Delta P$) was most strongly associated with survival even in patients receiving "protective plateau pressures and Vt".[2] Studies showed that children managed with $\Delta P$ under 15 $cmH_2O$ had lower duration of MV, ICU LOS, and more ventilator-free days at day 28.[3,4] Recently, in a cohort of 222 children with pediatric acute respiratory failure, higher driving pressure was independently associated with increased time to extubation, while patients with $\Delta P$ under 15 $cmH_2O$ had increase 28-day ventilator free days. Importantly, it was shown that dynamic airway pressure gradients overestimated driving pressure.[5]

Patients self-inflicted lung injury (P-SILI) can occur in patients with lung injury who have increased respiratory drive. Intense inspiratory effort that may worsen lung injury through different mechanisms (eg, overdistension, pendelluft, atelectrauma, increased vascular transmural pressure), likely aggravating preexisting lesions.[6] In patients on conventional mechanical ventilation (CMV), detection of a strong respiratory effort (through inspection of airway pressure wave forms or esophageal pressure monitoring) as well as patient-ventilator asynchrony (identification of breath stacking) should warrant immediate intervention by optimizing sedation, neuromuscular blockade, and PEEP levels.[6]

Additionally, high levels of inspired oxygen can be damaging to the lung. Arterial saturations should be maintained between 88-92% in moderate to severe ARDS by titration of $FiO_2$. This becomes particularly relevant when inhaled nitric oxide (iNO) is used in patients with suspected pulmonary hypertension because production of peroxynitrite can aggravate lung injury and promote fibrosis, especially in younger infants where postnatal alveolarization may be impaired. Persistent requirement of $FiO_2$ >60% should be avoided.[7] Not only does high $FiO_2$ potentially exacerbate lung injury but it also worsens ventilation-perfusion ($V_A$/Q) mismatch and may destabilize low $V_A$/Q units, resulting in absorption atelectasis. Permissive hypercapnia with serum pH goals between 7.15-7.30 has been recommended for patients with severe lung disease. Bicarbonate infusion to improve pH, however, is not recommended. Persistent acidosis, especially with hemodynamic or cardiac compromise, may indicate the need for ECLS.

### Pre-ECLS Patient Management

Currently, for children with moderate to severe PARDS (Table 13-1), data to guide the choice of CMV mode are lacking.[8] When employing CMV, data in the adult population show improved outcomes when limiting tidal volume to 6 cc/kg ideal bodyweight (IBW), compared to 12 cc/kg.[7] In the absence of comparable data in children, limiting Vt seems logical. The PALICC guidelines suggest keeping Vt below 8 cc/kg IBW and limiting inspiratory pressure to 28 cm $H_2O$ unless there is increased chest wall elastance (increase to 29-32 cm $H_2O$).[7]

PEEP adjustment to optimize gas exchange is an important component of ventilator management prior to ECLS—following the ARDSnet PEEP/$FIO_2$ table can be helpful (although not well applied in pediatrics).[9] Lower PEEP than recommended has been associated with increased mortality in children with severe respiratory failure. One study compared observed PEEP in 1134 children vs. suggested PEEP according to the $FiO_2$ from the ARDSnet graph. Outcomes were based on severity of PARDS.[9] Clinicians tended to use higher PEEP than suggested when the $FiO_2$ surpassed 0.5. PEEP set below that recommended by the ARDSnet protocol was associated with greater mortality, consistent across all initial $PaO_2$/$FiO_2$ subgroups. When PEEP exceeded protocol levels by 1 to 4 cm $H_2O$, mortality was lowest. Lung recruitment maneuvers are not routinely recommended. However, when

| NONINVASIVE MECHANICAL VENTILATION* | INVASIVE MECHANICAL VENTILATION | | |
|---|---|---|---|
| | Mild | Moderate | Severe |
| $PaO_2$/$FiO_2$ ≤ 300 | 4≤ OI <8  5≤ OSI <7.5 | 8≤ OI <16  7.5≤ OSI <12.3 | OI ≥16  OSI ≥12.3 |
| *Facemask, BiPAP, or CPAP ≥5 cmH2O  Oxygenation Index (OI)=Mean Airway pressure x FiO2 / PaO2 (post ductal)  Oxygen Saturation Index (OSI): Use SpO2 in place of PaO2 | | | |

**Table 13-1.** Severity of illness scores for pediatric acute respiratory distress syndrome (PARDS).

used they should include PEEP assessment for oxygenation improvement, avoiding barotrauma.

High frequency oscillatory ventilation (HFOV) has been used with success in children with severe ARDS, but no studies demonstrate its superiority to CMV. The same holds true for high frequency jet or percussive ventilation (HFJV, HFPV, respectively). PALICC recommends considering HFJV with severe airleak disease and to consider HFPV in PARDS with secretion-induced atelectasis.[7] Also, airway pressure release ventilation *(APRV)* can be considered, but no evidence suggests that it decreases mortality or progression to ECLS.[7] We recommend that clinicians employ ventilator modes with which they are most experienced when managing children with severe respiratory failure.

Data on prone positioning in children have shown enhanced gas exchange with improved ventilation-perfusion (V/Q) matching but not better outcomes. Prone positioning also produces more homogeneously distributed stress and strain.[4,10] However, the strong outcome data in adults and the physiologic underpinnings of prone positioning support the use of this maneuver whenever safe prior to ECLS.[10] Complications related to prone positioning are few.

Conflicting evidence exists for the use of inhaled nitric oxide (iNO) before ECLS. In a multicenter study of 55 children, iNO was associated with increased ECLS-free survival (92% vs. 52%)[11] while in another study, responders to iNO (≥20% improvement in oxygenation by 6 hours) had lower use of ECLS but not improved survival.[12] In a retrospective, propensity matched study not limited to children with moderate to severe PARDS, iNO was not associated with decreased mortality.[13] PALICC recommend a pre-ECLS trial of iNO, especially in those with pulmonary hypertension or RV dysfunction, but in unstable patients the use of iNO should not delay cannulation.[7]

Neuromuscular blockade (NMB) has been employed with improved outcomes early in adults with severe ARDS. In a small prospective, case-control study, children with PARDS treated with NMB had lower mortality than those not so treated.[14] NMB should be considered early in the course of severe hypoxemic respiratory failure, especially when sedation alone does not adequately aid ventilatory management.[7]

Other adjunctive therapies, including surfactant and corticosteroids, lack sufficient data to support their use in children with severe hypoxemic respiratory failure.

Children with respiratory failure are considered for ECLS candidacy when conventional support does not provide adequate gas exchange, if they are receiving dangerous levels of ventilator support, or if they have severe barotrauma. ECLS may also be employed to facilitate other procedures (eg, airway surgery) (Table 13-2).[15,16] Updated recommendations from the Pediatric Acute Lung Injury Consensus

| NEONATAL | SURVIVAL |
|---|---|
| CDH | 55% |
| MAS | 91% |
| PPHN/PFC | 73% |
| Sepsis | 51% |
| Pneumonia | 41% |
| Air Leak | 66% |
| Other | 72% |
| **PEDIATRIC** | **SURVIVAL** |
| Viral pneumonia | 71% |
| Bacterial pneumonia | 74% |
| Pneumocystis | 80% |
| Aspiration | 70% |
| ARDS/postop, trauma | 70% |
| ARDS/not postop/trauma | 69% |
| Acute resp failure | 67% |
| CDH=congenital diaphragmatic hernia; MAS=meconium aspiration syndrome; PPHN=persistent pulmonary hypertension of newborn; PFC=persistent fetal circulation; ARDS=acute respiratory distress syndrome | |

**Table 13-2.** Outcomes with ECMO by diagnosis (Data adapted from International ELSO Registry, April 2021, 2016-2020).

Conference (PALICC 2) for care of PARDS and for ECLS are available.[7] Due to a lack of high-quality published studies, recommendations remain general and outline the need for future studies.

ECLS recommendations include: 1) ECLS should be considered to support children with severe PARDS where the cause of the respiratory failure is believed to be reversible, or the child may be a candidate for transplantation or other destination therapies; 2) Children with severe PARDS should be evaluated for ECLS when lung protective strategies result in inadequate gas exchange; 3) Serial evaluation of ECLS eligibility is more useful than single-point assessment; 4) Decisions to institute ECLS should be based on a structured evaluation of case history and clinical status by an established expert team; 5) Current evidence does not support extracorporeal carbon dioxide removal ($ECCO_2R$) technology in children but it may be appropriate in select patients.

PALICC recommendations for respiratory failure include evaluating oxygenation indices ($PaO_2/FiO_2$, $Sat/FiO_2$, OI, OSI) every six hours from onset of PARDS for the first 24h and serially thereafter as clinically indicated to stratify PARDS severity, risk of mortality, and illness trajectory.[16] Severity of illness measures are shown in Table 13-2.[17] Despite evidence that OI levels <16-20 are associated with increased death, values at ECLS initiation remain above 30-40 in most reports. When patients have OI levels >16-20, it is recommended that they be cared for in a center where ECLS can be applied in a timely fashion.

**Overview of ECLS for Respiratory Support**

Among children outside of the neonatal period (between 28 days and 18 years), ECLS use increased with 600-800 cases per year between 2015 and 2020.[17-19] There are no randomized clinical trials informing care of children beyond the neonatal period, but clinical trials in neonates and adults support ECLS in acute respiratory failure.[20-22] ECLS is used in a complex and diverse group of pediatric patients (Table 13-3).[23,24] Children with respiratory failure may be supported with either VA or VV ECMO. Roughly one-third of children have their carotid artery cannulated for respiratory ECMO.[18]

***Pediatric Acute Respiratory Distress Syndrome (PARDS) and Acute Respiratory Failure***

There are no established thresholds for initiating ECLS in PARDS or acute respiratory failure.[25,26] Observed clinician practice suggests this transition commonly occurs at a median oxygenation of index of 40 (despite evidence that lower levels of OI are also associated with

| CATEGORY | EXAMPLES |
|---|---|
| Infectious | |
| | Viral infection Adenovirus, Enterovirus human metapneumovirus, cytomegalovirus, herpes simplex virus, SARS-CoV-19, etc |
| | Bacterial infections Pertussis, legionella, etc |
| | Fungal infections |
| Malignancy | Parasitic infections *Pneumocystis jirovecii* pneumonia |
| Malignancy/Immune Dysfunction | |
| | Common pediatric malignancies |
| | Hematopoietic stem cell transplantation |
| | Chimeric antigen T-cell (CAR-T) therapy |
| | Human immunodeficiency virus (virus) |
| | Hemophagocytic lymphohistiocytosis (HLH) |
| | Langerhans cell histiocytosis |
| | Multi-inflammatory syndrome in children (MIS-C) |
| Pulmonary Hemorrhage | |
| | Diffuse alveolar hemorrhage |
| Diffuse Lung Injury | |
| | Toxin exposure |
| | Drug overdose |
| | Vaping injury |
| | Amniotic fluid embolism |
| | Gas inhalation |
| Special Pulmonary Pathologies | |
| | Acute chest syndrome/sickle cell disease |
| | Hepatopulmonary syndrome |
| | Plastic bronchitis |
| | Cystic fibrosis |
| | Lung transplantation |
| Trauma/Burn | |
| Airway Surgeries | |
| | Airway reconstruction/slide tracheoplasty |
| | Endobronchial tumor |

**Table 13-3.** Examples of successful use of respiratory ECMO in children.

increased mortality) and a $PaO_2/FiO_2$ ratio of approximately 60.[24,27] Outcomes among children with acute respiratory failure are favorable relative to other indications of ECLS support, with reported mortality rates from multicenter studies ranging between 25 and 40%.[23,28,29] ECLS support was delivered on average for 13 days to children with acute respiratory failure.[28]

### Status Asthmaticus

ECLS has been applied to children with refractory status asthmaticus with survival approaching 90% and an average ECLS run of 6 days.[24] A review of the ELSO Registry data from 1986-2007 and separately 2009-2014 found 60/64 (94%) and 72/84 (86%) children with asthma survived to hospital discharge, respectively.[24,30] Patients typically had severe hypercarbic respiratory failure with median pH 6.96 (IQR 6.78-7.28) and $PaCO_2$ 123 mmHg (IQR 70-237 mmHg).[30] ECLS was used generally as a rescue after other asthma therapies failed. Once on ELCS, experts suggested severe hypercarbia should be reduced by 10-20 mmHg per hour[30] to avoid cerebral complications from acute changes in cerebral blood flow.[31]

### Respiratory ECLS in Complex Conditions

Respiratory ECLS is increasingly employed in complicated conditions ranging from chronic respiratory failure to malignancy and burn injury. In a ELSO Registry report, 35/59 (59%) of children receiving ECLS in the setting of chronic respiratory failure survived to hospital discharge.[24] ECLS was also used as a bridge to lung transplant in 68 children from 2004-2019, although numbers may be increasing as lung transplant in children expands overall.[32] Pediatric lung transplant was most often offered for chronic respiratory diseases such as cystic fibrosis, but 7 (10%) children had acute respiratory failure.[32] Among children successfully bridged to lung transplant with ECLS, 11/68 (16%) died prior

to hospital discharge and the estimated 5-year survival was 54% (95% confidence interval 39-66%).

ECLS has also been used to support respiratory failure in cancer, hemophagocytic lymphohistiocytosis (HLH), after hematopoietic stem cell transplant (HSCT), and in numerous other immunocompromised states as well.[34,35] Estimated survival to hospital discharge has ranged from approximately 40-50% in cancer,[24,33] 35-40% in HLH,[35] and 15-20% in HSCT.[34]

Severe pulmonary hemorrhage represents a significant risk given the need for anticoagulation, but ECLS has been successfully employed for children with this condition, with survival rates of 60% or more.[23,24] Case series reported reducing anticoagulation targets to address the bleeding risk.[36,37] Children with severe airway abnormalities have also been supported with ECLS prior to surgical repair for physiologic stabilization, and postoperatively for optimal healing of the surgical site without mechanical irritation from endotracheal tubes or positive airway pressure.[37-39] ECLS has been used in the setting of burns or smoke inhalation injury with survival rates of 56%, but complications were common.[40]

### Prolonged Respiratory ECLS

Prolonged ECLS, defined as greater than 21 days of ECLS support, was reported in 12% of respiratory ECLS in a 1993-2007 review of the ELSO Registry, with survival rates of 38%.[41] Survival gradually declines with increasing duration of ECLS, but prognostication in prolonged ECLS support remains difficult. Consequently, it is prudent not to discontinue care based on prognostication, but rather if major complications arise that preclude adequate long-term quality of life. Recent data has reported that lung regeneration seems to occur, even in adults, and prolongation of ECLS duration is now occurring for months to allow lung recovery.

# References

1. Bhalla AK, Klein MJ, Modesto I, et al. Mechanical power in pediatric acute respiratory distress syndrome: a PARDIE study. Crit Care. 2022;26(1):2.
2. Amato MB, Meade MO, Slutsky AS, et al. Driving pressure and survival in acute respiratory distress syndrome. N Engl J Med 2015;372(8):747-755.
3. Yehya N, Hodgson CL, Amato MB et al. Response to ventilator adjustments foe predicting acute respiratory distress syndrome mortality. Driving pressure versus oxygenation. Ann Am Thorac Soc 2021;18(5):857-864.
4. Rauf A, Sachdev A, Venkataraman ST, et al: Dynamic airway driving pressure and outcomes in children with acute hypoxemic respiratory failure. Respir Care 2021; 66:403–409.
5. van Schelven P, Koopman AA, Burgerhof JGM, et al. Driving pressure Is associated with outcome in pediatric acute respiratory failure. Pediatr Crit Care Med. 2022 Mar 1;23(3):e136-e144.
6. Carteaux G, Parfait M, Combet M, et al. Patient-self inflicted lung injury: A practical review. J Clin Med. 2021;10(12):2738.
7. The Pediatric Acute Lung Injury Consensus Conference Group. Pediatric acute respiratory distress syndrome: Consensus recommendation from the Pediatric Acute Lung Injury Consensus Conference. Pediatr Crit Care Med 2015: 16(5):428-429.
8. Cheifetz IM. Pediatric ARDS. Respir Care. 2017 Jun;62(6):718-731.
9. Khemani RG, Parvathaneni K, Yehya N, et al. Positive End-Expiratory Pressure Lower Than the ARDS Network Protocol Is Associated with Higher Pediatric Acute Respiratory Distress Syndrome Mortality. Am J Respir Crit Care Med. 2018 Jul 1;198(1):77-89.
10. Gattinoni L, Taccone P, Carlesso E, et al. Prone positioning in acute respiratory distress syndrome. Rational, indications, and limits. Am J Respir Crit Care Med 2013;188(11):1286-1293.
11. Bronicki RA, Fortenberry J, Schreiber M, et al. Multicenter randomized controlled trial of inhaled nitric oxide for pediatric acute respiratory distress syndrome. J Pediatr. 2015;166(2):365-369.
12. Dowell JC, Thomas NJ, Yehya N. Association of response to inhaled nitric oxide and duration of mechanical ventilation in pediatric acute respiratory distress syndrome. Pediatr Crit Care Med 2017;18(11):1019-1126.
13. Bhalla A, Yehya N, Mack WJ, et al. The association between inhaled nitric oxide treatment and ICU mortality and 28-day ventilator-free days in pediatric acute respiratory distress syndrome. Crit Care Med 2018;46(11):1803-1810.
14. Chandra S, Goel S, Dawra R. Early neuromuscular blockade in children with pediatric acute respiratory distress syndrome. J Pediatr Intensive Care 2020;9(3):201-206.
15. Torre M, Carlucci M, Avanzini S, et al. Gaslini's tracheal team: preliminary experience after one year of paediatric airway reconstructive surgery. Ital J Pediatr 2011;37:51.
16. Khemani RG, Smith L, Lopez-Fernandez YM, et al, Pediatric Acute Respiratory Distress syndrome Incidence and Epidemiology (PARDIE) Investigators; Pediatric Acute Lung Injury and Sepsis Investigators (PALISI) Network. Paediatric acute respiratory distress syndrome incidence and epidemiology (PARDIE): an international, observational study. Lancet Respir Med. 2019 Feb;7(2):115-128.
17. Organization ELS. The ELSO Registry Dashboard. Accessed April 1, 2020, https://www.elso.org/Registry/FullCOVID19RegistryDashboard.aspx.
18. Barbaro RP, Brodie D, MacLaren G. Bridging the Gap Between Intensivists and Primary Care Clinicians in Extracorporeal Membrane Oxygenation for Respiratory Failure in Children: A Review. JAMA Pediatr. 2021;175(5):510-517.
19. Barbaro RP, MacLaren G, Boonstra PS, et al. Extracorporeal membrane oxygenation for COVID-19: evolving outcomes from the international Extracorporeal Life Support Organization Registry. Lancet. 2021;398(10307):1230-1238.
20. UK collaborative randomised trial of neonatal extracorporeal membrane oxygenation. UK Collaborative ECMO Trail Group. Lancet. 1996;348(9020):75-82.
21. Peek GJ, Mugford M, Tiruvoipati R, et al. Efficacy and economic assessment of conventional ventilatory support versus extracorporeal membrane oxygenation for severe adult respiratory failure (CESAR): a multicentre randomised controlled trial. Lancet. 2009;374(9698):1351-1363.
22. Combes A, Hajage D, Capellier G, et al. Extracorporeal membrane oxygenation for severe acute respiratory distress syndrome. N Engl J Med 2018;378(21):1965-1975.
23. Zabrocki LA, Brogan TV, Statler KD, et al. Extracorporeal membrane oxygenation for pediatric respiratory failure: Survival and predictors of mortality. Crit Care Med. 2011;39(2):364-370.
24. Barbaro RP, Boonstra PS, Paden ML, et al. Development and validation of the pediatric risk estimate score for children using extracorporeal respiratory support (Ped-RESCUERS). Intensive Care Med 2016;42(5):879-888.
25. Dalton HJ, Reeder R, Garcia-Filion P, et al. Factors Associated with bleeding and thrombosis in children receiving extracorporeal membrane xygenation. Am J Resp Crit Care Med. 2017;196(6):762-771.

26. Erickson S. Extra-corporeal membrane oxygenation in paediatric acute respiratory distress syndrome: overrated or underutilized? Ann Transl Med. Oct 2019;7(19):512.

27. Barbaro RP, Boonstra PS, Kuo KW, et al. Evaluating mortality risk adjustment among children receiving extracorporeal support for respiratory failure. ASAIO J 2019;65(3):277-284.

28. Barbaro RP, Paden ML, Guner YS, et al. Pediatric Extracorporeal Life Support Organization Registry International Report 2016. ASAIO J 2017;63(4):456-463.

29. Barbaro RP, Xu Y, Borasino S, et al, RESTORE Study Investigators. Does extracorporeal membrane oxygenation improve survival in pediatric acute respiratory failure? Am JRespir Crit Care Med 2018;197(9):1177-1186.

30. Hebbar KB, Petrillo-Albarano T, Coto-Puckett W, et al. Experience with use of extracorporeal life support for severe refractory status asthmaticus in children. Crit Care. 2009;13(2):R29.

31. Cavayas YA, Munshi L, Del Sorbo L, Fan E. The early change in PaCO2 after extracorporeal membrane oxygenation initiation is associated with neurological complications. Am J Respir Crit Care Med 2020;201(12):1525-1535.

32. Thompson K, Staffa SJ, Nasr VG, et al. Mortality after lung transplantation for children bridged with extracorporeal membrane oxygenation. Ann Am Thorac Soc. 2022; 19:415-423.

33. Bridges BC, Kilbaugh TJ, Barbaro RP, et al. Veno-venous extracorporeal membrane oxygenation for children with cancer or hematopoietic cell transplant: A ten center cohort. ASAIO J 2021;67(8):923-929.

34. Zinter MS, McArthur J, Duncan C, et al. Candidacy for extracorporeal life support in children after hematopoietic cell transplantation: A position paper from the pediatric acute lung injury and sepsis investigators network's hematopoietic cell transplant and cancer immunotherapy subgroup. Pediatr Crit Care Med. 2022; 23:205-213.

35. Barreto JA, Mehta A, Thiagarajan RR, et al. The use of extracorporeal life support in children with immune-mediated diseases. Pediatr Crit Care Med. 2022; 23(1):e60-e65.

36. Abrams D, Agerstrand CL, Biscotti M, et al. Extracorporeal membrane oxygenation in the management of diffuse alveolar hemorrhage. ASAIO J 2015;61(2):216-218.

37. Kolovos NS, Schuerer DJ, Moler FW, et al. Extracorporal life support for pulmonary hemorrhage in children: a case series. Crit Care Med. 2002;30(3):577-580.

38. Hoetzenecker K, Klepetko W, Keshavjee S, et al. Extracorporeal support in airway surgery. J Thorac Dis. Jul 2017;9(7):2108-2117.

39. Raake J, Johnson B, Seger B, et al. Extracorporeal membrane oxygenation, extubation, and lung-recruitment maneuvers as rescue therapy in a patient with tracheal dehiscence following slide tracheoplasty. Respir Care. 2011;56(8):1198-202.

40. Thompson KB, Dawoud F, Castle S, et al. Extracorporeal membrane oxygenation support for pediatric burn patients: Is it worth the risk? Pediatr Crit Care Med. May 2020;21(5):469-476.

41. Brogan TV, Zabrocki LA, Thiagarajan RR, et al. Prolonged extracorporeal membrane oxygenation for children with respiratory failure. Pediatr Crit Care Med. 2012; 13(4):e249-e254.

# 14

## Management of Children with Respiratory Failure

*Mark Davidson, Micheal Heard, Gail Annich, Ira Cheifetz*

## Introduction

ECLS can be used to effectively support children with reversible severe pediatric acute respiratory distress syndrome (PARDS) who are refractory to conventional intensive care, providing the patient time for recovery of end-organ function. In this chapter, we focus on the many challenges faced by teams caring for pediatric patients with severe respiratory failure beyond the neonatal period and how the wider multidisciplinary team can best support the patient during an ECLS run. We will focus on specific management strategies as well as the essential holistic aspects of pediatric ECLS care.

## Predicting Outcomes

The indications for ECLS in children with respiratory failure have broadened over time as the technology, management techniques, and understanding of respiratory physiology have further developed (see Chapter 13).[1] Established PICU severity of illness scores, such as the pediatric risk of mortality score (PRISM III), pediatric index of mortality (PIM 2), and pediatric logistic organ dysfunction score (PELOD) perform poorly at predicting pediatric ECLS mortality.[2] Historically, the Oxygenation Index (OI) was used as a clinical indicator to guide timing to cannulation onto ECMO

support.[3-5] This approach has recently been challenged and may be less useful than previously thought.[5] OI is not routinely used in many well-established ECLS centers.

Experience in adult respiratory failure has backed the early deployment of ECLS, as used in the treatment algorithm of the EOLIA study,[7] as well as the adult respiratory failure scores such as RESP,[8] and PRESERVE.[9] However, a recent study highlighted the absence of a hard 'cutoff' in terms of pre-ECLS days of ventilation, emphasizing that the decision to initiate ECLS must be informed both by available evidence as well as institutional experience and knowledge.[10]

## Management of the ECLS Circuit

It is important to review all aspects of ECLS support for pediatric respiratory failure multiple times a day to ensure the settings are optimized and potential complications are prevented or detected and acted on early. Key areas to consider during an ECLS run for respiratory failure are blood flow, sweep gas flow, blender oxygen delivery, anticoagulation, and transfusion triggers. Excellent care of the circuit, including the membrane lung, is essential. Targets for $SaO_2$, $SvO_2$, and $PaCO_2$ must be established. These areas will be adjusted depending on the mode of ECLS utilized. In this section, we will focus on VV ECMO as the most common form of respiratory ECMO support.

When setting adequate blood flow targets on VV ECMO, it is important to consider the mode of cannulation. In patients with a poorly positioned double lumen ECMO cannula, recirculation of oxygenated blood from the return (or reinfusion limb) of the ECMO cannula into the drainage limb of the ECMO cannula may occur, especially when the ECMO flow is increased. If this occurs, the oxygen saturation of the blood from the drainage limb of the circuit will increase, while the patient's arterial and venous saturations may remain static or even fall. An easy, quick bedside check will be noting the color of the blood in the drainage ECMO tubing to be similar to the reinfusion or return tubing. The percentage of re-circulation can be estimated by calculating the recirculation fraction, where $S_{pre}O_2$ is the oxygen saturation of blood entering the membrane and $S_{post}O_2$ the saturation of blood leaving the membrane oxygenator. The $S_vO_2$ is not a true central venous saturation but often estimated from blood sampled from a central line placed in either the superior or inferior vena cava:

$$(S_{pre}O_2 - S_vO_2) / (S_{post}O_2 - S_vO_2) \times 100$$

If VV ECMO is utilized via a well-placed bicaval cannula, the potential impact of recirculation will be less and often negligible. If VV ECMO is deployed via a two-cannula approach, with a femoral venous drainage cannula and a jugular return, the potential recirculation will also be minimal as long as the drainage cannula is sited inferiorly to the right atrium and the tip of the return cannula is not directly in the right atrium.

Blood flow, $FsO_2$, and hemoglobin concentration directly affect a patient's oxygen arterial saturation. It should be remembered that in VV ECMO, an $SaO_2$ >75% may be adequate

as long as the patient's venous saturations and other markers of end organ function are adequate. One does not need to target $SaO_2$ >90% in patients on VV ECMO. There is evidence from all aspects of intensive care as to the deleterious impact of hyperoxia, and the field of ECLS is no different.[11]

Ensuring clear targets for $PaCO_2$ targets are essential. At initiation of ECMO, rapid or precipitous falls in $PaCO_2$ can increase cerebral vascular resistance and are associated with worse neurological outcomes.[12,13]

Management of the ECLS circuit also includes paying close attention to any increase in transmembrane pressures which may signify evolution of clots in the membrane and, if significant, would warrant a change out of the membrane lung (or potentially circuit) (see Chapter 7). Changes in transmembrane pressures tend to occur gradually and prior to any change in gas exchange, which is a late sign of this complication of ECMO. Early discussion with perfusion team members will guide this assessment.

Other aspects of ECMO circuit management, including cannula care and anticoagulation, are covered in the later sections of this chapter.

**Ventilatory Management**

Optimal ventilator management for patients supported with ECLS for respiratory failure is center-dependent and often based on anecdote rather than published evidence. Nonetheless, the overwhelming expert consensus is to avoid using damaging ventilator settings. The goals of ECLS support are to minimize barotrauma, volutrauma, atelectrauma, and biotrauma associated with injurious ventilator settings, in order to promote lung healing.

The current recommendations in the updated ELSO guidelines on pediatric respiratory ECMO management suggests initial ventilator settings with $FiO_2$ <50%, peak inspiratory pressure (PIP) of <25 cmH$_2$O, and

PEEP between 5-15 cmH$_2$O. Respiratory rate of 10-20 breaths per minute and inspiratory times of 0.8-1 second are recommended by the authors, depending on patient age and size. When adjusting the ventilator settings once the patient is on ECLS, the underlying pathology must be considered in determining how best to support the underlying lung pathology. For example, a patient with significant air leak and pneumothoraces may be best served by a period of complete lung rest without any positive pressure, merely ensuring some humidification at the end of the endotracheal tube. A patient in status asthmaticus will require reduced inspiratory times and respiratory rate to avoid gas trapping. Ventilator management strategies must be tailored to the underlying pathophysiology.

Perhaps the most important lesson for lung management during respiratory ECMO support, learned over many years by the authors, is to understand the underlying disease process and be patient to allow the necessary lung remodelling and recovery to occur. This may take weeks to months in certain disease states, and the key message is not to expect recovery too soon which could cause further secondary lung injury. This is very different than cardiac ECMO when early reintervention, if required, and weaning from ECMO is a primary focus. Long periods of respiratory ECMO support can be effective and enable patient recovery when delivered by a well-trained team.

To facilitate a lung protective strategy during a prolonged ECLS run, it is recommended to use lower ventilator settings including CPAP. Some centers, after a period of appropriate training, may choose to progress to extubation as part of an 'awake' period of ECMO support.[14,15] There are no clear data to guide the use of specific ventilation modes once the pediatric patient is on ECLS, (eg, pressure controlled or high frequency ventilation). Once again, institutional experience is important, and a patient-centered approach should be taken.

As part of a lung protective strategy, any significant pneumothoraces or hemothoraces should be drained in a timely fashion by a skilled team. If left untreated, a progressively enlarging pneumothorax or hemothorax may impair ECMO drainage, cardiac function, and/ or lung recovery. Should an air leak develop secondary to significant lung pathology, the patient should have a drain placed and positive pressure ventilation limited, or ceased all together, to allow the lung injury and air leak time to heal. Nonetheless, the decision to drain any pleural collection is an extremely important one which needs to factor in the risks and potential benefits of the procedure. Converting a small pleural effusion into a large hemothorax by inexpert chest drain insertion will not help the patient (see Chapter 51).

In an international survey of ventilation practices for pediatric and adult patients on ECLS, 27% of the pediatric centers queried would consider extubating their patients, 14% of whom would consider this in the first week of support.[16] In adult ECLS centers, 68% will extubate an ECLS patient, with 41% doing this in the first two weeks of support. This represents a major shift in respiratory support on ECLS in recent years; however, the challenges to managing an awake extubated patient on respiratory ECMO safely need to be weighed against the risks, not only at an institutional level but also at an individual patient level. In centers practicing extubation on ECLS, a clear pathway and training are essential, including the presence of well-trained staff required for rapid establishment of an airway in the event of a significant circuit complication or cardiovascular instability. There should be clear plans for patient management prior to decannulation or other procedures and other specifics should be outlined for each patient.[17]

A recent survey described the low frequency of the routine use of tracheostomy in ECMO patients, performed in only 12% of surveyed pediatric centers.[16] Tracheostomy is not seen as routine practice in pediatric respiratory ECMO patients.

Prone positioning in ARDS has become a part of routine management in many patients with severe respiratory failure.[18-20] However, whether it adds additional benefit to patients already on ECLS remains unclear.

The role of the physiotherapist/respiratory therapist is essential in any respiratory ECMO run (see Chapter 47). Their role is multifaceted and includes assessing and assisting in the optimization of the recovering lung, as well as the neuromuscular and neurodevelopmental aspects of a holistic ECLS care package. Respiratory physiotherapy input to patient care becomes essential as the patient progresses after the initial stages of care, when the lung injury is at its greatest. The importance of avoiding any secondary lung injury from exposure to high concentrations of inspired oxygen or significant inspiratory pressures on manual breaths are essential. The role of lung recruitment maneuvers is controversial and are not routinely recommended in adult patients with ARDS.[21,22]

Patients with pulmonary hypertension may receive therapies such as inhaled nitric oxide or intravenous pulmonary vasodilators prior to ECLS. Continuation of these medications once on ECLS is controversial. In general, routine discontinuation of inhaled nitric oxide or other vasodilator medications is recommended. The only caveat is for VV ECMO patients with severe right heart failure secondary to pulmonary hypertension, in whom pulmonary vasodilators may improve right heart function.

Flexible bronchoscopy is increasingly being used safely as a diagnostic tool in pediatric ECMO patients with a relatively high yield, eg, diagnosing airway anomalies, tube malposition, or microbiological confirmation of ventilator-associated pneumonia. Initial bronchoscopy findings often guide the need for future bronchoscopies during an ECLS run. Multiple case series have demonstrated the value of bronchoscopies in pediatric ECLS.[23-27]

In recent years, there has been a burgeoning interest in point of care ultrasound (POCUS) to assess lung pathology and illness. This has been followed by similar publications in patients supported with ECLS.[28-30]

Evidence from an experienced Swedish ECLS center demonstrated that CT imaging identified findings requiring interventions in 18% of their respiratory ECMO patients.[31] Similarly, in a small case series in pediatric patients, CT imaging led to interventions in 84% of patients.[32]

A pragmatic approach to investigating respiratory ECMO patients is to support the development of POCUS in any respiratory ECMO center and have a low threshold for undertaking both thoracic CT imaging and flexible bronchoscopy.

**Cardiovascular Management**

Many patients with severe respiratory failure will require vasoactive support prior to the initiation of ECLS. Unless intrinsic cardiac disease is present, much of this need relates to the underlying condition causing the hypoxia and/or hypercarbia and the high-pressure ventilatory support necessary to sustain life. Once ECLS is initiated, ventilator support can be reduced allowing for a reduction in mean airway pressure and, therefore, an improvement in systemic venous return. Additionally, with the improvement of oxygen delivery due to the membrane lung, the effect of hypoxia on the myocardium is resolved, leading to the return of normal cardiac function. Frequently, vasoactive/inotropic agents can be weaned off as both systemic blood pressure and peripheral perfusion improve.

## Renal and Fluid Management

Patients on ECLS require careful consideration of renal function and fluid balance due to the high risk of developing acute kidney injury, which is associated with increased hospital mortality.[33] A recent metaanalysis of pediatric ECLS patients reported a pooled estimated incidence of AKI and severe AKI requiring RRT of 61.9% and 40.9%, respectively.[33] The mechanism of AKI in patients on ECLS is multifactorial, with a combination of hemodynamic alterations associated with baseline disease, capillary leak, failure of renal homeostasis, fluid overload, and inadequate renal perfusion.[34] Fluid management options that are commonly utilized to maintain renal perfusion and manage extravascular fluid shifts include optimization of intravascular fluid volume, pharmacological therapies (eg, diuretics), and RRT.

Patients requiring ECLS often require fluid resuscitation to maintain their hemodynamic profile during resuscitation and stabilization. They may also continue to require volume replacement in the initial stages after cannulation to optimize venous return and facilitate adequate circuit flows. With ensuing capillary leak, volume resuscitation may result in significant tissue edema and reduced intravascular fluid volume, which can reduce renal perfusion. Fluid overload is associated with adverse outcomes, such as increased mortality in the pediatric ECLS population.[35] It is important, therefore, to ensure strict fluid balance with the aims of avoiding hypovolemia and ensuring renal perfusion while preventing tissue edema. Important considerations include specifying overall fluid allowance, including medication infusions and nutrition in intake calculations, concentrating medications were possible, and ensuring accuracy of outputs.

Diuretics can be administered via bolus doses or continuous infusions and are commonly used in ECLS patients to help manage evolving tissue edema. Loop diuretics are commonly used and have been shown to reduce volume overload and achieve adequate urine output. Care must be taken to titrate drug doses to clinical effect and prevent any nephrotoxicity.

Renal replacement therapy is used to maintain fluid balance, support renal function, maintain electrolyte balance, and potentially clear inflammatory cytokines (see Chapter 42).[36] The timing of initiation of RRT is often individualized for each patient based on fluid status and any biochemical derangement. Continuous renal replacement therapy (CRRT) is most commonly used due to a reduction in rapid fluid shifts. The provision of CRRT can be in a parallel system to the ECLS circuit or integrated within the circuit itself. The benefit of an integrated approach is that additional vascular access and anticoagulation are not needed; however, care must be taken to avoid potential disadvantages (eg, risk of air entrainment). High access or return pressures may be outside the alarm limits for the CRRT device, resulting in interruption of treatment.[37] The benefit to running parallel systems is that the difficulty in providing RRT related to pressure limits has been removed. On the other hand, there is a need to insert separate vascular access, which can carry substantial risks in children on ECLS support.

Pediatric data have reported improved accuracy with fluid management when CRRT is utilized, which may contribute to shorter ECLS runs.[35,38] In addition, a previous systematic review of 19 studies reported that ECLS survivors who had received CRRT had a lower fluid balance than those who did not.[39] This review concluded that the combination of CRRT and ECLS appeared to be safe and effective with regard to improving management of both fluids and electrolytes; however, this study noted an increased mortality in patients who required both ECLS and CRRT as opposed to ECLS alone (Odds Ratio: 5.89; 95%CI: 4.38-7.92. p<0.00001). This may reflect a potentially higher illness severity in patients requiring both ECLS and RRT. The review demonstrated that recovery of renal function appeared to be satisfactory, with no evidence of chronic renal failure in patients receiving CRRT on ECLS. A more recent metaanalysis of 43 studies with 21,624 patients reported that mortality rates for ECLS patients changed as the use of RRT increased. As RRT rates increased from 30% to 50%, total mortality tended to decrease. The risk ratio for mortality was also reported to increase the longer the initiation of RRT was delayed, suggesting benefit to earlier initiation of therapy.[40]

**Gastrointestinal and Nutrition Management**

Adequate nutrition is essential for healing during any acute illness and intensive care stay. This can be provided by enteral feeding, parenteral nutrition (PN), or a combination of both. Enteral feeding has been shown to be safe and effective during ECLS in all groups of patients and may limit the need for total parenteral nutrition and its associated complications.[41]

In patients unable to tolerate nasogastric (NG) feeds, the placement of a nasojejunal (NJ) feeding tube can be helpful in establishing enteral feeds. An NJ tube can be placed safely in a patient while on ECLS support if undertaken by a trained individual.

Recent evidence suggests that the use of early PN may be associated with poorer outcomes. The PEPaNIC trial demonstrated that late introduction of PN in a pediatric intensive care stay (day 8 of admission to PICU) was associated with a shorter duration of mechanical ventilation and a shorter intensive care stay when compared to early initiation of PN (started within 24 h of admission of admission to PICU).[42]

There is no strong evidence base to guide the caloric, protein, or other nutritional goals that should be targeted in pediatric patients

supported on ECLS. A recent study of adult ECLS patients demonstrated that they had a resting energy expenditure lower than traditional expectations.[43]

The early initiation of a bowel management strategy is essential in any ICU patient, including pediatric ECLS patients. A recent study showed an incidence of constipation in 33% of pediatric ECLS patients. The early use of laxatives or stool softeners is essential to encourage effective and safe enteral nutritional delivery.[44]

**Nursing Management**

*Awake Patients*

Maintaining normal sleep-wake cycles for patients is important. Intensive care units are noisy, and lights may be left on 24 hours a day.[45] The ECLS bedspace can be the busiest in the unit, with multiple caregivers, alarms, and procedures. Caregivers should be aware of the sleep-wake cycle and diminish these interruptions. Overhead lights should be turned off at night and localized lighting used to assist in the maintenance of a normal circadian rhythm. Consider the level of sound at the ECLS bedspace, including alarm levels, and decrease extraneous noise as much as possible. Noise levels have been associated with negative effects on sleep, thus contributing to delirium.[46] Ensuring that 'quiet time' is observed in the afternoon and an appropriate 'lights out for nighttime' ritual will aid in decreasing delirium and sleep-deprivation hallucinations, leading to a more suitable environment.

*Activities and Mobilization*

Awake patients require age-appropriate stimulation and activities. Pediatric institutions may have Child Life specialists—experts in child development who promote effective coping mechanisms through education, preparation, and play—or other similarly trained individuals who act as a valuable resource to determine the best activities for patients. A team that includes physical, speech, and occupational therapists should be created to support the ECLS center and establish specific protocols for the patient. Protocols should include both awake and somnolent patients, with the ability to alter therapy as needed. All sizes of patients must be considered. Mobilization of the ECLS patient should be considered when medically feasible. Patients may sit, walk, and even ride a tricycle while on ECMO, as long as cannulation strategies, medical stability, and the patient's abilities are included in the decision.[47] Early mobility may lead to decreased hospitalization duration and improved mental status of the ICU patient.[48,49]

## *Eye Care*

Patients who remain deeply sedated require frequent assessment of the eyes. Critically ill patients who are mechanically ventilated, sedated or unconscious have decreased tear production and reduced or absent blink reflexes. These patients are consequently at high risk for exposure keratopathy and other ophthalmic complications.[50] Intensive care nurses should perform a focused eye assessment at least once every 12 hours to evaluate for ability to maintain eye closure, eyelid swelling, conjunctival redness, corneal hazing, and discharge or crusting on the eyelid. These are the early signs of dry eye that may progress to corneal ulceration or eye infection.[51,52]

The inclusion of eye care into the routine care provided to all ICU patients is a key component of nursing care. Standard practice includes instillation of a lubricant every two hours. For patients who have an inability to maintain eyelid closure, one can use properly installed polyethylene covers which may be more effective at providing a barrier against tear evaporation and exposure to air currents.[53]

The nursing team should use normal saline soaked gauze to clean from the inner to the outer canthus at least every eight hours. Any sign of abnormality should be reported to the clinical care team with consideration of an ophthalmology consult.

## *Skin Care*

The ECLS patient is at considerable risk for pressure areas due to the critical nature of their illness, the use of anticoagulant therapy, and immobility. The head and neck are frequently edematous due to the lack of mobility. Large cannulas sutured in place, endotracheal/oronasal tubes, and other intensive care devices increase risk for pressure ulcers.[54] In 2007, the National Pressure Ulcer Advisory Panel made the prevention and treatment of pressure ulcers in infants and children a key priority.[55] The use of the Pediatric Braden Q Scale or other similar scores for pressure area staging can assist the nursing team in the early awareness and assessment of pressure ulcers, providing appropriate and timely interventions. Basic nursing interventions that may lower the risk of development of pressure ulcers, include avoiding injury due to shear forces, turning the patient every two hours, use of positioning aids, and changing dirty or wet linen accordingly. Pediatric patients should have soiled diapers changed as soon as possible. Avoiding the use of multiple layers and plastic lined protective barriers is recommended to assist in the flow of blood in the prevention of pressure ulcers. ECLS patients may also have a higher risk of pressure areas due to the use of paralytic medications. Additionally, difficulty in cannula positioning may make regular patient turning a challenging endeavor. In these cases, the nurse may use fluidized positioners for extremities, head, and shoulders. The careful manipulation of these positioners every two hours will serve to reposition the patient so that pressure areas are rotated. Finally, the ECLS patient may be placed on a special mattress such as an air-filled bed or action bed designed to reduce pressure on the skin.[56]

### Oral Care

Intensive care patients are at high risk for poor oral health. ECLS patients have additional risks of anticoagulation and possibly poor nutrition. Pediatric patients can present several different oral health dilemmas, including the presence of braces or other orthodontic devices and natural tooth loss. The nurse must perform a comprehensive oral assessment and provide mouth care as prescribed. Frequency of mouth care varies but is recommended hourly for high-risk patients, eg, unconscious ones, because lack of care between 2-6 hours can significantly reduce the benefits of any oral intervention previously performed.[57] Many mouthwashes contain alcohol, which can cause a burning sensation in the mouth, may increase existing inflammation, and are not recommended as part of an oral care protocol. Chlorhexidine gluconate (CHG) has been shown to be a very effective antibacterial mouthwash. Saline is a nonirritant mouthwash and can be useful in situations where other rinses are not available. Toothbrushes can effectively remove plaque when used correctly. If a patient is conscious and of a suitable age, allowing them to brush their own teeth is beneficial because nurses may have difficulty in assessing how hard to brush. ECLS patients are at risk for oral bleeding due to the need for anticoagulation so firm bristled brushes should be avoided. Foam swabs are useful for cleaning the oral cavity but only when soaked in CHG. Remove orthodontic devices when possible. If not, the use of dental wax to protect the inner lips may be beneficial. Finally, lip care is also a part of oral health. Lubricants (eg, petroleum jelly) are often recommended but should be avoided because they can increase tissue dryness. Water based or aloe based lip balms should preferably be used.[58]

### Wound Care

Most ECLS centers have an institutional protocol for dressing of intravascular devices as part of a Central Line-Associated Bloodstream Infection (CLABSI) policy. The protocol may include types of catheters, assessment tools, frequency and types of dressing changes, and prevention techniques. All breaks in the skin must be considered wounds and carry risks of hemorrhage or infection.

The nurse should routinely assess all cannulation sites, including integrity and type of dressing, drainage or bleeding, catheter position, stability, and security. Additionally, the skin around the cannula is assessed for redness, swelling and breakdown. Cleaning the cannula site is best done utilizing CHG. CHG swabs or pads may be used to gently clean the incision site. Other cleaning agents include betadine and sterile saline wipes. The types of dressing used on ECLS cannulas vary greatly but are typically considered dry dressings. They may be simple gauze or gauze pads. Transparent film dressings have a thin layer of plastic that covers a wound area, creating a barrier. They allow some oxygen exchange to reduce bacteria growth. These dressings are best for dry, nonexudative sites. Removal of transparent dressings can tear the underlying skin, so caution must be exercised. Once a site begins to bleed or drain, the use of these dressings is contraindicated due to the frequent removal that may result in skin tears. Stable bloody drainage is preferentially left alone until the dressing is required to be changed. This allows the clot to strengthen and prevent further blood loss. Foam dressings have an adsorptive and protective effect for at-risk sites or pressure ulcers. They are self-adherent and easily cut to fit for specific sites. Tape may be used to secure dressings in place. Available in paper, cloth, or plastic, selecting a type that best fits the need of the dressing, without putting the skin under unnecessary risk, is important. Many patients also have sensitivities to tape, which must be considered. Cannula sites, which are typically in the neck or groin, can be difficult to dress. Pediatric patients vary in size and movement, which also must be considered when choosing a dressing.[59]

## Pharmacology

ECLS and critical illness affect the pharmacokinetics and pharmacodynamics of many medications (see Chapter 49). Close consultation with critical care pharmacists and therapeutic drug monitoring should be undertaken when available, especially for medications which may cause acute kidney injury (eg, vancomycin, aminoglycosides).[60,-62] Sedation may be necessary in the ECLS patient to reduce the risk of cannula dislodgment and promote patient comfort. Nonetheless, ECLS per se does not mandate sedation. There are a multitude of reports supporting the maintenance of wakefulness during ECLS.[63- 66]

## Neurological Management

Neurological insults are a potential complication during ECLS in both adult and pediatric patients.[67,68] The mechanisms of neurological insult are multifactorial, including critical illness, inflammatory processes, metabolic disturbances, and hematological sequelae.[69] In a systematic review of 44 studies evaluating adult patients on ECLS, the median risk of acute neurological complications was 13%.[67] These complications included intracranial hemorrhage (5%), ischemic stroke (5%), and seizures (2%). The median mortality in patients with neurological complications during ECLS was significantly higher than those who did not experience an adverse neurological event (83% vs. 42%, p<0.001).[67] In the pediatric respiratory ECMO population, intracranial hemorrhage was reported in 5% of patients and was also associated with high mortality (79%).[70]

Performing a baseline clinical neurological examination of an ECLS patient is important to identify any changes on subsequent serial assessment. Concerning features include unstable hemodynamics, changes in pupillary reactions, seizures, identification of new focal neurological deficits, or changes identified on routine neuromonitoring (eg, near infrared spectroscopy [NIRS], electroencephalography [EEG]).

Cranial ultrasound has been used as a means of neuro surveillance in younger ECLS patients.[71] The benefits to performing cranial ultrasound scans, which are only possible in young children with an open fontanelle, are that it allows a fast, portable, low cost, no-radiation mode of assessment. This modality does not, however, predict neurodevelopmental outcomes and may have less inter-observer reliability when compared to other imaging modalities.[71,72]

In a survey of European ECMO centers, 73% of pediatric centers used cranial ultrasound as a form of routine monitoring.[73] The frequency of ultrasonography varied between centers, with reported frequency ranging from daily (25%), twice weekly (20%), thrice weekly (17%), to only when clinically concerned (15%). The majority of centers in this survey reported that they would undertake brain computed tomography (CT) if clinical concerns were identified (74%). The most commonly used modality of neuromonitoring in this survey, across both adult and pediatric populations, was NIRS (48% vs. 80%). A prospective study assessed the prognostic value of cerebral NIRS in infants less than three months of age on ECLS and determined that nonsurvivors had significantly lower NIRS readings than survivors.[74] Retrospective studies have also reported associations between cerebral desaturation detected by NIRS and neurological complications, reporting that 70% of patients who have an acute intracranial event have had a differential greater than 10% between left and right recordings of cerebral NIRS.[75]

Electroencephalography is another option for neuromonitoring of ECLS patients which can be used in an intermittent or continuous fashion. Retrospective, single-center studies have shown that 16-24% of children on ECLS who have continuous EEG monitoring show electrographic seizure activity, which was associated with intracranial hemorrhage. [76,-78] The severity of EEG findings was also felt to correlate with the severity of findings on follow-up neuroimaging.[78] A high proportion of pediatric centers offer predischarge neuroradiological assessment for patients.[73]

An important consideration for pediatric ECLS patients is neurodevelopmental followup (see Chapter 16). Pediatric studies have reported the potential for neuropsychological deficits and learning difficulties in ECLS survivors.[79,80] There are also reports of impaired executive functioning.[79] It is worth noting that neuropsychological dysfunction and lower psychomotor development scores are associated with reduced cerebral NIRS values. A nadir in cerebral NIRS of less than 35%, or less than 40% for more than 10 minutes, is of particular concern.[81,82]

**Anticoagulation, Thrombosis, and Bleeding Management**

Anticoagulation can be challenging in pediatric ECLS patients because of differences in developmental hemostasis and variability in factor levels.[83-85] Management of anticoagulation for pediatric respiratory failure patients follows the same guidelines as set out for all ECLS patients in ELSO's Anticoagulation Guidelines.[86] The choice of anticoagulant is usually unfractionated heparin, but direct thrombin inhibitors have recently become more popular. There is no good evidence that any of the present laboratory markers of anticoagulation are superior in preventing bleeding or thrombosis. Heparin effect is measured with ACT, aPTT, antiXa, or a combination of these, depending upon patient age and center practices. Anticoagulation in this patient population is generally initiated according to protocol but should later be individualized, with anticoagulation decisions being made according to patient response, not absolute numbers.[87,88]

Blood product replacement also requires a protocol within each center, but again needs to be customized for each patient depending upon existing requirements. A platelet count between $50-100 \times 10^9$/L is usually maintained in children receiving ECLS. A lower count can be safely maintained in adolescents who are not at high risk of bleeding. Red blood cell transfusions are also often required because oxygenation can be optimized either by increasing ECMO circuit blood flow or by raising hemoglobin concentrations to increase blood oxygen content. The adequacy of oxygenation is more important than adhering to a fixed number, but usual transfusion thresholds are between 8 to 10 g/dL, depending on the clinical circumstances, assessment of global oxygen delivery, and age.

Thrombi in the circuit are a common complication of ECLS (see Chapter 6).[89] These are generally small and of little significance but require close monitoring. If the circuit has a heavy clot burden—detectable by direct observation, failing oxygenator performance, or rising plasma free hemoglobin—then component or circuit exchange may be necessary. Bleeding is also common, with cannula or surgical site bleeding being the most frequent. This generally responds to blood product support and local measures. If not, withholding anticoagulation may become necessary, but this should be regarded as a last resort in children. The smaller the patient, the more concerning it is to withhold anticoagulation because it risks catastrophic circuit thrombosis.[90]

## End of Life Planning

ECLS is a lifesaving therapy and should only be deployed when there is a chance the patient will survive. However, complications may arise which preclude continuation of ECLS. In these challenging circumstances, goals of care change to providing the family time to prepare for, and be involved in, the final minutes, hours, or days of their child's life.[47] A careful end-of-life care plan must be agreed across the multidisciplinary team. Involvement of chaplaincy, pastoral care, and social work may also be beneficial during this difficult time.

Families will differ in their wishes but may wish to cuddle their child as they are extubated prior to cessation of ECLS support. Others may wish ECLS support to be ceased and the cannulas removed prior to extubation. A flexible patient- and family-centered approach is essential because some families will wish to be present for each step and others will not. Consideration of stabilization of the cannula sites is undertaken and methods such as bracing, wrapping, and supporting the patient while transitioning to a parent's lap will allow this to occur with minimal risk. Parents may wish to lie in bed with their child. Ideally, there should be no time limit as to how long the family may hold their child, as well as how many members of the family wish to hold them or spend time with them. While this may not be convenient to staff, the importance of recognizing what the family wishes for their child is paramount.

Removal of the ECLS circuit may be performed while the patient is in a parent's arms. Consider clamping the cannulas and leaving them in situ to avoid an unnecessary surgical procedure, which may not allow the family to be present at the time of death. Cutting away the ECMO circuit and capping the cannulas will allow the family to continue to hold as long as they wish. Specialists should be considerate of the potential for blood spillage during the cutting of the tubing. Pinching the ECMO tubing while applying the clamps can be very effective in reducing the spillage of blood at this time. Consider whether removing the endotracheal tube for a clear facial appearance is feasible. Additionally, cannulas and tubing may be tucked under a blanket or gown to allow a more 'natural' appearance of the child.

## Family Support

Communication with family members is a key challenge during any period of ECLS support. It is essential that there are transparent and timely discussions with the family and carers and that the ECLS team have a similar mental model for a communication strategy with the family. A recent paper by Moynihan et al[91] gives a very helpful overview of one particular communication strategy.

## Conclusion

Management of the child receiving respiratory ECMO requires meticulous attention to achieve optimal outcomes and limit the iatrogenic complications associated with intensive care. Minimization of ventilator induced lung injury or associated renal or myocardial injury is key to a successful outcome. A current area of focus is the limitation of sedation, allowing the patient to be in an 'awake' state which may facilitate extubation in highly selected patients. Aligned to this is the aggressive use of early neurorehabilitation, both in patients receiving ECLS and after decannulation. Excellent nursing care is essential to support the patient and the family.

## References

1. Maratta C, Potera RM, et al Extracorporeal life support organization (ELSO): 2020 Pediatric respiratory ELSO Guideline ASAIO 2021.
2. Barbaro RP, Boonstra PS, et al. Evaluating mortality risk adjustment among children receiving extracorporeal support for respiratory failure ASAIO 2019;65:277-284.
3. Trachsel D, McCrindle BW, et al. Oxygenation Index predicts outcome in children with acute hypoxemic respiratory failure Am J Resp Criti Care Med 2005;172:206-211.
4. Rowan CM, Hege KM, et al. Oxygenation Index predicts mortality in pediatric stem cell transplant patients requiring mechanical ventilation Pediatr Tranplant 2012;16:645-650.
5. Karimova A, Brown K, Ridout D, et al. Neonatal extracorporeal membrane oxygenation: practice parameters and predictors of outcome in the UK Arch Dis Child Fetal Neonatal Ed 2009;62:F129-132.
6. Polito A, Dupuis-Lozeron E, et al. Ventilation parameters before extra-corporeal membrane oxygenator and in-hospital mortality in children: a review of the ELSO registry ASAIO 2022;68:281-286.
7. Combes A, Hajag D, et al. Extracorporeal Membrane Oxygenation for Severe Acute Respiratory Distress Syndrome N Engl J Med 2018;378:1965-75.
8. Schmidt M, Bailey M, et al. Predicting survival after extracorporeal membrane oxygenation for severe acute respiratory failure. Am J Respir Crit Care Med 2014;189(11):1374-1382.
9. Schmidt M, Zogheib E, et al. The PRESERVE mortality risk score and analysis of long term outcomes after extracorporeal membrane oxygenation for severe acute respiratory failure Int Care Med 2013;39(10):1704-1713.
10. Hermann M, Laxar D, et al. Duration of invasive mechanical ventilation prior to Extracorporeal Membrane Oxygenation is not associated with survival in acute respiratory distress syndrome caused by coronavirus disease 2019. Annals of Int Care 2022;12(6).
11. Bonnemain J, Rusca M, Ltaief Z, et al. Hyperoxia during extracorporeal cardiopulmonary resuscitation for refractory cardiac arrest is associated with severe circulatory failure and increased mortality. BMC Cardiovasc Disord. 2021;21(1):542.
12. Joram N, Beqiri E, Pezzato S, et al. Impact of Arterial Carbon Dioxide and Oxygen Content on Cerebral Autoregulation Monitoring Among Children Supported by ECMO. Neurocrit Care. 2021 Oct;35(2):480-490.
13. Cavayas YA, Munshi L, Del Sorbo L, et al. The Early Change in PaCO2 after Extracorporeal Membrane Oxygenation Initiation Is Associated with Neurological Complications. Am J Respir Crit Care Med. 2020 Jun 15;201(12):1525-1535.
14. Raake J, Johnson B, Seger B, et al. Extracorporeal membrane oxygenation, extubation, and lung-recruitment maneuvers as rescue therapy in a patient with tracheal dehiscence following slide tracheoplasty. Respir Care. 2011;56(8):1198-1202.
15. MacLaren G, Combes A, Bartlett RH. Contemporary extracorporeal membrane oxygenation for adult respiratory failure: life support in the new era. Intensive Care Med. 2012;38(2):210-220.
16. Jenks CL, Tweed J, Gigli KH, et al. An International Survey on Ventilator Practices Among Extracorporeal Membrane Oxygenation Centers. ASAIO J. 2017 Nov/Dec;63(6):787-792.
17. Costa J, Dirnberger DR, Froehlich CD, et al. Awake Neonatal Extracorporeal Membrane Oxygenation. ASAIO J. 2020;66(5):e70-e73.
18. Guervilly C, Hraiech S, Gariboldi V, et al. Prone positioning during veno-venous extracorporeal membrane oxygenation for severe acute respiratory distress syndrome in adults. Minerva Anestesiol.2014;80(3):307-313.
19. Kimmoun A, Guerci P, Bridey C, et al. Prone positioning use to hasten veno-venous ECMO weaning in ARDS. Intensive Care Med. 2013;39(10):1877-1879.
20. Kimmoun A, Roche S, Bridey C, et al. Prolonged prone positioning under VVECMO is safe and improves oxygenation and respiratory compliance. Ann Intensive Care. 2015;5(1):35.
21. Turner DA, Cheifetz IM, Rehder KJ, et al. Active rehabilitation and physical therapy during extracorporeal membrane oxygenation while awaiting lung transplantation: A practical approach. Crit Care Med 39: 2593–2598, 2011.
22. Papazian L, Aubron C, Brochard L, et al formal guidelines: management of acute respiratory distress syndrome Ann Intensive Care 2019;9(1):69.
23. Kamat P et al. Use of Flexible Bronchoscopy in Paediatric Patients Receiving Extracorporeal Membrane Oxygenation (ECMO) Support. Paediatric Pulmonology 2011; 46:1108-1113.
24. Prentice E, Mastopietro C. Flexible bronchoscopy for children on extracorporeal membrane oxygenation for cardiac failure. Paediatric Critical Care Mediicne 2011; 12 (4): 422-425.
25. Field-Riley A, et al. Utility of flexible fiberoptic bronchoscopy for critically ill pediatric patients: A systematic review. World Journal of Critical Care Medicine 2015; 4(1): 77-88.
26. Valverde C, et al. use of flexible bronchoscopy (FB) in paediatric patients during the weaning of ECMO.

Pediatric Critical Care Medicine 2014; 15(4): Supplement 108-109.

27. Rosner E, et al. The Utility of Flexible Bronchoscopy in Pediatric VenoVenous ECMO: A Multicentre Study. Critical Care Medicine 2018; 47 (1): Supplement 1236.

28. Ntoumenopoulos G, Buscher H, Scott S. Lung ultrasound score as an indicator of dynamic lung compliance during veno-venous extra-corporeal membrane oxygenation. Int J Artif Organs. 2021 Mar;44(3):194-198.

29. Xiao Lu, Arbelot C, Schreiber A, et al. Ultrasound Assessment of Lung Aeration in Subjects Supported by Venovenous Extracorporeal Membrane Oxygenation Respiratory Care Dec 2019, 64 (12) 1478-1487.

30. Zhang X, Fu Y, Yue G, et al. Lung ultrasound for the assessment of lung recruitment in neonates with massive pneumothorax during extracorporeal membrane oxygenation: a case report. J Artif Organs. 2022 Jun;25(2):163-169.

31. Lidegran M, Palmer K, Jorulf H, et al. CT in the evaluation of patients on ECMO due to acute respiratory failure. Pediatr Radiol. 2002;32(8):567-574.

32. Goodwin SJ, Randle E, Iguchi A, et al. Chest computed tomography in children undergoing extracorporeal membrane oxygenation: a 9-year single-centre experience. Pediatr Radiol. 2014;44(6):750-760; quiz 747-759.

33. Hansrivijit P, Lertjitbanjong P, Thongprayoon C, et al. Acute Kidney Injury in Pediatric Patients on Extracorporeal Membrane Oxygenation: A Systematic Review and Meta-analysis. Medicines (Basel). 2019 Nov 1;6(4):109.

34. Villa G, Katz N, Ronco C. Extracorporeal Membrane Oxygenation and the Kidney. Cardiorenal Med. 2015;6(1):50-60.

35. Selewski DT, Askenazi DJ, Bridges BC, et al. The Impact of Fluid Overload on Outcomes in Children Treated With Extracorporeal Membrane Oxygenation: A Multicenter Retrospective Cohort Study. Pediatr Crit Care Med. 2017;18(12):1126-1135.

36. Zhang J, Tian J, Sun H, et al. How does continuous renal replacement therapy affect septic acute kidney injury? Blood Purif. 2018;46(4):326-331.

37. Ostermann M, Connor M, et al. Continuous renal replacement therapy during extracorporeal membrane oxygenation: why, when and how?, Current Opinion in Critical Care: December 2018 - Volume 24 - Issue 6 - p 493-503.

38. Symons JM, McMahon MW, Karamlou T, et al. Continuous renal replacement therapy with an automated monitor is superior to a free-flow system during extracorporeal life support. Pediatr Crit Care Med. 2013 Nov;14(9):e404-8.

39. Chen H, Yu RG, Yin NN, et al. Combination of extracorporeal membrane oxygenation and continuous renal replacement therapy in critically ill patients: a systematic review. Crit Care. 2014 Dec 8;18(6):675.

40. Han SS, Kim HJ, Lee SJ, et al. Effects of Renal Replacement Therapy in Patients Receiving Extracorporeal Membrane Oxygenation: A Meta-Analysis. Ann Thorac Surg. 2015 Oct;100(4):1485-95.

41. Perez G, Gonzalez E, et al. Early Enteral Nutrition and Gastrointestinal Complications in Pediatric Patients on Extracorporeal Membrane Oxygenation JPGN 2022;74: 110–115 .

42. Fivez T, Kerklaan D, Mesotten D, et al. Early versus late parenteral nutrition in critically ill children. N Engl J Med. (2016) 374:1111–22.

43. De Waele E, Jonckheer J, Pen JJ, et al. Energy expenditure of patients on ECMO: a prospective pilot study. Acta Anaesthesiol Scand. (2019) 63:360–4.

44. Perez G, Gonzalez E, et al. Early Enteral Nutrition and Gastrointestinal Complications in Pediatric Patients on Extracorporeal Membrane Oxygenation JPGN 2022;74: 110–115.

45. AL-Samsan RH, Cullen P. Clinical investigations: Sleep and adverse environmental factors in sedated mechanically ventilated pediatric intensive care patients. Pediatric Critical Care 2005;6(5):562–567.

46. Xie H, Kang J, Mills GH. Clinical review: The impact of noise on patients' sleep and the effectiveness of noise reduction strategies in intensive care units. Critical Care 2009;13(2):208.

47. Bergeron A, Holifield L. Extracorporeal membrane oxygenation: The nurse's role in patient care. Nursing Critical Care 2020;15(3):6-14.

48. Bergbower EAS, Herbst C, Cheng N, et al. A novel early mobility bundle improves length of stay and rates of readmission among hospitalized general medicine patients. J Community Hosp Intern Med Perspect. 2020;10(5):419-425. Published 2020 Sep 3.

49. Walker TC, Kudchadkar SR. Early mobilization in the pediatric intensive care unit. Transl Pediatr. 2018;7(4):308-313.

50. Marshall AP, Elliott R, Rolls K, et al. Eyecare in the critically ill: clinical practice guideline. Australian Critical Care 2008;21(2):97-109.

51. Hernandez EV, Mannis MJ. Superficial keratopathy in intensive care patients. American Journal of Ophthalmology 1997;124(2):212-216.

52. Joyce N. Eye care for the intensive care patients. A systematic review. The Joanna Briggs Institute for Evidence Based Nursing and Midwifery, Systematic Review. 2002; No. 21.

53. Shan H, Min D. Prevention of exposure keratopathy in intensive care unit. International Journal of Ophthalmology 2010;3(4):346-348.

54. Schindler CA, Mikhailov TA, Kuhn EM, et al. Protecting fragile skin: Nursing interventions to decrease development of pressure ulcers in pediatric intensive care. American Journal of Critical Care 2011;20(1):26–34.

55. Baharestani MN, Ratliff CR. Pressure ulcers in neonates and children: An NPUAP white paper. Advances in Skin and Wound Care 2007;20(4):208–220.

56. Butler CT. Pediatric skin care: Guidelines for assessment, prevention, and treatment. Pediatric Nursing 2006;32(5):443–450.

57. Murphy A. Clinical review - Oral hygiene a priority of care. Available at: https://www.inmo.ie/article/printarticle/2764. Accessed January 18, 2022.

58. DeKeyser-Ganz F, Fink NF, Asher O, et al. ICU nurses' oral-care practices and the current best evidence. Journal of Nursing Scholarship 2009;41(2):132–138.

59. Hess CT. Clinical Guide: Skin and Wound Care. 6th ed. Ambler, PA: Lippincott, Williams & Wilkins; 2008.

60. Cheng V, Abdul-Aziz MH, Roberts JA, et al. Optimising drug dosing in patients receiving extracorporeal membrane oxygenation. J Thorac Dis. 2018 Mar;10(Suppl 5):S629-S641.

61. Kühn D, Metz C, Seiler F, et al. Antibiotic therapeutic drug monitoring in intensive care patients treated with different modalities of extracorporeal membrane oxygenation (ECMO) and renal replacement therapy: a prospective, observational single-center study. Crit Care. 2020 Nov 25;24(1):664.

62. Di Nardo M, Wildschut ED. Drugs pharmacokinetics during veno-venous extracorporeal membrane oxygenation in pediatrics. J Thorac Dis. 2018 Mar;10(Suppl 5):S642-S652.

63. Turner DA, Cheifetz IM, Rehder KJ, et al. Active rehabilitation and physical therapy during extracorporeal membrane oxygenation while awaiting lung transplantation: a practical approach. Crit Care Med. 2011 Dec;39(12):2593-8.

64. Turner DA, Rehder KJ, Bonadonna D, et al. Ambulatory ECMO as a bridge to lung transplant in a previously well pediatric patient with ARDS. Pediatrics. 2014 Aug;134(2):e583-5.

65. Langer T, Santini A, Bottino N, et al. "Awake" extracorporeal membrane oxygenation (ECMO): pathophysiology, technical considerations, and clinical pioneering. Crit Care. 2016 Jun 30;20(1):150.

66. Costa J, Dirnberger DR, Froehlich CD, et al. Awake Neonatal Extracorporeal Membrane Oxygenation. ASAIO J. 2020 May;66(5):e70-e73.

67. Sutter Raoul, Tisljar Kai, Marsch, Stephan. Acute Neurologic Complications During Extracorporeal Membrane Oxygenation: A Systematic Review, Crit Care Med September 2018 - Volume 46 - Issue 9 - p 1506-1513.

68. Bembea MM, Felling RJ, Caprarola SD, et al. Neurologic Outcomes in a Two-Center Cohort of Neonatal and Pediatric Patients Supported on Extracorporeal Membrane Oxygenation. ASAIO J. 2020 Jan;66(1):79-88.

69. Said AS, Guilliams KP, Bembea MM. Neurological Monitoring and Complications of Pediatric Extracorporeal Membrane Oxygenation Support. Pediatr Neurol. 2020 Jul;108:31-39.

70. Barbaro RP, Paden ML, Guner YS, et al. Pediatric Extracorporeal Life Support Organization Registry International Report 2016. ASAIO J. 2017 Jul/Aug;63(4):456-463.

71. Lin N, Flibotte J, Licht DJ. Neuromonitoring in the neonatal ECMO patient. Semin Perinatol. 2018;42(2):111-121.

72. Blackenberg FG, Loh NN, Bracci P, et al. Sonography, CT, and MR Imaging: A prospective Comparison of Neonates with Suspected Intracranial Ischemia and Hemorrhage. Am J Neuroradiol. January 2000; 21(1):213-218.

73. Cvetkovic M, Chiarini G, Belliato M, et al. International survey of neuromonitoring and neurodevelopmental outcome in children and adults supported on extracorporeal membrane oxygenation in Europe. Perfusion. 2021 Sep 22:2676591211042563.

74. Clair MP, Rambaud J, Flahault A, et al. Prognostic value of cerebral tissue oxygen saturation during neonatal extracorporeal membrane oxygenation. PLoS One. 2017 Mar 9;12(3):e0172991.

75. Pozzebon S, Blandino Ortiz A, Franchi F, et al. Cerebral Near-Infrared Spectroscopy in Adult Patients Undergoing Veno-Arterial Extracorporeal Membrane Oxygenation. Neurocrit Care. 2018 Aug;29(1):94-104.

76. Sansevere AJ, DiBacco ML, Akhondi-Asl A, et al. EEG features of brain injury during extracorporeal membrane oxygenation in children. Neurology. 2020 Sep 8;95(10):e1372-e1380.

77. Cook RJ, Rau SM, Lester-Pelham SG, et al. Electrographic Seizures and Brain Injury in Children Requiring Extracorporeal Membrane Oxygenation. Pediatr Neurol. 2020 Jul;108:77-85.

78. Fox J, Jenks CL, Farhat A, et al. EEG is A Predictor of Neuroimaging Abnormalities in Pediatric Extracorporeal Membrane Oxygenation. J Clin Med. 2020 Aug 4;9(8):2512.

79. Madderom MJ, Schiller RM, Gischler SJ, et al. Growing up after critical illness: verbal, visual-spatial, and working memory problems in neonatal extracorporeal membrane oxygenation survivors. Crit Care Med 2016; 44: 1182–1190.

80. IJsselstijn H, Hunfeld M, Schiller RM, et al. Improving long-term outcomes after extracorporeal

membrane oxygenation: from observational follow-up programs toward risk stratification. Front Pediatr 2018; 6: 177.

81. Yao FS, Tseng CC, Ho CY, et al. Cerebral oxygen desaturation is associated with early postoperative neuropsychological dysfunction in patients undergoing cardiac surgery. J Cardiothorac Vasc Anesth. 2004 Oct;18(5):552-8.

82. Kussman BD, Wypij D, Laussen PC, et al. Relationship of intraoperative cerebral oxygen saturation to neurodevelopmental outcome and brain magnetic resonance imaging at 1 year of age in infants undergoing biventricular repair. Circulation 2010;122:245–54.

83. CHAPTER 6 of this Edition Adverse Effects of ECLS Lindsay Ryerson MD, Gail Annich MD, Andriy Batchinsky MD, Gennaro Martucci, Teryn Roberts PhD, Ravi Thiagarajan, Christophe Vandenbriele MD PhD, Graeme MacLaren MBBS MSc.

84. Attard C, Straaten Karlaftis, V, et al. Developmental hemostasis: age-specific differences in the levels of hemostatic proteins Journal of thrombosis and haemostasis, 2013-10, Vol.11 (10), p.1850-1854.

85. Toulon, P Developmental hemostasis: laboratory and clinical implications International Journal of laboratory hematology, 2016-05, Vol.38 (S1), p.66-77.

86. McMichael ABV, Ryerson LM, Ratano D, et al. 2021 ELSO Adult and Pediatric Anticoagulation Guidelines ASAIO journal (1992), 2022-03-01, Vol.68 (3), p.303-310.

87. Saini A, Spinella PC. Management of anticoagulation and hemostasis for pediatric extracorporeal membrane oxygenation. Clin Lab Med, 2014. 34(3): p. 655-73.

88. Ozmen C.P, et al. Anticoagulation and Transfusion Management During Neonatal and Pediatric Extracorporeal Membrane Oxygenation: A Survey of Medical Directors in the United States. Pediatr Crit Care Med, 2021.

89. Sivarajan VB, Best D, Brizard CP, et al. Improved outcomes of paediatric extracorporeal support associated with technology change. Interact Cardiovasc Thorac Surg 2010;11:400–5.

90. Deshpande SJ, Vitali S, Thiagarajan R, et al. Coagulations Studies Do Not Correlate With Each Other or With Hematologic Complications During Pediatric Extracorporeal Membrane Oxygenation. Pediatr Crit Care Med. 2021 Jun 1;22(6):542-552.

91. Moynihan KM, Purol N, Alexander PMA, et al .A communication guide for pediatric extracorporeal membrane oxygenation Ped Crit Care Med 2022;22(9):832-841.

# 15

## Weaning and Decannulation of Children with Respiratory Failure

*Thomas Pranikoff and Graeme MacLaren*

ECLS offers critically ill patients many benefits during their illness. Associated with these benefits are significant risks. Discontinuation of support should be considered when the risk:benefit ratio increases and patients are able to be cared for by less invasive techniques. After a period of initial stabilization, the question of whether discontinuation of ECLS is possible should be frequently evaluated as the patient's condition improves.

### Strategies to Expedite Withdrawal of ECLS

At the initiation of extracorporeal support, it should be estimated how long the patient will require support. When improvement of lung function begins to appear, a trial off ECLS may be attempted. In this way, patients are subjected to the potential risks of extracorporeal support for the least amount of time.

The need to avoid ventilator-induced lung injury has led many clinicians to utilize ventilatory strategies while on ECLS which are designed to minimize injury primarily by lowering airway pressure and $FiO_2$. An extreme offshoot of this strategy, now being used in some centers, is elective extubation while on ECLS. In one single-center study, extubation during ECLS permitted increased physical activity in cannulated pediatric patients and the opportunity to prevent the physical deconditioning associated with long ICU stays.[1] Spontaneous ventilation may have been effective in promoting spontaneous reaeration, cough, and secretion mobilization in patients with severe pulmonary consolidation. However, it remains unknown whether positive pressure of any sort is harmful or helpful in an injured lung. What this study did not answer is whether extubation speeds or delays resolution of lung injury and alveolar reinflation.[1]

One survey of international centers which participate in the ELSO Registry found that 27% of centers have a specific ventilation protocol for patients on VV ECMO. Lung rest was the primary goal in 77% of respondents and lung recruitment or a combination of both in 18% of respondents. Eighty percent of centers used a PEEP of greater than 5 $cmH_2O$. Most centers (90%) prioritized weaning from ECLS over the ventilator. Weaning from ECLS was accomplished by reduction of sweep gas in 43% and flow rates in 21%.[2]

Several strategies have been suggested by individual centers that may potentially decrease the duration of an ECLS run. In a matched pair analysis, Hermon et al. compared seven pediatric ECLS patients given porcine surfactant with seven who were not.[3] Groups were matched based on age, weight, and underlying diagnosis. The most common diagnosis in both groups was ARDS. Mean tidal volume improved significantly over time in the surfactant group (100% at baseline vs. 186.2% at 10 hours after surfactant application) compared to the control group (100% vs. 98.7%; p=0.0053). Similarly, mean compliance values increased significantly over time in the surfactant group (100% before vs. 176.1% at 10 hours after surfactant application) compared to the control group (100% vs. 97.6%; p=0.0067). Radiographic scores tended to decrease in the surfactant group within 48 hours following surfactant application. ECLS flow tended to decrease in this group within 10 hours following surfactant application but not in the control group. Mortality was not affected by treatment.[4] Two other studies showed an improvement in pulmonary mechanics and a decrease in ECLS duration in term neonates on ECLS who received multiple doses of surfactant.[4,5]

The use of prone positioning to redistribute pulmonary blood flow into regions of the lung that are better aerated and mobilize edema has been advocated for patients with ARDS but the efficacy remains controversial. Many centers that care for patients with ARDS with ECLS have used this technique safely (Chapter 47).[6,7]

## Weaning Support and Trialing

Indications of lung recovery on venovenous support include increasing saturation of venous blood returned to the circuit, increasing $PaO_2$, or decreasing $PaCO_2$ without changes in either extracorporeal flow or ventilator settings. Increasing lung compliance, clearing of the chest radiograph, and increased $VO_2$ and $VCO_2$ measured via the airway are also seen. When this process begins, it will usually continue until termination of extracorporeal support is possible unless a new problem, such as pneumonia or sepsis, intervenes.

When lung function begins to improve, weaning from support may be possible. It is important to understand that weaning is a diagnostic rather than a therapeutic maneuver.

The purpose of weaning is to obtain information to help make the decision of whether support can be discontinued and transitioned to mechanical ventilation alone. Since lung rest is the major benefit from venovenous support, the decision to terminate support must include careful consideration of the clinical situation. In the ideal situation, at the time of decannulation, ventilator support will be at a level considered to be safe (low inspiratory pressure and $FiO_2$). In some situations, these goals must be modified. For example, in a patient with bleeding (eg, postoperative, intracranial, gastrointestinal) which cannot be controlled by medical means, there needs to be an assessment of the risks of continuing with ECLS vs. discontinuing ECLS while utilizing mechanical ventilation at higher $FiO_2$ and airway pressures than otherwise might be desired.

Weaning can be accomplished in patients on venovenous support by setting the ventilator to acceptable levels (eg, Pplat <30 cmH$_2$O, PEEP 8-12 cmH$_2$O, $FiO_2$ <0.5-0.6), then discontinuing the sweep gas flow across the oxygenator while continuing blood flow. This is accomplished by simply turning off the sweep gas flow. If room air is allowed to flow across the membrane lung, this can provide ongoing gas transfer. During this time, the patient is closely monitored for changes in respiratory rate, $SaO_2$, agitation, heart rate, and blood pressure. Spontaneous ventilation usually augments lung function, but some patients may need additional sedation. Anticoagulation should be continued, except in percutaneously cannulated patients where it is generally favorable to cease anticoagulation one hour prior to removing the cannulas and putting pressure on the site. The ventilator is adjusted according to arterial blood gases. Often the goals of support should be modified to accept levels of $PaO_2$ in the 60-80 mmHg range and $PaCO_2$ in the 40-60 mmHg range. This will allow the use of lower airway pressures and $FiO_2$ to protect the recovering lungs. If the trial continues with stable blood gases at acceptable level of respiratory support for several hours, decannulation can be planned. In children with respiratory failure receiving VA ECMO, weaning and decannulation is performed similarly to patients receiving cardiac support (Chapter 19).

## Technique for Decannulation of Patients on VV ECMO

Most patients on VV ECMO will be cannulated percutaneously. Some patients, mostly newborns, may be cannulated by a surgical cutdown. For these patients, it is advisable to use a brief general anesthetic with neuromuscular blockade. This will ensure the optimal conditions and prevent negative pressure using a Valsalva maneuver which could cause air embolus when the vein is open or if the side holes are exposed while the cannula is being withdrawn. The wound is sterilely prepped and opened. The cannula cutdown site is exposed and clot is removed for visualization. A ligature is placed around the cannula and vein and left untied. The circuit is clamped and patient ventilator settings are adjusted to insure that support off ECLS will be tolerated. The skin sutures and sutures around the vein are divided and the cannula is rapidly removed by one person and the previously placed ligature is tied by a second person. The wound is closed after hemostasis is assured. Situations which make this more challenging include tearing of the vein with complete division and not enough stump left to control (usually the result of a long ECLS run). For the former, if the vein can be grasped with a forceps, it can then be either simply ligated or suture ligated. For the latter, it is sufficient to place a purse string suture in the tissue around the vein to close off the soft tissues since venous pressure is quite low and usually easy to control.

For percutaneously cannulated patients, either sedation or local anesthesia will usually suffice. The patient should be placed supine rather than in a sitting position to lower the risk of air embolus. The skin and cannula are sterilely prepped and draped. Two options are available for hemostasis. After clamping the circuit and dividing the skin sutures the cannula can be rapidly removed (so that air does not enter the side holes and exit the end hole into the vein) and direct pressure held over the cannulation site. Usually 5–10 minutes of pressure will provide hemostasis. The alternative is to place a purse string suture in the skin close to the cannula exit site in the skin. Monofilament suture (nylon or polypropylene) slides better and is easier to tie. One person can rapidly remove the cannula while another ties the purse string; it is unnecessary to hold pressure using this technique. Hematoma formation is unusual due to the relatively low venous pressure.

## Continuing Venous Access after Decannulation

Venous access is often challenging in critically ill children, especially after completing ECLS. When considering decannulation, future access needs should be assessed and a plan established. As children are often edematous at this point in their illness, using peripheral venous sites can be challenging. Establishing new central venous or dialysis catheter access may even be technically impossible, in which case a technique of guidewire exchange can be used. Although this carries risks of thrombosis and infection, it may be the only practical solution in some patients. The cannulation site, cannula, connector, and tubing are prepped and sterilely draped. A purse string suture is placed around the skin at the access site and left untied. The circuit and cannula are clamped, leaving room on the tubing between the clamp and the cannula connector. The line kit is opened and the guidewire is prepared. It is important to have a guidewire of at least twice the length of the ECLS cannula, which may not be in the kit and thus should be obtained separately. The introducer needle is then placed through the tubing until blood is aspirated and the guidewire is advanced through the connector and into the cannula lumen (Figure 15-1). A second person prepares to tie the purse string suture and places a single throw of the knot which is tightened to prevent hemorrhage as the cannula is withdrawn, being sure the guidewire remains. The line is then placed over the guidewire to the appropriate depth and the purse string suture is tied to provide hemostasis. The line is aspirated and flushed to assure patency and securely sutured to the skin.

## Approaches to Inadvertent Decannulation

If unplanned removal of the venous cannula occurs, immediate action is necessary. The bedside ECLS Specialist must be familiar with managing this emergency since they will often be the only team member at the bedside. Priorities in this situation are hemostasis and respiratory support. Direct pressure will provide hemostasis. Simultaneously, ventilation must be escalated to provide adequate respiratory support. Hand ventilation may provide this, but using a conventional or high-frequency ventilator is usually necessary. Depending on the amount of lung dysfunction that remains, two scenarios are possible. The first is that ventilation and oxygenation are adequate at acceptable levels of ventilation and FiO$_2$. In this case, mechanical ventilation should be continued and weaned as possible, utilizing a lung protective strategy. The second scenario is that, even with high levels of ventilation and FiO$_2$, the patient is not adequately supported. In this situation, ECLS should be reestablished expeditiously, while supporting the patient as best as possible. If possible, separate teams should be responsible for each of these tasks (Chapter 7).

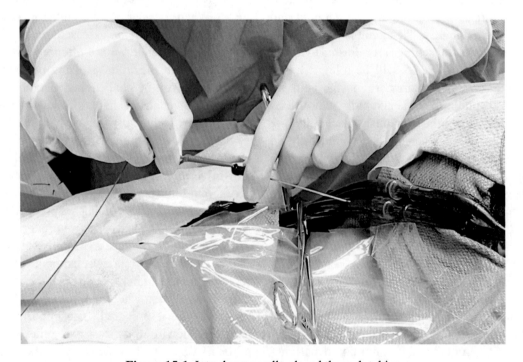

**Figure 15-1.** Introducer needle placed through tubing.

# References

1.  Anton-Martin P, Thompson MT, Sheeran PD, et al. Extubation During Pediatric Extracorporeal Membrane Oxygenation: A Single-Center Experience. Pediatr Crit Care Med 2014; 15(9):861-9.
2.  Marhong JD, Telesnicki T, Munshi L, et al. Mechanical Ventilation during Extracorporeal Membrane Oxygenation An International Survey. Ann Am Thorac Soc 2014; 11(6):956-61.
3.  Hermon M, Burda G, Male C, et al. Surfactant application during extracorporeal membrane oxygenation improves lung volume and pulmonary mechanics in children with respiratory failure. Crit Care 2005; 9(6):R718-24.
4.  Lotze A, Knight G, Martin G, et al. Improved pulmonary outcome after exogenous surfactant therapy for respiratory failure in term infants requiring extracorporeal membrane oxygenation. J Pediatr 1993; 122(2):261-8.
5.  Stillerman L, Gunn S, Hart J, et al. Effects of exogenous surfactant on neonates supported by extracorporeal membrane oxygenation. J Perinatol 1997; 17(4):262-5.
6.  Kimmoun A, Roche S, Bridey C, et al. Prolonged prone positioning under VV-ECMO is safe and improves oxygenation and respiratory compliance. Ann Intensive Care 2015; 5(1):35.
7.  Haefner S, Bratton S, Annich G, et al. Complications of intermittent prone positioning in pediatric patients receiving extracorporeal membrane oxygenation for respiratory failure. Chest 2003; 123(5):1589-94.

# 16

## Complications, Followup, and Outcomes of Pediatric Patients with Respiratory Failure

*Susan L. Bratton, Parthak Prodhan, Maayke Hunfeld, Lakshmi Raman*

## History

ECLS in children with respiratory failure was an accepted "rescue therapy" for decades before its use in adult patients.[1] However, attempts to directly demonstrate efficacy by a randomized trial comparing it to conventional ventilation and supportive care in children were hampered by both the lower incidence of hypoxic respiratory failure[2] and lower mortality in pediatric compared to adult patients. Concurrent improvement in survival rates with lower tidal volume ventilation and permissive hypercapnia made clinicians unwilling to predict sufficiently high expected mortality for potential subjects to meet eligibility for study randomization.[3,4] Currently, the strongest study design report of ELCS in pediatric respiratory failure comes from a secondary analysis of a prospective study,[5] comparing those who received ECLS as part of their care to those who did not. Ninety-day mortality was similar in both groups (25% for ECLS vs. 30% non-ECLS patients).[6]

ECLS is currently used to "rescue" pediatric patients (age groups defined by ELSO) as infants (>28 days to <1 year) and children (>1 to <18 years) with primary respiratory failure unresponsive to other therapies.[7] Survival with ECLS requires that: 1) the underlying pulmonary process is reversible or can be stabilized and rescued later by organ transplantation,[8] 2) additional organ injury and failure are prevented by ECLS support, and 3) rapid identification and correction of ECLS related complications associated with mortality are prevented or mitigated (eg, an atrial septostomy with left atrial hypertension causing pulmonary hemorrhage and poor coronary artery perfusion).

## Outcomes

### Hospital Survival

Survival has steadily improved from 56% in 2001 to 62% in 2014,[9-10] and more recently to 67%[11] to 70%, based on a report from North American Centers.[6] However, patient complexity has increased, with more comorbid conditions such as cancer or genetic conditions, and acute complications such as cardiac arrest and acute renal failure (ARF) noted.[6,12]

ECLS to treat pediatric respiratory failure is a relatively rare event, with the highest number of annual ECLS runs reported to ELSO in 2019 (n=870) internationally, with a median annual center volume for neonates and children for all indications of 8 (IQR 2.17) cases.[11] Thus, single-center studies have relatively small sample sizes, while most multicentered ECLS studies either use ELSO[13] or administrative databases.[14-15]

A limitation of such administrative data sources is that medical procedure codes (eg, renal replacement therapies [RRT]) that treat ARF do not meet criteria for ARF and the timing of diagnosis codes (eg, cardiac arrest) are not specified in relationship to ECLS deployment. Some diagnosis codes such as a cancer or genetic conditions likely reflect preexisting conditions.

### Demographic and Clinical Features Associated with Survival

Demographic and clinical features of ECLS for pediatric respiratory failure by hospital survival are shown in Table 16-1 using data provided by ELSO during 2001-2013.[9] Significantly lower hospital survival was noted in children ≥10 years (53%) and among those with severe acidosis and severe hypoxia (Table 16-1).

| FEATURES | SURVIVED* N (%) | DIED** N (%) | P-VALUE |
|---|---|---|---|
| Age in Years | | | p=0.003 |
| <1*** | 1139 (46) | 886 (48) | |
| 1-2 | 452 (18) | 271 (15) | |
| 3-5, 1 | 242 (10) | 165 (9) | |
| 6-9 | 185 (7) | 119 (6) | |
| >10 | 477 (19) | 416 (22) | |
| Mechanical Ventilation | | | p<0.001 |
| >14 Days | 157 (6) | 184 (10) | |
| pH prior to ECLS | | | p<0.001 |
| <7.11 | 647 (26) | 572 (31) | |
| 7.11-7.34 | 1172 (47) | 937 (50) | |
| >7.34 | 676 (27) | 348 (19) | |
| VV ECMO | 1239 (50) | 626 (34) | p<0.001 |
| Primary Pulmonary Diagnosis | | | p<0.001 |
| Other | 1645 (66) | 1260 (68) | |
| Asthma | 134 (5) | 30 (2) | |
| Aspiration | 100 (4) | 37 (2) | |
| RSV | 309 (12) | 152 (8) | |
| Sepsis ARDS | 276 (11) | 311 (17) | |
| Pertussis | 47 (2) | 93 (5) | |
| Coexisting Conditions | | | |
| Structural heart disease | 232 (9) | 193 (10) | p=NS |
| Chronic lung disease | 85 (3) | 76 (4) | p=NS |
| Cancer | 60 (2) | 101 (5) | p<0.001 |
| Immunodeficiency | 34 (1) | 42 (2) | p=0.027 |
| Myocarditis | 22 (1) | 29 (2) | p=0.046 |
| Cardiac arrest | 316 (13) | 335 (18) | p<0.001 |
| Acute renal failure | 301 (12) | 522 (28) | p<0.001 |
| Acute liver necrosis | 8 (0) | 68 (4) | p<0.001 |

*N=2495; **N=1857; ***excludes infants <30 days of age at ECLS initiation;
NS=not statistically significant; RSV=Respiratory syncytial virus; ARDS=Acute Respiratory Distress Syndrome

**Table 16-1.** Select demographic and clinical features reported to ELSO for pediatric respiratory failure patients. (Adapted from Bailly et al.[9])

### ECLS Mode

VA ECMO provides cardiorespiratory support while VV ECMO relies on the lungs to provide additional oxygenation and the patient's native cardiac function to sustain adequate blood pressure and perfusion. VA use is associated with greater organ failure at the time of ECLS initiation. In contrast, VV use is associated with greater protection from systemic air/clot embolization from the ECLS circuit, substantially lower central nervous system complications,[12] and lower hospital mortality compared to VA.[9]

A steady increase in VV ECMO and double-lumen VV catheters compared with V-A cannulation has been observed. From 1993 to 2007, VV increased from 35% to 46%, and use of double-lumen VV catheters from 1% to 19%.[12] The 2016-2020 ELSO International Report showed V-V cannulation in 55-63% of annual runs for pediatric respiratory failure.[11] Like patients initially treated with VA, those transitioned from VV to VA had similar mortality.[11,12,16]

### Prolonged Duration of Ventilation Before ECLS

Prolonged use of large tidal volume breaths and high airway pressures targeted to normalize $PaCO_2$ are well known to cause ventilator induced lung injury(VILI). ECLS when implemented after irreversible lung injury has occurred[17] will only extend time to death from multiorgan failure. Early reports of ECLS to rescue pediatric respiratory failure recommended less than 10 days of pre-ECLS mechanical ventilation for infants and no more than 5-7 days for older children.[10,18] The reported median duration of mechanical ventilation prior to ECLS was 6 days, but noted that 8% of children ventilated >14 days had significantly greater mortality.[9-10] However, the median duration of pre-ECLS mechanical ventilation has decreased to a median of 2.5 days (IQR 1-5 days) in a recent report among infants >2 weeks to 18 years of age.[6] Those patients being evaluated for ECLS after prolonged ventilatory support should be evaluated for the duration of potentially harmful ventilator settings.

## Comorbid Conditions

### Cancer and Hematopoietic Stem Cell Transplantation (HSCT)

Obviously, cancer care can be complex with infectious complications, organ failure due to regimen-associated toxicity, engraftment status, and varying long-term prognosis across different malignancy types. Survival after HSCT and ECLS (reported to ELSO from 1990-2019) has historically been low (19%), but over the last decade has increased to 26%.[19] A recent propensity matched study from 2011-2018 found that patients treated with ECLS to provide respiratory support compared to control subjects had 61% survival to hospital discharge, but the ECLS patients had lower platelet counts, received greater platelet transfusions, and suffered greater rates of new neurologic impairment. (46% vs. 20%).[20] A multidisciplinary panel provided "a clinical decision support tool for pediatric hematologists, oncologists, and critical care physicians during the difficult decisionmaking process of ECMO candidacy and management."[21] Cancer patients treated with ECLS had lower median platelet counts, received more platelet transfusions, and had a greater risk of thrombotic complications and death.[22] Maue et al.[23] reported oncology and HSCT patients had a higher mortality and received more blood products while on ECLS than general pediatric intensive care unit patients, despite similar pre-ECLS hypoxia.

### Primary Pulmonary Process

Among pulmonary diagnostic categories, hospital survival is significantly greater for status asthmaticus, aspiration pneumonia, and respiratory syncytial virus (RSV), bronchiolitis, or pneumonia, but significantly lower for pertussis and acute adult respiratory failure due to sepsis compared to "other" conditions, with a median mortality of 43% (Table 16-1).[9] Two models have been developed for mortality prediction among pediatric patients with severe respiratory failure.[9-10] Table 16-2 compares the two prediction models to aid in evaluation of candidates for ECLS, as well as for use in risk adjustment. The models are quite similar with use of blood gas measurements analyzed as either continuous or discrete grouped variables. Bailly et al.[9] used both receipt of renal replacement therapies (RRT) and diagnosis codes for ARF prior to ECLS, which made ARF much more common compared to Barbaro et al.[10] (19% vs. 2%), as well as pre-ECLS cardiac arrest (15% vs. 5%).

Such scores could be used to adjust for case mix and performance and may be useful for counselling parents about estimated mortality. A generalized model for mortality prediction risk regardless of indication and pediatric age, the PEP score,[24] was developed using data from the prospective observational study of bleeding and thrombosis during ECLS Study (BATE)[25] for all pediatric patients.

### Prolonged ECLS

Brogan et al.[26] reported an analysis that included first ECLS runs among children with acute respiratory failure reported to ELSO from 1993-2007. They found that 75% received ECLS for ≤14 days, with 12% supported for ≥21 days (38% survival). The survival to hospital discharge with 22-28 days of ECLS declined to 30%, and with 29-45 days of ECLS, survival was 25%. No patient with

>52 days of ECLS survived. No significant differences were found between survivors and non survivors among patients with prolonged ECLS for pre-ECLS clinical features; however, ECLS complications increased with duration of ECLS.[26] The 2016-2020 International ELSO Summary documented that the mean duration of ECLS was much lower (13 days), while the longest annual run ranged from 111 days to 250 day when compared to 2000-2005 data, when the longest annual run ranged from 36 to 101 days.[11] This suggests that technical support of acute respiratory failure with ECLS has improved over time and further analysis of prolonged ECLS support in more recent years regarding patient selection with survival and morbidity are needed.

A recent analysis of 1818 ELSO patients treated from 1998 to 2015 with multiple ECLS runs during the same hospital admission reported hospital survival of 37% for 2 runs and 29% for ≥3 runs. Pediatric patients had less mortality than adults (OR: 0.5 [95% CI: 0.02-0.8]). Cardiac support on the first run was associated with higher mortality than pulmonary support, regardless of final run indication [OR:1.4 (95%CI: 1.1-1.8)].[16] Recannulation poses technical challenges as many centers do not reconstruct the carotid if the ECLS run has been greater than 2-3 days because of the risk of delayed stroke. When the carotid arterial catheter is removed both the proximal and distal ends are ligated.

| CHARACTERISTICS | Peds RESCUERS[10] | P-PREP[9] |
|---|---|---|
| Blood gas values | pH, $PaCO_2$ | pH |
| | | 7.11-7.34 |
| | | >7.34 |
| $PaO_2/FiO_2$ | Not included | <100 |
| | | 101-200 |
| | | 201-300 |
| | | >300 |
| Mean Airway Pressure | | |
| | Conventional Ventilator | Not included |
| | High Frequency Oscillatory Ventilation | |
| Hours from admission to initiation of ECLS | Log transformed | Not included |
| Hours from starting mechanical ventilation | Log transformed | Days >14 |
| Milrinone prior to ECLS | Yes | Not included |
| Mode of ECLS | Not included | V-A vs. V-V |
| Year of ECLS | Not included | Year |
| Comorbid Conditions | Cancer | Cancer |
| | | Acute Renal Failure |
| | | Cardiac Arrest pre-ECLS |
| | | Acute Liver Necrosis |
| Primary Pulmonary Process | Asthma | Asthma |
| | Bronchiolitis | RSV |
| | Pertussis | Pertussis |
| | | Aspiration Pneumonia |
| | | Sepsis Acute Respiratory Failure |
| Area under the Receiver Operator Curve-development | 0.69 | 0.69 |
| Area under the Receiver Operator Curve-validation | 0.63 | 0.66 |

**Table 16-2.** Comparison of mortality prediction tools for pediatric respiratory failure.

## ECLS Complications and Mortality

### *Neurologic*

Neurologic complication rates reported by ELSO include determination of death based on neurologic criteria (2%), diffuse brain ischemia (1%), central nervous system hemorrhage (4%), brain infarction (4%), and clinical seizures (2%).[11] Table 16-3 lists the various complications collected by ELSO from 2016-2020. All neurologic complications are more frequent with VA than VV ECLS and pediatric respiratory failure patients with neurologic complications (excluding seizures) are less likely to survive to hospital discharge.

Daily neurologic assessments should be performed in all patients while on ECLS with sedating medications doses as low as possible. Multimodal neuromonitoring is recommended

| | |
|---|---|
| Membrane Lung Failure | Change indicated due to clot formation, gas exchange failure or blood leak |
| Blood Pump Failure | Change indicated due to equipment failure |
| Raceway Rupture | In a roller pump rupture of the raceway tubing |
| Other Tubing Rupture | Rupture of ECLS tubing |
| Circuit Change | Entire circuit (except cannulas) changed due to clot formation or mechanical failure |
| Cannula problems | Requiring intervention (reposition or exchange) for misplacement, dislodgement, replacement due to clots/fibrin, mechanical failure, or inappropriate position |
| Temp Regulator Malfunction | Malfunction of temperature regulation device leading to unintentional (< 35°) hypothermia or hyperthermia (> 39°) |
| Clots and Air Emboli | If a clot or an air embolus causes a mechanical failure or change out of a circuit component |
| Thrombosis/Clots: Circuit Component | Circuit component (eg, pigtails, connectors, bridge, arterial or venous tubing) requiring change due to clot formation or mechanical failure of the component |
| Clots in Hemofilter | Clots in hemofilter causing hemofilter to need to be changed or to fail |
| Air in Circuit | Requiring circuit intervention or circuit clamping for bubble detector alarm, visualized air, air entry into patient |
| GI Hemorrhage | Upper or lower GI hemorrhage requiring PRBC transfusion (>20ml/kg/24 hrs of PRBCS or >3U PRBCs/24 hrs in neonates and pediatrics, and/or, endoscopic intervention, and/or hemostatic agent deployment |
| Peripheral, Mediastinal Cannulation Site or Surgical Site Bleeding | Site bleeding requiring PRBC transfusion (>20ml/kg/24 hrs of PRBCS or >3U PRBCs/24 hrs in neonates and pediatric and/or, surgical intervention (includes intravascular hemostatic agent deployment). A reperfusion cannula is a type of peripheral cannulation site. |
| CNS Complications | Brain death; seizures (clinical vs. electrographic); CNS diffuse ischemia, localized ischemia, intraparenchymal, subdural or subarachnoid bleed, ≥ grade 2 intraventricular hemorrhage, Neurosurgical procedure performed during ECLS run (eg, intracranial pressure monitor, external ventricular drain, craniotomy) |
| Creatinine 1.5 – 3.0 or > 3.0 | After ECMO start time, patient has a new creatinine serum measurement of 1.5- 3.0 or > 3.0 mg/dL |
| Renal Replacement | Any form of dialysis or fluid removal |
| CV Complications | CPR, a treated dysrhythmia, tamponade treated for blood or other fluid |
| Pulmonary Complications | Pneumothorax treated with chest tube, hemorrhage requiring PRBC transfusion (>20ml/kg/24 hrs of PRBCS or >3U PRBCs/24 hrs in neonates and pediatric and/or, surgical intervention |

**Table 16-3.** Mechanical and patient complications during ECLS reported to ELSO.

to monitor brain function, consisting of near infrared spectroscopy and augmented electroencephalography (EEG), particularly in the setting where clinical parameters are limited because of sedation and use of muscle relaxants. For patients with open fontanelles, frequent ultrasonography of the head should be checked, particularly in the first 3 days of ECMO support. If there are any concerns for a change in mental status, or focal neurologic finding, then computed tomography of the head is indicated.[27]

In the future, neuromonitoring modalities will likely be expanded with techniques such as transcranial doppler, quantitative EEG, noninvasive cerebrovascular autoregulation monitoring, or plasma cerebral biomarkers.[28] It is recommended to perform brain MRI prior to hospital discharge.[27,28]

### Acute Renal Failure and Use of Renal Replacement Therapy

Exposure of blood to the oxygenator membrane is frequently associated with cytokine release and fluid overload (FO). Swaniker et al.[29] noted that surviving children with acute respiratory failure receiving ECLS had lower average FO of 9% when ECLS was initiated that decreased to 4% at the time when ECLS was discontinued. The mean FO when ECLS started among nonsurvivors was 25% and increased to 35% by the time of death.[29]

A secondary analysis of the Kidney Interventions During Membrane Oxygenation (KIDMO) Study Group[30] reevaluated FO in 256 neonates and older infants.[31] AKI was defined by serum creatinine-based criteria alone and FO was based on patient weight at ICU admission. During the ECLS course, 71% had FO and 51% had severe AKI. The authors evaluated FO when RRT was initiated and 63% of patients with <20% FO had lower hospital mortality (47%) but as FO increased (30 to <40%, 40 to <50% and ≥50%), hospital mortality increased

(63%, 74% and 68%, respectively). The authors concluded that patients in whom RRT was initiated when the FO% was lower had greater decreases in FO%, shorter duration of ECLS, and improved survival.[31] This requires further investigation as other reports present conflicting conclusions where the use of RRT is associated with longer duration of ECLS and greater odds of death during ECLS.[9,30]

### Hemorrhage, Hemolysis and Thrombosis

Variability in anticoagulation strategies for monitoring and treatment continues across various institutions. While on ECLS, it remains unclear what the optimal therapy and monitoring strategy is mitigating both hemorrhage and thrombosis. Hemorrhage is one of the most frequent complications during ECLS support and is associated with decreased survival.[32] Hemorrhagic complications defined as blood loss leading to a transfusion or an intracranial hemorrhage are more common in children (30%) compared to neonates (16%).[25] This higher rate of hemorrhage in older children compared to neonates occurs at these anatomic sites: cannula (11% vs. 5%), surgical (8% vs. 5%), gastrointestinal (4% vs. 1%), pulmonary (6% vs. 2%) and blood sampling for testing (55% vs. 75%). Blood sampling was the only bleeding source for at least one transfusion in 66% vs. 40%. The rate of overall thrombotic events was 11.0 per 100 days. Patient-related 4.5/100 days and circuit related thromboses was 7/100 days.[25]

Hemolysis was not associated with pump type but was associated with turbulent and greater flow rates. Hemolysis, typically defined as a plasma free hemoglobin >50 mg/dL, was present in 27% of pediatric vs. 40% of neonatal respiratory failure ECLS patients. Additionally, hemolysis was associated with use of a hemofilter, with RRT, and greater transfusion of blood products. Finally, it was associated with later thrombotic complications and duration of ECLS but not mortality.[25] During care of children >31 days and <18 years, Dalton et al. reported that 34% of respiratory failure pediatric patients had circuit related thrombosis or clot and required exchange of the entire circuit (15%), or its components (6% oxygenator; 5% bladder, 5% tubing, 4% clots in the arterial cannula, 4% hemofilter).[25]

### Mechanical Complications

Mechanical failure occurred in about 15% of ECLS courses reported to the ELSO Registry over a 20-year period,[29] with a decreasing trend in the current era. The prevalence of mechanical failure in pediatric respiratory failure were 7% oxygenator failure, 0.2% raceway rupture, 6% clots in hemofilter, 5% air in the circuit, 17% circuit change, 13% hemolysis, and 23% thrombosis or clot in circuit component.

### Infectious Complications

Patients are at high risk for nosocomial infections. Factors increasing the infection risk include a need for invasive procedures and prolonged use of support devices, including central venous, arterial, and urinary catheters. Furthermore, alterations in the immune response often accompany critical illness and exposure of the blood and surfaces of the ECLS circuit.[32,33] Infections are associated with a prolonged need for support, an increased risk of mechanical and patient-related complications, and increased hospital mortality.[33] Older children on ECLS for pulmonary indications have a higher prevalence of culture-proven infections compared to neonates (17% vs. 6%).[33] Infection prevalence almost doubles among patients who require ECLS for >14 days (30%) compared to those with shorter runs (8-14 days [16%] and ≤7 days [6%]).[34]

### Post Discharge Mortality and Morbidity

Pathan et al.[36] reported the one-year outcomes of children supported on ECLS for acute respiratory failure and found the severity of hypoxia and the presence of shock were associated with patient posthospital discharge mortality, whereas comorbid conditions were not. If shock complicated the initial ECLS run, one year later survival decreased to 46%.

In another single-center study, Gupta et al.[37] reported 22 ECLS runs ≥28 days. Only 45% (n=10) of cases were successfully decannulated from ECLS. Six patients (27%) were alive 30 days after decannulation, and only 4 patients (19%) survived to hospital discharge. Of the three living children, two had significant neurologic issues with brain atrophy and developmental delay, one awaited renal transplant, and all three survivors had chronic lung disease.

Decreased Health Related Quality of Life (QoL) after respiratory failure treated with mechanical ventilation (with only rare use of ECLS) occurred in 19% of infants and children and was associated with pre-PICU admission features, duration of mechanical ventilation, and inadequate pain and sedation management.[38] Long-term followup studies of pediatric patients (nonneonates) are largely lacking. A recent long-term study of survival after neonatal ECLS found that a third had either hypertension and/or chronic kidney disease.[39]

### Long Term Neurodevelopmental Outcomes

Data on long-term neurodevelopmental followup after pediatric respiratory ECLS are scarce. Kakat et al.[40] described one-year followup of 98 neonates (77%) and children (23%) after respiratory ECLS. Thirty survivors had neurologic problems, including seizures, motor or vision abnormalities (n=8), hearing problems (n=8), and behavior problems (n=6). Eight children had difficulties in multiple domains. Bembea et al.[41] assessed neurologic and neurocognitive outcomes in neonatal and pediatric cardiac and respiratory survivors at 6 months (n=31) and 12 months (n=34). Scores for adaptive behavior and cognitive, neurologic, and quality of life assessments were all below the general population norms. Jen et al.[42] reported that, among 87 nonneonatal cardiac and respiratory ECLS survivors, 56 (63%) of whom had a median followup of 3.7 years, 16% had neurologically debilitating conditions such as epilepsy (7%) and developmental delay (9%).[42]

Health related QoL of pediatric ECLS survivors was evaluated by surveying the patient and parent proxies (primary respiratory failure occurred in 81%).[43] Followup ranged from 1 to 7.5 years with an age range of 2 to 21 years. Four children required special education classes. Seventy percent indicated a normal QoL assessed with Pediatric Quality of Life Inventory (PesQL). However, psychosocial scores (a subscale of PedsQL) revealed impaired QoL in 50%.

**Followup**

ELSO long-term followup guidelines were revised in 2021.[44] It recommended that ECLS centers offer long-term followup as standard of care in a multidisciplinary, structured, and standardized way, promoting the early detection of neurologic and neurodevelopmental problems to trigger early interventions. ELSO is now recommending that all pediatric patients treated with ECLS have a structured followup with a multidisciplinary clinic to promote recovery, follow known organ dysfunction/recovery, and detect unanticipated problems such as learning impairments, long-term kidney disease complicating AKI and long-term pulmonary function (see Appendix, p.773). Children of multiple ages can receive ECLS for acute respiratory failure, so the initial timing of followup is related to hospital discharge while the later followup is related to the child's age (Figure 16-1).

In addition, structured followup creates the opportunity for evaluation of outcome data and effectiveness. This followup should begin predischarge with medical and neurologic evaluation and family education. After discharge, specific care for underlying or acquired diseases are needed with neurodevelopmental care, including school performance. Proposed followup times are at 3, 6, and 12 months. Followup through school age and adolescence should be individually tailored to patient needs. Health care providers should inform parents about possible sequelae and should advise parents to seek medical review in case of problems.

Challenges to followup of children treated with ECLS for respiratory failure include that it is a rare event in a very heterogenous population for both patient event age and etiology of respiratory failure. Patients frequently have co-existing conditions such as cancer, immune deficits, or genetic conditions that may also limit survival and quality of function. Although recent reports of followup for children at risk of neurologic injury after intensive care are more common,[38] traditionally pediatric critical care providers have not organized follow-up for ECLS patients. Additional challenges include barriers to followup at tertiary centers (distance, transportation), low reimbursement for follow-up after critical illness, and poor access to neuropsychology expertise for timely assessment and interventions.

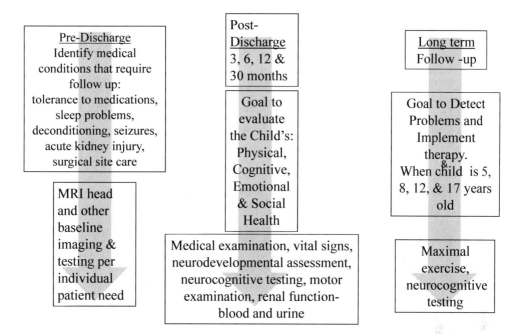

**Figure 16-1.** Recommended multidisciplinary followup of pediatric respiratory failure: assessments and suggested timing.

# References

1. Combes A, Hajage D, Capellier G, et al. Extracorporeal membrane oxygenation for severe acute respiratory distress syndrome. N Engl J Med. 2018; 378: 1965-1975.
2. Zimmerman JJ, Akhtar SR, Caldwell E, et al. Incidence and outcomes of pediatric acute lung injury. Pediatrics. 2009; 124: 87-95.
3. Green TP, Moler FW, Goodman DM et al. Probability of survival after prolonged extracorporeal membrane oxygenation in pediatric patients with acute respiratory failure. Extracorporeal Life Support Organization. Crit Care Med. 1995; 23: 1132-1139.
4. Green TP, Timmons OD, Fackler JC, et al. The impact of extracorporeal membrane oxygenation on survival in pediatric patients with acute respiratory failure. Pediatric Critical Care Study Group. Crit Care Med. 1996;24: 323-329.
5. Curley MA, Wypij D, Watson RS, et al. Protocolized sedation vs usual care in pediatric patients mechanically ventilated for acute respiratory failure: a randomized clinical trial. JAMA. 2015; 313: 379-389.
6. Barbaro RP, Xu Y, Borasino S, et al. Does extracorporeal membrane oxygenation improve survival in pediatric acute respiratory failure? Am J Respir Crit Care Med. 2017 197: 1177-1186.
7. Pediatric Acute Lung Injury Consensus Conference Group. Pediatric acute respiratory distress syndrome: Consensus recommendations from the Pediatric Acute Lung Injury Consensus Conference. Pediatr Crit Care Med. 2015; 16: 428-439.
8. Diso D, Anile M, Patella M, et al. Lung transplantation for cystic fibrosis: outcome of 101 single-center consecutive patients. Transplant Proc. 2013;45: 346-348.
9. Bailly DK, Reeder RW, Bratton SL et al. Development and validation of a score to predict mortality in children undergoing ECMO for respiratory failure: Pediatric pulmonary rescue with Extracorporeal Membrane Oxygenation Prediction (P-PREP) Score. Crit Care Med. 2017; 45: e58–e66.
10. Barbaro RP, Boonstra PS, Paden ML, et al. Development and validation of the pediatric risk estimate score for children using extracorporeal respiratory support (Ped-RESCUERS). Intensive Care Med. 2016; 42:879–888.
11. ELSO International Report 2016-2020. Extracorporeal Life Organization. Available @https://www.elso.org/Registry/ELSOLiveRegistryDashboard.aspx (accessed January 28, 2022).
12. Zabrocki LA, Brogan TV, Statler KD, et al. Extracorporeal membrane oxygenation for pediatric respiratory failure: Survival and predictors of mortality. Crit Care Med. 2011; 39: 364-370.
13. Tonna JE, Barbaro RP, Rycus PT, et al. On the academic value of 30 years of the Extracorporeal Life Support Organization Registry. ASAIO J. 2021; 67: 1–3.
14. Bokman CL, Tashiro J, Perez EA, et a. Determinants of survival and resource utilization for pediatric extracorporeal membrane oxygenation in the United States 1997-2009. J Pediatr Surg. 2015; 50: 809-814.
15. Freeman CL, Bennett TD, Casper CT, et al. Pediatric and neonatal extracorporeal membrane oxygenation: Does center volume impact mortality? Crit Care Med. 2014; 42: 512-519.
16. Cooper DS, Thiagarajan RR, Henry BM, et al. Outcomes of multiple runs of extracorporeal membrane oxygenation: An analysis of the Extracorporeal Life Support Registry. J Intensive Care Med. 2022; 37: 195-201.
17. Zapol WM, Snider MT, Hill JD, et al. Extracorporeal membrane oxygenation in severe acute respiratory failure. A randomized prospective study. JAMA. 1979; 242: 2193-2196.
18. Moler FW, Custer JR, Bartlett RH, et al. Extracorporeal life support for severe pediatric respiratory failure: an updated experience 1991-1993. J Pediatr. 1994; 124: 875-880.
19. Olson TA, O'Neil ER, Viamonte HK, et al. Improving outcomes for children requiring extracorporeal membrane oxygenation therapy following hematopoietic stem cell transplantation. Crit Care Med. 2021; 1;49:e381-e393.
20. Steppan DA, Coleman RD, Viamonte HK, et al. Outcomes of pediatric patients with oncologic disease or following hematopoietic stem cell transplant supported on extracorporeal membrane oxygenation: The PEDECOR experience. Pediatr Blood Cancer. 2020; 67: e28403.
21. Di Nardo M, Ahman AH, Merli P, et al. Extracorporeal membrane oxygenation in children receiving haematopoietic cell transplantation and immune effector cell therapy: an international and multidisciplinary consensus statement. Lancet Child Adolesc Health. 2021; 9;S2352-4642.
22. Cashen K, Dalton H, Reeder R, et al. Platelet transfusion practice and related outcomes in pediatric extracorporeal membrane oxygenation. Pediatr Crit Care Med. 2020; 21: 178–185.
23. Maue DK, Hobson MJ, Friedman ML, et al. Outcomes of pediatric oncology and hematopoietic cell transplant patients receiving extracorporeal membrane oxygenation. Perfusion. 2019;34:598-604.
24. Bailly DK, Reeder RW, Winder M et al. Development of the pediatric extracorporeal membrane oxygenation prediction model for risk-adjusting mortality. Pediatr Crit Care Med. 2019; 20:426-434.
25. Dalton HJ, Reeder R, Garcia-Filion P, et al. Factors associated with bleeding and thrombosis in children

receiving extracorporeal membrane oxygenation. Am J Respir Crit Care Med. 2017; 196: 762-771.

26. Brogan TV, Zabrocki L, Thiagarajan RR, et al. Prolonged extracorporeal membrane oxygenation for children with respiratory failure. Pediatr Crit Care Med 2012; 13: e249-e254.

27. Maratta C, Potera RM, Van Leeuwen G, et al. Extracorporeal Life Support Organization (ELSO): 2020 pediatric respiratory ELSO guideline. ASAIO J. 2020; 66:975-979.

28. Said AS, Guilliams KP, Bembea MM. Neurological monitoring and complications of pediatric extracorporeal membrane oxygenation support. Pediatr Neurol. 2020 ;108:31-39.

29. Swaniker F, Kolla S, Moler F, et al. Extracorporeal life support outcome for 128 pediatric patients with respiratory failure. J Pediatr Surg. 2000;35;197-202.

30. Fleming GM, Askenazi DJ, Bridges BC, et al. A multicenter international survey of renal supportive therapy during ECMO: the kidney intervention during extracorporeal membrane oxygenation (KIDMO) group. ASAIO J. 2012;58:407–414.

31. Gorga SM, Sahay RS, Askenazi DJ, et al. Fluid overload and fluid removal in pediatric patients on extracorporeal membrane oxygenation requiring continuous renal replacement therapy: A multicenter retrospective cohort study. Pediatr Nephrol. 2020; 35: 871–882.

32. Dalton HJ, Garcia-Filion P, Holubkov R, et al. Association of bleeding and thrombosis with outcome in extracorporeal life support. Pediatr Crit Care Med 2015;16: 167–174.

33. Biffi S. Di Bella S, Scaravilli V, et al. Infections during extracorporeal membrane oxygenation: epidemiology, risk factors, pathogenesis and prevention. Int J Antimicrob Agents. 2017; 50:9-16.

34. Bizzarro MJ , Conrad SA, Kaufman DA, et al. Infections acquired during extracorporeal membrane oxygenation in neonates, children, and adults. Pediatr Crit Care Med. 2011; 12:277-281.

35. Gardner AH, Prodhan P, Stovall SH. et al. Fungal infections and antifungal prophylaxis in pediatric cardiac extracorporeal life support. J Thorac Cardiovasc Surg. 2012 ;143:689-695.

36. Pathan N, Ridout DA, Smith E, et al. Predictors of outcome for children requiring respiratory extracorporeal life support: implications for inclusion and exclusion. Intensive Care Med. 2008; 34:2256–2263.

37. Gupta P, McDonald R, Chipman CW et al. 20-year experience of prolonged extracorporeal membrane oxygenation in critically ill children with cardiac or pulmonary failure. Ann Thorac Surg. 2012; 93:1584-1590.

38. Watson RS, Asaro LA, Hutchins L, et al. Risk factors for functional decline and impaired quality of life after pediatric respiratory failure. Am J Respir Crit Care Med. 2019; 1;200:900-909.

39. Zwiers AJM, Usselstjin H, van Rosmalen J, et al. CKD and hypertension during long-term follow-up in children and adolescents previously treated with extracorporeal membrane oxygenation. Clin J Am Soc Nephrol. 2014; 9:2070-2080.

40. Kakat S, O'Callaghan M, Smith L, et al. The 1-year follow-up clinic for neonates and children after respiratory extracorporeal membrane oxygenation support: A 10-year single institution experience. Pediatr Crit Care Med. 2017;18:1047-1054.

41. Bembea MM, Felling RJ, Caprarola SD, et al. Neurologic outcomes in a two-center cohort of neonatal and pediatric patients supported on extracorporeal membrane oxygenation. ASAIO J. 2020;66:79-88.

42. Jen HC, Shew S: Hospital readmissions and survival after nonneonatal pediatric ECMO. Pediatrics. 2010; 125:1217-1223.

43. Chandler HK, Teppa B, Johnson KA, et al. Determining comorbidities and quality of life among pediatric survivors of extracorporeal life support. J Crit Care. 2015; 30:1085-1089.

44. Ijsselstijn H, Schiller RM, Holder C, et al. Extracorporeal Life Support Organization (ELSO) guidelines for follow-up after neonatal and pediatric extracorporeal membrane oxygenation. ASAIO J. 2021;67:955-963.

# 17

## Initiating Extracorporeal Life Support for Cardiac Failure in Children

*Ravi R. Thiagarajan, Tanya Perry, Sarah Tabbutt, Timothy J. Jones, David S. Cooper*

### Introduction

ECLS has an established role for the management of acute decompensated heart failure in children with congenital (CHD) or acquired heart disease who fail to respond to conventional medical and surgical interventions. In the 1970s, modified CPB circuits were used to provide prolonged ECLS in children undergoing corrective and palliative cardiac surgical procedures for CHD.[1,2] These early experiences combined the growth of pediatric cardiac surgery for children with CHD to establish the importance of ECLS in children for managing refractory cardiopulmonary dysfunction in children with heart disease. With increasing familiarity and access, ECLS has grown substantially and is now commonplace in centers providing cardiac critical care and cardiac surgical services for children with heart disease.[3] Indeed, in some countries it has become a required standard of care for centers undertaking surgery for CHD.[4]

VA ECMO is the most common configuration used in children when cardiopulmonary recovery is expected following a short duration of ECLS.[5] For those in whom long-duration support is required, such as a bridge to heart transplantation, durable Ventricular Assist Device (VAD) is preferred.[5]

ECMO offers several advantages when used to support acute cardiorespiratory dysfunction in neonates and children with heart disease. These include speed and ease of deployment, deployment at the point of care, ability to provide respiratory in addition to cardiac support, and applicability across a broad range of patient sizes and intracardiac anatomy. Furthermore, familiarity and refinement of care based on vast experience with VA ECMO have helped ensure its successful and safe use.

Data from the ELSO Registry (October 2021), gathered from over 400 ECLS centers across the globe, reported that over a 5-year period (2016-2020), 7861 (11%) of a total 73,635 ECMO runs were used to support neonates and children for cardiac indications.[6] In this subgroup, survival to hospital discharge was 51% for neonates and 59% for older children. There is an increasing trend in the use of cardiac ECMO in both neonates and children (Figure 17-1), underlining the importance of ECMO in this population. In this chapter,

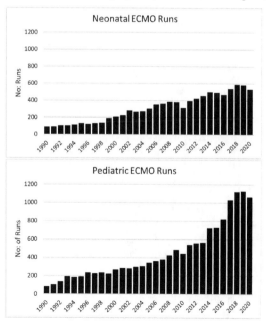

**Figure 17-1.** Trends in neonatal and pediatric ECMO utilization from ECLS Registry Report International Summary October 2021.

we provide the readers with an overview of indications and contraindications for ECLS use in children with congenital and acquired heart disease. We recognize that indications and contraindications will evolve over time with improvement in ECLS management and technology.

**General Indications and Contraindications for ECLS Support in Children with Heart Disease**

Table 17-1 shows common indications and contraindications for ECLS use in children with heart disease. ECLS to support children with severe cardiorespiratory dysfunction following surgery for congenital heart disease is a common indication for cardiac ECMO. In general, ECLS is deployed when conventional medical or surgical therapies have failed to reverse the trajectory of cardiopulmonary dysfunction, and cardiac arrest is imminent.

| INDICATIONS |
| --- |
| Congenital Heart Disease |
| • Preoperative Stabilization |
| • Postcardiotomy ECMO |
|   o Refractory cardiopulmonary failure |
|   o Failure to wean from cardiopulmonary bypass |
| Noncongenital and Acquired Cardiac Disease |
| • Refractory Acute Decompensated Heart Failure |
|   o Acute Viral Myocarditis |
|   o Cardiomyopathy |
|   o Sepsis |
|   o Noncardiac Systemic Disease |
| Both Congenital and Acquired Heart Diseases |
| • Refractory Cardiac Arrhythmia |
| • Pulmonary Hypertension |
| • Procedural Support |
| • Cardiac Arrest (ECPR) |
| • Bridge to Durable Ventricular Assist Device or Heart Transplantation |
| CONTRAINDICATIONS |
| Poor prognosis from primary disease |
| Established multiorgan failure |
| Severe pre-ECMO neurologic injury or intracranial hemorrhage |
| Severe surgical or visceral bleeding |
| Prematurity (<34 w gestation) |
| Size (<2 kg) |
| Family preference |

**Table 17-1.** Indications and contraindications for cardiac ECMO.

Although timing of ECLS deployment varies widely among providers, successful outcomes depend on early or timely ECLS deployment prior to the onset of permanent end-organ dysfunction or cardiac arrest.[7]

Contraindications for ECLS also vary widely among providers and have changed over time. When considering candidacy for any ECLS support, it is important to recognize that ECLS is merely a support modality and does not offer any therapeutic benefit. Thus, only those with a reversible cause and anticipated good prognosis for the primary disease-causing cardiopulmonary failure are likely to survive ECLS support and subsequent hospital discharge. Additionally, for children with heart disease, those who are candidates for heart transplantation in the setting of insufficient cardiac recovery may benefit from ECLS support. However, if it is determined that a patient would not be a candidate for longer term support such as a VAD or for transplantation, then ECLS may not be appropriate. Children in whom cardiopulmonary failure is nonrecoverable, those with poor prognosis from their primary disease, those with established multiorgan failure, or with pre-ECMO severe neurologic injury, may not benefit from ECLS. ECLS support in children with severe bleeding not amenable to medical or surgical interventions may not be possible. Similarly, providing adequate ECLS support through peripheral vessel cannulation (eg, internal jugular vein and carotid artery) in small sized neonates (body weight <2 kg) and those with multiple peripheral vessel occlusions may require central cannulation.[8] Finally, the high incidence of intracranial hemorrhage with anticoagulation used for ECLS in premature neonates (gestational age <34 weeks) requires very judicious use of ECLS.[9]

Treating clinicians should assess each potential ECLS candidate individually, weighing benefits, risks, technical challenges, and outcomes prior to recommending ECLS support.

Finally, and most importantly, a detailed and realistic discussion of the risks and benefits of ECLS with the family and caregivers should occur prior to deploying ECLS. However, as ECLS may be required emergently in the setting of acute decompensation or cardiac arrest, it is also important to recognize that an exhaustive discussion or assessment of risks and benefits of ECLS is not always possible. In these circumstances, ECLS can be deployed after a brief discussion to obtain consent, when possible. An in-depth discussion can then be held with the family regarding the pros and cons of continuing ECLS support after achieving stability. Furthermore, for high-risk surgical cases it is good practice to have discussions about the potential need for ECLS with the family before the surgery. Similarly, if the team believes ECLS would not be appropriate should the patient deteriorate, this should be discussed with the family and wider team and documented before surgical or catheter-based intervention is undertaken.

## ECLS for Congenital Heart Disease

Cardiac ECMO support for children with CHD, especially in the perioperative period following cardiac surgery, is not uncommon (Figure 17-2).[6] A recent publication using data from 41 U.S. children's hospitals reporting to the Pediatric Health Information System (PHIS) database estimated that 3% of all surgical procedures for repair or palliation of CHD required postoperative ECLS support (median ECMO utilization: 2.8% range 0-5.67%). As expected, ECLS was more commonly utilized in children undergoing complex surgical procedures.[9] Common indications for ECLS support in children with CHD are highlighted below.

### Preoperative Stabilization

ECLS can be used for preoperative stabilization in neonates and children with CHD presenting with refractory profound cyanosis, cardiogenic shock, or cardiac arrest as a bridge to a corrective or palliative procedures.[11] Brunetti et al., using data from 23 cardiac intensive care units in the United States reporting to the Pediatric Cardiac Critical Care Consortium, estimated that preoperative support was used in 10% of cardiac surgical patients requiring ECLS support.[11] Bautista-Hernandez et al. described ECLS use for preoperative stabilization in 26 children with CHD.[11] Refractory hypoxemia was the

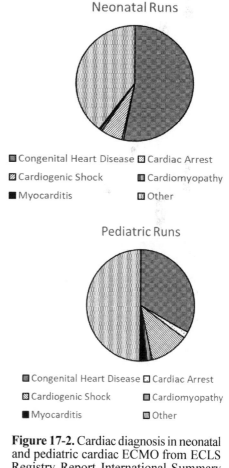

**Figure 17-2.** Cardiac diagnosis in neonatal and pediatric cardiac ECMO from ECLS Registry Report International Summary October 2021.

most frequent indication for ECLS support. Refractory hypoxemia can be seen in the setting of insufficient pulmonary blood flow and in neonates with obstructed total anomalous venous return. ECLS was used as a bridge to a corrective or palliative cardiac surgical procedure in all patients. Survival to hospital discharge was 62%. Little information exists about timing of cardiac surgery after stabilization with ECLS. However, early intervention prior to ECLS complications seems prudent.

### Postoperative ECLS Support

ECLS to support children with post-cardiotomy cardiopulmonary dysfunction following surgery for CHD is well established and a common indication for cardiac ECMO.[7,13-19] The indications for ECLS in the postoperative period after cardiac surgery are varied and include failure to separate from CPB, postoperative low cardiac output syndrome due to myocardial dysfunction, residual cardiac lesions, pulmonary hypertension, intractable arrhythmias, or to aid cardiopulmonary resuscitation (CPR) following cardiac arrest (ECPR). ECLS provides hemodynamic stability and end-organ perfusion while awaiting myocardial recovery, treatment of pulmonary hypertension, or the treatment of arrhythmia. In addition, it can provide the opportunity to investigate, diagnose, and intervene on significant residual lesions.[16,20] It is imperative to investigate residual lesions because cardiac catheterization and transcatheter interventions on ECLS have been shown to be performed with a low rate of complications, and earlier performance of cardiac catheterization in these patients is associated with higher survival.[21] ECLS use for failure to separate from CPB after surgery carries high mortality risk.[22] However, ECLS support in this situation can provide an opportunity to investigate and correct residual lesions or serve as a bridge to durable VAD or heart transplantation.

### Respiratory Failure

In children who develop respiratory failure after cardiac surgery due to primary lung disease, severe pulmonary hypertension, pulmonary hemorrhage, or insufficient pulmonary blood flow (eg, systemic to pulmonary artery shunt obstruction), ECLS provides excellent respiratory support until these issues are treated or resolved. In some cases, primary respiratory failure in children with CHD, including those with single ventricle CHD, can be supported successfully with VV ECMO.[23]

### Cardiac Arrest

Cardiac arrest in the postoperative period unresponsive to CPR can be rescued with rapid ECMO deployment (ECPR).[24] This indication is discussed in more detail later in this chapter.

### Postoperative Procedural Support

ECLS can be deployed prophylactically to provide safety for interventional cardiac catheterization procedures for residual lesions that cannot be addressed surgically. For example, an unstable patient with branch pulmonary artery obstruction after Tetralogy of Fallot repair can be considered for ECLS to provide stable perfusion and gas exchange for cardiac catheterization to dilate pulmonary arteries.

### ECLS in CHD Outcomes

Survival to hospital discharge for patients receiving ECLS following cardiac surgery ranges from 33-60%. Survival varies by age, indication for postcardiotomy cardiac ECMO, surgical complexity, bleeding complications, and duration of ECLS.[13,14,16,17,25] As previously mentioned, timing of ECLS deployment prior to the onset of multiorgan dysfunction or cardiac arrest is crucial to successful outcomes for postcardiotomy patients. Finally, residual lesions are common in children requiring cardiac ECMO after congenital cardiac surgery. Prompt diagnosis and intervention are crucial to successful ECLS support and survival in these patients.[20,26] Echocardiography can underestimate residual lesions once a patient is on ECLS, and consideration should be given for early cardiac catheterization or cross-sectional imaging to exclude residual lesions in any patient requiring ECLS following cardiac surgery.

## Extracorporeal Cardiopulmonary Resuscitation (ECPR)

ECLS can be rapidly deployed during CPR for cardiac arrest in children with cardiac disease when there is no return of spontaneous circulation (ROSC) despite ongoing high-quality conventional CPR.[24,27,28] In these situations, ECPR can provide stable systemic perfusion and gas exchange to enable diagnosis and treatment of conditions leading to cardiac arrest. Since the description of ECPR use in postoperative children with heart disease in 1992, it has now become a common indication for use of ECLS in children following cardiac surgery.[27-29] In postoperative patients, access to the right atrium and aorta via recent sternotomy provides an opportunity for rapid central cannulation for ECLS. ECPR can also be effectively utilized in children with nonsurgical acquired heart disease, such as acute fulminant viral myocarditis, typically via peripheral cannulation of the right internal jugular vein and carotid artery.[27] Although there is wide variability in ECPR utilization across ECLS centers, reports document 9–10% of in-hospital cardiac arrests are supported with ECPR.[29,30] Survival to hospital discharge for ECPR is reported to be 17-50%.[12,27,31,32] Lasa et al. demonstrated improved survival to hospital discharge with favorable neurologic outcome in children with ECPR compared

with conventional CPR in children after an in-hospital cardiac arrest, including cardiac surgical patients.[33] Ideal candidates for ECPR have sustained a witnessed cardiac arrest, have a reversible reason for the cardiac arrest, and have received immediate and effective CPR prior to ECLS deployment (see Chapter 21). Both ready access to ECLS equipment and team are required for successful ECPR. Children with CHD who have physiologic constraints that limit effective conventional CPR may be poor candidates for ECPR.[34]

## ECLS for Single Ventricle Congenital Heart Disease

Neonates with single ventricle congenital heart disease such as Hypoplastic Left Heart Syndrome (HLHS) are at increased risk for postcardiotomy ECLS support due to complex circulatory physiology posed by palliative procedures such as the Norwood operation for HLHS or systemic to pulmonary artery shunt operations for pulmonary atresia. Among patients undergoing the Norwood operation, it is reported that 9-17% of patients are supported with ECLS following surgery.[18,35,36] Indications for ECLS following the Norwood operation include failure to separate from CPB, refractory low cardiac output, cardiac arrest, and acute hypoxemia due to systemic to pulmonary artery shunt thrombosis or obstruction.[15] The Single Ventricle Reconstruction Trial, reflecting 549 patients following the Norwood operation across 15 centers, found birth weight less than 2.5 kg, older age at operation, and reoperations following the original operation were risk factors for ECLS.[37] A single-center study of neonates supported with ECLS after the Norwood operation found that birth weight <2.5 kg and longer duration of CPB, lactic acidosis, and the need for larger doses of inotropes were all associated with increased ECLS usage.[36,38] These factors can help identify neonates who may be at risk of requiring ECLS.

However, ECLS and ECPR are risk factors for poor survival in neonates requiring ECLS after the Norwood operation.[37] Survival to hospital discharge in neonates requiring ECLS after the Norwood operation is reported to be 31-44% in those placed on ECLS for failure to wean from CPB, and those placed on ECLS for cardiopulmonary dysfunction are at increased odds of death.[38,39]

ECLS can be considered for single ventricle patients with cavopulmonary circulations (Bidirectional Glenn [BDG] and Fontan), both in the immediate postoperative period and during subsequent admissions for cardiorespiratory failure.[40-42] Indications for ECLS in these patients include postcardiotomy or systolic and diastolic heart failure, atrioventricular valve regurgitation, hypoxemia due to lung disease including infections, or rarely plastic bronchitis. Providing adequate ECLS support in these patients may require transthoracic cannulation for the Glenn and multisite venous drainage for the Fontan circulation. Because patients with BDG or Fontan circulation presenting with acute decompensated heart failure have high systemic venous pressure, neurological and end-organ injury following CPR is common and may reduce good ECPR outcomes.[43] Evaluation for heart transplantation may be required in children with BDG or Fontan circulation presenting with acute decompensated heart failure who fail to promptly wean from ECLS. Survival to hospital discharge for children with BDG or Fontan circulation is poor because the need for ECLS often represents endstage cardiac failure. Issues related to longer term direction of therapy such as suitability or not for transplantation should be carefully considered when making decisions regarding candidacy for ECLS.[40-42]

**ECLS for Myocarditis and MIS-C**

ECLS can be effectively used to rescue children with acute fulminant myocarditis presenting with cardiogenic shock or cardiac arrest. These patients have the highest survival compared to any other group.[44,45] Cardiac recovery usually occurs in 7-10 days and patients can be successfully weaned off ECLS. Need for ECLS can be anticipated in patients with acute myocarditis with cardiogenic shock or malignant arrhythmias despite medical management. In a single center series of patients with acute fulminant myocarditis, Teele et al. reported those who were supported with ECLS presented with end-organ dysfunction and dysrhythmias.[45] Although forms of temporary VADs have emerged as alternative support modalities in patients with acute myocarditis, their use is limited by size and availability, and ECMO remains the mainstay of mechanical circulatory support for children with myocarditis.[5] In addition, ECMO cannulation for this population is generally peripheral, sparing myocardial cannulation. Children who do not recover cardiac function as expected in acute myocarditis should be evaluated and transitioned to a durable VAD as a bridge to recovery or heart transplantation. It is important to keep in mind that left atrial decompression is a protective factor for mortality in patients with myocarditis, and decompression of the left heart is essential for myocardial recovery.[46] This should be performed early after initiation of ECLS, given earlier time to decompression following ECLS cannulation is associated with shorter duration of ECLS and intensive care unit (ICU) length of stay.[47]

Acute cardiogenic shock and cardiac failure in children with SARS-CoV-2 associated Multisystem Inflammatory Syndrome (MIS-C) unresponsive to conventional medical management can be successfully supported with ECLS. Data on ECLS utilization in patients with MIS-C remains sparse, limited to case reports and small case series. Based on currently available reports, patients with MIS-C requiring ECLS recover within 7-10 days.[48,49] In addition, patients acutely ill with SARS-CoV-2 infection can present with respiratory or cardiac failure requiring ECLS support. For both types, early diagnosis and appropriate therapy can improve recovery.[50]

## ECLS for Procedural Support

ECLS can be deployed electively to provide hemodynamic support for critically ill children with heart disease requiring interventional cardiac catheterization for correction of structural defects or ablation of hemodynamically significant arrhythmias. The primary goal of ECLS in these instances is preservation of end-organ function and prevention of cardiac arrest. Zaleski et al. reported on the successful use of prophylactic ECLS for procedural support in a small series of children with heart disease from a single center experience.[51] The authors emphasized the need for multidisciplinary discussion to consider the risk and benefits ECLS prior to deployment. Planning for preprocedural support should include a plan for the proposed intervention, including technical, personnel, and equipment required for successful support. Many children requiring ECLS for procedural support can be weaned off ECLS soon after the successful intervention.

## ECLS for Intractable Arrhythmias

ECLS can be deployed in patients with acute decompensated heart failure from tachyarrhythmias unresponsive to medical therapies.[52] ECLS in these instances can help optimize antiarrhythmic medications and provide stability for ablation procedures. A recent study by Ghaleb and colleagues reported a 65% survival for children supported with ECLS for supraventricular arrhythmias.[53]

## ECLS in Pulmonary Hypertension

Pediatric pulmonary hypertension guidelines published by the American Heart Association/American Thoracic Society in 2015 recommended use of ECLS in children with CHD with refractory pulmonary hypertension and cardiac failure following cardiac surgery.[54,55] ECLS has also been used to bridge children with primary pulmonary hypertension to lung transplantation.[55]

## ECLS as a Bridge to Heart Transplantation

ECLS as a mechanical support modality for bridge to transplantation has been largely replaced with the availability of durable pediatric VADs, given survival to transplant is higher on durable VADs compared to ECLS or temporary VADs.[56] Durable VADs can provide the long duration of support required while waiting for organ availability, with the ability to provide physical and nutritional rehabilitation that are important to ensure good posttransplant outcomes.[50,57] Where possible, if the intent of ECLS in a patient with acute decompensated heart failure is bridge to heart transplantation, VAD should be chosen. In patients listed for heart transplantation, ECLS can be deployed to improve end-organ function in children with acute decompensated cardiac dysfunction with eventual transition to durable VAD once end-organs have recovered. Finally, ECLS can provide excellent support for cardiopulmonary dysfunction related to early graft failure following heart transplantation with good outcomes.[58]

In summary, ECLS is an invaluable support modality for children with congenital and acquired heart disease. Easy deployment in patients of all sizes and cardiac anatomical differences, and the vast experience with its use have established its importance in the management and rescue of critically ill children with heart disease. It is anticipated that indications and contraindications for use of cardiac ECMO will continue to evolve over time.

# References

1. Baffes TG, Fridman JL, Bicoff JP, et al: Extracorporeal circulation for support of palliative cardiac surgery in infants. Ann Thorac Surg 1970, 10(4):354-363.

2. Soeter JR, Mamiya RT, Sprague AY, et al: Prolonged extracorporeal oxygenation for cardiorespiratory failure after tetralogy correction. J Thorac Cardiovasc Surg 1973, 66(2):214-218.

3. Horak RV, Alexander PM, Amirnovin R, et al: Pediatric Cardiac Intensive Care Distribution, Service Delivery, and Staffing in the United States in 2018. Pediatr Crit Care Med 2020, 21(9):797-803.

4. Paediatric Congenital Heart Disease Standards: Level 1 - Specialist Children's Surgical Centres [www.england.nhs.uk/wp-content/uploads/2018/08/Congenital-Heart-Disease-Standards-Level-1-Specialist-Childrens-Surgical-Centres-Paediatric.pdf].

5. Hoskote A, Stiller B, Thiagarajan RR: What's new in mechanical support strategies for the intensivist in children with severe cardiac failure. Intensive Care Med 2021, 47(10):1152-1155.

6. ELSO International Summary, 2021.

7. Chaturvedi RR, Macrae D, Brown KL, et al: Cardiac ECMO for biventricular hearts after paediatric open heart surgery. Heart 2004, 90(5):545-551.

8. Ford MA, Gauvreau K, McMullan DM, et al: Factors Associated With Mortality in Neonates Requiring Extracorporeal Membrane Oxygenation for Cardiac Indications: Analysis of the Extracorporeal Life Support Organization Registry Data. Pediatr Crit Care Med 2016, 17(9):860-870.

9. Polito A, Barrett CS, Wypij D, et al: Neurologic complications in neonates supported with extracorporeal membrane oxygenation. An analysis of ELSO registry data. Intensive Care Med 2013, 39(9):1594-1601.

10. Bratton SL, Chan T, Barrett CS, et al: Metrics to Assess Extracorporeal Membrane Oxygenation Utilization in Pediatric Cardiac Surgery Programs. Pediatr Crit Care Med 2017, 18(8):779-786.

11. Bautista-Hernandez V, Thiagarajan RR, Fynn-Thompson F, et al: Preoperative extracorporeal membrane oxygenation as a bridge to cardiac surgery in children with congenital heart disease. Ann Thorac Surg 2009, 88(4):1306-1311.

12. Brunetti MA, Gaynor JW, Retzloff LB, et al: Characteristics, Risk Factors, and Outcomes of Extracorporeal Membrane Oxygenation Use in Pediatric Cardiac ICUs: A Report From the Pediatric Cardiac Critical Care Consortium Registry. Pediatr Crit Care Med 2018, 19(6):544-552.

13. Aharon AS, Drinkwater DC, Jr, Churchwell KB, et al: Extracorporeal membrane oxygenation in children after repair of congenital cardiac lesions. Ann Thorac Surg 2001, 72(6):2095-2101; discussion 2101-2092.

14. Alsoufi B, Shen I, Karamlou T, Giacomuzzi C, et al: Extracorporeal life support in neonates, infants, and children after repair of congenital heart disease: modern era results in a single institution. Ann Thorac Surg 2005, 80(1):15-21; discussion 21.

15. Brown KL, Ichord R, Marino BS, et al: Outcomes following extracorporeal membrane oxygenation in children with cardiac disease. Pediatr Crit Care Med 2013, 14(5 Suppl 1):S73-83.

16. Duncan BW, Hraska V, Jonas RA, et al: Mechanical circulatory support in children with cardiac disease. J Thorac Cardiovasc Surg 1999, 117(3):529-542.

17. Kolovos NS, Bratton SL, Moler FW, et al: Outcome of pediatric patients treated with extracorporeal life support after cardiac surgery. Ann Thorac Surg 2003, 76(5):1435-1441; discussion 1441-1432.

18. Mascio CE, Austin EH, 3rd, Jacobs JP, et al: Perioperative mechanical circulatory support in children: an analysis of the Society of Thoracic Surgeons Congenital Heart Surgery Database. J Thorac Cardiovasc Surg 2014, 147(2):658-664: discussion 664-655.

19. Walters HL, 3rd, Hakimi M, Rice MD, et al: Pediatric cardiac surgical ECMO: multivariate analysis of risk factors for hospital death. Ann Thorac Surg 1995, 60(2):329-336; discussion 336-327.

20. Howard TS, Kalish BT, Wigmore D, et al: Association of Extracorporeal Membrane Oxygenation Support Adequacy and Residual Lesions With Outcomes in Neonates Supported After Cardiac Surgery. Pediatr Crit Care Med 2016, 17(11):1045-1054.

21. Abraham BP, Gilliam E, Kim DW, et al: Early catheterization after initiation of extracorporeal membrane oxygenation support in children is associated with improved survival. Catheter Cardiovasc Interv 2016, 88(4):592-599.

22. Sperotto F, Cogo P, Amigoni A, et al: Extracorporeal Membrane Oxygenation Support for Failure to Wean From Cardiopulmonary Bypass After Pediatric Cardiac Surgery: Analysis of Extracorporeal Life Support Organization Registry Data. Crit Care Explor 2020, 2(9):e0183.

23. Aydin SI, Duffy M, Rodriguez D, et al: Venovenous extracorporeal membrane oxygenation for patients with single-ventricle anatomy: A registry report. J Thorac Cardiovasc Surg 2016, 151(6):1730-1736.

24. Chan T, Thiagarajan RR, Frank D, et al: Survival after extracorporeal cardiopulmonary resuscitation in infants and children with heart disease. J Thorac Cardiovasc Surg 2008, 136(4):984-992.

25. O'Halloran CP, Andren KG, Mecklosky J, et al: Mortality and Factors Associated With Hemorrhage During Pediatric Extracorporeal

Membrane Oxygenation. Pediatr Crit Care Med 2020, 21(1):75-81.

26. Agarwal HS, Hardison DC, Saville BR, et al: Residual lesions in postoperative pediatric cardiac surgery patients receiving extracorporeal membrane oxygenation support. J Thorac Cardiovasc Surg 2014, 147(1):434-441.

27. Thiagarajan RR, Laussen PC, Rycus PT, et al: Extracorporeal membrane oxygenation to aid cardiopulmonary resuscitation in infants and children. Circulation 2007, 116(15):1693-1700.

28. del Nido PJ, Dalton HJ, Thompson AE, et al: Extracorporeal membrane oxygenator rescue in children during cardiac arrest after cardiac surgery. Circulation 1992, 86(5 Suppl):II300-304.

29. Gupta P, Yan K, Chow V, et al: Variability of characteristics and outcomes following cardiopulmonary resuscitation events in diverse ICU settings in a single, tertiary care children's hospital. Pediatr Crit Care Med 2014, 15(3):e128-141.

30. Prodhan P, Fiser RT, Dyamenahalli U, et al: Outcomes after extracorporeal cardiopulmonary resuscitation (ECPR) following refractory pediatric cardiac arrest in the intensive care unit. Resuscitation 2009, 80(10):1124-1129.

31. Morris MC, Wernovsky G, Nadkarni VM: Survival outcomes after extracorporeal cardiopulmonary resuscitation instituted during active chest compressions following refractory in-hospital pediatric cardiac arrest. Pediatr Crit Care Med 2004, 5(5):440-446.

32. Kane DA, Thiagarajan RR, Wypij D, et al: Rapid-response extracorporeal membrane oxygenation to support cardiopulmonary resuscitation in children with cardiac disease. Circulation 2010, 122(11 Suppl):S241-248.

33. Lasa JJ, Rogers RS, Localio R, et al: Extracorporeal Cardiopulmonary Resuscitation (E-CPR) During Pediatric In-Hospital Cardiopulmonary Arrest Is Associated With Improved Survival to Discharge: A Report from the American Heart Association's Get With The Guidelines-Resuscitation (GWTG-R) Registry. Circulation 2016, 133(2):165-176.

34. Marino BS, Tabbutt S, MacLaren G, et al: Cardiopulmonary Resuscitation in Infants and Children With Cardiac Disease: A Scientific Statement From the American Heart Association. Circulation 2018, 137(22):e691-e782.

35. Hamzah M, Othman HF, Baloglu O, et al: Outcomes of hypoplastic left heart syndrome: analysis of National Inpatient Sample Database 1998-2004 versus 2005-2014. Eur J Pediatr 2020, 179(2):309-316.

36. Friedland-Little JM, Hirsch-Romano JC, Yu S, et al: Risk factors for requiring extracorporeal membrane oxygenation support after a Norwood operation. J Thorac Cardiovasc Surg 2014, 148(1):266-272.

37. Tabbutt S, Ghanayem N, Ravishankar C, et al: Risk factors for hospital morbidity and mortality after the Norwood procedure: A report from the Pediatric Heart Network Single Ventricle Reconstruction trial. J Thorac Cardiovasc Surg 2012, 144(4):882-895.

38. Sherwin ED, Gauvreau K, Scheurer MA, et al: Extracorporeal membrane oxygenation after stage 1 palliation for hypoplastic left heart syndrome. J Thorac Cardiovasc Surg 2012, 144(6):1337-1343.

39. Allan CK, Thiagarajan RR, del Nido PJ, et al: Indication for initiation of mechanical circulatory support impacts survival of infants with shunted single-ventricle circulation supported with extracorporeal membrane oxygenation. J Thorac Cardiovasc Surg 2007, 133(3):660-667.

40. Booth KL, Roth SJ, Thiagarajan RR, et al: Extracorporeal membrane oxygenation support of the Fontan and bidirectional Glenn circulations. Ann Thorac Surg 2004, 77(4):1341-1348.

41. Jolley M, Thiagarajan RR, Barrett CS, et al: Extracorporeal membrane oxygenation in patients undergoing superior cavopulmonary anastomosis. J Thorac Cardiovasc Surg 2014, 148(4):1512-1518.

42. Rood KL, Teele SA, Barrett CS, et al: Extracorporeal membrane oxygenation support after the Fontan operation. J Thorac Cardiovasc Surg 2011, 142(3):504-510.

43. Salvin JW, Laussen PC, Thiagarajan RR: Extracorporeal membrane oxygenation for postcardiotomy mechanical cardiovascular support in children with congenital heart disease. Paediatr Anaesth 2008, 18(12):1157-1162.

44. Rajagopal SK, Almond CS, Laussen PC, et al: Extracorporeal membrane oxygenation for the support of infants, children, and young adults with acute myocarditis: a review of the Extracorporeal Life Support Organization registry. Crit Care Med 2010, 38(2):382-387.

45. Teele SA, Allan CK, Laussen PC, et al: Management and outcomes in pediatric patients presenting with acute fulminant myocarditis. J Pediatr 2011, 158(4):638-643 e631.

46. Choudhury TA, Ofori-Amanfo G, Choi J, et al: Left Heart Decompression on Veno-Arterial Extracorporeal Membrane Oxygenation in Children With Dilated Cardiomyopathy and Myocarditis: An Extracorporeal Life Support Organization Registry Review. Pediatr Crit Care Med 2021, 22(12):1026-1032.

47. Zampi JD, Alghanem F, Yu S, et al: Relationship Between Time to Left Atrial Decompression and Outcomes in Patients Receiving Venoarterial Extracorporeal Membrane Oxygenation Support:

A Multicenter Pediatric Interventional Cardiology Early-Career Society Study. Pediatr Crit Care Med 2019, 20(8):728-736.

48. Kaushik S, Aydin SI, Derespina KR, et al: Multisystem Inflammatory Syndrome in Children Associated with Severe Acute Respiratory Syndrome Coronavirus 2 Infection (MIS-C): A Multi-institutional Study from New York City. J Pediatr 2020, 224:24-29.

49. Di Nardo M, Hoskote A, Thiruchelvam T, et al: Extracorporeal Membrane Oxygenation in Children with Coronavirus Disease 2019: Preliminary Report from the Collaborative European Chapter of the Extracorporeal Life Support Organization Prospective Survey. ASAIO J 2021, 67(2):121-124.

50. Barbaro RP, MacLaren G, Boonstra PS, et al: Extracorporeal membrane oxygenation support in COVID-19: an international cohort study of the Extracorporeal Life Support Organization registry. Lancet 2020, 396(10257):1071-1078.

51. Zaleski KL, Scholl RL, Thiagarajan RR, et al: Elective Extracorporeal Membrane Oxygenation Support for High-Risk Pediatric Cardiac Catheterization. J Cardiothorac Vasc Anesth 2019, 33(7):1932-1938.

52. Carmichael TB, Walsh EP, Roth SJ: Anticipatory use of venoarterial extracorporeal membrane oxygenation for a high-risk interventional cardiac procedure. Respir Care 2002, 47(9):1002-1006.

53. Ghaleb S, Thiagarajan RR, Cooper DS, et al: Outcomes of Pediatric Patients Treated With Extracorporeal Membrane Oxygenation for Intractable Supraventricular Arrhythmias. Pediatr Crit Care Med 2020, 21(8):e547-e556.

54. Abman SH, Hansmann G, Archer SL, et al: Pediatric Pulmonary Hypertension: Guidelines From the American Heart Association and American Thoracic Society. Circulation 2015, 132(21):2037-2099.

55. Thompson K, Staffa SJ, Nasr VG, et al: Mortality after Lung Transplantation for Children Bridged with Extracorporeal Membrane Oxygenation. Ann Am Thorac Soc 2021.

56. Dipchand AI, Kirk R, Naftel DC, et al: Ventricular Assist Device Support as a Bridge to Transplantation in Pediatric Patients. J Am Coll Cardiol 2018, 72(4):402-415.

57. Almond CS, Singh TP, Gauvreau K, et al: Extracorporeal membrane oxygenation for bridge to heart transplantation among children in the United States: analysis of data from the Organ Procurement and Transplant Network and Extracorporeal Life Support Organization Registry. Circulation 2011, 123(25):2975-2984.

58. Nair AG, Sleeper LA, Smoot LB, et al: Extracorporeal Membrane Oxygenation Support After Heart Transplantation in Children-Outcomes of a Single Center Cohort. Pediatr Crit Care Med 2020, 21(4):332-339.

# 18

## Management of Children with Cardiac Failure

*Steven M. Schwartz, Roxanne Kirsch, Hwa Jin Cho, Dorothy M. Beke, Peter P. Roeleveld, David J. Barron*

### Introduction

The medical care of the patient on ECLS or other forms of mechanical circulatory support (MCS) continues to be challenging. With ongoing evolution in technology and a growing variety of diseases for which ECLS is used, an in-depth understanding of unique patient anatomy, physiology, and the impact of ECLS physiology on patient physiology is essential for all team members.[1,2]

This chapter will address pertinent medical considerations for pediatric patients requiring ECLS for cardiovascular indications. Consideration of current clinical state, patient age, level of clinical stability, underlying disease, comorbidities related to that disease, knowledge of potential cardiac surgical interventions, potential for organ replacement, and type of durable MCS that might be possible are important aspects of caring for these patients.[3] The goals of medical care need to be tailored according to the indication for ECLS with attention to improving physiology, addressing common challenges, applying knowledge of outcomes where possible, and addressing the needs of the patient and family.

### Utilization of Cardiovascular ECLS

While this chapter is focused on the management rather than the initiation of ECLS for cardiac failure, management is often dictated by both the circumstances and goals of mechanical support. There are a few overarching pathways for which ECLS is used to support cardiac patients, which are important to provide context for any discussion of management while on ECLS. Most commonly, ECLS is used as a bridge to recovery. Failure to separate from cardiopulmonary bypass after surgery, or a subsequent unremitting low cardiac output state is a common scenario. Here, time for ventricular recovery, or opportunity for additional surgical or interventional therapies may allow successful separation from ECLS. ECLS may provide time for diseases such as myocarditis or intractable arrhythmias to improve while supporting vital organ function.[4] Stabilization with ECLS prior to surgical intervention may be necessary in certain cases with very unstable physiology. If recovery is unlikely despite ECLS support, or additional interventions to improve physiology are not possible, ECLS may be used to bridge to an alternate durable MCS or organ replacement therapy (Chapter 20). Finally, ECLS can be used as emergent rescue therapy in the setting of cardiopulmonary arrest (Chapter 21). Cardiac patients generally require a relatively short duration of ECLS, which affects the approach to managing the ECLS course. In all situations, management is directed at maximizing myocardial perfusion to aid cardiac recovery, addressing important residual lesions if present, and maintaining or improving end organ function.

## Management of Common Issues for the Cardiac ECLS Patient

Overall, evidence shows that some factors will be predictive of a good outcome, such as weight >3.3 kg, biventricular anatomy, low inotrope score, elective ECLS initiation rather than during CPR, pH >7.28, clearance of lactate within 24 hours of initiating ECLS, absence of renal failure, good hemostasis, absence of chromosomal disorders, and ability to separate from ECLS in <5 days.[5,6]

### *Myocardial Stun*

Although cardiac stun can happen with any initiation of ECLS, it is more likely to be seen in the patient with myocardial dysfunction prior to MCS. The sudden decrease in preload and increase in afterload to the poorly functioning heart will often induce a period of worsened cardiac function with minimal to no pulse pressure. This expected phenomenon requires diligent monitoring to ensure adequate myocardial perfusion and assurance of adequate ECLS flows to support end organ function and allow time for improvement. The generally expected time course for recovery of cardiac stun is 3-7 days.[7]

### *Ensuring Adequate Ventricular Decompression*

ECLS does not completely or automatically decompress the systemic ventricle in a two-ventricle circulation unless there is an atrial or ventricular communication or a specific cannula to vent the systemic atrium. Even with full VA support, there will be blood return to the left ventricle (LV). In the setting of a poorly functioning ventricle, either due to the underlying disease process or ventricular arrhythmias, the ventricle can no longer empty the blood returning to it and becomes increasingly distended with resultant left atrial (LA) hypertension and pulmonary edema. Importantly, the elevated intracavitary pressure will decrease myocardial perfusion pressure and cause subendocardial ischemia. This can further damage an already compromised myocardium. Adequate decompression is critical to myocardial recovery and reduction of myocardial injury on VA ECMO.

Signs of inadequate decompression include any of the following: 1) pulmonary edema on chest radiograph or lung ultrasound (US); 2) new bleeding from the endotracheal tube; 3) absence or loss of systemic pulse pressure that was previously present; 4) LV distension or lack of aortic valve opening on echocardiography; 5) spontaneous contrast in the LV and/or LA on echocardiography.

Appearance of spontaneous contrast in the ventricle on echocardiography indicates stasis of blood suggesting that decompression would be advantageous. Echocardiographic findings of LV or LA dilation, poor function, and transseptal gradients are all helpful, but the last of these can be misleading and underestimate LA pressure. Even if there is pulsatility of the arterial waveform, the LV end diastolic pressure (LVEDP) may be unacceptably high, so presence of a pulse pressure alone is inadequate to conclude that decompression is not needed in the absence of intracardiac shunt or a functioning LA vent. While there is a paucity of clear survival benefit, expert opinion advocates for LV decompression to maximize myocardial recovery for the above physiologic reasons. Also, there is clear evidence that decompression shortens the ECMO course.[8-11] It should be noted that long-term LV function, neurological function, and survival in patients with LA decompression for ECLS needs further study.

Options for LA decompression include a surgically placed vent cannula into the LA, catheter-based creation and dilation of an atrial septal communication, or use of a percutaneous micro-axial ventricular assist device (VAD) for those who are of adequate size.[10-15] Use of an LV vent has also been described.[8] A low flow probe on the tubing of the vent is recommended because it helps confirm that there is adequate decompression and that the vent is working. Thrombosis of the vent can easily occur due to its small size and low blood flow. Positioning of these vents are crucial and, if the vent adheres to the atrial wall, drainage can be impaired or cease and risk thrombus formation in the vent tubing due to stasis. If this occurs, the decompression of the atrium will no longer be adequate unless improvement in ventricular function has already occurred. Finally, an LA pressure monitor may be added surgically to provide monitoring of LA pressure if there is a concern about adequate decompression.

### *Bleeding*

Bleeding is common in patients on cardiac ECMO. In a multicenter analysis, nearly half of children with cardiac disease on ECLS had hemorrhagic complications, and this was associated with increased mortality risk.[16] Additionally, neonates who undergo CPB are at greater risk of needing ECLS if there is excess postoperative bleeding.[17] Risk factors for hemorrhagic complications during ECLS include mediastinal exploration prior to ECLS, greater surgical complexity, early postoperative cannulation, and longer bypass time.[16,18] Hemorrhage from surgical sites and generalized seepage puts patients at risk for tamponade, even with an open sternum. Bleeding also impedes the ability to provide appropriate ECLS flows. Early postoperative bleeding may resolve

over 12-24 hours with aggressive support for volume loss and meticulous attention to correcting factors contributing to bleeding, such as thrombocytopenia. Decisions regarding the need for or timing of mediastinal reexploration must consider the potential to disturb clot that is appropriately forming versus the importance of uncovering surgically correctable causes of bleeding. Anticoagulation targets are also commonly altered, and on occasion prothrombotic products, such as activated factor VII may be given but as a last resort, because it risks thrombus formation within the circuit. It is important to have the capability for rapid replacement of the ECLS circuit should circuit thrombosis result. Once better hemostasis has been achieved for several hours and patient hemodynamics are acceptable, anticoagulation is generally increased for circuit maintenance. It is not uncommon to have increased thrombus in the ECLS circuit or early membrane failure after large volume blood product replacement for bleeding, and this needs expectant monitoring.

### **Single Ventricle Physiology**

ECLS has been used in single ventricle circulations.[19-22] A multicenter database study suggested overall 59% weaned from ECLS, and 31% survived to hospital discharge. Risk factors for mortality in that study included black race, mechanical ventilation prior to ECLS, longer ECLS duration, and once on ECLS, development of multiorgan complications or acidosis. In addition, failure to separate from CPB as an indication for ECLS showed decreased survival.[19] This is generally consistent with previous series that have shown better outcomes with reversible problems (eg, shunt thrombosis) and a short ECLS course,[20,21] and perhaps early deployment and patient selection may be important determinants of outcome.[19,22] Although early initiation of ECLS may be helpful, the observation that ECLS initiated due to failure to separate from

CPB is associated with higher mortality[19] may reflect that the inability to ever separate from bypass sometimes results from a different set of problems than does the inability to maintain cardiac output several hours later. Use of ECLS for single ventricle patients has increased over time and is costly.[19,20] Further study to define the best use of ECLS in the single ventricle population is still required.

Regardless of the evolution of this data, understanding physiology in the single ventricle patient on ECLS is imperative to appropriately supporting the patient. Higher ECLS flows (150-200 mL/kg/min) are often required to support flow across the Blalock-Taussig-Thomas (BTT) shunt, open PDA (with or without stenting), and hybrid palliation strategies when present. This is to overcome the relatively higher volume of blood flow to the lower pressure bed of the lungs compared to the higher pressure bed of the systemic vascular system while the patient is on ECLS. The goal of ECLS flow is to provide adequate flow to maintain circulation rather than providing a specific amount of flow, which has systemic and pulmonary perfusion in parallel, rather than in series. It is also important to recognize that the mixed venous saturation from the ECLS circuit does not represent cardiac output, circuit function, or recirculation since the common atrial chamber is decompressing the systemic ventricle and generally contains fully mixed pulmonary and systemic venous return. If the lungs are healthy, the pulmonary venous return will be well oxygenated because of the flow from the arterial cannula through the BTT shunt to the lungs, and the "mixed" venous saturations in the venous drainage cannula are higher than in those with two-ventricle physiology. If the lungs and BTT shunt are working normally it is possible to support the patient using the ECLS circuit without a membrane oxygenator, sometimes called 'no-MO,' used as a paracorporeal VAD. Alternately, one can review shunt patency by 'capping' the

oxygenator and removing all gas exchange capability of the circuit. Thus, in the setting of good arterial cannula position, adequate lung volumes, and appropriate ventilation strategies blood gases should demonstrate appropriate $PaO_2$ and $PCO_2$ for a single ventricle circulation. If this trial is unsuccessful, shunt patency (or ductal patency) should be discussed and addressed as appropriate prior to attempts to separate from ECLS. Of note, outside of testing shunt function by functionally removing the oxygenator, the target blood gases and oxygenation should be as they are for any other VA ECMO patient. Another strategy to manage the parallel rather than in-series circulation present is to surgically constrict the BTT shunt. This approach adds some risk of shunt thrombosis, even after removing the constriction. It is now well understood that the shunt must be left open during ECLS as previous attempts to manage the shunt by totally occluding it resulted in 100% mortality, although partial occlusion can be effective to allow better systemic and myocardial perfusion at more manageable flows. For any patients with a BTT shunt cannulated for ECLS via the ipsilateral internal carotid artery, there is risk of slippage of the arterial cannula into the shunt, which will be reflected as sudden loss of all cardiac output supported by the circuit. In the event that a preoperative newborn with ductal dependent systemic, or even pulmonary circulation, is placed on ECLS and the ductus remains fully open, banding of the branch pulmonary arteries can be used to control pulmonary blood flow while on MCS.

As pulmonary blood flow supplied by a right ventricle to pulmonary artery (RVPA) conduit has become a more popular way to perform stage I single ventricle reconstruction for Hypoplastic Left Heart Syndrome (HLHS), it is important to understand that this type of circulatory pattern is inherently different than the BTT shunt in terms of accounting for pulmonary blood flow with ECMO flow rates. With a BTT shunt (or pulmonary artery bands), the flow to the lungs comes directly from the aorta and therefore must be accounted for as part of the ECMO flow, since the blood returned to the aorta by the ECMO circuit will directly perfuse the lungs as well as the body. With an RVPA conduit, blood flow to the lungs comes from the ventricle, which sits between the venous and arterial cannulas of the ECMO circuit. Therefore, one need only account for systemic blood flow with the ECMO circuit since any pulmonary blood flow will be supplied by whatever venous return is not taken up by the venous cannula. Therefore, there would generally be no benefit to restricting an RVPA conduit for a single ventricle patient on ECMO with this source of pulmonary blood flow. Similarly, this limits the ability to use ECMO without an oxygenator, as the ECMO circuit would serve as a direct right to left shunt as it would in a biventricular circulation.[23] Thus, in a patient with a BTT shunt the general goal should be to aim for high ECMO flows, whereas in patients with an RVPA conduit the aim should be to minimize ECMO flow to allow for antegrade flow through the RVPA conduit to promote pulmonary blood flow and minimize risk of clotting of the RVPA conduit.

RV-dependent coronary circulation in the setting of Pulmonary Atresia/Intact Ventricular Septum (PA/IVS) is worthy of special note. The myocardium is dependent on adequate preload, and efforts need to be made to keep the heart ejecting as a surrogate that the heart is adequately pre-loaded. Case reports have suggested the role of an aorto-RV shunt in extreme cases to try and maintain coronary perfusion during ECLS.[23]

ECLS support utilized in the cavopulmonary connection and Fontan circulation[21,22] has included: 1) VV support to provide improved oxygenation while awaiting a decrease in PVR and improved flow through the cavopulmonary connection(s), or 2) VA support more commonly used to stabilize the patient prior to take down of Fontan or Glenn connections. In both instances,

management of the patient requires vigilant observation for development of superior vena cava (SVC) syndrome, or venous congestion due to failure of flow through the pulmonary bed that can be difficult to recognize with maintenance of oxygenation by the membrane and/or support of cardiac output in the patient on VA ECMO. The anatomy of those with a bidirectional Glenn shunt requires a choice of the venous cannulation site for mechanical support. Use of the SVC can decompress the cerebral venous system and support oxygenation but may provide little cardiac output support. Cannulation of the atrium can support both oxygenation and cardiac output to a greater degree due to the larger amount of blood returning to the heart from the lower part of the body and is the generally recommended approach. It relies on passive flow through the lungs to decompress the SVC, so monitoring for SVC syndrome is still important. If there is obstruction of the pulmonary bed (eg, increased PVR or atelectasis in the setting of pulmonary infection), CVP elevation may worsen neurologic outcomes by reducing cerebral perfusion pressure. Atrial cannulation can be performed via a full sternotomy, a limited right 4th space anterior thoracotomy, or via the McEverdy approach to the IVC.

**Residual Cardiac Lesions**

When a postoperative cardiac patient requires ECLS, additional investigation for residual lesions is of utmost importance and early detection significantly improves survival.[24-26] Investigation with cardiac catheterization to clarify the physiologic impact of residual lesions should be pursued early in the postoperative patient. Echocardiography alone is usually insufficient to identify all residual lesions (as few as 20%) and cardiac catheterization can provide valuable detailed hemodynamic and anatomical data in conjunction with an opportunity to address residual burdens using catheter-based interventions. Negative studies can be helpful too, as defining a lack of significant residual lesion or physiologic burden aids in prognostication of cardiac and overall patient recovery.

The ECLS circuit can hamper the search for useful data, so studies need to consider the approach, ability to clamp the circuit at critical data collection points, and the correct interpretation in conjunction with other anatomic and physiologic investigations. Cardiac MRI is not technically possible. The presence of an open sternum, dressings, or cannula position can obscure echocardiographic windows. Furthermore, hemodynamic measurements by echocardiography or catheterization may be unreliable in the face of the limited intracardiac flows or ventricular filling on ECLS. Flow through the aortic cannula may produce or exacerbate aortic insufficiency. Therefore, certain diagnostic procedures or maneuvers may require temporary reduction or cessation of ECMO flow.

Despite these challenges in obtaining accurate data, it is important to acknowledge that residual lesions have been found in 70-80% of cases that require postoperative ECLS[24,27] and up to 75% of these patients benefit from subsequent surgical or catheter-based reintervention. Furthermore, those taken to the catheterization lab early (mean of 1.6 days after ECLS) had better outcomes.[28] Finally, the use of CT-angiography to identify residual lesions has been shown to improve survival.[25]

**Cardiovascular Assessment and Monitoring**

*Rhythm and Heart Rate*

Often during a period of cardiac stun, or in the inflamed heart, patients may experience low voltages on continuous telemetry or severe bradycardia. With adequate ECLS flows, these abnormalities should not prove problematic and return of appropriate heart rate or sinus rhythm can signal cardiac recovery. Additionally, and particularly in a postoperative patient, epicardial pacing may be required to demonstrate improvements in ventricular function that can be difficult to assess in the presence of atrioventricular dyssynchrony.

Arrhythmias that would otherwise cause hemodynamic instability or cardiovascular collapse are generally not as problematic while on ECLS. However, converting the patient back to sinus rhythm generally reduces myocardial demand and promotes ventricular recovery.[29] Decompressing the heart alone and the subsequent improvement in myocardial oxygen delivery may lead to resolution of the arrhythmias.

*Blood Pressure*

Patients on ECLS present challenges in blood pressure monitoring. Pulsatile MCS devices have a relatively normal arterial waveform, but continuous flow ventricular assist devices or ECLS with poor ventricular function show a flat waveform with little pulse pressure. It should, nonetheless, reflect mean arterial pressure. For the ECLS patient, arterial waveform changes can also reflect blood loss, impaired pump flow or function, hypertension related to volume overload or other issues.[29-31] For all MCS devices, determining adequacy of support is accomplished by assessing hemodynamic status, vital signs, capillary refill, warmth and color of extremities, urinary output, and neurological status.[29,32] Providing adequate systemic blood flow (which may or may not be represented by mean arterial pressure) minimizes secondary injury to tissues and organs. Normalizing elevated lactate within 24-48 hours is associated with improved outcomes.[33]

## Central Venous Pressure and Fluid Management

A simple way of estimating intravascular volume status is trending CVP in combination with ECLS inlet pressure. This is an important determination since MCS devices are dependent on adequate preload. If device flow is impaired, inlet pressures are very negative, and CVP is low, generally volume replacement is required. But when device flow falls with a high CVP in combination with more negative inlet pressures, a search for tamponade or right heart failure should ensue. If device flow is maintained with high CVP, hypervolemia may be present and should be treated. These generalizations must be qualified by recognizing the limitation of CVP. This number not only represents volume status but is also affected by cardiac and vascular compliance. Studies note the poor correlation between CVP and actual cardiac filling volume.[29] Fluid management therefore involves not only optimal goals for the patient, but attention to circuit function. Increasingly negative venous pressure, low flow, or circuit 'chattering' may occur in the circuit when the patient is intravascularly depleted. Volume repletion may improve circuit function, but a reassessment needs to be made not only of fluid status, but for potential causes of impaired venous return such as tamponade or cannula obstruction.[29]

## Echocardiography

Echocardiography should be performed to assess residual lesions and to monitor ventricular function and complications (eg, tamponade, signs of inadequate decompression). Serial studies are often indicated to correlate clinical findings, especially during clamp trials off ECLS, with detailed cardiac volume and functional status. Standard echocardiographic indices to assess ventricular function for children and neonates during ECLS are scant.

Assessments of RV and LV function including chamber size, ejection fraction, velocity-time integral of the LV outflow tract, tissue Doppler lateral mitral/tricuspid annular peak systolic velocity, tricuspid annular plane systolic excursion, and strain can be used during ECLS.[34] One particular caution in interpreting echocardiographic measurements of ventricular function while on ECLS is that function can change dramatically when the ventricle goes from unloaded to fully loaded during a clamp trial. This can occur when preload exposes good contractility via the Frank-Starling mechanism, or when afterload exposes poor contractility.

As mentioned previously, spontaneous contrast and a closed aortic valve may contribute to blood stasis or thrombosis in the LV or ascending aorta. Echocardiography should be repeated more frequently to recognize such clinical situations and may guide adjustment of flow rate, inotropic agents, and anticoagulation. The need for LV decompression can be considered for increased risk of pulmonary edema.[11,35]

The confirmation of cannula position by echocardiography ensures adequate venous drainage and optimal performance of ECLS because cannula malposition is associated with increased mortality and morbidity.[36] Echocardiography can help to detect other complications, such as pericardial effusion, tamponade, and hypovolemia (Chapter 48).

## Ventilator Management

### Cardiac and Pulmonary Considerations

Respiratory care of ECLS patients with an open lung strategy and good pulmonary toilet for patients with cardiovascular failure optimizes lung function and maintains the ability to separate from ECLS when cardiac recovery has occurred, generally within days. Patients may suffer pulmonary edema as a manifestation of inadequate LV decompression;

however, noncardiogenic lung edema from fluid retention and capillary leak after large volume blood product transfusions, inflammatory response to CPB, and reperfusion after periods of low output can occur. While many cardiac patients benefit from a lower positive end-expiratory pressure (PEEP) ventilation strategy, during ECLS support a higher PEEP (generally 10 cmH$_2$0) can maintain lung volume and prevent microatelectasis. This is utilized while being careful to avoid stretch and therefore a smaller tidal volume is beneficial. Whether using volume control or pressure control modes of ventilation, target tidal volume aims for a maximum of 6-8 mL/kg with peak inspiratory pressures <18-20 cmH$_2$0 and low rate (generally 10 breaths per minute), recognizing that the targeted values may be inappropriate in patients with an open sternum, or those with poor lung compliance secondary to atelectasis, pulmonary hemorrhage, or intrathoracic hematoma. Settings need to be reassessed on a continuous basis and adjusted based on evolving patient status and goals of ECLS.[29]

Most cardiac patients on ECLS have normal lung function and compliance and maintaining ventilator settings used in the absence of ECLS may prove optimal to improve cardiopulmonary interactions. Furthermore, the impact of ventilator strategies on venous return, PVR, and systemic ventricular afterload need to be carefully considered, and may dictate different targets in airway pressure or PaCO$_2$.[29] In select situations, it may be appropriate to extubate a patient without lung pathology or allow spontaneous breathing with pressure support.

## Inotrope/Vasoactive Medications

### *Supporting Cardiac Function*

Although the ECLS circuit effectively replaces cardiac function, it is important to support cardiac function and recovery beyond 'rest' on the circuit. As discussed earlier, maintaining LA decompression is important. Inotropic support such as with low-dose epinephrine (and/or milrinone or levosimendan) may be useful to promote native cardiac function. These need to be balanced with potential cardiac toxicities and consideration for increased myocardial oxygen demand, although their short-term use for ECLS patients has not been studied.[29] While there is very limited evidence to support any one specific approach, levosimendan has generally been used as a last resort and with very mixed outcomes, perhaps because of its more recent introduction to the list of available inotropic agents and its limited availability in North America.[37]

### *Supporting Organ Perfusion*

Vasoactive agents such as norepinephrine, vasopressin, phentolamine, and nitroprusside may serve as adjuncts to MCS to support blood pressure and organ perfusion. There is some support for use of nicardipine to treat hypertension on ECLS.[38] Particularly for centrifugal devices, increased afterload reduces pump flow, potentially necessitating vasodilator agents to ensure adequate flows and systemic support.

The rapid restoration of cerebral perfusion with VAD insertion has been associated with transient encephalopathy in adults; a condition improved by lowering device flow.[39] Similarly, severe hypertension occurs commonly upon initiation of MCS, at least in infants,[40,41] although linkage to intracranial hemorrhage has been variable. Alternatively, when flows are clearly adequate and the patient remains hypotensive, use of vasoconstricting agents often improve organ perfusion pressure.[29]

## Other Organ System Considerations Specific to the Cardiac ECLS Patient

### Infection

General considerations for appropriate monitoring and treatment of infection, renal dysfunction, or neurologic complications reflect those of the noncardiac ECLS population. However, a few specific issues should be mentioned. Leucopenia occurs commonly after large volume transfusion of packed red blood cells, platelets and plasma, and may not adequately reflect the presence (or absence) of infection, and blood temperature in the circuit can be manipulated by the heater-cooler, potentially masking a fever. Vigilant monitoring is required with attention to potential for endocarditis or endovascular infection, particularly in the presence of mechanical valves, synthetic grafts, or stents.

### Renal

Renal dysfunction may be exacerbated in the cardiac patient due to impaired renal blood flow prior to ECLS cannulation and use of nephrotoxic drugs. Mobilizing tissue edema and achieving fluid removal generally improves myocardial compliance and cardiopulmonary interactions, and so renal recovery and renal replacement therapy are an important priority in cardiac ECLS to allow for earlier separation from ECLS. Ongoing debate and much literature examines the association of poor outcomes and continuous renal replacement therapy (CRRT) in ECLS patients (see Chapter 42).[42-46]

### Neurologic

Neurologic monitoring with head ultrasound (for patients with open fontanelles) and assessing for risks of strokes or hemorrhage is important in cardiac ECLS patients. Neurologic complications may occur more commonly in the congenital heart disease patient population because many have baseline neurologic injury or dysfunction in association with their heart disease that can impact decisions about monitoring and investigations after ECLS initiation. Seizures during the postoperative phase are associated with poor late developmental outcome[47] and continuous (amplitude integrated) electroencephalogram (aEEG) monitoring may be considered in patients who underwent neonatal bypass, where seizures commonly follow.[48,49] Patients with a longer duration of hypotension and poorly perfused states, or those who have had cardiac arrest, may require EEG monitoring due to the risk of post-hypoxic seizures. However, no evidence exists that treatment of subclinical seizures changes neurologic outcome for these patients, and further investigation is required.

Near infrared spectroscopy can be used as an adjunct for monitoring adequate cerebral perfusion. Although use is variable, there is some evidence of predictive value in identifying changes in cerebral perfusion. [50,51]

### Analgesia and Sedation

Strategies for minimizing use of sedation allow spontaneous breathing, participation in care, and interaction with staff and family members.[3] Minimizing sedation is a growing trend for patients on ECLS, although occurring more commonly with VAD, where the expectation is often that the patient will be fully ambulatory or even go home with a device in place. In some centers, use of neuromuscular blocking agents commonly occurs for ECLS patients, but many are moving away from this practice. Potential benefits include better neurologic assessment and possibly less long-term muscle weakness.[1,3]

### Endocrine

Glycemic control has been the subject of several large trials in critically ill adults and children, but controversy regarding the optimal approach persists. With regard to pediatric patients on ECLS, a recent study revealed that both hyperglycemia and hypoglycemia, together recognized as dysglycemia, were not associated with increased mortality after adjustment for weight, severity of illness, pre-ECLS lactate, and ECLS indication.[52] The patients in this study were mostly neonates, and ECLS use suggested critical and unresolved medical issues. Other work has shown that the marginal contribution of hyperglycemia to adverse outcomes after pediatric heart surgery is less for neonates and those with residual cardiac lesions.[53] Taken together, these studies suggest that tight glycemic control for cardiac patients on ECLS is, at most, of secondary importance.

### Nutrition

Few data regarding appropriate caloric targets or optimal nutritional routes for patients on ECLS exist. Recent work suggests that early parenteral nutrition may be detrimental in critically ill children.[36] Studies have assessed the success of enteral rather than parenteral nutrition.[54-57] Hanekamp reported that 87% of neonates on VA ECMO received enteral nutrition and just over half of those achieved 40% of overall caloric goals by day 3 of support. In general, published reports suggest minimal risk to enteral feeding and potential benefit, as well as cost savings in adults on ECLS.[54,55]

### Skin Care and Immobility

Iatrogenic pressure injuries (PIs) are associated with increased morbidity, hospital length of stay (LOS), and increased expense in pediatric patients.[58-60] Various medical devices,[61] immobility, inadequate surface support, suboptimal nutrition, friction and shear, decreased tissue perfusion, and excess moisture have been implicated in PI formation in critically ill pediatric patients.[58,59 61] Each of these factors, along with immobility related to cannula position and safety concerns related to patient movement, is associated with a higher risk for the development of PI in patients supported by ECLS, with an incidence of 4.2%,[62] and overall incidence of 10.2% in critically ill infants and children, with those supported by ECLS noted to be at greatest risk.[63] Infants and young children who require prolonged immobilization and/or have neck cannulation for ECLS are particularly at risk for occipital PIs due to a larger surface area of the head,[62] while older children are more vulnerable to injuries of the buttocks, sacral, and coccyx regions.[59,61] Additionally, ears and heels are areas that are vulnerable to wound formation. A proactive approach should be instituted to decrease the incidence of PIs. Strategies to reduce the development of PIs in pediatric patients receiving ECLS include daily skin assessment, utilizing specialty support surfaces, managing moisture and protecting skin from cannulas with foam dressings, fluidized positioners to offload pressure from boney prominences and the occiput, floating heels off the bed surface, along with frequent changes in position (ideally, every two hours).[63-65] A bundled care approach of PI prevention has shown to be effective in reducing injury in pediatric patients receiving ECLS.[65] The use of mirrors is helpful to assess vulnerable areas that are not easily visible, or amenable to full body turns for inspection.[62]

Regardless of cannula position, most patients should tolerate listing (minor degrees of turning) without incident, to redistribute and relieve pressure from existing areas at risk for PI.[65] Bedrolls, fluidized positioners, pillows, and wedges may all be used for changing patient position; however, care must be taken to prevent accidental cannula dislodgement and any interruption in ECLS flow. Peripheral perfusion should be assessed with any position change to ensure adequate flow. Maintaining proper body alignment, especially with femoral cannulation, is crucial to decrease the risk of peripheral nerve injury. The institution of passive range of motion exercises and stretching muscles in immobilized patients as tolerated may be helpful (see Chapter 47). Measures to reduce contractures, such as the use of pressure-relieving boots to prevent foot drop and injury to heels, should be instituted whenever possible. Patients who require ECLS are prone to bone demineralization, muscle atrophy, motor dysfunction, and nerve injury requiring physical therapy and rehabilitation following the discontinuation of ECLS support, due to critical illness, prolonged immobility and body malalignment.[66]

*Eyes*

ECLS patients are at risk for corneal abrasion and eye injury due to critical illness and pharmacological muscle relaxants causing an inability to blink, close eyes, and produce natural tears. Administering eye lubricants, ensuring full closure of lids, and regular scheduled evaluations as indicated, will assist in decreasing deleterious effects of eye pain, infection, and impairment. Incorporating an eye care bundle that includes these elements of care can be useful in mitigating the incidence of injury for patients at risk during ECLS support.[67]

*Family Support*

Having a child in intensive care exacts an emotional toll on a family that may increase further with the need for ECLS support. Family members of patients who were on ECLS may experience anxiety and emotional distress lasting beyond the hospitalization.[68,69] Lewis et al.[68] found that 20% of parents whose children were on ECLS experienced ongoing posttraumatic stress symptoms months after ECLS decannulation, highlighting the need for psychological support for families of children with critical illness prior to cannulation, during an ECLS course, and beyond discharge or death. Curley and Meyer[70] reported that many parents expressed fears related to pain, suffering, and the possible death of their child during ECLS, and that daily conversations and details of progress with clinical team members helped to ameliorate concerns. It is important to maintain multidisciplinary support and open communication with the family to identify issues of significance to them. Goals of therapy should be discussed early and reviewed regularly.[29] Furthermore, the potential that ECLS proves unsuccessful for patient recovery needs to be communicated early. The involvement of palliative care services may assist in family support and aid in the identification of important care goals.

**Summary**

Managing children with cardiovascular disease using ECLS presents many challenges. With a thorough understanding of the problems unique to the population, knowledge of patient specific anatomy and physiology, combined with an understanding of ECLS and the interaction of this therapy with patient physiology, management is improved and the potential for successful decannulation maximized. The mainstay of cardiac ECMO is to ensure adequate systemic oxygen delivery while maximizing myocardial recovery by adequately offloading the heart, and to search for possible residual lesions as soon as possible.

# References

1. Van Meurs K, Lally KP, Peek G, et al. ECMO extracorporeal cardiopulmonary support in critical care. Ann Arbor, MI: Extracorporeal Life Support Organization. 2005;290.

2. Annich GM, Lynch WR, MacLaren G, et al. ECMO: extracorporeal cardiopulmonary support in critical care. Extracorporeal Life Support Organization; 2017.

3. Conrad SA, Dalton HJ. Extracorporeal life support. In: DG N, ed. Roger's Textbook of Pediatric Intensive Care 4th Ed. Lippincott Williams & Wilkins; 2008:544–563.

4. Rajagopal SK, Almond CS, Laussen PC, et al. Extracorporeal membrane oxygenation for the support of infants, children, and young adults with acute myocarditis: a review of the Extracorporeal Life Support Organization registry. Crit Care Med. 2010;38(2):382.

5. Roeleveld PP, Mendonca M. Neonatal Cardiac ECMO in 2019 and Beyond. Front Pediatr. 2019;7:327.

6. Merrill ED, Schoeneberg L, Sandesara P, et al. Outcomes after prolonged extracorporeal membrane oxygenation support in children with cardiac disease--Extracorporeal Life Support Organization registry study. J Thorac Cardiovasc Surg. Aug 2014;148(2):582-8.

7. Martin GR, Short BL, Abbott C, et al. Cardiac stun in infants undergoing extracorporeal membrane oxygenation. J Thorac Cardiovasc Surg. Apr 1991;101(4):607-11.

8. Brown G, Moynihan KM, Deatrick KB, et al. Extracorporeal Life Support Organization (ELSO): Guidelines for Pediatric Cardiac Failure. Asaio J. May 1 2021;67(5):463-475.

9. Eckhauser AW, Jones C, Witte MK, et al. Transthoracic echocardiographic predictors of left atrial hypertension in patients on venoarterial extracorporeal membrane oxygenation. World J Pedia Congenital Heart Surg. 2014;5(1):67-69.

10. Kotani Y, Chetan D, Rodrigues W, et al. Left atrial decompression during venoarterial extracorporeal membrane oxygenation for left ventricular failure in children: current strategy and clinical outcomes. Artificial organs. 2013;37(1):29-36.

11. Hacking DF, Best D, d'Udekem Y, et al. Elective decompression of the left ventricle in pediatric patients may reduce the duration of venoarterial extracorporeal membrane oxygenation. Artificial organs. 2015;39(4):319-326.

12. Di Molfetta A, Adachi I, Ferrari G, et al. Left ventricular unloading during extracorporeal membrane oxygenation - Impella versus atrial septal defect: A simulation study. Int J Artif Organs. Oct 2020;43(10):663-670.

13. Meuwese CL, de Haan M, Zwetsloot PP, et al. The hemodynamic effect of different left ventricular unloading techniques during veno-arterial extracorporeal life support: a systematic review and meta-analysis. Perfusion. Oct 2020;35(7):664-671.

14. Dominguez TE, del Olmo NL. Cardiac Extracorporeal Membrane Oxygenation: Dealing With What's Left After Cannulation. Pedia Crit Care Med. 2015;16(1):85-86.

15. Parekh D, Jeewa A, Tume SC, et al. Percutaneous Mechanical Circulatory Support Using Impella Devices for Decompensated Cardiogenic Shock: A Pediatric Heart Center Experience. Asaio J. Jan/Feb 2018;64(1):98-104.

16. Werho DK, Pasquali SK, Yu S, et al. Hemorrhagic complications in pediatric cardiac patients on extracorporeal membrane oxygenation: an analysis of the Extracorporeal Life Support Organization Registry. Pedia Crit Care Med. 2015;16(3):276.

17. Guzzetta NA, Allen NN, Wilson EC, et al. Excessive postoperative bleeding and outcomes in neonates undergoing cardiopulmonary bypass. Anesthesia & Analgesia. 2015;120(2):405-410.

18. Nardell K, Annich GM, Hirsch JC, et al. Risk factors for bleeding in pediatric post-cardiotomy patients requiring ECLS. Perfusion. 2009;24(3):191-197.

19. Sherwin ED, Gauvreau K, Scheurer MA, et al. Extracorporeal membrane oxygenation after stage 1 palliation for hypoplastic left heart syndrome. J Thorac Cardiovasc Surg. 2012;144(6):1337-1343.

20. Misfeldt AM, Kirsch RE, Goldberg DJ, et al. Outcomes of single-ventricle patients supported with extracorporeal membrane oxygenation. Pedia Crit Care Med.2016;17(3):194-202.

21. Allan CK, Thiagarajan RR, Pedro J, et al. Indication for initiation of mechanical circulatory support impacts survival of infants with shunted single-ventricle circulation supported with extracorporeal membrane oxygenation. J Thorac Cardiovasc Surg. 2007;133(3):660-667.

22. Hoskote A, Bohn D, Gruenwald C, et al. Extracorporeal life support after staged palliation of a functional single ventricle: subsequent morbidity and survival. J Thorac Cardiovasc Surg. 2006;131(5):1114-1121.

23. Said SM, Marey G, Greene R, et al. The double shunt technique as a bridge to heart transplantation in a patient with pulmonary atresia with intact septum and right ventricular-dependent coronary circulation. JTCVS Tech. Jun 2021;7:216-221.

24. Howard TS, Kalish BT, Wigmore D, et al. Association of Extracorporeal Membrane Oxygenation Support Adequacy and Residual Lesions With Outcomes in Neonates Supported After Cardiac Surgery. Pediatr Crit Care Med. Nov 2016;17(11):1045-1054.

25. Soynov IA, Kornilov IA, Kulyabin YY, et al. Residual Lesion Diagnostics in Pediatric Postcardiotomy Extracorporeal Membrane Oxygenation and Its Outcomes. World J Pediatr Congenit Heart Surg. Sep 2021;12(5):605-613.

26. Agarwal HS, Hardison DC, Saville BR, et al. Residual lesions in postoperative pediatric cardiac surgery patients receiving extracorporeal membrane oxygenation support. J Thorac Cardiovasc Surg. Jan 2014;147(1):434-41.

27. Kato A, Lo Rito M, Lee KJ, et al. Impacts of early cardiac catheterization for children with congenital heart disease supported by extracorporeal membrane oxygenation. Catheter Cardiovasc Interv. Apr 2017;89(5):898-905.

28. Abraham BP, Gilliam E, Kim DW, et al. Early catheterization after initiation of extracorporeal membrane oxygenation support in children is associated with improved survival. Catheter Cardiovasc Interv. Oct 2016;88(4):592-599.

29. Schwartz SM, Schmidt A. Medical and nursing care of the child on mechanical circulatory support. Pedia Crit Care Med. 2013;14(5_suppl):S43-S50.

30. O'Shea G. Ventricular assist devices: what intensive care unit nurses need to know about postoperative management. AACN advanced critical care. 2012;23(1):69-83.

31. Litton KA. Demystifying ventricular assist devices. Critical care nursing quarterly. 2011;34(3):200-207.

32. Pike N, Klee L, Zemetra B. Mechanical support of cardiopulmonary function: Extracorporeal membrane oxygenation, ventricular assist devices, and the intraaortic balloon pump. Nursing of the Critically Ill Child. 2013:155-184.

33. Alsoufi B, Awan A, Manlhiot C, et al. Results of rapid-response extracorporeal cardiopulmonary resuscitation in children with refractory cardiac arrest following cardiac surgery. European Journal of Cardio-Thoracic Surgery. 2014;45(2):268-275.

34. Bautista-Rodriguez C, Sanchez-de-Toledo J, Da Cruz EM. The Role of Echocardiography in Neonates and Pediatric Patients on Extracorporeal Membrane Oxygenation. Front Pediatr. 2018;6:297.

35. Unai S, Nguyen ML, Tanaka D, et al. Clinical Significance of Spontaneous Echo Contrast on Extracorporeal Membrane Oxygenation. Ann Thorac Surg. Mar 2017;103(3):773-778.

36. Barbaro RP, Paden ML, Guner YS, et al. Pediatric Extracorporeal Life Support Organization Registry International Report 2016. Asaio j. Jul/Aug 2017;63(4):456-463.

37. Pan KC, Shankar S, Millar J, et al. Role of levosimendan in weaning children requiring veno-arterial extracorporeal membrane oxygenation after cardiac surgery. Eur J Cardiothorac Surg. Jan 4 2021;59(1):262-268.

38. Liviskie CJ, DeAvilla KM, Zeller BN, et al. Nicardipine for the Treatment of Neonatal Hypertension During Extracorporeal Membrane Oxygenation. Pediatr Cardiol. Jun 2019;40(5):1041-1045.

39. Lietz K, Brown K, Ali SS, et al. The role of cerebral hyperperfusion in postoperative neurologic dysfunction after left ventricular assist device implantation for end-stage heart failure. J Thorac Cardiovasc Surg. 2009;137(4):1012-1019.

40. Boedy RF, Goldberg AK, Howell Jr CG, et al. Incidence of hypertension in infants on extracorporeal membrane oxygenation. J Pedia Surg. 1990;25(2):258-261.

41. Sell LL, Cullen ML, Lerner GR, et al. Hypertension during extracorporeal membrane oxygenation: cause, effect, and management. Surgery. 1987;102(4):724-730.

42. Chen Y-C, Tsai F-C, Chang C-H, et al. Prognosis of patients on extracorporeal membrane oxygenation: the impact of acute kidney injury on mortality. Annals Thorac Surg. 2011;91(1):137-142.

43. Askenazi DJ, Ambalavanan N, Hamilton K, et al. Acute kidney injury and renal replacement therapy independently predict mortality in neonatal and pediatric noncardiac patients on extracorporeal membrane oxygenation. Pedia Crit Care Med. 2011;12(1):e1-e6.

44. Paden ML, Warshaw BL, Heard ML, et a;. Recovery of renal function and survival after continuous renal replacement therapy during extracorporeal membrane oxygenation. Pediatric Crit Care Med. 2011;12(2):153.

45. Selewski DT, Cornell TT, Blatt NB, et al. Fluid overload and fluid removal in pediatric patients on extracorporeal membrane oxygenation requiring continuous renal replacement therapy. Crit Care Med. 2012;40(9):2694.

46. Han S-S, Kim HJ, Lee SJ, et al. Effects of renal replacement therapy in patients receiving extracorporeal membrane oxygenation: a meta-analysis. Annals Thorac Surg. 2015;100(4):1485-1495.

47. Bellinger DC, Wypij D, Rivkin MJ, et al. Adolescents with d-transposition of the great arteries corrected with the arterial switch procedure: neuropsychological assessment and structural brain imaging. Circulation. 2011;124(12):1361-1369.

48. Naim MY, Gaynor JW, Chen J, et al. Subclinical seizures identified by postoperative electroencephalographic monitoring are common after neonatal cardiac surgery. J Thorac Cardiovasc Surg. 2015;150(1):169-180.

49. Gaynor JW, Nicolson SC, Jarvik GP, et al. Increasing duration of deep hypothermic circulatory arrest

is associated with an increased incidence of postoperative electroencephalographic seizures. J Thorac Cardiovasc Surg. 2005;130(5):1278-1286.

50. Vedrenne-Cloquet M, Lévy R, Chareyre J, et al. Association of Cerebral Oxymetry with Short-Term Outcome in Critically ill Children Undergoing Extracorporeal Membrane Oxygenation. Neurocrit Care. Oct 2021;35(2):409-417.

51. Cvetkovic M, Chiarini G, Belliato M, et al. International survey of neuromonitoring and neurodevelopmental outcome in children and adults supported on extracorporeal membrane oxygenation in Europe. Perfusion. Sep 22 2021:2676591211042563.

52. Lou S, MacLaren G, Paul E, et al. Prevalence of dysglycemia and association with outcomes in pediatric extracorporeal membrane oxygenation. Pedia Crit Care Med. 2015;16(3):270-275.

53. Moga M-A, Manlhiot C, Marwali EM, et al. Hyperglycemia after pediatric cardiac surgery: impact of age and residual lesions. Crit Care Med. 2011;39(2):266-272.

54. Pettignano R, Heard M, Davis RM, et al. Total enteral nutrition versus total parenteral nutrition during pediatric extracorporeal membrane oxygenation. Crit Care Med. 1998;26(2):358-363.

55. Hanekamp MN, Spoel M, Sharman-Koendjbiharie I, et al. Routine enteral nutrition in neonates on extracorporeal membrane oxygenation. Pediatr Crit Care Med. May 2005;6(3):275-9.

56. Nellett M, Gregory MP, Lefaiver CA. Pilot study evaluates nutrition for patients receiving mechanical circulatory support in the intensive care unit. AACN Adv Crit Care. Jul-Sep 2012;23(3):258-69.

57. Umezawa Makikado LD, Flordelís Lasierra JL, Pérez-Vela JL, et al. Early enteral nutrition in adults receiving venoarterial extracorporeal membrane oxygenation: an observational case series. JPEN J Parenter Enteral Nutr. Mar 2013;37(2):281-4.

58. Curley MAQ, Hasbani NR, Quigley SM, et al. Predicting Pressure Injury Risk in Pediatric Patients: The Braden QD Scale. J Pediatr. Jan 2018;192:189-195.e2.

59. Delmore B, Deppisch M, Sylvia C, et al. Pressure Injuries in the Pediatric Population: A National Pressure Ulcer Advisory Panel White Paper. Adv Skin Wound Care. Sep 2019;32(9):394-408.

60. Quick Safety Issue 25: Preventing pressure injuries. The Joint Commission. https://www.jointcommission. org/resources/news-and-multimedia/newsletters/ newsletters/quick-safety/quick-safety-issue-25- preventing-pressure-injuries/.

61. Kulik LA, Hasbani NR, Stellar JJ, et al. Hospital-Acquired Pressure Injuries in Children With Congenital Heart Disease: Prevalence and Associated Factors. Pediatr Crit Care Med. Nov 2019;20(11):1048-1056.

62. Jackson JE, Kirkland-Kyhn H, Kenny L, et al. Reducing Hospital-acquired Pressure Injuries Among Pediatric Patients Receiving ECMO: A Retrospective Study Examining Quality Improvement Outcomes. Wound Manag Prev. Sep 2021;67(9):14-24.

63. Schindler CA, Mikhailov TA, Kuhn EM, et al. Protecting fragile skin: nursing interventions to decrease development of pressure ulcers in pediatric intensive care. Am J Crit Care. Jan 2011;20(1):26-34; quiz 35.

64. Courtwright SE, Mastro KA, Preuster C, et al. Reducing hospital-acquired pressure ulcers using bundle methodology in pediatric and neonatal patients receiving extracorporeal membrane oxygenation therapy: An integrative review and call to action. J Spec Pediatr Nurs. Oct 2017;22(4).

65. Pasek TA, Kitcho S, Fox S, et al. Preventing Hospital-Acquired Pressure Injuries by Using a Tiered Protocol in Children Receiving ECMO in the Pediatric Intensive Care Unit. Crit Care Nurse. Feb 1 2021;41(1):71-77.

66. Thiagarajan RR, Teele SA, Teele KP, et al. Physical therapy and rehabilitation issues for patients supported with extracorporeal membrane oxygenation. J Pediatr Rehabil Med. 2012;5(1):47-52.

67. McCall K, Hussin HM, Gregory ME, et al. A bundle improves eye care in PICU. Arch Dis Child. Sep 2016;101(9):832-5.

68. Lewis AR, Wray J, O'Callaghan M, et al. Parental symptoms of posttraumatic stress after pediatric extracorporeal membrane oxygenation. Pediatr Crit Care Med. Feb 2014;15(2):e80-8.

69. Tramm R, Ilic D, Murphy K, et al. Experience and needs of family members of patients treated with extracorporeal membrane oxygenation. J Clin Nurs. Jun 2017;26(11-12):1657-1668.

70. Curley MA, Meyer EC. Parental experience of highly technical therapy: survivors and nonsurvivors of extracorporeal membrane oxygenation support. Pediatr Crit Care Med. Apr 2003;4(2):214-9.

# 19

## Weaning and Decannulation of Children with Cardiac Failure

*D. Michael McMullan, Laurance Lequier, Lara Shekerdemian*

### Introduction

Successful ECLS weaning is generally defined as survival after discontinuation of ECLS without the need for reinitiating mechanical support.[1] Survival to decannulation after temporary pediatric cardiac ECLS occurs in 67% of patients,[2] and the outcome and overall survival are often influenced by factors unrelated to ECLS. In most instances, ECLS is removed at a stage when the patient remains fragile in their course of recovery but, in general, the risks of continuing support heavily outweigh the benefits of continuing. The timing and manner of weaning ECLS can significantly impact survival. There are only limited published data to guide clinicians as to which clinical parameters predict patient readiness for discontinuation of ECLS. ELSO has published a number of useful clinical practice guidelines on a variety of modes of ECLS based on expert opinion, informed by available evidence, with targeted clinical recommendations. The pediatric cardiac failure guideline is applicable to neonates and children with cardiac failure as an indication for ECLS and addresses patient selection, patient management, and pathways for weaning support or bridging to other durable, longer-term therapies.[3] While there are studies that have helped to prognosticate death after discontinuing ECLS, most of the identified parameters relate to underlying patient characteristics rather than factors associated with the weaning process itself. Therefore, ECLS weaning remains as much art as science and the clinician must rely on experience and expert opinion to navigate this process.

### Timing of Weaning of ECLS

Following ECLS cannulation, daily assessment of a patient's readiness to wean should occur. There are many factors to consider before weaning ECLS, including the original indication for support; assessment of myocardial and, where appropriate, pulmonary recovery; and adequacy of other end organ function. Discontinuation of ECLS for cardiac support is generally not considered during the first 48 hours of ECLS, and after a period of stable support with adequate tissue oxygen delivery, ventricular decompression, hemostasis, correction of metabolic disturbances, and exclusion of residual lesions.[4]

### Myocardial Injury and Recovery

Myocardial injury after open heart surgery with CPB results from a combination of inflammatory, ischemia-reperfusion, and surgical insults. Additionally, the intrinsic circulatory physiology, as well as the presence of residual lesions and pulmonary performance, will impact the ECLS course and ability to wean. The peak effect of CPB on myocardial function occurs within the first 24 hours postoperatively.[5] The clinical course of myocardial dysfunction is a major determinant of the expected timing of weaning and ultimate removal of ECLS. In the absence of other significant causes for post-cardiotomy myocardial failure, improvement in myocardial performance would be expected within a few days after CPB. The recovery may be more prolonged in the cases of primary myocardial dysfunction, prolonged preoperative myocardial ischemia or residual or new surgical concerns.[6] Early indicators of myocardial recovery include increasing pulse pressure, increasing systolic pressure, rising end-tidal $CO_2$, and improving ventricular systolic function on echocardiography.[7] However, it is important to note that recovery cannot be determined with confidence to be sufficiently present, or absent, without a formal trial of weaning.

While the cardiac ECLS is most often initiated for patients after cardiotomy, patients with primary myocardial dysfunction (eg, myocarditis) represent a group where the pattern and timing of recovery may be less predictable. Recovery after circulatory failure secondary to primary myocardial dysfunction (eg, myocarditis) may occur over weeks to months, or may not occur at all. A subset of these patients with profound and likely long term or even end stage myocardial failure may require conversion to a ventricular assist device (VAD) as a bridge to recovery or transplantation. An ELSO database review of 255 ECMO patients with an underlying diagnosis of myocarditis demonstrated that 61% survived to hospital discharge over a 10-year period.[8] Seven of the patients (3%) underwent heart transplantation and six survived to discharge. With the current commercially available VAD devices, it is increasingly clear that, in any age group, ECMO may not be the best form of mechanical circulatory support beyond two weeks when adequate myocardial recovery has not occurred.[9]

**Special Considerations**

*Residual Lesions:* Postoperative ECLS is at times required when preoperative physiology specifically predisposes to postoperative myocardial failure. Examples include late presentation of transposition of the great arteries with deconditioned left (systemic) ventricular function, congenital coronary abnormalities such as anomalous origin of the left coronary artery from the pulmonary artery (ALCAPA), and left heart obstruction with ventricular dysfunction. Some of these patients may benefit from longer support to facilitate myocardial recovery. ECLS can also be useful as a bridge to identify and repair of unrecognized lesions. Examples include undiagnosed critical aortic valve stenosis and intractable cyanosis despite balloon septostomy in patients with transposition of the great arteries and pulmonary hypertension. In the course of ECLS support after cardiac surgery, and particularly when weaning is not successful or possible, it is important to seek and intervene on residual lesions such as vessel or valvar obstruction or residual shunting. In these instances, the patient can often be immediately weaned after appropriate intervention. Early cardiac catheter evaluation has been shown to improve survival and reduce duration of ECLS when patients fail an attempt at weaning ECLS in the absence of echocardiographic evidence of a residual lesion or significant myocardial dysfunction.[10]

*Left atrial decompression:* In patients whose support includes a left atrial vent or atrial septostomy, lower vent flows coincident with a drop in circuit venous oxygenation may suggest left ventricular recovery. Initial steps in weaning ECLS should include occlusion and removal of the left atrial or left ventricular vent when ventricular recovery is observed.

*Systemic to pulmonary artery shunts:* Some patients undergo partial occlusion of a systemic to pulmonary artery shunt to achieve sufficient systemic perfusion and end-organ oxygen delivery while on ECLS. In these situations, it is essential to address this temporary intervention and ensure that shunt flow is optimized during weaning and trialing off ECLS.

*Recovery from postoperative events:* Sudden adverse events during the early postoperative period, such as bleeding, tamponade, shunt obstruction, airway compromise, refractory arrhythmias, or cardiac arrest may necessitate ECLS as part of the resuscitation. The timing of ECLS weaning in these challenging patients will depend on resolution of the insult and the degree of organ injury related to the event. When alternative vascular access sites for ECLS support are limited, such as may be the case in children who have had a remote sternotomy and have been supported for a prolonged period of time via cervical cannulation, successful recannulation of the cervical vessels may be challenging or impossible if vessels have previously been ligated. In this situation, greater certainty regarding successful weaning may be beneficial before discontinuing ECLS.

*Indeterminate Prognosis:* ECLS may be emergently initiated in the setting of pending or actual cardiopulmonary resuscitation, without a full understanding of the etiology of a patient's decompensations. When it becomes apparent that further support is futile based on the underlying disease or severe ECLS complications, the perception of prognosis and optimal clinical direction may differ between team members. Clear and consistent communication that elicits input from each member of the care team is very beneficial in these challenging situations.

**Predictors of Successful Weaning**

Weaning ECLS should only be considered when there are objective signs of myocardial recovery and adequate resolution of complicating factors, such as the systemic inflammatory response and pulmonary dysfunction. Myocardial function assessed by echocardiography during full ECLS support does not predict myocardial performance under preload and afterload conditions encountered after separation from ECLS. Because myocardial loading conditions impact the assessment of ventricular systolic function on ECLS, assessment of myocardial contractility during ECLS is most helpful when evaluated as a trend over time and under realistic loading conditions, with appropriate vasoactive support. Parameters such as aortic velocity time integral $\geq$10cm, left ventricular ejection fraction >20–25%, and lateral mitral annulus peak systolic velocity $\geq$6cm/s under low flow conditions have been demonstrated to be predict successful ECLS decannulation in adult patients with cardiogenic shock (Chapter 29).[11]

Echocardiography under low flow conditions as part of a weaning trial represents a cornerstone of most pediatric cardiac ECLS weaning protocols. The target is not near-normal or normal ventricular function but rather enough function to allow adequate organ oxygen delivery, a marker that remains ill-defined in the pediatric population and may vary between patients. In patients whose support includes a left atrial vent or atrial septostomy, the ability of the left ventricle to increase native ejection when the left atrial vent is clamped or removed is an important sign of myocardial recovery. Currently, no biomarkers have been shown to be predictive of myocardial recovery in patients on ECLS for cardiogenic shock.[12]

## Weaning and Trialing-off ECLS

Weaning is the term applied to the reduction of ECLS flow, which accompanies myocardial or cardiopulmonary recovery. It may be conducted over several hours to several days. The purpose of weaning ECLS flow is to determine if the patient is ready to trial off and eventually successfully be removed from ECLS. The weaning process varies according to institutional and patient factors but typically occurs over 4-12 hours. During this time ECLS flow should be gradually decreased while optimizing ventilation, intravascular volume status, and vasoactive medications. Vasoactive medications such as inotropes and vasopressors should be administered at low doses, and would typically include catecholamine inotropes, as well as inodilators (such as milrinone) and/or vasoconstrictors such as vasopressin or norepinephrine.[13] In addition, consideration should be given to the addition of inhaled nitric oxide for patients at risk of, or with, elevated or labile pulmonary vascular resistance.

Clinical examination, targeted echocardiography, and serial laboratory parameters should be used to assess the adequacy of cardiac output and ventricular function during ECLS weaning. Throughout the weaning process, adequacy of ventricular function is assessed by echocardiography, as well as clinical and biometric indicators of adequate cardiac output, oxygenation, and ventilation. When myocardial recovery is judged to be sufficient, the patient is optimized for decannulation. A recent study of pediatric cardiac ECLS patients revealed left ventricular outflow tract velocity time integral, divided by pulmonary artery wedge pressure (left atrial pressure) were a significant independent predictor of successful weaning from ECLS.[14] Qualitative assessment of ventricular function and dilatation by continuous transesophageal echocardiography during an extensive weaning protocol that included volume and inotropic challenges, has been shown to be predictive of successful decannulation in adult patients.[15] No other pediatric studies have examined echocardiographic predictors of successful ECLS weaning, and the applicability of adult findings is limited by differences in patient size, image acquisition challenges in small patients with an open sternum, and variable cardiac anatomy. Once a patient has demonstrated satisfactory hemodynamics on minimum ECLS flow of approximately 25-50 ml/kg/min (or for small infants, as low a flow as can be safely sustained on the pump), it is reasonable to trial off ECLS for a period of 30 minutes to 2 hours to determine whether the patient is ready for decannulation.

### Trial-off strategies

A clamp trial is the classic approach used in the majority of ECLS centers. Clamping the cannulas or circuit tubing distal (on the patient side) to a bridge connection allows complete separation of the patient from circuit support while circuit flow is maintained through the bridge connection. During the trial period, there is increased risk of thrombus formation due to reduced flow through the circuit and an increase in non-laminar flow through the bridge connection. The cannulas should be intermittently flushed by releasing the clamps and clamping the bridge for 15–30 seconds every 5–15 minutes. Careful inspection of the circuitry and cannulas should be performed through the trial-off period to prevent circuit embolism to the patient due to thrombus formation. In some centers, the use of an open bridge that regulates flow with an adjustable thumb clamp on the bridge allows patient flow to be decreased to low levels (10 ml/kg/min) and is used to test whether a patient is ready to be removed safely from ECLS.[16] This method avoids intermittent periods of clamping that may increase the risk for potential thrombus formation and thromboembolism to the patient.

Some programs advocate the use of a pump-controlled retrograde trial-off technique, which avoids manipulation of the ECLS circuit without insertion of an arteriovenous bridge and need for circuit clamping to reduce the risk of clot formation in the ECLS circuit.[17] An additional potential benefit of this technique is that it imposes additional afterload and therefore provides some reassurance that the patient has recovered sufficiently to decannulate.[18]

The main risk during a trial off ECLS is circuit thrombus formation and thromboembolism to the patient. This is particularly important in patients who are supported with central cannulation. ECLS flow should not be reduced below the lowest flow rate established for the circuit's oxygenator, and systemic anticoagulation should be adjusted preemptively. The overall risk of thrombus formation is dependent upon anticoagulation strategy, circuit size, existing clot burden, and circuit complexity. It is not uncommon for ECLS trial-off periods to last for 1-2 hours before decannulation. Ideally, full therapeutic anticoagulation during ECLS trial-off should be maintained.

## Rate of Weaning

The pace at which increasing myocardial loading conditions will affect the chances of successful weaning of an individual patient from ECLS can be very variable. Thus, the weaning strategy must be individualized for each patient based on duration and level of support, the underlying pathology, and subjective and objective evidence of myocardial recovery. Patients with longstanding ventricular dysfunction or chronically deconditioned ventricles may benefit from progressive increases in myocardial workload over longer periods of time, although objective evidence to support such an approach in ECLS patients has not been published. Conversely, patients who experience rapid recovery of ventricular function may successfully separate form

ECLS following a rapid wean. Patients with a systemic-to-pulmonary shunt that has been adjusted to optimize ECLS can be particularly challenging. In such cases, readiness to wean may have to be determined without reducing pump flow, as doing so may lead to significant desaturation. These important aspects of weaning are shown in Figure 19-1.[3]

## Preparing and Optimizing for Decannulation

Optimization of the patient should begin several hours prior to a weaning trial. Low-dose inotropes and vasopressors should be initiated with adequate time to ensure they are infusing into the patient. Ventilation settings should be adjusted and lung recruitment initiated to ensure adequate oxygenation and ventilation. Inhaled nitric oxide or other pulmonary vasodilator therapy should be initiated in patients at risk of pulmonary hypertensive crises. When possible, the patient should be euvolemic to optimize preloading conditions and volume expanders should be immediately available. Hematocrit should also be optimized according to the patient's underlying physiology. Metabolic abnormalities should be corrected, with special attention given to serum potassium, calcium, magnesium, phosphate, and glucose. All lines should be checked to ensure accurate intravascular pressure monitoring and drug delivery. Pacing wires should be attached to a pacemaker and tested to confirm appropriate function. Therapeutic anticoagulation should be continued to minimize the risk of thrombus formation within the circuit during periods of reduced flow. Thrombocytopenia and hypofibrinogenemia should be corrected and packed red blood cells should be available. Appropriate vascular access should be obtained in patients who have been supported with continuous renal replacement therapy via the ECLS circuit if post-ECLS renal support is anticipated. Anesthetic and resuscitation drugs should be prepared and available and, in general, patients should be fully sedated in preparation for, during, and for several hours after the wean, in order to minimize systemic and myocardial oxygen consumption.

## ECLS Decannulation

ECLS decannulation may be performed in the ICU or the operating room. Personnel, equipment, medications, and blood products are organized as detailed above for the decannulation procedure. Complications such as low cardiac output, pulmonary hypertension, bleeding, arrhythmias, and the need to reinitiate ECLS must all be anticipated and discussed in the 'time out'. A thorough, coordinated, and clearly defined plan of action should be developed in the event of clinical deterioration after discontinuation of ECLS, which would include preemptive planning as to candidacy for re-cannulation and plan of action in the event of cardiac arrest. The timing of decannulation

should take into consideration the availability of resources in the event that reinitiating of ECLS is required. When possible, decannulation procedures should occur early in the day to increase the likelihood of immediate availability of procedural personnel.

## Surgical Aspects of Decannulation

In preparation for a decannulation procedure, it is important to determine whether the patient will be a candidate for additional periods of ECLS. When possible, vascular structures should be reconstructed in such a way to facilitate recannulation in the future. Circulatory instability is common early after decannulation, and while this typically resolves with careful medical management, the ECLS circuit should be managed in such a way during this time that urgent re-cannulation and reinitiation of support is possible. As with any surgical procedure, a standardized procedural checklist should be

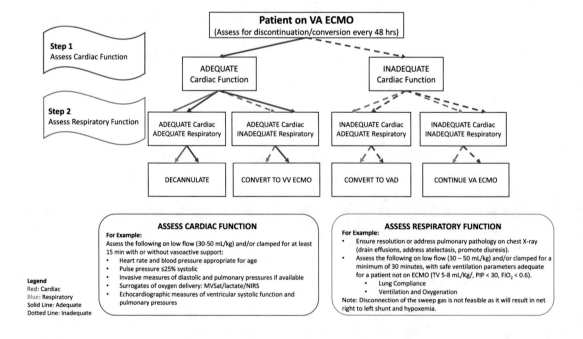

**Figure 19-1.** ECMO weaning flowsheet.

utilized and a pre-procedural 'time-out' should be performed. (Table 19-1).

*Central decannulation:* A portion of the circuit tubing beyond each cannula connector should be prepped and included in the sterile operative field. Heparin/direct thrombin inhibitor infusion is discontinued and circuit flow is gradually weaned. During this time, the surgical site is opened and the patient is observed for clinical evidence of inadequate end-organ oxygen delivery by evaluating the hemodynamic state (BP, HR, CVP), arterial blood gas, and blood lactate level. Direct visual inspection of the heart may provide useful estimations of contractility and intravascular volume status. At the time of decannulation from ECLS, the surgeon should take all measures possible to prevent bleeding, as hemorrhage can preclude decannulation in an otherwise 'ready' patient. Additionally, thrombus removal should be undertaken to gain unrestricted access to the arterial and venous cannulas, but excessive manipulation of the heart and extensive dissection should be avoided to prevent bleeding that may destabilize the patient. In patients who have a systemic-to-pulmonary shunt that has been partially or completely occluded with a surgical clip, the

clip should be removed and the shunt briefly compressed to confirm absence of occlusive thrombus. Once a consensus decision has been made about proceeding with decannulation, ECLS is fully discontinued and arterial and venous cannulas/tubing are clamped. ECLS cannulas are then sequentially removed and purse-strings may be either tied or secured with clips or buttons to facilitate urgent recannulation in patients who are at risk for early failure. The arterial and venous limbs of the circuit on the field can then be joined with a connector and recirculation of blood through the circuit can, if felt necessary, be initiated to preserve the circuit until the care team is satisfied that the patient will be capable of maintaining hemodynamic stability.

After decannulation from central ECLS, the mediastinum should be irrigated and chest tube patency should be confirmed. Standard chest closure may be performed in patients with adequate ventricular function, good markers of systemic perfusion, and good lung function. In all other cases, the chest should be left open and cannulation purse-strings should be snared and left in the chest. When leaving the chest open, debridement should be minimized until the time of chest closure to avoid blood loss and instability. Any visual evidence of purulent mediastinitis should be evaluated by culture, Gram- and fungal-stain. Some centers routinely send a mediastinal swab for microscopy and culture in all centrally cannulated patients at the time of decannulation.

*Peripheral decannulation:* The preparation and management of the ECLS circuit are similar to those already described for central decannulation. Surgical sites are opened and vessels are mobilized so that a length of vessel above and below the cannulation site are available for managing bleeding. Additional time for dissection and control of vessels may be necessary for those in whom percutaneous cannulation had been performed. Once a consensus decision has been made about

| DECANNULATION CHECKLIST |
| --- |
| Inotropes and vasopressors in line |
| Anesthetic and resuscitation drugs available |
| Temporary pacemaker attached to wires |
| Euvolemic state, volume expanders available |
| Packed red blood cells available |
| Platelets $80 \times 10^9$/L and fibrinogen 1.5g/L |
| Proper endotracheal tube placement |
| Adequate pulmonary recruitment |
| Normal electrolytes |
| Appropriate surgical instruments available |
| Established recannulation plan |
| Additional cannulae available |
| Additional ECMO circuit Available |

**Table 19-1.** Sample decannulation checklist.

267

proceeding with decannulation, ECLS can be discontinued and arterial and venous cannulas/tubing should be clamped. It is important to apply clamps to the cannula/tubing at each cannulation site to prevent exsanguination when two venous cannulae have been utilized. Vascular clamps or tourniquets are used to control each cannulation site. ECLS cannulas are then sequentially removed and the arterial and venous limbs of the ECLS circuit are connected for recirculation of blood. Cervical vessels may be repaired or ligated in neonates. There are risks and benefits in favor or against both repair and ligation, and long-term neurologic outcome data has not clearly defined which (if any) approach is optimal. While the long-term risk of cerebrovascular disease following carotid artery repair after neonatal ECMO is not known, it would appear that short-term carotid artery patency is excellent after reconstruction in neonates and approximately half of these patients have a normal carotid Doppler flow pattern four years after reconstruction.[19] Cervical vessel reconstruction at time of ECLS decannulation also facilitates subsequent recannulation if a patient requires ECLS at some point in the future.[20] Cervical and peripheral vessel reconstruction is recommended for non-neonatal patients. After cannulas have been removed, clamps/tourniquets are sequentially released for a brief moment to confirm patency of each vessel. Absence of bleeding from the proximal or distal segment of a vessel suggests thrombotic obstruction and thrombectomy should be performed. Depending on the cannulation technique utilized, vascular reconstruction may involve tying of the purse string suture, primary suture closure of the arteriotomy/venotomy site, or oblique incision with end-to-end anastomosis reconstruction. Vessel patency is recommended by palpation or Doppler before standard surgical site closure is performed. Careful routine evaluation of lower limb perfusion should be performed for 24

hours after femoral vessel decannulation has been performed.

**Failure to Wean**

When the trajectory of cardiovascular and/or pulmonary recovery appears to be inadequate to achieve successful separation from ECLS, early and aggressive investigation should be undertaken to identify and address residual lesions, unrecognized structural or functional abnormalities, inadequate support, infection, and pulmonary disease.[21] Echocardiography, chest ultrasound, CT angiography, cardiac catheterization, and electrophysiology studies can reveal lesions amenable to surgical or interventional correction, such as effusions, valvular regurgitation, outflow tract obstruction, coronary abnormalities, determinants of balance of pulmonary and systemic blood flow, and arrhythmias. Early cardiac catheterization has been shown to reduce ECLS duration and increase survival in children who fail an initial attempt at separation from ECLS without a clear reason for failure identified by echocardiography.[10] In a single-center series of patients supported on ECLS after cardiac surgery, one-third of patients had hemodynamically significant residual lesions that required correction for successful decannulation.[22] Additionally, the early detection of residual lesions within the first 3 days of ECLS is associated with a higher rate of successful decannulation and better survival to hospital discharge. Cardiac catheterization may detect many clinically important residual lesions that are not identified by echocardiography.[23] Timely diagnosis and correction of residual lesions reduces the likelihood an otherwise predictable trajectory of ECLS-related complications, multiorgan failure and death. Premature weaning and separation from ECLS in such patients increases the risk of end-organ damage secondary to low cardiac output, which may exclude them from future

VAD or transplant candidacy. Conversely, unnecessarily prolonged ECLS may expose patients to increased cumulative risk of ECLS-related complications.

Significant lung disease secondary to pneumonia, residual pulmonary edema, pneumothorax, atelectasis, or effusion can all delay successful weaning from cardiac ECLS. All efforts should be made to optimize pulmonary function prior to the weaning process. Consideration should be given to converting from VA ECMO to VV ECMO in patients who have evidence of complete or near-complete myocardial recovery in the setting of persistent severe pulmonary disease. This is particularly important in patients who are supported with peripheral VA ECMO cannulation in order to reduce the likelihood of inadequate cerebral and myocardial oxygen delivery (differential hypoxemia).

Frank and transparent discussions with family members and clinical decision-makers should occur on a regular basis so that they are aware of the increasing risk of mortality associated with longer duration ECLS. Expectations and goals of care in the event of failure of organ recovery should be established and revised throughout the course of ECLS, with a goal of shared values informing end-of-life care. A structured approach to end-of-life care encompasses preparatory family meetings, management of symptoms and discomfort, circuit management, and bereavement support.[24]

**Risk Factors for Mortality**

The hospital mortality associated with pediatric cardiac ECLS ranges between 45% and 50%, depending on the indication for support.[25] Risk factors for mortality in children on ECLS for cardiac disease include acute renal failure, bleeding, pre-ECLS lactic acidosis with delayed resolution post-ECLS initiation, and duration of ECLS.[26] Underlying cardiac pathology has a significant bearing on mortality. This is particularly evident in patients with single-ventricle physiology.[27] When myocardial function remains poor despite optimization of ECLS and identification and management of residual lesions, consideration may be given to transiting to longer-term device support strategies. Formal assessment for heart transplantation candidacy should occur when considering longer-term VAD support.[28] VAD support may be considered within 10 days in some patients, such as those with acute decompensation of chronic myocardial dysfunction (cardiomyopathy) or in patients with recalcitrant myocarditis.

**Conclusion**

Separating from ECLS is a complex process that is affected by multiple patient, circuit, and system factors. Careful planning and assessment for decannulation readiness should begin from the time of initiation of ECLS. Early initiation of ECLS and meticulous attention to the adequacy of support facilitates successful weaning and separation from ECLS. An early and aggressive approach to the diagnosis and management of residual lesions should be undertaken in children who fail to follow an expected course of myocardial recovery. Finally, children who fail to wean from ECLS should be considered for alternative forms of longer-term support to avoid ECLS-related complications. More experience is required to identify clinical parameters that predict successful weaning from ECLS and better define best practice in this area.

# References

1. ELSO Registry Committee: ELSO Registry Data Definitions. Ann Arbor, MI, Extracorporeal Life Support Organization, 2020, p. 113. Available at: https://www.elso.org/Portals/0/Files/PDF/ELSO/RegistryData/2001/Definitions. Accessed January 19, 2022.
2. Thiagarajan RR, Barbaro RP, Rycus PT, et al. Extracorporeal Life Support Organization International Registry Report 2016. ASAIO 2017; 63:456-63.
3. Brown G, Moynihan KM, Deatrick KB, et al. Extracorporeal Life Support Organization (ELSO): Guidelines for Pediatric Cardiac Failure. ASAIO J 2021; 67:463-475.
4. Di Nardo M, MacLaren G, Marano M, et al. ECLS in pediatric cardiac patients. Front Pediatr 2016; 4: 109.
5. Wernovsky G, Wypij D, Jonas RA, et al. Postoperative course and hemodynamic profile after the arterial switch operation in neonates and infants: A comparison of low flow cardiopulmonary bypass and circulatory arrest. Circulation. 1995; 92(8):2226-35.
6. Mascio CE, Austin EH, Jacobs JP, et al. Perioperative mechanical circulatory support in children: An analysis of the Society of Thoracic Surgeons Congenital Heart Surgery Database. J Thorac Cardiovasc Surg 2014; 147:658-64.
7. Fried JA, Masoumi A, Takeda K, et al. How I approach weaning from venoarterial ECMO. Crit Care 2020; 24: 307.
8. Raiagopal SK, Almond CS, Lausen PC, et al. Extracorporeal membrane oxygenation for the support of infants, children, and young adults with acute myocarditis: A review of the Extracorporeal Life Support Organization registry. Crit Care Med 2010; 38:382-7.
9. d'Udekem Y, Shime N, Lou S, et al. Recurrent or Prolonged Mechanical Circulatory Support. Pediatric Critical Care Medicine. 2013; 14:S69-S72.
10. Burke CR, Chan T, Rubio AE, et al. Early cardiac catheterization leads to shortened pediatric extracorporeal membrane oxygenation run duration. J Intervent Cardiol 2017; 30(2):170-176.
11. Aissaoui N, Luyt CE, Leprince P, et al. Predictors of successful extracorporeal membrane oxygenation (ECMO) weaning after assistance for refractory cardiogenic shock. Intensive Care Med 37: 1738–1745, 2011.
12. Howard TS, Kalish BT, Rajagopal SK, et al. Factors associated with mortality in children who successfully wean from extracorporeal membrane oxygenation. Pediatr Crit Care Med 19: 875–883, 2018.
13 Luyt C-E, Landivier A, Leprince P, et al. Usefulness of cardiac biomarkers to predict cardiac recovery in patients on extracorporeal membrane oxygenation support for refractory cardiogenic shock. Journal of Critical Care. 2012; 27(5):524.e7-e14.
14. Sawada K, Kawakami S, Marata S, et al. Predicting Paramaters for Success Weaning veno-arterial Extracorporeal Membrane Oxygenation in cardiogenic shock. ESC Heart Failure 2021; 8:471-80.
15. Cavarocchi NC, Pitcher HT, Yang Q, et al. Weaning of extracorporeal membrane oxygenation using continuous hemodynamic transesophageal echocardiography. J Thorac Cardiovasc Surg. 2013; 146(6):1474- 1479.
16. Lequier L, Horton SB, McMullan DM, et al. Extracorporeal Membrane Oxygenation Circuitry. PCCM 2013; 14:S7–S12.
17. Westrope C, Harvey C, Robinson S, et al. Pump controlled retrograde trial of from VA-ECMO. ASAIO J 2013; 59:517-9.
18. Pandya NR, Daley M, Mattke A, et al. A comparison of pump-controlled retrograde trial off to arteriovenous bridging for weaning from venoarterial extracorporeal membrane oxygenation. Eur J Cardiothorac Surg 2019; 56: 277–284.
19. Cheung PY, Vickar DB, Hallgren RA, et al. Carotid artery reconstruction in neonates receiving extracorporeal membrane oxygenation: a 4-year follow-up study. J Pediatr Surg 1997; 23(4):560-564.
20. Carpenter JC, Baker M, Sperberg K, et al. Common carotid artery imaging after vessel sparing decannulation from Extracorporeal Membrane Oxygenation (ECMO) support. J Pediatr Surg 2021; 56(12):2305-2310.
21. Howard TS, Kalish BT, Wigmore D, et al. Association of extracorporeal membrane oxygenation support adequacy and residual lesions with outcomes in neonates supported after cardiac surgery. Pediatr Crit Care Med 2016; 17: 1045–1054.
22. Agarwal HS, Hardison DC, Saville BR, et al. Residual lesions in postoperative pediatric cardiac surgery patients receiving extracorporeal membrane oxygenation support. J Thorac Cardiovasc Surg. 2014; 147(1):434- 441.
23. Callahan R, Trucco SM, Wearden PD, et al. Outcomes of pediatric patients undergoing cardiac catheterization while on extracorporeal membrane oxygenation. Pediatr Cardiol 2015; 36: 625–632.
24. Machado DS, Garros D, Montuno L, et al. Finishing well: Compassionate extracorporeal membrane oxygenation discontinuation. J Pain Symp Manage 2022; 63:e553-e562.
25. Brunetti MA, Gaynor JW, Retzloff LB, et al. Characteristics, risk factors, and outcomes of extracorporeal membrane oxygenation use in pediatric cardiac ICUs: A report from the pediatric

cardiac critical care consortium registry. Pediatr Crit Care Med 2018; 19: 544–552.

26.  Ford MA, Gauvreau K, McMullan DM, et al. Factors associated with mortality in neonates requiring extracorporeal membrane oxygenation for cardiac indications: Analysis of the extracorporeal life support organization registry Data. Pediatr Crit Care Med 2016; 17: 860–870.

27.  Kumar TK, Zurakowski D, Dalton H, et al. Extracorporeal membrane oxygenation in postcardiotomy patients: Factors influencing outcome. J Thorac Cardiovasc Surg 2010; 140:330–336.e2.

28.  Yarlagadda VV, Maeda K, Zhang Y, et al. Temporary circulatory support in U.S. children awaiting heart transplantation. J Am Coll Cardiol 2017;70: 2250–2260.

# 20

## Bridging Children with Cardiac Failure

*Peta M.A. Alexander, Sebastian C. Tume, Mark S. Bleiweis*

### Introduction

In contrast to adult patients, the pediatric population has a very wide spectrum of etiologies which can present with cardiac failure. Congenital heart disease and cardiomyopathies represent by far the most common causes. Frequently, children with symptomatic cardiac failure present in shock and when medical therapies fail to halt clinical deterioration, deployment of mechanical circulatory support is crucial to support organ systems. ECLS is the most utilized mechanical circulatory support in neonates and children with refractory cardiac failure, facilitating respiratory gas exchange and cardiac output for tissue oxygen delivery while allowing time for myocardial recovery or diagnosis and repair of anatomical lesions. Survival for children with heart disease supported with VA ECMO has improved over the past decade, despite expanding indications and increasing patient complexity. Institution of high-quality ECMO support for pediatric cardiac indications necessitates systems, protocols, interdisciplinary teams, and training (Figure 20-1, Figure 20-2). VA ECMO should

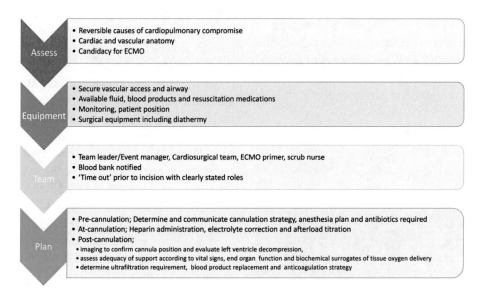

**Figure 20-1.** Cardiac ECMO cannulation preparation and planning.

be considered in patients with severe, refractory circulatory failure with four primary strategies for ECMO support:

- Bridge to recovery: In patients with reversible underlying disease processes where cardiac function recovery can occur with time, medical intervention, or surgical correction
- Bridge to bridge: In patients with acute single organ disease who can be supported with temporary or durable ventricular assist device (VAD)
- Bridge to decision: In patients who may recover end organ function, facilitate diagnosis, or determine candidacy for alternative support
- Bridge to organ transplantation: In patients who may require cardiopulmonary support until heart transplantation

In children supported with ECMO for cardiac indications, cannulation site and strategy are determined by the patient's size, underlying cardiac anatomy, the anatomy and surgical palliation of congenital heart disease (CHD) and any recent surgical intervention (Table 20-1).[1,2] This chapter is designed to give the reader an understanding of the issues associated with VA ECMO support of neonatal and pediatric patients with cardiac dysfunction and what might be realistic expectations for

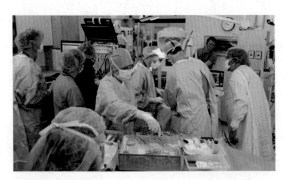

**Figure 20-2.** Cardiac ECMO cannulation at the CICU bedside. Image used with permission.

successful separation from VA ECMO. An attempt is also made to review related issues regarding patient support, highlighting common consequences of ECMO support that have significant bearing on outcomes.

**Bridge to Recovery**

The majority of neonatal and pediatric cardiac VA ECMO is commenced with the intention of bridging to cardiopulmonary recovery. Adequacy of VA ECMO support should be assessed by surrogates of tissue oxygen delivery (blood lactate, arteriovenous $O_2$ difference, mixed or central venous oxygen saturation, near-infrared spectroscopy [NIRS], measures of end-organ function eg, urine output, creatinine, liver function tests) and assessment of cardiac decompression (see Chapter 18).[3]

The clinical course of myocardial improvement may be rapid (eg, 24 hours to 5 days postcardiotomy, cardiopulmonary bypass, or acute rejection). Myocardial recovery can be more prolonged in the case of primary myocardial dysfunction such as primary cardiomyopathies, myocarditis, or prolonged ischemia before correction of cardiac lesion.[4-6] While the former may be well supported with VA ECMO, those with prolonged myocardial dysfunction (>7-10 days) should be considered for other forms of MCS as end-organs recover (Figure 20-3). For the subset of patients who are neither recovered or stable enough to undergo durable MCS or transplant, an option may be a temporary support device, often providing left ventricular support. When recovery appears unlikely, contraindications for advanced therapies may include significant acute brain injury, lung, liver, or kidney failure, or psychosocial factors such as lack of family support. Poor prognostic outlook should be disclosed to families, with iterative discussions to facilitate shared decision-making toward goal-concordant care.[7] Withdrawal of ECMO support occurs when care is futile, and families

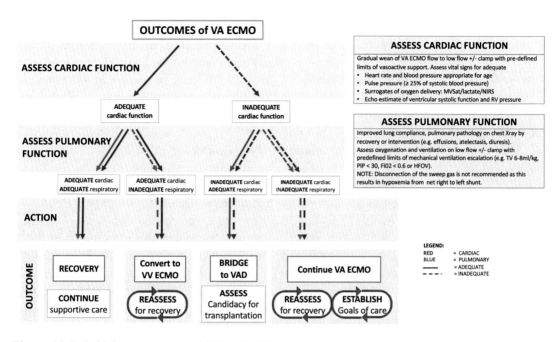

**Figure 20-3.** Bridging to recovery, bridge, decision or long-term support for patients supported on ECMO for cardiac disease.

| ANATOMY | CIRCULATION DESCRIPTION | CIRCULATION OF BLOOD FLOW | ANATOMICAL CANNULATION CONSIDERATIONS | FUNCTIONAL CANNULATION CONSIDERATIONS |
|---|---|---|---|---|
| **Normal cardiac anatomy or Biventricular Circulation** | Two-ventricles in series | Systemic venous blood returns via the right atrium, through lungs to left atrium to systemic circulation | Sized based cannulation considerations only<br>- carotid-internal jugular for small children<br>- femoral-femoral for larger children | Peripheral cannulation unless early post-operative (0 to ~10-14 days). Central cannulation standard right atrium to aorta.<br>Early assessment and consideration of left heart decompression. |
| **Single Ventricle Circulation:** Preoperative with patent ductus arteriosus, or post-Stage 1 palliation with systemic-to-pulmonary artery shunt | Single-ventricle parallel circulation with pulmonary blood flow dependent on patency of ductus arteriosus, shunt or conduit | Systemic venous blood to single ventricle, to systemic and pulmonary circulations | Small babies – carotid-internal jugular if peripheral. Concern for excess pulmonary blood flow and potential for systemic hypoperfusion | Peripheral cannulation unless early post-operative (0 to ~10-14 days). Central cannulation standard common or right atrium to aorta. If patent ductus or shunt based pulmonary blood flow, location of arterial return cannula may cross into pulmonary circulation – requires early assessment of cannula position |
| **Single Ventricle Circulation:** Post - bidirectional cavopulmonary connection (Glenn) or Hemi-Fontan circulation | Single-ventricle parallel circulation with pulmonary blood flow via superior vena cava | Inferior vena cava blood to single ventricle to systemic circulation; Superior vena cava blood through lungs passively, to single ventricle to systemic circulation | May require multiple venous drainage cannula to completely decompress (see Figure 4). If cannula in IVC or atria alone – Glenn circulation must be maintained through lungs in order for upper body (SVC) blood flow to return to atria | Peripheral cannulation unless early post-operative (0 to ~10-14 days). Central cannulation standard right atrium to aorta and may require SVC cannula to completely decompress. |
| **Single Ventricle Circulation:** Post- total cavopulmonary connection or Fontan circulation | Single-ventricle series circulation | Systemic venous return through lungs passively to single ventricle to systemic circulation | Either standard or may require multiple venous drainage cannula to completely decompress – depending on surgical anatomy | Peripheral cannulation unless early post-operative 0 to ~10-14 days). Central cannulation standard Fontan baffle to aorta and may require SVC cannula to completely decompress. |

**Table 20-1.** ECMO cannulation considerations for neonatal and pediatric patients, including congenital heart disease and surgically palliated anatomy.

are in agreement with this strategy. In these situations, communication with the family and other providers should reach consensus that ECMO support will not be reinitiated.

### Patients with Single Ventricle Circulation

Children post initial single-ventricle palliation for hypoplastic left heart syndrome (HLHS) are the most common pediatric population to receive postoperative ECMO support.[8] Particular attention should be paid to cannulation strategy when attempting to support this population (Table 20-1). The indication for initiation of ECMO in infants with single-ventricle physiology is associated with survival in 81% of patients cannulated for hypoxemia, but only 29% of those cannulated for hypotension survive to hospital discharge.[9] Children with single-ventricle circulation palliated with cavopulmonary connections (bidirectional Glenn and Fontan circulations) frequently need multisite cannulation for optimal venous drainage (Table 20-1, Figure 20-4). In

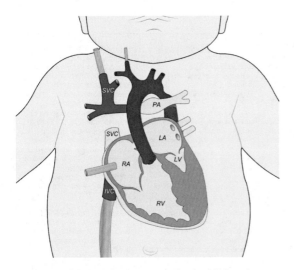

**Figure 20-4.** ECMO cannulation considerations for patient with single-ventricle circulation surgically palliated to bidirectional cavopulmonary connection (Glenn). Image Credit: Emily Harris, Boston Children's Hospital.

all stages of single-ventricle palliation, long-duration ECMO, inotropic support, and renal failure are associated with higher mortality. In rare instances when patients have adequate cardiac function and only require lung support, VV ECMO can be used, and the cannulas for drainage and return are both placed in the venous circulation.

### Postcardiotomy ECMO

Postcardiotomy ECMO is utilized in children with cardiac failure after CHD surgery for those who fail to wean from CPB due to significant compromise of ventricular function, suffer thrombosis of systemic-to-pulmonary artery shunts in patients with palliated single ventricle circulation, intractable arrhythmias, postoperative low cardiac output syndrome, and/or cardiopulmonary arrest. Of all neonates and children undergoing surgical repair or palliation for CHD, between 0.5-6% of patients receive ECMO support in the postoperative period.[8-10] Postcardiotomy ECMO may bridge patients to myocardial recovery, but in those with persistent myocardial or cardiopulmonary failure, may be used as a temporary bridge to decision for cardiac transplantation or durable MCS. VA ECMO has also been utilized as bridge to CHD surgery in the setting of profound preoperative cyanosis, cardiogenic shock, or preoperative cardiac arrest.[11]

Central cannulation is commonly used in the post-cardiopulmonary bypass period or in the presence of a recent sternotomy (ie, less than 10-14 days), with right atrial access for venous drainage and cannulation of the aorta for arterial return (Table 20-1). This strategy allows for direct left atrial decompression utilizing another venous drainage cannula if necessary for left heart decompression. Patients supported with ECLS in the postcardiotomy period should undergo thorough diagnostic evaluation to evaluate contributing factors including the presence of residual lesions, arrhythmias, or failure of normal sinus conduction.[5] Cardiac catheterization during ECMO support can be performed safely, and may exclude, confirm, or identify unexpected residual lesions.[12,13] Early diagnostic cardiac catheterization in this population has been associated with earlier decannulation from ECMO without increased complications or mortality.[14]

### *ECMO for Myocarditis or Cardiomyopathy*

Neonates and children presenting with myocardial failure, cardiogenic shock, or arrhythmias with or without cardiopulmonary arrest associated with cardiomyopathy or myocarditis comprise 8% and 5%, respectively, of the cardiac ECMO reported to the ELSO Registry.[11] Early assessment and management of ventricular function post-ECMO cannulation and adequacy of left heart decompression is essential for this population. Decompressing the hypertensive left atrium can be achieved by atrial septostomy, left atrial cannulation (directly or via catheter crossing the atrial septum), left ventricular venting via an open approach,[12] or an axial transaortic valve pump (Impella Abiomed, Danvers, MA) device.[15] Left atrial decompression performed early (<18h post cannulation) minimizes duration of ECMO and mechanical ventilation.

### Bridge to Decision

The goal of VA ECMO is to provide hemodynamic stability to facilitate recovery of end-organ and, ideally, cardiopulmonary function (Figure 20-3). This time period, where ECMO support is used for support of organ systems while allowing clinicians to more accurately determine the disease process or course, is often termed as 'bridging' to a decision. As the expectation of cardiac recovery recedes, an evaluation for heart transplantation or alternate support strategies, including durable VAD, may be necessary. However,

active infections, unknown neurologic status, neoplasms, as well as end-organ injury or failure can result in contraindications to listing for heart transplantation and LVAD. While some pediatric VAD programs offer destination support, the majority of children transitioned from ECMO to VAD support are considered as bridging to transplantation. A careful evaluation by the multidisciplinary team assessing patient risk factors, contraindications, complications prior to or during ECMO, and the center experience guides the decision making for the most appropriate therapy for the individual patient.

### Bridge to Bridge and Bridge to Transplantation

Patients considered for transplant or durable VAD normally proceed through a multidisciplinary evaluation process including a number of diagnostic studies and specialist consultations. Patients cannulated for ECMO are generally acutely decompensating, which precludes this thorough assessment of the patient prior to initiating support. Once stability has been achieved, a more thorough review of the patient's medical, surgical, and social situation can be undertaken to determine potential candidacy for cardiac transplantation.

VA ECMO provides excellent short-term support. However, consequences of support in the form of complications limit routine medium- or long-term use. The average duration of VA ECMO support for cardiac dysfunction is 6-7 days, with risks of complications increasing with duration of support.[11] Transplant waitlist survival for children attempting to bridge to heart transplantation with ECMO was only 45% in a study combining ELSO Registry data with the Organ Procurement Transplant Network database.[16] Further, VA ECMO utilization is consistently associated with poor post-transplantation outcomes.[17] Despite this, up to 8.6% of heart transplant recipients in past eras were bridged with ECMO (Table 20-2).[17] Importantly, while it is recognized that a prolonged ECMO run may negatively affect clinical outcomes of transplant recipients, a recent study demonstrates that some patients who receive ECMO and transition to VAD remain at risk of poor outcomes.[16] In this study of the International Society for Heart and Lung Transplantation (ISHLT) registry, survival for patients with CHD and dilated cardiomyopathy was similar in patients with VAD or no MCS prior to transplant, but pretransplant ECMO, even in those transitioned to VAD, was strongly associated with mortality after transplant, particularly in children with CHD.

The pretransplant risks of ECMO use are established within the pediatric heart transplantation community. The imperative for the treating clinical team is thus to ensure that potential bridge-to-transplantation patients are adequately resuscitated and rehabilitated to otherwise remain as optimal candidates for this therapy. Avoidance or management of renal injury and minimizing mechanical ventilation which both, along with prior cardiac surgery, affect complexity of posttransplantation management and survival.[17] In the USA, the United Network for Organ Sharing (UNOS) criteria for the most urgent waitlist criteria (Status 1A) changed for pediatric patients in 2016[19] As a result, patients awaiting heart transplantation for cardiomyopathy without hemodynamically significant CHD were only considered Status 1A when supported with mechanical ventilation, intraaortic balloon pump or MCS, while those patients with CHD would be eligible for Status 1A listing for these indications, as well as when receiving inotropic infusions as a hospital inpatient. While there was concern in the community for the safety of children with restrictive or hypertrophic cardiomyopathy on the waitlist, a recent review of ISHLT registry data demonstrated no change in wait-list times pre- and post- the change in policy for this group.[20]

Of note, adult patients supported with VA ECMO for cardiogenic shock and later transitioned to LVAD therapy prior to cardiac transplantation may have equivalent outcomes to those bridged without pre-VA ECMO support.[21] While this may be true for pediatric patients with cardiomyopathy, the same does not appear to be the case for pediatric patients with CHD bridged via ECMO to VAD support, with higher mortality associated with ECMO support persisting in this group through to post-transplantation mortality.[18]

| CHARACTERISTIC | 1992-2000 (n=3,666) | 2001-2009 (n=4,476) | 2010-JUN 2018 (n=5,307) | P-VALUE |
|---|---|---|---|---|
| No Mechanical Circulatory Support Used | - | 86.3% | 74.3% | <0.0001 |
| Extracorporeal Membrane Oxygenation | 4.4% | 8.6% | 4.4% | <0.0001 |
| Intraarterial Balloon Pump | 1.1% | 0.5% | 0.5% | 0.0114 |
| Ventricular Assist Device | - | 9.8% | 20.0% | <0.0001 |
| Biventricular Assist Device | - | 3.7% | 5.4% | <0.0001 |
| Total Artificial Heart | - | 0.2% | 0.3% | <0.0001 |

**Table 20-2.** Use of mechanical circulatory support bridging to pediatric heart transplant recipients. Adapted from The International Thoracic Organ Transplant Registry of the International Society for Heart and Lung Transplantation: Twenty-fourth pediatric heart transplantation report - 2021; focus on recipient characteristics.[17]

## Care of the ECLS Patient on the Transplant Waitlist

In addition to the general principles of management of the neonate or child supported with VA ECMO for cardiac indications,[3] the following considerations are specific to patients on the heart transplant waitlist.

### Preventing and Treating Pulmonary Edema on ECMO

In patients with biventricular circulation, VA ECMO increases systemic ventricular afterload which can exacerbate any prior cardiac insult and myocardial dysfunction, decreasing stroke volume, raising end diastolic pressure, resulting in pulmonary venous hypertension and pulmonary edema. Left ventricular distention leading to pulmonary edema and hemorrhage affects candidacy for alternative MCS strategies, as well as complicating posttransplant care, since lung injury may impact right ventricular function postoperatively. In patients with ECMO support for irreversible heart failure, strategies to prevent pulmonary compromise during support should be considered. Invasive or cardiac catheterization-based monitoring of LA pressures and maintaining the arterial pulse pressure >10 mmHg, as well as echocardiography assessment of aortic valve opening, left ventricular dimensions, and the presence of thrombus. Treatments for systemic ventricular distention include decreasing ECMO flow to facilitate ejection, intravenous inotropes to improve native contractility, and left atrial or ventricular venting (see section above, ECMO for Myocarditis or Cardiomyopathy).[15] To determine when weaning might be possible, assessment of hemodynamic parameters and cardiac function should be done throughout the duration of ECMO support (Figure 20-3).

### Preventing and Recognizing Neurological Injury on ECMO

Neurologic injury including ischemic and hemorrhagic strokes are feared complications in ECMO and smaller strokes may be silent but potentially pose a risk with the initiation of CPB during transplant.[22] Additionally, VA ECMO may be associated with hypoxic ischemic brain injury related to hyperoxia, reperfusion injury, and loss of pulsatile blood flow. Recommendations to identify and reduce brain injury include multimodal neurologic monitoring programs including clinical neurologic exams, transcranial Doppler, electroencephalography, and cranial ultrasound or computed tomography.[23]

### Renal Injury

Up to 50% of children supported with ECMO receive some form of renal replacement therapy.[24] Multiple mechanisms of injury are suspected to cause a reduction in renal oxygen delivery, including abnormal blood flow, lack of pulsatility, inflammation, disrupted renin-aldosterone hormonal system, and worsening volume overload. Renal injury is an independent risk factor for failure to wean from ECMO and mortality, in addition to being a relative contraindication for transplantation.

### Infection

Infection and sepsis are reported in over 40% of patients, associated with duration of ECMO, age, comorbidities, and cannulation site.[11] Unsurprisingly, infection increases mortality and is related to bacterial translocation from the gut and impairment of the immune system related to activation by the ECMO circuit. Infection may be challenging to identify since fever is blunted by the ECMO circuit and leukocytosis, leukopenia, thrombocytopenia, and other biomarkers do not correlate with infection in this population. Although it is common practice among ECMO centers, no strong data support antibiotic or antifungal prophylaxis, surveillance cultures, or deviation from standard ICU practices used in non-ECMO patients. Presence of risk factors such as open chest, immunocompromised state, and immunosuppression should be strongly considered when making therapeutic and prophylactic decisions.

### Blood Product Transfusion

Several factors increase the need for transfusions in this population. Multiple large bore vascular access sites, the often emergent nature of cannulation, and the need for systemic anticoagulation to prevent system clotting, combined with the inflammatory and prothrombotic response and hemolysis associated with the ECMO circuit, all contribute to blood loss and anemia while on VA ECMO.[25,26] No high quality data exist on targets for transfusion, but patient-specific transfusion thresholds may reduce unnecessary transfusion. Patients bridging to heart transplant with LVAD have higher sensitization with increased platelet transfusions (less so with leuko-reduced red blood cells transfusions).[27] Regardless, the goal of transfusion should be to maintain adequate oxygen delivery and perfusion while attempting to minimize overall transfusions and HLA sensitization.[28,29] There are not yet standardized methods for desensitization in this population, but intravenous immunoglobulin, plasmapheresis, and antibody therapy should be considered on an individual or center basis.

### Nutrition

Enteral nutrition should be initiated early via gastric or postpyloric routes unless there is shock and high vasopressor requirements. Concern for accelerated degradation of contemporary membrane lungs by the solutes within parenteral nutrition is not supported by data. Further, parenteral nutrition and supplements are not significantly sequestered by the ECMO tubing, suggesting administration can be effective when the enteral route is contraindicated.

### Ambulation and Rehabilitation

Muscle atrophy, neuromuscular weakness, and impairment of normal activity are common sequelae during treatment of the critically ill, especially those treated with ECLS. These can be further exacerbated in the setting of steroid and neuromuscular blockade use. Physical therapy and ambulation may be feasible for pediatric patients receiving ECLS support during bridging. Successful strategies for physical therapy and ambulation consist of a multidisciplinary approach, including occupational and physical therapy, respiratory therapy, providers, nursing, and ECMO specialists, and should be tailored based upon center experience and staff comfort. Development of early mobility protocols with dedicated teams allowing for the development of expertise can maximize rehabilitation time for appropriate patients and minimize adverse events (see Chapter 47).[30]

### Conclusion

The utilization of VA ECMO for bridging is core because ECMO is not an ultimate destination for the patient, but a transitional support to another therapeutic destination. In every instance of ECMO support, determination of the patient's strategy for liberation from ECMO is paramount. The majority of neonates and children supported with VA ECMO are expected to bridge to recovery; however, in a small proportion of children with prolonged myocardial or circulatory failure, bridging to heart transplant or a durable VAD can be considered.

# References

1. Marino BS, Tabbutt S, MacLaren G, et al. Cardiopulmonary Resuscitation in Infants and Children With Cardiac Disease: A Scientific Statement From the American Heart Association. Circulation. 2018;137(22):e691-e782.

2. MacLaren G, Dodge-Khatami A, Dalton HJ, et al. Joint statement on mechanical circulatory support in children: a consensus review from the Pediatric Cardiac Intensive Care Society and Extracorporeal Life Support Organization. Pediatr Crit Care Med. 2013;14(5 Suppl 1):S1-2.

3. Brown G, Moynihan KM, Deatrick KB, et al. Extracorporeal Life Support Organization (ELSO): Guidelines for Pediatric Cardiac Failure. ASAIO J. 2021;67(5):463-75.

4. Rossano JW, Lin KY. HAART for Kids' Hearts: The Long View. J Am Coll Cardiol. 2017;70(18):2248-9.

5. Lorusso R, Raffa GM, Kowalewski M, et al. Structured review of post-cardiotomy extracorporeal membrane oxygenation: Part 2-pediatric patients. J Heart Lung Transplant. 2019;38(11):1144-61.

6. Teele SA, Allan CK, Laussen PC, et al. Management and outcomes in pediatric patients presenting with acute fulminant myocarditis. J Pediatr. 2011;158(4):638-43 e1.

7. Moynihan KM, Purol N, Alexander PMA, et al. A Communication Guide for Pediatric Extracorporeal Membrane Oxygenation. Pediatr Crit Care Med. 2021;22(9):832-41.

8. Mascio CE, Austin EH, 3rd, Jacobs JP, et al. Perioperative mechanical circulatory support in children: an analysis of the Society of Thoracic Surgeons Congenital Heart Surgery Database. J Thorac Cardiovasc Surg. 2014;147(2):658-64: discussion 64-5.

9. Allan CK, Thiagarajan RR, del Nido PJ, et al. Indication for initiation of mechanical circulatory support impacts survival of infants with shunted single-ventricle circulation supported with extracorporeal membrane oxygenation. J Thorac Cardiovasc Surg. 2007;133(3):660-7.

10. Bratton SL, Chan T, Barrett CS, et al. Metrics to Assess Extracorporeal Membrane Oxygenation Utilization in Pediatric Cardiac Surgery Programs. Pediatr Crit Care Med. 2017;18(8):779-86.

11. Barbaro RP, Paden ML, Guner YS, et al. Pediatric Extracorporeal Life Support Organization Registry International Report 2016. ASAIO J. 2017;63(4):456-63.

12. Zampi JD, Alghanem F, Yu S, et al. Relationship Between Time to Left Atrial Decompression and Outcomes in Patients Receiving Venoarterial Extracorporeal Membrane Oxygenation Support: A Multicenter Pediatric Interventional Cardiology Early-Career Society Study. Pediatr Crit Care Med. 2019;20(8):728-36.

13. Callahan R, Trucco SM, Wearden PD, et al. Outcomes of pediatric patients undergoing cardiac catheterization while on extracorporeal membrane oxygenation. Pediatr Cardiol. 2015;36(3):625-32.

14. Boscamp NS, Turner ME, Crystal M, et al. Cardiac Catheterization in Pediatric Patients Supported by Extracorporeal Membrane Oxygenation: A 15-Year Experience. Pediatr Cardiol. 2017;38(2):332-7.

15. Parekh D, Jeewa A, Tume SC, et al. Percutaneous Mechanical Circulatory Support Using Impella Devices for Decompensated Cardiogenic Shock: A Pediatric Heart Center Experience. ASAIO J. 2018;64(1):98-104.

16. Almond CS, Singh TP, Gauvreau K, et al. Extracorporeal membrane oxygenation for bridge to heart transplantation among children in the United States: analysis of data from the Organ Procurement and Transplant Network and Extracorporeal Life Support Organization Registry. Circulation. 2011;123(25):2975-84.

17. Singh TP, Cherikh WS, Hsich E, et al. The International Thoracic Organ Transplant Registry of the International Society for Heart and Lung Transplantation: Twenty-fourth pediatric heart transplantation report - 2021; focus on recipient characteristics. J Heart Lung Transplant. 2021;40(10):1050-9.

18. Edelson JB, Huang Y, Griffis H, et al. The influence of mechanical Circulatory support on post-transplant outcomes in pediatric patients: A multicenter study from the International Society for Heart and Lung Transplantation (ISHLT) Registry. J Heart Lung Transplant. 2021;40(11):1443-53.

19. UNOS. Modification to the Pediatric Heart Allocation Policy [Webinar]. Available from: https://optn.transplant.hrsa.gov/media/1254/webinar_script_changes-to-pediatric-heart-policy.pdf.

20. Chouairi F, Mullan CW, Sen S, et al. Impact of the new heart allocation policy on patients with restrictive, hypertrophic, or congenital cardiomyopathies. PLoS One. 2021;16(3):e0247789.

21. Han JJ, Chung J, Chen CW, et al. Different Clinical Course and Complications in Interagency Registry for Mechanically Assisted Circulatory Support 1 (INTERMACS) Patients Managed With or Without Extracorporeal Membrane Oxygenation. ASAIO J. 2018;64(3):318-22.

22. Sansevere AJ, DiBacco ML, Akhondi-Asl A, et al. EEG features of brain injury during extracorporeal membrane oxygenation in children. Neurology. 2020;95(10):e1372-e80.

23. Farhat A, Li X, Huet B, Tweed J, et al. Routine Neuroimaging: Understanding Brain Injury in Pediatric Extracorporeal Membrane Oxygenation. Crit Care Med. 2022;50(3):480-90.

24. Gorga SM, Sahay RD, Askenazi DJ, et al. Fluid overload and fluid removal in pediatric patients on extracorporeal membrane oxygenation requiring continuous renal replacement therapy: a multicenter retrospective cohort study. Pediatr Nephrol. 2020;35(5):871-82.

25. O'Halloran CP, Alexander PMA, Andren KG, et al. RBC Exposure in Pediatric Extracorporeal Membrane Oxygenation: Epidemiology and Factors Associated With Large Blood Transfusion Volume. Pediatr Crit Care Med. 2018;19(8):767-74.

26. Bailly DK, Reeder RW, Muszynski JA, et al. Anticoagulation practices associated with bleeding and thrombosis in pediatric extracorporeal membrane oxygenation; a multi-center secondary analysis. Perfusion. 2022:2676591211056562.

27. Colvin MM, Cook JL, Chang PP, et al. Sensitization in Heart Transplantation: Emerging Knowledge: A Scientific Statement From the American Heart Association. Circulation. 2019;139(12):e553-e78.

28. Bembea MM, Cheifetz IM, Fortenberry JD, et al. Recommendations on the Indications for RBC Transfusion for the Critically Ill Child Receiving Support From Extracorporeal Membrane Oxygenation, Ventricular Assist, and Renal Replacement Therapy Devices From the Pediatric Critical Care Transfusion and Anemia Expertise Initiative. Pediatr Crit Care Med. 2018;19(9S Suppl 1):S157-S62.

29. Cholette JM, Muszynski JA, Ibla JC, et al. Plasma and Platelet Transfusions Strategies in Neonates and Children Undergoing Cardiac Surgery With Cardiopulmonary Bypass or Neonates and Children Supported by Extracorporeal Membrane Oxygenation: From the Transfusion and Anemia EXpertise Initiative-Control/Avoidance of Bleeding. Pediatr Crit Care Med. 2022;23(13 Supple 1 1S):e25-e36.

30. Abrams D, Javidfar J, Farrand E, et al. Early mobilization of patients receiving extracorporeal membrane oxygenation: a retrospective cohort study. Crit Care. 2014;18(1):R38.

# 21

## Extracorporeal Cardiopulmonary Resuscitation in Children

*Anne-Marie Guerguerian, Jeffrey P. Jacobs, Peter C. Laussen, Ravi R. Thiagarajan*

## Introduction

Outcomes following in-hospital cardiopulmonary arrests treated with conventional cardiopulmonary resuscitation (CPR) have improved, in part due to more arrests happening in PICU settings, where survival to hospital discharge is 32% in pulseless, and up to 63% in bradycardic, CPR events.[1,2] Survival has not changed for out-of-hospital arrest and remains <25%.[3,4] ELSO has reported the use of ECLS with CPR (ECPR) in children since 1992.[5,6] Since then, ECPR use has steadily increased in neonates and children (Figures 21-1 and 21-2). Of 1828 neonatal and pediatric ECPR cases in the ELSO Registry (2011-2015), 94% were witnessed and over 75% occurred in highly monitored environments such as the ICU (72%) or operating room (6%), while <2% were for out-of-hospital arrests.[7] Recently, the American Heart Association Emergency Cardiovascular Care (AHA ECC) guidelines proposed that *"ECPR may be considered as an intervention for selected infants and children (e.g., pediatric cardiac populations) with IHCA refractory to conventional CPR in settings where resuscitation systems allow ECPR to be well performed and implemented (weak recommendation, very low-quality evidence). There is insufficient evidence in pediatric OHCA*

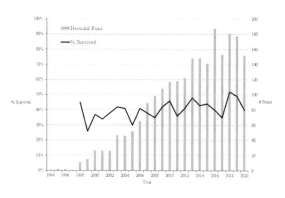

**Figure 21-1.** Neonatal ECPR Runs reported to the ELSO International Registry in October 2021 with the % survival to hospital discharge on the left axis and black line and the number of runs (#) reported annually in grey bars.

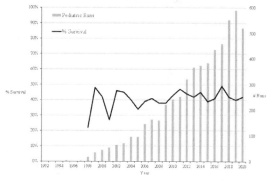

**Figure 21-2.** Pediatric ECPR Runs reported to the ELSO International Registry in October 2021 with the % survival to hospital discharge on the left axis and black line and the number of runs (#) reported annually in grey bars.

to formulate a treatment recommendation for the use of ECPR."[8-10] ELSO Guidelines for ECPR in children and adults were published in 2021.[11,12]

## Definition of ECPR

ECPR is the rapid deployment of V-A ECMO or cardiopulmonary bypass to provide cardiopulmonary support during cardiopulmonary arrest when conventional CPR is ongoing but unsuccessful in achieving sustained return of spontaneous circulation (ROSC). Sustained ROSC is deemed to have occurred when chest compressions are not required for 20 consecutive minutes and signs of circulation persist.[13] In 2018, ECPR was additionally defined to include ECLS within 20 min of ROSC without ongoing compressions.[14]

## Objectives of ECPR

The objective of ECPR is to reduce ischemic injury to organs, especially the brain and heart.[15] High quality conventional CPR only provides partial blood flow to organs. By providing more flow and better gas exchange, ECPR may permit return of circulation in circumstances where CPR alone cannot. ECPR can serve as a bridge to recovery, therapy, transition to a ventricular assist device, transplantation, or palliative care. ECPR or ECLS may be used to assist in rewarming patients with cold exposure associated deep hypothermia (see below).[16]

## Epidemiology, Utilization, and Outcomes

The ELSO Registry October 2021 report included 2,261 neonatal ECPR runs (70% survived to decannulation, 42% survived to hospital discharge) and 5,682 pediatric ECPR runs (59% survived to decannulation, 42% survived to hospital discharge).[17] Only cases that successfully achieve ECLS flows are included in the registry.

### Survival after ECPR

Survival data from registries, administrative databases, and trials is reported at decannulation, ICU discharge, and/or hospital discharge. Only recently have some studies reported long-term outcomes. In the initial ELSO Registry paper from 2007, survival to hospital discharge was 38%.[18] A 2014 ELSO Registry neonatal ECPR study reported hospital discharge rates of 39% in term neonates and 25% in preterm neonates.[19] Analysis of the Asia Pacific ELSO Registry for two periods during the years spanning 1999-2016 of 321 ECPR cases found survival to hospital discharge increased to 51% in the most recent era.[20] A study of 593 cases from the ELSO Registry (2010-2014) linked with the American Heart Association Get With the Guidelines-Resuscitation Registry (76% were postcardiac surgery) reported 41% survival to hospital discharge.[21] Noncardiac diagnoses, preexisting renal insufficiency, longer CPR duration before ECLS, and adverse events during ECLS were all associated with worse outcomes. Other reports of mostly retrospective series in predominantly cardiac patients have variable survival rates of 35%-65%.[22-25]

### Neurologic Outcomes

Data from ELSO reports that 22% of ECPR patients had acute neurologic injury: 11% brain death, 7% cerebral infarction, and 7% intracranial hemorrhage.[26] Hospital mortality in patients with acute neurologic injury was 89%. After adjustment, pre-ECLS factors such as a diagnosis of cardiac disease and less acidosis were associated with decreased probability of neurologic injury. ECLS factors associated with neurologic injury included pulmonary hemorrhage, CPR during ECLS, and use of dialysis.[17] The highest risk of death was associated with neurologic complications during ECLS over any other system.[21] ECPR patients who survive to hospital discharge have good neurological outcomes, with 84% discharged to home rather than to inpatient rehabilitation.

### Long-term Outcomes

Secondary analyses of the THAPCA trials have allowed better understanding of the functional and neurologic outcomes of ECPR survivors.[27] Of 147 children receiving ECPR, 85% had a cardiac condition and 51% were postcardiac surgery. Of these 61/147 (41%) survived to 12 months, 55% had Vineland Adaptive Behavior Scales II (VABS II) scores $\geq$70 and on neurologic examination, and 60% had no or mild impairment. Many ECPR survivors had favourable functional outcome at 12 months, but many showed a decline from prearrest baseline in all domains. Neurocognitive outcome scores remote from the hospitalization are lower than population means despite favorable global outcomes at discharge. Quality of life reported by parents is reasonably good in ECPR survivors.

## Patient Selection

### ECPR in Children with Cardiac Disease

High quality ECPR is a complex intervention and should not be applied in patients as an ad-hoc procedure. ECPR is best suited in select populations when delivered by organized systems.[5,6] ECLS deployment prior to cardiac arrest may be preferred in patients for whom CPR is likely to be ineffective such as patients with[28] : 1) limited stroke volume with chest compressions, 2) limited effective pulmonary blood flow and oxygenation with compressions, 3) limited cerebral perfusion with compressions.

### Cardiac Surgical

The most common indication for ECPR remains the period after cardiac surgery.[29]

Because the risk of cardiac arrest is high in neonates with univentricular physiology undergoing cardiac surgery, ECPR is frequently used to support these neonates.[30]

### Cardiac Medical

Patients with medical cardiac disease such as acute fulminant myocarditis, or dysrhythmias are ideal candidates for ECPR.[31] CPR duration before ECPR deployment is longer in medical cardiac patients compared to surgical cardiac patients.

### Periprocedural Support

ECPR can be used to rescue children who have cardiac arrest during cardiac catheterization. Preprocedural evaluation of high-risk patients and their suitability for elective ECLS to support the procedure are valuable for both clinicians and families.

### ECPR in Children with Noncardiac Disease

### Medical and Surgical Diseases

Acute respiratory failure, sepsis, or pneumonia were the most frequent diagnosis in a study of ECPR.[32] ECPR outcomes are universally worse in children without cardiac disease compared to children with cardiac disease. Some patients have underlying physiology making conventional CPR ineffective; early ECPR should be part of a predefined cardiopulmonary arrest care plan in these cases. Examples include patients with:

- obstructed pulmonary blood flow from a large pulmonary embolus,
- severe hyperkalemia with new onset leukemia or lymphoma and tumor lysis syndrome,
- terminal respiratory failure listed for lung transplantation, and
- severe forms of pulmonary hypertension.

In patients with pulmonary hypertension, preventing cardiopulmonary arrest is key, as the pulmonary circulation will not be effective for gas exchange and perfusion, and right ventricular hypertension impedes coronary perfusion during compressions. A recent ELSO Registry study of 106 ECPR of 605 ECLS runs (2007-2018) for pulmonary hypertension documented 27% survival.[24] Cardiopulmonary arrests that have a higher likelihood of being refractory to conventional CPR include those associated with poisoning from channel calcium blockers and those associated with severe rhabdomyolysis-associated overdoses and concomitant hyperkaliemia.[33] ECPR is rarely used in children with noncardiac surgical diagnosis.[18] ECPR may be applied in trauma patients or in general surgery patients suffering anesthetic or perioperative complications (eg, patients with refractory hyperkaliemia in malignant hyperthermia, congenital diaphragmatic hernia, other congenital thoracic anomalies).

### ECPR in Children with Out-of-Hospital Cardiac Arrest

There are insufficient data to support a recommendation for the use of ECPR in out-of-hospital cardiopulmonary arrest in children.[22] In a recent ELSO Registry analysis, <2% of ECPR (2011-2015) were from out-of-hospital arrest.

### ECPR in Accidental Hypothermia

Severe hypothermia defined with core temperatures <28°C may occur with drowning, cold outdoor exposure, or snow burial. Some organizations include ECLS in their algorithms for rewarming in cases of outdoor exposure and severe hypothermia with absent signs of life or cardiopulmonary arrest; however, pediatric specific guidelines are lacking. Survival to hospital discharge for pediatric and adult drowning was reported as 23% in a study from the ELSO Registry. Those with pre-ECLS cardiac arrest had worse survival compared to those without. ECPR may be beneficial in patients where hypothermia is the cause of the arrest, rather than the consequence of it.

### Equipment

### *Circuit and Equipment*

An ECLS circuit must be readily available (dry or wet primed), self-contained, and easily portable. Centrifugal pumps are the most frequently used for ECPR. Polymethylpentene or polypropylene are the membranes commonly used.[7] Heat exchangers can provide targeted temperature management (TTM).

### *Anticoagulation*

Anticoagulation before cannulation and connection to the ECLS system for ECPR should follow local ECLS protocols (Chapter 4).

### *Prime and Transfusion Therapies*

Blood or crystalloid solution can be used for priming. The majority of circuits used in pediatric ECPR cases are blood primed according to ELSO.[7] Delays in ECLS deployment while awaiting blood should be avoided.

### System and Team

### *Decision and Initiation*

The decision to initiate ECPR and the timing of ECPR initiation should be separate steps. The decision to initiate ECPR or not should be made early; it can also be made in anticipation of a high-risk event in a specific patient. Patients at high risk for needing ECPR should be evaluated for possible ECPR initiation in detail. This evaluation includes formal ultrasonographic assessment of the patency of all vessels that may be potentially used for cannulation. Timing of ECPR initiation should also be based on the expected time needed to achieve extracorporeal blood flow if sustained ROSC does not occur. The ELSO Registry reports that 30% of cases are cannulated <30 minutes after start of compressions and the median time to achieve ECLS flow is 40 minutes.[7] Some organizations set process benchmarks at <30 minutes or <40 minutes to ECLS flow and expect clinicians to make the decision to deploy within 5 and launch within 10 minutes following start of compressions.

## The Team

ECPR requires a well-coordinated team whose roles and responsibilities are defined in advance. Standard resuscitation measures should be initiated by the first team who focus on high quality CPR with minimal interruptions before and during ECLS deployment. A second group of individuals are dedicated to ECPR with rapid priming and cannulation. A paging system is useful to mobilize the ECPR team and resources. Because ECPR is a low-frequency, high-risk event, medical simulation training is helpful (Chapter 54). In some organizations, ECPR teams are available 24/7. This approach may not be sustainable for all organizations.

## Resuscitation Measures

Three key discrete *times* $(t_0, t_1, t_2)$ and four *intervals* $(i_1, i_2, i_3, i_4)$ delineate phases of care when applying ECPR. Conducting each step while optimizing the duration of each phase is critical for success (Figure 21-3):

- **Interval 1** ($i_1$): Interval from time of cardiopulmonary arrest $(t_0)$ to start of CPR $(t_1)$, where $(i_1=t_1-t_0)$.
- **Interval 2** ($i_2$): From start of CPR $(t_1)$ to launching ECPR $(t_2)$, where $(i_2=t_2-t_1)$.

- **Interval 3** ($i_3$): From ECPR Launch $(t_2)$ to achieving adequate ECLS perfusion $(t_3)$, where $(i_3=t_3-t_2)$.
- **Interval 4** ($i_4$): Interval from establishment on ECLS $(t_3)$ to on-going targeted post-cardiac arrest care on ECLS (E-PCAC) where $(i_4=t_x-t_3)$. This is not uniform or predictable; it may occur when the patient is separated from ECLS or when post-cardiac arrest care interventions are completed while still on ECLS i.e., which ever comes first at time x $(t_x)$.

### *Approaches to Minimize Ischemia and Reperfusion Injury*

Current high-quality CPR metrics apply to high quality ECPR (compression-to-breath ratios, diastolic blood pressure, and $ETCO_2$) and should be used to guide CPR during ECLS cannulation:

- **Limiting Interval 1:** Witnessed and in-hospital events offer the best conditions where the period of no-flow prior to starting conventional CPR is kept to a minimum to increase the chance of myocardial recovery and reduce the risk of brain injury. Ideally, Interval 1 is < 1 minute ($i_1=t_1-t_0$ <1 min). Unwitnessed arrests may not be suited for ECPR as the duration of ischemia from the no-flow Interval is unknown.

- **High quality conventional CPR during Intervals 2+3:** Ensured by close monitoring of the effectiveness of delivering airway management, compressions, defibrillation and/or medications, and additional interventions focused on reversing the cardiopulmonary arrest. In hospital, this monitoring includes:
  - continuous monitoring of ECG,
  - plethysmography,
  - pulse oxymetry,
  - capnography,

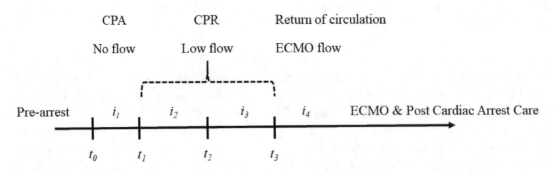

**Figure 21-3.** Key times and intervals of a cardiopulmonary arrest and resuscitation measures with ECPR.

---

*Legend:*

**Interval 1 ($i_1$)** Interval from the start time of cardiopulmonary arrest ($t_0$) to the start of conventional CPR ($t_1$) where ($i_1=t_1-t_0$).

- Recognize cardiopulmonary arrest and initial rhythm

**Interval 2 ($i_2$):** Interval from start time of conventional CPR ($t_1$) to launching the ECPR system ($t_2$) where ($i_2=t_2-t_1$).

- Start CPR measures
- Call Code Resuscitation Team
- Maintain high quality CPR with intra-arrest monitoring
- Anticipate refractory CPA response to conventional CPR
- Determine if patient may be suitable to resuscitate with ECPR
- Make decision that patient is suitable for ECPR
- No ROSC
- Launch ECPR system

**Interval 3 ($i_3$):** Interval from time of launch of ECPR system ($t_2$) to achieving return of circulation ($t_3$) with adequate flow and perfusion where ($i_3=t_3-t_2$).

- Patient in cannulation location: continue to optimize high quality CPR
- Patient not in a cannulation location: transport to cannulation location with CPR

- Team members assemble at cannulation location
- Notify Blood Bank
- Assemble equipment and prime at cannulation location
- Position patient and maintain high quality CPR
- Reconnect to bedside intra-arrest monitoring if arrives from arrest location
- Patient identification verified and clock timed (Time out #1)
- Heparin bolus delivered
- Cannulation plan verified
- Cannulation start (+/- sternotomy)
- Cannulation completed
- Cannulas matched to drainage and return tubing of circuit (Time out #2)
- Cannulas connected to ECMO system
- Pump flows increased to 100 ml/kg/min as default or 2-3 L/min
- Gas flow meter and FdO2 adjusted

**Interval 4 ($i_4$):** Interval from time of return of circulation ($t_3$) to on-going targeted post cardiac arrest care on ECMO (E-PCAC) where ($i_4=t_x-t_3$).

- Pump flows adjusted to target mean blood pressure
- Ventilator adjusted and FiO2 weaned
- Circuit and patient arterial blood gas measured
- Lactate and Complete Blood Count
- Inotropes and inhaled nitric oxide wean
- Point of care testing for anticoagulation
- Temperature target verified

- ◆ intra-arterial blood pressure,
- ◆ cerebral near infrared spectroscopy,
- ◆ minimal interruptions to compressions, and
- ◆ prompt recognition of rhythms that may require defibrilliation.

Delivery of resuscitation medications and documentation of interventions are essential.

- **High quality ECPR:** During Interval 3, the team prepares for ECPR without compromising the quality of CPR. The transition may involve:

  - ◆ intra-hospital transport to the cannulation location,
  - ◆ positioning the patient with rolls under the shoulders or under the pelvis, and
  - ◆ turning the head to the side, or preparation for chest re-opening and providing open chest CPR (OC-CPR).

In this context, it becomes important to have protocols in place that assign roles and responsibilities for resuscitation, priming and cannulation.

### *Cannulation Location*

The patient, equipment, and team members involved in ECPR require a large amount of space. A *space map* helps to organize team members and equipment around the bed. Cannulation locations and transport protocols should be preapproved (eg, ICU or Catheterization Laboratory). CPR quality must not be compromised during transport.[34] The location chosen is a compromise between the difficulties of transporting during CPR and cannulating in an austere environment. When the arrest location can be immediately transformed to deliver ECPR, Interval 3 is most

often shorter ($i_3 = t_3 - t_2$) than when transport is necessary.[35]

### Cannulation

Cannulation for ECPR must be rapid and effective (Chapter 4). In children with vessels accessed previously, it is essential to have easily available documentation of occluded vessels to prevent delays in cannulation. A cannulation strategy should be planned in high-risk patients.[36]

### *Vascular Approach and Impact on CPR Quality*

Peripheral and transthoracic cannulation will affect resuscitation differently. The impact of transitioning from conventional CPR measures to ECPR preparation has an effect on mean compression numbers, End-Tidal Carbon dioxide ($ETCO_2$) during resuscitation and need for interruptions in the ECPR phase.[37] Peripheral approaches are less likely to interfere with chest compressions than chest cannulation, where there may be more interruptions while reopening the chest and initiating open-chest CPR (OC-CPR). Little is known about the impact of head rotation on cerebral perfusion pressure during neck cannulation. No data exists to inform which cannulation approach provides the best cardiopulmonary and cerebral perfusion in general.[38] The need to have an immobile surgical field during cannulation will interrupt compressions. During these interruptions, clear calm communication between cannulators and the resuscitation team leader is important. Counting seconds of no CPR out loud can be helpful. Restarting CPR without the surgeon being ready can result in a complete failure of cannulation and can be avoided by good teamwork and communication. Transthoracic cannulation may be faster than peripheral cannulations, especially in postoperative patients.[35] In postoperative patients, it is difficult to untangle the relationship between their more favorable outcomes, shorter duration of $i_1+i_2+i_3$, the use of central cannulation, and the application of OC-CPR.[27] Transthoracic central cannulation may also be used in the context of penetrating trauma of the heart and great vessels, intra-operative cardiopulmonary arrest, or refractory severe septic shock (Chapter 36).[39]

## ECPR Protocols

A written protocol enhances performance and minimizes disruptive variability. Such protocols define roles and responsibilities, order tasks, and provide individual and shared checklists with process algorithms. The protocol should address location for cannulation (as discussed above) and should also include general patient selection and initiation criteria (Figure 21-3). The algorithm should also contain 'time-outs' to verify safety checks and a target total duration $(i_1+i_2+i_3)$ to attain full ECLS flows as an important benchmark.

## Quality Measures

Institutions should establish internal quality measures to assess the safety and efficacy of all ECPR events, whether they resulted in a successful cannulation or not (Chapter 55). These quality measures serve as an important mechanism to detect vulnerable areas in the algorithm (eg, decisionmaking vs. cannulation procedure vs. circuit readiness). No universally accepted time-to-cannulation benchmarks for in-hospital events formally exist; however, given the increase in ECPR, some measure similar to the best practices recommended in adult out-of-hospital ECPR are emerging.[40] Prolonged times to attaining return of extracorporeal circulation with ECPR blood flow are associated with worse outcomes.[21] For in-hospital cardiopulmonary arrests, some organizations aim to have processes in place to achieve return of circulation within 30 minutes

either by initiation of extracorporeal circulation or ROSC. If ROSC occurs within 30 minutes, the responsible physician decides whether or not to pursue extracorporeal circulation. Understanding the process lag times and the Intervals required to launch the ECPR helps the team leader direct care. Benchmarks can be used for performance review and for team and system training using simulation. Debriefing after all ECPR events is necessary to understand what worked well and what deficiencies need to be fixed.[41] Debriefs should be conducted as a team immediately after real and simulated events ('hot') or later ('cold'), as team and individual debriefs.

## Early ECLS Postcardiac Arrest Care (E-PCAC)

Postcardiac arrest care in patients who receive ECPR begins immediately after ECLS flow is established at $t_3$. ECLS blood flow must be adjusted, and end-organ perfusion restored to optimize tissue oxygen delivery. Adequate ECLS flow may be indicated by:

- improved clinical perfusion and neurologic function,
- improvement and resolution of laboratory markers of ischemia (eg, metabolic acidosis or lactate), and
- restoration of urine output.

E-PCAC is focused on minimizing ongoing ischemia reperfusion injury, particularly in the brain, heart, and lungs.[42,43] Diagnostic or therapeutic procedures may include radiological imaging and interventional cardiac catheterization, which should be safely undertaken without delay. Children with signs of left atrial hypertension and pulmonary edema or hemorrhage require prompt diagnosis and emergent left ventricular decompression (Chapters 4,18). Adequate coronary perfusion is a key target. Institutions who offer ECPR must be able to optimize patients once cannulated or transfer them to another institution that can.[44] The risk of neurological injury is greater with ECPR patients compared to ECLS patients thus the means to assess, monitor, and image the brain is paramount during $i_4$. Neurologic assessment includes:

- sedation hold with awakening and clinical assessment,
- neuromonitoring (cerebral near infrared spectroscopy, continuous EEG),
- neuroimaging,
- consultation with a neurologist, and
- repeat neuroimaging as necessary, both before and after decannulation.

## ECLS Blood Flow, Gas Exchange, Temperature, and Blood Pressure

### ECLS Flow

ECLS flow is guided by the resolution of markers of ischemia such as lactate, $MVO_2$ and NIRS. Inotropes should be weaned as tolerated to decrease afterload and allow ECLS flow to be increased. Repeated epinephrine boluses pre-cannulation may be associated with:

- increased afterload from increased systemic and cerebral vascular resistance, impairing the increase in ECLS flows, and/or
- increased cerebral ischemia and worse neurologic outcomes.

While we do not advocate changing established CPR protocols, it is sensible to avoid giving a timed epinephrine dose a few seconds before ECLS flow is established. Pulmonary vasodilators can also be weaned. Setting daily hemodynamic perfusion pressure goals (systolic, diastolic, and mean pressure in the absence of pulsatility) is necessary to enhance myocardial recovery.

### Gas Exchange

No published clinical evidence exists to guide membrane gas management during or after ECPR deployment in children, but retrospective research in adult ECPR suggests that hyperoxia may be associated with worse neurologic outcomes.[45] Most pediatric centers use blended gases on their standard ECLS circuits ($O_2$ and Air) to titrate $FsO_2$ and attempt to minimize hyperoxia because it may worsen ischemia-reperfusion injury. From published work in pediatric ECLS,[46] out-of-hospital adult ECPR,[47] and pediatric preclinical[48] and clinical resuscitation literature,[49] an association exists between postresuscitation hyperoxia and mortality. NIRS devices do not require pulsatility to estimate the oximetry of the underlying tissue, making them more useful than standard pulse oximetry when pulsatility disappears. Bilateral probes may be applied to the prefrontal area and/or to the calf muscles (when femoral cannulation is used) to monitor for asymmetry, hyperoxemia, and ischemia. In pediatric ECLS, hypocapnia in the first 48 hours may be associated with increased risk of a neurologic event.[46] Sweep gas flow when initiating ECLS should therefore be carefully controlled to prevent profound and rapid hypocapnia, which may be associated with cerebral ischemia at a time when the cerebral vascular reactivity is altered by ischemia and acidosis. Sweep flow should not exceed blood flow initially and early measurement of arterial blood gases is essential to avoid inadvertent hypocapnia or hypercapnia, which may influence neurologic outcome.

### Temperature

The ELSO Registry reports therapeutic hypothermia use in more than half of neonatal and pediatric ECPR cases.[7] No comparative trials suggest an optimal target temperature, and no randomized control trials support one target temperature versus another. Nevertheless, the target temperature should be deliberate and defined by the responsible physician based on patient factors and/or institutional protocols; hyperthermia should not be tolerated. When a heat exchanger device is not used, a patient monitoring device must be used to measure continuous core or central temperature (ie, esophageal, rectal, or bladder temperature). External or skin temperature measurements are not sufficient post-resuscitation due to poor peripheral perfusion.

**Other Pharmacological Cointerventions and Aseptic Technique**

Aseptic technique is used for cannulation and OC-CPR. Little guidance exists about the standard use of surgical antimicrobial prophylaxis for ECPR and for transthoracic cannulation. No specific guidance exists about the use of steroids during ECPR. Dosing of prostaglandins to maintain ductal patency and other vasoactive agents are center-specific and guided by individualized patient physiology.

**Anticipating End-of-Life Care in the ECPR Patient and Their Family**

The probability of death and new neurological injury is high for children who require ECPR. Accordingly, well integrated end-of-life practices are an essential component of an ECPR program.[50] Patient- and family-centered care plans should encompass gradual end-of-life discussions and communication. The large proportion of ECPR patients who survive to decannulation but die before discharge highlights the importance of starting end-of-life communication during ECLS.

**Duration of CPR and Time to ECLS Flow**

The ELSO Registry reports that the median duration of CPR prior to ECLS flow was 40 minutes (IQR=25–61 minutes) and 73% received CPR <60 minutes.[7] In a study completed with merged registry data, the median duration of CPR prior to ECLS initiation was 48 minutes (IQR=28–70 minutes).[21] In this study, a longer duration of CPR before initiation of ECLS was associated with decreased odds of survival. However, they also reported that half of survivors had CPR duration of ≥42 minutes prior to ECLS initiation, and 30% of survivors had CPR duration >1 hour.[21] Esangbedo et al. examined the relationship between CPR duration before achieving flows and mortality.[23] Of 46 studies that analyzed CPR duration, only 15 showed an increase in risk of mortality with increasing CPR duration. Long-term neurologic outcomes at 12 months are worse with longer CPR duration.[27] Organizations should monitor the duration of Intervals 1, 2, and 3 to understand the source of delays and solve each specifically. Unwitnessed events in most settings have a poor prognosis and are considered a relative contraindication for ECPR, given the unknown duration of Interval 1. Ideally, Interval 1 is <1 minute if the event is witnessed. Interval 2 with high quality CPR would ideally be long enough to provide time for interventions to reverse the cardiopulmonary arrest, anticipate the likelihood of the refractory nature of the event, make the decision about suitability of ECPR, and obtain return of circulation. Most systems know their average duration required to transition from conventional CPR to achieving ECLS flows with transthoracic or peripheral cannulation. Based on this knowledge, some centers pre-set the duration of Interval 2 to 3-10 minutes, to prompt ECPR launch and achieve ECLS flows within 30-60 minutes. In events that occur in locations of the hospital where cannulations cannot be performed, the system needs to build in the time to transport to the cannulation location during Interval 3.

## Resources

An ECPR system has significant costs and resource implications. In systems that already care for high-risk cardiac surgical children, the additional resources necessary to build an ECPR system may be less compared to an institution that does not. On average, 12-15 skilled individuals are deployed, and they must interrupt their responsibilities to focus on ECPR. Additionally, an ECPR system requires response systems across the hospital such as a strong resuscitation team, an efficient blood bank, and sufficient redundant resources and expertise to ensure that these skilled individuals can be emergently reallocated for an unplanned ECLS cannulation and initiation that may require 1-2 hours of stabilization, all without impacting the care of other patients. Institutions which do not offer cardiac surgery or interventional cardiology and opt to offer ECPR should form part of a hub-and-spoke network to allow safe transfer on ECLS during Interval 4 to a center that can provide comprehensive E-PCAC.

## Ethics and Informed Consent

Because of the rapid nature of ECPR deployment, obtaining informed consent for ECPR while the process is unfolding is challenging. In high volume cardiac surgical centers, information is given, and consent secured at the time as the preoperative consent. Oversight for informed consent should follow the process for conventional CPR rather than ECLS. Patients eligible for ECLS may not be automatically suited for ECPR. The subtle differences in indication should be explained to guardians of children with complex conditions (eg, patients with severe pulmonary hypertension before a cardiac catheterization laboratory study) or listed for solid organ transplantation (eg, heart or lung). These special circumstances illustrate that a single recommendation is not sufficient to serve all these situations and their local context. In unexpected ECPR events, parents should be informed as soon as possible and when reasonable. These conversations ideally include:

- potential reasons for the arrest;
- the time-limited purpose for ECLS based on institutional bridging options;
- the care plan that involves the possibilities of survival, survival with morbidities, and of death; and
- prognosis.

These conversations are best conducted on a frequent regular or daily basis, which allows guardians to be aware of the changes in condition and the evolving status of the child.[51]

## Summary

ECPR utilization has increased in neonatal and pediatric resuscitation. Offering ECPR requires institutions to commit to sustaining a system able to provide additional expertise and resources to ensure that high quality ECPR is followed by comprehensive E-PCAC and family centered end-of-life care. Data about short- and long-term outcomes of survivors and their families are emerging and will guide further research on how to improve outcomes. Patient selection must continue to be one of the key topics of inquiry. As we develop the ability to predict and anticipate which patients may be at risk of cardiopulmonary arrest, clinicians need data to inform their decisions. If the patient is suitable for resuscitation, the clinician must contemplate the following five scenarios when their patient deteriorates:

1. responds to clinical management (no ECLS, no cardiopulmonary arrest);
2. be cannulated for ECLS before a cardiopulmonary arrest;

3. have a cardiopulmonary arrest, followed by sustained ROSC, and be cannulated later for ECLS;
4. have a cardiopulmonary arrest and undergo successful ECPR; or
5. have a cardiopulmonary arrest and undergo unsuccessful ECPR.

A robust ECPR system will ensure that patient selection includes deciding when to deploy ECPR, but also includes upstream decisionmaking about the management needed to prevent cardiopulmonary arrest. Such upstream decisionmaking may involve elective ECLS or undertaking other interventions that may help reverse the driver of the deteriorating physiology.

# References

1. Holmberg MJ, Wiberg S, Ross CE, et al. American Heart Association's Get With The Guidelines-Resuscitation I. Trends in Survival after Pediatric In-Hospital Cardiac Arrest in the United States. Circulation 2019.

2. Berg RA, Nadkarni VM, Clark AE, et al. Eunice Kennedy Shriver National Institute of Child H, Human Development Collaborative Pediatric Critical Care Research N. Incidence and Outcomes of Cardiopulmonary Resuscitation in PICUs. Crit Care Med 2016;44:798-808.

3. Tijssen JA, Prince DK, Morrison LJ, et al. Resuscitation Outcomes C. Time on the scene and interventions are associated with improved survival in pediatric out-of-hospital cardiac arrest. Resuscitation 2015;94:1-7.

4. Fink EL, Prince DK, Kaltman JR, et al. Unchanged pediatric out-of-hospital cardiac arrest incidence and survival rates with regional variation in North America. Resuscitation 2016;107:121-8.

5. del Nido PJ, Dalton HJ, Thompson AE, et al. Extracorporeal membrane oxygenator rescue in children during cardiac arrest after cardiac surgery. Circulation 1992;86:II300-4.

6. Dalton HJ, Siewers RD, Fuhrman BP, et al. Extracorporeal membrane oxygenation for cardiac rescue in children with severe myocardial dysfunction. Crit Care Med 1993;21:1020-8.

7. Barbaro RP, Paden ML, Guner YS, et al. Pediatric Extracorporeal Life Support Organization Registry International Report 2016. ASAIO journal 2017;63:456-63.

8. Duff JP, Topjian AA, Berg MD, et al. 2019 American Heart Association Focused Update on Pediatric Advanced Life Support: An Update to the American Heart Association Guidelines for Cardiopulmonary Resuscitation and Emergency Cardiovascular Care. Circulation 2019;140:e904-e14.

9. Maconochie IK, Aickin R, Hazinski MF, et al. Pediatric Life Support: 2020 International Consensus on Cardiopulmonary Resuscitation and Emergency Cardiovascular Care Science With Treatment Recommendations. Resuscitation 2020;156:A120-a55.

10. Topjian AA, Raymond TT, Atkins D, et al. 2020 American Heart Association Guidelines for Cardiopulmonary Resuscitation and Emergency Cardiovascular Care. Pediatrics 2020.

11. Guerguerian AM, Sano M, Todd M, et al. Pediatric Extracorporeal Cardiopulmonary Resuscitation ELSO Guidelines. ASAIO journal 2021;67:229-37.

12. Richardson ASC, Tonna JE, Nanjayya V, et al. Extracorporeal Cardiopulmonary Resuscitation in Adults. Interim Guideline Consensus Statement From the Extracorporeal Life Support Organization. ASAIO journal 2021;67:221-8.

13. Jacobs I, Nadkarni V, Bahr J, et al. International Liason Committee on R. Cardiac arrest and cardiopulmonary resuscitation outcome reports: update and simplification of the Utstein templates for resuscitation registries. A statement for healthcare professionals from a task force of the international liaison committee on resuscitation (American Heart Association, European Resuscitation Council, Australian Resuscitation Council, New Zealand Resuscitation Council, Heart and Stroke Foundation of Canada, InterAmerican Heart Foundation, Resuscitation Council of Southern Africa). Resuscitation 2004;63:233-49.

14. ELSO. ELSO Registry ECPR Addenda Definitions April 2019. 07/23/2020 Version ed2021:47.

15. Tisherman SA, Grenvik A, Safar P. Cardiopulmonary-cerebral resuscitation: advanced and prolonged life support with emergency cardiopulmonary bypass. Acta Anaesthesiol Scand Suppl 1990;94:63-72.

16. Bauman BD, Louiselle A, Nygaard RM, et al. Treatment of Hypothermic Cardiac Arrest in the Pediatric Drowning Victim, a Case Report, and Systematic Review. Pediatr Emerg Care 2021;37:e653-e9.

17. International Summary ECLS Registry Report. Ann Arbor, MI: Extracorporeal Life Support Organization; 2021 October 2021.

18. Thiagarajan RR, Laussen PC, Rycus PT, et al. Extracorporeal membrane oxygenation to aid cardiopulmonary resuscitation in infants and children. Circulation 2007;116:1693-700.

19. McMullan DM, Thiagarajan RR, Smith KM, et al. Extracorporeal cardiopulmonary resuscitation outcomes in term and premature neonates. Pediatric critical care medicine 2014;15:e9-e16.

20. Chen G-L, Qiao Y-R, Ma J-H, et al. Extracorporeal Cardiopulmonary Resuscitation in Children of Asia Pacific: A Retrospective Analysis of Extracorporeal Life Support Organization Registry. Chinese medical journal 2018;131:1436-43.

21. Bembea MM, Ng DK, Rizkalla N, Rycus P, et al. Outcomes After Extracorporeal Cardiopulmonary Resuscitation of Pediatric In-Hospital Cardiac Arrest: A Report From the Get With the Guidelines-Resuscitation and the Extracorporeal Life Support Organization Registries. Crit Care Med 2019;47:e278-e85.

22. Holmberg MJ, Geri G, Wiberg S, et al. Extracorporeal cardiopulmonary resuscitation for cardiac arrest: A systematic review. Resuscitation 2018;131:91-100.

23. Esangbedo ID, Brunetti MA, Campbell FM, Lasa JJ. Pediatric Extracorporeal Cardiopulmonary Resuscitation: A Systematic Review*. Pediatr Crit Care Med 2020:E934-E43.

24. Morell E, Rajagopal SK, Oishi P, et al. Extracorporeal membrane oxygenation in pediatric pulmonary hypertension. Pediatr Crit Care Med 2020:256-66.

25. Farhat A, Ling RR, Jenks CL, et al. Outcomes of Pediatric Extracorporeal Cardiopulmonary Resuscitation: A Systematic Review and Meta-Analysis. Crit Care Med 2021;49:682-92.

26. Barrett CS, Bratton SL, Salvin JW, et al. Neurological injury after extracorporeal membrane oxygenation use to aid pediatric cardiopulmonary resuscitation. Pediatric critical care medicine 2009;10:445-51.

27. Meert KL, Guerguerian AM, Barbaro R, et al. Extracorporeal Cardiopulmonary Resuscitation: One-Year Survival and Neurobehavioral Outcome among Infants and Children with In-Hospital Cardiac Arrest. Critical care medicine 2019;47:393-402.

28. Marino BS, Tabbutt S, MacLaren G, et al. American Heart Association Congenital Cardiac Defects Committee of the Council on Cardiovascular Disease in the Y, Council on Clinical C, Council on C, Stroke N, Council on Cardiovascular S, Anesthesia, Emergency Cardiovascular Care C. Cardiopulmonary Resuscitation in Infants and Children With Cardiac Disease: A Scientific Statement From the American Heart Association. Circulation 2018;137:e691-e782.

29. Melvan JN, Davis J, Heard M, et al. Factors Associated With Survival Following Extracorporeal Cardiopulmonary Resuscitation in Children. World Journal for Pediatric and Congenital Heart Surgery 2020;11:265-74.

30. Jolley M, Yarlagadda VV, Rajagopal SK, et al. Extracorporeal membrane oxygenation-supported cardiopulmonary resuscitation following stage 1 palliation for hypoplastic left heart syndrome. Pediatric critical care medicine 2014;15:538-45.

31. Teele SA, Allan CK, Laussen PC, et al. Management and outcomes in pediatric patients presenting with acute fulminant myocarditis. J Pediatr 2011;158:638-43 e1.

32. Conrad SJ, Bridges BC, Kalra Y, et al. Extracorporeal Cardiopulmonary Resuscitation Among Patients with Structurally Normal Hearts. ASAIO journal 2017;63:781-6.

33. Koshel CK, Alexander PMA, Rycus P, et al. Extracorporeal Membrane Oxygenation for Pediatric Toxin Exposures: Review of the Extracorporeal Life Support Organization Registry. ASAIO journal 2021.

34. Loaec M, Himebauch AS, Kilbaugh TJ, et al. Pediatric cardiopulmonary resuscitation quality during intra-hospital transport. Resuscitation 2020;152:123-30.

35. Marquez AM, Vargas-Gutierrez M, Todd M, et al. Abstract 13945: Central Cannulation During Pediatric Extracorporeal Cardiopulmonary Resuscitation is Faster Than Peripheral Approaches. Circulation 2021;144:A13945-A.

36. Alsoufi B, Trivedi J, Rycus P, et al. Repeat Extracorporeal Membrane Oxygenation Support Is Appropriate in Selected Children With Cardiac Disease: An Extracorporeal Life Support Organization Study. World J Pediatr Congenit Heart Surg 2021;12:597-604.

37. Taeb M, Levin AB, Spaeder MC, et al. Comparison of Pediatric Cardiopulmonary Resuscitation Quality in Classic Cardiopulmonary Resuscitation and Extracorporeal Cardiopulmonary Resuscitation Events Using Video Review. Pediatric critical care medicine 2018;19:831-8.

38. Chenouard A, Liet JM, Maminirina P, et al. Neurological Outcome According to the Site of Cannulation in Septic Children Supported by Venoarterial Extracorporeal Membrane Oxygenation. ASAIO journal 2021;67:1349-55.

39. Ruth A, Vogel AM, Adachi I, et al. Central venoarterial extracorporeal life support in pediatric refractory septic shock: a single center experience. Perfusion 2021:026765912110017.

40. Hutin A, Abu-Habsa M, Burns B, et al. Early ECPR for out-of-hospital cardiac arrest: Best practice in 2018. Resuscitation 2018;130:44-8. 10.1016/j.resuscitation.2018.05.004.

41. Lirette M, Dahan M, Pisesky A, et al. ACED it! Acute Critical Event Debriefing to improve performance and patient safety. IPSSV2021 International Pediatric Simulation Symposia and Worshops2021.

42. Lasa JJ, Jain P, Raymond TT, et al. Extracorporeal Cardiopulmonary Resuscitation in the Pediatric Cardiac Population: In Search of a Standard of Care. Pediatric critical care medicine 2017.

43. Topjian AA, de Caen A, Wainwright MS, et al. Pediatric Post-Cardiac Arrest Care: A Scientific Statement From the American Heart Association. Circulation. 2019 Aug 6;140(6):e194-e233.

44. Zampi JD, Alghanem F, Yu S, et al. Relationship Between Time to Left Atrial Decompression and Outcomes in Patients Receiving Venoarterial Extracorporeal Membrane Oxygenation Support: A Multicenter Pediatric Interventional Cardiology Early-Career Society Study. Pediatric critical care medicine 2019;20:728-36.

45. Chang WT, Wang CH, Lai CH, et al. Optimal Arterial Blood Oxygen Tension in the Early Postresuscitation Phase of Extracorporeal Cardiopulmonary Resuscitation: A 15-Year Retrospective Observational Study. Crit Care Med 2019;47:1549-56.

46. Cashen K, Reeder R, Dalton HJ, et al. Hyperoxia and Hypocapnia During Pediatric Extracorporeal Membrane Oxygenation: Associations With Complications, Mortality, and Functional Status Among Survivors. Pediatric critical care medicine 2018;19:245-53.

47. Halter M, Jouffroy R, Saade A, et al. Association between hyperoxemia and mortality in patients treated by eCPR after out-of-hospital cardiac arrest. Am J Emerg Med 2019.

48. Marquez AM, Morgan RW, Ko T, et al. Oxygen Exposure During Cardiopulmonary Resuscitation Is Associated With Cerebral Oxidative Injury in a Randomized, Blinded, Controlled, Preclinical Trial. J Am Heart Assoc 2020;9:e015032.

49. Guerra-Wallace MM, Casey FL 3rd, Bell MJ, et al. Hyperoxia and hypoxia in children resuscitated from cardiac arrest. Pediatric critical care medicine 2013;14:e143-8.

50. Moynihan KM, Jansen M, Siegel BD, et al. Extracorporeal Membrane Oxygenation Candidacy Decisions: An Argument for a Process-Based Longitudinal Approach. Pediatr Crit Care Med. 2022 May 25.

51. Suzuki Y, Cass SH, Kugelmann A, et al. Outcome of Extracorporeal Membrane Oxygenation for Pediatric Patients With Neoplasm: An Extracorporeal Life Support Organization Database Study (2000-2019). Pediatric critical care medicine 2022.

# 22

## Complications, Followup, and Outcomes of Children with Cardiac Failure

*Michele Domico, Malaika H. Mendonca, Francis Fynn-Thompson, Katherine L. Brown, Aparna Hoskote*

## Introduction

The most common indications for ECLS in children with heart disease are acute postcardiotomy failure, refractory cardiac arrest, severe cardiac dysfunction, cardiogenic shock, or arrhythmias unresponsive to conventional medical therapy.[1] Over the last decade, the use of ECLS to support children with cardiovascular disease has increased[2,3] relative to respiratory indications, particularly in neonates.[4,5] ECLS utilization within congenital heart surgery programs is on average 2-3% of cardiac surgical cases.[6] Congenital heart disease (CHD) remains the most common neonatal and pediatric cardiac diagnosis requiring support.[5] The overall survival to discharge is currently at 43% for neonates and 53% for children,[4] and has remained relatively unchanged over the last decade.[4,7]

In this chapter, we will review complications linked to worse outcomes that are frequently seen in children with cardiovascular diseases, namely, bleeding and thrombosis,[8] renal failure,[9] and acute neurological events.[10] Particular attention to long-term neurodevelopmental outcome, and quality of life will be presented. Awareness, early intervention, and protocolized followup of these potential complications in the ICU setting may enable the use of protective measures.

## Common Complications During ECLS

Acquired comorbidities during ECLS can impact in-hospital mortality and contribute to longer-term morbidity. Although many types of complications can occur, some of the most devastating are neurologic events, acute kidney injury (AKI), bleeding, and thrombosis.

### Bleeding, Thrombosis, and Hemolysis

Bleeding and thrombosis remain significant complications despite advancements in technology, circuitry, and monitoring. Hemorrhage commonly occurs at the cannulation site, surgical site, in the central nervous system, and gastrointestinal tract. The prevalence of hemorrhagic complications on ECLS ranges from 12-70%,[11,12] with bleeding most commonly noted at the surgical (17%) and cannulation site (14%).[8] Dalton et al. reported 37.5% of ECLS patients had a thrombotic event, with the majority occurring in the circuit as compared to the patient.[12] Hemolysis (defined by plasma-free hemoglobin >50 mg/dl) occurs in 7-41% of children and neonates receiving cardiac ECMO support.[4, 8,12]

ECLS necessitates the contact of blood and a nonendothelial surface, which results in coagulation and fibrinolytic pathway activation plus an inflammatory response (Chapter 6).[13] The prothrombotic state requires vigilant monitoring of anticoagulation not only to prevent clotting but avoid bleeding complications. In 2022, ELSO published updated anticoagulation guidelines.[14] Both bleeding and clotting often coexist in the same patient and contribute to significant morbidity and mortality.[8,11,15] In a subset analysis of 727 cardiac failure patients, Dalton et al. described bleeding events during cardiac ECMO, which were associated with reduced survival by 33% in neonates and 32% in children.[8] A similar decrease in survival likelihood was associated with thrombotic complications for both neonatal (RR 0.56; 95% CI, 0.38–0.82) and pediatric cardiac failure patients (RR 0.63; 95% CI, 0.49–0.82).[8]

Children with cardiac disease may be more susceptible to bleeding events, particularly those postcardiotomy. In a subset analysis, Werho et al. reviewed 8905 children with cardiac disease and showed a significantly higher rate of on-ECMO hemorrhage in cardiac patients as compared to noncardiac patients (49% vs. 32%). The highest group was cardiac surgical patients, with a 57% rate of hemorrhage as compared to cardiac medical patients (38%).[11] A Pediatric Cardiac Critical Care Consortium (PC[4]) Registry analysis revealed that 83 of 329 (25%) of cardiac surgical ECMO patients experienced bleeding requiring reoperation, and those with a bleeding event on ECMO had significantly increased mortality rates (34% with hemorrhage versus 20% without hemorrhage).[16]

Oxidative damage from hemolysis can cause an increase in vascular resistance, induce renal tubular toxicity, and contribute to abnormal coagulation.[17] A major source of hemolysis is the pump head, with data to suggest centrifugal pumps create less hemolysis,[18] but this remains controversial.[19,20] Elevated plasma free hemoglobin levels are associated with mortality,[21] predictive of a subsequent thrombotic event,[12] and may trigger blood product transfusion. Increased transfusion of blood products has also been associated with worse outcomes.[22,23] Identifying anticoagulation targets, unifying their measurements, understanding effects of circuit design,[24] and developing evidenced based guidelines is critical to reduce the risk of bleeding and thrombosis.

## *Acute Kidney Injury (AKI)*

Renal failure during ECLS is a frequently associated with mortality. AKI is common in children treated with ECLS[25] and reported as high as 90% in postcardiotomy patients based on pRIFLE scoring,[26] with cardiac surgery as an independent risk factor for development of AKI.[9] The need for renal replacement therapy (RRT) during ECLS is also associated with increased mortality,[9,21,25,27-30] identifying RRT as an independent factor associated with poor survival.[31] Gupta et al. reported on 3502 cardiac surgical ECMO patients from the Pediatric Health Information System database, with 484 (14%) receiving RRT.[9] Significantly increased mortality was noted in patients receiving RRT compared with no RRT (70% vs. 38%).[9] Although the presence of AKI is associated with worse outcome, it is potentially recoverable in the majority of survivors.[32] However, 'recovery of renal function' commonly refers to normalization of serum creatinine or return of native urine output, whereas attention must be paid to true long-term recovery.

## *Neurologic Events*

Acute neurologic events (ANE) are relatively common in the cardiac ICU. Nearly 8% of all children admitted to the cardiac ICU may experience neurologic injury, with the need for ECLS independently associated with the presence of an ANE.[33] Given that central nervous system (CNS) complications on ECLS are associated with the use of ECPR, LVAD, VA ECMO, bicarbonate, and inotropes,[34] such complications are inherently more likely in children with cardiovascular disease. The neurological complications commonly seen during ECLS include clinical or encephalographic (EEG) seizures, hypoxic-ischemic injury, thromboembolic stroke, and intracranial hemorrhage.[11,34-38] The reported incidence of any type of neurologic event on ECLS was 24% in neonates and 20% in children, as compared to 9% in adult cardiac patients.[4] In neonates and children supported for cardiac indications, ELSO Registry data show that over a 5-year period from 2016 to 2020, seizures were reported in 6-8%, cerebral infarction or ischemia in 4-7%, and intracranial hemorrhage in 6-11%.[4] Postcardiotomy pediatric patients supported with ECLS have a high (12%) incidence of stroke.[35] CNS complications reported to the ELSO Registry should be viewed as minimal estimates because the registry data is inherently limited by the voluntary nature of reporting, the methods of evaluation are not systematic, and the context in which data are collected is acute, intensive care based, and short term.

Protecting the brain and mitigating any injury are of paramount importance to any critically unwell child supported on ECLS. Early identification and intervention to minimize neurological morbidity may be masked by sedative medications and muscle relaxants, which can hinder neurological assessment, particularly for seizures. Recent studies utilizing continuous EEG monitoring have shown that nonconvulsive seizures including status epilepticus may be more common on ECLS than previously reported, ranging from 17% to 23%.[38-41] Seizures on ECLS have been shown to correlate with lower IQ scores, cerebral palsy, and increased mortality.[38,40,42]

Additional neuromonitoring modalities on ECLS include near-infrared spectroscopy (NIRS), cranial ultrasound scan (CUS), cerebral function analysis monitor, transcranial doppler, computed tomography (CT), and brain injury biomarkers.[36,40,43-47] Brain magnetic resonance imaging (MRI) is a superior imaging modality but is incompatible with ECMO circuitry. A systematic review of neuromonitoring during ECLS reported a large variability in the timing and definitions of the neurological event and the outcome measure.[48] No single modality can reliably, continuously, and safely predict neurological events; however, a combination of modalities may yield a higher chance of early detection of ANE during and after ECLS.[46,49]

In-hospital mortality is higher in neonates and children who have suffered an ANE as compared to those without.[10,33,50] An ELSO Registry study published in 2015 demonstrated a mortality rate of 73% in neonates who suffered an ANE as compared to 53% in those without neurologic injury, with higher risk in low weight babies, those with worse acidosis and following ECPR.[10] Multiple studies have shown that neurological complications on ECLS in the form of an ANE are closely linked to neurodevelopmental morbidity.[37,51-54] Furthermore, there may be subtle neurological concerns that may not be identified as an ANE, yet have an impact on the neurodevelopmental profile.[52] Hence, all children supported on ECLS, including those supported for cardiac disease, need follow up and targeted outpatient neurologic evaluation.[55-57]

**Early Survival Outcomes**

Survival to hospital discharge in children with cardiovascular disease supported with ECLS varies by age, indication for mechanical support, the type of cardiac defect, and the operative intervention that the child has undergone.[6] An ELSO Registry publication describing 4471 neonates supported on ECLS for cardiac indications from 2001-2011 reported an overall survival rate of 41%.[7] In a recent summary of ECLS outcomes from ELSO in 2020, there were 531 neonates and 1064 children who received cardiac support, with 52% of neonates and 60% of children surviving to hospital discharge.[4] Right-sided obstructive lesions were associated with shorter runs and higher survival (up to 68%),[5] as compared to children supported for failure to wean from cardiopulmonary bypass, who had a survival rate of 45%.[58]

## Risk Factors for Early Morbidity and Mortality

Cardiac ECMO outcomes are influenced by several factors, such as the specific indication for support, patient age, timing of initiation, type of cardiac pathology being supported (eg, single ventricle vs. biventricular circulation), and presence of underlying genetic or congenital abnormalities (Chapter 11). Prenatal brain development and challenges with critical illness in early life further augment the risk for neurodevelopmental difficulties. Embedded in these are a series of composite patient and case-specific risk factors associated with worse outcomes that must be highlighted. These include palliated single ventricle anatomy,[7,59-64] prolonged duration of ECLS,[30, 61, 66-68] associated AKI, [9,30,59,64,69] and postcardiotomy cardiac failure with residual lesions.[70] Additionally, several studies have demonstrated an association between mortality and lower pre- and post-canulation pH;[7,10,61,62,65] failure to clear lactate on support;[61,64,65,71] prematurity or birth weight <3 kg;[7,10,31,60,61,72] and the need for ongoing inotrope support,[68] emphasizing not only the need for high-quality resuscitation but attention to the adequacy of systemic perfusion on ECLS.[73] Notably, a large database study of 2908 children, showed that the duration of time from cardiac surgery to ECLS initiation is not in itself associated with increased mortality, but rather with prolonged ECLS duration and ICU stay.[74]

Early recognition of residual lesions in postoperative patients, particularly neonates, is crucial to improving survival in the postcardiotomy ECLS population.[75] It is critical to investigate and characterize the extent, nature, and, when possible, the hemodynamic burden of residual cardiac lesions. It has been reported that residual lesions are present in approximately 25% of postcardiotomy patients receiving ECLS. The impact of such residual lesions on all postoperative cardiac surgical patients are now well recognized.[76] Early recognition (within 72 hours) and intervention on such lesions can improve survival after postcardiotomy ECLS.[61] The decision to intervene and the optimal timing of this can be difficult and should be based on the specific clinical situation, with a goal to mitigate the ongoing hemodynamic burden as rapidly as possible.

## Specific Populations

There are important considerations that can influence outcome regarding disease specific factors which are discussed below.

### *Single Ventricle*

According to the Society of Thoracic Surgeons (STS) database, the most frequent postcardiotomy ECLS indication is hypoplastic left heart syndrome (HLHS) after stage one palliation (S1P), at 17%. These infants also have a high early mortality rate up to 57%.[5] The indication for support is typically to support progressive low cardiac output or acute hypoxemia, with poorer outcomes linked to cardiac failure, organ dysfunction and ECLS complications.[65,77,78] Survival appears to be influenced mainly by the particular indication and the duration to full flow ECLS deployment.[70] The overall management of these patients is complicated by the challenge of striking the right balance between promoting systemic blood flow and the runoff through either an aortopulmonary shunt or a right-ventricular-to-pulmonary-artery shunt. Any evidence of inadequate systemic oxygen delivery requires early recognition and should prompt consideration of physical restriction of the shunt to limit runoff and thereby increase systemic blood flow.[73]

Outcomes for patients with single ventricle circulation are substantially worse that those with biventricular circulations[7,59,62,64] even after the Glenn and Fontan operations.[79] Much of this risk is related to technical challenges of cannulating multiple venous sites to provide adequate cardiac decompression and ECLS flow, along with the persistence of systemic venous hypertension in the face of seemingly adequate support.[70] Based on ELSO Registry data, 230 patients with Fontan circulation supported on ECLS experienced 35% survival to discharge[80] and 103 patients with Glenn circulation supported on ECLS experienced 41% survival to discharge.[60] A recent, more encouraging study of 40 single ventricle ECLS patients—the majority being HLHS patients after S1P—reported a survival rate of 53%.[81]

## Myocarditis

Consistently higher survival rates ranging from 60% to 83% are noted in children supported with myocarditis,[2,5,82-85] one exception being neonatal enteroviral myocarditis (survival rate 33%).[86] The reversible nature of myocardial dysfunction and short time frame for recovery makes ECLS a very suitable mechanical support strategy for patients with cardiogenic shock from fulminant myocarditis. Longer-term survival outcomes in myocarditis patients successfully weaned from mechanical circulatory support are high. One center reported 95% (46 of 48) of survivors were alive at a mean of 5.5 years post discharge.[87] In children with myocardial dysfunction that does not recover, ECMO has been used as a bridge to transplantation (Chapter 20).

## Multisystem Inflammatory Syndrome in Children (MIS-C)

Coronavirus disease 2019 (COVID-19) can later develop into a life-threatening inflammatory disease with manifestations similar to toxic shock syndrome or Kawasaki disease, now known as multisystem inflammatory syndrome in children (MIS-C).[88,89] Cardiac manifestations are common with MIS-C and include ventricular dysfunction, coronary artery dilation and aneurysms, arrythmias, and conduction abnormalities.[88-90] Severe cases can present as vasodilatory or cardiogenic shock,[89,91] even progressing to ECLS.[92] A systematic review of the literature described 917 children with MIS-C including 58 that received ECLS. Overall mortality rate (those with and without ECMO) was 1.9%.[89] As of October 2021, there were 222 children with MIS-C reported to the ELSO Registry, with 114 surviving to hospital discharge (51% survival rate) (Peter Rycus, personal communication).

## Long-Term Survival

To compound a relatively high early mortality rate faced by children with cardiovascular disease on ECLS, there is evidence of additional late mortality of 4% to 12%.[62,63,93-98] A cohort of 169 children with various types of heart disease supported on ECLS had a 5-year survival rate of 32%, with 6% post discharge mortality.[99] The authors demonstrated a significantly increased rate of late death in children with cardiac disease as compared to meconium aspiration.[99] The Children's Hospital of Philadelphia reviewed 396 cardiac ECMO patients, with only 43% (n=170) surviving to discharge. At 6-year median follow up, 66% of the children were deceased.[100] Longer-term outcomes may be worse in single ventricle patients. For example, of 15 neonates with functional single ventricle surviving postcardiotomy ECPR, late cardiac attrition was noted as 5 infants (33%) died before followup at a median age of 22 months.[71] In a cohort of 64 infants with HLHS supported on ECLS after a Norwood operation, only 16 (25%) survived to their Fontan operation.[30]

**Long-Term Neurodevelopmental Outcomes**

Published studies related to longer-term neurodevelopmental outcomes of children supported on ECLS for cardiac indications are displayed in Table 22-1. A significant amount of pathology is present in survivors, with the incidence of neurodevelopmental deficits ranging from 20% to 73%, depending on the study design, type of test used, inherent case mix, and local practice variations.[62,93,94,99-104] The neurodevelopmental difficulties described in this population vary across different domains including deficits in gross and fine motor skills, cognitive function, language, visual perception, processing speed, sustained attention, verbal, visuospatial, and working memory, academic achievement, executive functioning, behavior, and psychosocial adjustment.[103] The majority of studies are single center, incorporate mixed age and mixed diagnosis cohorts, are followed up at a wide range of time intervals post support, use a range of evaluation methods, and present variable thresholds to determine a favorable neurologic outcome, all of which limits interpretation of the results. Recent studies support a neurobiologic correlate for critical illness in early life in the form of reduced hippocampal volumes and white matter microstructural abnormalities,[105] and impairment of perioperative brain volumes in children with CHD (d-Transposition of Great Arteries and single ventricle physiology) who had exposure to ECMO, worse in those with multiple exposures.[106]

ECPR survivors represent a unique subset who potentially have a higher incidence of neurological complications on ECLS and are at risk of neurodevelopmental sequelae. An ELSO Registry study on ECPR outcomes reported a high incidence (22%) of neurological complications on ECLS.[50] As a secondary analysis of hypothermia after cardiac arrest, Meert et al. reported the 1-year survival and neurobehavioral outcomes using Vineland Adaptive Behavior Scales (VABS, Second Edition) at baseline and at 1-year followup in survivors of ECPR for in-hospital arrest.[54] While comparing baseline VABS score with the 1-year score, they found that one-third (30.5%) had VABS ≥70 points (good neurobehavioral outcome) while it was decreased by ≤15 points in 22.1%.[54] Importantly, many cardiac ECMO outcome studies include a significant proportion of children supported with ECPR, which may impact on the overall neurodevelopmental outcome findings.[69,100,104]

**Post ECMO Quality of Life (QoL)**

The evaluation of QoL has gained increased emphasis in recent years, with the development of new methods for assessment in children and growing interest in the functional outcomes of patients with congenital heart disease.[107-109] The assessment of QoL remains challenging in young children and in those with significant cognitive delays because the child needs to complete the questionnaire themselves. The most commonly used child self-report and parent proxy-reported questionnaire is PedsQL 4.0 (Pediatric Quality of Life Inventory)[110] and the Pediatric Cardiac Quality of Life Inventory (PCQLI).[109] The PedsQL 4.0 was designed to measure the core health dimensions (physical, mental, social and school functioning) in children aged 2 to 18 years[110] and the PCQLI was developed as a disease-specific pediatric cardiac QoL measurement for children aged 8-18 years.[109]

Available studies documenting quality of life in children after being supported for cardiac indications are harder to come by than mixed populations or respiratory cases and are listed in Table 22-2. These studies report 18% to 53%

of cardiac ECMO survivors had significantly diminished QoL scores as compared to age-matched, healthy peers.[100,111-116] It is unclear if the QoL outcomes are associated with ECLS itself or the patients' underlying cardiac disease, their prior hospitalizations, and complications preceding ECLS. In comparison to children with CHD who have had no exposure to ECLS, children supported on ECLS have worse QoL. In prospective, multicenter studies in a heterogeneous CHD cohort at 6 weeks and 6 months after cardiac surgery,[117] and in the single ventricle population at 6 years of age,[118] worse QoL scores were reported. Worse physical scores[117] and adaptive behavior[118] in the ECLS treated children indicate that these are a high-risk group that need screening and intervention with potential for improvement as noted in psychosocial and total scores at 6 months.[117]

**Followup**

It is well known that children growing up with congenital heart disease have a significantly increased risk for neurodevelopmental disabilities in the areas of intelligence, academic achievement, language (development, expressive and receptive), visual construction and perception, attention, executive functioning, fine motor skills, gross motor skills, and psychosocial maladjustment (internalizing and externalizing problems). Similar neurodevelopmental issues may be found in survivors after ECLS. The '2012 American Heart Association (AHA) scientific statement on the evaluation and management of neurodevelopmental outcomes in children with congenital heart disease' lists ECLS as an important high-risk group for neurodevelopmental followup and recommends that all ECLS patients should be referred for formal medical and developmental evaluation and future reevaluation, whether or not any developmental concerns are present.[57] Longitudinal followup that supports assessment

at regular intervals is of paramount importance because neurodevelopmental problems can manifest late, often after the child has started school. Neurodevelopmental status may be evaluated through CNS imaging, EEG, and the assessment of intelligence quotient (IQ), academic achievement, neuropsychological outcome, and motor skills. In addition, evaluation of speech and language, auditory abilities, as well as behavioral and emotional functioning is useful in this high-risk population. A 2021 ELSO publication outlines recommendations for medical and specialist followup for neonatal and pediatric ECLS survivors from hospital discharge until adolescence, individualized depending on clinical status and neurodevelopmental morbidities.[56] A proposed model for long-term followup in children after ECLS is shown in the Appendix (p.773). Although described as an example after ECLS in neonates, this is generalizable to all children supported on ECLS. In addition, the 2012 AHA scientific statement describes a proposed screening and surveillance algorithm with age-specific tests at regular intervals. The recommended assessments are 6 months, 9 months or at 1 year, 18 months, 24 months, 30 months and 4 years, 8 years, middle school (11-14 years of age), and high school (15-18 years of age), with referral to early intervention services and/or special education services. These should be applied to children with cardiac disease who have been supported on ECLS.

**Conclusions**

Given the complex and high-risk nature of ECLS and underlying diverse health care needs of children with cardiac failure, the evaluation of complications and outcomes is a crucial part of patient care. Around half of children undergoing cardiac ECMO will survive to hospital discharge, with a significant proportion of the survivors experiencing longer-term neurodevelopmental problems. A clearer understanding of the precise mechanisms, timing and consequences of the diverse brain injuries in these children is essential to the development of interventions aimed at preventing them or mitigating their effects. Due to the variability of outpatient surveillance between ECLS centers, ELSO has recently published international guidelines for followup after neonatal and pediatric ECLS with recommendations from hospital discharge until adolescence.[56] We recommend that ECLS programs should adapt and apply these recommendations to improve the ultimate outcomes for cardiac ECMO survivors.

| REFERENCE | SURVIVAL TO HOSPITAL DISCHARGE | PROPORTION AVAILABLE AT FOLLOWUP | TIMEFRAME OF FOLLOWUP AFTER ECMO SUPPORT | METHOD OF OUTCOME EVALUATION AS APPROPRIATE FOR AGE | OUTCOME DESCRIPTION |
|---|---|---|---|---|---|
| Ibrahim 2000[93] | 27/67 (40%) | 25/67 (37%) One late death Of 67, 11 VAD patients | Median: 43 months Range: 11- 92 months | Telephone questionnaire to parents, neurologic outcome questionnaire to pediatricians | Parent report: 80% Good or excellent health status. 12% fair and 8% poor Pediatrician report: 59% with mod- severe neurologic impairment |
| Hamrick 2003[94] | 17/53 (32%) | 14/53 (26%) Two late deaths | Assessment at 1, 1.5, 2.5 and 4.5 years | Administered: BSID, SBIS, MSCA, WPPSI | 72% normal motor outcome 50% normal cognitive outcome |
| Chow 2004[95] | 31/90 (34%) | 28/90 (31%) Three late deaths | Mean 4.5 years Range 4 months to 9 years | Telephone questionnaire to parents | 54% normal neurological outcome |
| Wagner 2007[101] | 25/49 (51%) | 22/49 (45%) Three late deaths 13 of 22 were cardiac | Mean 4.6 years Range 0.7 to 11.1 years for cardiac patients only | Administered: Neurologic exam by pediatric neurologist, BSID, WPSSI, NEPSY | Overall 73% and 9 of 13 cardiac patients (69%) moderate to severe cognitive impairment |
| Taylor 2007[119] | 69/211 (33%) | 69/211 (33%) | Median 7.2 years Range 3.9 months to 12.6 years | Administered: POPC Telephone questionnaire to parents for quality of life | Only 105 cardiac patients in cohort with 24 surviving (23% survival), five with mod - severe disability (21%) |
| Lequier 2008[62] | 18/39 (46%) | 16/39 (41%) Two late deaths | 2 years | Administered: BSID, WPPSI Hearing evaluation Questionnaire: ABAS, MAHSC | Behavioral concerns in 88% Mental delay in 50% Motor or sensory disability in 12% |
| Chrysostomou 2013[63] | 69/95 (73%) | 63/95 (66%) Six late deaths | 1.7 years Range: 1 to 4 years | Administered: POPC and PCPC | 66% good outcome 22% mild disability 10% moderate and 2% severe |
| Ryerson 2015[98] | 64/98 (65%) | 50/98 (51%) Fourteen late deaths | Median of 48 months Range: 39 to 52 months | Administered: WPPSI, BB-VMI, FSIQ, VIQ, PIQ Visual and Hearing testing performed Parent Questionnaire: ABAS | Mean IQ in 41 survivors without chromosomal abnormalities was 79.7 25% had IQ > 2SD below mean Hearing loss in 8% |
| GarciaGuerra 2015[121] | 25/51 (49%) | 17/51 (33%) | Median 4.5 years of age Minimum 6 months post ECPR | Administered: WPPSI, BB-VMI Visual and Hearing evaluation | Mean full scale intelligence quotient 76.5 (lower than the population mean) with 24% having intellectual disability |
| Kuraim 2018[122] | 13/20 (65%) | 9/20 (45%) | Assessment 2 years post | Parent Questionnaire: ABAS-II | General adaptive function median score of 65 (score of < 70 is 2 SD below the mean) |
| Sadhwani 2019[104] | 82/184 (45%) | 28/184 (15%) Six late deaths | Median: 19 months Range: 13-28 months | Administered: BSID-III Parent Questionnaire : BSEAB, ITSEA or BASC-2 | ND scores at least 1 SD below mean for gross motor skills (61%), language (43%), and cognitive (29%) |
| Meert 2019[54] | 55 ECPR survivors in THAPCA study | N/A | 12 months | Administered: VABS=II, MSEL, WASI | 71% had VABS-II scores ≥ 70 (mean=100, SD=15) 54% had cognitive testing scores ≥ 70 |
| Bembea 2020[53] | 57/99 (57%) entire cohort | 40/99 (40%) Three late deaths 19 of 40 survivors were "cardiac failure" | Within 12 months | Administered: VABS-II, MSEL or WISC-IV, PSOM-NSE, PCPC | Only 39 cardiac failure patients in cohort with 19 surviving (49%). Of those 19, 37% (n=7) with adaptive behavior function >1 SD below the mean |

**Table 22-1.** Long-term neurological outcome studies in pediatric cardiac ECMO patients. Abbreviations are defined below.

| Neurodevelopment Tests | |
|---|---|
| Bayley Scales of Infant Development II (BSID) | Pediatric Stroke Outcome Measure – Short Neurologic Exam (PSOM-NSE) |
| Beery-Butenica Developmental Test of Visual-Motor Integration- fifth edition (BB-VMI) | Performance intelligence quotient (PIQ) |
| Full-scale intelligence quotient (FSIQ) | Stanford Binet Intelligence Scale (SBIS) |
| McCarthy Scales of Children's Abilities (MSCA) | Verbal intelligence quotient (VIQ) |
| Mullen Scales of Early Learning (MSEL) | Vineland Adaptive Behavior Scales-II (VABS-II) |
| Neuropsychological assessment (NEPSY) | Weshler Abbreviated Scale of Intelligence (WASI) |
| Pediatric Cerebral Performance Category (PCPC) | Weshler intelligence scale for children IV (WISC-IV) |
| Pediatric Overall Performance Category (POPC) | Weschler Preschool and Primary Scale of Intelligence III (WPPSI) |
| Parental Questionnaires | |
| Adaptive Behavior Assessment System (ABAS) | Infant-Toddler Social and Emotional Assessment (ITSEA) |
| Bayley Social-Emotional and Adaptive Behavior Questionnaire (BSEAB) | Multiattribute Health Status Classification System (MAHSC) |
| Behavior Assessment System for Children- second edition (BASC-2) | |

| REFERENCE | POPULATION & PROPORTION AVAILABLE AT FOLLOWUP* | TIMEFRAME OF FOLLOWUP | METHOD OF OUTCOME EVALUATION | OUTCOME DESCRIPTION |
|---|---|---|---|---|
| Mahle 2005 [96] | Children with CHD supported on ECMO 14/32 (44%) | 1-year post support | Health Utilities Index 2 | Quality of life mean score 0.75 (+/- 0.19) compared to full score of 1.0 |
| Taylor 2007[119] | Children receiving ECMO – mixed cohort 69/211 (33%) | Median 7.2 yrs post support (range 3.9 mo to 12.6 yrs) | Health State Utility Index | 71% good 23% moderate 6% poor quality of life |
| Costello 2012[111] | Children with CHD supported on ECMO 41/397 (10%) 94 eligible patients 41 parent proxies | Median age 7 years (range 1.1 to 14 years) | Child Health Questionnaire | Physical summary scores lower than mean: 42.4 (+16.4) |
| Wray2012 [115] | Children with cardiomyopathy bridged to transplant 26/33 (79%) | Median 3.1 years post-transplant (range 1-6.3 yrs) | Pediatric Quality of Life Inventory (PedsQL) 4.0 | Physical and psychosocial scores equivalent to non-bridged transplant (slightly lower than normal). |
| Garcia Guerra 2014[112] | Children who received ECLS for cardiac reasons 47/98 (47%) | Median age 3.2 years post support | Peds QL 4.0 | Mean summary scores 64.9, significantly lower than chronic health conditions and treated with ECMO |
| Elias 2017[100] | Children receiving ECLS, majority (92%) with cardiac disease 98/396 (25%) 65 phone survey 33 written survey | Median age 7.3 years post support | Peds QL 4.0 | Child and parent reported mean scores were significantly lower (63.6 and 68.3) than normative scored (86.2 and 84.9) |
| Fleck 2017[116] | Children receiving MCS, predominantly cardiac disease 19/50 (38%) | Median 4.5 years (range 0.3-11.3 years) post support | KINDL Questionnaires, SF -36 Health Survey | Parent-reported health-related QoL is lower than healthy children |
| Friedland-Little 2017[114] | Children who received ECMO after Norwood operation (n=12) | Median 7 years (range 3-12 yrs) post support | Peds QL 4.0 Peds QL 3.0 cardiac module | Patient reported QoL at or below threshold for significantly impaired |
| Torres-Andres 2018[123] | ECPR majority (79%) with cardiac disease 36/56 (64%) | Median 3 years (IQR 1.5-4.5 yr) post support | Peds QL McMaster Family Assessment | Median Peds QL score was 84 (76-89) and MMFAD was 1.62 (1.33-1.83) which is similar to heathy controls |
| Wray 2021[117] | 27 children who received ECLS after cardiac surgery | At 6 weeks and 6 months post-surgery | Peds QoL 4.0 | At both time points, physical HRQoL was significantly worse in ECLS patients as compared to a morbidity-free control |
| Meenaghan 2021[120] | Children who received ECMO for cardiac reasons (n=39) | Range 5 months to 12 years post support | Peds QoL 4.0 | ECMO patients had significantly lower QoL scores in every domain as compared to healthy cohort, lowest being school functioning |

*Unless stated the patients not assessed were reported deceased.

**Table 22-2.** Quality of Life (QoL) studies in pediatric cardiac ECMO patients.

## References

1. Brown G, Moynihan KM, Deatrick KB, et al. Extracorporeal Life Support Organization (ELSO): Guidelines for Pediatric Cardiac Failure. ASAIO J. 2021;67(5):463-475.

2. Di Nardo M, MacLaren G, Marano M, et al. ECLS in Pediatric Cardiac Patients. Front Pediatr. 2016;4:109.

3. Lorusso R, Raffa GM, Kowalewski M, et al. Structured review of post-cardiotomy extracorporeal membrane oxygenation: Part 2-pediatric patients. J Heart Lung Transplant. 2019;38(11):1144-1161.

4. ELSO. https://www.elso.org/Registry/ELSOLiveRegistryDashboard.aspx. International Registry Report Accessed October 2021.

5. Barbaro RP, Paden ML, Guner YS, et al. Pediatric Extracorporeal Life Support Organization Registry International Report 2016. ASAIO J. 2017;63(4):456-463.

6. Mascio CE, Austin EH, 3rd, Jacobs JP, et al. Perioperative mechanical circulatory support in children: an analysis of the Society of Thoracic Surgeons Congenital Heart Surgery Database. J Thorac Cardiovasc Surg. 2014;147(2):658-664.

7. Ford MA, Gauvreau K, McMullan DM, et al. Factors Associated With Mortality in Neonates Requiring Extracorporeal Membrane Oxygenation for Cardiac Indications: Analysis of the Extracorporeal Life Support Organization Registry Data. Pediatr Crit Care Med. 2016;17(9):860-870.

8. Dalton HJ, Garcia-Filion P, Holubkov R, et al. Association of bleeding and thrombosis with outcome in extracorporeal life support. Pediatr Crit Care Med. 2015;16(2):167-174.

9. Gupta P, Beam B, Schmitz ML. Outcomes associated with the use of renal replacement therapy in children receiving extracorporeal membrane oxygenation after heart surgery: a multi-institutional analysis. Pediatr Nephrol. 2015;30(6):1019-1026.

10. Polito A, Barrett CS, Rycus PT, et al. Neurologic injury in neonates with congenital heart disease during extracorporeal membrane oxygenation: an analysis of extracorporeal life support organization registry data. ASAIO J. 2015;61(1):43-48.

11. Werho DK, Pasquali SK, Yu S, et al. Hemorrhagic complications in pediatric cardiac patients on extracorporeal membrane oxygenation: an analysis of the Extracorporeal Life Support Organization Registry. Pediatr Crit Care Med. 2015;16(3):276-288.

12. Dalton HJ, Reeder R, Garcia-Filion P, et al. Factors Associated with Bleeding and Thrombosis in Children Receiving Extracorporeal Membrane Oxygenation. Am J Respir Crit Care Med. 2017;196(6):762-771.

13. Annich GM. Extracorporeal life support: the precarious balance of hemostasis. J Thromb Haemost. 2015;13 Suppl 1:S336-342.

14. McMichael ABV, Ryerson LM, Ratano D, et al. 2021 ELSO Adult and Pediatric Anticoagulation Guidelines. ASAIO J. 2022; 68:303-310.

15. Murphy DA, Hockings LE, Andrews RK, et al. Extracorporeal membrane oxygenation-hemostatic complications. Transfus Med Rev. 2015;29(2):90-101.

16. Brunetti MA, Gaynor JW, Retzloff LB, et al. Characteristics, Risk Factors, and Outcomes of Extracorporeal Membrane Oxygenation Use in Pediatric Cardiac ICUs: A Report From the Pediatric Cardiac Critical Care Consortium Registry. Pediatr Crit Care Med. 2018;19(6):544-552.

17. Dufour N, Radjou A, Thuong M. Hemolysis and Plasma Free Hemoglobin During Extracorporeal Membrane Oxygenation Support: From Clinical Implications to Laboratory Details. ASAIO J. 2020;66(3):239-246.

18. Johnson KN, Carr B, Mychaliska GB, et al. Switching to centrifugal pumps may decrease hemolysis rates among pediatric ECMO patients. Perfusion. 2022 Mar;37(2):123-127.

19. O'Halloran CP, Thiagarajan RR, Yarlagadda VV, et al. Outcomes of Infants Supported With Extracorporeal Membrane Oxygenation Using Centrifugal Versus Roller Pumps: An Analysis From the Extracorporeal Life Support Organization Registry. Pediatr Crit Care Med. 2019;20(12):1177-1184.

20. Dalton HJ, Hoskote A. There and Back Again: Roller Pumps Versus Centrifugal Technology in Infants on Extracorporeal Membrane Oxygenation. Pediatr Crit Care Med. 2019;20(12):1195-1196.

21. Borasino S, Kalra Y, Elam AR, et al. Impact of Hemolysis on Acute Kidney Injury and Mortality in Children Supported with Cardiac Extracorporeal Membrane Oxygenation. J Extra Corpor Technol. 2018;50(4):217-224.

22. O'Halloran CP, Alexander PMA, Andren KG, et al. RBC Exposure in Pediatric Extracorporeal Membrane Oxygenation: Epidemiology and Factors Associated With Large Blood Transfusion Volume. Pediatr Crit Care Med. 2018;19(8):767-774.

23. Qin CX, Yesantharao LV, Merkel KR, et al. Blood Utilization and Clinical Outcomes in Extracorporeal Membrane Oxygenation Patients. Anesth Analg. 2020;131(3):901-908.

24. Maul TM, Aspenleiter M, Palmer D, et al. Impact of Circuit Size on Coagulation and Hemolysis Complications in Pediatric Extracorporeal Membrane Oxygenation. ASAIO J. 2020;66(9):1048-1053.

25. Fleming GM, Sahay R, Zappitelli M, et al. The Incidence of Acute Kidney Injury and Its Effect on Neonatal and Pediatric Extracorporeal Membrane

Oxygenation Outcomes: A Multicenter Report From the Kidney Intervention During Extracorporeal Membrane Oxygenation Study Group. Pediatr Crit Care Med. 2016;17(12):1157-1169.

26. Elella RA, Habib E, Mokrusova P, et al. Incidence and outcome of acute kidney injury by the pRIFLE criteria for children receiving extracorporeal membrane oxygenation after heart surgery. Ann Saudi Med. 2017;37(3):201-206.

27. Wolf MJ, Chanani NK, Heard ML, et al. Early renal replacement therapy during pediatric cardiac extracorporeal support increases mortality. Ann Thorac Surg. 2013;96(3):917-922.

28. Hansrivijit P, Lertjitbanjong P, Thongprayoon C, et al. Acute Kidney Injury in Pediatric Patients on Extracorporeal Membrane Oxygenation: A Systematic Review and Meta-analysis. Medicines (Basel). 2019;6(4).

29. Alsoufi B, Al-Radi OO, Gruenwald C, et al. Extracorporeal life support following cardiac surgery in children: analysis of risk factors and survival in a single institution. Eur J Cardiothorac Surg. 2009;35(6):1004-1011.

30. Friedland-Little JM, Aiyagari R, Yu S, et al. Survival through staged palliation: fate of infants supported by extracorporeal membrane oxygenation after the Norwood operation. Ann Thorac Surg. 2014;97(2):659-665.

31. Bhat P, Hirsch JC, Gelehrter S, et al. Outcomes of infants weighing three kilograms or less requiring extracorporeal membrane oxygenation after cardiac surgery. Ann Thorac Surg. 2013;95(2):656-661.

32. Gupta P, Carlson J, Wells D, et al. Relationship between renal function and extracorporeal membrane oxygenation use: a single-center experience. Artif Organs. 2015;39(4):369-374.

33. Bell JL, Saenz L, Domnina Y, et al. Acute Neurologic Injury in Children Admitted to the Cardiac Intensive Care Unit. Ann Thorac Surg. 2019;107(6):1831-1837.

34. Cengiz P, Seidel K, Rycus PT, et al. Central nervous system complications during pediatric extracorporeal life support: incidence and risk factors. Crit Care Med. 2005;33(12):2817-2824.

35. Werho DK, Pasquali SK, Yu S, et al. Epidemiology of Stroke in Pediatric Cardiac Surgical Patients Supported with Extracorporeal Membrane Oxygenation. Ann Thorac Surg. 2015;100(5):1751-1757.

36. LaRovere KL, Vonberg FW, Prabhu SP, et al. Patterns of Head Computed Tomography Abnormalities During Pediatric Extracorporeal Membrane Oxygenation and Association With Outcomes. Pediatr Neurol. 2017;73:64-70.

37. Nasr DM, Rabinstein AA. Neurologic Complications of Extracorporeal Membrane Oxygenation. J Clin Neurol. 2015;11(4):383-389.

38. Lin JJ, Banwell BL, Berg RA, et al. Electrographic Seizures in Children and Neonates Undergoing Extracorporeal Membrane Oxygenation. Pediatr Crit Care Med. 2017;18(3):249-257.

39. Piantino JA, Wainwright MS, Grimason M, et al. Nonconvulsive seizures are common in children treated with extracorporeal cardiac life support. Pediatr Crit Care Med. 2013;14(6):601-609.

40. Okochi S, Shakoor A, Barton S, et al. Prevalence of Seizures in Pediatric Extracorporeal Membrane Oxygenation Patients as Measured by Continuous Electroencephalography. Pediatr Crit Care Med. 2018;19(12):1162-1167.

41. Yuliati A, Federman M, Rao LM, et al. Prevalence of Seizures and Risk Factors for Mortality in a Continuous Cohort of Pediatric Extracorporeal Membrane Oxygenation Patients. Ped Crit Care Med. 2020;21(11):949-958.

42. Parish AP, Bunyapen C, Cohen MJ, et al. Seizures as a predictor of long-term neurodevelopmental outcome in survivors of neonatal extracorporeal membrane oxygenation (ECMO). J Child Neurol. 2004;19(12):930-934.

43. Maldonado Y, Singh S, Taylor MA. Cerebral near-infrared spectroscopy in perioperative management of left ventricular assist device and extracorporeal membrane oxygenation patients. Curr Opin Anaesthesiol. 2014;27(1):81-88.

44. Rollins MD, Yoder BA, Moore KR, et al. Utility of neuroradiographic imaging in predicting outcomes after neonatal extracorporeal membrane oxygenation. J Pediatr Surg. 2012;47(1):76-80.

45. Bembea MM. Neuromonitoring of neonatal extracorporeal membrane oxygenation patients using serial cranial ultrasounds. Pediatr Crit Care Med. 2013;14(9):903-904.

46. Lorusso R, Taccone FS, Belliato M, et al. Brain monitoring in adult and pediatric ECMO patients: the importance of early and late assessments. Minerva Anestesiol. 2017;83(10):1061-1074.

47. Svrckova P, Meshaka R, Holtrup M, et al. Imaging of cerebral complications of extracorporeal membrane oxygenation in infants with congenital heart disease - ultrasound with multimodality correlation. Pediatr Radiol. 2020;50(7):997-1009.

48. Bembea MM, Rizkalla N, Freedy J, et al. Plasma Biomarkers of Brain Injury as Diagnostic Tools and Outcome Predictors After Extracorporeal Membrane Oxygenation. Crit Care Med. 2015;43(10):2202-2211.

49. Gannon CM, Kornhauser MS, Gross GW, et al. When combined, early bedside head ultrasound and electroencephalography predict abnormal computerized tomography or magnetic resonance brain images obtained after extracorporeal

membrane oxygenation treatment. J Perinatol. 2001;21(7):451-455.

50. Barrett CS, Bratton SL, Salvin JW, et al. Neurological injury after extracorporeal membrane oxygenation use to aid pediatric cardiopulmonary resuscitation. Pediatr Crit Care Med. 2009;10(4):445-451.

51. Chrysostomou C, Morell VO, Kuch BA, et al. Short- and intermediate-term survival after extracorporeal membrane oxygenation in children with cardiac disease. J Thorac Cardiovasc Surg. 2012.

52. Kakat S, O'Callaghan M, Smith L, et al. The 1-Year Follow-Up Clinic for Neonates and Children After Respiratory Extracorporeal Membrane Oxygenation Support: A 10-Year Single Institution Experience. Pediatr Crit Care Med. 2017;18(11):1047-1054.

53. Bembea MM, Felling RJ, Caprarola SD, et al. Neurologic Outcomes in a Two-Center Cohort of Neonatal and Pediatric Patients Supported on Extracorporeal Membrane Oxygenation. ASAIO J. 2020;66(1):79-88.

54. Meert K, Slomine BS, Silverstein FS, et al; Therapeutic Hypothermia after Paediatric Cardiac Arrest (THAPCA) Trial Investigators: One-year cognitive and neurologic outcomes in survivors of paediatric extracorporeal cardiopulmonary resuscitation. Resuscitation. 2019; 139: 299–307.

55. Ijsselstijn H, Hunfeld M, Schiller RM, et al. Improving Long-Term Outcomes After Extracorporeal Membrane Oxygenation: From Observational Follow-Up Programs Toward Risk Stratification. Front Pediatr. 2018;6:177.

56. Ijsselstijn H, Schiller RM, Holder C, et al. Extracorporeal Life Support Organization (ELSO) Guidelines for Follow-up After Neonatal and Pediatric Extracorporeal Membrane Oxygenation. ASAIO J. 2021;67(9):955-963.

57. Marino BS, Lipkin PH, Newburger JW, et al. Neurodevelopmental Outcomes in Children With Congenital Heart Disease: Evaluation and Management: A Scientific Statement From the American Heart Association. Circulation. 2012;126(9):1143-1172.

58. Sperotto F, Cogo P, Amigoni A, et al. Extracorporeal Membrane Oxygenation Support for Failure to Wean From Cardiopulmonary Bypass After Pediatric Cardiac Surgery: Analysis of Extracorporeal Life Support Organization Registry Data. Crit Care Explor. 2020;2(9):e0183.

59. Kolovos NS, Bratton SL, Moler FW, et al. Outcome of pediatric patients treated with extracorporeal life support after cardiac surgery. Ann Thorac Surg. 2003;76(5):1435-1441.

60. Jolley M, Thiagarajan RR, Barrett CS, et al. Extracorporeal membrane oxygenation in patients undergoing superior cavopulmonary anastomosis. J Thorac Cardiovasc Surg. 2014;148(4):1512-1518.

61. Howard TS, Kalish BT, Wigmore D, et al. Association of Extracorporeal Membrane Oxygenation Support Adequacy and Residual Lesions With Outcomes in Neonates Supported After Cardiac Surgery. Pediatr Crit Care Med. 2016;17(11):1045-1054.

62. Lequier L, Joffe AR, Robertson CM, et al. Two-year survival, mental, and motor outcomes after cardiac extracorporeal life support at less than five years of age. J Thorac Cardiovasc Surg. 2008;136(4):976-983 e973.

63. Chrysostomou C, Maul T, Callahan PM, et al. Neurodevelopmental Outcomes after Pediatric Cardiac ECMO Support. Front Pediatr. 2013;(19)1:47.

64. Kumar TK, Zurakowski D, Dalton H, et al. Extracorporeal membrane oxygenation in postcardiotomy patients: factors influencing outcome. J Thorac Cardiovasc Surg. 2010;140(2):330-336 e332.

65. Allan CK, Thiagarajan RR, del Nido PJ, et al. Indication for initiation of mechanical circulatory support impacts survival of infants with shunted single-ventricle circulation supported with extracorporeal membrane oxygenation. J Thorac Cardiovasc Surg. 2007;133(3):660-667.

66. Merrill ED, Schoeneberg L, Sandesara P, et al. Outcomes after prolonged extracorporeal membrane oxygenation support in children with cardiac disease--Extracorporeal Life Support Organization registry study. J Thorac Cardiovasc Surg. 2014;148(2):582-588.

67. Gupta P, Robertson MJ, Beam B, et al. Relationship of ECMO duration with outcomes after pediatric cardiac surgery: a multi-institutional analysis. Minerva Anestesiol. 2015;81(6):619-627.

68. Sherwin ED, Gauvreau K, Scheurer MA, et al. Extracorporeal membrane oxygenation after stage 1 palliation for hypoplastic left heart syndrome. J Thorac Cardiovasc Surg. 2012;144(6):1337-1343.

69. Cashen K, Reeder R, Dalton HJ, et al. Functional Status of Neonatal and Pediatric Patients After Extracorporeal Membrane Oxygenation. Pediatr Crit Care Med. 2017;18(6):561-570.

70. Brown KL, Ichord R, Marino BS, et al. Outcomes following extracorporeal membrane oxygenation in children with cardiac disease. Pediatr Crit Care Med. 2013 Jun;14(5): S73-83.

71. Polimenakos AC, Rizzo V, El-Zein CF, et al. Post-cardiotomy Rescue Extracorporeal Cardiopulmonary Resuscitation in Neonates with Single Ventricle After Intractable Cardiac Arrest: Attrition After Hospital Discharge and Predictors of Outcome. Pediatr Cardiol. 2017;38(2):314-323.

72. Sasaki T, Asou T, Takeda Y, et al. Extracorporeal life support after cardiac surgery in children:

outcomes from a single institution. Artif Organs. 2014;38(1):34-40.

73. Allen KY, Allan CK, Su L, et al. Extracorporeal membrane oxygenation in congenital heart disease. Semin Perinatol. 2018; 42(2):104-110.

74. Gupta P, Robertson MJ, Rettiganti M, et al. Impact of Timing of ECMO Initiation on Outcomes After Pediatric Heart Surgery: A Multi-Institutional Analysis. Pediatr Cardiol. 2016; 37(5):971-8.

75. Melvan JN, Davis J, Heard M, et al. Factors Associated with Survival Following Extracorporeal Cardiopulmonary Resuscitation in Children. World J Ped Congen Heart Surg. 2020;11(3):265-274.

76. Nathan M, Levine JC, Van Rompay MI, et al. Impact of Major Residual Lesions on Outcomes After Surgery for Congenital Heart Disease. J Am Coll Cardiol. 2021;77(19):2382-2394.

77. Ravishankar C, Gaynor JW. Mechanical support of the functionally single ventricle. Cardiol Young. 2006;16 Suppl 1:55-60.

78. Hoskote A, Bohn D, Gruenwald C, et al. Extracorporeal life support after staged palliation of a functional single ventricle: subsequent morbidity and survival. J Thorac Cardiovasc Surg. 2006;131(5):1114-1121.

79. Booth KL, Roth SJ, Thiagarajan RR, et al. Extracorporeal membrane oxygenation support of the Fontan and bidirectional Glenn circulations. Ann Thorac Surg. 2004;77(4):1341-1348.

80. Rood KL, Teele SA, Barrett CS, et al. Extracorporeal membrane oxygenation support after the Fontan operation. J Thorac Cardiovasc Surg. 2011;142(3):504-510.

81. Stephens EH, Shakoor A, Jacobs SE, et al. Characterization of Extracorporeal Membrane Oxygenation Support for Single Ventricle Patients. World J Pediatr Congenit Heart Surg. 2020;11(2):183-191.

82. Rajagopal SK, Almond CS, Laussen PC, et al. Extracorporeal membrane oxygenation for the support of infants, children, and young adults with acute myocarditis: a review of the Extracorporeal Life Support Organization registry. Crit Care Med. 2010;38(2):382-387.

83. Duncan BW, Bohn DJ, Atz AM, et al. Mechanical circulatory support for the treatment of children with acute fulminant myocarditis. J Thorac Cardiovasc Surg. 2001;122(3):440-448.

84. Nosaka N, Muguruma T, Fujiwara T, et al. Effects of the elective introduction of extracorporeal membrane oxygenation on outcomes in pediatric myocarditis cases. Acute Med Surg. 2015;2(2):92-97.

85. Xiong H, Xia B, Zhu J, et al. Clinical Outcomes in Pediatric Patients Hospitalized with Fulminant Myocarditis Requiring Extracorporeal Membrane Oxygenation: A Meta-analysis. Pediatr Cardiol. 2017;38(2):209-214.

86. Madden K, Thiagarajan RR, Rycus PT, et al. Survival of neonates with enteroviral myocarditis requiring extracorporeal membrane oxygenation. Pediatr Crit Care Med. 2011; 12:314-318.

87. Hsu KH, Chi NH, Yu HY, et al. Extracorporeal membranous oxygenation support for acute fulminant myocarditis: analysis of a single center's experience. Eur J Cardiothorac Surg. 2011;40(3):682-688.

88. Alsaied T, Tremoulet AH, Burns JC, et al. Review of Cardiac Involvement in Multisystem Inflammatory Syndrome in Children. Circulation. 2021;143(1):78-88.

89. Yasuhara J, Kuno T, Takagi H, et al. Clinical characteristics of COVID-19 in children: A systematic review. Pediatr Pulmonol. 2020;55(10):2565-2575.

90. Domico M, McCanta AC, Hunt JL, et al. High-grade heart block requiring transvenous pacing associated with multisystem inflammatory syndrome in children during the COVID-19 pandemic. HeartRhythm Case Rep. 2020;6(11):811-814.

91. Simpson JM, Newburger JW. Multisystem Inflammatory Syndrome in Children in Association With COVID-19. Circulation. 2020;142(5):437-440.

92. Radia T, Williams N, Agrawal P, et al. Multi-system inflammatory syndrome in children & adolescents (MIS-C): A systematic review of clinical features and presentation. Paediatr Respir Rev. 2021;38:51-57

93. Ibrahim AE, Duncan BW, Blume ED, et al. Long-term follow-up of pediatric cardiac patients requiring mechanical circulatory support. Ann Thorac Surg. 2000;69(1):186-192.

94. Hamrick SE, Gremmels DB, Keet CA, et al. Neurodevelopmental outcome of infants supported with extracorporeal membrane oxygenation after cardiac surgery. Pediatrics. 2003;111(6 Pt 1):e671-675.

95. Chow G, Koirala B, Armstrong D, et al. Predictors of mortality and neurological morbidity in children undergoing extracorporeal life support for cardiac disease. Eur J Cardiothorac Surg. 2004;26(1):38-43.

96. Mahle WT, Forbess JM, Kirshbom PM, et al. Cost-utility analysis of salvage cardiac extracorporeal membrane oxygenation in children. J Thorac Cardiovasc Surg. 2005;129(5):1084-1090.

97. Chaturvedi RR, Macrae D, Brown KL, et al. Cardiac ECMO for biventricular hearts after paediatric open heart surgery. Heart. 2004;90(5):545-551.

98. Ryerson LM, Guerra GG, Joffe AR, et al. Survival and neurocognitive outcomes after cardiac extracorporeal life support in children less than 5 years of age: a ten-year cohort. Circulation Heart failure. 2015;8(2):312-321.

99. Iguchi A, Ridout DA, Galan S, et al. Long-term survival outcomes and causes of late death in neonates,

infants, and children treated with extracorporeal life support. Pediatr Crit Care Med. 2013;14(6):580-586.

100. Elias MD, Achuff BJ, Ittenbach RF, et al. Long-Term Outcomes of Pediatric Cardiac Patients Supported by Extracorporeal Membrane Oxygenation. Pediatr Crit Care Med. 2017;18(8):787-794.

101. Wagner K, Risnes I, Berntsen T, et al. Clinical and psychosocial follow-up study of children treated with extracorporeal membrane oxygenation. Ann Thorac Surg. 2007;84(4):1349-1355.

102. Brown KL, Miles F, Sullivan ID, et al. Outcome in neonates with congenital heart disease referred for respiratory extracorporeal membrane oxygenation. Acta Paediatr. 2005;94(9):1280-1284

103. Marino BS, Cassedy A, Drotar D, et al. The Impact of Neurodevelopmental and Psychosocial Outcomes on Health-Related Quality of Life in Survivors of Congenital Heart Disease. J Pediatr. 2016;174:11-22 e12.

104. Sadhwani A, Cheng H, Stopp C, et al. Early Neurodevelopmental Outcomes in Children Supported with ECMO for Cardiac Indications. Pediatr Cardiol. 2019;40(5):1072-1083.

105. Schiller RM, Ijsselstijn H, Madderom MJ, et al. Neurobiologic Correlates of Attention and Memory Deficits Following Critical Illness in Early Life. Crit Care Med. 2017;45(10):1742-1750.

106. Chao B, Claessens N, Lim JM, et al. Decreased Brain Volumes and Infants With Congenital Heart Disease Undergoing Venoarterial Extracorporeal Membrane Oxygenation. Pediatr Crit Care Med. 2020; 21:738-745.

107. Robson VK, Stopp C, Wypij D, et al. Longitudinal Associations between Neurodevelopment and Psychosocial Health Status in Patients with Repaired D-Transposition of the Great Arteries. J Pediatr. 2019;204:38-45 e31.

108. Ernst MM, Marino BS, Cassedy A, et al. Biopsychosocial Predictors of Quality of Life Outcomes in Pediatric Congenital Heart Disease. Pediatr Cardiol. 2018;39(1):79-88.

109. Marino BS, Shera D, Wernovsky G, et al. The development of the pediatric cardiac quality of life inventory: a quality of life measure for children and adolescents with heart disease. Qual Life Res. 2008;17(4):613-626.

110. Varni JW, Seid M, Kurtin PS. PedsQL 4.0: reliability and validity of the Pediatric Quality of Life Inventory version 4.0 generic core scales in healthy patient populations. Med Care. 2001;39(8):800-812.

111. Costello JM, O'Brien M, Wypij D, et al. Quality of life of pediatric cardiac patients who previously required extracorporeal membrane oxygenation. Pediatr Crit Care Med. 2012;13(4):428-434.

112. Garcia Guerra G, Robertson CM, Alton GY, et al. Health-related quality of life in pediatric cardiac extracorporeal life support survivors. Pediatr Crit Care Med. 2014;15(8):720-727.

113. Boyle K, Felling R, Yiu A, et al. Neurologic Outcomes After Extracorporeal Membrane Oxygenation: A Systematic Review. Pediatr Crit Care Med. 2018;19(8):760-766.

114. Friedland-Little JM, Uzark K, Yu S, et al. Functional Status and Quality of Life in Survivors of Extracorporeal Membrane Oxygenation After the Norwood Operation. Ann Thorac Surg. 2017;103(6):1950-1955.

115. Wray J, Lunnon-Wood T, Smith L, et al. Perceived quality of life of children after successful bridging to heart transplantation. J Heart Lung Transplant. 2012;31(4):381-386.

116. Fleck TP, Dangel G, Bachle F, et al. Long-Term Follow-Up on Health-Related Quality of Life After Mechanical Circulatory Support in Children. Pediatr Crit Care Med. 2017;18(2):176-182.

117. Wray J, Ridout D, Jones A, et al. Morbidities after cardiac surgery: Impact on Children's Quality of Life and Parents' mental health. Ann Thorac Surg. 2021;112:2055-62.

118. Goldberg CS, Hu C, Brosig C, et al. Behavior and Quality of Life at 6 Years for Children With Hypoplastic Left Heart Syndrome. Pediatrics. 2019;144(5).

119. Taylor AK, Cousins R, Butt WW. The long-term outcome of children managed with extracorporeal life support: an institutional experience. Crit Care Resusc. 2007; 9(2):172-177.

120. Meenaghan SM, Nugent GM, Dee EC, et al. Health Related Quality of Life in pediatric cardiac patients after extracorporeal life support. Ped Cardiol. 2021; 42:1433-1441.

121. Garcia Guerra G, Zorzela L, Robertson CM, et al. Survival and Neurocognitive outcomes in pediatric extracorporeal-cardiopulmonary resuscitation. Resus. 2015; 96:208-13.

122. Kuraim GA, Garros D, Ryerson L, et al. Predictors and outcomes of early post-operative veno-arterial extracorporeal membrane oxygenation following infant cardiac surgery. J Intensive Care. 2018; 6(56).

123. Torres-Andres F, Fink EL, Bell MJ, et al. Survival and Long Term Function Outcome for Children with Cardiac Arrest Treated with Extracorporeal Cardiopulmonary Resuscitation. Pediatr Crit Care Med. 2018; 19:451-458.

# 23

## Initiating Extracorporeal Life Support for Adult Respiratory Failure

*Purnema Madahar, Giacomo Grasselli, Daniel Brodie, Eddy Fan*

## Introduction

The role of ECLS as a supportive therapy for respiratory failure has expanded since its first successful use in 1971 in an adult patient with acute respiratory distress syndrome (ARDS),[1] both due to advances in ECLS technology and the findings of several clinical studies.[2,3] Recent trials on ECLS for severe ARDS suggest a potential trend towards improved mortality in a highly-selected patient population.[4-7] However, for most other types of respiratory failure, ECLS has little evidence base with a lack of randomized control trials demonstrating a mortality benefit compared to conventional treatments. ECLS is also resource-intensive and has a high rate of complications related to the device. Initiating ECLS for respiratory failure should be considered on a case-by-case basis as part of a specialized, multidisciplinary assessment for patients who have a) failed conventional therapies despite optimization and remain at high risk for death, b) a potentially reversible cause of respiratory failure without comorbidities that limit short-term life expectancy, and c) no contraindications to ECLS. This chapter will focus on elucidating these principles based on current literature, guidelines and expert opinion.

## Rationale for ECLS in Respiratory Failure

Respiratory failure may lead to severe gas exchange abnormalities, often necessitating support with invasive mechanical ventilation, with known sequelae of developing ventilator-induced lung injury (VILI), particularly in the setting of poor lung mechanics and low compliance. In this setting, ECLS can potentially a) manage derangements in gas exchange using the artificial membrane lung (which itself mimics the role of the pulmonary-alveolar capillary membrane), thereby serving to bridge a patient with refractory hypoxemia and/or severe respiratory acidemia and, b) particularly in the case of ARDS, reduce the risk of VILI by allowing the use of lower ventilator pressures, volumes and respiratory rates than would be possible without ECLS.

## Modes of Support for Respiratory Failure

VV ECMO is the most common mode for supporting respiratory failure. If concomitant vasodilatory shock or hypoxemia-induced right ventricular (RV) dysfunction is present, VV ECMO may still be the appropriate initial strategy since RV dysfunction and shock may improve once gas exchange is corrected. However, if other shock states, including RV failure due to chronic pulmonary hypertension are present, VA or VVA ECMO should be considered and are discussed separately in Chapter 27.[3,8,9]

## Clinical Conditions Considered for ECLS in Respiratory Failure

Establishing whether the underlying disease process is potentially reversible is the guiding principle when considering which clinical entities are suitable for ECLS as a bridge to recovery. Acute hypoxemic respiratory failure and ARDS are the most common etiologies for initiating ECLS for acute respiratory failure,

and is often triggered by bacterial, viral or aspiration pneumonias.[10] Other diagnoses that are considered reversible and that may be supported with ECLS as a bridge to recovery include acute eosinophilic pneumonia, status asthmaticus, pulmonary hemorrhage syndromes, traumatic lung injury, inhalational injury, large bronchopleural fistula, and primary graft dysfunction after lung transplantation.[3,11] If the underlying lung disease is chronic or irreversible, ECLS can still be considered, but only if eligible as a bridge to lung transplantation.

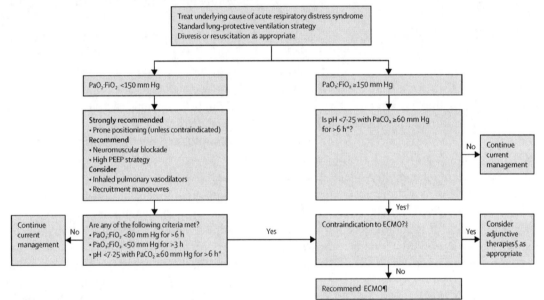

**Figure 23-1.** Algorithm for management of acute respiratory distress syndrome, including indications for ECMO. Reproduced with permission: Abrams et al.[20]
*With respiratory rate increased to 35 breaths per minute and mechanical ventilation settings adjusted to keep a plateau airway pressure of <32 cmH2O.
†Consider neuromuscular blockade.
‡There are no absolute contraindications that are agreed upon except end-stage respiratory failure when lung transplantation will not be considered; exclusion used in the EOLIA trial can be taken as a conservative approach to ECMO contraindications.
§For example, neuromuscular blockade, high PEEP strategy, inhaled pulmonary vasodilators, recruitment maneuvers, and high-frequency oscillatory ventilation.
¶Recommend early ECMO as per EOLIA trial criteria; salvage ECMO, which involves deferral of ECMO initiation until further decompensation (as in the crossovers to ECMO in the EOLIA control group), is not supported by the evidence but might be preferable to not initiating ECMO at all in such patients.
ECMO, extracorporeal membrane oxygenation; EOLIA, Extracorporeal Membrane Oxygenation to Rescue Lung Injury in Severe Acute Respiratory Distress Syndrome; PaCO2, partial pressure of carbon dioxide in arterial blood; PaO2:FiO2, ratio of partial pressure of oxygen in arterial blood to the fractional concentration of oxygen in inspired air; PEEP, positive end-expiratory pressure.

## Initiating ECMO for Refractory Hypoxemia

### ECMO for ARDS

Early referral for ECMO is crucial in order to allow for appropriate patient assessment, medical optimization, and commencement of ECMO in appropriate candidates. The optimal timing of initiation of ECMO remains unclear, but it is generally accepted up to the first 7 days of invasive mechanical ventilation, as prolonged duration of mechanical ventilation prior to ECMO is associated with increased mortality before and after ECMO.[11–14] Strategies to optimize gas exchange and lung mechanics should be trialed first, according to the evidence-based algorithm for managing patients with ARDS.[2,15–21] Early and appropriate use of these interventions can often improve gas exchange sufficiently to obviate the need for ECMO; particularly, a trial of prone positioning, which should be strongly considered prior to evaluation for ECMO (Figure 23-1).[20]

If gas exchange remains inadequate or substantial ongoing injurious lung ventilation persists despite maximal medical optimization, ECMO should be considered in appropriate candidates. Recent studies suggest early initiation of VV ECMO for severe ARDS may have a potential mortality benefit.[5–7] Commonly accepted criteria for initiating ECMO for severe ARDS are based on the inclusion criteria from the ECMO to Rescue Lung Injury in Severe ARDS (EOLIA) study, an international, multicenter randomized controlled trial, and are comprised of the following.[5]

- $PaO_2:F_iO_2$ ratio <50 mmHg for >3 hours despite optimization of mechanical ventilation ($F_iO_2 \geq 80\%$, tidal volume = 6 cc/kg and trial of PEEP $\geq 10$ cmH$_2$O); or,
- $PaO_2:F_iO_2$ ratio <80 mmHg for >6 hours despite optimization of mechanical ventilation as listed above; or,

- Arterial blood pH <7.25 with $PaCO_2$ $\geq 60$ mmHg for >6 hours despite an optimized respiratory rate of at least 35 breaths per minute and optimization of ventilation settings to maintain a plateau pressure $\leq 32$ cmH$_2$O.

Earlier studies prior to EOLIA, such as the Conventional ventilation or ECMO for Severe Adult Respiratory failure (CESAR) randomized controlled trial, which compared conventional mechanical ventilation strategies to care at a specialized center for consideration of ECMO, and the current extracorporeal life support organization (ELSO) guidelines, have overall similar criteria and are equally acceptable (Table 23-1).[4,11] Initiation of ECMO outside of these criteria may be considered when a patient is unstable and cannot safely progress through the ARDS algorithm because conventional strategies (eg, prone positioning) cannot safely be performed or are unavailable at the treating center, and ECMO is required for safe transport to an experienced center, known as "rescue" ECMO.[20] Similarly, if a patient has progressed beyond the standard criteria and the decision to initiate ECMO is delayed, ECMO might still be considered as a "salvage" therapy.[5,20]

### ECMO for ARDS due to Coronavirus Disease 2019

The use of ECMO for severe ARDS due to coronavirus disease 2019 (COVID-19) continues to expand as the pandemic evolves, despite its resource-intensive setup. Given the multiple shortages, capacity limitations and finite resources available during a pandemic, patient selection for ECMO should be judicious and focus on patients who carry the best possible prognosis.[22,23] Minimum criteria to initiate ECMO for ARDS due to COVID-19 remains the same as the currently accepted recommendations listed above.[3,5,24] More stringent contraindications are now being considered for initiating ECMO, based on a growing body of evidence revealing worsening outcomes in patients supported with ECMO for COVID-19-related ARDS as the pandemic progresses based on analyses comparing outcomes from the first and later waves.[25,26] The most recent report from the international ELSO Registry noted a 90-day in-hospital mortality rate of 51.9% (95% CI 50-53.8) in those supported with ECMO after May $1^{st}$, 2020, compared to 36.9% (95% CI 34.1-39.7) prior to May $1^{st}$, 2020, at centers which provided ECMO support throughout the pandemic. Centers that adopted ECMO later in the pandemic (after May $1^{st}$, 2020) had 90-day in-hospital mortality rates of 58.9% (95% CI 55.4-62.3). Advanced age, multiple pre-ECMO comorbidities - particularly malignancy, cardiac arrest prior to ECMO and acute kidney injury - were associated with increased risk of mortality.[25] The 2021 ELSO guidelines for ECMO for COVID-19 recommend identifying patients who meet standard ECMO criteria and are not at high risk for mortality despite ECMO support (ie, chronic organ failure, acute multi-organ failure, severe neurologic injury with poor prognosis for recovery, etc.) while balancing capacity and resources available at the treating center.[24]

| EXPERT SOCIETY OR CLINICAL TRIAL GROUP | CESAR[4] | EOLIA[5] | ELSO[11] |
|---|---|---|---|
| Inclusion Criteria/ Considerations for ECMO | ▪ Age 18-65 years<br>▪ Potentially reversible severe respiratory failure<br>▪ Murray score ≥ 3*, or<br>▪ pH < 7.20 after ventilator optimization | ▪ Age ≥ 18 years<br>▪ $PaO_2$:$FiO_2$ < 50 mmHg > 3 hours,¶ or<br>▪ $PaO_2$:$FiO_2$ < 80 mmHg > 6 hours,¶ or<br>▪ pH <7.25 with $PaCO_2$ ≥ 60† | ▪ $PaO_2$:$FiO_2$ < 80 mmHg,¶ or<br>▪ pH <7.25,† or<br>▪ Ventilatory support as bridge to lung transplantation |
| Exclusion Criteria/ Contraindications for ECMO | ▪ Mechanical ventilation > 7 days with peak inspiratory pressures > 30 $cmH_2O$ and $FiO_2$ > 80%<br>▪ CNS hemorrhage<br>▪ Contraindications to anticoagulation<br>▪ Planned limitation of life sustaining treatment | ▪ Mechanical ventilation ≥ 7 days<br>▪ Pregnancy<br>▪ BMI > 45 kg/m²<br>▪ Chronic lung disease requiring oxygen or noninvasive ventilation<br>▪ HIT Malignancy with fatal prognosis in < 5 years<br>▪ Need for VA-ECMO<br>▪ SAPS II >90<br>▪ Non-drug-induced coma following cardiac arrest<br>▪ Irreversible neurologic injury<br>▪ ECMO cannulation not possible due to vascular access or device availability<br>▪ Planned limitation of life sustaining treatment | *Absolute:*<br>▪ Irreversible underlying condition and anticipated nonrecovery<br><br>*Relative:*<br>▪ CNS hemorrhage<br>▪ Significant CNS injury<br>▪ Irreversible and incapacitating CNS pathology<br>▪ Systemic bleeding<br>▪ Contraindications to anticoagulation<br>▪ Immunosuppression<br>▪ Older age<br>▪ Mechanical ventilation > 7 days with plateau pressures > 30 cm H2O and FiO2 > 90% |

*Murray score is a composite score including imaging characteristics, $PaO_2$:$FiO_2$ ratio, PEEP and compliance. Higher scores are associated with more severe respiratory failure.[12]
¶ Despite optimization of mechanical ventilation: $F_1O_2$ ≥80%, tidal volume = 6 cc/kg and trial of PEEP ≥10 cm $H_2O$, including a trial of proning if feasible
† Despite a respiratory rate of at least 35 breaths per minute and optimization of ventilation settings to maintain a plateau pressure ≤ 32 cm $H_2O$ for EOLIA and ≤30 $cmH_2O$ for ELSO.
ARDS=acute respiratory distress syndrome; BMI=body mass index; CNS=central nervous system; CESAR=conventional ventilatory support versus extracorporeal membrane oxygenation for severe adult respiratory failure; EOLIA=extracorporeal membrane oxygenation to rescue lung injury in severe acute respiratory distress syndrome; HIT=heparin induced thrombocytopenia; $PaCO_2$=partial pressure of carbon dioxide in arterial blood; $PaO_2$:$FiO_2$,=ratio of partial pressure of oxygen in arterial blood to the fractional concentration of oxygen in inspired air; PEEP=positive end-expiratory pressure; SAPS II=simplified acute physiology score; VA=venoarterial; VV=venovenous.

**Table 23-1.** Criteria for initiating VV ECMO for patients with severe ARDS according to expert society and clinical trial groups.

## ECMO for Other Types of Hypoxemic Respiratory Failure

Limited data exist to support the use of ECMO for other forms of respiratory failure and patient selection should be considered on a case-by-case basis for the clinical entities discussed in this section.

Primary graft dysfunction (PGD) is a type of acute lung injury that occurs within 72 hours of lung transplantation and its severity is graded similarly to ARDS, based on extent of alveolar infiltrates and $PaO_2:FiO_2$ ratio, with the most severe form (grade 3) defined as a $PaO_2:FiO_2$ ratio less than 200.[27] ECMO has been utilized at several transplant centers for management of grade 3 PGD and small, mostly retrospective, single-center studies have shown comparable rates of 30-day survival, bronchiolitis obliterans syndrome-free survival, and acute rejection episodes, to post-transplant patients who did not require ECMO.[28–30]

Select cases of hemoptysis and bleeding due to pulmonary hemorrhage syndromes, including diffuse alveolar hemorrhage (DAH) and associated-vasculitides, have been supported with ECMO.[31–34] Often these cases will require holding or lower levels of anticoagulation while accepting the potentially increased risk of device-related complications. A recent systemic review looking at ECMO for DAH, primarily caused by autoimmune syndromes, demonstrated a 30-day mortality rate of 10.5%.[33] Patient selection is crucial and the ability to bridge to recovery via alternate treatments is necessary in order to have a potentially successful outcome, which may include management with embolization, immunosuppression, or surgery, depending on the underlying etiology for bleeding.

Other potential roles for ECMO include airway obstruction or large bronchopleural fistula pending definitive treatment, unilateral pneumonia, acute eosinophilic pneumonia or lung injury due to trauma or inhalational exposure, leading to severe hypoxemia despite conventional therapies.[11,34–38]

## Contraindications to ECLS for Respiratory Failure

The only absolute contraindication to initiate ECLS for respiratory failure is the presence of an irreversible underlying condition and anticipated non-recovery in patients ineligible for lung transplantation.[3,11] Potential relative contraindications relate to risk factors associated with overall poor prognosis despite initiation of ECLS, and to a lesser extent, pre-ECLS comorbidities that would hinder device-related access or management. Irreversible neurologic injury, moribund status, untreatable metastatic cancer, uncontrollable systemic bleeding (particularly in the central nervous system), contraindications to anticoagulation, prolonged mechanical ventilation with high airway pressures and $F_iO_2$, and advanced age should be assessed as part of patient selection criteria and discussed with a multi-disciplinary team specializing in ECLS. Similar contraindications were exclusion criteria in the major randomized-controlled trials for ECLS (Table 23-1).[4,5,39,40]

## Summary

ECLS can effectively support a variety of conditions that lead to respiratory failure. Recent evidence favors early initiation of VV ECMO in severe ARDS when conventional therapies are failing. Criteria for initiating ECMO for COVID-19 related ARDS remains the same, if not more stringent, than currently accepted recommendations. The role of ECLS for other types of respiratory failure should be considered on a case-by-case basis at experienced ECLS centers. Appropriate candidate selection and assessment of the risk to benefit ratio due to device-related complications is crucial in achieving improved patient outcomes when considering this resource-intensive intervention.

# References

1. Hill JD, O'Brien TG, Murray JJ, et al. Prolonged Extracorporeal Oxygenation for Acute Post-Traumatic Respiratory Failure (Shock-Lung Syndrome) — Use of the Bramson Membrane Lung. New Engl J Medicine. 1972;286(12):629-634.
2. Fan E, Brodie D, Slutsky AS. Acute Respiratory Distress Syndrome: Advances in Diagnosis and Treatment. Jama. 2018;319(7):698-710.
3. Brodie D, Slutsky AS, Combes A. Extracorporeal Life Support for Adults With Respiratory Failure and Related Indications. Jama. 2019;322(6):557-568.
4. Peek GJ, Mugford M, Tiruvoipati R, et al. Efficacy and economic assessment of conventional ventilatory support versus extracorporeal membrane oxygenation for severe adult respiratory failure (CESAR): a multicentre randomised controlled trial. Lancet. 2009;374(9698):1351-1363.
5. Combes A, Hajage D, Capellier G, et al. Extracorporeal Membrane Oxygenation for Severe Acute Respiratory Distress Syndrome. New Engl J Med. 2018;378(21):1965-1975.
6. Goligher EC, Tomlinson G, Hajage D, et al. Extracorporeal Membrane Oxygenation for Severe Acute Respiratory Distress Syndrome and Posterior Probability of Mortality Benefit in a Post Hoc Bayesian Analysis of a Randomized Clinical Trial. Jama. 2018;320(21):2251.
7. Munshi L, Walkey A, Goligher E, Pham T, Uleryk EM, Fan E. Venovenous extracorporeal membrane oxygenation for acute respiratory distress syndrome: a systematic review and meta-analysis. Lancet Respir Medicine. 2019;7(2):163-172.
8. Bréchot N, Hajage D, Kimmoun A, et al. Venoarterial extracorporeal membrane oxygenation to rescue sepsis-induced cardiogenic shock: a retrospective, multicentre, international cohort study. Lancet. 2020;396(10250):545-552.
9. Ling RR, Ramanathan K, Poon WH, et al. Venoarterial extracorporeal membrane oxygenation as mechanical circulatory support in adult septic shock: a systematic review and meta-analysis with individual participant data meta-regression analysis. Crit Care. 2021;25(1):246.
10. Group O behalf of the LSI and the ET, Bellani G, Laffey JG, Pham T, Fan E. The LUNG SAFE study: a presentation of the prevalence of ARDS according to the Berlin Definition! Crit Care. 2016;20(1):268.
11. Tonna JE, Abrams D, Brodie D, et al. Management of Adult Patients Supported with Venovenous Extracorporeal Membrane Oxygenation (VV ECMO): Guideline from the Extracorporeal Life Support Organization (ELSO). Asaio J. 2021;67(6):601-610.
12. Murray JF, Matthay MA, Luce JM, Flick MR. An Expanded Definition of the Adult Respiratory Distress Syndrome. Am Rev Respir Dis. 1988;138(3):720-723.
13. Schmidt M, Zogheib E, Rozé H, et al. The PRESERVE mortality risk score and analysis of long-term outcomes after extracorporeal membrane oxygenation for severe acute respiratory distress syndrome. Intens Care Med. 2013;39(10):1704-1713.
14. Schmidt M, Bailey M, Sheldrake J, et al. Predicting Survival after Extracorporeal Membrane Oxygenation for Severe Acute Respiratory Failure. The Respiratory Extracorporeal Membrane Oxygenation Survival Prediction (RESP) Score. Am J Resp Crit Care. 2014;189(11):1374-1382.
15. Ventilation with Lower Tidal Volumes as Compared with Traditional Tidal Volumes for Acute Lung Injury and the Acute Respiratory Distress Syndrome. New Engl J Medicine. 2000;342(18):1301-1308.
16. Papazian L, Forel JM, Gacouin A, et al. Neuromuscular Blockers in Early Acute Respiratory Distress Syndrome. New Engl J Medicine. 2010;363(12):1107-1116.
17. Guérin C, Reignier J, Richard JC, et al. Prone Positioning in Severe Acute Respiratory Distress Syndrome. New Engl J Medicine. 2013;368(23):2159-2168.
18. Fan E, Sorbo LD, Goligher EC, et al. An Official American Thoracic Society/European Society of Intensive Care Medicine/Society of Critical Care Medicine Clinical Practice Guideline: Mechanical Ventilation in Adult Patients with Acute Respiratory Distress Syndrome. Am J Resp Crit Care. 2017;195(9):1253-1263.
19. Network NH Lung, and Blood Institute PETAL Clinical Trials, Moss M, Huang DT, et al. Early Neuromuscular Blockade in the Acute Respiratory Distress Syndrome. New Engl J Med. 2019;380(21):1997-2008.
20. Abrams D, Ferguson ND, Brochard L, et al. ECMO for ARDS: from salvage to standard of care? Lancet Respir Medicine. 2019;7(2):108-110.
21. Duggal A, Rezoagli E, Pham T, et al. Patterns of Use of Adjunctive Therapies in Patients With Early Moderate to Severe ARDS Insights From the LUNG SAFE Study. Chest. 2020;157(6):1497-1505.
22. Abrams D, Lorusso R, Vincent JL, Brodie D. ECMO during the COVID-19 pandemic: when is it unjustified? Crit Care. 2020;24(1):507.
23. Supady A, Curtis JR, Abrams D, et al. Allocating scarce intensive care resources during the COVID-19 pandemic: practical challenges to theoretical frameworks. Lancet Respir Med. 2021 Apr;9(4):430-434.
24. Badulak J, Antonini MV, Stead CM, et al. Extracorporeal Membrane Oxygenation for COVID-19: Updated 2021 Guidelines from the

Extracorporeal Life Support Organization. ASAIO J. 2021;67(5):485-495.

25. Barbaro RP, MacLaren G, Boonstra PS, et al. Extracorporeal membrane oxygenation for COVID-19: evolving outcomes from the international Extracorporeal Life Support Organization Registry. Lancet. 2021;398(10307):1230-1238.

26. Broman LM, Eksborg S, Coco VL, et al. Extracorporeal membrane oxygenation for COVID-19 during first and second waves. Lancet Respir Medicine. 2021;9(8):e80-e81.

27. Snell GI, Yusen RD, Weill D, et al. Report of the ISHLT Working Group on Primary Lung Graft Dysfunction, part I: Definition and grading—A 2016 Consensus Group statement of the International Society for Heart and Lung Transplantation. J Hear Lung Transplant. 2017;36(10):1097-1103.

28. Wigfield CH, Lindsey JD, Steffens TG, Edwards NM, Love RB. Early Institution of Extracorporeal Membrane Oxygenation for Primary Graft Dysfunction After Lung Transplantation Improves Outcome. J Hear Lung Transplant. 2007;26(4):331-338.

29. Hartwig MG, Walczak R, Lin SS, Davis RD. Improved Survival but Marginal Allograft Function in Patients Treated With Extracorporeal Membrane Oxygenation After Lung Transplantation. Ann Thorac Surg. 2012;93(2):366-371.

30. Bellier J, Lhommet P, Bonnette P, et al. Extracorporeal membrane oxygenation for grade 3 primary graft dysfunction after lung transplantation: Long-term outcomes. Clin Transplant. 2019;33(3):e13480.

31. Yusuff H, Malagon I, Robson K, Parmar J, Hamilton P, Falter F. Extracorporeal membrane oxygenation for Life-threatening ANCA-positive pulmonary capillaritis. A review of UK experience. Hear Lung Vessel. 2015;7(2):159-167.

32. Delvino P, Monti S, Balduzzi S, Belliato M, Montecucco C, Caporali R. The role of extracorporeal membrane oxygenation (ECMO) in the treatment of diffuse alveolar haemorrhage secondary to ANCA-associated vasculitis: report of two cases and review of the literature. Rheumatol Int. 2019;39(2):367-375.

33. Reddy HG, Maynes EJ, Saxena A, et al. Utilization of extracorporeal life support for diffuse alveolar damage and diffuse alveolar hemorrhage: A systematic review. Artif Organs. 2021;45(6):559-568.

34. Kim CW, Kim DH, Son BS, et al. The Feasibility of Extracorporeal Membrane Oxygenation in the Variant Airway Problems. Ann Thorac Cardiovas. 2015;21(6):517-522.

35. Hong Y, Jo KW, Lyu J, et al. Use of venovenous extracorporeal membrane oxygenation in central airway obstruction to facilitate interventions leading to definitive airway security. J Crit Care. 2013;28(5):669-674.

36. Lin J, Frye L. The intersection of bronchoscopy and extracorporeal membrane oxygenation. J Thorac Dis. 2021 Aug;13(8):5176-5182.

37. Akkanti B, Gentry B, Kesavan R, Kar B. Acute eosinophilic pneumonia. Bmj Case Reports. 2016;2016:bcr2015212899.

38. Dougherty SC, Ghaus S, Debesa O. Extracorporeal Membrane Oxygenation in Severe Acute Eosinophilic Pneumonia. Frontiers Medicine. 2019;6:65. doi:10.3389/fmed.2019.00065

39. Combes A, Fanelli V, Pham T, Ranieri VM; European Society of Intensive Care Medicine Trials Group and the "Strategy of Ultra-Protective lung ventilation with Extracorporeal CO2 Removal for New-Onset moderate to severe ARDS" (SUPERNOVA) investigators. Feasibility and safety of extracorporeal CO2 removal to enhance protective ventilation in acute respiratory distress syndrome: the SUPERNOVA study. Intensive Care Med. 2019 May;45(5):592-600.

40. McNamee JJ, Gillies MA, Barrett NA, et al. Effect of Lower Tidal Volume Ventilation Facilitated by Extracorporeal Carbon Dioxide Removal vs Standard Care Ventilation on 90-Day Mortality in Patients With Acute Hypoxemic Respiratory Failure. JAMA. 2021;326(11):1013-1023.

# 24

## Management of Adult Patients with Respiratory Failure

*David Furfaro, Jayne Sheldrake, Graeme MacLaren, Daniel L. Herr, Cara Agerstrand*

### General Principles

Medical management of adult patients with respiratory failure supported on VV ECMO is complex. Ideally, patients should be treated at experienced centers with established protocols and sufficient case volume.[1,2] Increased ECLS center volume is associated with lower mortality due to protocolized evaluation of candidates, decreased complication rates, and adherence to evidenced-based care principles for ARDS.[3,4] Additionally, these centers often employ multidisciplinary care teams, which have also been shown to improve outcomes.[5]

### Physiologic Optimization

The main treatment goals for patients on VV ECMO are to utilize the circuit to optimize oxygenation and carbon dioxide ($CO_2$) clearance, treat reversible causes of respiratory failure, promote lung rest, minimize ventilator-induced lung injury (VILI), and avoid or minimize harm from complications.[6,7] Additional aims are to minimize sedation, promote safe spontaneous breathing when possible, and mobilize patients.[8] Blood flow through the circuit should be adjusted to maintain adequate oxygen delivery ($DO_2$). The initial oxygenation goal is an arterial oxygen saturation ($SaO_2$) 80–90%, although this varies considerably between centers.[9] Lower $SaO_2$ may be tolerable if there are signs of adequate systemic $DO_2$, including preserved tissue perfusion, normal lactic acid levels, and intact end-organ function. Carbon dioxide ($CO_2$) removal is primarily determined by sweep gas flow rate. While initial settings are often targeted to maintain an arterial partial pressure of carbon dioxide ($PaCO_2$) in the normal range, the primary aim of sweep gas is to correct acidemia. The sweep gas flow rate should be adjusted to target a physiologic pH of at least ≥7.30, although it may not be possible to offset severe metabolic acidosis.[9,10] Of note, rapid decreases in $PaCO_2$ are associated with neurological complications, likely due to alterations in cerebral blood flow, so hypercapnia should be corrected slowly (eg, over 4–8 hours) after ECLS initiation.

### Respiratory Support and Ventilator Management

#### Lung Protective Ventilation

Lung protective ventilation is the cornerstone of ARDS management and all patients with respiratory failure on VV ECMO should receive low tidal volume ventilation (≤6 ml/kg or ideal body weight [IBW]) with airway plateau pressures ≤30 cmH₂O. More recent studies in ARDS have emphasized the importance of optimizing PEEP, minimizing driving pressure, and reducing mechanical power. The gas exchange provided by VV ECMO facilitates ultraprotective ventilator settings to provide lung rest.[11] Lung rest entails minimizing the risk of VILI by utilizing lower driving pressure, plateau pressure, and respiratory rate, and decreasing the fraction of inspired oxygen ($FiO_2$) to reduce oxygen toxicity.[12]

Ultraprotective lung ventilation, or 'lung rest' ventilation, is a widely adopted approach to mechanical ventilation in ECMO-supported patients. While the optimal ventilator strategy is unproven, certain targets are considered best practice.[13] The use of moderate to high PEEP (eg, 10-15 $cmH_2O$) is associated with decreased mortality.[14] PEEP should be titrated to maintain alveolar recruitment and respiratory system compliance while avoiding alveolar overdistention. Low tidal volume ventilation ($\leq$4–6 ml/kg of IBW) should target inspiratory plateau pressures of $\leq$24 $cmH_2O$ and minimization of driving pressure.[15] Transpulmonary pressure measurement can be used to adjust ventilator settings where appropriate expertise is available, and may be particularly helpful in severely obese patients. $CO_2$ clearance should be achieved primarily via ECLS, allowing for a low respiratory rate of 4–10 breaths/minute to decrease mechanical power. $FiO_2$ should be reduced as low as possible while maintaining $DO_2$, with a goal $FiO_2$ <50% to avoid oxygen toxicity.

Multiple ventilator modes can be utilized to achieve lung rest. Pressured-control ventilation is most common, but volume assist control ventilation, and airway pressure release ventilation (APRV) with enhanced lung protective approaches are also acceptable strategies.[13,14] These modes were utilized in the two randomized controlled trials of VV ECMO for severe respiratory failure, and those protocols can provide guidance for initial ventilator management (Table 24-1).[2,15] Once 'lung rest' is achieved, oxygenation and $CO_2$ targets should be maintained by adjusting the ECLS settings, not by increasing ventilator support.

### Spontaneous Breathing and Awake Extubation

There is increasing evidence that one of the main benefits of ECMO in respiratory failure is mitigating or avoiding VILI.[8] Patients with ARDS may be additionally at risk for patient self-induced lung injury (P-SILI), both when they are not intubated, and when breathing spontaneously on mechanical ventilation.[16,17] However, after the initial phase of ARDS, a degree of spontaneous breathing may be beneficial for improving lung function, maintaining respiratory muscle strength, and preventing diaphragm atrophy.[16]

| | PRESSURE CONTROLLED VENTILATION | VOLUME ASSIST CONTROL VENTILATION | AIRWAY PRESSURE RELEASE VENTILATION |
|---|---|---|---|
| Trial protocol | CESAR[3] | EOLIA[27] | EOLIA[27] |
| Lung protective ventilator setting | Inspiratory pressure of 10 cm $H_2O$ | Tidal volume targeted for plateau pressure $\leq$24 cm $H_2O$ | High pressure $\leq$24 cm $H_2O$ |
| PEEP (cm $H_2O$) | 10 | $\geq$10 | $\geq$10 |
| Respiratory rate (breaths/minute) | 10 | 10–30 | Spontaneous |
| Fraction of inspired $O_2$ | 0.30 | 0.30–0.50 | 0.30–0.50 |

**Table 24-1.** Modes of mechanical ventilation used in trials of ECMO.

For patients supported on ECLS as a bridge-to-lung transplantation, endotracheal extubation with spontaneous breathing is often safe and desirable to promote ambulation and nutritional support.[8,18] While endotracheal extubation in patients with ARDS is possible, it is often more challenging due to high respiratory drive and low pulmonary compliance.[19] When invasive mechanical ventilation remains necessary to minimize ongoing lung injury, efforts should be made to keep patients awake with gentle spontaneous breathing rather than accepting prolonged periods of deep sedation or neuromuscular blockade.[10,12]

## Bronchoscopy

Bronchoscopy is performed frequently in patients on VV ECMO for airway clearance, investigation for infection, and diagnosis and treatment of airway bleeding.[20] Flexible bronchoscopy is safe in patients on ECLS and anticoagulation generally does not need to be interrupted. It may be performed routinely during the ECLS run, particularly when found to be effective at secretion clearance or if respiratory cultures are required. In cases of airway hemorrhage, a cryoprobe can be safely and effectively used for blood clot extraction where expertise is available.

## Tracheostomy

Tracheostomy is commonly performed in patients supported with ECLS, although the optimal timing remains controversial.[20] The goals of tracheostomy are to provide a secure airway, decrease airway resistance, facilitate secretion clearance and oral hygiene, and decrease the need for sedative agents. Tracheostomy can be performed safely for patients on ECLS. Anticoagulation should be held 6 hours prior to the procedure, and resumed 6-12 hours afterwards, depending on the extent of any bleeding. Percutaneous dilatational

tracheostomy is the preferred technique. While major complications are rare, local bleeding and the need for transfusion are common.

## *Refractory Hypoxemia and Prone Positioning*

In patients that remain hypoxemic despite VV ECMO support, efforts should be made to improve oxygenation while maintaining lung rest. The main strategy for improving systemic oxygenation to increase the ratio of VV ECMO flow to native cardiac output. This is typically achieved by increasing ECMO blood flow, provided this can be done without worsening recirculation or causing hemolysis. If sufficient blood flow cannot be achieved with the existing ECMO configuration, an additional drainage cannula with conversion to VV-V ECMO cannula configuration can be considered.

An alternative strategy to increase blood oxygen content and therefore $DO_2$ is through red blood cell transfusion and an increased hemoglobin target. However, any putative benefit needs to be balanced against the potential harms of transfused blood, which can include increased mortality, infection, volume overload, and transfusion-related acute lung injury.[21,21] Therapeutic hypothermia to 33° C can be used to improve oxygenation by decreasing metabolic demand. Neuromuscular blockade can similarly improve oxygenation by decreasing metabolic demand and promoting ventilator synchrony. Beta-blockade, most commonly achieved with esmolol due to its short half-life, can be used to decrease native cardiac output and improve oxygenation saturation. However, as the consequent reduction in cardiac output may reduce systemic $DO_2$, this method must be used cautiously, if at all, with close monitoring for signs of tissue hypoxia.

Prone positioning during ECLS is the subject of much interest, given the survival benefit demonstrated in ARDS for patients who are not receiving ECLS. Retrospective studies have found that prone positioning on ECLS is safe, improves oxygenation, and potentially reduces in-hospital mortality.[23,24] Based on this, prone positioning for ECLS-supported patients with ARDS can be considered where expertise is available, pending more robust evidence (Chapter 47).

**Sedation and Analgesia**

Sedation targets should be set using the Richmond Agitation-Sedation Scale (RASS), or similarly validated scales, and medications should be titrated to the desired sedation level.[25] In the initial period after ECLS initiation, deep sedation is favored to maintain lung rest and ventilator synchrony, and neuromuscular blockade is frequently required.[9] The most common pharmacologic agents used are propofol, benzodiazepines, and opioids.[26] Neuromuscular blockade should be weaned shortly after cannulation to minimize the risk of critical illness myopathy, accurately titrate sedation, and monitor for seizure activity. However, partial neuromuscular blockade can be used to achieve lung protective ventilation in patients with excessive respiratory drive and high sedation requirements.[27] Given evidence that benzodiazepine use is correlated with worse outcomes in critically ill patients, nonbenzodiazepine sedation regimens are recommended when appropriate.[28]

A robust body of evidence suggests that minimizing sedation use is beneficial for critically ill patients, and these same principles should be applied to appropriate patients supported on VV ECMO. After an initial stabilization period of 24-48 hours, a RASS goal of 0 to -1 should be targeted to promote gentle spontaneous breathing and early mobilization. In addition to analgesia, sedatives that can be used for lighter sedation are oral antipsychotics, dexmedetomidine, and ketamine. Additionally, respiratory drive can be decreased by titrating sweep.

**Hemodynamic Monitoring and Management**

*Monitoring*

All patients on VV ECMO should have continuous telemetry, central venous access, and an arterial line for blood pressure monitoring and sampling. All patients ideally should have echocardiographic evaluation prior to the initiation of ECLS to determine the optimal mode of hemodynamic support. Once a patient is on VV ECMO, echocardiography can be used to assess ventricular function, volume status, cannula position, and for evaluation of inadequate flow. Pulmonary artery catheters are not routinely recommended.

*Cardiovascular Impact of VV ECMO and Hemodynamic Management*

VV ECMO does not provide direct cardiovascular support. Following initiation of VV ECMO, fluid and electrolyte shifts can lead to hypotension and intravenous fluids or vasopressors may be required. If a patient supported on VV ECMO suffers a cardiac arrest, ACLS should be initiated and emergent conversion to either VV-A or V-VA ECMO should be considered, when appropriate.

After cannulation and the initial stabilization period, there is usually improvement in cardiovascular function due to correction of acidosis and hypoxemia resulting in improved cardiac contractility and vascular tone.[29] Additionally, VV ECMO leads to a reduction in pulmonary vascular resistance—due to reversal of hypoxic pulmonary vasoconstriction and reduction in mechanical ventilation pressures which decreases right ventricular (RV) afterload. These effects lead to a decrease in pulmonary artery pressure after ECLS initiation, and improved RV function and cardiac output.

## Fluid Status and Renal Support

In patients with ARDS, a conservative fluid management strategy is associated with improved outcomes, and similar principles should be applied to patients with respiratory failure on ECLS. Immediately following initiation of VV ECMO, intravenous fluids may be needed for hemodynamic stabilization and achieve adequate blood flow; however, following this, efforts should be made for fluid removal with the goal of returning patients to their dry weight and minimizing the risk of pulmonary edema.[10] Positive fluid balance early in the ECLS course is associated with increased mortality, so diuresis should begin as soon as is feasible.[30]

Acute kidney injury in ECLS-supported patients is associated with worse outcomes.[31] For patients with severe kidney injury who cannot maintain electrolyte homeostasis or volume control with diuretics, renal replacement therapy is safe and effective. Continuous renal replacement therapy (CRRT) is favored over intermittent hemodialysis. CRRT can be integrated into the ECMO circuit (postpump) or run in parallel via separate access.[31] The decision of which CRRT method to use should be based on the patient's risk profile and institutional experience.

## Infection Diagnosis and Treatment

### *Infectious Causes of Respiratory Failure*

Identification and treatment of the underlying etiology of respiratory failure is essential, so all patients should have a thorough infectious evaluation, unless the cause for respiratory failure is already known (eg, traumatic pulmonary contusion or asthma). This includes obtaining broad diagnostic testing for all patients and expanding the workup based on exposure history and for immunocompromised patients (Table 24-2).[32] For patients without a clear etiology of

|  | MICROBIOLOGIC TESTING IN ALL PATIENTS | ADDITONAL TESTING BASED ON EXPOSURE AND IMMUNE STATUS |
|---|---|---|
| Respiratory tract | • Sputum/BAL gram stain and culture<br>• Respiratory viral PCR test<br>• SARS-CoV-2 PCR<br>• MRSA nasal swab PCR screening<br>• TB microscopy, culture, and PCR testing. | • Fungal culture / staining<br>• PCP staining and PCR<br>• BAL cell count<br>• BAL cytology<br>• Transbronchial or open lung biopsy<br>• Testing for local specific pathogens |
| Blood | • Bacterial aerobic / anaerobic cultures<br>• HIV testing | • Beta D Glucan<br>• Galactomannan<br>• CMV and EBV PCR<br>• Herpes Virus PCR<br>• Thin / thick smear<br>• Tick borne illness testing<br>• Testing for local specific pathogens |
| Urine | • Urinalysis<br>• Urine culture<br>• Urine Streptococcal antigen<br>• Urine Legionella antigen | • Urine Histoplasmosis antigen<br>• Testing for local pathogens |
| BAL=bronchoalveolar lavage, CMV=cytomegalovirus, EBV=Epstein-Barr virus, MRSA=methicillin resistant *Staphylococcus aureus*, PCP=pneumocystis pneumonia=*Pneumocystis jirovecii* pneumonia, PCR=polymerase chain reaction, SARS-CoV-2=severe acute respiratory syndrome coronavirus 2 | | |

**Table 24-2.** Initial infectious evaluation for adults with respiratory failure requiring extracorporeal life support. Broad recommendations for infectious evaluation of adult patients with respiratory failure should be tailored based on the individual patient and treatment setting.

respiratory failure, cross-sectional imaging and bedside ultrasound is generally warranted.[32] In patients with pneumonia without an isolated organism, empiric broad-spectrum antibiotics, including coverage for atypical organisms, is recommended based on the local microbiome, and the patient's risk factors. Antibiotics should be narrowed based on culture data.

### Infection as a Complication of ECLS

The incidence of infection in adults is approximately 30/1000 ECLS days, and infections are associated with increased mortality (Chapter 6).[8,33] The most common types of infections are ventilator-associated pneumonia, bloodstream infections, and infections related to indwelling catheters and cannulas. Based on ELSO Registry data, the most common isolated organisms are *Staphylococcus* species, *Pseudomonas* species, and Enterobacterales.[34] Fungal infection should also be considered and there is an increased risk for aspergillosis.

Close monitoring for signs of sepsis is necessary. When an infection is suspected, repeat broad cultures are recommended. If there is suspicion for indwelling catheter infection, the line should be removed when feasible. While ECLS cannulas can become infected, this is relatively rare. Therefore, changing cannula sites for suspected infection is not routinely recommended given the inherent risks. Until a pathogen is identified, patients should be treated with broad spectrum antibiotics and antifungal agents should be considered. Despite the serious nature of infectious complications on ECLS, prophylactic antimicrobials should not be used unless an alternate indication is present.[35]

## Hematologic Monitoring and Management

### Anticoagulation

The hematological management of patients on VV ECMO is an important aspect of care. The coagulation process is dysregulated both by critical illness and the blood-circuit interaction of ECLS, placing the patient at increased risk of both bleeding and thrombosis (Chapter 6). The goal is to lower the risk of thrombosis while minimizing the risk of major bleeding. There are no randomized controlled trials to inform selection of anticoagulant or method of monitoring and practices vary widely by center. Heparin is the most used anticoagulant and has the longest history of use, although direct thrombin inhibitors are gaining popularity.[36]

Direct Thrombin Inhibitors (DTIs), such as argatroban and bivalirudin, represent an alternative to heparin as anticoagulation in ECLS. DTIs are indicated in patients with heparin induced thrombocytopenia (HIT) but may also be used in patients who appear to be resistant to heparin therapy or for patients with thrombocytopenia of unknown etiology. Additionally, there is increasing experience for using DTIs as the primary method of anticoagulation. These drugs may be safer in ECLS patients because of their short half-life and fewer necessary titrations.

### Coagulation Monitoring

A consistent and protocolized approach to anticoagulation monitoring based on institutional practices is recommended. In an international survey of heparin monitoring, 42% of centers used partial thromboplastin time monitoring, 30.0% used activated clotting time (ACT), and 22.7% used anti-Xa activity.[36] While all of these are reasonable methods, they are performed differently and measure distinct aspects of the clotting process.

Activated partial thromboplastin time (aPTT) is considered the standard measurement for the titration of unfractionated heparin. It is important for the laboratory to result aPTTs within an hour, and to not adjust heparin more than every 6 hours. In general, VV ECMO can be managed with lower levels of anticoagulation than VA ECMO (eg, target aPTT 40-60 seconds).[15] These targets should be individualized as necessary in complex cases (eg, in COVID-19 patients or those with specific comorbidities).

Anti-Xa level monitoring is gaining popularity as an alternative to aPTT in patients anticoagulated with heparin at centers where it can be reliably and efficiently performed. Anti-Xa levels measure the heparin-antithrombin complex and are thus specific to the anticoagulation effect of heparin and may be more accurate than aPTT. Of note, high levels of elevated free hemoglobin and hyperbilirubinemia, both markers of hemolysis, can artificially lower the anti-Xa value. The usual goal for anti-Xa level is 0.2 to 0.3 units/ml.[15]

### Thrombotic Complications

Venous thromboembolism (VTE) and circuit thrombosis are the common clotting complications associated with VV ECMO. Given the frequency of venous thrombosis, there should be a low threshold to screen for deep venous thrombosis or evaluate for pulmonary embolism. One common contributing factor to VTE is HIT, which should be considered when a patient receiving heparin develops thrombocytopenia. When detected, the treatment for HIT is stopping heparin and initiation of DTIs.

Clot formation within the ECLS system can lead to decreased gas transfer efficiency, impaired blood flow, and increased hemolysis. Even with adequate anticoagulation, clot can form in small gauge tubing, low flow zones, and at areas of turbulent flow such as kinks or connection points. Direct visualization of the oxygenator and circuit tubing with a high intensity flashlight can help in detecting fibrin deposition and thrombosis. Clinically significant oxygenator clot burden should be suspected with transmembrane pressures >60 mmHg, consistently rising transmembrane pressures without changes in flow rate, or with decreases in the gas transfer efficiency.

### Hemolysis

Hemolysis in patients on ECLS can be related to underlying medical conditions but is most commonly relate to the ECMO circuit. Red cell damage from shear stress is worsened by high flow rates, increased membrane pressure gradients, very negative drainage pressure, fibrin deposition, and suction events. Plasma free hemoglobin is the gold standard for identifying intravascular hemolysis on ECLS and a level >0.5 g/L is diagnostic.[37] However, as plasma free hemoglobin tests can have a long turnaround time, and levels may be elevated in sepsis, additional laboratory markers of hemolysis including lactate dehydrogenase, indirect bilirubin, haptoglobin and urinalysis (to detect hemoglobinuria) should also be obtained. When hemolysis is identified, measures should be taken to decrease contributing factors. This may include decreasing pump flow and minimizing oscillations in drainage pressure. Changing the oxygenator or entire circuit may also be required, particularly if there is accumulation of fibrin and clot, or in the setting of massive hemolysis. Transfusion goals should be similar to those used for critically ill patients not supported with ECMO.[15]

### Bleeding Complications

Bleeding complications on ECLS are common due to anticoagulation, underlying critical illness, and a high occurrence of conditions with bleeding diatheses (eg, renal failure, sepsis, thrombocytopenia, acquired von Willebrand factor deficiency). Bleeding can also occur with procedures, such as chest tube placement, or from excessive inline suctioning, so all procedures should be performed with caution. Minor cannula-site bleeding is the most common bleeding complication. However, serious bleeding complications do occur, including oropharyngeal and gastrointestinal bleeding, pulmonary hemorrhage, and hemothorax.[8] The most significant bleeding complication is intracranial hemorrhage (ICH), although studies show a high rate of neurologically intact survival.[38] When significant bleeding or ICH is identified, anticoagulation should be immediately stopped, coagulopathy should be reversed, and platelets should be maintained >50,000/mm³. Anticoagulation can be safely held for prolonged periods, particularly if blood flow is >2.5–3 L/min, and should be resumed only when the bleeding is controlled. Any change in neurologic exam should prompt evaluation for ICH, and if identified, neurosurgery consultation is recommended.

## Nutrition

Nutritional recommendations for patients on ECLS do not differ than those for critically ill patients with ARDS, and society guidelines are recommended.[39] Nutrition can be provided enterally or parenterally, but the former is preferred to reduce infectious complications. The use of neuromuscular blockade or prone positioning should not interrupt enteral feeding. Early enteral nutrition, and reaching caloric and protein goals by the second week of ECLS support, are factors associated with improved survival.[40]

## Physical Therapy

Physical therapy is an important component of care for patients with respiratory failure as data

suggests it may improve functional outcomes, decrease rates of delirium, and potentially reduce the duration of mechanical ventilation. Multiple studies have demonstrated the safety and feasibility of early mobilization for patients on ECLS.[41] It is particularly important for patients bridging to lung transplant to maintain conditioning. Physical therapy is not always possible if patients are severely hypoxemic, hemodynamically unstable, or heavily sedated, but it is recommended if feasible. For a detailed discussion, Chapter 47.

## Integument and Eye Care

Skin and eye care is an important aspect of treatment in critically ill patients in order to prevent pressure ulcers, dermatitis, skin breakdown, and exposure keratitis.[42,43] Patients on ECLS are at increased risk for skin and eye complications due to their long courses of critical illness, immobility, and increased number of access points. Cannula dressing and suture integrity should be assessed as a component of routine care and dressing changes or reinforcement of sutures should be performed in a sterile manner. Minimizing complications from pressure injury development can have a significant role in decreased morbidity and mortality. The movement and repositioning of a patient should be a key component in the routine care, with a coordinated team of all disciplines to insure stable cannula positions. This patient group often requires eye protection to maintain ocular surface integrity. Prevention of ocular surface disease is important in minimizing complications and patient discomfort.

## Psychosocial Support

The care team should communicate regularly with patients' family members. Involving palliative care services early may be beneficial for collaboration, symptom management, and support.[44] For patients that survive ECLS, there is a high incidence of anxiety, depression, and posttraumatic stress disorder (Chapter 26), so follow-up in a post-ICU clinic is recommended.[45] The use of ICU diaries may be an effective strategy to improve survivors' health-related quality of life.

Patients on VV ECMO often have prolonged ICU stays, with high rates of morbidity and mortality, and this can have a detrimental impact on caregivers and providers. The challenge of a successful ECLS program is to not only care for patients' and family members' psychological wellbeing, but also ICU staff. A program should strive to have a support system that can monitor for potential burnout and provide stress management tools and psychological support.

# References

1. Combes A, Brodie D, Bartlett R, et al. Position paper for the organization of extracorporeal membrane oxygenation programs for acute respiratory failure in adult patients. Am J Respir Crit Care Med. 2014;190(5):488-496.
2. Peek GJ, Mugford M, Tiruvoipati R, et al. Efficacy and economic assessment of conventional ventilatory support versus extracorporeal membrane oxygenation for severe adult respiratory failure (CESAR): a multicentre randomised controlled trial. Lancet. 2009;374(9698):1351-1363.
3. Na SJ, Jeon K. Extracorporeal membrane oxygenation support in adult patients with acute respiratory distress syndrome. Expert Review of Respiratory Medicine. 2020;14(5):511-519.
4. Barbaro RP, Odetola FO, Kidwell KM, et al. Association of hospital-level volume of extracorporeal membrane oxygenation cases and mortality. Analysis of the extracorporeal life support organization registry. Am J Respir Crit Care Med. 2015;191(8):894-901.
5. Na SJ, Chung CR, Choi HJ, et al. The effect of multidisciplinary extracorporeal membrane oxygenation team on clinical outcomes in patients with severe acute respiratory failure. Ann Intensive Care. 2018;8(1):31.
6. Tonna JE, Abrams D, Brodie D, et al. Management of Adult Patients Supported with Venovenous Extracorporeal Membrane Oxygenation (VV ECMO): Guideline from the Extracorporeal Life Support Organization (ELSO). ASAIO Journal. 2021;67(6):601-610.
7. Combes A, Schmidt M, Hodgson CL, et al. Extracorporeal life support for adults with acute respiratory distress syndrome. Intensive Care Med. Online November 2, 2020:1-13.
8. Brodie D, Slutsky AS, Combes A. Extracorporeal Life Support for Adults With Respiratory Failure and Related Indications: A Review. JAMA. 2019;322(6):557-568.
9. Brodie D, Bacchetta M. Extracorporeal Membrane Oxygenation for ARDS in Adults. New England Journal of Medicine. 2011;365(20):1905-1914.
10. MacLaren G, Combes A, Bartlett RH. Contemporary extracorporeal membrane oxygenation for adult respiratory failure: life support in the new era. Intensive Care Med. 2012;38(2):210-220.
11. Marhong JD, Munshi L, Detsky M, et al. Mechanical ventilation during extracorporeal life support (ECLS): a systematic review. Intensive Care Med. 2015;41(6):994-1003.
12. Fan E, Gattinoni L, Combes A, et al. Venovenous extracorporeal membrane oxygenation for acute respiratory failure : A clinical review from an international group of experts. Intensive Care Med. 2016;42(5):712-724.
13. Schmidt M, Pham T, Arcadipane A, et al. Mechanical Ventilation Management during Extracorporeal Membrane Oxygenation for Acute Respiratory Distress Syndrome. An International Multicenter Prospective Cohort. Am J Respir Crit Care Med. 2019;200(8):1002-1012.
14. Schmidt M, Stewart C, Bailey M, et al. Mechanical ventilation management during extracorporeal membrane oxygenation for acute respiratory distress syndrome: a retrospective international multicenter study. Crit Care Med. 2015;43(3):654-664.
15. Combes A, Hajage D, Capellier G, et al. Extracorporeal Membrane Oxygenation for Severe Acute Respiratory Distress Syndrome. N Engl J Med. 2018;378(21):1965-1975.
16. Yoshida T, Amato MBP, Kavanagh BP, et al. Impact of spontaneous breathing during mechanical ventilation in acute respiratory distress syndrome. Curr Opin Crit Care. 2019;25(2):192-198.
17. Grieco DL, Menga LS, Eleuteri D, et al. Patient self-inflicted lung injury: implications for acute hypoxemic respiratory failure and ARDS patients on non-invasive support. Minerva Anestesiol. 2019;85(9):1014-1023.
18. Tipograf Y, Salna M, Minko E, et al. Outcomes of Extracorporeal Membrane Oxygenation as a Bridge to Lung Transplantation. Ann Thorac Surg. 2019;107(5):1456-1463.
19. Kurihara C, Walter JM, Singer BD, et al. Extracorporeal Membrane Oxygenation Can Successfully Support Patients With Severe Acute Respiratory Distress Syndrome in Lieu of Mechanical Ventilation. Critical Care Medicine. 2018;46(11):e1070.
20. Jenks CL, Tweed J, Gigli KH, et al. An International Survey on Ventilator Practices Among Extracorporeal Membrane Oxygenation Centers. ASAIO J. 2017;63(6):787-792.
21. Vincent JL, Baron JF, Reinhart K, et al. Anemia and Blood Transfusion in Critically Ill Patients. JAMA. 2002;288(12):1499-1507.
22. Corwin HL, Gettinger A, Pearl RG, et al. The CRIT Study: Anemia and blood transfusion in the critically ill-current clinical practice in the United States. Crit Care Med. 2004;32(1):39-52.
23. Giani M, Martucci G, Madotto F, et al. Prone Positioning during Venovenous Extracorporeal Membrane Oxygenation in Acute Respiratory Distress Syndrome. A Multicenter Cohort Study and Propensity-matched Analysis. Annals ATS. 2021;18(3):495-501.
24. Poon WH, Ramanathan K, Ling RR, et al. Prone positioning during venovenous extracorporeal membrane oxygenation for acute respiratory distress

syndrome: a systematic review and meta-analysis. Critical Care. 2021;25(1):292.

25. Sessler CN, Gosnell MS, Grap MJ, et al. The Richmond Agitation-Sedation Scale: validity and reliability in adult intensive care unit patients. Am J Respir Crit Care Med. 2002;166(10):1338-1344.

26. deBacker J, Tamberg E, Munshi L, et al. Sedation Practice in Extracorporeal Membrane Oxygenation-Treated Patients with Acute Respiratory Distress Syndrome: A Retrospective Study. ASAIO J. 2018;64(4):544-551.

27. Goligher EC, Jonkman AH, Dianti J, et al. Clinical strategies for implementing lung and diaphragm-protective ventilation: avoiding insufficient and excessive effort. Intensive Care Med. 2020;46(12):2314-2326.

28. Barr J, Fraser GL, Puntillo K, et al. Clinical Practice Guidelines for the Management of Pain, Agitation, and Delirium in Adult Patients in the Intensive Care Unit. Critical Care Medicine. 2013;41(1):263-306.

29. Bunge JJH, Caliskan K, Gommers D, et al. Right ventricular dysfunction during acute respiratory distress syndrome and veno-venous extracorporeal membrane oxygenation. J Thorac Dis. 2018;10(Suppl 5):S674-S682.

30. Schmidt M, Bailey M, Kelly J, et al. Impact of fluid balance on outcome of adult patients treated with extracorporeal membrane oxygenation. Intensive Care Med. 2014;40(9):1256-1266.

31. Zeidman AD. Extracorporeal Membrane Oxygenation and Continuous Kidney Replacement Therapy: Technology and Outcomes - A Narrative Review. Adv Chronic Kidney Dis. 2021;28(1):29-36.

32. Papazian L, Calfee CS, Chiumello D, et al. Diagnostic workup for ARDS patients. Intensive Care Med. 2016;42(5):674-685.

33. Biffi S, Di Bella S, Scaravilli V, et al. Infections during extracorporeal membrane oxygenation: epidemiology, risk factors, pathogenesis and prevention. International Journal of Antimicrobial Agents. 2017;50(1):9-16.

34. Abrams D, Grasselli G, Schmidt M, et al. ECLS-associated infections in adults: what we know and what we don't yet know. Intensive Care Med. 2020;46(2):182-191.

35. O'Horo JC, Cawcutt KA, De Moraes AG, et al. The Evidence Base for Prophylactic Antibiotics in Patients Receiving Extracorporeal Membrane Oxygenation. ASAIO J. 2016;62(1):6-10.

36. Protti A, Iapichino GE, Di Nardo M, et al. Anticoagulation Management and Antithrombin Supplementation Practice during Veno-venous Extracorporeal Membrane Oxygenation: A Worldwide Survey. Anesthesiology. 2020;132(3):562-570.

37. Murphy DA, Hockings LE, Andrews RK, et al. Extracorporeal membrane oxygenation-hemostatic complications. Transfus Med Rev. 2015;29(2):90-101.

38. Lockie CJA, Gillon SA, Barrett NA, et al. Severe Respiratory Failure, Extracorporeal Membrane Oxygenation, and Intracranial Hemorrhage. Crit Care Med. 2017;45(10):1642-1649.

39. Krzak A, Pleva M, Napolitano LM. Nutrition therapy for ALI and ARDS. Crit Care Clin. 2011;27(3):647-659.

40. Davis RC, Durham LA, Kiraly L, et al. Safety, Tolerability, and Outcomes of Enteral Nutrition in Extracorporeal Membrane Oxygenation. Nutr Clin Pract. 2021;36(1):98-104.

41. Abrams D, Javidfar J, Farrand E, et al. Early mobilization of patients receiving extracorporeal membrane oxygenation: a retrospective cohort study. Crit Care. 2014;18(1):R38.

42. Rosenberg JB, Eisen LA. Eye care in the intensive care unit: Narrative review and meta-analysis. Critical Care Medicine. 2008;36(12):3151-3155.

43. de Laat E h. e. w., Schoonhoven L, Pickkers P, et al. Epidemiology, risk and prevention of pressure ulcers in critically ill patients: a literature review. J Wound Care. 2006;15(6):269-275.

44. Rao A, Zaaqoq AM, Kang IG, et al. Palliative Care for Patients on Extracorporeal Membrane Oxygenation for COVID-19 Infection. Am J Hosp Palliat Care. 2021;38(7):854-860.

45. Rajajee V, Fung CMC, Seagly KS, et al. One-Year Functional, Cognitive, and Psychological Outcomes Following the Use of Extracorporeal Membrane Oxygenation in Coronavirus Disease 2019: A Prospective Study. Critical Care Explorations. 2021;3(9):e0537.

# 25

# Weaning and Decannulation in Adult Respiratory Failure

*Brian E. Malley, Raj Ramanan, Vin Pellegrino, Chris Harvey*

## Introduction

VV ECMO is the modality of extracorporeal support most used for isolated adult respiratory failure. Clear criteria for the initiation of VV ECMO have been published in ELSO guidelines.[1] These are based on the CESAR and EOLIA randomized trials and are widely accepted among ECLS centers.[2,3]

In general terms, weaning a patient off VV ECMO consists of the following: 1) recognition of lung recovery, 2) decreasing the oxygenation and $CO_2$ removal provided by the ECMO circuit as the patient's native lung function improves, 3) performing a sweep gas trial off, and 4) decannulation following a successful trial. Weaning ECLS can consist of reducing some or all of the extracorporeal blood flow (EBF), sweep gas flow (SGF), and fraction of delivered oxygen in the sweep gas ($FsO_2$).

Within the aforementioned general constraints, there are multiple reasonable approaches to weaning and decannulation in VV ECMO which are based on expert opinion.[4-6] No prospective randomized trials aimed at comparing methods have been conducted to date. However, recent evidence does suggest that instituting a systematic approach to weaning and decannulation—analogous to the spontaneous breathing trial in mechanical ventilation—may allow for earlier safe liberation of patients from extracorporeal support.[5,7-11] As there is not a single universally accepted method, in this chapter we will focus on the major concepts that are part of the four steps of weaning and decannulation listed above.

## Appropriateness for Liberation Trials and Indicators of Recovery

Evaluating if a patient can begin the process of liberation from VV ECMO can be broken down into the following: 1) Is the patient generally clinically appropriate for liberation trials? and 2) Are there indicators of adequate native lung function?

The first question of general appropriateness depends strongly on the indication for ECLS. We will mostly address acute respiratory failure requiring VV ECMO support as a bridge-to-recovery. To be appropriate for liberation trials, these patients should first be in the expected recovery phase of the process which initially caused their respiratory failure (eg, viral or bacterial pneumonia, traumatic pulmonary contusion, inhalational injury, etc.). Additionally, a patient should be generally stable aside from their respiratory failure, without any ongoing processes which would foreseeably cause severe worsening of respiratory function. Specifically, patients should be hemodynamically stable (minimal or no vasopressor support), should not have evidence of untreated active pulmonary superinfections, and should not have signs of sepsis. Recovery of renal function often takes longer than recovery of the lungs and the continued need for renal replacement should not preclude attempts to liberate the patient from ECLS. For patients receiving ECMO circuit-based renal replacement, planning for alternative access should precede decannulation. In the case of other indications for VV ECMO such as support during surgical procedures (eg, tracheobronchial reconstruction) or as bridge-to-transplant in endstage respiratory disease, the timing of general appropriateness for weaning is largely determined by the outcome of the therapeutic procedure. In rare instances, the risks of ongoing extracorporeal support outweigh the benefits, such as in uncontrolled bleeding or recalcitrant blood stream infections. In these cases, premature ECMO separation may be judged to be in the best interests of the patient, sometimes with the possibility of subsequent re-cannulation if required.

The second factor to consider in readiness for liberation is recovery of lung function. In the case of VV ECMO as a bridge-to-recovery, the goal of ECLS is to mitigate ventilator-induced lung injury (VILI), facilitate lung rest, and replace native lung function. In respiratory failure, the forces exerted on the lung by either patient effort or mechanical ventilation can further exacerbate lung injury. We will focus mainly on patients who remain on mechanical ventilation during VV ECMO because this is the most common scenario.[12,13] Detailed discussion of ventilator management for patients on VV ECMO is covered elsewhere in this book. However, as a brief recap, studies of ECMO ventilator management show that the majority of centers use what are termed "lung protective" or "ultra-protective" ventilator settings, consistent with ELSO guidelines.[12,14,15] These guidelines include targeting positive end-expiratory pressure (PEEP) ≥10 cmH$_2$O,

tidal volume (V$_t$) of no more than 4-6 mL/kg of predicted body weight (PBW), inspiratory plateau pressure (P$_{plat}$) <25 cmH$_2$O (though further reductions may improve outcomes), respiratory rate (RR) 4-15 breaths per minute or spontaneous breathing, and fraction of inspired oxygen (FiO$_2$) 30-50% (but as low as possible).[1] Studies have shown that higher PEEP and lower mechanical power delivered to the lungs during the early course of an ECMO run are associated with improved outcomes, so there may be a point at which it is too early to begin weaning ECLS.[15-17]

Indicators of lung recovery include improved compliance (indicated by increased V$_t$ on pressure control mode or decreased P$_{plat}$ on volume control mode), improvement radiographic appearance of the lungs, and either improvement in PaO$_2$ and PaCO$_2$ on unchanged ECMO support or unchanged blood gas values on reduced ECMO support.[18,19] The exact indicators for a given patient will vary depending on the mode of ventilation in use and which ECLS parameters (EBF, SGF, FsO$_2$) are adjusted during routine daily care. Individual centers have also investigated quantitative comparisons of native and membrane lung CO$_2$ clearance, protocolized lung ultrasound, and transpulmonary pressure targeted ventilator titration.[17,20,21] No single set of indicators of lung recovery has shown to be superior in predicting readiness for weaning from VV ECMO in adult respiratory failure.

## Weaning

### Clinical Assessment

Traditionally, readiness has generally been determined by the treating physicians' judgment of indicators of recovery. More recently, multiple centers have trialed structured protocols analogous to the spontaneous awakening trials (SAT) and spontaneous breathing trials (SBT) that are standard of care in management of sedation and mechanical ventilation. This includes both protocols driven by physicians and protocols driven by respiratory therapists or perfusionists, just as with SAT and SBT protocols.[9] These methods have shown promise with reductions in both time to first sweep gas off trial and time to decannulation without increased adverse events.[8,9,11] These trials have even shown success with liberating patients from VV ECMO safely at higher levels of support than traditionally would have indicated a sweep gas off trial was warranted. While no single protocol has shown to be superior to others, current evidence suggests that institutions should implement a local standardized VV ECMO liberation protocol.

### *Ventilator Management During Weaning*

When the patient's native lung function improves and allows for weaning ECLS, ventilatory support will need to be augmented from "ultra-protective" to traditional lung protective settings. Regardless of the ventilator mode, the $FiO_2$ should remain at 30-60%, PEEP should remain at least 5-10 $cmH_2O$, and RR $\leq$30 breaths/min. For volume control mode, the $V_t$ can be increased in increments of 1-2 mL/kg of PBW to a maximum of 6-8 mL/kg of PBW with acceptable plateau pressures ($P_{plat} \leq$28 $cmH_2O$). For pressure control or pressure support modes, the driving pressure can be increased to no more than 15-20 $cmH_2O$ with delivered $V_t$ in the 6-8 mL/kg of PBW range.[1] The majority of patients will still be on mechanical ventilation when weaning, and if a patient is breathing spontaneously, they should be monitored for signs of respiratory distress or increased work of breathing because patient self-inflicted lung injury (P-SILI) is possible, regardless of whether they are intubated or not.[1,12]

### *Sweep Gas Management*

Sweep gas management consists of sweep gas flow (SGF) and sweep gas composition (primarily $FsO_2$). The SGF should be weaned with the goal of maintaining safe lung ventilation, systemic oxygenation, and adequate $CO_2$ clearance. Many centers judge adequate $CO_2$ clearance based off a normal arterial blood pH rather than a normal arterial $CO_2$ because metabolic compensation of hypercapnia is seen frequently in patients requiring VV ECMO.

Because the proportion of total $CO_2$ clearance performed by the membrane is not routinely measured, and may not be represented solely by SGF setting, the effects of any reduction in SGF are somewhat uncertain.[20,22] For this reason, weaning SGF is an important part of routine care for stable or improving patients. This can be done either in a gradual set stepwise fashion (over hours/days) in response to signs of lung recovery, or more rapidly as a sweep gas off trial with close observation (and reintroduction if required) when local criteria are met. Irrespective of the extracorporeal blood flow (EBF), once the SGF ceases, ECMO support effectively ceases.

VV ECMO weaning using the titration of $FsO_2$ is more complex. The sweep gas provides the oxygen which is transferred in the membrane lung. However, in a properly functioning membrane lung even very low flows (SGF=1-2 LPM or less) of unenriched air as sweep gas ($FsO_2$=0.21) should result in a saturation close to 100% in the blood leaving the membrane lung.[7] Therefore, it is the ECMO blood flow rate and the patient's hemoglobin which are the major drivers of oxygen delivery and these along with the patient's total cardiac output which determine arterial blood oxygen saturation ($SaO_2$).[1,7,10] This physiology is discussed in greater detail in Chapter 5. Although some centers do titrate $FsO_2$, it is not considered necessary to titrate the sweep gas $FsO_2$ at any time (or for the purposes of weaning) and some centers always use oxygen ($FsO_2=1.0$) as the sweep gas for VV ECMO for safety and simplicity.

### Extracorporeal Blood Flow (EBF) Management

The extracorporeal blood low (EBF) is directly related to the oxygen delivered to the patient by VV ECMO. EBF is determined by multiple factors as discussed elsewhere in this book (see Chapters 3 and 5). Higher pump speeds and higher EBF are associated with hemolysis, while very low flow rates raise concern for stagnation and blood clot formation.[10] The exact range of safe EBF rates will vary with equipment and patient factors, although for general adult patients EBF of 3-6L is a safe range. EBF need not be adjusted outside this range to perform a weaning trial.

Some centers treat the EBF as a largely fixed parameter unless a patient has inadequate oxygenation and requires increased flow.[5,6] Other centers have more recently advocated for an approach of routine adjustment of EBF to meet patient needs during daily care.[10] This can be protocolized and performed on daily rounds or more frequently. Primarily, the benefit of this approach is that in order to maintain higher EBF, patients require some combination of larger cannulas (associated with greater thrombosis), additional cannulas (associated with increased complications), higher pump speeds (associated with greater hemolysis), increased intravascular volume (associated with worsened native lung function), and/or decreased mobility and increased sedation (associated with worse outcomes).[1,7,10,23] In summary, conservative EBF settings which maintain oxygenation may reduce these complications and a decreasing EBF requirement implies lung recovery and suggests the patient is appropriate for a weaning trial.

### Anticoagulation Management

Anticoagulation on VV ECMO is covered in Chapter 24. However, there are a few points particularly relevant to the weaning and decannulation process that we will address. First, although some anticoagulation is usual in VV ECMO care, it is possible to manage VV ECMO patients completely off anticoagulation and this remains true in the weaning and decannulation period. Secondly, reducing EBF rates likely increases the risk of circuit thrombosis and the need for anticoagulation. There are not clear cutoffs for safe blood flow rates on and off anticoagulation because this depends on multiple patient and equipment factors, but sources estimate a minimum EBF of 1-2 L as a bare minimum for safety and, more commonly, most centers do not drop flows below 2-3 L.[10,24] There is currently wide practice variation in regards to anticoagulation management, from centers that rarely use anticoagulation with VV ECMO to centers that keep patients on therapeutic anticoagulation throughout the weaning process, including the decannulation procedure itself. For patients on anticoagulation, current guidelines state that it is prudent to hold anticoagulation for at least 30-60 minutes prior to decannulation.[1] Local practices may vary, guided by the clinicians performing the procedure.

### Decannulation

The first step toward safely decannulating a patient from VV ECMO is the sweep gas off trial in which the gas flow is turned fully off or even disconnected. Functionally, this completely eliminates all extracorporeal support because no oxygen is added, or carbon dioxide removed despite blood still moving through the circuit. It is important to emphasize that the simple sweep gas off trial applies only to VV ECMO and would be dangerous in the V-A or V-VA ECMO configurations. The sweep gas off trial is the standard of care for predicting successful VV ECMO decannulation. Other methods such as SGF thresholds or a 100% oxygen challenge test on the ventilator have been shown to be less reliable.[19] During the trial the patient is closely monitored for hypoxia, hypercarbia, or unsafe increase in work of breathing. Monitoring normally consists of standard clinical observation, cardiac monitoring, and pulse oximetry as well as serial ABGs. Exact cutoffs vary between institutions but patients should remain within the bounds of lung protective ventilation as described above, should have adequate oxygenation with $SpO_2$ $\geq$88-92% and $PaO_2 \geq$70 mmHg, and should have pH $\geq$7.30.[1,5,6,8,9] In addition, patients should not have significant new tachycardia, hypertension, hypotension, or increased work of breathing.[1,6] Ultimately, it is up to the treating clinician to determine if a patient has passed their sweep gas off trial and should proceed to decannulation. Various lengths of time for sweep gas off trials have been used, ranging from 2-24 hours. In a study of 192 sweep gas off trials from VV ECMO, no significant changes in blood gas parameters were found after 2 hours from the time sweep gas was turned off.[25] ELSO guidelines recommend a minimum of 2-3 hours for a sweep gas off trial.[1] Longer trials are rarely necessary.

Most patients will still be mechanically ventilated at the time of decannulation.[13] For spontaneously breathing patients, there are variations within accepted practice. Some centers perform decannulations on awake spontaneously breathing patients, while other centers routinely reintubate patients for the decannulation procedure to facilitate sedation and lower the risk of entraining air during cannula removal. Particularly for patients with long ECLS runs, it is advisable to formally reassess pulmonary compliance prior to decannulation to ensure that safe, controlled positive pressure ventilation is possible in the event it is required following decannulation.

After the decision has been made to decannulate the patient, the procedure is relatively straightforward. If a cannula was placed using a surgical cutdown approach then it should be removed surgically and the vessel ligated or repaired.[26] However, most VV ECMO cannulas are placed percutaneously and can be removed at the bedside. The same general technique can be used to remove single-lumen, multistage single-lumen, and double-lumen cannulas. Usual preparations include having an active blood type and screen, making preparations for sedation/paralysis if needed, and in extubated patients ensuring *nil per os* (NPO) status in accordance with local protocols.[1] Patients reliant on renal replacement therapy via the ECMO circuit should have plans made for ongoing renal replacement access. As discussed previously, a decision on anticoagulation management should be made ahead of time, with usual guidelines recommended holding for at least 30-60 minutes prior to the procedure. Plans for hemostasis should be made in advance, with the most common methods being sutures and direct pressure. There is some variation in practice regarding methods of bleeding control, with some centers advocating for extended direct pressure of 20-60 minutes alone, some for placement of sutures without any direct pressure for hemostasis, and some for sutures followed by extended pressure. Sutures assist with hemostasis and shorten the period of venous compression, which may help reduce the risk of local venous thrombosis. Conversely, there are risks to placing sutures near a nonsterile active ECMO cannula. We will describe the decannulation procedure below as if both extended pressure and sutures are being used, but providers may choose to omit one or the other in their routine local practice.

The decannulation procedure is generally performed in a semi-sterile fashion as complete sterility is not possible with the existing cannulas. Experienced providers familiar with the procedure and capable of managing acute bleeding should be at the bedside and staff trained to manage the ECMO circuit, often certified perfusionists, should be present. If one of the cannulas being removed is in the internal jugular (IJ) vein, then the patient should be placed in the Trendelenburg position as with any IJ central catheter removal. Generally, both cannulas are removed in a coordinated fashion by two operators. First, if sutures are to be used, a suture of strong material is placed but not tied down. The sutures are placed around each cannula where it enters the skin using 0 silk and either a pursestring or mattress suture. Extreme care must be taken when suturing near any ECMO cannula. Then any other sutures or devices securing the cannulas should be removed and the operators should hold the cannulas in place. Pressure is held over the entry sites with gauze either by the operators or by assistants. If an IJ cannula is present, then at this point the ventilator should be placed on a brief inspiratory hold. If the patient is spontaneously breathing, they should bear down, hold exhalation, or hum. Then in a coordinated fashion, the circuit is clamped near the cannula at the return limb and then the drain limb, the pump is stopped, and then each operator removes their cannula by withdrawing it with a smooth, rapid, single movement. At this point, the ventilator or patient may resume normal respiration. If sutures are being used, they are then tied down securely. Pressure should then be held either just until hemostasis is achieved or for an extended period depending on operator preference.[7]

Decannulation is generally well tolerated but there is the possibility of immediate complications. Sudden hemodynamic or respiratory decompensation should prompt rapid evaluation for life-threatening complications including pulmonary embolism, air embolism, and bleeding. Pulmonary embolism can occur when a cannula associated deep vein thrombus is dislodged. Similarly, removal of cannulas (particularly multistage drains) can lead to

entraining air resulting in air embolus. Bleeding is possible but normally controlled with sutures and local pressure as described above.

There is a case report of modifying the above procedure to prevent the loss of the blood in the circuit for an anemic patient who could not receive blood due to religious restrictions. In this case, the drain limb of the circuit was clamped first and sterile saline infused into the circuit until the blood in the circuit had been returned to the patient, then the return limb was clamped and the cannulas removed.[27] This process is not usually required but has been described as a safe option in exceptional cases.

## Immediate Post-ECLS Management

### *Post-Decannulation Systemic Inflammatory Response Syndrome (SIRS)*

The phenomenon of fever, leukocytosis, and vasodilation leading to tachycardia or vasopressor use has been described in the 24-48 hours after decannulation. There are limited studies in this area, but there is an estimated incidence of fever or SIRS of 50-60% in the 48 hours after decannulation.[28,29] Limited evidence and anecdote suggests this may be more common after longer ECMO runs. In this critically ill patient population, these symptoms frequently prompt an infectious workup, and studies have shown various rates of confirmed infection ranging from 8-35% of febrile patients.[28,29] In the above studies, the presence of post-decannulation fever or SIRS in the absence of diagnosed infection was not associated with increased mortality. Currently there is no clear evidence for prophylactic antibiotic use around the time of VV ECMO decannulation.

### *Post-Decannulation Venous Thromboembolism*

Cannula-associated venous thrombus is a very frequent complication in adult VV ECMO patients. Multiple studies using CT venography or Doppler ultrasound for surveillance have estimated the prevalence of deep vein thrombosis (DVT) to be over 60% post decannulation, even in patients anticoagulated while on ECLS.[23,30] One small study of VV ECMO patients with COVID-19 showed 100% had evidence of DVT or pulmonary embolism.[31] Risk factors for DVT include femoral cannulation site, larger cannula size (eg, dual lumen cannulas), and lower aPTT values on anticoagulation.[23,30] Given the very high rates of cannula-associated DVT, routine surveillance of all patients decannulated from VV ECMO is warranted. Some centers obtain ultrasounds of all limbs given that VV ECMO patients are critically ill, relatively immobile, and at high risk of venous thromboembolism. Doppler ultrasound assessment of at least the cannulated vessels should be performed 24 hours after decannulation from VV ECMO for all patients.[1]

## Conclusion

There are multiple reasonable approaches to liberation of patients from VV ECMO, and while randomized studies have not been conducted, it is unlikely that different approaches within the above framework will result in significant enduring outcome differences. Recent studies appear to show some benefits from establishing a standardized approach at least at the local level, with protocols for weaning analogous to spontaneous breathing trials in mechanical ventilation, but clinical efficacy trials are lacking. Such protocols should address the safety of attempted weaning by including criteria regarding which patients are appropriate for possible liberation. The general approach to weaning can consist of ongoing (daily) weaning of ECLS leading up to eventual qualification for a sweep gas off trial or a more rapid approach to weaning ECLS triggered by indications of lung recovery. Weaning of oxygenation support generally means decreasing blood flow, it

can also involve $FsO_2$ titration but this is not required. Weaning of $CO_2$ removal is done by decreasing the sweep gas flow rate. The hallmark of VV ECMO weaning is the sweep gas off trial once a patient has reached a low enough level of extracorporeal support that their native lungs can attempt to provide all needed oxygenation and $CO_2$ removal. Passing a sweep gas off trial should include a patient maintaining adequate oxygenation and ventilation while not exceeding lung protective levels of ventilator support. Finally, safe decannulation from VV ECMO can generally be done at the bedside and bleeding controlled with sutures and/or pressure. After decannulation, the ECLS team should be vigilant for rare serious complications and systems should be in place to handle common complications such as SIRS and DVT.

## References

1. Tonna JE, Abrams D, Brodie D, et al. Management of Adult Patients Supported with Venovenous Extracorporeal Membrane Oxygenation (VV ECMO): Guideline from the Extracorporeal Life Support Organization (ELSO). Asaio J. 2021;67(6):601-610.
2. Combes A, Slutsky AS, Brodie D. ECMO for Severe Acute Respiratory Distress Syndrome. N Engl J Med. Sep 13 2018;379(11):1091-2.
3. Peek GJ, Mugford M, Tiruvoipati R, et al. Efficacy and economic assessment of conventional ventilatory support versus extracorporeal membrane oxygenation for severe adult respiratory failure (CESAR): a multicentre randomised controlled trial. Lancet. Oct 17 2009;374(9698):1351-63.
4. Broman LM, Malfertheiner MV, Montisci A, et al. Weaning from veno-venous extracorporeal membrane oxygenation: how I do it. J Thorac Dis. 2017;10(5):S692-S697.
5. Grant AA, Hart VJ, Lineen EB, et al. A Weaning Protocol for Venovenous Extracorporeal Membrane Oxygenation With a Review of the Literature. Artif Organs. 2018;42(6):605-610.
6. Vasques F, Romitti F, Gattinoni L, et al. How I wean patients from veno-venous extra-corporeal membrane oxygenation. Crit Care. 2019;23(1):316.
7. Extracorporeal life support : The ELSO Red Book 5th Edition. 5th ed. Extracorporeal Life Support Organization; 2017.
8. Gannon WD, Stokes JW, Bloom S, et al. Safety and Feasibility of a Protocolized Daily Assessment of Readiness for Liberation From Venovenous Extracorporeal Membrane Oxygenation. Chest. 2021;160(5):1693-1703.
9. Pratt EH, Mausert S, Wilson MD, et al. A Daily, Respiratory Therapist Assessment of Readiness to Liberate From Venovenous Extracorporeal Membrane Oxygenation in Patients With Acute Respiratory Distress Syndrome. Critical Care Explor. 2021;3(12):e0584.
10. Shekar K, Buscher H, Brodie D. Protocol-driven daily optimisation of venovenous extracorporeal membrane oxygenation blood flows: an alternate paradigm? J Thorac Dis. 2020;12(11):6854-6860.
11. Teijeiro-Paradis R, Tiwari P, Spriel A, et al. Standardized liberation trials in patients with COVID-19 ARDS treated with venovenous extracorporeal membrane oxygenation: when ready, let them breathe! Intens Care Med. 2021;47(12):1-3.
12. Marhong JD, Telesnicki T, Munshi L, et al. Mechanical Ventilation during Extracorporeal Membrane Oxygenation. An International Survey. Ann Am Thorac Soc. 2014;11(6):956-961.
13. Swol J, Shekar K, Protti A, et al. Extubate Before Venovenous Extracorporeal Membranous Oxygenation Decannulation or Decannulate While Remaining on the Ventilator? The EuroELSO 2019 Weaning Survey. Asaio J. 2020;67(4):e86-e89.
14. Gattinoni L, Tonetti T, Quintel M. How best to set the ventilator on extracorporeal membrane lung oxygenation. Curr Opin Crit Care. 2017;23(1):66-72.
15. Schmidt M, Stewart C, Bailey M, et al. Mechanical Ventilation Management During Extracorporeal Membrane Oxygenation for Acute Respiratory Distress Syndrome. Crit Care Med. 2015;43(3):654-664.
16. Chiu L-C, Lin S-W, Chuang L-P, et al. Mechanical power during extracorporeal membrane oxygenation and hospital mortality in patients with acute respiratory distress syndrome. Crit Care. 2021;25(1):13.
17. Wang R, Sun B, Li X, et al. Mechanical Ventilation Strategy Guided by Transpulmonary Pressure in Severe Acute Respiratory Distress Syndrome Treated With Venovenous Extracorporeal Membrane Oxygenation. Crit Care Med. 2020;48(9):1280-1288.
18. Al-Fares AA, Ferguson ND, Ma J, et al. Achieving Safe Liberation During Weaning From VV-ECMO in Patients With Severe ARDS The Role of Tidal Volume and Inspiratory Effort. Chest. 2021;160(5):1704-1713.
19. Hartley EL, Sanderson B, Vasques F, et al. Prediction of readiness to decannulation from venovenous extracorporeal membrane oxygenation. Perfusion. 2020;35(1_suppl):57-64.
20. Belliato M, Cremascoli L, Epis F, et al. Carbon Dioxide Elimination During Veno-Venous Extracorporeal Membrane Oxygenation Weaning: A Pilot Study. Asaio J. 2020;67(6):700-708.
21. Lu X, Arbelot C, Schreiber A, et al. Ultrasound Assessment of Lung Aeration in Subjects Supported by Venovenous Extracorporeal Membrane Oxygenation. Respir Care. 2019;64(12):1478-1487.
22. Epis F, Belliato M. Oxygenator performance and artificial-native lung interaction. J Thorac Dis. Mar 2018;10(Suppl 5):S596-S605.
23. Fisser C, Reichenbächer C, Müller T, et al. Incidence and Risk Factors for Cannula-Related Venous Thrombosis After Venovenous Extracorporeal Membrane Oxygenation in Adult Patients With Acute Respiratory Failure. Crit Care Med. 2019 Apr;47(4):e332-e339.
24. Krishnan S, Schmidt GA. Extracorporeal Life Support for Adults. Resp Med. 2016:223-232.
25. Na SJ, Choi HJ, Chung CR, et al. Duration of sweep gas off trial for weaning from venovenous extracorporeal membrane oxygenation. Ther Adv Respir Dis. 2019;13:1753466619888131.

26. Extracorporeal Life Support Organization (ELSO) General Guidelines for all ECLS Cases Version 1.4. Extracorporeal Life Support Organization; 2017.

27. Park SM, Lee B, Kim CY. Blood-sparing removal technique of extracorporeal membrane oxygenation circuit in a Jehovah Witness patient. Medicine. 2019;98(31):e16740.

28. Esposito EC, Jones KM, Galvagno SM Jr, et al. Incidence of healthcare-associated infections in patients with fever during the first 48 hours after decannulation from veno-venous extracorporeal membrane oxygenation. Perfusion. May 2021;36(4):421-428.

29. Thangappan K, Cavarocchi NC, Baram M, et al. Systemic inflammatory response syndrome (SIRS) after extracorporeal membrane oxygenation (ECMO): Incidence, risks and survivals. Heart Lung. Sep-Oct 2016;45(5):449-53.

30. Parzy G, Daviet F, Persico N, et al. Prevalence and Risk Factors for Thrombotic Complications Following Venovenous Extracorporeal Membrane Oxygenation: A CT Scan Study*. Crit Care Med. 2020;48(2):192-199.

31. Parzy G, Daviet F, Puech B, et al. Venous Thromboembolism Events Following Venovenous Extracorporeal Membrane Oxygenation for Severe Acute Respiratory Syndrome Coronavirus 2 Based on CT Scans. Crit Care Med. 2020 Oct;48(10):e971-e975.

# 26

## Complications, Followup, and Outcomes of Adults with Respiratory Failure

*Nicholas A. Barrett, Thomas Müller, Alain Vuylsteke, Carol L. Hodgson*

### Short Term Outcomes

Survival from severe ARDS has progressively improved over the last 20-30 years.[1] According to data from the ELSO Registry, survival for patients managed with ECLS for severe ARDS has steadily improved, with approximately two-thirds of patients surviving to decannulation and 55-60% being discharged from hospital alive.[2] The attributable survival benefit from ECLS has been explored in two randomized controlled trials, CESAR and EOLIA.[3,4] A recent metaanalysis combined the data from these two trials and demonstrated that ECLS was associated with improved outcomes for patients with severe ARDS over conventional ventilation, with a relative risk of death when receiving ECLS of 0.75, 95% confidence interval 0.6-0.94; p=0.013).[5]

Outcomes from ECLS for severe respiratory failure are known to be impacted by several factors. The etiology of respiratory failure is particularly important. It is well established that infective causes of ARDS, including viral or bacterial pneumonia, have a better outcome than noninfectious aetiologies (60-65% survival vs. 50-57% survival).[2] Severe asthma requiring ECLS has a survival of approximately 95%.[6] The patient characteristics at the onset of ECLS impact outcome, with higher degree of severity of illness and having three or more organ

failures, or undergoing cardiac arrest all being associated with lower survival.[5,7] Patient factors associated with better survival are younger age (18-49 years vs. others, OR 3.15 [2.17-4.15]) and higher weight (OR 0.67 [0.31-10.2]), while immunocompromise is associated with worse outcomes (OR 0.53 [0.35-0.85]).[7] Medical management prior to commencement of ECLS is of prognostic importance. Increased duration of mechanical ventilation before ECLS of 5-7 days or more is associated with reduced survival (OR 0.58 [0.31-0.81]) while undertaking therapies proven to provide lung protective ventilation, including limiting plateau pressures and tidal volumes, using neuromuscular blockade and ventilation in the prone position, all are associated with improved survival.[7,8] Another factor is clinician and team experience and there is a well-documented association between higher volume centers and improved survival.[9]

Short term (90 day) survival from COVID-19-related ARDS requiring ECLS have worsened during the pandemic.[10] Mortality prior to May 2020 (first wave) was reported as 36% and this rose to 52% during the second wave (May-December 2020).[10,11] The reasons for this are unclear but it may be due to changes in the dominant variant of the virus, response to or complications from therapies prior to ECMO, or clinicians offering ECLS to patients with intractable conditions. In later waves, patients had progressed to needing ECLS despite receiving therapies associated with an improved outcome and this may have placed them in a poorer prognostic group. Patients in later waves were more likely to have additional bacterial coinfections, possibly as a consequence of immunosuppression for COVID-19 and these infective complications were associated with increased mortality.[12,13]

Mortality prediction tools including the RESP and PRESERVE score have been developed for patients with severe ARDS using the associations described above.[8,14] These tools, similar to other population level scoring systems, may be able to help guide clinicians and families about prognosis but are not necessarily predictive on an individual level. It is important to appreciate that these scores were generated with data from patients who had been commenced on ECLS, therefore their ability to be used as a predictive tool prior to the decision to cannulate is unclear.

## Complications of VV ECMO

The morbidity and mortality of extracorporeal respiratory support is significant even as techniques and clinical management are improving. Complications directly related to using VV ECMO impact patient outcomes, with one metaanalysis estimating that the mortality due to complications during VV ECMO is around 6.9%.[15] The iatrogenic insult caused by the ECMO circuit explains why VV ECMO is not used as soon as possible in adult patients with acute reversible respiratory failure but only after failure of conventional support. Awareness and early recognition of complications related to the use of VV ECMO allow prompt treatment, improved outcome, and support the development of new technical or clinical preventative strategies. Complications of VV ECMO can be divided into circuit-related

complications, complications associated with cannulation, and coagulation-related issues.

### *Circuit-related Complications*

Early ECLS systems were prone to catastrophic mechanical failures, including rupture of tubing, plasma leak, or over heating of pumps. The development of polymethylpentene membrane oxygenators and centrifugal pumps reduced the occurrence of these issues. Mechanical or electrical failure are still possible and result in a life-threatening event requiring emergent pump or circuit exchange (Chapter 7). Backup components and trained staff must therefore be immediately available.

There are no standard and agreed indications to change components or a circuit at regular intervals during VV ECMO. The level of systemic anticoagulation, duration of support, configuration of the circuit, make of components, and patient physiopathology will affect how often or how quickly a component may fail. Progressive clotting of the membrane lung with accompanying hyperfibrinolysis and reduction in gas transfer was reported in an ELSO Registry analysis in 16.8 % of 7579 adult patients (noting that patients with preexisting coagulopathy, disseminated intravascular coagulation, active bleeding, or stroke had been excluded).[16] A single center analysis in 265 adult patients on VV ECMO devices found that at least one component needed changing in 83 patients, with 45% acute and 55% elective interventions.[17] Reasons included pump head thrombosis, acute oxygenator thrombosis, progressive clot formation, worsening of gas exchange, ongoing device-associated coagulation disorder, or suspected circuit infection. Progressive clot formation in the membrane oxygenator can be monitored by serial measurement of D-dimers in the plasma,[18-20] although no cutoff value is indicative of a need to change the circuit. Levels of D-dimers can be influenced by other clinical conditions (eg, deep vein thrombosis) or pharmacological interventions (eg, antifibrinolytic medications). Contamination and colonization by bacteria of membrane oxygenators in septic patients have been described and can be associated with hyperfibrinolysis and bleeding.[21]

A small amount of hemolysis commonly occurs during VV ECMO, and previous studies often did not differentiate between VA and VV ECMO. Hemolysis, defined by plasma free hemoglobin greater than 500 mg/L within 24 hours after cannulation, occurred in 3.9% of survivors and 15.9% of nonsurvivors in a study of 154 adult patients receiving VA and VV ECMO.[22] A Cox proportional hazard analysis identified hemolysis as an independent predictor of mortality (OR 3.4, 95% confidence interval: 1.3-8.8, p=0.01).[22] A retrospective, single-center study of 318 adult patients with acute respiratory failure concluded that marked hemolysis was not common in VV ECMO with modern devices.[23] Several studies suggested a link between degree of hemolysis and outcome. In 2022, Nunez et al. reported a prevalence of 5.3% hemolysis and this was associated with increased mortality (adjusted OR 1.38 (1.05, 1.81).[16] Multiple trauma, need for renal replacement therapy, increased daily red blood cell transfusion requirements, and high blood flow rates (3.0–4.5 L/min) through small-sized cannulas significantly increased hemolysis. Clinically relevant hemolysis can be caused by pumphead thrombosis.[23] Hemolysis was observed in 1063 adult consecutive patients with VA and VV ECMO and was significantly more frequent in VA ECMO when compared with VV ECMO (4% vs. 2%). Hemolysis due to pumphead thrombosis was more frequent in VV ECMO compared with VA ECMO (9% vs. 2%). ECPR and cardiac surgery are both associated with an increase in the incidence of hemolysis, irrespective of the use of ECLS.[24] Hemolysis may be more frequent in the pediatric and neonatal population. Hemolysis in VV ECMO can be decreased by ensuring the circuit access

pressures are above -100 mmHg and avoiding turbulent flow and high flow velocity. Routine monitoring of hemolysis might help to detect clot formation in the pumphead.

Air entrainment in the ECMO circuit is a complication that can cause the pump to fail to propel blood. Air will be entrained by the negative pressure generated on the drainage side and may originate from any intravascular access located in a major vein, or partial decannulation. Access ports to the circuit before the pump are a risk and should only be used by teams trained in detecting and correcting any air entrainment immediately.

### Complications of Cannulation

Complications related to the insertion of a cannula are similar to those encountered with any central venous cannulation but are likely magnified as the cannula size increases (Chapter 4). A combined analysis of the EOLIA and CESAR trials reported a fatal complication rate related to cannulation in 3 of 225 patients (1.3%).[5] The ELSO Registry (April 2021) reported cannula problems in 5.5% of adult patients with respiratory support,[25] while Nunez et al. described 9.8% of cannulation site bleeding.[16] The cannula or guidewire can lead to cardiac perforation with associated tamponade, or major blood vessel injury resulting in retroperitoneal bleed or hemothorax. Cannulation using ultrasound guidance and fluoroscopy or transoesophageal echocardiography decreases the risk of major cannulation complications.[26] Ischemia of the cannulated limb is common in arterial cannulation (VA ECMO) and can occasionally occur in VV ECMO by compression of the adjacent artery, hematoma at the insertion site, or injury of the artery during cannulation.[27]

The team should be prepared to deal with a perforation at the time of cannulation, including but not limited to the immediate availability of red blood cell concentrates. Experience in central venous cannulation is required, and adjuvants such as fluoroscopy while inserting cannulae might prove useful.

Deep vein thrombosis (DVT) during or after ECLS has been underdiagnosed for many years. Rastan et al. in 2006 described 25 clinically unrecognized DVT or pulmonary embolism (PE) in 78 postmortem examinations of patients who were supported with ECLS after cardiotomy.[28] The prevalence of DVT in cannulated vessels has been reported at 8.1/1,000 cannula days.[29] In a prospective study of 172 patients who were still alive after ECLS decannulation, any thrombosis was identified in 106 patients (62%), with 48 (28%) being deemed clinically significant.[30] The incidence of DVT was higher in patients with a mean aPTT of ≤50 seconds (odds ratio, 1.02; p=0.013) and in patients with a sustained elevation of D-dimers following decannulation.[30] Routine venous Doppler ultrasound following decannulation might inform subsequent anticoagulation management, although no randomized control trial has established the risk/benefit ratio of this. Attempting to decrease the incidence of DVTs is one of the reasons to continue using systemic anticoagulation in patients supported with ECLS.

Cannulas should be secured with care and attention, as dislodgement would be life threatening. Infection at the cannula insertion site was seen in 14% of patients supported with ECLS in the EOLIA trial.[3] Percutaneous insertion is preferrable to decrease the risk of infection. Meticulous fixation and nursing care are required.

### Coagulation-related Issues

The coagulation system is affected during VV ECMO. This activation is part of a wider inflammatory response initiated by the exposure of blood to a foreign surface. It is in part mitigated by the administration of heparin or other anticoagulants. All patients supported with extracorporeal circulation usually develop an acquired von Willebrand syndrome, at least partially explaining the increased incidence of bleeding.[31] This disturbance recovers quickly after discontinuation of ECLS.

In the EOLIA trial, patients supported with ECLS had significantly higher rates of very severe thrombocytopenia than those in the control group (<20,000 platelets per cubic millimeter; 27% vs. 16%; absolute risk difference, 11 percentage points; 95% CI, 0 to 21) and more bleeding events leading to packed red-cell transfusion (46% vs. 28%; absolute risk difference, 18 percentage points; 95% CI, 6 to 30).[3] The rate of ischemic stroke was lower in the ECLS group than in the control group (no patients vs. 5%; absolute risk difference, -5 percentage points; 95% CI, -10 to -2), and the rate of hemorrhagic stroke was similar in the two groups. Among all the patients who were treated with ECLS, the rate of bleeding was 53% and the rate of hematoma at the cannula insertion site was 6%.[3]

The most commonly observed coagulation issue while on VV ECMO is the activation and destruction of platelets. Thrombocytopenia appears to be an important risk factor for intracranial bleeding while on ECLS.[32] In a meta-analysis and systematic review, Jiritano et al. found a prevalence of severe thrombocytopenia (defined as less than 50 000/µl) of 25.4% in VV ECMO (95% CI 10.6-61.4; 4 studies).[33] A similar incidence has been reported by others.[34] APACHE II score and platelet count at the time of ECLS initiation were predictors for severe thrombocytopenia but the duration of ECLS was not.[3] Lebreton et al. reported a lower incidence of 18% of severe thrombocytopenia in a series of patients with COVID-19.[35] Weingart et al. found a decrease in the platelet count to 60% of the platelet counts measured prior to ECLS.[36] This decrease was not observed in patients treated with interventional lung assist, a pumpless arteriovenous $CO_2$ removal device. There is no consensus on the platelet count at which transfusion is recommended, although some have advised a liberal platelet transfusion strategy (Chapter 24).[32] Platelet counts usually recover rapidly after discontinuation of ECLS.[36,37]

Thrombocytopenia can be the result of heparin-induced thrombocytopenia (HIT). HIT is a clinical syndrome that can occur in patients treated with heparin and can have devastating consequences. Antibodies against heparin-platelet factor 4 complexes lead to the formation of arterial and venous thrombus and thrombocytopenia. The diagnosis of HIT in ECLS patients is difficult. The incidence of HIT during ECLS range widely between studies, perhaps because of a lack a standardized diagnostic workup, merging different types of ECLS, or various patient populations. Jiritano et al. reported a prevalence of HIT of 3.7% (95% CI 1.8-5.5; 12 studies) in VV ECMO[33]; whereas, Choi et al. found an incidence of confirmed HIT of 17% in an analysis of 309 patients in 6 retrospective studies.[38] Arachchillage et al. described an incidence of 5.1% of HIT in 156 patients on VV ECMO, which was not different to VA ECMO (11 HIT/142 patients).[37]

Thrombocytopenia and the presence of thromboembolic complications should trigger a detailed workup with hematologists to confirm or exclude heparin induced thrombocytopenia (HIT). Using an alternative anticoagulant such as argatroban or bivalirudin is advisable while HIT testing is performed. A platelet aggregation test or serotonin release assay are required to confirm the diagnosis in the presence of clinical signs. The ELISA test for platelet-factor-4 antibodies is not reliable due to a high false positive rate but might be useful when negative in the presence of a high clinical suspicion (ie, HIT can be excluded if the test is negative when the clinical presumption is high). It is not clear if heparin-coated circuits should be replaced in patients with HIT. A single center experience in 455 patients with confirmed HIT in 14 patients demonstrated no increased mortality when continuing with heparin-coated circuits despite discontinuing systemic heparin.[39]

### Infection and ECLS

Infections are common in patients receiving ECLS for severe respiratory failure, either as the primary initiating event or as a secondary complication.[2,40] *Staphylococcus aureus*, Enterobacterales, and yeasts are the most commonly reported cultured organisms. Infections are associated with an increased duration of ECLS support and increased mortality.[12,40] Patients with severe asthma, influenza, or COVID-19 are more likely to be supported with ECLS if they have a bacterial or fungal infection at presentation.[10,13]

Secondary infections while on ECMO are more likely in older age, with underlying immunodeficiency, and with increasing severity of illness.[40] Exposure of blood to circuit components may cause immune dysfunction leading to an increased risk of infections,[41] but in one randomized trial, blood stream infections, ventilator associated pneumonia, and other nosocomial infections were not more frequent than in patients with a similar severity of illness not supported with ECLS.[3] Similarly, the incidence of fungal infections is not higher than in the general ICU population, even if associated with a high mortality for patients supported on ECLS.[42] Nonetheless, source control can be harder to achieve during ECLS (Chapter 6).

Reports describe infection of the cannula site and/or the ECMO membrane,[21,43] including some shown through culture or DNA analysis of removed circuit components. The true incidence of cannula or circuit infections is unknown and is hampered by the lack of an accepted definition.[40] The impact of circuit component infection on patient outcome is not known.

## Followup and Long-term Outcomes after ECLS

Advances in critical care medicine have resulted in an increased number of patients surviving after a severe illness requiring ECLS support. However, survival is associated with long-term morbidity and healthcare utilization.[44] Patients on VV ECMO may have prolonged ICU and hospital length of stay, often exceeding a month.[45] Evaluation of the impact of ECMO on long-term recovery, including pulmonary function, quality of life (QoL) and physical, psychological and cognitive functioning, is crucial for clinical decisions about use of the therapy. The current evidence is limited due to the large number of single-center studies with small sample sizes, the lack of information about the level of functioning prior to the critical illness, and the lack of standardized definitions.[44,46]

In a recent systematic review of the QoL of adult patients on VV ECMO for ARDS, eight studies were eligible for inclusion, including one randomized controlled trial (n=441[47]). Regardless of the followup time, all included studies showed a decrease in the health-related QoL (HRQoL) score of patients with ARDS after VV ECMO. Compared to a matched general population, HRQoL was lower in patients with ARDS after VV ECMO. However, in survivors of ARDS, HRQoL was similar between ARDS patients treated with VV ECMO and conventional ventilatory support. In one single-center study, survival was similar in patients managed on ECLS compared to conventional ventilatory support at one year (22/33 vs. 28/47, 66% vs. 59%), and pulmonary function and computed tomography were almost normal in both groups.[48] Patients managed on conventional ventilatory support had lower HRQoL scores and higher rates of posttraumatic stress disorder, although this may have been due to baseline differences in comorbidities, which were more common in patients on conventional

ventilatory support. One of the largest studies published to date reported outcomes of 84 survivors at 6 months.[14] In that cohort, 36% reported exertional dyspnea and 30% were still receiving pulmonary treatment at a median of 17 months followup. HRQoL in 80% of the survivors revealed satisfactory mental health but persistent problems with physical and psychological function.

The COVID-19 pandemic has resulted in a large number of adults being managed with ARDS on ECLS, raising questions about the long-term outcomes of this group. A recent international multicenter retrospective review of 132 patients with severe COVID-19-related ARDS supported with ECLS reported six-month mortality of 53% (70 of 132[49]). Importantly, pre-ECLS cannulation determinants of six-month outcomes were identified. Patients ≥60 years of age and patients with a pH <7.23 were found to have a higher six-month mortality. This study provided insight into the long-term outcomes (six months) of patients requiring ECLS for COVID-19 related ARDS.

# References

1.  Pham T, Rubenfeld GD. Fifty Years of Research in ARDS. The Epidemiology of Acute Respiratory Distress Syndrome. A 50th Birthday Review. American journal of respiratory and critical care medicine. Apr 1 2017;195(7):860-870.

2.  Thiagarajan RR, Barbaro RP, Rycus PT, et al. Extracorporeal Life Support Organization Registry International Report 2016. ASAIO Journal. 2017;63(1):60-67.

3.  Combes A, Hajage D, Capellier G, et al. Extracorporeal Membrane Oxygenation for Severe Acute Respiratory Distress Syndrome. The New England journal of medicine. May 24 2018;378(21):1965-1975.

4.  Peek GJ, Mugford M, Tiruvoipati R, et al. Efficacy and economic assessment of conventional ventilatory support versus extracorporeal membrane oxygenation for severe adult respiratory failure (CESAR): a multicentre randomised controlled trial. Lancet (London, England). Oct 17 2009;374(9698):1351-63.

5.  Combes A, Peek GJ, Hajage D, et al. ECMO for severe ARDS: systematic review and individual patient data meta-analysis. Intensive care medicine. Nov 2020;46(11):2048-2057.

6.  Warren A, Chiu YD, Villar SS, et al. Outcomes of the NHS England National Extracorporeal Membrane Oxygenation Service for adults with respiratory failure: a multicentre observational cohort study. Br J Anaesth. Sep 2020;125(3):259-266.

7.  O'Neil ER, Lin H, Li M, et al. Extracorporeal Membrane Oxygenation Support for Influenza A: Retrospective Review of the Extracorporeal Life Support Organization Registry Comparing H1N1 With Other Subtypes. Crit Care Explor. Dec 2021;3(12):e0598.

8.  Schmidt M, Bailey M, Sheldrake J, et al. Predicting survival after extracorporeal membrane oxygenation for severe acute respiratory failure. The Respiratory Extracorporeal Membrane Oxygenation Survival Prediction (RESP) score. American journal of respiratory and critical care medicine. Jun 1 2014;189(11):1374-82.

9.  Barbaro RP, Odetola FO, Kidwell KM, et al. Association of hospital-level volume of extracorporeal membrane oxygenation cases and mortality. Analysis of the extracorporeal life support organization registry. American journal of respiratory and critical care medicine. Apr 15 2015;191(8):894-901.

10. Barbaro RP, MacLaren G, Boonstra PS, et al. Extracorporeal membrane oxygenation for COVID-19: evolving outcomes from the international Extracorporeal Life Support Organization Registry. Lancet (London, England). Oct 2 2021;398(10307):1230-1238.

11. Schmidt M, Langouet E, Hajage D, et al. Evolving outcomes of extracorporeal membrane oxygenation support for severe COVID-19 ARDS in Sorbonne hospitals, Paris. Critical care (London, England). Oct 9 2021;25(1):355.

12. Dognon N, Gaudet A, Parmentier-Decrucq E, et al. Extracorporeal Membrane Oxygenation for COVID 2019-Acute Respiratory Distress Syndrome: Comparison between First and Second Waves (Stage 2). J Clin Med. Oct 21 2021;10(21).

13. Bergman ZR, Wothe JK, Alwan FS, et al. Risk Factors of Mortality for Patients Receiving Venovenous Extracorporeal Membrane Oxygenation for COVID-19 Acute Respiratory Distress Syndrome. Surg Infect (Larchmt). Dec 2021;22(10):1086-1092.

14. Schmidt M, Zogheib E, Rozé H, et al. The PRESERVE mortality risk score and analysis of long-term outcomes after extracorporeal membrane oxygenation for severe acute respiratory distress syndrome. Intensive care medicine. Oct 2013;39(10):1704-13.

15. Vaquer S, de Haro C, Peruga P, Oliva JC, Artigas A. Systematic review and meta-analysis of complications and mortality of veno-venous extracorporeal membrane oxygenation for refractory acute respiratory distress syndrome. Ann Intensive Care. Dec 2017;7(1):51.

16. Nunez JI, Gosling AF, O'Gara B, et al. Bleeding and thrombotic events in adults supported with venovenous extracorporeal membrane oxygenation: an ELSO registry analysis. Intensive care medicine. Feb 2022;48(2):213-224.

17. Lubnow M, Philipp A, Foltan M, et al. Technical complications during veno-venous extracorporeal membrane oxygenation and their relevance predicting a system-exchange--retrospective analysis of 265 cases. PLoS One. 2014;9(12):e112316.

18. Dornia C, Philipp A, Bauer S, et al. D-dimers Are a Predictor of Clot Volume Inside Membrane Oxygenators During Extracorporeal Membrane Oxygenation. Artif Organs. Sep 2015;39(9):782-7.

19. Basken R, Cosgrove R, Malo J, et al. Predictors of Oxygenator Exchange in Patients Receiving Extracorporeal Membrane Oxygenation. J Extra Corpor Technol. Jun 2019;51(2):61-66.

20. Lubnow M, Philipp A, Dornia C, et al. D-dimers as an early marker for oxygenator exchange in extracorporeal membrane oxygenation. J Crit Care. Jun 2014;29(3):473.e1-5.

21. Müller T, Lubnow M, Philipp A, et al. Risk of circuit infection in septic patients on extracorporeal membrane oxygenation: a preliminary study. Artif Organs. Apr 2011;35(4):E84-90.

22. Omar HR, Mirsaeidi M, Socias S, et al. Plasma Free Hemoglobin Is an Independent Predictor of Mortality among Patients on Extracorporeal

Membrane Oxygenation Support. PLoS One. 2015;10(4):e0124034.

23. Lehle K, Philipp A, Zeman F, et al. Technical-Induced Hemolysis in Patients with Respiratory Failure Supported with Veno-Venous ECMO - Prevalence and Risk Factors. PLoS One. 2015;10(11):e0143527.

24. Appelt H, Philipp A, Mueller T, et al. Factors associated with hemolysis during extracorporeal membrane oxygenation (ECMO)-Comparison of VA-versus VV ECMO. PLoS One. 2020;15(1):e0227793.

25. ELSO. Extracorporeal Life Support Organisation Registry International Report 2021. https://www.elso.org/Portals/0/Files/Reports/2021_April/International%20Report%20April_page1.pdf

26. Burns J, Cooper E, Salt G, et al. Retrospective Observational Review of Percutaneous Cannulation for Extracorporeal Membrane Oxygenation. Asaio J. May-Jun 2016;62(3):325-8.

27. Wang L, Yang F, Zhang S, et al. Percutaneous versus surgical cannulation for femoro-femoral VA-ECMO in patients with cardiogenic shock: Results from the Extracorporeal Life Support Organization Registry. J Heart Lung Transplant. Jan 10 2022.

28. Rastan AJ, Lachmann N, Walther T, et al. Autopsy findings in patients on postcardiotomy extracorporeal membrane oxygenation (ECMO). Int J Artif Organs. Dec 2006;29(12):1121-31.

29. Cooper E, Burns J, Retter A, et al. Prevalence of Venous Thrombosis Following Venovenous Extracorporeal Membrane Oxygenation in Patients With Severe Respiratory Failure. Crit Care Med. Dec 2015;43(12):e581-4.

30. Fisser C, Reichenbächer C, Müller T, et al. Incidence and Risk Factors for Cannula-Related Venous Thrombosis After Venovenous Extracorporeal Membrane Oxygenation in Adult Patients With Acute Respiratory Failure. Crit Care Med. Apr 2019;47(4):e332-e339.

31. Kalbhenn J, Schlagenhauf A, Rosenfelder S, Schmutz A, Zieger B. Acquired von Willebrand syndrome and impaired platelet function during venovenous extracorporeal membrane oxygenation: Rapid onset and fast recovery. J Heart Lung Transplant. Aug 2018;37(8):985-991.

32. Cavayas YA, Del Sorbo L, Fan E. Intracranial hemorrhage in adults on ECMO. Perfusion. May 2018;33(1_suppl):42-50.

33. Jiritano F, Serraino GF, Ten Cate H, et al. Platelets and extra-corporeal membrane oxygenation in adult patients: a systematic review and meta-analysis. Intensive care medicine. Jun 2020;46(6):1154-1169.

34. Abrams D, Baldwin MR, Champion M, et al. Thrombocytopenia and extracorporeal membrane oxygenation in adults with acute respiratory

35. Lebreton G, Schmidt M, Ponnaiah M, et al. Extracorporeal membrane oxygenation network organisation and clinical outcomes during the COVID-19 pandemic in Greater Paris, France: a multicentre cohort study. Lancet Respir Med. Aug 2021;9(8):851-862.

36. Weingart C, Lubnow M, Philipp A, Bein T, Camboni D, Müller T. Comparison of Coagulation Parameters, Anticoagulation, and Need for Transfusion in Patients on Interventional Lung Assist or Veno-Venous Extracorporeal Membrane Oxygenation. Artif Organs. Sep 2015;39(9):765-73.

37. Arachchillage DRJ, Laffan M, Khanna S, et al. Frequency of Thrombocytopenia and Heparin-Induced Thrombocytopenia in Patients Receiving Extracorporeal Membrane Oxygenation Compared With Cardiopulmonary Bypass and the Limited Sensitivity of Pretest Probability Score. Crit Care Med. May 2020;48(5):e371-e379.

38. Choi JH, Luc JGY, Weber MP, et al. Heparin-induced thrombocytopenia during extracorporeal life support: incidence, management and outcomes. Ann Cardiothorac Surg. Jan 2019;8(1):19-31.

39. Pabst D, Boone JB, Soleimani B, Brehm CE. Heparin-induced thrombocytopenia in patients on extracorporeal membrane oxygenation and the role of a heparin-bonded circuit. Perfusion. 2019;34(7):584-589.

40. Abrams D, Grasselli G, Schmidt M, Mueller T, Brodie D. ECLS-associated infections in adults: what we know and what we don't yet know. Intensive care medicine. Feb 2020;46(2):182-191.

41. Ki KK, Millar JE, Langguth D, et al. Current Understanding of Leukocyte Phenotypic and Functional Modulation During Extracorporeal Membrane Oxygenation: A Narrative Review. Front Immunol. 2020;11:600684.

42. Cavayas YA, Yusuff H, Porter R. Fungal infections in adult patients on extracorporeal life support. Critical care (London, England). Apr 17 2018;22(1):98.

43. Winiszewski H, Boyadjian C, Besch G, et al. Extracorporeal Membrane Oxygenation Cannula-Related Infections: Epidemiology and Risk Factors. Asaio j. Jun 1 2021.

44. Wilcox ME, Jaramillo-Rocha V, Hodgson C, Taglione MS, Ferguson ND, Fan E. Long-Term Quality of Life After Extracorporeal Membrane Oxygenation in ARDS Survivors: Systematic Review and Meta-Analysis. J Intensive Care Med. Mar 2020;35(3):233-243.

45. Schmidt M, Pham T, Arcadipane A, et al. Mechanical Ventilation Management during Extracorporeal Membrane Oxygenation for Acute Respiratory Distress

Syndrome. An International Multicenter Prospective Cohort. American journal of respiratory and critical care medicine. Oct 15 2019;200(8):1002-1012.

46. Hodgson CL, Fulcher B, Mariajoseph FP, et al. A Core Outcome Set for Research in Patients on Extracorporeal Membrane Oxygenation. Crit Care Med. Dec 1 2021;49(12):e1252-e1254.

47. Kurniawati ER, Rutjens VGH, Vranken NPA, et al. Quality of life following adult veno-venous extracorporeal membrane oxygenation for acute respiratory distress syndrome: a systematic review. Qual Life Res. Aug 2021;30(8):2123-2135.

48. Grasselli G, Scaravilli V, Tubiolo D, et al. Quality of Life and Lung Function in Survivors of Extracorporeal Membrane Oxygenation for Acute Respiratory Distress Syndrome. Anesthesiology. Apr 2019;130(4):572-580.

49. Biancari F, Mariscalco G, Dalén M, et al. Six-Month Survival After Extracorporeal Membrane Oxygenation for Severe COVID-19. J Cardiothorac Vasc Anesth. Jul 2021;35(7):1999-2006.

# 27

## Initiating Extracorporeal Life Support for Adult Cardiac Failure

*Silvia Mariani, Joseph E. Tonna, Hergen Buscher, Justin A. Fried, Katarzyna Hryniewicz, Roberto Lorusso*

## Introduction

### *Cardiogenic Shock: Definition, Epidemiology, and Pathophysiology*

Cardiogenic shock (CS) is a life-threatening clinical syndrome characterized by cardiac dysfunction resulting in end-organ hypoperfusion and tissue hypoxia.[1] The diagnosis of CS is marked by clinical signs of hypoperfusion, such as cold sweated extremities, oliguria, confusion, dizziness, and narrow pulse pressure. Additionally, hypoperfusion, tissue hypoxia and organ dysfunction are evident through metabolic acidosis and elevated serum lactate.[1,2] Despite the fact that previous definitions of CS included hemodynamic parameters, such as hypotension (systolic blood pressure <90 mmHg for more than 30 min), reduced cardiac index (CI <2.2 L/min/m2), elevated pulmonary capillary wedge pressure (PCWP) or the need for catecholamines, compensatory mechanisms may preserve blood pressure through vasoconstriction, even as tissue perfusion and oxygenation are significantly decreased.[1,2]

The precipitating causes of CS are diverse and include acute events such as acute myocardial infarction, myocarditis or malignant arrhythmias, as well as the progression of chronic heart failure. CS can also result as a complication of cardiac surgery, coronary angioplasty, pulmonary embolism or pulmonary diseases. Cardiac arrest represents the most extreme cardiac compromise (Chapter 32).

CS accounts for 2-5% of all patients presenting with acute heart failure (AHF) and is associated with an in-hospital mortality of 30-60%.[1] About half of in-hospital deaths occur within the first 24 hours of presentation.[1] Historically, the most common cause of CS has been acute coronary syndrome (ACS). Indeed, 5-10% of patients with a myocardial infarction may develop CS.[3-8] However, the contribution of ACS has declined over the past two decades and the incidence of other etiologies, such as acute decompensated chronic heart failure, are increasing.[9,10] Overall, CS resulting from causes other than ACS are often more complex to treat but may have a better or at least comparable short-term outcome.[1]

The pathophysiology of CS begins with an initial cardiac insult which impairs myocardial contractility and consequently cardiac output, leading to elevated cardiac filling pressures and hypotension.[1] After this first trigger event, the pathological spiral of cardiogenic shock can rapidly result in multiorgan systemic dysfunction and death (Figure 27-1).

### Classification of Cardiogenic Shock and Role of ECLS

CS management must simultaneously target the underlying cardiac condition and stop the consequent negative cascade which can be described according to the Society for Cardiovascular Angiography and Interventions[11] classification (Figure 27-2). Stage C is characterized by hypoperfusion, which may include signs of organ failure and the requirement for inotropes, vasopressors, or mechanical support, including ECLS. In stage D the patient deteriorates despite these initial interventions, with a mortality rate higher than 40%.[12] The threshold for the use of ECLS has so far not been clearly defined but it seems reasonable to consider ECLS from stage D or, if modified by cardiac arrest, from stage C. Overall, ECLS should be considered in case of refractory CS within 6 hours of its occurrence,

and in patients with reversible circulatory collapse or eligibility for durable ventricular assist device (VAD) or transplantation.[13] Ideally, VA ECMO should be initiated before the onset of irreversible end-organ damage and anaerobic metabolism. Indeed, arterial lactate equal or greater than 10 mmol/L (90.1 mg/dL) at ECLS initiation and its delayed clearance in the first 12-24 hours identifies patients with poor outcomes.[14-16] Etiologies compromising appropriate ECLS function should be considered as potential contraindications (Table 27-1). Poor life expectancy, severe liver disease, acute brain injury, vascular disease, and immunocompromise represent exclusion criteria for ECLS application.[13]

### Acute Coronary Syndrome

ACS remains the leading cause of morbidity and mortality worldwide, despite significant

## Pathophysiological Response to Cardiogenic Shock

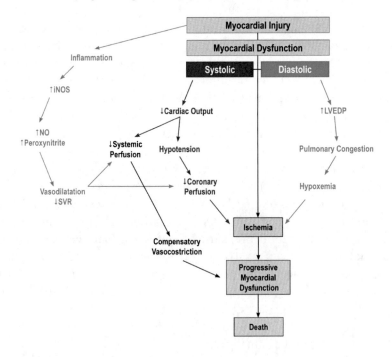

**Figure 27-1.** Pathophysiological Response to Cardiogenic Shock. LVEDP=left ventricular end-diastolic pressure; NO=nitric oxide; SVR=systemic vascular resistance.

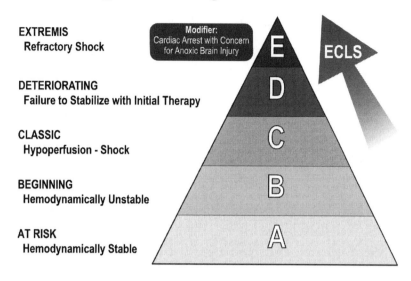

# SCAI Stages of Cardiogenic Shock and ECLS

**EXTREMIS**
Refractory Shock

Modifier:
Cardiac Arrest with Concern
for Anoxic Brain Injury

E

ECLS

**DETERIORATING**
Failure to Stabilize with Initial Therapy

D

**CLASSIC**
Hypoperfusion - Shock

C

**BEGINNING**
Hemodynamically Unstable

B

**AT RISK**
Hemodynamically Stable

A

| E | A patient with refractory shock or actual/impeding circulatory collapse. |
|---|---|
| D | A patient who has clinical evidence of shock that worsens or fails to improve despite escalation of therapy |
| C | A patient who has clinical evidence of hypoperfusion that initially requires pharmacologic or **mechanical support**. Hypotension is usually present |
| B | A patient who has clinical evidence of hemodynamic instability (hypotension, tachycardia or abnormal systemic hemodynamics) without hypoperfusion |
| A | A hemodynamically stable patient who is not experiencing signs or symptoms of CS, but is at risk for its development |

**Figure 27-2.** Society for Cardiovascular Angiography and Interventions (SCAI) staging for cardiogenic shock. CS=cardiogenic shock.

---

- Cardiac recovery unlikely and no indication for heart transplant or durable left ventricular (LV) assist device

- Poor life expectancy (end-stage peripheral organ disease, malignant tumor, massive pulmonary emboli in cancer patients, chemotherapy-induced chronic cardiomyopathy, etc.)

- Severe aortic valve regurgitation

- Severe vascular disease with extensive aortic and peripheral vessel involvement (calcification, stenosis, and closure), including axillary arteries

- Acute Type A or B aortic dissection with extensive aortic branch (ascending, supra-aortic and femoral) involvement (pre-operatively)

- Severe neurologic impairment (eg, prolonged anoxic brain damage, extensive trauma and bleeding)

- Severe immunologic disease with marked blood and coagulation disorders

- Liver cirrhosis (Child-Pugh class B and C)

---

**Table 27-1.** Contraindications to ECLS initiation for cardiac failure in adult patients. Adapted with permission from Lorusso et al.[13]

improvements in access to medical care and revascularization.[17-19] Indeed, the 30-day mortality of patients suffering from ST-segment–elevation myocardial infarction (STEMI) is around 14%, with the highest mortality of patients experiencing CS. Of the 5-10% of myocardial infarction patients affected by CS, 30–40% of cases develop it at admission, while 60–70% occur later during the hospitalization.[1] Overall, the prevalence of CS following STEMI has decreased in the last few decades, but in-hospital mortality has remained unchanged at 35–50%.[1,17-19]

Initial evaluation of CS following STEMI (STEMI-CS) should include a Swan-Ganz catheter, lactate, calculation of cardiac output, cardiac power output (CPO, with normal values >0.6) and pulmonary artery pulsatility index (PAPI, with a normal value >1.85), which is strongly associated with in-hospital mortality and right ventricular dysfunction.[20] Further mortality predictors are presented in Table 27-2.[21-23]

Although primary percutaneous coronary intervention (PCI) of the culprit vessel is a Class 1 ACC/AHA recommendation for treatment of STEMI, recent data suggests that, in patients with STEMI-CS, restoration of circulation with mechanical circulatory support (MCS) may be beneficial prior to revascularization[24] and may be considered depending on patient age, comorbidities, neurological function, and the prospects for long-term survival and quality of life (2021 ESC guidelines: Class IIb, Level of evidence C).[2,18]

In patients with isolated left ventricular dysfunction, temporary left ventricular assist device (eg, Impella, Abiomed, Danvers, USA) can be considered as first line MCS.[25] In patients with advanced, SCAI D or E shock, including patients in cardiac arrest, VA ECMO is the only device that can provide full cardiopulmonary support and should be implemented prior to revascularization.[26,27] In addition, percutaneous right ventricular assist device (RVAD) can be considered in isolated right ventricular failure due to inferior STEMI. Finally, in patients suffering from STEMI-CS and supported with peripheral VA ECMO with LVEF <30%, low pulse pressures (<20 mmHg) and/or elevated pulmonary capillary wedge pressure (PCWP >18 mmHg), it is recommended to consider further LV unloading as described in Chapter 44.

### Acute Decompensated Chronic Heart Failure

In parallel with the decrease in the overall incidence of STEMI-CS,[19] non-ACS etiologies such as acute decompensated heart failure (ADHF) have become more frequent. In an analysis of 2093 patients admitted to North American cardiac care units from 2017 to 2020, 67% percent of patients had CS unrelated to ACS.[28]

There is growing evidence that ADHF-CS may have distinct characteristics to ACS, and it necessitates a unique approach.[29-33] In contrast to patients with AHF or STEMI-CS, patients with preexisting cardiomyopathy are less likely to achieve sufficient ventricular recovery to liberate from ECLS support without the need for heart replacement therapy (eg, durable VAD or heart transplantation). In a study of 52 patients with chronic heart failure that

| CLINICAL PARAMETER | |
|---|---|
| Age >73 years | 1 |
| Prior stroke | 2 |
| Glucose >10.6 mmol/L (191 mg/dl) | 1 |
| Creatinine >132.6 μmol/L (1.5 mg/dl) | 1 |
| TIMI <3 after PCI | 2 |
| Lactate >5 mmol/L | 2 |

**Table 27-2.** IABP-SHOCK II trial predictors of 30-day mortality in acute coronary syndrome related cardiogenic shock.[21,23]

underwent ECLS for cardiogenic shock, 44.2% underwent durable VAD placement during the index hospitalization with a survival to discharge of 82.6%, while of the 29 patients who did not receive durable VAD, the survival to discharge was only 17.2%.[30] This emphasizes the need for early evaluation for VAD (ECLS as bridge-to-VAD) or heart transplantation (ECLS as bridge-to-transplantation) in patients with ADHF-CS who are placed on ECLS. Their potential candidacy for heart replacement therapies should be considered in the decision to initiate ECLS support (Chapter 30).

Historically, posttransplant outcomes of patients bridged with ECLS have been poor,[34] although high volume ECLS and heart transplant centers may be able to achieve better outcomes.[35] While heart transplantation after ECLS has increased, it remains a viable option for only a small minority of adults, given donor organ scarcity.[36] At the same time, the use of ECLS as bridge to durable VAD has significantly increased in the new VAD era.[37-39] ECLS is an option for select ADHF-CS patients who are not candidates for heart transplant, as well as patients who are eligible for transplant but at high risk for further decompensation and mortality during the waiting time. ECLS provides systemic perfusion and can facilitate preoperative optimization before VAD implantation. Despite this, preoperative use of ECLS has been associated with higher rates of mortality and adverse event rates in the early postoperative period following durable VAD implantation.[40] As the complication rate of ECLS tends to increase with duration of support, transition to durable VAD should occur in a timely fashion after recovery of end-organ function is achieved in suitable candidates. It is important to note that while one of the major benefits of ECLS is its capacity to unload the right ventricle, assessment of native RV function and risk of postoperative RV failure after VAD implantation may be challenging while patients are supported with ECLS.

## Isolated Right Ventricular Failure

### Pathophysiology and Etiology of Right Ventricular Failure

In adults the RV shape and function is profoundly related to the interplay with the LV, based on the role of the interventricular septum which intrudes into the RV. Vice versa, a failing RV negatively impacts on the LV through a distortion of its functional capacity as well as through a reduction in preload. This is the basic pathophysiological pattern which can develop in case of RV failure due to increased pulmonary resistance, fulminant acute RV disease, or decompensation of chronic conditions as listed in Table 27-3.[41] Furthermore, most of these conditions require mechanical ventilation which

| ACUTE CONDITIONS | DECOMPENSATED CHRONIC CONDITION |
|---|---|
| Acute core pulmonale | Chronic core pulmonale |
| - Pulmonary embolism | - Interstitial lung disease |
|   o Thromboembolic | - Obstructive lung disease |
|   o Fat embolism | - Alveolar hypoventilation |
|   o Air embolism | - Primary pulmonary hypertension |
|   o Amniotic fluid | Congenital cardiac disease |
| - ARDS | Intra-cardiac shunt |
| - LV failure | Connective tissue disease |
| Primary RV failure | Chronic cardiomyopathy |
| - RV myocardial infarct | Post implantation of left ventricular assist |
| - Valvular regurgitation | devices |
| ARDS=acute respiratory distress syndrome; LV=left ventricle; RV=right ventricle. | |

**Table 27-3.** Etiology of right ventricular failure.

by itself increases RV afterload and reduces preload.[42]

In all these cases, ECLS should only be considered if first-line treatments fail, are not available or contraindicated, and the underlying condition can be treated. In case of acute decompensation of chronic RV failure, very poor long-term outcomes are expected.[43] Thus, ECLS should only be considered if a bridge to a heart transplantation or durable VAD is possible. A special group of patients who might experience RV failure are those suffering from severe COVID-19, as discussed below.

### Options for MCS of the Right Heart

Mechanical RV circulatory support can be subdivided in options which only support the right heart and those providing biventricular support (Table 27-4). While the latter always provides oxygenation, RV support can be initiated without an oxygenator. However, many of the conditions listed in Table 27-3 have an intrinsic respiratory failure component and may require extracorporeal oxygenation.

Although VV ECMO does not provide direct circulatory support, it does have an indirect effect on RV function favoring the reduction of pulmonary vascular resistance and facilitating lung protective ventilation. However, judging if this indirect effect is sufficient in cases of RV failure requires a case-specific discussion within the interdisciplinary ECMO team. VA ECMO provides excellent support for the RV but requires arterial cannulation and may be complicated by differential hypoxia. However, it is the modality of choice whenever biventricular failure is present. Alternative configurations such as venovenoarterial (VVA) ECMO may provide the benefits mentioned for VV and VA ECMO and can avoid differential hypoxia. Venopulmonary ($V_{RA}$-$V_{PA}$) ECMO avoids the negative effect of an increase in LV afterload but requires direct access to the pulmonary artery via a sternotomy or through the use of a ProtekDuo® double lumen cannula.[44] In specific situations such as fixed pulmonary hypertension, right atrium-left atrium ($V_{RA}$-$A_{LA}$) ECMO could be considered.

Finally, an intracardiac placed pump such as the Impella RP® (Abiomed, Danvers, USA) drains blood directly from the RV and returns it into the pulmonary artery without the addition of an oxygenator (Chapter 44).[44]

### ECLS in Cardiac Surgery

ECLS is increasingly utilized to provide biventricular support for patients prior to, during or after surgical procedures (Figure 27-3) as prophylactic or rescue treatment. These patients are characterized by specific comorbidities and

| | VV ECMO | VA ECMO | VV-A ECMO | $V_{RA}$-$V_{PA}$ ECMO | $V_{RA}$-$A_{LA}$ ECMO | ProtekDuo | Impella RP |
|---|---|---|---|---|---|---|---|
| Venous cannulation | ++ | + | ++ | + | + | + | + |
| Arterial cannulation | | + | + | + | + | | |
| Oxygenation | ++ | (+) | + | ++ | ++ | + | |
| RV support | (+) | ++ | + | ++ | ++ | ++ | ++ |
| LV support | | ++ | + | | | | |
| Recirculation | + | | | | | | |
| LV=left ventricle; RV=right ventricle; VA=venoarterial; VPA=venopulmonary; VV=venovenous; VV-A=venovenoarterial; RA=right atrium; LA=left atrium; PA=pulmonary artery | | | | | | | |

**Table 27-4.** Options for mechanical circulatory support of the right heart.

conditions that should be considered in the ECLS management and outcomes (Table 27-5).

The application of ECLS before surgery might be considered in patients with poor organ perfusion, acidosis, or cardiac arrest to improve the preoperative condition and enhance the intraoperative and postoperative outcomes (2020 EACTS/ELSO/STS/AATS expert consensus: Class IIb, Level C).[45] Most patients requiring preoperative ECLS suffer from ACS with multivessel disease, acute valvular diseases, acute progression of chronic valve diseases, traumatic lesions and endocarditis. Additionally, in the presence of STEMI-related ventricular septal defect, surgery might be delayed allowing partial myocardial healing and fibrotic tissue formation while the patient is supported with ECLS, conditions that aid in achieving a better surgical result and successful outcome (2020 EACTS/ELSO/STS/AATS expert consensus: Class IIb, Level C).[45]

The use of prophylactic, intraoperative ECLS to allow for gradual recovery of myocardial function after cardiac surgery has gained importance in high-risk patients with impaired general condition, severely reduced cardiac function, or when a complex perioperative course is anticipated (2020 EACTS/ELSO/STS/AATS expert consensus: Class IIb, Level C).[45] The main advantage of this prophylactic approach is the initiation of ECLS in a logistically favorable condition while weaning off cardiopulmonary bypass (CPB) weaning, preventing implantation in an emergency situation.

Besides the abovementioned cases, most ECLS cannulation in cardiac surgery occurs in patients suffering from postcardiotomy cardiogenic shock (PC-CS).[46] ECLS for PC-CS should be initiated prior to end-organ injury or onset of anaerobic metabolism (lactate <4 mmol/l) in the absence of uncontrollable bleeding (2020 EACTS/ELSO/STS/AATS expert consensus: Class I, Level B).[45] Also, ECLS should be considered in the following situations:

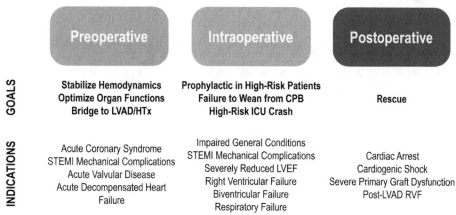

**Figure 27-3.** Summary of goals and indications for the use of extracorporeal life support in cardiac surgery. CPB=cardiopulmonary bypass; HTx=heart transplantation; LVAD=left ventricular assist device; LVEF=left ventricular ejection fraction; RVF=right ventricular failure; STEMI=ST-elevation myocardial infarction.

- Patients supported with an IABP and optimal medical therapy but experiencing a failure to wean from CPB or marginal hemodynamics (2020 EACTS/ELSO/STS/AATS expert consensus: Class I, Level B).[45]
- Severe primary graft dysfunction (PGD) following a heart transplant (2020 EACTS/ELSO/STS/AATS expert consensus: Class IIa, Level B).[45]
- Severe refractory RV failure after durable VAD implantation (2020 EACTS/ELSO/STS/AATS expert consensus: Class IIb, Level C).[45]

An Oxy-RVAD may be considered in patients with isolated RV dysfunction and concomitant respiratory compromise or in patients undergoing pulmonary artery embolectomy and suffering from RV failure.

Despite the increasing use of postcardiotomy ECLS, survival rates to discharge have not improved over time, ranging from 20-40%.[45,47-49] Mortality is particularly high in patients with significant comorbidities, advanced age, elevated lactate level, and renal injury. All these risk factors are associated with death and should be carefully considered prior to ECLS initiation (2020 EACTS/ELSO/STS/AATS expert consensus: Class IIa, Level B).[45]

**Interventional and Transcatheter Procedures**

The field of interventional cardiology and transcatheter procedures has grown as one of the emerging indications for ECLS, including transcatheter aortic valve implantation (TAVI) patients, patients with advanced heart failure requiring MitraClip (Abbott Laboratories, Abbot Park, USA) implantation, or ventricular tachycardia (VT) ablation. All these patients are at risk of hypotension, decompensated heart failure, shock, or arrhythmias that may lead

| BASELINE CHARACTERISTICS | - Older patient age<br>- Higher rate of comorbidities and organ damage before surgery<br>- Higher number of pre-ECLS medications (anticoagulants, antiplatelets, diuretics, cardioactive drugs)<br>- Type, duration and prognosis of the underlying disease<br>- Previous cardiac surgery<br>- Infection at the time of surgery (eg, endocarditis) |
|---|---|
| OPERATION-RELATED CHARACTERISTICS | - Complex procedures (eg, multiple valves operation, aortic dissection)<br>- Cardiopulmonary bypass +/- circulatory arrest<br>- Myocardial ischemia<br>- Vasoplegia<br>- Bleeding<br>- Presence of other mechanical circulatory supports (eg, IABP, Impella, VAD) |
| POSTOPERATIVE CHARACTERISTICS | - Central vs. peripheral cannulation<br>- Delayed chest closure<br>- Wound infections<br>- Re-operations |
| ECLS=post-cardiotomy extracorporeal life support; IABP=intra-aortic balloon pump; VAD=ventricular assist device. | |

**Table 27-5.** Specific characteristics of the postcardiotomy patient that might differ from other cardiogenic shock etiologies.

to rapid hemodynamic deterioration, cardiac arrest, or death.

One of the most common interventional procedures for which ECLS support might be indicated is high-risk PCI (2021 ACC/AHA/ SCAI guidelines: Class IIb, Level B-R).[17] It refers to PCIs performed in patients with one or more of the following features: unprotected left main coronary artery disease, intervention of the last patent vessel with reduced left ventricular ejection fraction (<35%), complex 3-vessel disease, or comorbidities including severe aortic stenosis or mitral regurgitation.[50,51] In these patients, elective placement of MCS with either an IABP, Impella (Abiomed, Danvers, USA), TandemHeart (CardiacAssist, Pittsburgh, USA), or VA ECMO may be reasonable to prevent hemodynamic compromise during PCI.[50,51]

Similarly, patients with severely reduced LV ejection fraction undergoing VT ablation might benefit from the use of temporary MCS to avoid acute decompensation during the procedure (2019 HRS/EHRA/APHRS/LAHRS expert consensus: Class of recommendation IIa)[52] and to allow mapping and ablation of unstable VTs in selected cases (2019 HRS/EHRA/ APHRS/LAHRS expert consensus: Class of recommendation IIb).[52] It is estimated that up to 11% of patients undergoing VT ablation develop intraprocedural acute hemodynamic decompensation due to altered preload and afterload caused by volume resuscitation and repetitive electrical instability.[53] To better identify high-risk patients who might benefit from prophylactic MCS, a PAINESD risk score ≥15 might be used.[54,55] Moreover, patients with biventricular failure with elevated filling pressures or suffering from CS before the VT ablation and patients with heterogenous ventricular tachycardia and undergoing prolonged procedures should be considered for MCS. Continuous hemodynamic monitoring with a Swan-Ganz catheter is advised and awake VA ECMO with monitored anesthesia

care should be the first choice, but endotracheal intubation should be considered in case of CS.

A similar situation can be identified for TAVI procedures where the prophylactic use of ECLS has demonstrated better survival compared to emergent implantation.[56,57] Patients might benefit from the use of MCS during TAVI in case of preprocedural heart failure requiring hospitalization and stabilization, moderate or severe LV and/or RV failure, hemodynamic instability during balloon aortic valvuloplasty, borderline hemodynamics during procedures with central venous pressure/pulmonary capillary wedge pressure >20 mmHg, mean pulmonary artery pressure >40 mmHg and cardiac index <2.0 with no improvement with inotropes, slow recovery from rapid LV pacing, high vasopressor requirements during general anesthesia, and concomitant high-risk percutaneous coronary intervention.[56]

The use of temporary MCS has also been described in association with MitraClip implantation in a few cases.[58]

## Myocarditis, Infection, and Non-Infection-Related Indications

Myocarditis is an inflammatory cardiac disease that may be caused by infection, exposure to toxic substances, and immune system activation.[59] Its clinical presentation includes both acute and chronic forms, with recovery of cardiac function in about 50% of cases.[60] Among the acute forms, 26.6% of patients might be affected by LV systolic dysfunction, ventricular arrhythmias, or cardiogenic shock,[59] while fulminant myocarditis (FM) accounts for 8.6% of total cases. In such patients, inotropes such as milrinone, levosimendan, or dobutamine, and temporary MCS may be considered as bridge to durable MCS, transplant or recovery.[59,60] In these patients, an MCS strategy that decreases afterload may increase the likelihood of ventricular recovery or remission while reducing myocardial inflammation.[59,60] Therefore, peripheral VA ECMO should always mandate consideration of LV venting. Alternatively, IABP or intraaortic axial pumps (eg, Impella) could be considered. If no weaning from MCS is possible after 2-3 weeks of support, durable VAD implantation or urgent heart transplant should be considered.[59]

A unique type of infection-related myocardial disease requiring MCS is the one derived from COVID-19. Although respiratory symptoms have dominated COVID-19 clinical presentation, up to 20-25% of overall patients show cardiac involvement.[61-65] The underlying mechanisms for cardiac failure are severe immune system over-reaction, thrombosis, pulmonary embolism, direct damage to the cardiomyocytes and arrhythmias.[66] The right heart might be particularly affected by increased pulmonary afterload and loss of RV radial function.[67] Lastly, COVID-19 patients suffering from severe systemic hypoxia are at risk of type 2 myocardial infarction.[68] VV ECMO has been the most used configuration in COVID-19 patients,[69,70] while VA ECMO or other ECLS configurations have been used in 4-5% and 2-3% of patients, respectively.[69-71] Despite this, 3-4% of COVID-19 patients supported with ECLS require conversion to a different configuration such as hybrid ECLS[72] to provide full cardiorespiratory support.[73] Successful experiences with the use of an OxyRVAD in COVID-19 patients have been described, with a survival rate ranging from 61-75%.[74-76] As a general guide, the use of cardiac support including VA ECMO, hybrid ECLS configurations, and OxyRVAD in COVID-19 patients is recommended for patients with COVID-19 and severe cardiopulmonary failure who meet the traditional criteria for MCS in cardiac arrest and CS.[77,78]

## Cardiogenic Shock from Other Nonsurgical Etiologies

Situations of severe unstable arrhythmias such as ventricular tachycardia or electrical storm might result in CS for which the traditional criteria for ECLS can be applied. However, clinical and scientific experience with this specific use of ECLS are still limited and ECLS is mainly applied in case of ventricular arrhythmias related to myocarditis or unstable acute coronary syndromes.[79-80] Arrhythmias might also complicate events such as hypothermia or poisoning (Chapter 37).

A further indication for ECLS is represented by the Takotsubo syndrome (TS), which is a form of acute heart failure characterized by wall motion abnormalities of one or both cardiac ventricles, dynamic LV outflow tract obstruction (LVOTO), LVOTO-related severe mitral regurgitation, and severe reduction of cardiac function, which typically recovers within days to weeks.[81-83] In Takotsubo patients, 10–15% develop cardiogenic shock[82,84-86] and 5-10% experience cardiac arrest or require cardiopulmonary resuscitation.[84,85] The pathogenesis of this disorder is not well understood but a role of the sympathetic nervous system and circulating endogenous catecholamines has been proposed.[82,83,85,87] Hence, catecholamines, and especially inotropes, should be avoided and MCS should be considered as a valid bridge-to-recovery option.[82-83] Of note, IABP potentially worsens LVOTO and should be avoided in TS patients.[88] Thus, VA ECMO, intraaortic axial pumps, or the combination of both are the supports of choice.

## Pregnancy, Trauma, Sepsis, Poisoning, and Malignancy

For further discussion of ECLS indications associated with pregnancy (including postpartum cardiomyopathy), trauma, sepsis, poisoning, and malignancy, please refer to Chapter 34-37 and 39.

**Conclusions**

The application of ECLS for cardiac etiologies is increasing both in terms of the number of treated patients and involved centers. Indeed, advances in technology, expertise, and transport of critically ill patients, has further expanded the population of possible ECLS candidates (Figure 27-4). The combination of devices and hybrid ECLS forms have also contributed to the continuous expansion of ECLS indications. Finally, the prophylactic use or the performance of so called "protected procedures" in interventional cardiology and cardiac surgery has promoted the idea of using ECLS to prevent hemodynamic compromise during high-risk interventions. New indications are also constantly emerging (intoxication, TS, infections, etc.), indicating that ECLS represents a reliable intervention to improve CS outcomes. Timing, however, is also increasingly considered as one of the most critical aspects for successful ECLS. Initiating support prior to profound CS or within a few hours from the onset of cardiac compromise must be always considered, avoiding the application of ECLS as a last resort when any possible recovery is unlikely.

ECLS is gaining a pivotal role to optimize patients' conditions prior to interventions, prevent hemodynamic deterioration, or bridge patients to cardiac recovery or advanced therapies in cases where the acute damage and/or the underlying disease hamper any attempt to restore the pre-acute injury cardiac state. The right system, at the right time, at the appropriate place represent the most effective triad in the decision-making. Ongoing studies will most likely provide additional and critical information to indicate the actual role and efficacy of ECLS in cardiogenic shock.

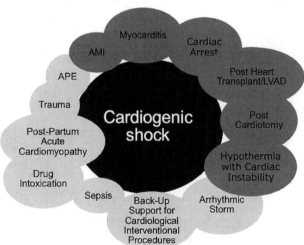

**Figure 27-4.** Common (dark gray) and emerging situations (light gray) for extracorporeal life support in the context of cardiogenic shock. AMI=acute myocardial infarction; APE=massive pulmonary embolism; LVAD=left ventricular assist device; Sepsis=sepsis-associated cardiomyopathy. Adapted with permission from Lorusso et al.[13]

# References

1. Chioncel O, Parissis J, Mebazaa A et al. Epidemiology, pathophysiology and contemporary management of cardiogenic shock - a position statement from the heart failure association of the european society of cardiology. Eur J Heart Fail 2020;22(8):1315-1341.
2. McDonagh TA, Metra M, Adamo M et al. 2021 esc guidelines for the diagnosis and treatment of acute and chronic heart failure. Eur Heart J 2021;42(36):3599-3726.
3. Samsky MD, Morrow DA, Proudfoot AG, Hochman JS, Thiele H, Rao SV. Cardiogenic shock after acute myocardial infarction: A review. Jama 2021;326(18):1840-1850.
4. Fox KA, Steg PG, Eagle KA et al. Decline in rates of death and heart failure in acute coronary syndromes, 1999-2006. Jama 2007;297(17):1892-1900.
5. Samsky M, Krucoff M, Althouse AD et al. Clinical and regulatory landscape for cardiogenic shock: A report from the cardiac safety research consortium thinktank on cardiogenic shock. Am Heart J 2020;219:1-8.
6. Samsky MD, Krucoff MW, Morrow DA et al. Cardiac safety research consortium "shock ii" think tank report: Advancing practical approaches to generating evidence for the treatment of cardiogenic shock. Am Heart J 2020;230:93-97.
7. Thiele H, Ohman EM, de Waha-Thiele S, et al. Management of cardiogenic shock complicating myocardial infarction: An update 2019. Eur Heart J 2019;40(32):2671-2683.
8. Khalid L, Dhakam SH. A review of cardiogenic shock in acute myocardial infarction. Curr Cardiol Rev 2008;4(1):34-40.
9. Berg DD, Bohula EA, van Diepen S et al. Epidemiology of shock in contemporary cardiac intensive care units. Circ Cardiovasc Qual Outcomes 2019;12(3):e005618.
10. Yandrapalli S, Sanaani A, Harikrishnan P et al. Cardiogenic shock during heart failure hospitalizations: Age-, sex-, and race-stratified trends in incidence and outcomes. Am Heart J 2019;213:18-29.
11. Baran DA, Grines CL, Bailey S et al. Scai clinical expert consensus statement on the classification of cardiogenic shock: This document was endorsed by the american college of cardiology (acc), the american heart association (aha), the society of critical care medicine (sccm), and the society of thoracic surgeons (sts) in april 2019. Catheter Cardiovasc Interv 2019;94(1):29-37.
12. Jentzer JC, van Diepen S, Barsness GW et al. Cardiogenic shock classification to predict mortality in the cardiac intensive care unit. J Am Coll Cardiol 2019;74(17):2117-2128.
13. Lorusso R, Shekar K, MacLaren G et al. Elso interim guidelines for venoarterial extracorporeal membrane oxygenation in adult cardiac patients. Asaio j 2021;67(8):827-844.
14. Fux T, Holm M, van der Linden J. Arterial lactate before initiation of venoarterial extracorporeal membrane oxygenation for postcardiotomy shock improves postimplant outcome prediction. J Thorac Cardiovasc Surg 2019;157(5):e266-e267.
15. Biancari F, Fiore A, Jonsson K et al. Prognostic significance of arterial lactate levels at weaning from postcardiotomy venoarterial extracorporeal membrane oxygenation. J Clin Med 2019;8(12).
16. Li CL, Wang H, Jia M, et al. The early dynamic behavior of lactate is linked to mortality in postcardiotomy patients with extracorporeal membrane oxygenation support: A retrospective observational study. J Thorac Cardiovasc Surg 2015;149(5):1445-1450.
17. Writing Committee M, Lawton JS, Tamis-Holland JE et al. 2021 acc/aha/scai guideline for coronary artery revascularization: A report of the american college of cardiology/american heart association joint committee on clinical practice guidelines. J Am Coll Cardiol 2022;79(2):e21-e129.
18. Neumann FJ, Sousa-Uva M, Ahlsson A et al. 2018 esc/eacts guidelines on myocardial revascularization. Eur Heart J 2019;40(2):87-165.
19. Virani SS, Alonso A, Aparicio HJ et al. Heart disease and stroke statistics-2021 update: A report from the american heart association. Circulation 2021;143(8):e254-e743.
20. Fincke R, Hochman JS, Lowe AM et al. Cardiac power is the strongest hemodynamic correlate of mortality in cardiogenic shock: A report from the shock trial registry. J Am Coll Cardiol 2004;44(2):340-348.
21. Pöss J, Köster J, Fuernau G et al. Risk stratification for patients in cardiogenic shock after acute myocardial infarction. J Am Coll Cardiol 2017;69(15):1913-1920.
22. Basir MB, Kapur NK, Patel K et al. Improved outcomes associated with the use of shock protocols: Updates from the national cardiogenic shock initiative. Catheter ,Cardiovasc Interv 2019;93(7):1173-1183.
23. Thiele H, Zeymer U, Neumann FJ et al. Intraaortic balloon support for myocardial infarction with cardiogenic shock. N Engl J Med 2012;367(14):1287-1296.
24. Karami M, den Uil CA, Ouweneel DM et al. Mechanical circulatory support in cardiogenic shock from acute myocardial infarction: Impella cp/5.0 versus ecmo. Eur Heart J Acute Cardiovasc Care 2020;9(2):164-172.
25. van den Brink FS, Magan AD, Noordzij PG et al. Veno-arterial extracorporeal membrane oxygenation in addition to primary pci in patients presenting with

st-elevation myocardial infarction. Neth Heart J 2018;26(2):76-84.

26. Hryniewicz K, Sandoval Y, Samara M et al. Percutaneous venoarterial extracorporeal membrane oxygenation for refractory cardiogenic shock is associated with improved short- and long-term survival. Asaio j 2016;62(4):397-402.

27. Kapur NK, Alkhouli MA, DeMartini TJ et al. Unloading the left ventricle before reperfusion in patients with anterior st-segment-elevation myocardial infarction. Circulation 2019;139(3):337-346.

28. Bhatt AS, Berg DD, Bohula EA et al. De novo vs acute-on-chronic presentations of heart failure-related cardiogenic shock: Insights from the critical care cardiology trials network registry. J Card Fail 2021;27(10):1073-1081.

29. Lawler PR, Mehra MR. Advancing from a "hemodynamic model" to a "mechanistic disease-modifying model" of cardiogenic shock. J Heart Lung Transplant 2018;37(11):1285-1288.

30. Garan AR, Malick WA, Habal M et al. Predictors of survival for patients with acute decompensated heart failure requiring extra-corporeal membrane oxygenation therapy. Asaio j 2019;65(8):781-787.

31. Morici N, Viola G, Antolini L et al. Predicting survival in patients with acute decompensated heart failure complicated by cardiogenic shock. Int J Cardiol Heart Vasc 2021;34:100809.

32. Truby L, Mundy L, Kalesan B et al. Contemporary outcomes of venoarterial extracorporeal membrane oxygenation for refractory cardiogenic shock at a large tertiary care center. Asaio j 2015;61(4):403-409.

33. Schmidt M, Burrell A, Roberts L et al. Predicting survival after ecmo for refractory cardiogenic shock: The survival after veno-arterial-ecmo (save)-score. Eur Heart J 2015;36(33):2246-2256.

34. Zalawadiya S, Fudim M, Bhat G et al. Extracorporeal membrane oxygenation support and post-heart transplant outcomes among united states adults. J Heart Lung Transplant 2017;36(1):77-81.

35. Coutance G, Jacob N, Demondion P et al. Favorable outcomes of a direct heart transplantation strategy in selected patients on extracorporeal membrane oxygenation support. Crit Care Med 2020;48(4):498-506.

36. Parker WF, Chung K, Anderson AS et al. Practice changes at u.S. transplant centers after the new adult heart allocation policy. J Am Coll Cardiol 2020;75(23):2906-2916.

37. Molina EJ, Shah P, Kiernan MS et al. The society of thoracic surgeons intermacs 2020 annual report. Ann Thorac Surg 2021;111(3):778-792.

38. Shah P, Yuzefpolskaya M, Hickey GW et al. Twelfth Interagency Registry for Mechanically Assisted Circulatory Support Report: Readmissions After Left Ventricular Assist Device. Ann Thorac Surg. 2022 Mar;113(3):722-737.

39. Saeed D, Potapov E, Loforte A et al. Transition from temporary to durable circulatory support systems. J Am Coll Cardiol 2020;76(25):2956-2964.

40. Ton VK, Xie R, Hernandez-Montfort JA et al. Short- and long-term adverse events in patients on temporary circulatory support before durable ventricular assist device: An imacs registry analysis. J Heart Lung Transplant 2020;39(4):342-352.

41. Vieillard-Baron A, Naeije R, Haddad F et al. Diagnostic workup, etiologies and management of acute right ventricle failure : A state-of-the-art paper. Intensive Care Med 2018;44(6):774-790.

42. Repesse X, Charron C, Vieillard-Baron A. Acute respiratory distress syndrome: The heart side of the moon. Curr Opin Crit Care 2016;22(1):38-44.

43. Savale L, Vuillard C, Pichon J et al. Five-year survival after an acute episode of decompensated pulmonary arterial hypertension in the modern management era of right heart failure. Eur Respir J 2021;58(3).

44. Kapur NK, Esposito ML, Bader Y et al. Mechanical circulatory support devices for acute right ventricular failure. Circulation 2017;136(3):314-326.

45. Lorusso R, Whitman G, Milojevic M et al. 2020 eacts/elso/sts/aats expert consensus on post-cardiotomy extracorporeal life support in adult patients. J Thorac Cardiovasc Surg 2021;161(4):1287-1331.

46. Lorusso R, Raffa GM, Alenizy K et al. Structured review of post-cardiotomy extracorporeal membrane oxygenation: Part 1-adult patients. J Heart Lung Transplant 2019;38(11):1125-1143.

47. Kowalewski M, Zielinski K, Brodie D et al. Venoarterial extracorporeal membrane oxygenation for postcardiotomy shock-analysis of the extracorporeal life support organization registry. Crit Care Med 2021.

48. Whitman GJ. Extracorporeal membrane oxygenation for the treatment of postcardiotomy shock. J Thorac Cardiovasc Surg 2017;153(1):95-101.

49. Vallabhajosyula S, Arora S, Sakhuja A et al. Trends, predictors, and outcomes of temporary mechanical circulatory support for postcardiac surgery cardiogenic shock. Am J Cardiol 2019;123(3):489-497.

50. Levine GN, Bates ER, Blankenship JC et al. 2011 accf/aha/scai guideline for percutaneous coronary intervention: Executive summary: A report of the american college of cardiology foundation/american heart association task force on practice guidelines and the society for cardiovascular angiography and interventions. Circulation 2011;124(23):2574-2609.

51. Atkinson TM, Ohman EM, O'Neill WW et al. A practical approach to mechanical circulatory support in patients undergoing percutaneous coronary

intervention: An interventional perspective. JACC Cardiovasc Interv 2016;9(9):871-883.

52. Cronin EM, Bogun FM, Maury P et al. 2019 hrs/ehra/aphrs/lahrs expert consensus statement on catheter ablation of ventricular arrhythmias: Executive summary. J Arrhythm 2020;36(1):1-58.

53. Santangeli P, Muser D, Zado ES et al. Acute hemodynamic decompensation during catheter ablation of scar-related ventricular tachycardia: Incidence, predictors, and impact on mortality. Circ Arrhythm Electrophysiol 2015;8(1):68-75.

54. Mariani S, Napp LC, Kraaier K et al. Prophylactic mechanical circulatory support for protected ventricular tachycardia ablation: A meta-analysis of the literature. Artif Organs 2021;45(9):987-997.

55. Mariani S, Napp LC, Lo Coco V et al. Mechanical circulatory support for life-threatening arrhythmia: A systematic review. Int J Cardiol 2020;308:42-49.

56. Raffa GM, Kowalewski M, Meani P et al. In-hospital outcomes after emergency or prophylactic veno-arterial extracorporeal membrane oxygenation during transcatheter aortic valve implantation: A comprehensive review of the literature. Perfusion 2019;34(5):354-363.

57. Orvin K, Perl L, Landes U et al. Percutaneous mechanical circulatory support from the collaborative multicenter mechanical unusual support in tavi (must) registry. Catheter Cardiovasc Interv 2021;98(6):E862-e869.

58. Jung RG, Simard T, Kovach C et al. Transcatheter mitral valve repair in cardiogenic shock and mitral regurgitation: A patient-level, multicenter analysis. JACC Cardiovasc Interv 2021;14(1):1-11.

59. Ammirati E, Frigerio M, Adler ED et al. Management of acute myocarditis and chronic inflammatory cardiomyopathy: An expert consensus document. Circ Heart Fail 2020;13(11):e007405.

60. Tschope C, Cooper LT, Torre-Amione G et al. Management of myocarditis-related cardiomyopathy in adults. Circ Res 2019;124(11):1568-1583.

61. Guzik TJ, Mohiddin SA, Dimarco A et al. Covid-19 and the cardiovascular system: Implications for risk assessment, diagnosis, and treatment options. Cardiovasc Res 2020;116(10):1666-1687.

62. Basso C, Leone O, Rizzo S et al. Pathological features of covid-19-associated myocardial injury: A multicentre cardiovascular pathology study. Eur Heart J 2020;41(39):3827-3835.

63. Ramadan MS, Bertolino L, Zampino R et al. Cardiac sequelae after covid-19 recovery: A systematic review. Clin Microbiol Infect 2021.

64. Richardson S, Hirsch JS, Narasimhan M et al. Presenting characteristics, comorbidities, and outcomes among 5700 patients hospitalized with covid-19 in the new york city area. JAMA 2020;323(20):2052-2059.

65. Shi S, Qin M, Shen B et al. Association of cardiac injury with mortality in hospitalized patients with covid-19 in wuhan, china. JAMA Cardiol 2020;5(7):802-810.

66. Shafi AMA, Shaikh SA, Shirke MM et al. Cardiac manifestations in covid-19 patients-a systematic review. J Card Surg 2020;35(8):1988-2008.

67. Bleakley C, Singh S, Garfield B et al. Right ventricular dysfunction in critically ill covid-19 ards. Int J Cardiol 2021;327:251-258.

68. Musher DM, Abers MS, Corrales-Medina VF. Acute infection and myocardial infarction. N Engl J Med 2019;380(2):171-176.

69. Barbaro RP, MacLaren G, Boonstra PS et al. Extracorporeal membrane oxygenation for covid-19: Evolving outcomes from the international extracorporeal life support organization registry. The Lancet 2021;398(10307):1230-1238.

70. Lorusso R, Combes A, Coco VL et al. Ecmo for covid-19 patients in europe and israel. Intensive Care Med 2021;47(3):344-348.

71. Barbaro RP, MacLaren G, Boonstra PS et al. Extracorporeal membrane oxygenation support in covid-19: An international cohort study of the extracorporeal life support organization registry. Lancet 2020;396(10257):1071-1078.

72. Lo Coco V, Swol J, De Piero ME et al. Dynamic extracorporeal life support: A novel management modality in temporary cardio-circulatory assistance. Artif Organs 2020.

73. Kowalewski M, Fina D, Slomka A et al. Covid-19 and ecmo: The interplay between coagulation and inflammation-a narrative review. Crit Care 2020;24(1):205.

74. Mustafa AK, Alexander PJ, Joshi DJ et al. Extracorporeal membrane oxygenation for patients with covid-19 in severe respiratory failure. JAMA Surg 2020;155(10):990-992.

75. Mustafa AK, Joshi DJ, Alexander PJ et al. Comparative propensity matched outcomes in severe covid-19 respiratory failure-extracorporeal membrane oxygenation or maximum ventilation alone. Ann Surg 2021;274(5):e388-e394.

76. Cain MT, Smith NJ, Barash M et al. Extracorporeal membrane oxygenation with right ventricular assist device for covid-19 ards. J Surg Res 2021;264:81-89.

77. Badulak J, Antonini MV, Stead CM et al. Extracorporeal membrane oxygenation for covid-19: Updated 2021 guidelines from the extracorporeal life support organization. ASAIO J 2021;67(5):485-495.

78. Shekar K, Badulak J, Peek G et al. Extracorporeal life support organization coronavirus disease 2019 interim guidelines: A consensus document

from an international group of interdisciplinary extracorporeal membrane oxygenation providers. ASAIO J 2020;66(7):707-721.

79. Al-Khatib SM, Stevenson WG, Ackerman MJ et al. 2017 aha/acc/hrs guideline for management of patients with ventricular arrhythmias and the prevention of sudden cardiac death: Executive summary: A report of the american college of cardiology/american heart association task force on clinical practice guidelines and the heart rhythm society. Heart Rhythm 2018;15(10):e190-e252.

80. Priori SG, Blomström-Lundqvist C, Mazzanti A et al. 2015 esc guidelines for the management of patients with ventricular arrhythmias and the prevention of sudden cardiac death: The task force for the management of patients with ventricular arrhythmias and the prevention of sudden cardiac death of the european society of cardiology (esc). Endorsed by: Association for european paediatric and congenital cardiology (aepc). Eur Heart J 2015;36(41):2793-2867.

81. Jurisic S, Gili S, Cammann VL et al. Clinical predictors and prognostic impact of recovery of wall motion abnormalities in takotsubo syndrome: Results from the international takotsubo registry. J Am Heart Assoc 2019;8(21):e011194.

82. Lyon AR, Bossone E, Schneider B et al. Current state of knowledge on takotsubo syndrome: A position statement from the taskforce on takotsubo syndrome of the heart failure association of the european society of cardiology. Eur J Heart Fail 2016;18(1):8-27.

83. Ghadri JR, Wittstein IS, Prasad A et al. International expert consensus document on takotsubo syndrome (part i): Clinical characteristics, diagnostic criteria, and pathophysiology. Eur Heart J 2018;39(22):2032-2046.

84. Di Vece D, Citro R, Cammann VL et al. Outcomes associated with cardiogenic shock in takotsubo syndrome. Circulation 2019;139(3):413-415.

85. Sharkey SW, Pink VR, Lesser JR et al. Clinical profile of patients with high-risk tako-tsubo cardiomyopathy. Am J Cardiol 2015;116(5):765-772.

86. Templin C, Ghadri JR, Diekmann J et al. Clinical features and outcomes of takotsubo (stress) cardiomyopathy. N Engl J Med 2015;373(10):929-938.

87. Wittstein IS, Thiemann DR, Lima JA et al. Neurohumoral features of myocardial stunning due to sudden emotional stress. N Engl J Med 2005;352(6):539-548.

88. Mariani S, Richter J, Pappalardo F et al. Mechanical circulatory support for takotsubo syndrome: A systematic review and meta-analysis. Int J Cardiol 2020;316:31-39.

# 28

## Management of Adult Patients with Cardiac Failure

*Bhavesh Patel, Jose Alfonso Rubio Mateo-Sidron, Benjamin Bongiorno, Kai Singbartl, Ayan Sen,
Dirk W. Donker*

Venoarterial ECMO is a widely accepted short-term hemodynamic support modality for cardiogenic shock and its implementation depends upon close attention to interprofessional collaboration and multifaceted clinical management to achieve optimal outcomes.

### Patient and Circuit Monitoring

Patients undergoing VA ECMO will receive standard hemodynamic and respiratory ICU monitoring (Figure 28-1 and Table 28-1). The primary goal of VA ECMO is to stabilize the systemic circulation and promote myocardial recovery by ensuring acceptable cardiac loading conditions. Therefore, specific hemodynamic monitoring to assess cardiac load and residual transpulmonary flow is often warranted and a pulmonary artery catheter and/or repeated echocardiography can provide valuable information to timely recognize potentially detrimental cardiac overload or other unfavorable hemodynamic conditions.

To identify worsening of a patient's clinical status or impending complications from VA ECMO early, regular, and careful evaluation of the patient's condition (Table 28-1)[1] include:

- Changes in arterial pulsatility, development of pulmonary edema, and systemic or local hypoperfusion with an emphasis on limb ischemia,
- Neurological assessment regarding consciousness, pupillary reaction, and focal deficits,
- Check of devices, pumps, IV lines, and tubing,
- Check of mechanical ventilator for changes in lung compliance, oxygenation and ventilation,
- Adequacy of end-organ perfusion and related functions (eg, liver, kidney, bowel).

Regular circuit checks are mandatory and must include:

- Safe position and good visibility of the device (display),
- Connection to (emergency) power supply,
- Gas connections ($O_2$ and air) to blender,
- Cannulas and tubing (no kinks), sutures, tie-bands, and connectors,
- Entire circuit (tubing and oxygenator) inspection for clots and/or fibrin,
- Gas blender settings, blood color difference between arterial and venous circuit limb,
- Pump parameters and alarms: minimum pump speed and blood flow rate,
- Emergency equipment: clamps, emergency hand crank, appropriately sized connectors,

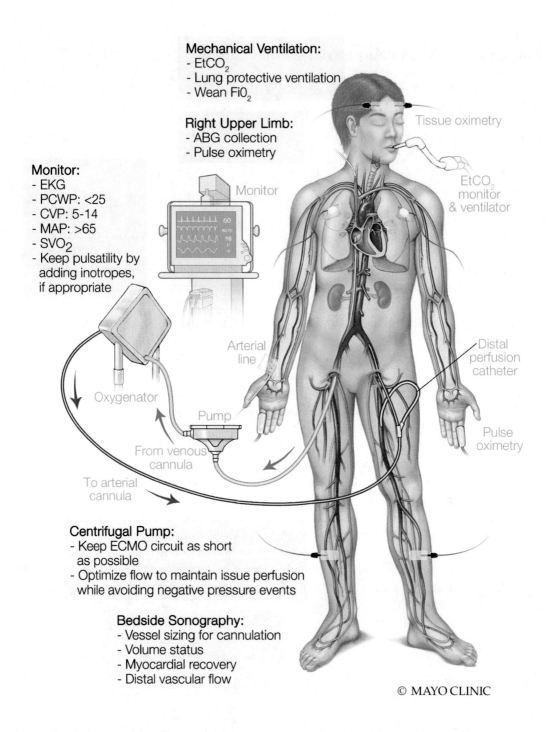

**Mechanical Ventilation:**
- $EtCO_2$
- Lung protective ventilation
- Wean $FiO_2$

**Right Upper Limb:**
- ABG collection
- Pulse oximetry

Tissue oximetry

$EtCO_2$ monitor & ventilator

**Monitor:**
- EKG
- PCWP: <25
- CVP: 5-14
- MAP: >65
- $SVO_2$
- Keep pulsatility by adding inotropes, if appropriate

Monitor

Arterial line

Distal perfusion catheter

Oxygenator

Pump

From venous cannula

To arterial cannula

Pulse oximetry

**Centrifugal Pump:**
- Keep ECMO circuit as short as possible
- Optimize flow to maintain issue perfusion while avoiding negative pressure events

**Bedside Sonography:**
- Vessel sizing for cannulation
- Volume status
- Myocardial recovery
- Distal vascular flow

© MAYO CLINIC

**Figure 28-1.** ICU monitoring for VA ECMO patients; reproduced with permission from the Mayo Foundation for Education and Research.

| | MONITOR FOR | TREATMENT |
|---|---|---|
| **Rhythm** | Dysrhythmias such as ventricular fibrillation that may prevent ventricular ejection | Antiarrhythmics<br>Cardioversion<br>Pacing<br>Ablation |
| **MAP** | Hypotension (MAP ≈ CO × SVR)<br>(i) Inadequate VA ECMO flow<br>(ii) Inadequate SVR | (i) See 'Flow' below<br>(ii) Start vasoconstrictor |
| **Pulsatility** | Lack of pulsatility on arterial waveform caused by<br>    (i) poor myocardial function<br>    (ii) excessive VA ECMO support<br>    (iii) Inadequate preload<br>    (iv) RV failure<br>May result in<br>    (i) thrombus<br>    (ii) myocardial ischemia<br>    (iii) pulmonary edema (CXR, wedge) | If poor myocardial function, consider:<br>    decreasing VA ECMO flow<br>    starting or increasing inotrope<br>    starting or increasing vasodilator<br>    IABP<br>    myocardial decompression (venting) |
| **Flow (liters/min)** | Low flows (assuming centrifugal pump)<br>    (i) Inadequate preload<br>    (a) Hypovolemia (may see hemolysis, circuit chattering)<br>    (b) Mechanical obstruction<br>    (ii) Excessive afterload (thrombus, kink, SVR)<br>    (iii) Inadequate RPM | (i) Volume: crystalloid/colloid/transfusion<br>    Release of mechanical obstruction<br>(ii) Exchange oxygenator, relieve cannula kink, vasodilator to decrease SVR<br>(iii) Increase RPM |
| **Gas exchange** | Inadequate $PaO_2$<br>Inadequate or excessive $CO_2$ elimination<br>    (i) VA ECMO settings<br>    (a) $FsO_2$<br>    (b) Blood flow<br>    (c) Sweep gas flow rate<br>    (ii) Oxygenator function<br>    (a) Pre- and post-membrane pressures<br>    (b) Pre- and post-oxygenator gases<br>    (iii) Upper body hypoxemia (femoral-femoral cannulation) | (i) If hypoxemia, increase $FsO_2$ or flow.<br>If hypercarbia, increase sweep.<br>If hypocarbia, decrease sweep or add $CO_2$.<br>(ii) Increased and inadequate arterialization of post-oxygenator gases suggests oxygenator malfunction<br>(iii) Increase pulmonary venous $O_2$ content<br>    Adjust $FiO_2$ and/or PEEP<br>    Treat etiology of pulmonary dysfunction<br>    Increase VA ECMO flow<br>    Change to axillary/carotid cannulation<br>    V-VA ECMO<br>    VV ECMO |
| **Oxygen delivery: $SvO_2$ and lactate** | Decreased $SvO_2$ and increasing lactate suggest inadequate oxygen delivery ($DO_2 = CO \times CaO_2$)<br>    (i) VA ECMO flow<br>    (ii) Hemoglobin<br>    (iii) $SaO_2$<br>Excessive oxygen consumption ($ER = VO_2/DO_2$)<br>    (i) Febrile<br>    (ii) Shivering | (i) Increase VA ECMO flow<br>(ii) Transfuse<br>(iii) Ensure adequate gas exchange<br><br>(i) Antipyretics<br>(ii) Consider agents such as meperidine or dexmedetomidine |
| **Distal limb ischemia** | Loss of pulses<br>Cyanosis and coolness of limb | Femoral-femoral cannulation:<br>DP or PT anterograde perfusion catheter |
| **Anticoagulation** | Adequate heparinization by PTT | |
| **Temperature** | Normothermia unless therapeutic hypothermia | |

**Table 28-1.** Approach to Monitoring and Managing the VA ECMO Patient, adapted from Chung.[1]

tubing, shears, rapid access line, tie-gun/ straps and a primed backup circuit,

- Position and performance of associated devices (eg, IABP, Impella).

**Cardiovascular Management**

Widely accepted hemodynamic targets are a mean arterial blood pressure (MAP) >65 mmHg, a systolic blood pressure >90 mmHg and, when additionally using a pulmonary artery catheter, a cardiac index of >2.2 $L/min/m^2$ and a pulmonary capillary wedge pressure <15 mmHg. Importantly, the measurement of cardiac output using a pulmonary artery catheter only accounts for the native pulmonary circulation. Moreover, correct thermodilution of transpulmonary flow depends on proper catheter position and may interfere with dynamically changing venous flows around the drainage cannula. End-tidal $CO_2$ monitoring can be a useful surrogate estimate of transpulmonary blood flow. Thresholds of an end-tidal $CO_2$ <14 mmHg in conjunction with a pulse pressure <15 mmHg may predict a low native cardiac output <1L/min with good accuracy.[2]

Achieving these hemodynamic goals can be challenging and strongly positive fluid balances are associated with poor outcome, while high-dose vasopressors can impede the microcirculation, and liberal use of inotropes may hamper myocardial recovery.[3] However, patients supported by VA ECMO for refractory shock are typically in need of well-tailored fluid resuscitation and vasopressors to manage the vasoplegic aspects of shock, while inotropes aid to stimulate the myocardial contractile reserve and insure cardiac flow and ejection. Pulsatility on the arterial waveform in the presence of an IABP may provide false reassurance. Assessing aortic valve opening with echocardiography is important.

In some patients, it may be necessary to increase VA ECMO flow to higher blood flow rates, eg, >4 L/min. However, higher VA ECMO flows increase the risks of certain adverse effects, including impaired cardiac ejection, left ventricular overload, and pulmonary congestion. This occurs because VA ECMO constitutes partial cardiopulmonary bypass. Blood flow not captured by the venous drainage cannula continues as native cardiac output and residual transpulmonary blood flow through the right ventricle (RV) to the left ventricle (LV). With a competent aortic valve and poor LV function, peripheral VA ECMO pressurizes the aorta resulting in proportionally excessive LV afterload, more so when right ventricular contractility is preserved.[4] Without adequate LV ejection into the aorta, the LV overdistends, which may rapidly culminate in severe pulmonary edema, pulmonary hemorrhage, and increased risk of LV cavity and aortic root thrombosis. Detection of these phenomena requires careful assessment of reduced arterial line pulsatility possibly indicating LV overload, bedside echocardiography to evaluate LV in- and outflow,[5-7] elevated pulmonary capillary wedge pressures, decreased end-tidal $CO_2$,[2,8] and reduced lung compliance and oxygenation. This last point can lead to hypoxemic blood entering the left heart. Upon LV ejection, the hypoxemic blood reaches the proximal aorta and its branches including the coronary and cerebral arteries, potentially causing significant ischemia to heart and brain. This phenomenon, differential hypoxemia, is more pronounced with poor pulmonary gas exchange and preserved or improving left ventricular ejection upon cardiac recovery. Therefore, timely detection of evolving differential hypoxemia is essential and easily monitored by pulse-oximetry on the right arm, as an accessible branch of the proximal aorta, and near-infrared spectroscopy (NIRS) on the forehead (Figure 28-1). Differential hypoxemia should be managed by adequate pulmonary oxygenation and may require switching peripheral VA ECMO to venovenoarterial (V-VA), subclavian V-A, or central V-A cannulation. Alternatively, strictly draining deoxygenated venous blood from the superior vena cava has been proposed to mitigate differential hypoxemia.[9,10] The dynamic balance between systemic support and cardiac protection should always be borne in mind while meeting the circulatory and respiratory needs of the patient through tailoring of VA ECMO support (Chapter 5).[4,11,12]

## Mechanical Ventilation Management

Although there is limited evidence to guide the practice of invasive mechanical ventilation while on VA ECMO, the goal is to optimize support of gas exchange, decrease workload of breathing, and minimize ventilator induced lung injury (VILI), while maintaining cardiac performance for oxygen delivery to organs perfused with native cardiac output. Achieving these goals is not only dependent upon mechanical ventilatory support and native cardiopulmonary function but also cannulation strategy, ECMO support, transfusion thresholds, and hemodynamic targets.

The prevalence of radiologic pulmonary edema during peripheral VA ECMO is reported to be 18-32% in small cohorts of patients in cardiogenic shock,[13,14] compared to up to 80% with moderate or severe pulmonary edema in postcardiotomy shock.[15] Postmortem pulmonary histopathologic evaluation of patients who received ECMO for cardiac support revealed pulmonary hemorrhage (68%), thromboembolic disease (48%), hemorrhagic infarct (23%) and diffuse alveolar damage (20%).[16]

In addition to the hydrostatic alveolar-capillary barrier damage directly attributable to heart failure, the lung injury related to VA ECMO is a dynamically changing, complex mix of hydrostatic pulmonary edema, pulmonary hemorrhage, inflammatory infiltration, and lung embolism and/or ischemia (Figure 28-2).[17] Indistinguishable from simple fluid overload on chest radiography, this heterogenous pattern of lung injury also contributes to altered regional distribution of energy imposed on the lung tissue during each mechanically ventilated breath, which is believed to contribute to VILI and hypoxemia from ventilation-perfusion mismatch.[18] Additionally, the decreased transpulmonary blood flow, increased physiologic dead space, decreased lung compliance, and increased work of breathing may result in hypercapnia, ventilator asynchrony,[19,20] and increased oxygen consumption.[21]

A well-grounded mechanical ventilation strategy, in concert with proper ECMO and critical care management, has important implications for recovery of this cardiopulmonary injury but there is a paucity of research in this area.[22,23] There are over 30 different commercially available ventilators with approximately 500 names for 50 different modes[24] of mechanical ventilation, hence we recommend a control mode selection most familiar to the local care team because no one mode has proven superiority during VA ECMO. Lung protective mechanical ventilation, ie, tidal volume 3-6 ml/kg, plateau pressure <27 $cmH_2O$,[22,25] low driving pressure <14 $cmH_2O$,[26,27] and moderate positive end-expiratory pressure (PEEP) (8-10 $cmH_2O$), when no obstructive shock or severe right ventricular dysfunction is suspected,[28-30] are generally acceptable initial settings. Additionally, a respiratory rate of 6-12/min with a minute ventilation proportional to transpulmonary blood flow, while monitoring for intrinsic PEEP and non-injurious $FiO_2$ settings, can be adopted from the ARDS literature.[31,32] Most $CO_2$ clearance should occur extracorporeally in order to minimize the risk of VILI.

Special attention should be directed to optimal PEEP selection considering the complex interaction between intrathoracic pressures,[33] visceral and renal perfusion,[34,35] lung recruitment,[36] transpulmonary blood flow, ventilation, and native cardiac output[33,36,37] (Figure 28-3). PEEP will affect biventricular load with disproportionate effects on right ventricular function and transpulmonary blood flow.[19,38,39] Critically low transpulmonary blood flow (<1 L/min), as indicated by arterial pulse pressure <15 mmHg or end-tidal $CO_2$ <14 mmHg[2], should prompt adjustments in minute ventilation and PEEP to avoid blood flow stagnation and severe alkalosis of natively ejected blood.

Generic targets for $SaO_2$, $PaO_2$, $PaCO_2$, and pH are challenging to recommend and can be difficult for clinicians to manage due to regional variations in oxygen delivery,[40] based on cannula configuration and competing native and VA ECMO circulations.[41,42] It is important to individualize these targets based on individual clinical settings. Factors

determining patient $PaO_2$ and $PaCO_2$ include where the measurement is taken, native heart function, native lung function, transpulmonary blood flow, mechanical ventilator settings (mean airway pressure, $FiO_2$ and minute ventilation), ECMO settings (blood flow rate, sweep gas flow rate, $FSO_2$), cannula configuration[9] and left ventricular venting strategy, where relevant. Despite the known potential adverse effects of tissue hyperoxia ($PaO_2$ >100-300 mmHg) and hypocarbia ($PaCO_2$ <30), these are common on VA ECMO[23,43] and may have deleterious side effects, including poor neurologic outcomes.[52,44-47] Likewise, hypercarbia ($PaCO_2$ >45) is well known to promote pulmonary vasoconstriction and thereby increasing pulmonary vascular

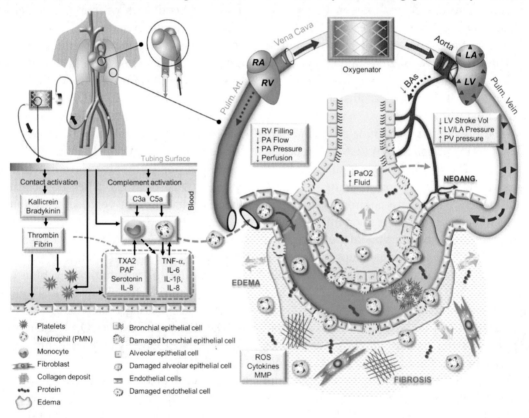

**Figure 28-2.** Lung injury related to VA ECMO; reproduced with permission from Mayo Foundation for Education and Research.

resistance and right ventricular afterload. Future practice may be informed by results of studies to evaluate the effect of conservative versus liberal oxygen strategy during VA ECMO (Blender-ClinicalTrials.gov Identifier: NCT038410840).

### Complications During Mechanical Ventilation

Mechanical ventilation management of differential hypoxemia is an important aspect of VA ECMO care. As myocardial recovery is dependent upon adequate myocardial oxygen delivery, appropriate oxygenation and ventilation of transpulmonary blood flow is crucial. Ventilator adjustments for differential hypoxemia include $FiO_2$ and PEEP titration, potentially guided by an esophageal balloon for transpulmonary pressure measurements,[48] and assessment of lung recruitability.[49] Additional interventions which have been employed include neuromuscular blockage,[50] optimal patient positioning, inhaled pulmonary vasodilators such as inhaled nitric oxide (iNO), inhaled prostacyclin/analogs (eg, epoprostenol, iloprost, treprostinil), inhaled phosphodiesterase III inhibitors (milrinone) or inhaled levosimendan,[51] beta-blockers to decrease transpulmonary blood flow when intrapulmonary shunt is excessive, the addition of a venous return cannula for hybrid V-VA ECMO, conversion to central or axillary VA ECMO, or specific positioning of the drainage cannula in the superior caval vein.[9] While some of these simpler interventions may be worth

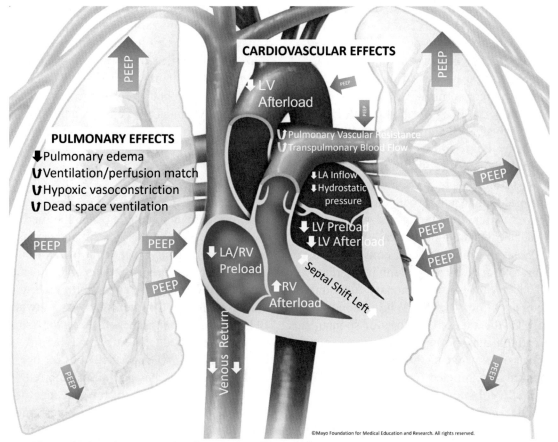

**Figure 28-3.** Pulmonary and cadiovascular effects subject to PEEP management; reproduced with permission from Mayo Foundation for Education and Research.

attempting in selected patients, they are often ineffective or of marginal utility. Sustained, worsening differential hypoxemia should usually prompt cannula reconfiguration.

Optimal mechanical ventilator management is also relevant with respect to LV overdistention. When promoting LV ejection or initiating adjunct venting strategies, it is important to maintain proper oxygenation of the ejected blood using strategies outlined above on differential hypoxemia, with an emphasis on PEEP titration in concert with an adequate $FiO_2$.

Ventilator associated pneumonia occurs frequently on VA ECMO and can be challenging to diagnose.[52] Potentially effective strategies to decrease this include reducing duration of mechanical ventilation, avoiding over-sedation and prolonged paralytics, maintaining oral hygiene (see ENT section), and semi recumbent body position (head of bed 30-45 degrees). Bronchoscopy may be necessary to establish the diagnosis of pneumonia, assess radiographic abnormalities and clear secretions, and can be safely performed on VA ECMO.[53] Chest physical therapy and mobilization are also effective techniques at clearing retained secretions[54] and reserving tracheal suctioning when indicated to <15 sec may decrease mucosal trauma and associated tracheitis.[55,56]

Ventilator asynchrony and weaning from mechanical ventilation generally increase work of breathing and oxygen consumption,[57,58] thus tolerance is dependent upon recovery of underlying cardiopulmonary function and hemodynamic stability. While supported on ECMO, the excessive efforts of spontaneous breathing may be better tolerated,[59] but the threats of lung and diaphragm injury by patient induced self-inflicted lung injury (P-SILI) as well as ventilator induced diaphragm injury (VIDI) require careful monitoring.[60,61]

In summary, mechanical ventilation management on VA ECMO requires an awareness of the complex interaction between ECMO-associated changes in lung condition, pulmonary blood flow, and the cardiopulmonary effects of mechanical ventilation. Early management of congestive pulmonary edema, pulmonary hemorrhage, ventilator associated pneumonia and minimizing transfusions while optimizing gas exchange using lung protective mechanical ventilation are reasonable strategies while comprehensively monitoring and awaiting cardiac recovery on VA ECMO.

**Analgo-sedation, Neurologic Monitoring, Physical Therapy and Mobility**

Optimal sedation management in patients on ECLS is complex because of specific ECLS-related, pharmacokinetic, and pharmacodynamic considerations.[62] In general, analgo-sedative drugs must be administered in a very targeted manner to allow rapid discontinuation of sedation and promote rehabilitation, while maximizing patient comfort and minimizing the risk of delirium. However, ECLS can significantly alter both the pharmacokinetics and pharmacodynamics of commonly administered drugs. For example, fentanyl, midazolam, propofol, and dexmedetomidine may require high dosages to achieve desired therapeutic effects (Chapter 49). [82,63]

The so called *awake* VA ECMO approach is a very demanding strategy for the medical and nursing team because it requires increased monitoring during patient mobilization to ensure safety and proper fixation of the devices, but has proven feasible and safe in otherwise stable patients (Chapter 47).[64,74,153] Awake ECMO has been successfully established in well-selected patients as a bridge to lung transplant[65] (Chapter 40) but its use in cardiogenic shock has also been reported.[66,67] It can allow patients to actively perform physical therapy, express themselves freely, and facilitates easier neurological assessment. In addition, mobilizing and maintaining spontaneous breathing can prevent diaphragm dysfunction, pneumonia, and other negative sequelae of controlled mechanical ventilation and immobilization.[68,153]

Although standardized neuromonitoring on ECLS may improve outcomes,[69] there is no widely accepted standard. Cranial computed tomography (CT), NIRS, brain ultrasound and transcranial doppler (TCD), electroencephalogram (EEG) and serum biomarkers can help to reveal brain injury. Some centers perform cranial CT before initiating ECLS, but, in general, its use is limited to a clinical indication and requires intrahospital transport of a patient on ECLS, with all inherent risks and challenges. Newer, portable CT scanners may make this easier in the future.

NIRS is widely used as a monitoring system for early detection of cerebral hypoxemia, eg, as a result of differential hypoxemia.[70] The absolute regional brain oxygen saturation ($rScO_2$) value varies significantly between individuals and has not sufficiently been validated; however, a drop of >25% from baseline may be sensitive to reflect acute brain injury, which emphasizes the importance to monitor trends.[71]

Transcranial Doppler (TCD) can detect microemboli.[72] However, its interpretation can be difficult because the specificity of TCD tracings for different types of circulatory assistance (ECMO, Impella, etc.) need to be considered.[73]

EEG, continuously or upon clinical indication, can be used for the detection of seizures but also as a diagnostic and prognostic tool in the setting of post cardiac arrest care and to detect cerebral ischemia.[74,75] Neuromonitoring of the critically ill remains an important, challenging field which is rapidly evolving.[76]

## Eyes, Ears, Nose and Throat Care

Care for the eyes, ears, nose, and throat requires diligent attention to prevent complications, maintain comfort, and promote functional recovery. In ECLS patients, orogastric tube insertion may be preferred over NGT when possible due to the high incidence of epistaxis.[77,78] Conservative bedside management with external nasal pinching or nasal packing typically suffices to control bleeding but otolaryngology consultation and surgical packing using temporary hemostatic gauze may be necessary in more severe situations.[79,80,81]

Although no consensus exists on optimal oral healthcare in the critically ill and the use of chlorhexidine is falling out of favor, it seems pragmatic that comprehensive oral hygiene be performed routinely and gently to avoid gingival trauma and bleeding.[82,83]

## Nutrition and Gastrointestinal Dysmotility

Enteral nutrition (EN) confers a survival benefit in critically ill patients and is an accepted standard of care when patients are unable to meet their nutritional needs after seven days.[84]

EN is frequently withheld in patients receiving VA ECMO based on safety concerns, such as EN intolerance or acute mesenteric ischemia. Both may not be directly related to EN but are rather a reflection of the severity of the underlying disease.[85] Nonetheless, mounting evidence has demonstrated the safety of early EN in patients undergoing VA ECMO. Recent data even point to a reduced risk of mesenteric ischemia and survival benefits with early initiation of EN in these patients.[86,87] Prokinetic agents, eg, metoclopramide or erythromycin, can be helpful to overcome EN intolerance but care has to be taken because of their effects on the QT interval.[88]

Patients typically exhibit a significant catabolic stress response, thus determination of energy requirements usually follow established recommendations with 20–25 kcal/kg/d for caloric intake and 1.5 g/kg/d for protein.[89] Vitamin and micronutrients monitoring may be of value during prolonged ECMO runs.[90]

## Renal Management

Acute kidney injury (AKI) occurs in an estimated 47-56% of patients supported by VA ECMO and has an associated mortality of 33%.[91] ELSO Registry data demonstrated a 3% prevalence of chronic kidney disease (CKD)[91] and a 14% prevalence of preexisting AKI (defined as a serum creatinine >1.5 mg/dL (>132 umol/L) with or without renal replacement therapy).[92] While the exact mechanism of VA ECMO-associated AKI is not well understood, factors including systemic hypoperfusion as a result of the shock state requiring ECLS and premorbid kidney disease are major contributors. VA ECMO-related renal injury may occasionally be the result of hemolysis byproducts, hemoglobinuria, microemboli, and inflammatory effects of blood exposure to the circuit and membrane.[93-97]

Defining and monitoring the degree of AKI during VA ECMO can be done using RIFLE,[98] AKIN,[99] or KDIGO[96] criteria, which largely utilize urine output and serum creatinine change over time. All of these demonstrate that a worse outcome is associated with worsening AKI. Treatment and prevention of AKI requires avoiding renal congestion, optimizing renal perfusion pressure and optimizing oxygen delivery by maintaining an adequate hemoglobin, oxygen saturation and renal blood flow. Optimizing the patient's fluid status remains challenging even with the use of serial echocardiograms and ultrasound assessments of the inferior vena cava (IVC). Ultrasound assessment of volume responsiveness to improve perfusion can overcome the challenges of using the traditionally unreliable central venous pressure (CVP).[100,101] Empiric fluid challenges may be expeditious and pragmatic but detrimental, as increasing evidence underscores that excessive fluid is harmful.[3,101] In situations of IVC congestion, the use of diuretics may be helpful.[102] Local blood flow and renal perfusion may be affected by cannula positioning and point of care Doppler ultrasound can be used to monitor changes.[103] Using the lowest possible VA ECMO flow and pump speed with appropriately sized and positioned cannulas to maintain adequate end organ oxygen delivery, as indicated by central venous oxygen saturation, lactate clearance, and an adequate urine output, minimizes the detrimental effects of VA ECMO-associated hemolysis and blood shear stress.[96,104,105]

CKD patients may need a higher MAP (70-85 mmHg) to ensure adequate renal perfusion.[106] Nephrotoxic medications should be avoided if possible and dose adjustments should be undertaken.

## Hematological and Coagulation Management

VA ECMO protocols routinely include the use of therapeutic systemic anticoagulation, with the primary goal of minimizing circuit thrombosis and avoiding thromboembolic complications. Unfractionated heparin (UFH) is widely used due to its ease of titration, monitoring, and rapid reversal with protamine. When heparin-induced thrombocytopenia (HIT) or heparin resistance develops, a direct thrombin inhibitor (DTI) such as bivalirudin or argatroban may be used.[77] Although evidence is growing in support of primary use of DTIs, large clinical trials are still necessary.[107-109]

The optimal anticoagulation strategy for VA ECMO has not been established[110] and ideally requires the integration of multiple laboratory measures of hemostasis (Table 28-2) with the clinical hemostatic state of the patient.[107]

### *Hemorrhage*

The cumulative incidence of any bleeding in VA ECMO patients in the ELSO Registry was 33%, with a significant impact on outcome.[111] Major bleeding is a less common but serious complication and may occur at various sites that require specific actions.[112,113]

| LABORATORY TEST | FREQUENCY | COMMENTS |
|---|---|---|
| ACT | Q1H-Q2H | q1 hr until heparin dose unchanged for 6 hours, then q2 hr |
| aPTT | Q6H-Q12H | |
| Anti-factor Xa Assay | Q6H-Q12H | or 4 hours after each heparin change |
| Platelets | Q6H-Q12H | |
| INR | Q12H-Q24H | |
| Fibrinogen | Q12H-Q24H | |
| CBC | Q12H-Q24H | |
| Antithrombin level | Daily-PRN | |
| Plasma free hemoglobin | Daily | |
| Thromboelastometry | Daily- PRN bleeding or thrombotic complications | |
| ACT=activated clotting time; aPTT=activated partial thromboplastin time; CBC=complete blood count; INR=international normalized ratio | | |

**Table 28-2.** Coagulation Test and Lab Monitoring Frequency, adapted from McMichael[112]

Management of bleeding involves rapid diagnosis and control at the site of bleeding in parallel with estimating the degree of hemorrhage, rate of loss, and control of anticoagulation intensity. Major bleeding with hemodynamic compromise should prompt urgent volume resuscitation including packed red blood cells, fresh frozen plasma and platelets as necessary, corrective surgery where indicated, discontinuation of systemic anticoagulation infusion, consideration of reversal agents, and tranexamic acid. In the more extreme cases, activated factor VII, prothrombin complex concentrate, and mechanical compression packing may be necessary.[114,115]

Determining the presence of any associated clotting defect is a cornerstone of medical bleeding management for which laboratory testing and thromboelastography may guide therapy[116] (Table 28-2).

The decision to continue transfusion of red blood cells should be based on active clinical bleeding and/or evidence of decreased systemic or regional oxygen delivery, rather than a fixed hemoglobin level. However, insufficient evidence is available to define a safe lower threshold in VA ECMO.[117] The target platelet count should be increased to 50,000-100,000/$mm^3$ and fibrinogen concentrations should be maintained >1.5 g/L (150 mg/dL) (Table 28-3).[107]

Management of the patient's hematological system during VA ECMO can be complicated. Low levels of factor XIII [118] and acquired von Willebrand syndrome[119] are common. Some centers have a dedicated team to oversee anticoagulation and blood product management.[120]

### Thrombosis

A 15.6% incidence of circuit thrombosis on VA ECMO has been described, 8.2% of which were oxygenator thrombosis.[121] Small fibrin deposits (white) and clot (dark) formation on the pre-oxygenator side of the circuit are common and pose little risk to the patient because embolized material will be captured

| | GOAL | PRODUCT TO TRANSFUSE |
|---|---|---|
| **Platelets** | >50,000-100,000 x $10^9$/L (bleeding patient) >20,000-50,000 x $10^9$/L (non-bleeding patient) | Platelets 10ml/kg (max 2 units) |
| **INR** | <1.5 (bleeding patient) <3 (non-bleeding patient) | Fresh frozen plasma 10ml/kg (max 2 units) |
| **Fibrinogen** | >1.5 g/L (bleeding patient or before surgical intervention) >1 g/L (non-bleeding) | Cryoprecipitate 1 Unit/5kg (max 6 units) |
| **Hemoglobin** | >70-90 g/L (consider higher goal for unstable patient, lower goal for stable patient) | Packed RBC 10ml/kg (max 2 units) |
| RBCs=red blood cells; INR=international normalized ratio; UFH=unfractionated heparin | | |

**Table 28-3.** Transfusion Thresholds and Targets, adapted from McMichael[112]

by the oxygenator. Clinical practice guidelines recommend regular monitoring of the circuit and oxygenator with a flashlight and measurement of pre- and post-oxygenator pressures and blood gases. Declines in oxygenator efficiency and worsening trans-oxygenator pressure gradients may necessitate oxygenator exchange.[122]

Thrombotic complications may also induce a consumptive coagulopathy based on a complex interplay of a multitude of pro- and anticoagulant factors. Consequently, an increased thrombotic and bleeding risk may arise. In order to control this balance between thrombotic and hemorrhagic diathesis, the degree of such a consumptive coagulopathy should carefully be monitored by checking D-dimer, markers of hemolysis (plasma free hemoglobin, LDH), decreasing fibrinogen and platelet count, and/or changes in viscoelastic testing. Significant consumptive coagulopathy may arise rapidly after initiation of ECLS despite therapeutic levels of anticoagulation and should prompt evaluation for ECMO component or circuit exchange.[123]

## Nosocomial Infection

Nosocomial infection is one of the most frequent complications during ECLS, with reported rates between 9-65% and associated with increased mortality, duration of ECMO support, mechanical ventilation, and ICU and hospital lengths of stay.[124,125] Risk factors for developing infections during VA ECMO are highlighted in Chapter 6.[124] The most common infections are lower respiratory tract infections, bloodstream infections (BSI), and surgical site infections.[126,127]

It can be difficult for clinicians to differentiate infection from systemic inflammatory syndromes in patients on ECLS.[128] Moreover, fever as a clinical sign will be absent because the blood temperature is regulated by an efficient extracorporeal heater/cooler system. At present, traditional microbiological approaches

alongside innovative molecular techniques may facilitate rapid identification of the etiological agent of BSIs.[129,130]

The most frequent infective agents during ECLS are coagulase-negative staphylococcus (CoNS), Candida species (spp.), *Pseudomonas aeruginosa*, Enterobacterales, *Staphylococcus aureus*, and Enterococcus spp.[131] When infection is clinically suspected during ECLS, empiric broad-spectrum antibiotic therapy is administered immediately after collecting samples for microbiology.[132]

Prevention of infections in the critically ill should follow locally supported bundled interventions for central line associated bloodstream infection, catheter associated urinary tract infection, ventilator associated pneumonia and surgical site infections.[133] There is no current data to support the use of routine antibiotic prophylaxis in ECLS patients.[127,134,135] Therapeutic drug monitoring is discussed in Chapter 49.

## Skin and Cannula Site Management

Cardiogenic shock is associated with cutaneous hypoperfusion, increasing the incidence of deep cutaneous ulcers and associated tissue injury.[136,137] Hemodynamic instability may lead to apprehension in turning patients, increasing the risk of hospital-acquired pressure ulcers. Special attention should be given to patients at high risk (Braden Scale score <15).[138] Impaired tissue perfusion and skin dysfunction may contribute to the 18% incidence of percutaneous cannulation site infection.[139] Prevention strategies are therefore important and include a bundled cannula insertion plan with full sterile barrier precautions and dressings method. This can be augmented by daily chlorhexidine baths for skin decontamination and at least a daily change of dressings depending on the amount of serous or serosanguineous discharge at the cannula insertion site. Transparent semipermeable dressings which permit visual inspection of the insertion site for bleeding, erythema, purulence, securement, and migration are used in a majority of ECLS centers and also allow to check and document a stable cannula position and recognize possible gradual migration over time.[140] Theoretically, chlorhexidine-impregnated dressings could help to further reduce the risk of infection although there is currently insufficient evidence for routine use in ECLS patients. To prevent pressure ulcers and injury at the cannula insertion site, hydrocolloid or foam pads can be placed beneath the cannula. Hydrocolloid pads equipped with a cannula attachment device have the advantage of adding fixation points to secure the cannula position without the risks of skin lesions.

The potentially life-threatening consequences of limb ischemia make monitoring of distal limb perfusion during VA ECMO of utmost importance. Although there is no standardized approach to monitoring, current practices focus on dedicated clinical observation including monitoring of clinical findings (decreasing skin temperature, discoloration of the skin and increasing stiffness of the ankle joint, increasing calf stiffness and circumference, rising creatine kinase), in conjunction with tissue oxygenation as monitored by NIRS,[141,142] and Doppler ultrasonography. If clinical observation and/or NIRS suggest limb ischemia, more invasive diagnostic measures, eg, angiography, and expert consultation will become necessary (Chapter 4).[141] If ischemia is irreversible, limb amputation must be considered early to avoid additional life-threatening complications from release of toxic metabolites or development of gangrene.

**Special Considerations for Acute Coronary Ischemia Post Percutaneous Coronary Intervention (PCI) ECLS**

Management of VA ECMO support initiated directly before or after percutaneous coronary intervention (PCI) requires special attention to antithrombotic or anticoagulation strategy, myocardial protection, and hemodynamic monitoring.

Antithrombotic and anticoagulation therapy are an essential part of post-PCI and VA ECMO care to prevent potentially deleterious thromboembolic events, eg, in-stent thrombosis, membrane thrombosis, left ventricular and aortic root thrombus formation. Hemorrhagic complications are a major concern, especially with triple therapy, ie. dual antiplatelet therapy (DAPT) and systemic anticoagulation on VA ECMO.[143,144]

Although data is limited, it is reasonable for acute coronary syndrome (ACS) patients post-PCI on VA ECMO support without active bleeding to receive systemic anticoagulation with heparin or bivalirudin, and antithrombotic therapy with aspirin and a P2Y12 receptor inhibitor such as cangrelor (considering its parenteral route and rapid onset), which can be switched to clopidogrel once enteral absorption is assured.[144-146]

ACS patients demand careful monitoring for myocardial ischemia while on VA ECMO. Serial or continuous multilead electrocardiography and the regular assessment of biomarkers reflecting the success of coronary revascularization and or relapsing myocardial ischemia are pivotal elements of bedside monitoring. Clinical signs of gradual or progressive hemodynamic deterioration such as a disproportionate need for fluid resuscitation, significant increase of vasopressive or inotropic support, a higher degree of VA ECMO blood flow, or a decrease of arterial pulsatility should always prompt urgent diagnostics. Although the differential diagnosis is inherently broad, consideration should be given to extensive myocardial ischemia, late complications of an acute or subacute myocardial infarction (eg, interventricular septal or papillary muscle rupture), cardiac tamponade, and complications related to cardiac catheterization such as retroperitoneal hematoma. Here, echocardiography and point of care ultrasound play important roles for early diagnostics (Chapter 48).[7] Pulmonary artery catheters may be useful, but specifically in inferior and inferoposterior myocardial infarction, right ventricular involvement should be excluded because manipulation of a catheter within an ischemic right ventricular cavity may promote troublesome ventricular arrhythmias and increase the risk of perforation.

Unresolved issues in the care of these patients include the optimal anticoagulation and antithrombotic strategies, hemoglobin transfusion targets,[147] and the role of IABP or transaortic microaxial pumps to optimize coronary artery flow and reduce subendocardial ischemia.[11,148,149]

## Special Considerations for Postcardiotomy ECLS

Postcardiotomy VA ECMO is being increasingly used with a prevalence reported between 0.4% and 3.7%.[150] The most common indication for postcardiotomy ECLS implementation is intraoperative failure to wean from cardiopulmonary bypass. It may also be implemented for delayed refractory cardiogenic shock or postoperative cardiac arrest in the ICU.[151] Postcardiotomy VA ECMO can be considered as a standard-of-care in postcardiac transplant graft dysfunction (Chapter 41).

Possible predictors of the need for temporary postcardiotomy ECLS include old age, renal failure, prior myocardial infarction, left main coronary artery disease, left ventricular dysfunction, and redo cardiac surgery.[152,153] In the absence of early cardiac recovery (48-72 hours), LVAD or cardiac transplantation may be pursued for appropriate candidates.[154] Determining that a patient has reached a therapeutic ceiling with irrefutable evidence of medical futility should be considered in a timely manner and be based on clear criteria that demonstrate a lack of recovery, noncandidacy

for durable mechanical circulatory support, or progression to an unsurvivable condition. Currently, the following factors negatively influence survival after postcardiotomy ECLS: lactate levels immediately prior to ECLS, as well as its highest level 12-48 hours post-ECLS initiation; renal, liver or respiratory failure; and the duration of ECLS support.[151]

Peripheral cannulation may be preferred to reduce the risks of infection and bleeding.[127,155,156] Published experience demonstrates a weaning rate of around 50%. Survival to hospital discharge is far less common (<40%), although the majority who survive to discharge are still alive at 1-year followup. The survival of patients who received postcardiotomy ECLS for postcardiac transplant graft dysfunction is better because post-graft dysfunction is frequently reversible.[157]

## Special Considerations for Acute Massive Pulmonary Embolus

Massive acute pulmonary embolism (MAPE), defined as pulmonary embolism (PE) with cardiogenic shock refractory to supportive measures, is associated with high mortality rates of up to 50%.[158] If MAPE decompensates to cardiac arrest, mortality is >80%.[159]

VA ECMO is a reliable, fast way to reduce right ventricle (RV) overload and restore tissue perfusion and oxygenation, while awaiting resolution of the pulmonary vascular thrombus load by initiation of systemic thrombolysis, catheter based therapy, and/or surgical embolectomy.[160,161] In MAPE patients supported with VA ECMO, higher survival was associated with those aged <61 years old and those treated with surgical embolectomy.[162]

Although poorer outcomes result when ECLS was instituted during cardiopulmonary arrest and worsened further if initiated greater than 30 min from the time of arrest, short-term survival rates of 34% is a significant improvement from thrombolysis alone.[162,163]

Frequently, patients with MAPE are placed on ECLS as a salvage intervention. However, a protocolized strategy involving early institution of VA ECMO appears to be an effective method to optimize outcomes in patients with MAPE, thereby serving as a bridge to recovery or facilitating the implementation of other advanced interventions.[164] Current data show that ECLS with anticoagulation alone can eventually lead to sufficient RV recovery to allow decannulation.[165] However, RV strain markedly improves in 24 to 48 hours with percutaneous interventions, faster than with anticoagulation alone.[166,167] Major bleeding post thrombolysis for PE is 9% and intracranial bleeding 1.5%,[168] which increases in the setting of VA ECMO with percutaneous catheter-directed therapy or surgical thrombectomy. Therapeutic strategies should be individualized.[162,169] Major bleeding within 24 hours of systemic thrombolytic administration can be treated with cryoprecipitate and tranexamic acid.

Given the heterogeneity in regard to management of PE, an increasing number of institutions are establishing multidisciplinary pulmonary embolism response teams (PERTs) in an effort to providing optimal acute and long-term care.[161]

# References

1. Chung M, Shiloh AL, Carlese A. Monitoring of the Adult Patient on Venoarterial Extracorporeal Membrane Oxygenation. The Scientific World Journal. 2014;2014:10.

2. Mourad M, Eliet J, Zeroual N, et al. Pulse pressure and end-tidal carbon dioxide for monitoring low native cardiac output during veno-arterial ECLS: a prospective observational study. Critical Care. 2020;24(1):569.

3. Schmidt M, Bailey M, Kelly J, et al. Impact of fluid balance on outcome of adult patients treated with extracorporeal membrane oxygenation. Intensive care medicine. 2014;40(9):1256-1266.

4. Donker DW, Sallisalmi M, Broome M. Right-Left Ventricular Interaction in Left-Sided Heart Failure With and Without Venoarterial Extracorporeal Membrane Oxygenation Support-A Simulation Study. Asaio J. 2021;67(3):297-305.

5. Douflé G, Roscoe A, Billia F, Fan E. Erratum to: Echocardiography for adult patients supported with extracorporeal membrane oxygenation. Critical care (London, England). 2016;20:34-34.

6. Nanjayya VB MD. Ultrasound guidance for extracorporeal membrane oxygenation: general guidelines. ELSO. Published 2015. Accessed January 5, 2022.

7. Donker DW, Meuwese CL, Braithwaite SA, et al. Echocardiography in extracorporeal life support: A key player in procedural guidance, tailoring and monitoring. Perfusion. 2018;33(1_suppl):31-41.

8. Naruke T, Inomata T, Imai H, et al. End-tidal carbon dioxide concentration can estimate the appropriate timing for weaning off from extracorporeal membrane oxygenation for refractory circulatory failure. International Heart Journal. 2010;51(2):116-120.

9. Frenckner B, Broman M, Broome M. Position of draining venous cannula in extracorporeal membrane oxygenation for respiratory and respiratory/circulatory support in adult patients. Crit Care. 2018;22(1):163.

10. Lindfors M, Frenckner B, Sartipy U, et al. Venous Cannula Positioning in Arterial Deoxygenation During Veno-Arterial Extracorporeal Membrane Oxygenation-A Simulation Study and Case Report. Artif Organs. 2017;41(1):75-81.

11. Donker DW, Brodie D, Henriques JPS, et al. Left Ventricular Unloading During Veno-Arterial ECMO: A Simulation Study. Asaio J. 2019;65(1):11-20.

12. Burkhoff D, Sayer G, Doshi D, et al. Hemodynamics of Mechanical Circulatory Support. J Am Coll Cardiol. 2015;66(23):2663-2674.

13. Demondion P, Fournel L, Golmard J-L, et al. Predictors of 30-day mortality and outcome in cases of myocardial infarction with cardiogenic shock treated by extracorporeal life support. European Journal of Cardio-Thoracic Surgery. 2013;45(1):47-54.

14. Boulate D, Luyt C-E, Pozzi M, et al. Acute lung injury after mechanical circulatory support implantation in patients on extracorporeal life support: an unrecognized problem†. European Journal of Cardio-Thoracic Surgery. 2013;44(3):544-550.

15. Distelmaier K, Wiedemann D, Lampichler K, et al. Interdependence of VA-ECMO output, pulmonary congestion and outcome after cardiac surgery. European Journal of Internal Medicine. 2020;81:67-70.

16. Lee HE, Yi ES, Rabatin JT, et al. Histopathologic Findings in Lungs of Patients Treated With Extracorporeal Membrane Oxygenation. Chest. 2018;153(4):825-833.

17. Roumy A, Liaudet L, Rusca M, et al. Pulmonary complications associated with veno-arterial extra-corporeal membrane oxygenation: a comprehensive review. Critical Care. 2020;24(1):212.

18. Gattinoni L, Tonetti T, Cressoni M, et al. Ventilator-related causes of lung injury: the mechanical power. Intensive Care Med. 2016;42(10):1567-1575.

19. Fessler HE. Heart-lung interactions: applications in the critically ill. Eur Respir J. 1997;10(1):226-237.

20. Figueroa-Casas JB, Montoya R. Effect of Tidal Volume Size and Its Delivery Mode on Patient-Ventilator Dyssynchrony. Ann Am Thorac Soc. 2016;13(12):2207-2214.

21. Cheifetz IM. Cardiorespiratory Interactions: The Relationship Between Mechanical Ventilation and Hemodynamics. Respir Care. 2014;59(12):1937.

22. Amado-Rodríguez L, Del Busto C, López-Alonso I, et al. Biotrauma during ultra-low tidal volume ventilation and venoarterial extracorporeal membrane oxygenation in cardiogenic shock: a randomized crossover clinical trial. Ann Intensive Care. 2021;11(1):132.

23. Justus A, Burrell A, Anstey C, et al. The Association of Oxygenation, Carbon Dioxide Removal, and Mechanical Ventilation Practices on Survival During Venoarterial Extracorporeal Membrane Oxygenation. Front Med (Lausanne). 2021;8:756280.

24. Chatburn RL, El-Khatib M, Mireles-Cabodevila E. A Taxonomy for Mechanical Ventilation: 10 Fundamental Maxims. Respir Care. 2014;59(11):1747.

25. Brower RG MM, Morris A, Schoenfeld D, et al. Ventilation with Lower Tidal Volumes as Compared with Traditional Tidal Volumes for Acute Lung Injury and the Acute Respiratory Distress Syndrome. New England Journal of Medicine. 2000;342(18):1301-1308.

26. Amato MBP, Meade MO, Slutsky AS, et al. Driving Pressure and Survival in the Acute Respiratory

Distress Syndrome. New England Journal of Medicine. 2015;372(8):747-755.

27. Del Sorbo L, Goffi A, Tomlinson G, et al. Effect of Driving Pressure Change During Extracorporeal Membrane Oxygenation in Adults With Acute Respiratory Distress Syndrome: A Randomized Crossover Physiologic Study. Crit Care Med. 2020;48(12):1771-1778.

28. Mercat A, Richard JC, Vielle B, et al. Positive end-expiratory pressure setting in adults with acute lung injury and acute respiratory distress syndrome: a randomized controlled trial. JAMA. 2008;299(6):646-655.

29. Guo L, Xie J, Huang Y, et al. Higher PEEP improves outcomes in ARDS patients with clinically objective positive oxygenation response to PEEP: a systematic review and meta-analysis. BMC Anesthesiol. 2018;18(1):172.

30. Wiesen J, Ornstein M, Tonelli AR, et al. State of the evidence: mechanical ventilation with PEEP in patients with cardiogenic shock. Heart. 2013;99(24):1812-1817.

31. Bellani G, Laffey JG, Pham T, et al. Epidemiology, Patterns of Care, and Mortality for Patients With Acute Respiratory Distress Syndrome in Intensive Care Units in 50 Countries. Jama. 2016;315(8):788-800.

32. ELSO. ELSO Guidelines for Cardiopulmonary Extracorporeal Life Support. 2017. https://www.elso.org/Portals/0/ELSO%20Guidelines%20General%20All%20ECLS%20Version%201_4.pdf. Published Version 1.4. Published August 2017. Accessed January 3, 2022.

33. Sarge T, Baedorf-Kassis E, Banner-Goodspeed V, et al. Effect of Esophageal Pressure-guided Positive End-Expiratory Pressure on Survival from Acute Respiratory Distress Syndrome: A Risk-based and Mechanistic Reanalysis of the EPVent-2 Trial. Am J Respir Crit Care Med. 2021;204(10):1153-1163.

34. Putensen C, Wrigge H, Hering R. The effects of mechanical ventilation on the gut and abdomen. Curr Opin Crit Care. 2006;12(2):160-165.

35. Koyner JL, Murray PT. Mechanical Ventilation and the Kidney. Blood Purif. 2010;29(1):52-68.

36. Goligher EC, Hodgson CL, Adhikari NKJ, et al. Lung Recruitment Maneuvers for Adult Patients with Acute Respiratory Distress Syndrome. A Systematic Review and Meta-Analysis. Ann Am Thorac Soc. 2017;14(Supplement_4):S304-S311.

37. Alviar CL, Miller PE, McAreavey D, et al. Positive Pressure Ventilation in the Cardiac Intensive Care Unit. J Am Coll Cardiol. 2018;72(13):1532-1553.

38. Luecke T, Pelosi P. Clinical review: Positive end-expiratory pressure and cardiac output. Crit Care. 2005;9(6):607-621.

39. Pinsky MR. Cardiopulmonary Interactions: Physiologic Basis and Clinical Applications. Ann Am Thorac Soc. 2018;15(Suppl 1):S45-S48.

40. Avgerinos DV, DeBois W, Voevidko L, et al. Regional variation in arterial saturation and oxygen delivery during venoarterial extracorporeal membrane oxygenation. J Extra Corpor Technol. 2013;45(3):183-186.

41. Alwardt CM, Patel BM, Lowell A, et al. Regional perfusion during venoarterial extracorporeal membrane oxygenation: a case report and educational modules on the concept of dual circulations. The Journal of extra-corporeal technology. 2013;45(3):187-194.

42. Joyce CJ, Anderson C, Shekar K. Hyperoxia on Venoarterial Extracorporeal Membrane Oxygenation: A Modifiable Risk? Crit Care Med. 2022;50(1):e99-e100.

43. Munshi L, Kiss A, Cypel M, et al. Oxygen Thresholds and Mortality During Extracorporeal Life Support in Adult Patients. Crit Care Med. 2017;45(12):1997-2005.

44. Al-Kawaz MN, Canner J, Caturegli G, et al. Duration of Hyperoxia and Neurologic Outcomes in Patients Undergoing Extracorporeal Membrane Oxygenation. Crit Care Med. 2021;49(10):e968-e977.

45. Hayes R, Shekar K, Fraser J. Is hyperoxaemia helping or hurting patients during extracorporeal membrane oxygenation? Review of a complex problem. Perfusion. 2013;28(3):184-193.

46. Cavayas YA, Munshi L, del Sorbo L, Fan E. The Early Change in Pa-CO2 after Extracorporeal Membrane Oxygenation Initiation Is Associated with Neurological Complications. American Journal of Respiratory and Critical Care Medicine. 2020;201(12):1525-1535.

47. Diehl A, Burrell AJC, Udy AA, et al. Association Between Arterial Carbon Dioxide Tension and Clinical Outcomes in Venoarterial Extracorporeal Membrane Oxygenation. Crit Care Med. 2020;48(7):977-984.

48. Beitler JR, Sarge T, Banner-Goodspeed VM, et al. Effect of Titrating Positive End-Expiratory Pressure (PEEP) With an Esophageal Pressure–Guided Strategy vs an Empirical High PEEP-Fio2 Strategy on Death and Days Free From Mechanical Ventilation Among Patients With Acute Respiratory Distress Syndrome: A Randomized Clinical Trial. JAMA. 2019;321(9):846-857.

49. Chen L, Del Sorbo L, Grieco DL, et al. Potential for Lung Recruitment Estimated by the Recruitment-to-Inflation Ratio in Acute Respiratory Distress Syndrome. A Clinical Trial. Am J Respir Crit Care Med. 2020;201(2):178-187.

50. Ho ATN, Patolia S, Guervilly C. Neuromuscular blockade in acute respiratory distress syndrome: a

systematic review and meta-analysis of randomized controlled trials. J Intensive Care. 2020;8:12.

51. Kundra TS, Prabhakar V, Kaur P, et al. The Effect of Inhaled Milrinone Versus Inhaled Levosimendan in Pulmonary Hypertension Patients Undergoing Mitral Valve Surgery - A Pilot Randomized Double-Blind Study. J Cardiothorac Vasc Anesth. 2018;32(5):2123-2129.

52. Bouglé A, Bombled C, Margetis D, et al. Ventilator-associated pneumonia in patients assisted by veno-arterial extracorporeal membrane oxygenation support: Epidemiology and risk factors of treatment failure. PLoS One. 2018;13(4):e0194976-e0194976.

53. Sharma NS, Peters T, Kulkarni T, et al. Flexible Bronchoscopy Is Safe and Effective in Adult Subjects Supported With Extracorporeal Membrane Oxygenation. Respir Care. 2016;61(5):646.

54. Berry MP, Martí JD. Clinical management of secretion retention in critically ill patients who are intubated and mechanically ventilated. Current Respiratory Medicine Reviews. 2014;10(3):163-175.

55. Shott SR. American Academy of Otolaryngology—Head and Neck Surgery: Free Papers: Otolaryngolic Complications of Extracorporeal Membrane Oxygenation (ECMO). Archives of Otolaryngology–Head & Neck Surgery. 1992;118(11):1153-1153.

56. AARC Clinical Practice Guidelines. Endotracheal suctioning of mechanically ventilated patients with artificial airways 2010. Respir Care. 2010;55(6):758-764.

57. Pinsky MR. Breathing as exercise: the cardiovascular response to weaning from mechanical ventilation. Intensive Care Med. 2000;26(9):1164-1166.

58. Zhou Y, Holets SR, Li M, et al. Etiology, incidence, and outcomes of patient-ventilator asynchrony in critically-ill patients undergoing invasive mechanical ventilation. Sci Rep. 2021;11(1):12390.

59. Vignon P. Cardiovascular failure and weaning. Ann Transl Med. 2018;6(18):354-354.

60. Brochard L, Slutsky A, Pesenti A. Mechanical Ventilation to Minimize Progression of Lung Injury in Acute Respiratory Failure. Am J Respir Crit Care Med. 2017;195(4):438-442.

61. Goligher EC, Dres M, Patel BK, et al. Lung- and Diaphragm-Protective Ventilation. Am J Respir Crit Care Med. 2020;202(7):950-961.

62. Shekar K, Roberts JA, McDonald CI, et al. Sequestration of drugs in the circuit may lead to therapeutic failure during extracorporeal membrane oxygenation. Critical care. 2012;16(5):R194.

63. Cheng V, Abdul-Aziz MH, Roberts JA, et al. Optimising drug dosing in patients receiving extracorporeal membrane oxygenation. J Thorac Dis. 2018;10(Suppl 5):S629-S641.

64. van Houte J, Donker DW, Wagenaar LJ, et al. Non-intubated recovery from refractory cardiogenic shock on percutaneous VA-extracorporeal membrane oxygenation. Neth Heart J. 2015;23(7-8):386-388.

65. Biscotti M, Gannon WD, Agerstrand C, et al. Awake Extracorporeal Membrane Oxygenation as Bridge to Lung Transplantation: A 9-Year Experience. Ann Thorac Surg. 2017;104(2):412-419.

66. Kim HA, Kim YS, Cho YH, et al. Implementation of Venoarterial Extracorporeal Membrane Oxygenation in Nonintubated Patients. J Chest Surg. 2021;54(1):17-24.

67. Montero S, Huang F, Rivas-Lasarte M, et al. Awake venoarterial extracorporeal membrane oxygenation for refractory cardiogenic shock. Eur Heart J Acute Cardiovasc Care. 2021;10(6):585-594.

68. Deng L, Xia Q, Chi C, Hu G. Awake veno-arterial extracorporeal membrane oxygenation in patients with perioperative period acute heart failure in cardiac surgery. J Thorac Dis. 2020;12(5):2179-2187.

69. Ong CS, Etchill E, Dong J, et al. Neuromonitoring detects brain injury in patients receiving extracorporeal membrane oxygenation support. J Thorac Cardiovasc Surg. 2021 Oct 30:S0022-5223(21)01508-7.

70. Cvetkovic M, Chiarini G, Belliato M, et al. International survey of neuromonitoring and neurodevelopmental outcome in children and adults supported on extracorporeal membrane oxygenation in Europe. Perfusion. 2021:2676591211042563.

71. Hunt MF, Clark KT, Whitman G, et al. The Use of Cerebral NIRS Monitoring to Identify Acute Brain Injury in Patients With VA-ECMO. J Intensive Care Med. 2021;36(12):1403-1409.

72. Marinoni M, Migliaccio ML, Trapani S, et al. Cerebral microemboli detected by transcranial doppler in patients treated with extracorporeal membrane oxygenation. Acta Anaesthesiol Scand. 2016;60(7):934-944.

73. Marinoni M, Cianchi G, Trapani S, et al. Retrospective Analysis of Transcranial Doppler Patterns in Veno-Arterial Extracorporeal Membrane Oxygenation Patients: Feasibility of Cerebral Circulatory Arrest Diagnosis. Asaio J. 2018;64(2):175-182.

74. Astrup J, Siesjo BK, Symon L. Thresholds in cerebral ischemia - the ischemic penumbra. Stroke. 1981;12(6):723-725.

75. Sinnah F, Dalloz MA, Magalhaes E, et al. Early Electroencephalography Findings in Cardiogenic Shock Patients Treated by Venoarterial Extracorporeal Membrane Oxygenation. Crit Care Med. 2018;46(5):e389-e394.

76. Musick S, Alberico A. Neurologic Assessment of the Neurocritical Care Patient. Front Neurol. 2021 Mar 22;12:588989.

77. Thomas J, Kostousov V, Teruya J. Bleeding and Thrombotic Complications in the Use of Extracorporeal Membrane Oxygenation. Seminars in Thrombosis and Hemostasis. 2018;44(1):20-29.

78. Zangrillo A, Landoni G, Biondi-Zoccai G, et al. A meta-analysis of complications and mortality of extracorporeal membrane oxygenation. Crit Care Resusc. 2013;15(3):172-178.

79. Mazzeffi M, Kiefer J, Kon Z, Wolf J. Severe epistaxis during adult extracorporeal membrane oxygenation: not your average nosebleed. Journal of Thoracic Disease. 2015;7(11):E564-E565.

80. Harrison MA, Baker AL, Roy S, et al. Management of upper aerodigestive tract bleeding on extracorporeal membrane oxygenation. Mechanical Circulatory Support. 2013;4(1):11826580.

81. Seikaly H. Epistaxis. New England Journal of Medicine. 2021;384(10):944-951.

82. Dennesen P, van der Ven A, Vlasveld M, et al. Inadequate salivary flow and poor oral mucosal status in intubated intensive care unit patients. Crit Care Med. 2003;31(3):781-786.

83. Dale CM, Rose L, Carbone S, et al. Effect of oral chlorhexidine de-adoption and implementation of an oral care bundle on mortality for mechanically ventilated patients in the intensive care unit (CHORAL): a multi-center stepped wedge cluster-randomized controlled trial. Intensive Care Med. 2021;47(11):1295-1302.

84. Taylor BE, McClave SA, Martindale RG, et al. Guidelines for the Provision and Assessment of Nutrition Support Therapy in the Adult Critically Ill Patient: Society of Critical Care Medicine (SCCM) and American Society for Parenteral and Enteral Nutrition (A.S.P.E.N.). Crit Care Med. 2016;44(2):390-438.

85. Reintam Blaser A, Preiser JC, Fruhwald S, et al. Gastrointestinal dysfunction in the critically ill: a systematic scoping review and research agenda proposed by the Section of Metabolism, Endocrinology and Nutrition of the European Society of Intensive Care Medicine. Crit Care. 2020;24(1):224.

86. Ohbe H, Jo T, Yamana H, et al. Early enteral nutrition for cardiogenic or obstructive shock requiring venoarterial extracorporeal membrane oxygenation: a nationwide inpatient database study. Intensive Care Med. 2018;44(8):1258-1265.

87. Renaudier M, de Roux Q, Bougouin W, et al. Acute mesenteric ischaemia in refractory shock on veno-arterial extracorporeal membrane oxygenation. Eur Heart J Acute Cardiovasc Care. 2020;10(1):62-70.

88. Singer P, Blaser AR, Berger MM, et al. ESPEN guideline on clinical nutrition in the intensive care unit. Clin Nutr. 2019;38(1):48-79.

89. Bear DE, Haslam J, Camporota L, et al. An international survey of nutrition practices in adult patients receiving veno-venous ECMO. Intensive Care Med Exp. 2015;3(Suppl 1):A295.

90. Lindberg BR, Videm V, Dahl T, et al. Influence of the ECMO circuit on the concentration of nutritional supplements. Scientific Reports. 2020;10(1):19275.

91. Cheng R, Hachamovitch R, Kittleson M, et al. Complications of extracorporeal membrane oxygenation for treatment of cardiogenic shock and cardiac arrest: A meta-analysis of 1,866 adult patients. Annals of Thoracic Surgery. 2014;97(2):610-616.

92. Schmidt M, Burrell A, Roberts L, et al. Predicting survival after ECMO for refractory cardiogenic shock: the survival after veno-arterial-ECMO (SAVE)-score. European heart journal. 2015;36(33):2246-2256.

93. Zanatta P, Forti A, Bosco E, et al. Microembolic signals and strategy to prevent gas embolism during extracorporeal membrane oxygenation. J Cardiothorac Surg. 2010;5:5.

94. Williams DC, Turi JL, Hornik CP, et al. Circuit oxygenator contributes to extracorporeal membrane oxygenation-induced hemolysis. ASAIO journal. 2015;61(2):190-195.

95. McILwain RB, Timpa JG, Kurundkar AR, et al. Plasma concentrations of inflammatory cytokines rise rapidly during ECMO-related SIRS due to the release of preformed stores in the intestine. Lab Invest. 2010;90(1):128-139.

96. Lee SW, Yu MY, Lee H, et al. Risk Factors for Acute Kidney Injury and In-Hospital Mortality in Patients Receiving Extracorporeal Membrane Oxygenation. PLoS One. 2015;10(10):e0140674.

97. Villa G, Katz N, Ronco C. Extracorporeal Membrane Oxygenation and the Kidney. Cardiorenal Medicine. 2016;6(1):50-60.

98. Lin C, Chen Y, Tsai F, et al. RIFLE classification is predictive of short-term prognosis in critically ill patients with acute renal failure supported by extracorporeal membrane oxygenation. Nephrology, dialysis, transplantation : official publication of the European Dialysis and Transplant Association - European Renal Association. 2006;21:2867 - 2873.

99. Chen YC, Tsai FC, Fang JT, et al. Acute kidney injury in adults receiving extracorporeal membrane oxygenation. J Formos Med Assoc. 2014;113(11):778-785.

100. Marik PE, Cavallazzi R. Does the central venous pressure predict fluid responsiveness? An updated meta-analysis and a plea for some common sense. Critical care medicine. 2013;41(7):1774-1781.

101. Benes J, Kirov M, Kuzkov V, et al. Fluid Therapy: Double-Edged Sword during Critical Care? Biomed Res Int. 2015;2015:729075.

102. Kingma JG, Simard D, Rouleau JR. Renocardiac syndromes: physiopathology and treatment stratagems. Canadian Journal of Kidney Health and Disease. 2015;2(1):1-10.

103. Hermansen JL, Pettey G, Sorensen HT, et al. Perioperative Doppler measurements of renal perfusion are associated with acute kidney injury in patients undergoing cardiac surgery. Sci Rep. 2021;11(1):19738.

104. Toomasian JM, Bartlett RH. Hemolysis and ECMO pumps in the 21st Century. Perfusion. 2011;26(1):5-6.

105. Lehle K, Philipp A, Zeman F, et al. Technical-Induced Hemolysis in Patients with Respiratory Failure Supported with Veno-Venous ECMO - Prevalence and Risk Factors. PLoS One. 2015;10(11):e0143527.

106. DellaVolpe JD, Moore JE, Pinsky MR. Arterial blood pressure and heart rate regulation in shock state. Current opinion in critical care. 2015;21(5):376-380.

107. McMichael ABV, Ryerson LM, Ratano D, et al. 2021 ELSO Adult and Pediatric Anticoagulation Guidelines. Asaio J. 2022;68(3):303-310.

108. Sheridan EA, Sekela ME, Pandya KA, et al. Comparison of Bivalirudin Versus Unfractionated Heparin for Anticoagulation in Adult Patients on Extracorporeal Membrane Oxygenation. ASAIO J. 2022 Jul 1;68(7):920-924.

109. Seelhammer TG, Bohman JK, Schulte PJ, et al. Comparison of Bivalirudin Versus Heparin for Maintenance Systemic Anticoagulation During Adult and Pediatric Extracorporeal Membrane Oxygenation. Crit Care Med. 2021;49(9):1481-1492.

110. Ranucci M. The conundrum of anticoagulation and hemostatic management in ECMO patients. Minerva Anestesiol. 2016;82(2):147-148.

111. Sy E, Sklar MC, Lequier L, et al. Anticoagulation practices and the prevalence of major bleeding, thromboembolic events, and mortality in venoarterial extracorporeal membrane oxygenation: A systematic review and meta-analysis. J Crit Care. 2017;39:87-96.

112. Aubron C, DePuydt J, Belon F, et al. Predictive factors of bleeding events in adults undergoing extracorporeal membrane oxygenation. Ann Intensive Care. 2016;6(1):97.

113. Le Guennec L, Cholet C, Huang F, et al. Ischemic and hemorrhagic brain injury during venoarterial-extracorporeal membrane oxygenation. Ann Intensive Care. 2018;8(1):129.

114. Anselmi A, Guinet P, Ruggieri VG, et al. Safety of recombinant factor VIIa in patients under extracorporeal membrane oxygenation. European journal of cardio-thoracic surgery : official journal of the European Association for Cardio-thoracic Surgery. 2016;49(1):78-84.

115. Repesse X, Au SM, Brechot N, et al. Recombinant factor VIIa for uncontrollable bleeding in patients with extracorporeal membrane oxygenation: report on 15 cases and literature review. Crit Care. 2013;17(2):R55.

116. Nair P, Hoechter DJ, Buscher H, et al. Prospective observational study of hemostatic alterations during adult extracorporeal membrane oxygenation (ECMO) using point-of-care thromboelastometry and platelet aggregometry. J Cardiothorac Vasc Anesth. 2015;29(2):288-296.

117. Bembea MM, Cheifetz IM, Fortenberry JD, et al. Recommendations on the Indications for RBC Transfusion for the Critically Ill Child Receiving Support From Extracorporeal Membrane Oxygenation, Ventricular Assist, and Renal Replacement Therapy Devices From the Pediatric Critical Care Transfusion and Anemia Expertise Initiative. Pediatr Crit Care Med. 2018;19(9S Suppl 1):S157-S162.

118. Kalbhenn J, Wittau N, Schmutz A, et al. Identification of acquired coagulation disorders and effects of target-controlled coagulation factor substitution on the incidence and severity of spontaneous intracranial bleeding during veno-venous ECMO therapy. Perfusion. 2015;30(8):675-682.

119. Heilmann C, Geisen U, Beyersdorf F, et al. Acquired von Willebrand syndrome in patients with extracorporeal life support (ECLS). Intensive Care Med. 2012;38(1):62-68.

120. Chlebowski MM, Baltagi S, Carlson M, et al. Clinical controversies in anticoagulation monitoring and antithrombin supplementation for ECMO. Crit Care. 2020;24(1):19.

121. Thiagarajan RR, Barbaro RP, Rycus PT, et al. Extracorporeal Life Support Organization Registry International Report 2016. ASAIO J. 2017;63(1):60-67.

122. Eckman PM, Katz JN, El Banayosy A, et al. Veno-Arterial Extracorporeal Membrane Oxygenation for Cardiogenic Shock: An Introduction for the Busy Clinician. Circulation. 2019;140(24):2019-2037.

123. Basken R, Cosgrove R, Malo J, et al. Predictors of Oxygenator Exchange in Patients Receiving Extracorporeal Membrane Oxygenation. J Extra Corpor Technol. 2019;51(2):61-66.

124. Abrams D, Grasselli G, Schmidt M, et al. ECLS-associated infections in adults: what we know and what we don't yet know. Intensive Care Medicine. 2020;46(2):182-191.

125. Schmidt M, Brechot N, Hariri S, et al. Nosocomial infections in adult cardiogenic shock patients supported by venoarterial extracorporeal membrane oxygenation. Clin Infect Dis. 2012;55(12):1633-1641.

126. Biffi S, Di Bella S, Scaravilli V, et al. Infections during extracorporeal membrane oxygenation: epidemiology, risk factors, pathogenesis and prevention. Int J Antimicrob Agents. 2017;50(1):9-16.

127. Lorusso R, Whitman G, Milojevic M, et al. 2020 EACTS/ELSO/STS/AATS expert consensus on post-cardiotomy extracorporeal life support in adult patients. Eur J Cardiothorac Surg. 2021;59(1):12-53.

128. Tanaka D, Pitcher HT, Cavarocchi NC, et al. Can procalcitonin differentiate infection from systemic inflammatory reaction in patients on extracorporeal membrane oxygenation? J Heart Lung Transplant. 2014;33(11):1186-1188.

129. Afshari A, Schrenzel J, Ieven M, et al. Bench-to-bedside review: Rapid molecular diagnostics for bloodstream infection--a new frontier? Crit Care. 2012;16(3):222.

130. Orszag P, Disque C, Keim S, et al. Monitoring of patients supported by extracorporeal membrane oxygenation for systemic infections by broad-range rRNA gene PCR amplification and sequence analysis. J Clin Microbiol. 2014;52(1):307-311.

131. Husain-Syed F, Ricci Z, Brodie D, et al. Extracorporeal organ support (ECOS) in critical illness and acute kidney injury: from native to artificial organ crosstalk. Intensive Care Med. 2018;44(9):1447-1459.

132. Pieri M, Greco T, De Bonis M, et al. Diagnosis of infection in patients undergoing extracorporeal membrane oxygenation: a case-control study. The Journal of thoracic and cardiovascular surgery. 2012;143(6):1411-1416.

133. Chang BH, Hsu YJ, Rosen MA, et al. Reducing Three Infections Across Cardiac Surgery Programs: A Multisite Cross-Unit Collaboration. Am J Med Qual. 2020;35(1):37-45.

134. Gopalakrishnan R, Vashisht R. Sepsis and ECMO. Indian J Thorac Cardiovasc Surg. 2020:1-8.

135. O'Horo JC, Cawcutt KA, De Moraes AG, et al. The evidence base for prophylactic antibiotics in patients receiving extracorporeal membrane oxygenation. ASAIO journal. 2016;62(1):6-10.

136. Brueske BS, Sidhu MS, Chang IY, et al. Braden skin score sub-domains predict mortality among cardiac intensive care patients. Am J Med. 2022 Jun;135(6):730-736.e5.

137. Rao AD, Preston AM, Strauss R, et al. Risk Factors Associated With Pressure Ulcer Formation in Critically Ill Cardiac Surgery Patients: A Systematic Review. J Wound Ostomy Continence Nurs. 2016;43(3):242-247.

138. Swafford K, Culpepper R, Dunn C. Use of a Comprehensive Program to Reduce the Incidence of Hospital-Acquired Pressure Ulcers in an Intensive Care Unit. Am J Crit Care. 2016;25(2):152-155.

139. Allou N, Lo Pinto H, Persichini R, et al. Cannula-Related Infection in Patients Supported by Peripheral ECMO: Clinical and Microbiological Characteristics. Asaio J. 2019;65(2):180-186.

140. Bull T, Corley A, Lye I, et al. Cannula and circuit management in peripheral extracorporeal membrane oxygenation: An international survey of 45 countries. PLoS One. 2019;14(12):e0227248.

141. Bonicolini E, Martucci G, Simons J, et al. Limb ischemia in peripheral veno-arterial extracorporeal membrane oxygenation: a narrative review of incidence, prevention, monitoring, and treatment. Crit Care. 2019;23(1):266.

142. Patton-Rivera K, Beck J, Fung K, et al. Using near-infrared reflectance spectroscopy (NIRS) to assess distal-limb perfusion on venoarterial (V-A) extracorporeal membrane oxygenation (ECMO) patients with femoral cannulation. Perfusion. 2018;33(8):618-623.

143. Oude Lansink-Hartgring A, de Vries AJ, Droogh JM, van den Bergh WM. Hemorrhagic complications during extracorporeal membrane oxygenation - The role of anticoagulation and platelets. J Crit Care. 2019;54:239-243.

144. Katz A, Lewis TC, Arnouk S, et al. Clinical Use of Cangrelor After Percutaneous Coronary Intervention in Patients Requiring Mechanical Circulatory Support. Ann Pharmacother. 2021;55(10):1215-1222.

145. Gorog DA, Price S, Sibbing D, et al. Antithrombotic therapy in patients with acute coronary syndrome complicated by cardiogenic shock or out-of-hospital cardiac arrest: a joint position paper from the European Society of Cardiology (ESC) Working Group on Thrombosis, in association with the Acute Cardiovascular Care Association (ACCA) and European Association of Percutaneous Cardiovascular Interventions (EAPCI). Eur Heart J Cardiovasc Pharmacother. 2021;7(2):125-140.

146. Radu RI, Ben Gal T, Abdelhamid M, et al. Antithrombotic and anticoagulation therapies in cardiogenic shock: a critical review of the published literature. ESC Heart Fail. 2021;8(6):4717-4736.

147. Ducrocq G, Gonzalez-Juanatey JR, Puymirat E, et al. Effect of a Restrictive vs Liberal Blood Transfusion Strategy on Major Cardiovascular Events Among Patients With Acute Myocardial Infarction and Anemia: The REALITY Randomized Clinical Trial. Jama. 2021;325(6):552-560.

148. Donker DW, Brodie D, Henriques JPS, et al. Left ventricular unloading during veno-arterial ECMO: a review of percutaneous and surgical unloading interventions. Perfusion. 2019;34(2):98-105.

149. Kapur NK, Reyelt L, Swain L, et al. Mechanical Left Ventricular Unloading to Reduce Infarct Size During Acute Myocardial Infarction: Insight from Preclinical and Clinical Studies. J Cardiovasc Transl Res. 2019;12(2):87-94.

150. Raffa GM, Gelsomino S, Sluijpers N, et al. In-hospital outcome of post-cardiotomy extracorporeal life

support in adult patients: the 2007-2017 Maastricht experience. Crit Care Resusc. 2017;19(Suppl 1):53-61.

151. Lorusso R, Raffa GM, Alenizy K, et al. Structured review of post-cardiotomy extracorporeal membrane oxygenation: part 1-Adult patients. J Heart Lung Transplant. 2019;38(11):1125-1143.

152. Zaaqoq AM, Pottash M, Ahlstrom E, et al. Postcardiotomy Extracorporeal Membrane Oxygenation: Narrative Review Navigating the Ethical Issues. J Cardiothorac Vasc Anesth. 2022 Aug;36(8 Pt A):2628-2635.

153. Smedira NG, Blackstone EH. Postcardiotomy mechanical support: risk factors and outcomes. Ann Thorac Surg. 2001;71(3 Suppl):S60-66; discussion S82-65.

154. Slottosch I, Liakopoulos O, Kuhn E, et al. Outcomes after peripheral extracorporeal membrane oxygenation therapy for postcardiotomy cardiogenic shock: a single-center experience. J Surg Res. 2013;181(2):e47-55.

155. Bakhtiary F, Keller H, Dogan S, et al. Venoarterial extracorporeal membrane oxygenation for treatment of cardiogenic shock: clinical experiences in 45 adult patients. J Thorac Cardiovasc Surg. 2008;135(2):382-388.

156. Hsu PS, Chen JL, Hong GJ, et al. Extracorporeal membrane oxygenation for refractory cardiogenic shock after cardiac surgery: predictors of early mortality and outcome from 51 adult patients. Eur J Cardiothorac Surg. 2010;37(2):328-333.

157. Marasco SF, Vale M, Pellegrino V, et al. Extracorporeal membrane oxygenation in primary graft failure after heart transplantation. Ann Thorac Surg. 2010;90(5):1541-1546.

158. Kucher N, Rossi E, De Rosa M, et al. Massive pulmonary embolism. Circulation. 2006;113(4):577-582.

159. Soar J, Berg KM, Andersen LW, et al. Adult Advanced Life Support: 2020 International Consensus on Cardiopulmonary Resuscitation and Emergency Cardiovascular Care Science with Treatment Recommendations. Resuscitation. 2020;156:A80-A119.

160. Giri J, Sista AK, Weinberg I, et al. Interventional Therapies for Acute Pulmonary Embolism: Current Status and Principles for the Development of Novel Evidence: A Scientific Statement From the American Heart Association. Circulation. 2019;140(20):e774-e801.

161. Konstantinides SV, Meyer G. The 2019 ESC Guidelines on the Diagnosis and Management of Acute Pulmonary Embolism. Eur Heart J. 2019;40(42):3453-3455.

162. Karami M, Mandigers L, Miranda DDR, et al. Survival of patients with acute pulmonary embolism treated with venoarterial extracorporeal membrane oxygenation: A systematic review and meta-analysis. J Crit Care. 2021;64:245-254.

163. Yusuff HO, Zochios V, Vuylsteke A. Extracorporeal membrane oxygenation in acute massive pulmonary embolism: a systematic review. Perfusion. 2015;30(8):611-616.

164. Ain DL, Albaghdadi M, Giri J, et al. Extra-corporeal membrane oxygenation and outcomes in massive pulmonary embolism: Two eras at an urban tertiary care hospital. Vasc Med. 2018;23(1):60-64.

165. Pasrija C, Kronfli A, George P, et al. Utilization of Veno-Arterial Extracorporeal Membrane Oxygenation for Massive Pulmonary Embolism. Ann Thorac Surg. 2018;105(2):498-504.

166. Tu T, Toma C, Tapson VF, et al. A Prospective, Single-Arm, Multicenter Trial of Catheter-Directed Mechanical Thrombectomy for Intermediate-Risk Acute Pulmonary Embolism: The FLARE Study. JACC Cardiovasc Interv. 2019;12(9):859-869.

167. Kucher N, Boekstegers P, Muller OJ, et al. Randomized, controlled trial of ultrasound-assisted catheter-directed thrombolysis for acute intermediate-risk pulmonary embolism. Circulation. 2014;129(4):479-486.

168. Chatterjee S, Chakraborty A, Weinberg I, et al. Thrombolysis for pulmonary embolism and risk of all-cause mortality, major bleeding, and intracranial hemorrhage: a meta-analysis. Jama. 2014;311(23):2414-2421.

169. Goldberg JB, Spevack DM, Ahsan S, et al. Survival and Right Ventricular Function After Surgical Management of Acute Pulmonary Embolism. J Am Coll Cardiol. 2020;76(8):903-911.

# 29

## Weaning and Decannulation in Adult Cardiac Failure

*Vinodh Bhagyalakshmi Nanjayya, Jae Seung Jung, Guillaume Lebreton, Kiran Shekar*

### Introduction

VA ECMO is used as a bridge to recovery, surgery, durable mechanical circulatory support (MCS), heart transplantation (HTx), or decision in selected patients with cardiogenic shock (CS) or refractory cardiac arrest (CA). Timely weaning assessment is critical to the success of VA ECMO. Premature weaning without allowing time for cardiac and end-organ function recovery may lead to worsening organ dysfunction and death. Delayed weaning prolongs the support duration and exposes patients to the risk of complications and mortality.[1] Once the patients pass the weaning assessment, decannulation occurs to liberate patients from VA ECMO.

### Pathophysiology of Weaning VA ECMO

Bypassing of blood from the right atrium (RA) leads to reduced right ventricular (RV) preload, RV ejection fraction (EF), RV cardiac output (CO), and left ventricular (LV) preload. Simultaneously, returning blood into the arterial system increases LV afterload, which leads to a reduction in LV stroke volume, increased myocardial oxygen demand, and increased LV filling pressure.[2] Decreases in preload and increases in afterload reduce LVEF and CO. In patients with severe LV dysfunction, the increased afterload may lead to LV distension causing myocardial edema, worsening LV dysfunction, and delaying ventricular recovery. Therefore, it is important to reduce VA ECMO blood flow and assess the impact of increasing RV and LV preload and reducing LV afterload on hemodynamics and cardiac contractility. When the cardiac function has sufficiently recovered to meet physiologic requirements at an acceptable level of pharmacological support, the patient can be liberated from ECLS.

### Tools to Assess Cardiac Recovery

A combination of parameters is used. The clinical parameters include evaluation of peripheral perfusion, CVP, MAP, pulsatility, pulse pressure (PP), and extent of vasoactive support. Invasive hemodynamic monitoring devices such as pulmonary artery (PA) catheters can provide additional parameters, eg, PA systolic and diastolic pressures, mean PA pressure, PA pulsatility, pulmonary capillary wedge pressure, and CO. However, due to suction pressure in the RA by the access cannula, these parameters need to be carefully interpreted.

Echocardiography is a valuable, noninvasive, bedside evaluation tool to assess cardiac recovery.[3,4] It provides information about ventricular size and function, CO, valvular function, and pericardial effusion. It can also provide estimates of PA pressure and LAP. Generally, transthoracic echocardiography (TTE) is used as first-line, and transesophageal echocardiography (TEE) as second-line modality because TEE is more invasive. Only when the transthoracic acoustic windows are inadequate should TEE be used.

Biomarkers such as lactate can help assess organ function and cardiac recovery time.[5-7] Microcirculation monitoring using incident dark-field imaging of sublingual microcirculation has also been attempted.[8]

**Prerequisites for VA ECMO Weaning**

Allowing sufficient duration for stabilization of end-organ function and resolution of the etiology of CS in important before a weaning trial (Table 29-1). Generally, weaning trials

are performed 48-72 hours after initiation.[7,9-13] The duration might be less than 48 hours in specific etiologies such as drug toxicity and ECPR. Patients in a stable rhythm with MAP >60-65 mmHg on low dose vasoactive agents with good and consistent pulsatility on the arterial line trace have stable hemodynamic parameters for weaning. In patients with LV distension, weaning trials should be considered only after LV unloading. If the patient is intubated, the patient should be well oxygenated on safe mechanical ventilation settings with $FiO_2$ <0.6. In some centers, $FsO_2$ is also set to 0.5 during the weaning trial. A clear chest x-ray generally indicates resolution of any pulmonary edema and no focus of early sepsis. Generally, metabolic parameters such as lactate should be normalized before the weaning study. If there is evidence of significant hypovolemia on echocardiography, patients may need a fluid

| PRECONDITIONS |
|---|
| **1. Cardiac pathology consistent with weaning*** |
| **2. Appropriate time frame for recovery from the etiology** |
| • Depends on the etiology of CS/CA |
| • Shorter in patients with drug toxicity, ECPR |
| • Longer in patients with AMI with myocardial stunning |
| **3. Stable hemodynamics on no or low dose vaso-active agents**** |
| • Stable rhythm (If in AF, rate well controlled) |
| • Good and consistent pulsatility on arterial line trace |
| • MAP > 60 mmHg |
| • Appropriate LV venting, in case of LV distension |
| **4. Stable or recovering organ function** |
| • Lung function |
|    ▪ Good oxygenation on safe lung ventilation with FiO2 < 0.6 |
|    ▪ Clear chest X-ray |
| • Liver function recovered |
| • Normal lactate level |
| • Renal function stable with or without continuous renal replacement therapy |
| • Optimal fluid balance |
| **5. Multidisciplinary team consensus on prognosis** |
| CS=Cardiogenic shock, CA=cardiac arrest, ECPR=ECMO assisted cardiopulmonary resuscitation, AMI=Acute myocardial infarction, AF=Atrial fibrillation, MAP=Mean Arterial Pressure, LV=Left ventricle, FiO2=Fraction of inspired oxygen. *Examples include myocarditis, primary graft dysfunction post-orthotopic heart transplantation, pulmonary embolism, acute myocardial infarction, arrhythmia induced cardiomyopathy, post cardiotomy, drug toxicity, ECPR. **Epinephrine <0.05 µg/kg/min, Dobutamine <5 µg/kg/min, Milrinone <0.375 µg/kg/min, Norepinephrine <0.05 µg/min, or Vasopressin <0.02 U/min. Vasoactive inotropic score (VIS) <10 can also be used as low dose support [VIS= Dopamine dose (µg/kg/min)+Dobutamine dose (µg/kg/min)+100 x epinephrine dose (µg/kg/min) +100 X norepinephrine dose (µg/kg/min)+ 10,000 x vasopressin dose (U/kg/min)+ 10 x milrinone dose (µg/kg/min)] |

**Table 29-1.** Preconditions for weaning from VA ECMO.

bolus to optimise ventricular preload before weaning assessment.

In some situations, weaning assessment may need to be initiated earlier. For example, in patients with irreversible severe LV dysfunction who are ineligible for HTx or durable MCS, clinicians may proceed with a one-way wean after optimizing as many potentially reversible conditions as possible. Also, in patients with multiple ECMO-related complications, weaning may need to be attempted earlier.

**Weaning Techniques**

All the VA ECMO weaning techniques are based on strategies to reduce ECMO flow to improve ventricular preload and reduce LV afterload to assess cardiac recovery. However, flow reduction increases circuit thrombosis risk. Hence, adequate anticoagulation is essential. Several weaning protocols are described.[14-18] They are:

1. Reduction of blood flow and assessment of cardiac recovery using clinical and echocardiography parameters.[5,7-13,19-24]
2. Addition of an arteriovenous (AV) bridge in the circuit.[25]
3. Pump-controlled retrograde trial off (PCRTO).[26,27]

*1) Reduction of ECMO Blood Flow and Cardiac Assessment*

In this method, circuit flow is reduced stepwise with cardiac assessment at each stage. The flow decrement can be done in 0.5-1 L/min intervals or as a percentage of ECMO blood flow at baseline (eg, 66% and 33%).[7,10,13,19] This can be done over 10-15 minutes at each step or gradually over several hours.[9,12,20,28] The principle is to allow sufficient time for cardiorespiratory adaptations and assessment at each step. If using echocardiography, 10-15 minutes is adequate to demonstrate LV and

RV changes. In the final stage, the flow is reduced to the minimum possible rate and cardiorespiratory assessment is made. If the patient meets the criteria for weaning at low flow (eg, 0.5-1 L/min), then the process of decannulation can begin.

Clinical parameters of hemodynamic stability include pulsatility and MAP ≥60 mmHg on low vasoactive agent support. On echocardiography, the general LV function parameters which are shown to be associated with successful weaning are LVEF >20-25%, LV outflow tract velocity time integral (LVOT VTI) ≥10 cm using pulsed wave Doppler, and lateral mitral annulus peak systolic velocity (TDSa) ≥6 cm/s.[10,28] The main RV parameters associated with successful weaning are RVEF >25% estimated using 3D echocardiography,[22] absence of significant RV dilatation with concurrent reduction in LV size,[29] and absence of severe tricuspid regurgitation.[20] In a weaning protocol that used a unique system called hemodynamic TEE (hTEE), lack of LV or RV distension at the end of the weaning protocol was associated with successful weaning.[19] Recently, lateral tricuspid annulus systolic peak velocity (RV S')/RV systolic pressure >0.33 measured at a median VA ECMO flow of 3.2 L/min has been described to be a better predictor than the traditional echocardiography parameters in a single-center study.[30] Any change in lateral mitral annulus early diastolic peak myocardial velocity (lateral e' velocity) and >10% change in the RV S' when the ECMO flow is reduced to 30-50% of baseline for 15 minutes has also been proposed as more sensitive than LVEF, LVOT VTI and TDSa for predicting successful weaning.[11] However, most of these tests require further validation.

The main advantage of this technique is that it is easy to do at the bedside without any circuit manipulation. The main caveat is that evidence for this technique is mostly from retrospective single-center studies with small sample sizes. There was significant heterogeneity in the diagnostic groups with a substantial risk of selection bias. For example, not all the patients who met the weaning criteria were weaned in the prospective studies.[10] Therefore, prospectively validation of these parameters is needed. The other caveat is that full RV loading is not achieved for accurate RV assessment. In addition, echocardiography parameters are based on Doppler techniques and care is needed with Doppler alignment and range gate placement during image acquisition. In pathologies sparing or involving only the basal anterolateral wall segments, TDSa will not be a good predictor of weaning. The weaning studies using this technique require a significant time commitment from echocardiography personnel. If TTE is inadequate, TEE is needed, which may not be readily accessible in all ECMO centers.

### 2) Use of AV Bridge in the Circuit

This technique, used in pediatric ECMO weaning, has been recently described in adult VA ECMO weaning.[25,31,32] An AV bridge is created by adding a length of tubing connecting three-way taps between the arterial and venous limbs of the circuit. Patient blood flow is then reduced gradually over an extended period. This is usually accomplished using a releasable clamp (eg, Hoffman clamp) on the bridge or return tubing after the y-connector towards the arterial cannula. If hemodynamics remain stable when there is low flow in the circuit, both the access and return cannulae are isolated by turning the three-way taps off to the cannulae. Heparin flush lines are added to both access and return cannulae or the cannulae are manually flushed using heparinized saline intermittently to prevent thrombus formation. As the blood is diverted through the bridge, the circuit flow is kept high to avoid clot formation in the circuit. Full RV loading can be achieved using this method, and both LV and RV assessment can be done independently of the ECMO circuit. Also, in patients with hypoxia, this can help determine whether the patient needs to be reconfigured from VA to VV ECMO. If the hemodynamics remain stable and echocardiography shows adequate contractility and CO with low vasoactive agent support, decannulation may proceed.

The main advantage of this technique is that patients can be kept off the ECMO circuit to assess LV and RV accurately. The main risk is the risk of air entrainment during circuit manipulation. Also, adequate anticoagulation is still needed because thrombus can still form in areas in the bridge close to the three-way taps. The blood flow through the bridge needs to be monitored to prevent thrombus formation in the bridge. The evidence for this strategy is again based on small, single-center studies.

### 3) PCRTO Technique

This technique was first demonstrated in neonatal and pediatric ECMO weaning.[32,33] Once the patient is ready for weaning, the RPM is gradually reduced. If the hemodynamics remain stable, the blood is allowed to flow retrograde to the circuit flow by decreasing the pump speed to <1000 RPM to achieve around 0.5-1.0 L/min flow to create a left to right shunt.[26,27] Slow titration of the RPM is done to avoid an abrupt drop in LV afterload due to flow reversal with concomitant vasopressor support requirement. During PCRTO, the oxygen to the circuit is removed. This helps in the assessment of the native lung function independent of ECMO. Also, the distal perfusion cannula is disconnected, and a heparin flush line is connected to the distal perfusion to avoid thrombus formation. If the hemodynamics remain stable on a low to moderate dose of vasoactive agent support and echocardiography shows good biventricular contractility without any worsening lactate levels, the patient is deemed suitable for weaning. Anticoagulation is essential to prevent circuit thrombosis.

The main advantage of this technique is that there is full RV loading, and therefore, RV assessment can be done. If hemodynamics do not change even with the additional resistance offered by the circuit, the patient is most likely to wean from ECMO. However, this creates an AV shunt ("systemic flow steal"), and the amount of shunting needs to be regulated. Otherwise, patients may go into RV failure or high cardiac output failure. Only two small, single-center studies have been conducted in adults so far.[26,27] Although the results are encouraging, further validation is required.

## Predictors of Successful ECMO Wean

No single factor can predict successful weaning from VA ECMO. It is a conglomeration of multiple factors, and the results need to be interpreted in the context of the overall CS and heart failure trajectory (Table 29-2).

## Weaning in Special Situations

### 1) Mechanically Unloaded LV

Weaning is complicated in the presence of an LV vent because it further reduces LV preload. Patients could have LA or LV vents

| PREDICTORS |
|---|
| **Hemodynamic parameters on no or low vasoactive agent support\*** |
| MAP ≥60 mmHg |
| CVP <15 mmHg or CVP rise <5 mmHg |
| **Echocardiography Parameters** |
| *On minimal ECMO flow* |
| • LV |
| ❖ No significant LV dilatation |
| ❖ LVEF > 20-25%[10] |
| ❖ LVOT VTI > 10 cm[10] |
| ❖ TDSa ≥6 cm/sec[10] |
| • RV |
| ❖ Less than 2 of RVEDD ≥35 mm, TAPSE <1.5 cm, RVS'<10 cm/sec, Poor RVEF, Severe TR[20]\*\* |
| ❖ 3D RVEF >24.6%[22]\*\* |
| ❖ RV dilatation with reduction in LVEDV\*\* |
| *On reduction of ECMO flow by 30-50%[11]\*\** |
| • Any change in lateral e' (cm/sec) |
| • >10% change in RVS' |
| *On Full ECMO support[30]\** |
| • RVS'/RVSP >0.33 |
| VA ECMO=Venoarterial extracorporeal membrane oxygenation, MAP=Mean arterial pressure, CVP=Central venous pressure, LV=Left ventricle, LVEF=Left ventricular ejection fraction, LVOT VTI=Left ventricular outflow tract velocity time integral, TDSa=Lateral mitral annulus peak systolic velocity, RV=Right ventricle, RVEDD=Right ventricular end diastolic dimension, TAPSE=Tricuspid annular plane systolic excursion, RVS'=Lateral tricuspid annulus systolic peak velocity, RVEF=Right ventricular ejection fraction, TR=Tricuspid regurgitation, 3D RVEF=3D derived Right ventricular ejection fraction, LVEDV=Left ventricular end-diastolic volume, Lateral e'=Lateral mitral annulus early diastolic peak myocardial velocity, RVSP=Right ventricular systolic pressure (also called Pulmonary artery systolic pressure). \*Epinephrine <0.05 µg/kg/min, Dobutamine <5 µg/kg/min, Milrinone <0.375 µg/kg/min, Norepinephrine <0.05 µg/min, or Vasopressin <0.02 U/min. Vasoactive inotropic score (VIS) <30 was used in one study [VIS= Dopamine dose (µg/kg/min)+Dobutamine dose (µg/kg/min)+100 x epinephrine dose (µg/kg/min) +100 X norepinephrine dose (µg/kg/min)+ 10,000 x vasopressin dose (U/kg/min)+ 10 x milrinone dose (µg/kg/min)]. #Based on small single or two-center studies. Need external validation. |

**Table 29-2.** Summary of predictors of successful weaning from VA ECMO.

(Chapter 4).[34] During weaning, when the ECMO flow is reduced, the venting cannulas will still be accessing blood from the LA or LV, and the LV preload will not be optimized. The effect on LV preload of a transapical LV vent is greater because the cannula is shorter and broader. Therefore, even at lower ECMO flow, more blood may be drained from LV than the RA. Gate clamps may need to be used to reduce the flow through the vent during weaning. However, this increases the risk of thrombus formation in the vent. Hence, anticoagulation needs to be optimized. Cases in which Impella (Abiomed, Danvers, MA) is used for LV venting, the minimum flow setting is P2, and the estimated blood flow is around 1-2 L/min. Hence, weaning assessment using normal echocardiography parameters is further complicated. One may need to consider removing these devices before performing weaning studies or consider a transition to a single device strategy (eg, Impella alone) and then wean the patient. When an intraaortic balloon pump (IABP) is used as a venting strategy, it is easier to perform the regular weaning study because there is minimal impact on LV preload.[35]

### 2) Isolated RV Failure

Another notable group to consider is patients with isolated RV failure, such as massive pulmonary embolism (PE), RV infarction, or severe pulmonary hypertension (PHT). Failure to wean such patients generally manifests with progressive RV dilatation, worsening tricuspid regurgitation, elevations in PA pressure and CVP, and hypotension during weaning. With PE, there is improvement in RV function following thrombolysis or systemic anticoagulation, and successful weaning is possible. Similarly, in patients with RV infarction, timely revascularisation may restore some RV function, and the patient may be weaned. If the patients fail recurrent

weaning trials, then options of RV assist devices (RVAD) may need to be explored. Generally, patients with severe PHT are challenging to wean because the RV distends and fails during weaning. VA ECMO is instituted usually as a bridge to surgical intervention such as pulmonary thromboendarterectomy in patients with chronic thromboembolic pulmonary hypertension, or heart-lung transplantation. Another group that develops RV failure is patients with severe ARDS on VV ECMO. These patients may need VVA ECMO or oxyRVAD. Once RV function recovers, weaning parameters are generally very similar to the weaning of patients with isolated RV failure (Table 29-3). Generally, VVA patients are reconfigured to VV ECMO once RV function recovers, and then VV ECMO is weaned.[36]

### 3) Differential Hypoxemia

The main question in patients with differential hypoxemia is whether reconfiguration to VV ECMO from VA ECMO or VVA ECMO is needed. In one study, these patients were identified by reducing the $FsO_2$ to 0.21 and titrating ventilator $FiO_2$.[10] Occurrence of hypoxia with significant elevation in ventilator $FiO_2$ was deemed an indication for reconfiguring to VV ECMO. In our practice, we generally identify these patients with worsening hypoxia by noting a considerable increase in $FiO_2$ (eg, $FiO_2$ >0.7) during the weaning study without reducing $FsO_2$. In the AV bridge and PCRTO techniques discussed above, lung assessment is done independently of the circuit because the blender oxygen is disconnected from the circuit.

### Adjuncts to VA ECMO Weaning

In patients who have failed a weaning study, IABP and levosimendan have been proposed to increase the success of further weaning attempts. Evidence for IABP is conflicting and limited to observational studies (Chapter 44).

In these studies, IABP was inserted before or after ECMO cannulation to reduce LV afterload rather than at the time of weaning. Therefore, it is difficult to tease out whether IABP has an adjuvant role in patients who have failed ECMO weaning. Evidence for levosimendan comes from several observational studies with or without propensity matching.[37] Results from a large, double-blind, randomized placebo control trial are awaited to further elucidate its role in weaning.[38]

| SUMMARY OF WEANING |
|---|
| **1. Prerequisites** |
| • Ensure adequate time for resolution of pathology (eg, resolution of pneumonia) or definitive surgical intervention (eg, Lung transplantation, Pulmonary thromboendarterectomy) |
| • Ensure adequate time for organ function stabilization |
| **2. Ensure safe lung ventilation and oxygenation** |
| • For Oxy-RVAD-turn off fresh gas flow for more than 2 hours and check ABG[36] |
| • For VA ECMO-ensure FiO2 ≤0.6 |
| • Check ABG for adequate systemic oxygenation, and normal $PaCO_2$ level or adequate metabolic compensation, if patient has hypercapnia |
| **3. Ensure adequate anticoagulation** |
| **4. Reduction of Oxy-RVAD/ VA ECMO blood flow** |
| • Stepwise reduction of blood flow 0.5-1.0 L/min to 2.0 L/min with monitoring of hemodynamics and vasoactive support |
| • Ensure stable hemodynamic parameters on low vasoactive support* for at least 24 hours with flow at 2.0 L/min prior to the next step |
| • Final echocardiography guided stepwise reduction of blood flow at 0.5 L/min every 15 minutes to the minimum acceptable blood flow (usually 0.5-1 L/min) |
| • Leave at minimum acceptable flow for <15 minutes only to prevent circuit thrombosis |
| **4. Acceptable hemodynamic parameters on low vasoactive agent support*** |
| • MAP ≥60 mmHg |
| • CVP <15 mmHg or CVP rise <5 mmHg |
| **5. Acceptable echocardiography parameters** |
| *On minimal ECMO flow* |
| • LV parameters similar to the once shown in Table 2.** |
| • RV parameters[#] |
| ❖ No RV dilatation with reduction in LVEDV |
| ❖ Recruitment of right ventricular systolic function to normal or mild RV dysfunction |
| ❖ TAPSE >10 mm[36##] |
| ❖ No worsening of tricuspid regurgitation |
| ❖ Increment in RVOT VTI |
| VA ECMO=Venoarterial extracorporeal membrane oxygenation, Oxy-RVAD=Oxygenated right ventricular assist device, ABG=Arterial blood gas, FiO2=Fraction of inspired oxygen, RV=Right Ventricle, MAP=Mean arterial pressure, CVP=Central venous pressure, LV=Left ventricle, LVEDV=Left ventricular end-diastolic volume, TAPSE=Tricuspid annular plane systolic excursion, RVOT VTI=Right ventricular outflow tract velocity time integral. <br> *Epinephrine <0.05 µg/kg/min, Dobutamine <5 µg/kg/min, Milrinone <0.375 µg/kg/min, Norepinephrine <0.05 µg/kg/min, or Vasopressin <0.02 U/min. Vasoactive inotropic score (VIS) <30 was used in one study [VIS= Dopamine dose (µg/kg/min)+Dobutamine dose (µg/kg/min)+100 x epinephrine dose (µg/kg/min) +100 X norepinephrine dose (µg/kg/min)+ 10,000 x vasopressin dose (U/kg/min)+ 10 x milrinone dose (µg/kg/min)]. <br> **Particularly important in patients with severe long-term pulmonary hypertension who might have a small LV cavity with coexistent LV dysfunction. <br> #Based on authors' personal experience. For RVOT VTI, no cut-off value has been defined. <br> ##TAPSE is normally reduced in patients after lung transplantation and cardiac surgery. Therefore, it is not reliable in the assessment of weaning of RV support in these patient groups. |

Table 29-3. Summary of weaning from VA ECMO or Oxy-RVAD in isolated RV failure.

## Proposed Weaning Strategy

The proposed weaning strategy is summarised in Figure 29-1. Based on current evidence, we recommend hemodynamic and echocardiography guidance for VA ECMO weaning.

## Failure to Wean from VA ECMO

Despite treatment optimization, some patients cannot be weaned and require further evaluation for durable MCS or HTx (Chapter 30). One of the primary considerations in patients eligible for LVAD is RV function, to determine whether the patient needs RVAD (temporary or durable) along with LVAD. Therefore, determining RV function on echocardiography during the weaning study is critical. No one parameter can predict this. Clinicians must depend on serial hemodynamic and echocardiography evaluation of the RV to determine the need for temporary or durable RVAD.[39,40,41] In patients deemed ineligible for long-term MCS, clinicians must decide about a one-way wean from VA ECMO or palliative care measures, after discussions with patients and families.

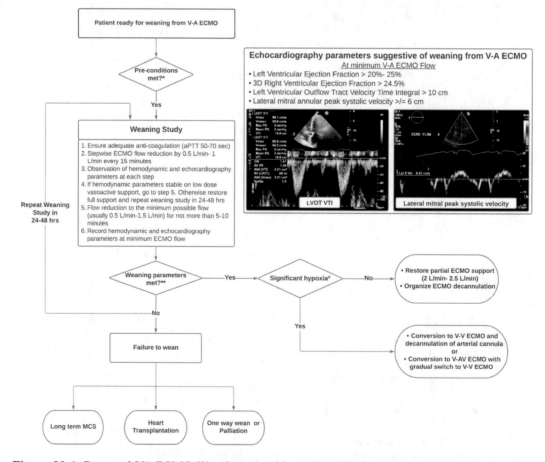

**Figure 29-1.** Proposed VA ECMO Weaning Algorithm. (VA ECMO=Venoarterial Extracorporeal Membrane Oxygenation, aPTT=Activated partial thromboplastin clotting time. Refer to Table 3 for VA ECMO in isolated RV failure. *Refer to Table 1 for preconditions. **Refer to Table 2 for weaning parameters. #Significant hypoxia-Requiring FiO2 >0.7 to maintain oxygenation.)

## Decannulation

After a successful weaning study, patients are left on partial VA ECMO support while awaiting decannulation. During decannulation, the cannula is disconnected from the circuit, flushed with heparinized saline, and kept clamped for some time (usually 15 min). Decannulation is done if the patient remains stable (Figure 29-2). Some patients will fail decannulation despite optimization for weaning. Therefore, patient suitability for re-instituting VA ECMO always needs to be made before decannulation.

In the case of surgical cannulation, cannulas must be removed using open surgical techniques. For percutaneously placed femoral cannula removal, open surgical removal is commonly performed because the size of the arterial cannula is large, and patients may need vascular patch repair.[7,10,12,19,22] In addition, some patients may need embolectomy to prevent lower limb

ischemia due to distal embolization of residual thrombus. However, surgical decannulation generally requires operating theater access. Also, surgical decannulation has associated risks such as wound infection, bleeding, scar formation, and wound breakdown. An alternative approach is the application of manual compression after cannula removal followed by prolonged compression using a femoral artery compression device. However, this procedure is associated with a higher risk of vascular complications needing open repair. In a retrospective, propensity-matched study, percutaneous decannulation was associated with 15% vascular complications compared to 3% of surgical decannulations.[42]

The use of percutaneous vascular closure devices for femoro-femoral VA ECMO decannulation has increased recently.[43] The main advantage of these devices is avoidance of surgical incision and the resulting complications. However, this requires a trained clinician to

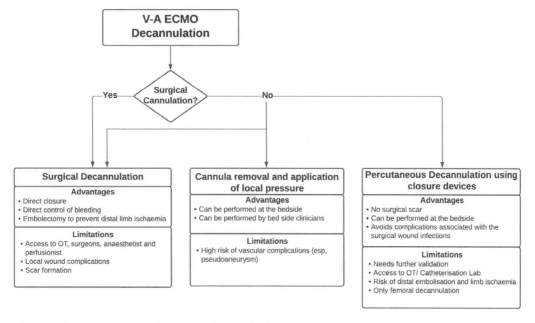

**Figure 29-2.** VA ECMO decannulation techniques. VA-ECMO=Venoarterial Extracorporeal Membrane Oxygenation, OT=Operation theater

perform the procedure in the interventional cardiology suite, operating theatre, or at the bedside, depending on the operator's preference. Also, some of the closure devices need the suture to be placed in the vessel at the time of cannulation which raises the possibility of infection in patients with long ECMO runs.[44] In some devices, the cannula is punctured to insert the guidewire of the closure devices before decannulation. Again, this could lead to infection. Also, the possibility of distal embolization remains with these closure devices, particularly in patients with distal perfusion catheters in the superficial femoral artery because thrombus can form in the zone between the arterial cannula and the distal perfusion cannula.[45] Patients may need angiography to confirm that the closure devices are appropriately positioned and there is no leak or pseudoaneurysm. Vascular ultrasound after decannulation to show perfusion in the distal limbs is also essential. Recently published small, single-center case series show the feasibility of these devices for ECMO decannulation.[45-50] However, there are no large, randomized controlled trials currently comparing the vascular closure device with surgical decannulation. More evidence demonstrating the safety of this approach is needed before widespread adoption of this technology, particularly the risk of infection and the possible need for operative interventions after decannulation.

### *Monitoring Post-ECMO Decannulation*

Due to the risk of distal embolization following arterial cannula removal, it is recommended to monitor lower limb perfusion. This could be done using clinical parameters and handheld Doppler ultrasound devices by bedside clinicians. Vascular ultrasound evaluation of the lower limb vessels following decannulation would identify thrombus in arteries and cannula-related deep vein thrombosis. Monitoring upper limb perfusion in patients with subclavian artery

cannulation is also recommended for early identification of limb ischemia.

About 60% of patients after ECMO decannulation develop post-decannulation systemic inflammatory syndrome (SIRS) with new-onset fever, leucocytosis, or worsening vasopressor requirement.[51] In some patients, SIRS may last for a week after decannulation. Those with SIRS related to an underlying infection seem to have worse outcomes.

### Conclusions

Weaning is a crucial stage in the management of patients on VA ECMO. In general, once end-organ function has stabilized, pulsatility is restored, fluid status is optimized, and inotropic support is minimized, weaning should be attempted. All the weaning strategies reduce ECMO support and assess hemodynamics and echocardiography parameters. Decannulation, done after a successful weaning study, can be done using open surgical techniques, percutaneously, or with percutaneous closure devices. The evidence for percutaneous closure devices is steadily accumulating.

# References

1. Smith M, Vukomanovic A, Brodie D, et al. Duration of veno-arterial extracorporeal life support (VA ECMO) and outcome: an analysis of the Extracorporeal Life Support Organization (ELSO) registry. Crit Care. 2017;21(1):45.
2. Ostadal P, Mlcek M, Kruger A, et al. Increasing venoarterial extracorporeal membrane oxygenation flow negatively affects left ventricular performance in a porcine model of cardiogenic shock. Journal of Translational Medicine. 2015;13(1):266.
3. Douflé G, Roscoe A, Billia F, Fan E. Echocardiography for adult patients supported with extracorporeal membrane oxygenation. Critical care (London, England). Crit Care. 2015 Oct 2;19:326.
4. Nanjayya VB, Murphy D. Extracorporeal Life Support Organization (ELSO) Ultrasound guidance for extra-corporeal membrane oxygenation veno-arterial ECMO specific guidelines. Extracorporeal Life Support Organization. Accessed 30 January, 2022. https://www.elso.org/Portals/0/Files/elso_Ultrasoundguidance_vaecmo_guidelines_May2015.pdf.
5. Slottosch I, Liakopoulos O, Kuhn E, et al. Lactate and lactate clearance as valuable tool to evaluate ECMO therapy in cardiogenic shock. J Crit Care. 2017;42:35-41.
6. Biancari F, Fiore A, Jónsson K, et al. Prognostic Significance of Arterial Lactate Levels at Weaning from Postcardiotomy Venoarterial Extracorporeal Membrane Oxygenation. J Clin Med. 2019;8(12):2218.
7. Luyt CE, Landivier A, Leprince P, et al. Usefulness of cardiac biomarkers to predict cardiac recovery in patients on extracorporeal membrane oxygenation support for refractory cardiogenic shock. J Crit Care. 2012;27(5):524.e7-14.
8. Akin S, Dos Reis Miranda D, Caliskan K, et al. Functional evaluation of sublingual microcirculation indicates successful weaning from VA-ECMO in cardiogenic shock. Crit Care. 2017;21(1):265.
9. Rastan AJ, Dege A, Mohr M, et al. Early and late outcomes of 517 consecutive adult patients treated with extracorporeal membrane oxygenation for refractory postcardiotomy cardiogenic shock. J Thorac Cardiovasc Surg. 2010;139(2):302-11, 311.e1.
10. Aissaoui N, Luyt CE, Leprince P, et al. Predictors of successful extracorporeal membrane oxygenation (ECMO) weaning after assistance for refractory cardiogenic shock. Intensive Care Med. 2011;37(11):1738-45.
11. Kim D, Jang WJ, Park TK, et al. Echocardiographic Predictors of Successful Extracorporeal Membrane Oxygenation Weaning After Refractory Cardiogenic Shock. J Am Soc Echocardiogr. 2021;34(4):414-422.e4.
12. Guihaire J, Dang Van S, Rouze S, et al. Clinical outcomes in patients after extracorporeal membrane oxygenation support for post-cardiotomy cardiogenic shock: a single-centre experience of 92 cases. Interact Cardiovasc Thorac Surg. 2017;25(3):363-369.
13. Lee W, Kim Y, Choi H, et al. Advanced Age as a Predictor of Survival and Weaning in Venoarterial Extracorporeal Oxygenation: A Retrospective Observational Study. BioMed Research International. 2017;2017:3505784.
14. Brahmbhatt DH, Daly AL, Luk AC, et al. Liberation From Venoarterial Extracorporeal Membrane Oxygenation: A Review. Circ Heart Fail. 2021;14(7):e007679.
15. Ortuno S, Delmas C, Diehl JL, et al. Weaning from veno-arterial extra-corporeal membrane oxygenation: which strategy to use? Ann Cardiothorac Surg. 2019;8(1):E1-e8.
16. Lüsebrink E, Stremmel C, Stark K, et al. Update on Weaning from Veno-Arterial Extracorporeal Membrane Oxygenation. J Clin Med. 2020;9(4):992.
17. Trahanas JM, Li SS, Crowley JC, et al. How to Turn It Down: The Evidence and Opinions Behind Adult Venoarterial Extracorporeal Membrane Oxygenation Weaning. ASAIO Journal. 2021;67(9):964-972.
18. Singh G, Hudson D, Shaw A. Medical Optimization and Liberation of Adult Patients From VA-ECMO. Can J Cardiol. 2020;36(2):280-290.
19. Cavarocchi NC, Pitcher HT, Yang Q, et al. Weaning of extracorporeal membrane oxygenation using continuous hemodynamic transesophageal echocardiography. J Thorac Cardiovasc Surg. 2013;146(6):1474-9.
20. Pappalardo F, Pieri M, Arnaez Corada B, et al. Timing and Strategy for Weaning From Venoarterial ECMO are Complex Issues. J Cardiothorac Vasc Anesth. 2015;29(4):906-11.
21. Slottosch I, Liakopoulos O, Kuhn E, et al. Outcomes after peripheral extracorporeal membrane oxygenation therapy for postcardiotomy cardiogenic shock: a single-center experience. J Surg Res. 2013;181(2):e47-55.
22. Huang KC, Lin LY, Chen YS, et al. Three-Dimensional Echocardiography-Derived Right Ventricular Ejection Fraction Correlates with Success of Decannulation and Prognosis in Patients Stabilized by Venoarterial Extracorporeal Life Support. J Am Soc Echocardiogr. 2018;31(2):169-179.
23. Matsumoto M, Asaumi Y, Nakamura Y, et al. Clinical determinants of successful weaning from extracorporeal membrane oxygenation in patients with fulminant myocarditis. ESC Heart Fail. 2018;5(4):675-684.

24. Sertic F, Chavez L, Diagne D, et al. Predictors of in-hospital mortality and midterm outcomes of patients successfully weaned from venoarterial extracorporeal membrane oxygenation. J Thorac Cardiovasc Surg. 2021;161(2):666-678.e3.

25. Babar ZUD, Sharma AS, Ganushchak YM, et al. An arterio-venous bridge for gradual weaning from adult veno-arterial extracorporeal life support. Perfusion. 2015;30(8):683-688.

26. Ju MH, Lim MH, Lee SY, et al. Early experience of pump-controlled retrograde trial off for weaning from veno-arterial extracorporeal membrane oxygenation in adult patients with cardiogenic shock. Perfusion. 2021;36(4):401-406.

27. Ling L, Chan KM. Weaning adult patients with cardiogenic shock on veno-arterial extracorporeal membrane oxygenation by pump-controlled retrograde trial off. Perfusion. 2018;33(5):339-345.

28. Aissaoui N, El-Banayosy A, Combes A. How to wean a patient from veno-arterial extracorporeal membrane oxygenation. Intensive Care Med. 2015;41(5):902-905.

29. Aissaoui N, Caudron J, Leprince P, et al. Right-left ventricular interdependence: a promising predictor of successful extracorporeal membrane oxygenation (ECMO) weaning after assistance for refractory cardiogenic shock. Intensive Care Med. 2017;43(4):592-594.

30. Kim D, Park Y, Choi KH, et al. Prognostic Implication of RV Coupling to Pulmonary Circulation for Successful Weaning From Extracorporeal Membrane Oxygenation. JACC Cardiovasc Imaging. 2021;14(8):1523-1531.

31. Holgren SE, Frede RT, Crumley JP, et al. Novel Utilization of the Bridge During Weaning Off Venoarterial ECMO: The Hoffman Clamp Method. Innovations (Phila). 2016;11(3):229-31.

32. Mattke CA, Haisz E, Pandya N, et al. Creating a Controlled Arterio-Venous Shunt by Reversing the Extracorporeal Membrane Oxygenation Blood Flow: A Strategy for Weaning Patients Off Veno-Arterial Extracorporeal Membrane Oxygenation. Pediatr Crit Care Med. 2017;18(10):973-976.

33. Westrope C, Harvey C, Robinson S, et al. Pump controlled retrograde trial off from VA-ECMO. ASAIO Journal. 2013;59(5):517-9.

34. Rajagopal K. Left Ventricular Distension in Veno-arterial Extracorporeal Membrane Oxygenation: From Mechanics to Therapies. ASAIO Journal. 2019;65(1):1-10.

35. Fried JA, Masoumi A, Takeda K, et al. How I approach weaning from venoarterial ECMO. Crit Care. 2020;24(1):307.

36. Lorusso R, Whitman G, Milojevic M, et al. 2020 EACTS/ELSO/STS/AATS expert consensus on post-cardiotomy extracorporeal life support in adult patients. Eur J Cardiothorac Surg. 2021;59(1):12-53.

37. Burgos LM, Seoane L, Furmento JF, et al. Effects of levosimendan on weaning and survival in adult cardiogenic shock patients with veno-arterial extracorporeal membrane oxygenation: systematic review and meta-analysis. Perfusion. 2020;35(6):484-491.

38. Ellouze O, Soudry Faure A, Radhouani M, et al. Levosimendan in venoarterial ECMO weaning. Rational and design of a randomized double blind multicentre trial. ESC Heart Fail. 2021;8(4):3339-3347.

39. Kiernan MS, French AL, DeNofrio D, et al. Preoperative three-dimensional echocardiography to assess risk of right ventricular failure after left ventricular assist device surgery. J Card Fail. 2015;21(3):189-97.

40. Raina A, Seetha Rammohan HR, Gertz ZM, et al. Postoperative right ventricular failure after left ventricular assist device placement is predicted by preoperative echocardiographic structural, hemodynamic, and functional parameters. J Card Fail. 2013;19(1):16-24.

41. Gudejko MD, Gebhardt BR, Zahedi F, et al. Intraoperative Hemodynamic and Echocardiographic Measurements Associated With Severe Right Ventricular Failure After Left Ventricular Assist Device Implantation. Anesth Analg. 2019;128(1):25-32.

42. Danial P, Hajage D, Nguyen LS, et al. Percutaneous versus surgical femoro-femoral veno-arterial ECMO: a propensity score matched study. Intensive Care Med. 2018;44(12):2153-2161.

43. Majunke N, Mangner N, Linke A, et al. Comparison of Percutaneous Closure Versus Surgical Femoral Cutdown for Decannulation of Large-Sized Arterial and Venous Access Sites in Adults After Successful Weaning of Veno-Arterial Extracorporeal Membrane Oxygenation. J Invasive Cardiol. 2016;28(10):415-419.

44. Martin-Tuffreau A-S, Bagate F, Boukantar M, et al. Complete percutaneous angio-guided approach using preclosing for venoarterial extracorporeal membrane oxygenation implantation and explantation in patients with refractory cardiogenic shock or cardiac arrest. Crit Care. 2021;25(1):93.

45. Shah A, Ghoreishi M, Taylor BS, et al. Complete percutaneous decannulation from femoral venoarterial extracorporeal membrane oxygenation. JTCVS Tech. 2020;6:75-81.

46. Lüsebrink E, Stremmel C, Stark K, et al. Percutaneous Decannulation Instead of Surgical Removal for Weaning After Venoarterial Extracorporeal Membrane Oxygenation—A Crossed Perclose ProGlide Closure Device Technique Using a

Hemostasis Valve Y Connector. Critical Care Explorations. 2019;1(6): e0018.

47. Chandel A, Desai M, Ryan LP, et al. Preclosure technique versus arterial cutdown after percutaneous cannulation for venoarterial extracorporeal membrane oxygenation. JTCVS Tech. 2021;10:322-330.

48. Hwang JW, Yang JH, Sung K, et al. Percutaneous removal using Perclose ProGlide closure devices versus surgical removal for weaning after percutaneous cannulation for venoarterial extracorporeal membrane oxygenation. J Vasc Surg. 2016;63(4):998-1003.e1.

49. Au SY, Chan KS, Fong KM, et al. One-year experience of bedside percutaneous VA-ECMO decannulation in a high-ECMO-volume center in Hong Kong. Perfusion. 2021;36(8):803-807.

50. Liu Z, Xu Y, Xu X, et al. Comparison of Success Rate and Complications of Totally Percutaneous Decannulation in Patients With Veno-Arterial Extracorporeal Membrane Oxygenation and Endovascular Aneurysm Repair. Front Med (Lausanne). 2021;8:724427.

51. Thangappan K, Cavarocchi NC, Baram M, Thoma B, Hirose H. Systemic inflammatory response syndrome (SIRS) after extracorporeal membrane oxygenation (ECMO): Incidence, risks and survivals. Heart & Lung. 2016;45(5):449-453.

# 30

## Bridging Adult Patients with Cardiac Failure

*Christopher Wilcox, Glenn J.R. Whitman, Amy E. Hackmann, Leonardo Salazar, Alain Combes*

## Introduction

As ECLS is increasingly utilized in emergent lifesaving situations, caregivers are recognizing the pitfalls of its institution when performed without consideration for an exit strategy. Prior to supporting patients with ECLS, it is incumbent upon the ECLS team to determine the pathways that the patient might follow that would allow for ECLS discontinuation. In every case, one can consider ECLS as a "bridge" to an outcome, as follows:

- to cardiac surgery,
- to recovery,
- to decision, where the ECLS team gains time to facilitate an evaluation to determine if any of the following pathways are options, or whether ECLS should be withdrawn,
- to transplantation, directly off ECLS,
- to durable mechanical circulatory support,
- to temporary mechanical support in preparation for transplantation.

The chapter that follows is designed to give the reader an understanding of the issues associated with bridging and what might be a realistic expectation for successful separation from VA ECMO. An attempt is also made to review related issues regarding patient support, while highlighting common complications

encountered during ECLS support that can have a significant bearing on outcomes. Refer to the accompanying algorithm which gives an overview of how to approach these patients. (Figure 30-1).

## ECLS in Preparation for Cardiac Surgery

A number of cardiac surgical emergencies carry profound mortality risks despite intervention, due in part to the hemodynamic instability and subsequent multiorgan dysfunction accompanying that condition at initial presentation. In certain instances, VA ECMO can be used to stabilize these patients prior to definitive surgical correction.

For some patients, support may only be required for a relatively short period, such as those presenting with shock from acute mitral regurgitation, coronary dissection as a cardiac catheterization laboratory complication, or acute mitral regurgitation after balloon valvuloplasty for mitral stenosis.[1] Use of ECLS in these situations stabilizes the hemodynamics to allow patient transfer to the appropriate operating room facility, recovery of organ perfusion, and then intraoperative support prior to cannulation.

Acute cardiogenic shock after myocardial infarction (MI) carries a 40-67% in-hospital mortality in patients who fail to respond to inotropic and less invasive mechanical circulatory support (eg, intraaortic balloon pump).[2,3] In these patients presenting in cardiogenic shock with systemic hypoperfusion, VA ECMO as a bridge to revascularization may lessen the degree of multi-system organ failure pre-operatively.[4] Overall, outcomes in acute MI shock supported with ECLS tend to be worse than other more reversible causes of heart failure.[5]

Complications of acute MI such as papillary muscle rupture causing severe mitral regurgitation or postinfarction ventricular septal defect (VSD) are relatively rare and associated with high mortality.[6] Use of VA ECMO prior to operative repair may allow recovery of severe hypoxemia and pulmonary edema, acute renal insufficiency, and shock liver. In VSDs, ECMO can be used to allow healing of the ventricular muscle prior to attempted repair. Outcomes improve significantly if repair is performed

more than seven days after acute MI, however, waiting would not be feasible in many patients without ECMO support.[7]

The management of pulmonary embolism (PE) with hemodynamic instability can include VA ECMO support as a bridge to definitive management of the clot. More commonly, endovascular therapies such as mechanical thrombectomy or catheter-directed thrombolytics or thrombus suction are used to treat significant or massive PEs. Patients who fail these therapies and have central thrombus or clot in transit may be surgical embolectomy candidates.[8]

In the setting of ischemic stage D-E cardiogenic shock, outcomes are abysmal, and ECLS should be strongly considered, if an exit strategy exists. In general, severe aortic valve insufficiency (AI) is a contraindication because retrograde flow from the ECMO circuit will further distend the compromised left

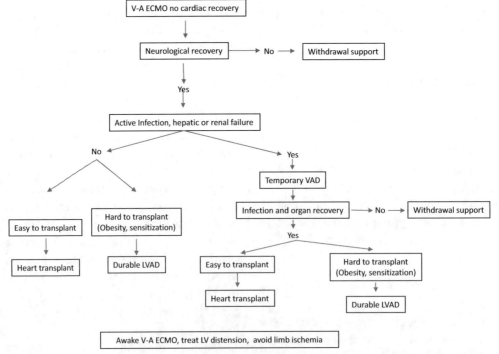

**Figure 30-1.** A proposed algorithm for the VA ECMO patient without expected cardiac recovery regarding a) cessation of ECMO, b) bridging to heart transplant or a durable VAD directly, or c) bridging to temporary mechanical circulatory support, to bridge to transplant or VAD.

ventricle. Aortic dissection might also represent a contraindication (although no conclusive evidence exists in this respect) because ECMO may propagate the dissection further and is commonly associated with acute AI. However, a recent successful salvage with ECPR of a type A aortic dissection challenges this approach.[9]

The timing of decannulation from ECLS in these settings is variable. ECLS is transitioned to traditional cardiopulmonary bypass for the operative procedure, and in many cases, patients can be weaned off bypass as with routine operations. After VSD repair specifically, ECLS support postoperatively may allow improved repair durability by decreasing ventricular wall tension, although this aspect requires further elucidation based on the known effect of retrograde flow against LV ejection.[10] The addition of direct LV decompression with an Impella device may also facilitate recovery by decreasing pressure on the repair as well as unloading the left ventricle.

**Bridge to Recovery**

Cardiac recovery on VA ECMO may occur at different time points based on the disease process for which support was initiated. In a mixed cohort, the median duration of support was 8 days in one review.[11] At approximately three days of support, patients with viral myocarditis, primary graft dysfunction posttransplant, or postcardiotomy shock from poor LV protection intraoperatively may have sufficient recovery to begin weaning. By seven days of support, lack of recovery should prompt consideration of other advanced therapies, the evaluation for which could have been started at the commencement of ECLS. Thus, in almost all cases, by 10-14 days of VA ECMO support, a definitive plan for the patient can be created. In a subset of patients who have not recovered and are not stable enough to undergo durable MCS or transplant, an option may be another temporary support device, often providing univentricular support.

This may include percutaneous LVAD or RVAD support but could initially involve changing the ECMO cannulation strategy to allow more prolonged weaning attempts.

When recovery appears unlikely, contraindications for advanced therapies may include significant acute brain injury (frequently associated with ECPR), lung, liver, or kidney failure, medical contraindications such as poorly controlled diabetes or a recent cancer diagnosis, or psychosocial factors such as substance abuse or lack of family support. Families and patients, when possible, need to be kept aware of the trajectory of the patient on ECLS and the decision making that occurs when recovery has not occurred. Withdrawal of ECLS is common when care is futile, and families often support this strategy. In these situations, communication with the family and other providers should reach consensus that ECLS will not be reinitiated.

**Bridge to Decision**

The goal of VA ECMO is to provide hemodynamic stability while a patient's therapeutic options are determined. This time period, after ECMO has been instituted but with no clarity as to what are appropriate options, can be viewed as "bridging" to a decision. If the possibility of cardiac recovery has been excluded, evaluation for heart transplantation (HTx) or a durable, Left Ventricular Assist Device (LVAD) is required. However, neurologic compromise, active infections, as well as hepatic and renal failure all can result in absolute contraindications for HTx and LVAD.[12] A careful evaluation by the multidisciplinary team assessing patient risk factors, contraindications, complications prior to or during ECLS, and the center experience guides the decision making as to the most appropriate therapy for the individual patient.

## Bridging to Transplantation or Durable Mechanical Support

Patients considered for transplant or LVAD normally proceed through a complex evaluation process, including a number of diagnostic studies and specialist consultations. Patients placed on ECLS are generally acutely decompensating, which precludes this thorough assessment of the patient prior to initiating support. Once stability has been achieved, a more thorough review of the patient's medical, surgical, and social situation can occur. 5-20% of VA ECMO patients may proceed to LVAD or transplantation, but recovery is the only option for the majority of patients placed emergently on VA ECMO.[13]

VA ECMO provides excellent short-term support. However, inevitable complications prevent its use for the medium or long term.[14] Data from the ELSO Registry suggests that the average duration of VA ECMO support is 5-9 days, with the risk of complications beginning within days of its initiation and increasing with duration of support. A prolonged VA ECMO run negatively affects clinical outcomes.[15] Hence, the goals for a patient's clinical course is to bridge to a modality that allows separation from ECMO as rapidly as possible prior to complications developing.

Regarding transplantation, renal insufficiency is associated with reduced posttransplant graft survival,[16,17] while mechanical ventilation at the time of transplant confers a roughly 2.5 times higher 1-year mortality[18] and dramatically complicates early postoperative recovery due to nosocomial infections and higher primary graft dysfunction. Extubation while on VA ECMO prior to transplantation has led to excellent outcomes, as recently reported by a large European transplant center.[19]

Nevertheless, VA ECMO has been historically associated with poor outcomes, with a 1-year posttransplant survival of only 57.8%.[16] However, with the change in transplant allocation in 2018, ECMO as a bridge to transplantation has increased.[20] In the old allocation system, VA ECMO patients had the same priority status as more stable patients (eg, those supported with LVADs). However, it was felt that the system disadvantaged ECMO and temporary support patients who had long wait list times with high wait list mortality. The new allocation system gives higher wait list priority to these patients.[21] As a corollary, VAD patients are now disadvantaged such that far fewer (21%) patients are transplanted from VAD, while those bridged on temporary support devices have increased, as follows: VA ECMO (+5 %), intraaortic balloon pump (+21%), and temporary ventricular assist devices (+5 %). Gratifyingly, waitlist mortality has dropped from 37% to 16.2%.

As mentioned above, a high-volume French transplant center has recently reported that with careful selection, minimizing ECMO complications, increasing pre-transplant extubation, and continuing ECMO support after HTx, transplantation with or without ECMO as a bridge showed no difference in survival (1-yr: 85.5% and 3-yr: 80.3% vs non-ECMO patients, 1-yr: 80.7%; 3-yr: 72%).[19] In short, the strategy-bridge cardiogenic shock to HTx is changing from durable LVADs to short term MCS, mostly VA ECMO.

When the duration of support is long due to donor scarcity or patient complications, ECMO to heart transplantation should be avoided, but rather transitioning to temporary ventricular assist devices for support. VA ECMO patients without cardiac recovery and with contraindications to transplant but not to durable support should obviously be bridged to LVAD.

Implanting a durable LVAD as a mechanical circulatory device in an INTERMACS 1 profile patient is associated with increased mortality and morbidity.[22,23] However, VA ECMO as a strategy to improve organ function before durable LVAD implantation in cardiogenic shock patients has been reported.[24] ECMO was shown to improve hemodynamic profiles and creatinine and bilirubin levels by the time of VAD implant. One-year survival in VA ECMO bridged to LVAD therapy should now be viewed as comparable to the general population (77% vs. 88%, p 0.6).[25]

## ICU Care of Candidates Bridging to MCS or Transplant

### Preventing and Treating Pulmonary Edema during ECLS

VA ECMO increases LV afterload, which can exacerbate the prior cardiac insult, decreasing stroke volume, raising LV end diastolic pressure, causing pulmonary venous hypertension and pulmonary edema. In cases of ECMO support for irreversible heart failure, clinicians caring for VA ECMO patients must take this into consideration to prevent pulmonary compromise during support. In these cases, comprehensive consideration of other strategies (eg, IABP, Impella, direct LV venting) is essential for successful clinical support so as to bridge to transplantation or durable LV support.

Left ventricular distention leading to pulmonary edema and pulmonary hemorrhage affects candidacy for advanced therapies because lung injury may impact right ventricular function postoperatively. This can be done by monitoring LA pressures with pulmonary artery catheterization and maintaining the arterial pulse pressure >10 mmHg. Echocardiography is an important adjunct to this assessment, with a focus on aortic valve opening, LV size, and the presence of any sign of LV blood stasis or thrombus. Treatments for LV distention include decreasing ECLS flow to facilitate ejection, intravenous inotropes to improve native contractility, and left ventricular venting by IABP or percutaneous LVAD, direct surgical

vent placement, or atrial septostomy. To determine when weaning might be possible, assessment of hemodynamic parameters and cardiac function should be done throughout the duration of ECMO support at relatively standard intervals.

### Limb Ischemia

There is significant risk of limb ischemia ipsilateral to the femoral artery cannulated, whether by a percutaneous access or cut-down technique. Contralateral vein cannulation to avoid venous hypertension along with antegrade distal limb perfusion is recommended to reduce the risk of limb ischemia.[26-28] Early monitoring of the distal limbs with near-infrared spectroscopy in addition to bedside Doppler and clinical examination can detect early malperfusion and allow timely intervention where necessary. This has been shown to decrease the need for fasciotomy or amputation.[29]

### Organ System Considerations While Bridging

Neurologic injury including ischemic and hemorrhagic strokes are feared complications of ECLS. Smaller strokes may be silent but potentially pose a risk with the initiation of cardiopulmonary bypass during transplantation.[30] Additionally, VA ECMO is associated with hypoxic ischemic brain injury related to hyperoxia, reperfusion injury, loss of pulsatile blood flow, and differential oxygenation.[31,32] Recommendations to reduce brain injury include targeting a $PaO_2$ at or less than 120 mmHg with a right radial arterial line and cerebral near infrared spectroscopy monitoring to detect low or discordant cerebral oxygenation.[33] Additionally, multimodal neurologic monitoring programs including clinical neurologic exams, transcranial Doppler, electroencephalography, brain-injury specific blood biomarkers, somatosensory evoked potentials, and computed tomography are feasible and detect a high percentage of neurologic complications.[34]

Mechanical ventilation is associated with ventilator-induced lung injury and risk for ventilator associated pneumonia.[35] In order to reduce volutrauma, low tidal volume ventilation, typically 6 ml/kg ideal body weight, is recommended.[35] Liver dysfunction is common and can be identified by elevations in aspartate transaminase, alanine aminotransferase, and alkaline phosphatase, however higher peak bilirubin is most associated with increased mortality.[36,37] Bilirubin elevation is not typically associated with ischemia and the mechanism of injury may be related to complex organ interplay and abnormal hormonal response.[38]

Renal failure requiring dialysis occurs in 30-50% of patients supported with VA ECMO.[39,40] Multiple mechanisms of injury are suspected to cause a reduction in renal oxygen delivery including abnormal blood flow, lack of pulsatility, inflammation, disrupted renin-aldosterone hormonal system, and worsening volume overload.[40] Renal replacement therapy is an independent risk factor for failure to wean from ECMO and mortality, in addition to being a relative contraindication for transplantation.[40,41]

Infection and sepsis are reported in over 40% of patients, associated with duration of ECLS, age, comorbidities, and cannulation site.[42,43] Unsurprisingly, infection is associated with increased mortality (Chapter 6). Cannulas themselves are less likely to be infected than indwelling central lines.[44] Although it is common practice amongst ECLS centers, no strong data support antibiotic or antifungal prophylaxis, surveillance cultures, or deviation from standard ICU practice used in non-ECMO patients.[42,43]

Regarding transfusions, several factors increase the need for transfusions in this population. Multiple large bore vascular access sites, the often emergent nature of cannulation, and the need for systemic anticoagulation to prevent system clotting, combined with the inflammatory and prothrombotic response and hemolysis associated with the ECMO circuit, all contribute to blood loss and anemia during VA ECMO.[45] In fact, bleeding is one of the most common complications of VA ECMO, leading to the need for transfusions in virtually 100% of patients. Central cannulation is associated with even greater transfusion requirements. No high-quality data exist on targets for transfusion specific to this population and patient specific transfusion thresholds may reduce unnecessary transfusion. Patients bridging to transplant with LVAD have higher sensitization with increased platelet transfusions (less so with leuko-reduced red blood cells transfusions).[46,47] Regardless, the goal of transfusion should be to maintain adequate oxygen delivery and perfusion while attempting to minimize overall transfusions and HLA sensitization. There are not yet standardized methods for desensitization in this population, but intravenous immunoglobulin, plasmapheresis, and antibody therapy should be considered on an individual or center basis.[46]

### Nutrition

Multiple trials have shown enteral nutrition (EN) initiated within 24 hours of cannulation is safe and reduces in-hospital mortality.[48] EN should begin as early as possible via the gastric or postpyloric route unless there is shock and high vasopressor requirements, in which case parenteral nutrition should be considered to reduce the risk of bowel ischemia. Concern for accelerated degradation of the oxygenator membrane by the solutes within parenteral nutrition is not supported by data. Furthermore, parenteral nutrition and supplements are not significantly sequestered by the ECMO tubing or oxygenator.[49]

In VA ECMO, patients are frequently underfed and increasing caloric and protein intake to meet actual energy expenditure has been associated with decreased mortality.[50] Indirect calorimetry can be used to measure oxygen uptake as well as $CO_2$ elimination, both across the ventilator and the ECMO circuit oxygenator, and values applied to the Weir equation to calculate individual energy expenditure.[51] Energy expenditure calculations using pre- and post- oxygenator blood gases may represent a straightforward, universally applicable approach to calculate energy expenditure and optimize nutrition, but requires further validation.[51]

### *Ambulation and Rehabilitation*

Patient functional and nutritional status at the time of surgery are directly related to both candidacy and outcome in heart transplantation and durable LVAD implantation.[52] Muscle atrophy, neuromuscular weakness, and impairment of normal activities are common sequelae during treatment of the critically ill, especially those treated with ECLS. Physical therapy and ambulation are feasible for patients receiving ECLS support during bridging (Chapter 47).[53] An important consideration for VA ECMO is cannula positioning. Often implanted with urgency due to cardiogenic shock, the femoral artery and vein are frequent sites for cannulation which may limit, but not necessarily preclude, therapy and ambulation. If the situation allows, consideration should be given for other cannulation strategies including central catheters or a venous jugular cannula with subclavian, axillary, or innominate arterial access.[54]

Successful strategies for physical therapy and ambulation consist of a multidisciplinary approach including occupational and physical therapy, respiratory therapy, providers, nursing, and ECLS specialists, and should be tailored based upon site experience and staff comfort. Development of early mobility protocols with dedicated teams allowing for the development of expertise can maximize rehabilitation time for appropriate patients and minimize adverse events.[53]

### *Evaluation and Prevention of Fragility and Deconditioning*

Evaluation of a patient's fragility may identify patients that will benefit most from intensive nutritional and rehabilitation interventions while bridging. Traditional methods of assessing the neuromuscular junction and strength, such as electromyography, may be limited initially by sedation or be less available in the ICU setting. Bedside ultrasound of quadriceps echogenicity provides a potential assessment for muscle atrophy and can be compared over time to determine the effectiveness of interventions.[55] Additionally, assessing the quality of skeletal muscle has been demonstrated by reviewing the fatty muscle fraction within paraspinal muscles, with increasing percentages associated with significantly higher 1-year mortality.[56] Although further clinical data is needed, these non-invasive measures can be considered to monitor anabolic states in response to physical therapy and nutrition, and possibly to predict success in bridging to definitive therapy.

### Conclusion

The concept of VA ECMO for bridging is central because it is never a destination in and of itself, but always a support to another destination. In every instance of ECMO support, determination of the patient's strategy for liberation from ECMO is the first order of care. When a patient presents in extremis with a cardiac structural or vascular insufficiency problem, ECLS may be used to stabilize the patient hemodynamically and to allow any organ insult to resolve prior to a definitive procedure (eg, open heart surgery or a catheter-based solution). However, in many situations, ECMO is placed urgently in the face of cardiac collapse with no therapeutic cardiac procedure as an option. In these cases, there are only 3 choices: recovery, heart transplant, or a durable ventricular assist device. In no situation is successful bridging guaranteed because the mortality associated with achieving any one of these outcomes is significant.

# References

1. Watanabe N. Acute mitral regurgitation. Heart. 2019;105(9):671-677.
2. Baran DA, Grines CL, Bailey S, et al. SCAI clinical expert consensus statement on the classification of cardiogenic shock: This document was endorsed by the American College of Cardiology (ACC), the American Heart Association (AHA), the Society of Critical Care Medicine (SCCM), and the Society of Thoracic Surgeons (STS) in April 2019. Catheter Cardiovasc Interv. 2019;94(1):29-37.
3. Jentzer JC, van Diepen S, Barsness GW, et al. Cardiogenic Shock Classification to Predict Mortality in the Cardiac Intensive Care Unit. J Am Coll Cardiol. 2019;74(17):2117-2128.
4. Kapur NK, Davila CD. Timing, timing, timing: the emerging concept of the "door to support"time for cardiogenic shock. Eur Heart J. 2017;38(47):3532-3534.
5. Gariboldi V, Grisoli D, Tarmiz A, et al. Mobile extracorporeal membrane oxygenation unit expands cardiac assist surgical programs. Ann Thorac Surg. 2010;90(5):1548-1552.
6. Obadia B, Théron A, Gariboldi V, et al. Extracorporeal membrane oxygenation as a bridge to surgery for ischemic papillary muscle rupture. J Thorac Cardiovasc Surg. 2014;147(6):e82-e84.
7. Arnaoutakis GJ, Zhao Y, George TJ, et al. Surgical repair of ventricular septal defect after myocardial infarction: outcomes from the Society of Thoracic Surgeons National Database. Ann Thorac Surg. 2012;94(2):436-443; discussion 443-444.
8. Poterucha TJ, Bergmark B, Aranki S, et al. Surgical Pulmonary Embolectomy. Circulation. 2015;132(12):1146-1151.
9. Shinar Z. Contraindicated? - Aortic dissection and ECPR. Resuscitation. 2020;156:268-269.
10. Kwon J, Lee D. The effectiveness of extracorporeal membrane oxygenation in a patient with post myocardial infarct ventricular septal defect. J Cardiothorac Surg. 2016;11(1):143.
11. Rousse N, Juthier F, Pinçon C, et al. ECMO as a bridge to decision: Recovery, VAD, or heart transplantation? Int J Cardiol. 2015;187:620-627.
12. Mehra MR. Guidelines for Listing Candidates for Heart Transplant: A 10-Year Update. JAMA Cardiol. 2017;2(1):98-99.
13. Cheng R, Hachamovitch R, Kittleson M, et al. Complications of extracorporeal membrane oxygenation for treatment of cardiogenic shock and cardiac arrest: a meta-analysis of 1,866 adult patients. Ann Thorac Surg. 2014;97(2):610-616.
14. Aissaoui N, Luyt CE, Leprince P, et al. Predictors of successful extracorporeal membrane oxygen-ation (ECMO) weaning after assistance for refractory cardiogenic shock. Intensive Care Med. 2011;37(11):1738-1745.
15. Pappalardo F, Pieri M, Arnaez Corada B, et al. Timing and Strategy for Weaning From Venoarterial ECMO are Complex Issues. J Cardiothorac Vasc Anesth. 2015;29(4):906-911.
16. Zalawadiya S, Fudim M, Bhat G, et al. Extracorporeal membrane oxygenation support and post-heart transplant outcomes among United States adults. J Heart Lung Transplant. 2017;36(1):77-81.
17. Haglund NA, Feurer ID, Dwyer JP, et al. Does renal dysfunction and method of bridging support influence heart transplant graft survival? Ann Thorac Surg. 2014;98(3):835-841.
18. Miller PE, Jentzer J, Katz JN. Are Unselected Risk Scores in the Cardiac Intensive Care Unit Needed? J Am Heart Assoc. 2021;10(21):e021940.
19. Coutance G, Jacob N, Demondion P, et al. Favorable Outcomes of a Direct Heart Transplantation Strategy in Selected Patients on Extracorporeal Membrane Oxygenation Support. Crit Care Med. 2020;48(4):498-506.
20. Ohira S, Spielvogel D, Gass AL, et al. Direct Advanced Therapy Off Veno-Arterial Extracorporeal Membrane Oxygenation Support: Impact of New Heart Allocation Policy on Early Outcomes. J Heart Lung Transplant. 2021;40(4, Supplement):S132.
21. Nordan T, Critsinelis AC, Mahrokhian SH, et al. Bridging With Extracorporeal Membrane Oxygenation Under the New Heart Allocation System: A United Network for Organ Sharing Database Analysis. Circ Heart Fail. 2021;14(5):e007966.
22. Maltais S, Haglund NA, Davis ME, et al. Does INTERMACS Classification Predict Outcomes after LVAD Implantation? J Heart Lung Transplant. 2016;35(4):S376.
23. Cowger J, Shah P, Stulak J, et al. INTERMACS profiles and modifiers: Heterogeneity of patient classification and the impact of modifiers on predicting patient outcome. J Heart Lung Transplant. 2016;35(4):440-448.
24. Soleimani B, Brehm C, Stephenson E, Pae W. Application of Extracorporeal Membrane Oxygenator (ECMO) Support in Adult Patients with Cardiogenic Shock as a Bridge to Implantable Left Ventricular Assist Device (LVAD). J Heart Lung Transplant. 2016;35(4):S335-S336.
25. Han JJ, Chen C, Chung J, et al. ECMO-Bridge to LVAD Therapy Is a Safe and Effective Strategy for Critically Ill Patients. The Journal of Heart and Lung Transplantation. 2017;36(4):S328.
26. Lamb KM, DiMuzio PJ, Johnson A, et al. Arterial protocol including prophylactic distal perfusion catheter decreases limb ischemia complications

in patients undergoing extracorporeal membrane oxygenation. J Vasc Surg. 2017;65(4):1074-1079.

27. Lorusso R, Shekar K, MacLaren G, et al. ELSO Interim Guidelines for Venoarterial Extracorporeal Membrane Oxygenation in Adult Cardiac Patients. ASAIO J. 2021;67(8):827-844.

28. Zangrillo A, Biondi-Zoccai G, Landoni G, et al. Extracorporeal membrane oxygenation (ECMO) in patients with H1N1 influenza infection: a systematic review and meta-analysis including 8 studies and 266 patients receiving ECMO. Critical Care. 2013;17(1):R30. doi:10.1186/cc12512.

29. Kim DJ, Cho YJ, Park SH, et al. Near-Infrared Spectroscopy Monitoring for Early Detection of Limb Ischemia in Patients on Veno-Arterial Extracorporeal Membrane Oxygenation. ASAIO J. 2017;63(5):613-617.

30. Lockie CJA, Gillon SA, Barrett NA, et al. Severe Respiratory Failure, Extracorporeal Membrane Oxygenation, and Intracranial Hemorrhage. Crit Care Med. 2017;45(10):1642-1649.

31. Wilcox C, Choi CW, Cho SM. Brain injury in extracorporeal cardiopulmonary resuscitation: translational to clinical research. J Neurocrit Care. 2021;14(2):63-77.

32. Al-Kawaz MN, Canner J, Caturegli G, et al. Duration of Hyperoxia and Neurologic Outcomes in Patients Undergoing Extracorporeal Membrane Oxygenation. Crit Care Med. 2021;49(10):e968-e977.

33. Hunt MF, Clark KT, Whitman G, et al. The Use of Cerebral NIRS Monitoring to Identify Acute Brain Injury in Patients With VA-ECMO. J Intensive Care Med. 2021;36(12):1403-1409.

34. Cho SM, Ziai W, Mayasi Y, et al. Noninvasive Neurological Monitoring in Extracorporeal Membrane Oxygenation. ASAIO J. 2020;66(4):388-393.

35. Zhang Z, Gu WJ, Chen K, Ni H. Mechanical Ventilation during Extracorporeal Membrane Oxygenation in Patients with Acute Severe Respiratory Failure. Can Respir J. 2017;2017:1783857.

36. Dobrilovic N, March R, Yin K, et al. Liver Dysfunction Associated With In-Hospital Mortality in Adult Extracorporeal Membrane Oxygenation Support. Crit Care Explor. 2021;3(7):e0484.

37. Masha L, Peerbhai S, Boone D, et al. Yellow Means Caution: Correlations Between Liver Injury and Mortality with the Use of VA-ECMO. ASAIO J. 2019;65(8):812-818.

38. Jung C, Kelm M, Westenfeld R. Liver function during mechanical circulatory support: from witness to prognostic determinant. Crit Care. 2016;20(1):134.

39. Lorusso R, Raffa GM, Alenizy K, et al. Structured review of post-cardiotomy extracorporeal membrane oxygenation: part 1-Adult patients. J Heart Lung Transplant. 2019;38(11):1125-1143.

40. Villa G, Katz N, Ronco C. Extracorporeal Membrane Oxygenation and the Kidney. Cardiorenal Med. 2015;6(1):50-60.

41. Ostermann M, Lumlertgul N. Acute kidney injury in ECMO patients. Crit Care. 2021;25(1):313.

42. Biffi S, Di Bella S, Scaravilli V, et al. Infections during extracorporeal membrane oxygenation: epidemiology, risk factors, pathogenesis and prevention. Int J Antimicrob Agents. 2017;50(1):9-16.

43. Gopalakrishnan R, Vashisht R. Sepsis and ECMO. Indian J Thorac Cardiovasc Surg. Published online May 14, 2020:1-8.

44. Manerikar A, Watanabe S, Kandula V, et al. Indwelling Central Venous Catheters Drive Bloodstream Infection During Veno-venous Extracorporeal Membrane Oxygenation Support. ASAIO J. 2022 Jun 1;68(6):859-864.

45. Firstenberg MS. Advances in Extracorporeal Membrane Oxygenation: Volume 3. BoD – Books on Demand; 2019.

46. Colvin MM, Cook JL, Chang PP, et al. Sensitization in Heart Transplantation: Emerging Knowledge: A Scientific Statement From the American Heart Association. Circulation. 2019;139(12):e553-e578.

47. Massad MG, Cook DJ, Schmitt SK, et al. Factors influencing HLA sensitization in implantable LVAD recipients. Ann Thorac Surg. 1997;64(4):1120-1125.

48. Bear DE, Smith E, Barrett NA. Nutrition Support in Adult Patients Receiving Extracorporeal Membrane Oxygenation. Nutr Clin Pract. 2018;33(6):738-746.

49. Lindberg BR, Videm V, Dahl T, et al. Influence of the ECMO circuit on the concentration of nutritional supplements. Sci Rep. 2020;10(1):19275.

50. Park J, Heo E, Song IA, et al. Nutritional support and clinical outcomes in critically ill patients supported with veno-arterial extracorporeal membrane oxygenation. Clin Nutr. 2020;39(8):2617-2623.

51. Wollersheim T, Frank S, Müller MC, et al. Measuring Energy Expenditure in extracorporeal lung support Patients (MEEP) - Protocol, feasibility and pilot trial. Clin Nutr. 2018;37(1):301-307.

52. Copeland H, Lirette S, Mohammed A, et al. Functional Status of Heart Transplant Recipients Predicts Survival. J Heart Lung Transplant. 2021;40(4, Supplement):S278.

53. Abrams D, Javidfar J, Farrand E, et al. Early mobilization of patients receiving extracorporeal membrane oxygenation: a retrospective cohort study. Crit Care. 2014;18(1):R38.

54. Salna M, Abrams D, Brodie D. Physical rehabilitation in the awake patient receiving extracorporeal circulatory or gas exchange support. Ann Transl Med. 2020;8(13):834.

55. Hayes K, Holland AE, Pellegrino VA, et al. Acute skeletal muscle wasting and relation to physical

function in patients requiring extracorporeal membrane oxygenation (ECMO). J Crit Care. 2018;48:1-8.

56. Faron A, Kreyer S, Sprinkart AM, et al. CT fatty muscle fraction as a new parameter for muscle quality assessment predicts outcome in venovenous extracorporeal membrane oxygenation. Sci Rep. 2020;10(1):22391.

# 31

## Extracorporeal Life Support for Adult Congenital Heart Disease

*Omar M. Sharaf, Graeme MacLaren, Erika B. Rosenzweig, Anne Marie Valente, Gregory Schears,*
*Joseph Dearani, Giles J. Peek, Mark S. Bleiweis, Jeffrey P. Jacobs*

### Introduction

From the year 2000, more adults than children are alive with congenital heart disease (CHD).[1-5] Each year, more of these adults with congenital heart disease (ACHD) undergo surgery. Furthermore, many of these operations are reoperations in ACHD and are associated with unique risks.[2]

Increased long-term survival after complex neonatal heart surgery has resulted in a rapidly growing population of ACHD.[3-5] This increased survival of neonates with CHD is attributable to advances in multiple domains, including: diagnostic imaging, preoperative care, surgical technique, cardiopulmonary bypass, postoperative care, ECLS, and VAD use.

Nevertheless, many ACHD suffer from progression of their disease or late sequelae of their childhood repair. Furthermore, ACHD may develop any of the myriad diseases that otherwise healthy adults can acquire. Consequently, many ACHD require surgical or transcatheter intervention or both. Analysis of The Society of Thoracic Surgeons Congenital Heart Surgery Database (STS CHSD) reveals that "a history of previous cardiac surgery does not independently confer a significant incremental risk of operative mortality, but that patients with greater number of previous operations appear to be at higher risk."[2]

Approximately 20% of ACHD undergo cardiac surgery in adulthood to treat a combination of congenital and acquired lesions.[6,7] Surgery in ACHD is marked by unique challenges and risks, including operative complexity coupled with adult-onset comorbidities.[8,9] ACHD may require ECLS in a variety of settings including: preoperative, intraoperative, postoperative, and nonoperative. In this chapter, we explore some of the unique challenges related to ECLS in ACHD.

### Scores and Tools for Evaluating Need for and Risk of ECLS in ACHD

Multiple tools and scoring systems are available to assess the need for and risk of ECLS in both children and adults, and many of these scoring systems can be applied to ACHD. In this section, we discuss important limitations and considerations needed when using these scoring tools for ACHD.

ACHD often have different baseline arterial and mixed venous oxygen saturations secondary to congenital or acquired intracardiac shunts and/or systemic and pulmonary circulations that are partially or completely parallel rather than in series. Examples include patients with functionally univentricular circulations, patients with systemic-to-pulmonary artery shunts, patients with superior cavopulmonary anastomosis(es) (Glenn), and patients with fenestrated Fontan circulations. Such challenging patients present important issues in multiple areas:

- Indications for ECLS
- Expected outcomes from ECLS
- Cannulation strategies for ECLS
- Strategies for initiating ECLS
- Strategies for weaning from ECLS
- Strategies for bridging to more durable support.

It must be remembered that most scoring systems were fundamentally designed to assess the need for and risk of ECLS in patients without CHD. Their application to ACHD must be modified to account for the circulation of a given patient, as well as their baseline arterial and mixed venous oxygen saturations.

### Scoring Systems for Isolated Respiratory Failure and Potential VV ECMO

Selection of ACHD for VV ECMO in hypoxic respiratory failure is similar to patients without ACHD, with the exception that the baseline saturation of ACHD may be different. The aim is to select patients with a potentially reversible etiology of their respiratory failure. Additionally, the purpose of VV ECMO in

respiratory failure is to allow a patient's lungs to recover without the barotrauma of high-pressure mechanical ventilation. ACHD may develop isolated respiratory failure and ARDS independent of their congenital cardiac disease. ACHD may also develop isolated respiratory failure and ARDS after surgical or transcatheter intervention for their CHD in the postoperative or postinterventional setting.[10]

ECLS became an established modality for treating respiratory failure in neonates before adults; thus, the first ECLS scoring system, oxygenation index (OI), was developed for neonates with hypoxic respiratory failure (Figure 31-1).[11,12] An OI >40 despite optimal medical therapy is accepted as an indication for initiation of ECLS in term or late preterm neonates.[13,14] However, in adults with hypoxic respiratory failure due to ARDS, OI alone is not a strong predictor of mortality.[15] Thus, multiple tools and scoring systems have been developed and evaluated for use in adults.

Combining OI with age, the age-adjusted oxygenation index (AOI), is a stronger predictor of mortality in adults with severe respiratory failure, with a C-index (or AUC) of 0.72-0.75.[15] However, AOI score is calculated using plateau pressure rather than mean airway pressure because mean airway pressure was not routinely reported in the databases used to create this score. Specifically, it is calculated by

$$Oxygenation\ Index\ (OI) = \frac{P_{AW}\ (mmHg) \times FiO_2\ (\%) \times 100}{PaO_2\ (mmHg)}$$

**Figure 31-1.** Oxygenation Index (OI) Formula. FiO$_2$, fraction of inspired oxygen; PAW, mean airway pressure; PaO$_2$, partial pressure of arterial oxygen.

$$Age\text{-}Adjusted\ Oxygenation\ Index\ (AOI) = \frac{P_{plateau}\ (cm\ H_2O) \times FiO_2\ (\%) \times 100}{PaO_2\ (mmHg)}$$

**Figure 31-2.** Age-Adjusted Oxygenation Index (AOI) Formula. FiO$_2$, fraction of inspired oxygen; PaO$_2$, partial pressure of arterial oxygen; Pplateau, plateau pressure.

multiplying plateau pressure ($cmH_2O$) by $FiO_2$ as a whole number divided by $PaO_2$ (mmHg) (Figure 31-2). Adjusted for age, an AOI >80 is an indication for initiating ECLS in adults with respiratory failure. When AOI is ≥60 but <80, mortality risk is greater than 50%, and ECLS should be considered.

Another tool for assessing the severity of acute lung injury in adult respiratory failure is the Murray Score.[16] This score was validated by Peek and colleagues in a randomized controlled trial (the CESAR trial)[17] and is calculated as the average of four variables graded 0-4 (Figure 31-3): 1) consolidation on chest x-ray (CXR), 2) $PaO_2/FiO_2$ ratio, 3) positive end-expiratory pressure (PEEP, cm $H_2O$), and 4) lung compliance (mL/cm $H_2O$). A Murray Score of 0 suggests no lung injury,

0.1-2.5 suggests mild to moderate lung injury, and >2.5 suggests severe lung injury. A Murray Score of ≥3.0 is an indication for ECLS, while patients with scores between 2.0-3.0 should be considered for ECLS.

The Age, $PaO_2/FiO_2$, and Plateau Pressure Score (APPS) is another tool that may be used to stratify the severity of respiratory failure in adults.[18] The APPS was derived and validated in two separate cohorts of 300 patients with ARDS and was predictive of in-hospital mortality. This score is calculated at 24 hours after a diagnosis of ARDS while on mechanical ventilation using three variables: 1) age (years), 2) $PaO_2/FiO_2$, and 3) plateau pressure (cm $H_2O$). Each variable is graded as 1-3 and added together with a minimum total score of 3 and a maximum score of 9 (Figure 31-4). An APPS of 8 or higher is

| | Point Allocation | | |
|---|---|---|---|
| | 1 Point | 2 Points | 3 Points |
| Age (years) | < 47 | 47 – 66 | > 66 |
| $PaO_2/FiO_2$ Ratio | > 158 | 105 – 158 | < 105 |
| $P_{plateau}$ (cm $H_2O$) | < 27 | 27 – 30 | > 30 |

*Age, $PaO_2/FiO_2$, and Plateau Pressure Score (APPS)*
*= Age Points + $PaO_2/FiO_2$ Points + $P_{plateau}$ Points*

**Figure 31-3.** Murray Score. $C_L$, lung compliance; CXR, chest x-ray; $FiO_2$, fraction of inspired oxygen; $PaO_2$, partial pressure of arterial oxygen; PEEP, positive end-expiratory pressure; PIP, peak inspiratory pressure; $V_T$, tidal volume.

| | Point Allocation | | |
|---|---|---|---|
| | 1 Point | 2 Points | 3 Points |
| Age (years) | < 47 | 47 – 66 | > 66 |
| $PaO_2/FiO_2$ Ratio | > 158 | 105 – 158 | < 105 |
| $P_{plateau}$ (cm $H_2O$) | < 27 | 27 – 30 | > 30 |

*Age, $PaO_2/FiO_2$, and Plateau Pressure Score (APPS)*
*= Age Points + $PaO_2/FiO_2$ Points + $P_{plateau}$ Points*

**Figure 31-4.** Age, $PaO_2/FiO_2$, and Plateau Pressure Score (APPS). $FiO_2$, fraction of inspired oxygen; $PaO_2$, partial pressure of arterial oxygen; $P_{plateau}$, plateau pressure.

$$Horovitz\ Index = \frac{PaO_2\ (mmHg)}{FiO_2\ (\%) \times 100}$$

**Figure 31-5.** Horovitz Index. $FiO_2$, fraction of inspired oxygen; $PaO_2$, partial pressure of arterial oxygen.

associated with greater than 80% mortality and is thus an indication for ECLS.

A simpler tool is the Horovitz index, also known as the P/F ratio, which only requires two variables but is not as strongly predictive of mortality as other scoring tools.[19] The P/F ratio was validated by the ARDS Definition Task Force to develop the Berlin definition, predicting mortality with an AUC of 0.577.[20] The Horovitz index is calculated by dividing $PaO_2$ (mmHg) by $FiO_2$ as a whole number (Figure 31-5). Using the P/F ratio, ARDS is stratified by severity as follows:

- >300 is not ARDS,
- >200-300 is mild ARDS,
- >100-200 is moderate ARDS, and
- ≤100 is severe ARDS and may be considered an indication for ECMO if $FiO_2$ >90% (Chapter 23).

### Scoring Systems for Cardiac Failure and Potential VA ECMO

While the previously described scores have been created and evaluated among patients with isolated respiratory failure, cardiac failure resulting in cardiogenic shock is a separate entity that requires separate scoring systems to predict survival with and without VA ECMO. Notably, there are no established cutoffs for initiating VA ECMO using these scoring systems, and multiple other measures should be attempted prior to consideration for ECMO, including: volume administration, inotropic support, mechanical ventilation, other pharmacological therapies, and potentially intraaortic balloon counterpulsation.

Additionally, the following scores were developed without considering patients not supported with ECMO and are thus not appropriate for guiding initiation of VA ECMO but rather for predicting survival after VA ECMO is initiated. The decision to initiate VA ECMO should be based on clinical judgment in patients with refractory cardiogenic shock. In patients who are deemed to be good candidates for VA ECMO, the following scores may help predict survival. Once again, these scoring systems have not been validated in ACHD. Thus, their application to ACHD must be performed with consideration of the pathway of the flow of blood in a given patient, as well as their baseline arterial and mixed venous oxygen saturations.

The Survival after VA ECMO (SAVE) score was created based on a group of 3,846 patients with refractory cardiogenic shock to identify pre-ECMO factors affecting hospital survival.[21] It was internally validated with an AUC of 0.68 and externally validated in a group of 161 patients with an AUC of 0.90.[21] The score incorporates 12 variables to stratify patients into one of five risk classes. To calculate the SAVE score, each of the 12 variables is scored as displayed in Table 31-1. Etiology of acute cardiogenic shock should be scored as one of five groups, including: myocarditis (3 points), refractory ventricular tachycardia or fibrillation (2 points), post heart or lung transplantation (3 points), CHD (-3 points), and other diagnoses (0 points).

Mortality increases with increasing SAVE risk classification, with a SAVE-score of 0 representing approximately 50% mortality. These SAVE scores are further classified:

- SAVE risk class I: score > 5 and is associated with 25% mortality.
- SAVE risk class II: score of 1 to 5 and is associated with 42% mortality.
- SAVE risk class III: score of -4 to 0 and is associated with 58% mortality.
- SAVE risk class IV: score of -9 to -5 and is associated with 70% mortality.
- SAVE risk class V: score ≤ -10 and is associated with 82% mortality.

Of note, patients who received post-cardiotomy ECLS or ECPR were excluded from this study. Importantly, the SAVE score

| PARAMETER | POINT ALLOCATION |
|---|---|
| ***Acute Cardiogenic Shock Diagnosis Group*** *(may select multiple)* | |
| Myocarditis | 3 |
| Refractory VT/VF | 2 |
| Post Heart or Lung Transplantation | 3 |
| Congenital Heart Disease | -3 |
| Other | 0 |
| ***Age*** *(years)* | |
| 18 – 38 | 7 |
| 39 – 52 | 4 |
| 53 – 62 | 3 |
| ≥ 63 | 0 |
| ***Weight*** *(kg)* | |
| ≤ 65 | 1 |
| 65 – 89 | 2 |
| ≥ 90 | 0 |
| ***Acute Pre-ECMO Organ Failures*** *(may select multiple)* | |
| Liver Failure[1] | -3 |
| Central Nervous System Dysfunction[2] | -3 |
| Renal Failure[3] | -3 |
| ***Chronic Renal Failure***[4] | |
| Yes | -6 |
| No | 0 |
| ***Duration of Intubation Prior to Initiation of ECMO*** *(hours)* | |
| ≤ 10 | 0 |
| 11 – 29 | -2 |
| ≥ 30 | -4 |
| ***PIP ≤ 20 cm $H_2O$*** | 3 |
| ***Pre-ECMO Cardiac Arrest*** | -2 |
| ***Pre-ECMO Diastolic Blood Pressure ≥ 40 mmHg***[5] | 3 |
| ***Pre-ECMO Pulse Pressure ≤ 20 mmHg***[5] | -2 |
| ***Pre-ECMO Bicarbonate ≤ 15 mmol/L***[5] | -3 |
| ***Constant Value Added to All Calculations*** | -6 |
| **Total SAVE Score** | -35 to 17 |

| RISK CLASS | TOTAL SAVE SCORE |
|---|---|
| I | > 5 |
| II | 1 – 5 |
| III | -4 – 0 |
| IV | -9 – -5 |
| V | ≤ -10 |

PIP=peak inspiratory pressure; VT=ventricular tachycardia; VF=ventricular fibrillation.
[1] Defined as bilirubin ≥ 33 μmol/L or elevation of serum aminotransferases (AST or ALT) > 70 UI/L.
[2] Includes neurotrauma, stroke, encephalopathy, cerebral embolism, seizure, and epileptic syndromes.
[3] Defined as acute renal insufficiency (creatinine > 1.5 mg/dL) with or without renal replacement therapy.
[4] Defined as either kidney damage or glomerular filtration rate < 60 mL/min/1.73 m$^2$ for ≥ 3 months.
[5] Any recorded value within 6 hours prior to ECMO cannulation.

**Table 31-1.** Survival after venoarterial extracorporeal membrane oxygenation (SAVE) Score and classification. Adapted from original article.[21]

recognizes and accounts for the increased risk of the presence of CHD; in fact, CHD is recognized and valued as the highest risk etiology of cardiac failure in this system, with a value of negative three points.

Another potential scoring tool that predicts survival after initiation of VA ECMO is the prEdictioN of Cardiogenic shock OUtcome foR AMI patients salvaGed by VA-ECMO (ENCOURAGE) risk score.[22] The ENCOURAGE risk score predicts 30-day and 6-month survival after ECMO initiation. The score was developed among 138 patients with cardiogenic shock secondary to acute myocardial infarction who were treated with VA ECMO. The ENCOURAGE risk score was internally validated with an AUC of 0.84. It accounts for seven pre-ECMO parameters and classifies patients into one of five groups (Table 31-2). Variables required to calculate the ENCOURAGE mortality risk score are

| PARAMETER | POINT ALLOCATION |
|---|---|
| **Age *(years)*** | |
| ≤60 | 0 |
| >60 | 5 |
| **Sex** | |
| Male | 0 |
| Female | 7 |
| **Body Mass Index *(kg/m²)*** | |
| ≤25 | 0 |
| >25 | 6 |
| **Glasgow Coma Score** | |
| ≥6 | 0 |
| <6 | 6 |
| **Creatinine *(μmol/L)*** | |
| ≤150 | 0 |
| >150 | 5 |
| **Serum Lactate *(mmol/L)*** | |
| <2 | 0 |
| 2–8 | 8 |
| >8 | 11 |
| **Prothrombin Activity *(%)*** | |
| ≥50 | 0 |
| <50 | 5 |

**Table 31-2.** Prediction of Cardiogenic Shock Outcome for Acute Myocardial Infarction Patients Salvaged by Venoarterial Extracorporeal Membrane Oxygenation (ENCOURAGE) risk score.

measured prior to the initiation of ECMO and include: age, sex, body mass index (BMI), Glasgow coma score, creatinine, lactate, and prothrombin activity. The ENCOURAGE risk score is unique among VA ECMO scores in that it predicts long-term survival. However, it is limited to use in cardiogenic shock secondary to acute myocardial infarction and does not account for the presence or absence of CHD.

While the SAVE score and ENCOURAGE score provide helpful prognostic information in patients supported with VA ECMO, these scores are static. The PREDICT VA ECMO score was developed as a dynamic prognostic model among a group of 205 patients treated with VA ECMO and included patients undergoing cannulation for VA ECMO during CPR.[23] The PREDICT VA ECMO score may be calculated at six and 12 hours after initiation of ECMO to predict hospital survival. In an external validation cohort, the AUC was 0.718 for the six-hour PREDICT VA ECMO score and 0.735 for the 12-hour PREDICT VA ECMO score. The scoring system is based on point-of-care biomarkers including lactate, blood pH, and standard bicarbonate concentration. The six-hour PREDICT VA ECMO score relies on labs drawn at six hours only, while the 12-hour score requires lab measurements at one hour, six hours, and 12 hours after ECMO initiation. Labs may be collected within 30 minutes of each respective time point. Although the PREDICT VA ECMO score was evaluated in patients with cardiogenic shock and patients who received ECPR, it performs better in patients with cardiogenic shock. Notably, the PREDICT VA ECMO does not account for the presence or absence of CHD.

Each of these scoring systems can provide useful information. However, it is critical to contextualize the information derived from these scoring systems with the unique pathological and physiological features of ACHD.

## Evidence-Based Medicine and Randomized Trials Related to ECLS

Although ECLS was first successfully used in an adult[24] and then later in a neonate[25] (in 1971 and 1974, respectively), the first randomized, controlled study of ECLS was published in 1979.[26] The use of ECLS in adults subsequently decreased in the following years; however, several studies subsequently evaluated ECLS in both adult and pediatric populations, popularizing its use. Although congenital heart surgeons were among the first to conduct randomized controlled trials of ECLS, none of these studies focused on the use of ECLS in ACHD. Nevertheless, it is important to understand the evidence base in order to comprehend the rationale for the use of ECLS in ACHD.

The first randomized, controlled study of ECLS was conducted by Zapol et al. in adults with acute respiratory failure.[26] In this multicenter study across nine medical centers, patients were randomized to undergo VA ECMO or conventional medical therapy. After enrollment of 90 patients, the study was prematurely suspended because of high mortality of 90% in both groups. Zapol et al. concluded that ECLS was not associated with improved survival in adults with acute respiratory failure. The use of ECLS in adult patients essentially ceased after this report[27]; however, Bartlett and colleagues in Michigan continued to support neonates with ECLS.[28]

### Neonatal Randomized ECLS Trials

Subsequent randomized studies of ECLS were conducted in neonates. Bartlett and O'Rourke designed innovative "play the winner" studies, which showed benefit.[20,23,29,30] These trials were followed by Field and the United Kingdom (UK) Collaborative ECMO Trial Group, who performed a conventional randomized study of neonatal ECMO[31] that

was stopped early due to a significantly higher survival of 70% in those supported with ECMO vs. 41% among patients treated with conventional management. This trial paved the way for the widespread use of ECLS in neonates with respiratory failure, eventually prompting the reevaluation of the use of ECLS in adults.

### Randomized ECLS Trials in Adults

In 2009, Peek et al published the CESAR trial, which compared ECMO to conventional ventilatory support in adults with severe respiratory failure using a design similar to that used by the United Kingdom (UK) Collaborative ECMO Trial Group.[17] Patients randomized to ECMO had higher survival at 6-month followup compared to those allocated to conventional management. Based on their findings, Peek et al. recommended that adult patients with severe, potentially reversible respiratory failure with a Murray Score >3.0 or a pH <7.20 despite optimal conventional management be considered for support with ECLS.

Combes et al. conducted the ECMO to Rescue Lung Injury in Severe ARDS (EOLIA) trial[32] to address some of the shortcomings of the CESAR trial. The crossover design meant that there was no significant difference in mortality between the ECMO and control arms; however, there was a difference in treatment failure, favoring ECMO. An individual patient metaanalysis of the 429 patients in both CESAR and EOLIA showed a significant increase in survival in the ECMO patients.[33]

### Insights in the Use of ECLS in Patients with COVID-19 Infection

ECLS is increasingly utilized to support patients with COVID-19. As described above, none of the previously described randomized trials focused on the use of ECLS in ACHD. Similarly, ACHD may develop COVID-19, and it is important to understand the evidence base for using ECLS to support patients with COVID-19, even although this evidence base does not specifically analyze the impact of COVID-19 on ACHD.

The COVID-19 pandemic has had a far-reaching impact on society and has been associated with significant mortality. As of December 31, 2021, 287,365,929 patients had been diagnosed with COVID-19 worldwide, with 5,433,469 deaths (1.9% mortality).[34] In the United States alone over the same period, the mortality rate has been 1.5%, with a total of 54,443,678 cases and 824,630 deaths.[34] Early experience in Wuhan was not promising, with only 1 of 6 patients surviving ECMO.[35] However, subsequent reports were more promising.[36-44] Compared to nonsurvivors of COVID-19 supported with ECMO, survivors were younger and intubated sooner after diagnosis, and those who required VV ECMO rather than VA ECMO had higher survival. Older age and obesity appear to be risk factors, and prone positioning appears to be beneficial. Overall, it appears that between 35%-50% of patients with COVID-19 supported with ECMO ultimately survive and are discharged home.[36-44] This information may be useful when considering ECMO support for COVID-19 in ACHD.

**Respiratory ECMO for ACHD**

Some ACHD may have isolated respiratory failure and benefit from VV ECMO.[10] Multiple unique challenges exist with providing VV ECMO in ACHD. As discussed above, ACHD often have different baseline arterial and mixed venous oxygen saturations secondary to congenital or acquired intracardiac shunts and/or systemic and pulmonary circulations that are partially or completely parallel rather than in series. When contemplating VV ECMO in ACHD, baseline arterial and mixed venous oxygen saturations must be considered when setting goals and expectations. The anatomy,

morphology, pathology, and pathophysiology of the congenital cardiac malformation must be thoroughly understood. Cannulation can be extremely challenging in ACHD secondary to multiple factors including congenitally abnormal systemic and pulmonary venous connections, surgically altered systemic and pulmonary venous connections, residual systemic-to-pulmonary communications, and the loss of patent blood vessels secondary to multiple cardiac catheterizations and cardiac surgical procedures. All ACHD should undergo detailed ultrasound as soon as the team starts to consider ECLS, in order to assess the patency of femoral and neck vessels. The conduct of ECLS can be challenging secondary to residual systemic-to- pulmonary shunts and should only be undertaken by those with experience in managing ACHD. In patients with residual systemic-to-pulmonary communications, return cannula position relative to the shunt is critical to avoid residual shunting of deoxygenated blood in the setting of pulmonary hypertension and/or right ventricular failure. In ACHD with pulmonary hypertension, utilization of respiratory ECMO with creation of an oxygenated right-to-left shunt may be adequate vs. VA ECMO, in cases with respiratory failure, a patent shunt, and preserved left ventricular function.[45]

- In patients with superior cavopulmonary connections (Glenn), the superior vena cava (or bilateral superior vena cavae) is not connected to the heart but is instead connected to the pulmonary artery.
- In patients with total cavopulmonary connection (TCPC) type Fontan connections, blood in the inferior vena cava does not drain into the systemic venous atrium but instead drains to the pulmonary artery. Patients with a 'classic' atriopulmonary Fontan, however, may use the right atrium as part of the Fontan pathway.

- In patients with interrupted inferior vena cava, the femoral vein will not drain in the usual pathway through the inferior vena cava to the heart. Instead, the inferior vena cava is interrupted and femoral venous blood will drain to the heart via an azygous continuation.

**Cardiac ECMO for ACHD**

As ACHD age, there is an increased prevalence of heart failure, as well as other noncardiac comorbidities. In fact, health care utilization among ACHD has grown steadily in both inpatient and outpatient settings, and those with complex forms of CHD have the highest rates of emergency department utilization, hospitalization, and critical care needs.[46] In parallel with survivorship, the complexity of CHD in ACHD has increased substantially over the past two decades, and there is an increased need for options of mechanical circulatory support.[47]

Multiple indications for ECLS in ACHD exist:

- ECLS may be a useful tool in stabilizing ACHD who present with cardiogenic shock, low cardiac output state, or cardiomyopathies due to acute coronary injury.
- ECLS may be used as a rescue therapy in ACHD unable to wean from cardiopulmonary bypass or those who need peri-procedural support.
- ECLS is appropriate in cases where there are reversible causes of ventricular dysfunction and may serve as a bridge-to-decision or bridge-to-transplant.[48]
- ECLS may be appropriate during cardiac arrest in patients with CHD and should be considered early in resuscitation efforts.[49]
- Table 31-3 lists potential indications and relative contraindications for ECLS in ACHD.

As discussed above, ACHD often have complex anatomy and may have undergone multiple prior interventions, resulting in limitations to vascular access. It is also important to consider potential comorbidities which may be present in ACHD, because renal, neurologic, and pulmonary complications are associated with worse survival following ECLS. The prevalence of renal disease is higher in ACHD than in the general population, and 9% of ACHD have at least moderately decreased renal function (ie, glomerular filtration rate <60 ml/min/1.73 $m^2$) which is associated with a three-fold increase in overall mortality.[50] ACHD are also at an increased risk of stroke, neurodevelopmental disorders, cognitive impairment, psychiatric disease, and epilepsy.[51] Patients who have undergone prior thoracotomy may have restrictive lung disease, and obstructive sleep apnea is underdiagnosed

| POTENTIAL INDICATIONS | RELATIVE CONTRAINDICATIONS |
|---|---|
| Mean arterial pressure < 60 mmHg | Multi-system organ failure |
| Left atrial pressure >20 mmHg | Sepsis with systemic vasoplegia |
| Low cardiac index (<2 L/min/m²) | Neurologic damage |
| Rising lactate | Severe aortic regurgitation |
| Failure to respond to vasoactive agents | Unwitnessed arrest |
| Failure to wean from cardiopulmonary bypass | Prolonged resuscitation (>60 min) |
| Evidence of end-organ damage | No hope of recovery or transplant option |

**Table 31-3.** Potential indications and relative contraindications for ECMO in ACHD.

and undertreated in ACHD. Pulmonary arterial hypertension related to CHD affects 5%-10% of ACHD and is associated with significant morbidity and mortality.[52] ACHD may also have hepatic dysfunction.[53] ACHD with the highest prevalence of liver disease include: Fontan circulation, congestive heart failure, and other conditions associated with chronically elevated right atrial pressures, such as tricuspid valve disease, tetralogy of Fallot with severe pulmonary regurgitation, transposition of the great arteries with atrial switch repair, and Eisenmenger syndrome.

Hematologic issues in ACHD include: coagulopathies, iron deficiency, and bleeding disorders.

Dolgner et al. examined predictors of ECLS support after cardiac surgery in ACHD from the Pediatric Health Information Systems database from 2003 to 2014.[54] During that time, 4665 ACHD underwent cardiac surgery in 39 pediatric hospitals. Fifty-one patients (1.1%) were supported with ECLS and 64 (1.4%) died without it. Of the 51 patients who were supported with ECLS, 34 (67%) died. Risk factors for death included older age, increased surgical complexity, functionally univentricular physiology, preoperative hospitalization, and the presence of noncardiac complex chronic conditions.

The same group of investigators have more recently reported on outcomes of ACHD from the ELSO Registry from 1994-2016.[54] They identified 368 ACHD who received ECLS after cardiac surgery, with an overall mortality of 61%. Pre-cannulation risk factors for mortality included[55]: Fontan physiology, weight >100 kg, female gender, delayed cannulation, and neuromuscular blockade. After adding post-cannulation features into the multivariate model, the following factors were associated with increased mortality[55]: renal complications, neurological complications, and pulmonary hemorrhage.

Adults with Fontan physiology have notably poor outcomes after ECPR. Multiple potential reasons exist for the poor outcomes in these patients, one of which is difficulty in administering CPR, as chest compressions result in increased intrathoracic pressure which may limit effective pulmonary blood flow and therefore oxygenation. Compressions also result in increased cerebral venous pressure, which may impair cerebral perfusion. By the time cannulation occurs, irreversible end-organ damage may have occurred. Many contributing factors to poor outcomes in these patients relate to the inability to maintain adequate venous drainage and systemic perfusion, which results in neurologic injury. Use of more than one cannula from more than one site should augment venous return, yet, unfortunately, many of these patients have central venous occlusions from multiple prior interventions.

## ECLS and VAD as a Bridge to Heart, Lung, or Heart and Lung Transplantation

The use of ECLS or VAD to bridge patients to transplantation is described in detail in the following chapters:

- Chapter 30 (Bridging adult patients with cardiac failure),
- Chapter 40 (Lung transplantation), and
- Chapter 41 (Cardiac transplantation).

Specific issues related to ACHD are highlighted in this section.

In general, ACHD are a challenging group to bridge to transplantation. They typically have undergone multiple operations, placing them at substantial risk of mediastinal adhesions and vascular complications, such as venous stenosis or thrombosis. These factors increase the technical complexity and risks of inserting mechanical circulatory support devices, as can specific anatomic diagnoses and the nature of previous operations. For example, in patients with Transposition of the Great Arteries palliated with a Senning or Mustard operation, the atria are unlikely to accommodate venous drainage cannulas. ACHD have often received multiple blood product transfusions and been exposed to allograft material.[56-58] The consequent alloimmunization may delay finding a suitable donor organ and thus prolong the duration of mechanical circulatory support.

While ECLS has the advantage of providing support to both the lungs and the pulmonary and/or systemic ventricle, survival to transplantation is higher with the use of VAD in most circumstances.[59-61] ECLS is typically used as a bridge to transplantation in ACHD when VAD insertion is technically difficult or impossible,[62] there is significant concomitant lung disease or pulmonary hypertension, or waitlist times are short.

The regional or national mechanisms for determining the priority of allocation for cardiac transplantation may have an important influence on outcomes when comparing ECLS to VAD. Recent data from the Interagency Registry for Mechanically Assisted Circulatory Support (INTERMACS) and the United Network for Organ Sharing (UNOS) databases demonstrated no difference in posttransplant mortality whether ECLS was used as a bridge directly to cardiac transplantation or as a bridge to VAD.[63] Other variables such as age, the degree of critical illness, and mechanical ventilation can influence the choice of mechanical support device, making unadjusted comparisons between outcomes associated with ECLS and VAD unhelpful.[64] Fundamentally, the decision whether to bridge an ACHD to transplantation with ECLS or VAD is influenced by a number of factors, including waitlist times and local surgical expertise, and needs to be individualized to the needs of the patient and the expertise of the center.

Detailed planning as to the most appropriate form of mechanical circulatory support and how it should be inserted is critically important.[65] Some intensive care units have standardized workflows where the candidacy of each patient for ECLS is documented on admission, and the relevant vessels and cannula sizes are charted at the bedside. As discussed above, this documentation should include the status of the patency of each of the relevant vessels. The axillary artery may be one valuable approach because it can be surgically accessed without a need to dissect mediastinal adhesions and its use can facilitate extubation and mobilization, thus providing optimal conditions for bridging to transplantation. In patients with cavopulmonary connections in whom ECLS is needed, consideration should be given to drainage of both vena cavae.

## ECLS and VAD as a Bridge to Combined Heart-Liver and Heart-Liver-Kidney Transplantation in ACHD

Improvements in surgical technique and perioperative management have resulted in patients with CHD surviving well into adulthood.[1-5,66] Patients with functionally univentricular physiology and the Fontan palliation are a subgroup of patients with CHD that are more vulnerable than most to late complications and have limited life expectancy, with less than 50% alive at 30 years.[67] These patients are prone to heart failure as they get older, often with concurrent severe liver and/or kidney failure. The reasons for this end-organ failure are believed to be related to chronic, elevated systemic venous pressures secondary to the absence of a functional right ventricle, chronic low cardiac output, and organ injury that may have occurred over the complex surgical and medical course.[68]

The liver failure seen with Fontan physiology differs from that seen in typical congestive heart failure because these patients with functionally univentricular circulation develop extensive fibrosis secondary to a fibroinflammatory response, making it a nonreversible form of hepatic failure that progresses to cirrhosis at times.[69] Thus, the need for combined heart-liver (HLT) or heart-liver-kidney (HLKT) transplantation is necessary if this subgroup of patients with CHD is to survive longer term and have a satisfactory quality of life.

The first heart-liver transplant occurred in 1984.[70] Between 1987 and 2015, the UNOS database showed that only 41 patients with CHD underwent HLT.[71] A more recent analysis from 2009 to 2020 showed a 5-fold increase in HLT in patients with CHD, which now surpasses the group of patients without CHD.[72] There are several reasons for this recent increase in HLT in patients with CHD.

- Over 1,000 Fontan operations are performed each year in the United States.[73]
- With improved surgical techniques, perioperative care, and long-term outpatient management, these patients are living into adulthood, though in a chronic state of compensated heart failure.[74]
- By 20 years, 21% of these patients require cardiac transplantation.[75]
- Because these ACHD are relatively younger compared to adult patients needing transplant for acquired heart disease or cardiomyopathy, they are often in better physical condition, so transplant teams are more willing to take a risk on using more than one organ in a single patient to try to extend the life of these patients with CHD.
- In addition, the 5-year survival of patients with CHD undergoing HLT is identical to patients with CHD undergoing cardiac transplantation alone (~85% [72]), making HLT in ACHD a reasonable risk with little controversy in a suitable candidate.
- Lastly, transplanting a heart with the liver confers a degree of protection from rejection for the heart.[76]

The use of VA ECMO to support patients with Fontan circulation beyond the original acute postoperative period is very challenging.

VA ECMO requires adequate capture of venous drainage to help pump output to the systemic circulation. Because the Fontan circulation is in series and does not have a typical right atrial reservoir, dual upper and lower peripheral venous cannulation may be necessary if peripheral V-A cannulation is being used.[77] In some patients with Fontan circulation, a compliance chamber such as the BetterBladder™ is necessary to compensate for the lack of a native systemic venous atrium. In the largest, retrospective series from the ELSO database, the outcome of 230 patients with Fontan circulation supported with ECMO between 1987 and 2009 was analyzed.[78] The overall survival to discharge was only 35%, and when looking at the most recent two years of data (30 patients), only 36% survived despite advances in the practice of ECMO. In the largest single center study that included 20 patients from 1984 to 2002, 50% of the patients survived to discharge, although only 5 patients (25%) were alive at a median follow up of 35 months.[79]

Given our current experience with supporting patients with Fontan circulation with ECLS, the limited availability of organs, and the length of time for organs to become available, ECLS as a bridge to a combined HLT or HLKT does not appear to be a prudent approach with a predictably favorable outcome. Instead, VA ECMO may serve a role as a very temporary bridge to a durable VAD if a VAD is not immediately available or feasible. Experience with mechanical circulatory support of patients with Fontan physiology with successful HLT or HLKT at the time of writing is extremely limited and not reported in the literature. Based on current evidence, Fontan HLT or HLKT should be limited to high volume centers that can optimize the selection of patients, preferably without the need for ECLS, and have the capability to provide mechanical circulatory support in the perioperative setting if necessary. Nevertheless, as these techniques evolve and improve, it is highly likely that indications will expand.

## The Future of ECLS in ACHD

It is likely that the growing population of complex ACHD will stimulate increasing use of ECLS for perioperative support; intercurrent illnesses; and bridge to decision, device, or transplantation. Gene therapy,[80] stem cell treatments,[81] use of non-heart beating organ donors,[82] and transgenic porcine heart transplantation[83] will all require patients with endstage disease to have physiologic support while awaiting definitive treatment. ECLS will remain one of the central pillars of this support. Technological improvements in circuit design with improvements in surface coating and more intelligent servo regulation may make ECLS support for ACHD safer, easier, and less labor intensive. As such, ECLS is becoming an increasingly used tool rather than an extraordinary last-ditch measure.

## Summary

ACHD represent a highly challenging cohort of patients. Supporting ACHD with ECLS involves multiple unique challenges but also saves many lives. Many of the techniques available to support ACHD with ECLS in the current era were simply unavailable 20 years ago. As the art and science of ECLS evolves, it is likely that many new techniques will evolve over the next decade and that these techniques will save more lives.

# References

1. Dearani JA, Mavroudis C, Quintessenza J, et al. Surgical advances in the treatment of adults with congenital heart disease. Curr Opin Pediatr. 2009 Oct;21(5):565-72.

2. Jacobs JP, Mavroudis C, Quintessenza JA, et al. Reoperations for Pediatric and Congenital Heart Disease: An Analysis of the Society of Thoracic Surgeons (STS) Congenital Heart Surgery Database. Semin Thorac Cardiovasc Surg Pediatr Card Surg Annu. 2014;17(1):2-8.

3. Marelli AJ, Ionescu-Ittu R, Mackie AS, et al. Lifetime prevalence of congenital heart disease in the general population from 2000 to 2010. Circulation. 2014;130:749-56.

4. Warnes CA, et al. Task force 1: the changing profile of congenital heart disease in adult life. J Am Coll Cardiol, 2001. 37(5): p. 1170-5.

5. Hoffmann A, et al. Cerebrovascular accidents in adult patients with congenital heart disease. Heart, 2010. 96(15): p. 1223-6.

6. Burchill LJ, et al. Hospitalization Trends and Health Resource Use for Adult Congenital Heart Disease-Related Heart Failure. J Am Heart Assoc, 2018. 7(15): p. e008775.

7. Zomer AC, et al. Surgery in adults with congenital heart disease. Circulation, 2011. 124(20): p. 2195-201.

8. Cusimano RJ, Guest C. Coronary artery disease following repair of tetralogy of Fallot: implications and management. Can J Cardiol, 1996. 12(2): p. 172-4.

9. Fuller SM, et al. Estimating Mortality Risk for Adult Congenital Heart Surgery: An Analysis of The Society of Thoracic Surgeons Congenital Heart Surgery Database. Ann Thorac Surg, 2015. 100(5): p. 1728-35; discussion 1735-6.

10. Yuriy Stukov, Jeffery P Jacobs, Jessica Cornman. Repeated extracorporeal membrane oxygenation for support of an adult with congenital heart disease and reperfusion pulmonary oedema. Cardiol Young. 2022 Apr 25:1-5.

11. Heiss KF, Bartlett RH. Extracorporeal membrane oxygenation: an experimental protocol becomes a clinical service. Adv Pediatr. 1989;36:117-35.

12. Bayrakci B, Josephson C, Fackler J. Oxygenation index for extracorporeal membrane oxygenation: is there predictive significance? J Artif Organs. 2007;10(1):6-9.

13. O'Rourke PP, Crone RK, Vacanti JP, et al. Extracorporeal membrane oxygenation and conventional medical therapy in neonates with persistent pulmonary hypertension of the newborn: a prospective randomized study. Pediatrics. Dec 1989;84(6):957-63.

14. Fletcher K, Chapman R, Keene S. An overview of medical ECMO for neonates. Semin Perinatol. Mar 2018;42(2):68-79.

15. Dechert RE, Park PK, Bartlett RH. Evaluation of the oxygenation index in adult respiratory failure. J Trauma Acute Care Surg. Feb 2014;76(2):469-73.

16. Murray JF, Matthay MA, Luce JM, et al. An expanded definition of the adult respiratory distress syndrome. Am Rev Respir Dis. Sep 1988;138(3):720-3.

17. Peek GJ, Mugford M, Tiruvoipati R, et al. Efficacy and economic assessment of conventional ventilatory support versus extracorporeal membrane oxygenation for severe adult respiratory failure (CESAR): a multicentre randomised controlled trial. Lancet. Oct 17 2009;374(9698):1351-63.

18. Villar J, Ambrós A, Soler JA, et al. Age, PaO2/FIO2, and Plateau Pressure Score: A Proposal for a Simple Outcome Score in Patients With the Acute Respiratory Distress Syndrome. Crit Care Med. Jul 2016;44(7):1361-9.

19. Horovitz JH, Carrico CJ, Shires GT. Pulmonary response to major injury. Arch Surg. Mar 1974;108(3):349-55.

20. Ranieri VM, Rubenfeld GD, Thompson BT, et al. Acute respiratory distress syndrome: the Berlin Definition. JAMA. Jun 20 2012;307(23):2526-33.

21. Schmidt M, Burrell A, Roberts L, et al. Predicting survival after ECMO for refractory cardiogenic shock: the survival after veno-arterial-ECMO (SAVE)-score. Eur Heart J. Sep 01 2015;36(33):2246-56.

22. Muller G, Flecher E, Lebreton G, et al. The ENCOURAGE mortality risk score and analysis of long-term outcomes after VA-ECMO for acute myocardial infarction with cardiogenic shock. Intensive Care Med. Mar 2016;42(3):370-378.

23. Wengenmayer T, Duerschmied D, Graf E, et al. Development and validation of a prognostic model for survival in patients treated with venoarterial extracorporeal membrane oxygenation: the PREDICT VA-ECMO score. Eur Heart J Acute Cardiovasc Care. Jun 2019;8(4):350-359.

24. Hill JD, O'Brien TG, Murray JJ, et al. Prolonged extracorporeal oxygenation for acute post-traumatic respiratory failure (shock-lung syndrome). Use of the Bramson membrane lung. N Engl J Med. Mar 23 1972;286(12):629-34.

25. Bartlett RH. Esperanza. Presidential address. Trans Am Soc Artif Intern Organs. 1985;31:723-6.

26. Zapol WM, Snider MT, Hill JD, et al. Extracorporeal membrane oxygenation in severe acute respiratory failure. A randomized prospective study. JAMA. Nov 16 1979;242(20):2193-6.

27. Wolfson PJ. The development and use of extracorporeal membrane oxygenation in neonates. Ann Thorac Surg. Dec 2003;76(6):S2224-9.

28. Bartlett RH, Gazzaniga AB, Toomasian J, et al. Extracorporeal membrane oxygenation (ECMO) in neonatal respiratory failure. 100 cases. Ann Surg. Sep 1986;204(3):236-45.

29. Bartlett RH, Roloff DW, Cornell RG, et al. Extracorporeal circulation in neonatal respiratory failure: a prospective randomized study. Pediatrics. Oct 1985;76(4):479-87.

30. Zelen M. The randomization and stratification of patients to clinical trials. J Chronic Dis. Sep 1974;27(7-8):365-75.

31. UK collaborative randomised trial of neonatal extracorporeal membrane oxygenation. UK Collaborative ECMO Trail Group. Lancet. Jul 13 1996;348(9020):75-82.

32. Combes A, Hajage D, Capellier G, et al; EOLIA Trial Group, REVA, and ECMONet. Extracorporeal Membrane Oxygenation for Severe Acute Respiratory Distress Syndrome. N Engl J Med. 2018 May 24;378(21):1965-1975.

33. Combes A, Peek GJ, Hajage D, et al. ECMO for severe ARDS: systematic review and individual patient data meta-analysis. Intensive Care Med. 2020 Nov;46(11):2048-2057.

34. Coronavirus COVID-19 Global Cases by the Center for Systems Science and Engineering (CSSE). Accessed December 31, 2021. https://coronavirus.jhu.edu/map.html.

35. Yang X, Yu Y, Xu J, et al. Clinical course and outcomes of critically ill patients with SARS-CoV-2 pneumonia in Wuhan, China: a single-centered, retrospective, observational study. Lancet Respir Med. 05 2020;8(5):475-481.

36. Jacobs JP, Stammers AH, St Louis J, et al. Extracorporeal Membrane Oxygenation in the Treatment of Severe Pulmonary and Cardiac Compromise in Coronavirus Disease 2019: Experience with 32 Patients. ASAIO J. 2020 Jul;66(7):722-730.

37. Jacobs JP, Stammers AH, St Louis J, et al. Multi-institutional Analysis of 100 Consecutive Patients with COVID-19 and Severe Pulmonary Compromise Treated with Extracorporeal Membrane Oxygenation: Outcomes and Trends Over Time. ASAIO J. 2021 May 1;67(5):496-502.

38. Stammers AH, Mongero LB, Tesdahl EA, et al. The assessment of patients undergoing cardiac surgery for Covid-19: Complications occuring during cardiopulmonary bypass. Perfusion. 2022 May;37(4):350-358.

39. Jacobs JP, Stammers AH, St Louis JD, et al. Multi-institutional Analysis of 200 COVID-19 Patients treated with ECMO: Outcomes and Trends. Ann Thorac Surg. 2022 May;113(5):1452-1460.

40. Zaaqoq AM, Barnett AG, Griffee MJ, et al; COVID-19 Critical Care Consortium (COVID Critical). Beneficial Effect of Prone Positioning During Venovenous Extracorporeal Membrane Oxygenation for Coronavirus Disease 2019. Crit Care Med. 2022 Feb 1;50(2):275-285.

41. Barbaro RP, MacLaren G, Boonstra PS, et al; Extracorporeal Life Support Organization. Extracorporeal membrane oxygenation for COVID-19: evolving outcomes from the international Extracorporeal Life Support Organization Registry. Lancet. 2021 Oct 2;398(10307):1230-1238.

42. Mongero LB, Stammers AH, Tesdahl EA, et al. The Use of Extracorporeal Membrane Oxygenation in COVID-19 Patients with Severe Cardiorespiratory Failure: The Influence of Obesity on Outcomes. J Extra Corpor Technol. 2021 Dec;53(4):293-298.

43. Javidfar J, Zaaqoq AM, Yamashita MH, et al. Venovenous extracorporeal membrane oxygenation in obese patients. JJTCVS Tech. 2021 Dec;10:335-348.

44. Celeste A. Hall, Jeffrey P. Jacobs, MD, Alfred H. Stammers, MSA, et al. Multi-institutional Analysis of 505 COVID-19 Patients supported with ECMO: Predictors of Survival. Ann Thorac Surg. 2022 Jul;114(1):61-68.

45. Rosenzweig EB, Brodie D, Abrams DC, et al. Extracorporeal membrane oxygenation as a novel bridging strategy for acute right heart failure in group 1 pulmonary arterial hypertension. ASAIO J. 2014 Jan-Feb;60(1):129-33.

46. Briston DA, Bradley EA, Sabanayagam A, et al. Health Care Costs for Adults With Congenital Heart Disease in the United States 2002 to 2012. Am J Cardiol. 2016;118:590-6.

47. Ross HJ, Law Y, Book WM, et al, American Heart Association Adults With Congenital Heart Disease Committee of the Council on Clinical C, Council on Cardiovascular Disease in the Young tCoCR, Intervention, the Council on Functional G and Translational B. Transplantation and Mechanical Circulatory Support in Congenital Heart Disease: A Scientific Statement From the American Heart Association. Circulation. 2016;133:802-20.

48. Belohlavek J, Rohn V, Jansa P, et al. Veno-arterial ECMO in severe acute right ventricular failure with pulmonary obstructive hemodynamic pattern. J Invasive Cardiol. 2010;22:365-9.

49. Turbendian HK, Gebhardt J, Scherkenbach P, et al. A novel approach to delivery of extracorporeal support using a modified continuous flow ventricular assist device in a mid-volume congenital heart program. Artif Organs. 2021;45:55-62.

50. Dimopoulos K, Diller GP, Koltsida E, et al. Prevalence, predictors, and prognostic value of renal

dysfunction in adults with congenital heart disease. Circulation. 2008;117:2320-8.

51. Goldstein SA, Goldstein LB. Neurologic complications of congenital heart disease in adults. Handb Clin Neurol. 2021;177:15-22.

52. Goldstein SA, Krasuski RA. Pulmonary Hypertension in Adults with Congenital Heart Disease. Cardiol Clin. 2022;40:55-67.

53. Konno R, Tatebe S, Sugimura K, et al. Prognostic value of the model for end-stage liver disease excluding INR score (MELD-XI) in patients with adult congenital heart disease. PLoS One. 2019;14:e0225403.

54. Dolgner SJ, Krieger EV, Wilkes J, et al. Predictors of extracorporeal membrane oxygenation support after surgery for adult congenital heart disease in children's hospitals. Congenit Heart Dis. 2019;14:559-570.

55. Dolgner SJ, Nguyen VP, Krieger EV, et al. Long-term adult congenital heart disease survival after heart transplantation: A restricted mean survival time analysis. J Heart Lung Transplant. 2021;40:698-706.

56. Jacobs JP, Quintessenza JA, Boucek RJ, et al. Pediatric Cardiac Transplantation in Children with High Panel Reactive Antibody. Ann Thorac Surg. 2004 Nov; 78(5):1703-9.

57. Asante-Korang A, Jacobs JP, Ringewald J, et al. Management of children undergoing cardiac transplantation with high Panel Reactive Antibodies. Cardiol Young. 2011 Dec;21 Suppl 2:124-32. In: Jacobs JP, DeCampli, WM, Cooper DS, et al (Eds). 2011 Supplement to Cardiology in the Young: Annual Heart Week in Florida Supplement Number 9 - Hypoplastic Left Heart Syndrome And Other Challenges Related To Pediatric And Congenital Cardiac Disease: An Interdisciplinary Approach. Cardiology in the Young. 2011 Dec; 21(Suppl 2):1–176.

58. Bleiweis MS, Fricker FJ, Peek GJ, et al. An analysis of 183 Heart Transplants for Pediatric or Congenital Heart Disease: The Impact of High Panel-Reactive Antibody. The Annals of Thoracic Surgery. In Review.

59. Fraser CD, Jaquiss RD, Rosenthal DN, et al. Prospective trial of a pediatric ventricular assist device. New Engl J Med 2012; 367:532-41.

60. Das BB, Kogon B, Deshpande SR, et al. Contemporary outcomes of durable ventricular assist devices in adults with congenital heart disease as a bridge to heart transplantation. Artif Organs 2022 Apr;46(4):697-704.

61. Edelson JB, Huang Y, Griffis H, et al. The influence of mechanical circulatory support on post-transplant outcomes in pediatric patients: A multicenter study from the International Society for Heart and Lung Transplantation (ISHLT) Registry. J Heart Lung Transplant 2021; 40:1443-1453.

62. Shanefield SC, Knewitz D, Philip J, et al. Support with extracorporeal membrane oxygenation for over 1 year duration as a bridge to cardiac transplantation: a case report and review of the literature. Cardiol Young. 2021 Sep;31(9):1495-1497.

63. DeFilippis EM, Clerkin K, Truby LK, et al. ECMO as a bridge to left ventricular assist device or heart transplantation. JACC Heart Fail 2021; 9:281-289.

64. Fukuhara S, Takeda K, Kurlansky PA, et al. Extracorporeal membrane oxygenation as a direct bridge to heart transplantation in adults. J Thorac Cardiovasc Surg 2018; 155:1607-1618.

65. Cooper DS, Prêtre R. Clinical management of pediatric ventricular assist devices. Pediatr Crit Care Med 2013; 14:S27-36.

66. Gilboa SM, Devine OJ, Kucik JE, et al. Congenital heart defects in the United States: Estimating the magnitude of the affected population in 2020. Circulation 2016;134:101-109.

67. Pundi KN, Johnson JN, Dearani JA, et al. 40-year follow-up after the Fontan operation: long-term outcomes of 1,052 patients. J Am Coll Cardiol 2015;66:1700-1710.

68. de Leval MR. The Fontan circulation: a challenge to William Harvey? Nat Clin Pract Cardiovasc Med 2005;2:202-208.

69. Wu FM, Ukomadu C, Odze RD, et al. Liver disease in the patient with Fontan circulation. Congenit Heart Dis 2011;6:190-201.

70. Starzl TE, Bahnson HT, Hardesty Rl, et al. Heart–liver transplantation in a patient with familial hypercholesterolaemia. Lancet 1984;1:1382-1383.

71. Bryant R, Rizwan R, Safar F, et al. Contemporary outcomes of combined heart-liver transplant in patients with congenital heart disease. Transplantation 2018;102(2):e67-e73.

72. Cotter TG, Wang J, Peeraphatdit T, et al. Simultaneous heart-liver transplantation for congenital heart disease in the United States: Rapidly increasing with acceptable outcomes. Hepatology 2021;73(4):1464-1477.

73. Jacobs JP, Mayer JE Jr, Pasquali SK, et al. The Society of Thoracic Surgeons Congenital Heart Surgery Database: 2019 Update on Outcomes and Quality. Ann Thorac Surg. 2019 Mar;107(3):691-704. doi: 10.1016/j.athoracsur.2018.12.016. Epub 2019 Jan 11. PMID: 30641069.

74. Akintoye E, Miranda WR, Veldtman GR, et al. National trends in Fontan operation and in-hospital outcomes in the USA. Heart 2019;105:708-714.

75. Atz AM, Zak V, Mahony L, et al. Longitudinal outcomes of patients with single ventricle after the Fontan procedure. J Am Coll Cardiol 2017;69:2735-2744.

76. Ortega-Legaspi JM, Hoteit M, Wald J. Immune benefit of combined heart and liver transplantation. Current Opinion in Organ Transplantation 2020;25(5):513-518.

77. Bacon MK, Gray SB, Schwartz SM, et al. Extracorporeal membrane oxygenation (ECMO) support in special patient populations-The bidirectional Glenn and Fontan circulations. Frontiers in Pediatrics 2018;6:299.

78. Rood KL, Teele SA, Barrett CS, et al. Extracorporeal membrane oxygenation support after the Fontan operation. J Thor Cardiovasc Surg. (2011) 142:504–10.

79. Booth KL, Roth SJ, Thiagarajan RR, et al. Extracorporeal membrane oxygenation support of the Fontan and bidirectional Glenn circulations. Ann Thor Surgery (2004) 77:1341–8.

80. Mendell JR, Al-Zaidy SA, Rodino-Klapac LR, et al. Current Clinical Applications of In Vivo Gene Therapy with AAVs. Mol Ther. 2021 Feb 3;29(2):464-488.

81. Fisher SA, Doree C, Mathur A, et al. Stem cell therapy for chronic ischaemic heart disease and congestive heart failure. Cochrane Database Syst Rev. 2016 Dec 24;12(12):CD007888.

82. White CW, Messer SJ, Large SR, et al. Transplantation of Hearts Donated after Circulatory Death. Front Cardiovasc Med. 2018 Feb 13;5:8.

83. Xenotransplantation. The science behind the first successful pig-to-human heart transplant. The Economist. Science and Technology Edition. Pub The Economist Group, London, United Kingdom. January 15, 2022. https://www.economist.com/science-and-technology/2022/01/15/the-science-behind-the-first-successful-pig-to-human-heart-transplant. Accessed February 3, 2022.

# 32

## Extracorporeal Cardiopulmonary Resuscitation in Adult Patients

*Susanna Price, Jan Bělohlávek, Yih-Sharng Chen, Demetris Yannopoulos*

The incidence of sudden cardiac arrest is substantial, with in-hospital (IHCA) and out-of-hospital cardiac arrest (OHCA) estimated at 200 and 140 individuals per 100,000 adult multiday admission/population, respectively, and significant variation between countries, regions, and hospitals. Survival to hospital discharge after cardiac arrest is low; IHCA 6-26% and OHCA typically <10%,[1] but in well-organized systems this can be as high as 27% for OHCA.[2,3] The most important interventions that improve outcome in cardiac arrest are high-quality, uninterrupted chest compressions, and early defibrillation.[4] When an arrest proves refractory to these interventions, the chances of survival fall and extracorporeal cardiopulmonary resuscitation (ECPR) may be considered when the appropriate expertise and system infrastructure is available and established.

ECPR is the application of rapid-deployment VA ECMO to provide circulatory support in patients with cardiac arrest in whom conventional CPR (CPR) is unsuccessful in achieving sustained return of spontaneous circulation (ROSC).[5] Through a return of assisted circulation, ECPR can provide precious time for diagnosis, therapy, and recovery. ECPR is a time-sensitive, complex intervention that requires teamwork, clearly defined roles, optimal logistics, and well-trained health care providers.

Despite the lack of high-quality evidence supporting its use, the deployment of ECPR has increased for both in- and out-of-hospital cardiac in recent years (<100 in 2009 to >1500 in 2019),[5] and is recommended to be considered in specific circumstances for particular patient populations in both National and International guidelines.[6-8] This chapter will provide a summary of current evidence surrounding the use of ECPR, practical guidance regarding its implementation, and outline key areas regarding post-ECPR management.

### Evidence for ECPR

In the first published report on ECPR, eight cardiac arrest patients managed with ECPR resulted in one patient surviving to hospital discharge, neurologically intact.[9] This initial publication highlighted the requirement for readily available teams able to rapidly establish assisted circulation, and the vital role of CPR as the basis for successful resuscitation. Key areas of subsequent research include identification of which patients are most likely to benefit, timing of implementation, the site of cannulation, and how to optimize cannulation and postarrest strategies.

## Patient Selection

Optimal patient selection for ECPR remains to be determined. Protocols and guidelines suggest identifying those most likely to survive with favorable neurological outcomes and with very low chance of survival with conventional means. For each, therefore, the potential benefits must be weighed against complications (individual risk vs. benefit) and resource implications (societal risk vs. benefit).

A number of selection criteria have been published, in line with the inclusion criteria for the major randomized trials in OHCA (Table 32-1). For IHCA, the relation with initial rhythm may be less stringent, as shown in a large registry study where more than 50% of patients had an initial rhythm of PEA or asystole.[10] Indeed, PEA may have a better prognosis during IHCA than OHCA because many events occur in monitored areas, with immediate high-quality CPR, and the possibility of pseudo-PEA (reflecting merely profound hypotension/low cardiac output state rather than cardiac arrest with electromechanical dissociation). Since

ECPR can only act as a bridge to recovery or longer-term therapy, patients with potentially reversible etiologies should be targeted. These may include acute myocardial infarction, tachyarrhythmias, pulmonary embolism, deep hypothermia, myocarditis, and drug toxicity.

A risk score (RESCUE-IHCA) has been published intended to predict hospital mortality for adult ECPR in IHCA. Here, preexisting patient characteristics (patient type, presenting rhythm, time of day, age, and renal insufficiency) together with the potentially modifiable event characteristic (duration of arrest) demonstrated a score performance of 72% prediction ability (external validation 68% prediction ability).

## Timing of ECPR Initiation

Central to ECPR stands the definition of a refractory arrest. However, definitions differ (ranging between 10-60 mins) within the literature. Numerous studies have demonstrated that survival declines after 10 minutes of CPR without ROSC, and in these patients ECPR may be beneficial, even if overall resuscitation times

| EXAMPLE OF INCLUSION CRITERIA FOR ECPR |
|---|
| Age <70 years |
| Witnessed arrest |
| Arrest to first CPR ("no-flow interval") <5 minutes (ie, bystander CPR) |
| Initial cardiac rhythm of VF/pVT/PEA |
| Arrest to ECMO flow <60 minutes "low flow interval"* |
| ETCO$_2$ >10 mmHg (1.3 kPA) during CPR before annulation for ECMO |
| Intermittent ROSC or recurrent VF |
| "Signs of Life" during conventional CPR may be a positive predictive factor for survival |
| The absence of previously known life limiting comorbidities (eg, endstage heart failure/chronic obstructive pulmonary disease/endstage renal failure/liver failure/terminal illness) and consistent with patient's goals of care |
| No known aortic valve incompetence (>mild aortic valve incompetence should be excluded) |
| *Unless other favorable prognostic features are present: eg, periods of intermittent ROSC/hypothermia prearrest/young age/signs of life during CPR. CPR=cardiopulmonary resuscitation; ECMO=extracorporeal membrane oxygenation; ECPR=extracorporeal cardiopulmonary resuscitation; ROSC=return of spontaneous circulation. |

**Table 32-1.** Inclusion criteria of three randomized trials on ECPR in OHCA.[5]

are prolonged.[12,15] Prolonged CPR in patients who undergo ECPR is, however, consistently associated with worse outcomes and thus 10-20 minutes of CPR without ROSC is often quoted as the point where ECPR should be considered.[2,16,17] As rapidity of establishing ECPR is a main determent of survival[6]; based on available evidence the goal is to implement ECPR on average within 60 minutes and ideally within 45 minutes of the cardiac arrest. It appears that after 30 minutes of CPR, every additional minute without ECPR initiation adds ~2-2.5% mortality rate.

**Outcomes in ECPR**

There is little high-quality data supporting the use of ECPR in IHCA, and emerging data regarding its use in OHCA. Key studies in ECPR are summarized in Table 32-2.

*IHCA*

There are currently no randomized controlled trials addressing ECPR in the in-hospital setting. Single-center, retrospective, and observational studies showing ECPR in IHCA is feasible and may improve outcomes. A study by Chen and colleagues reported almost a third of 135 patients with neurological successful outcome with an average of 55.7 (+/-27 min) of CPR before ECMO initiation.[6]

Time-to-ECMO was directly related to survival. Two propensity matched studies and a meta-analysis provide further observational evidence to the potential of ECPR in IHCA.[14,18]

*OHCA*

There are currently two published randomized trials on ECPR in OHCA with mixed results. The ARREST trial was a Phase 2, single-center open label RCT where patients with a shockable rhythm were randomized on hospital arrival to CPR vs. ECPR. The trial was stopped early due to protocol based prespecified superiority criteria after enrollment of 30 patients.[11] It demonstrated a significantly higher survival to discharge in the ECPR group (43% vs. 7%, HR 0.16 [CI 0.06-0.41]). The second trial randomized adults with witnessed refractory OHCA of presumed cardiac origin to either invasive (intra-arrest transport to a center for ECPR and invasive assessment and treatment) or a standard (continued CPR delivered on site) strategy. This trial was stopped prematurely because of futility, demonstrating a nonsignificant difference in primary outcome (6-month survival neurologically intact 31.5% (ECPR) vs. 22% (CPR), p=0.09).[12] The study also showed that 6- month survival was statistically superior with ECPR. The Prague trial, similar to the ARREST trial, provided further evidence that for prolonged duration

| | ARREST[11] | PRAGUE[12] | INCEPTION[13] |
|---|---|---|---|
| **Age** | 18-75 years | 18-65 years | 18-70 years |
| **Initial rhythm** | VF/pVT[1] | Witnessed, presumed cardiac etiology | Witnessed, VF/pVT, bystander CPR |
| **Resuscitation** | No ROSC after 3 shocks | >5 min ALS[2] | No ROSC after 3 rounds of ALS CPR[2] |
| **Timing** | Transfer time to ED <30min | | Arrival ED <50 min of arrest |
| [1]pulseless ventricular tachycardia. [2]Advanced Life Support (ie, ambulance protocol) | | | |

**Table 32-2.** Key studies in ECPR.

of resuscitation, ECPR may improve survival compared to standard CPR. In the subgroup with neurologically intact survival after CPR duration >45 min, 24/26 patients had received ECPR, including 4 crossovers from the standard therapy arm, indicating that there may still be benefit from ECPR despite prolonged resuscitation in certain patient populations.

## Practicalities and Techniques

Current international guidelines offer a weak recommendation for ECPR as a rescue strategy for select patients with cardiac arrest of a potentially reversible etiology in whom CPR is failing, undertaken within established, highly functioning systems of care.[19-22]

### *Initiation of ECPR*

**Who:** There are no absolute inclusion/exclusion criteria for patients to be considered for ECPR; however, based on current evidence, examples of inclusion criteria are shown in Table 32-1. In IHCA, established scores may be used to attempt to predict in-hospital death, but each case should be considered on an individual basis.[14] Patients with shockable presenting rhythms (reflective of a high prevalence of coronary artery disease) between 18-75 years old, who have had intermittent ROSC and can be supported within 60 minutes from their initial arrest, should be strongly considered in capable and organized systems.

**When:** Considering initiation of ECPR, there are time-lags inherent in all systems of care, each of which must be minimized for optimal outcomes within organised systems of care. These include:

- cardiac arrest → CPR (no flow),
- CPR start → ECPR decision,
- CPR start → ECPR initiation (low flow),
- ECPR decision to return of assisted circulation with VA support,
- ECMO.

Assessment for ECPR candidacy should occur early, with current recommendations suggesting cannulation be considered in suitable patients after 10-20 mins of failed resuscitation, aiming to establish adequate ECMO flow at least within 60 mins of cardiac arrest onset and to minimise the low flow duration once the decision is made to initiate ECMO.[5]

**Where:** The optimal place to initiate ECPR has not yet been determined. In OHCA, data does not demonstrate superiority or inferiority of prehospital ECPR vs. transportation under CPR to an ECPR center. Within hospitals, successful practice has been demonstrated in the emergency department, the cardiac catheterization laboratory, and the intensive care unit. The optimal location will depend on local infrastructure, staffing, and logistical considerations. A preprimed circuit is a significant asset in achieving fast on pump times and should be considered within a system. Availability of fluoroscopy and/or echocardiography may facilitate faster and more precise cannulation (Chapter 4).

**By whom:** Whether for IHCA or OHCA, ECPR will be provided by a trained multidisciplinary ECMO team with 24/7 coverage, and delivered withing a highly functioning specialist unit.[9,23-25] Successful cannulation for ECPR has been demonstrated in numerous different models, including by cardiovascular surgeons, emergency department clinicians, intensivists, and trained ECPR cardiologists.[26,27] Mobile teams consisting of highly trained resuscitation physicians and paramedics that serve a larger population in multiple health care systems have been successfully deployed in Minneapolis and Paris.[28]

**How:** The aim is to minimize both low-flow time and complications related to cannulation. Percutaneous peripheral cannulation is the most frequently used approach (except immediately postcardiotomy). After determining suitability for ECPR, the next preparatory steps include identification of the code leader (not engaged in the cannulation process, but providing oversight of the parallel ongoing CPR and preparation and initiation of ECPR), undertaking a team brief (determining all essential equipment and team members are immediately available), ensuring the circuit is primed and ready, that the femoral vessels are adequately visualized using ultrasound, and the patient is draped in a sterile fashion. Key stages to consider include the following.

**External cardiac massage** must continue throughout cannulation, potentially assisted by use of an automated mechanical compression device, taking care to avoid device migration towards the abdomen or the upper chest.[29] Throughout cannulation, pauses in chest compressions must be kept to a minimum. CPR should be continued as defined by the code leader and according to standard ACLS protocols. The only modifications to ACLS include: 1) in the event of refractory VT/VF, defibrillation attempts are temporarily suspended during guidewire insertion until established on VA ECMO support, and 2) discontinuing adrenaline boluses when the circuit is being connected to the cannulas (to avoid inadvertent hypertension).

**Choice of cannula size** should be determined by the vessel size and flow required (generally arterial 15-17 Fr and venous 25-27 Fr multistage, although a single-stage drainage cannula is acceptable).[30] In larger males, a 17-19 Fr arterial return cannula may be used.

**Cannulation** is most usually via the common femoral artery and vein using a modified Seldinger technique.[31-33] As unsuccessful cannulation is potentially fatal, cannulators must be meticulous in their approach, ensuring: 1) Identification of the target vessels for cannulation. This is determined by vessel size and operator(s) and may be unilateral or bilateral. Unilateral cannulation can help localization of the second vessel to be found and punctured for guidewire insertion; 2) Imaging

the vessels in real-time during cannulation. US guidance is highly recommended to avoid multiple punctures and vascular complications. Fluoroscopy with angiography can also be useful, facilitating guidewire insertion, followed by cannulation using the angiography introducer. Aim at the common femoral artery above the bifurcation. Visualization of venous and arterial guidewires (ultrasound, transthoracic/transesophageal echo/fluoroscopy) to confirm correct cannulation is very important and avoid liver lacerations or perforations. Verify freedom of the wire tip to assure proper placement of the cannulas intravascularly. Aim the venous cannula at mid right atrial position. Flushing the first cannula with heparinized saline (or intermittently backflushed) to prevent clot formation. In the event of pulmonary embolism, ultrasound visualisation is mandatory to avoid inadvertent cannulation of a thrombosed vein.

*Please see www.elso.org for two videos of cannulation for ECPR to show steps needed for cannulation. Videos provided by D. Yannopoulus.*

**Connection of circuit and cannulas**: Despite time pressures, as with every VA ECMO initiation, all air should be purged during connection and final checks should be undertaken to avoid risk of embolization. RPMs are gradually increased to generate adequate positive pressure in the return limb of the circuit. Finally, clamps are removed to ensure antegrade ECMO flow, at which stage mechanical chest compressions can be discontinued. The code leader should anticipate that vasopressor/inotrope infusions may need to be rapidly weaned to avoid hypertension. A heparin bolus can be given as soon as the system is connected and adjusted accordingly per institutional protocols. This may be omitted in hypothermic or near-drowning victims because of the risk of hemorrhage. Many patients initially develop vasoplegia and require 2-3 vasopressors and large intravenous volume resuscitation. Consider progressive correction of acid base balance and regulate pressors to maintain a mean arterial pressure of >60-65 mmHg.

Cardioversion is not emergent after ECLS initiation and waiting for a few minutes to establish perfusion seems to lead to more successful and sustained organized cardiac rhythm.

The patient will require a right radial arterial pressure line to assess right innominate arterial saturation and oxygen content as cardiac function recovers, and a distal perfusion catheter inserted in the superficial femoral artery to avoid leg ischemia and necrosis. NIRS may also be useful to monitor for this complication. An intraaortic balloon pump, intravenous cooling catheters, or other supporting devices can be considered based on local practices.

## Immediate Steps Post-initiation of VA ECMO

Key steps in immediate postarrest management that are specific (or particularly key) in ECPR are shown in Table 32-3. Where femoral cannulation has been used and a distal perfusion cannula has not already been positioned, this should be undertaken (ideally within 4 hours) to reduce the risk of limb ischemia.[34]

## Post-resuscitation Care

Key to successful management of a patient with cardiac arrest (once resuscitated) is reversal of any potential underlying cause. In particular, as studies using protocolized catheterisation post-ECPR initiation demonstrated increased

| ISSUE | ACTION | NOTES |
|---|---|---|
| **Access cannula** | • Confirm position (echo and/or fluoroscopy)<br>• Secure<br>• Dress | • Drainage cannula tip in RA (SVC-RA junction) |
| **Mean arterial pressure** | • Measure right-upper limb arterial line<br>• Although no optimal MAP demonstrated, aim 60-80 mmHg | • May need to rapidly down-titrate/hold pressors/inotropes |
| **PaO₂** | • Measure from right-sided arterial line | • Avoid hyperoxia if possible<br>• If hypoxemia, consider differential hypoxia |
| **Arterial blood gases** | • Titrate sweep gas flow & mechanical ventilation if ROSC has occurred | • Aim to avoid hypocarbia |
| **Ensure adequate drainage & flows** | • If drainage insufficiency despite appropriate placement, consider fluids/transfusion | • If flow (VA + native) excessive, may consider reducing VA-ECMO flow |
| **Cardiac pathology/LV decompression** | • Echocardiography<br>• 12-lead ECG | • Comprehensive study by experienced imager<br>• ? failure of LV decompression |
| **General measures** | • ETT placement & end-tidal CO₂<br>• Establish central access (if not already<br>• Review sedation/analgesia<br>• CXR | • To assess native cardiopulmonary circulation |
| **Formal laboratory investigations** | • Standard post-arrest including cardiac biomarkers | • Anticoagulation profile/targets must consider increased bleeding risk post-arrest +/- PCI[35,36] |

**Table 32-3.** CPR-specific immediate postarrest management (minutes).

survival, emergent coronary angiography should be undertaken for all ECPR patients without an obvious noncardiac cause, independent of age and presenting rhythm. Other potentially reversible cardiac causes for cardiac arrest should be addressed according to standard international guidelines. Further ECPR-specific post-resuscitation care after initial stabilisation includes that of standard post-arrest management. Additional key considerations are shown in Table 32-4.

Where the cause of cardiac arrest is unclear, additional investigations may include CT brain, abdomen/pelvis, and CT pulmonary angiography.

## Ongoing Management

Further management will be as with any patient receiving VA ECMO and in the postarrest, critical care setting, with a typical VA run of 3-4 days (Chapter 28).[37] Similarly, patients who survive ECPR neurologically intact, but fail to recover sufficient cardiac function to be successfully weaned from VA ECMO should be discussed early with a referral centre with transplant and durable VAD capability as soon as this situation becomes apparent. The prevalence of brainstem death is significantly higher in patients undergoing ECPR vs. CPR, but without significant differences in rates of organ donation.[38] A number of challenges exist around decisionmaking in these patients, including timing of withdrawal, and mechanisms by which brainstem death may be declared. The protocols around withdrawal of life-sustaining therapies and brainstem death testing are, however, the same as any patient receiving VA ECMO.

## Additional Organizational Considerations

Provision of ECPR is highly resource-intensive, and depends upon coordination of a trained multidisciplinary team working within an appropriate organisational infrastructure in a service that is experienced in ECMO provision.[5,39] Prehospital EMS/ECPR team/hospital communications, operational pathways, cost, and outcomes sharing are of fundamental importance for a successful program.[28] A successful program should include rigorous training, quality improvement, and governance, ideally with all patients either part of a formal clinical trial or registry. A number of factors are mandatory to ensure optimal outcomes (Table 32-5).

## Conclusion

ECPR offers the promise of improving rates of survival after cardiac arrest with functional and neurological recovery. Sufficient data exist to support initiation as an extension to CPR in select individuals, with reversible aetiology, minimal (no) no-flow time, and minimal low-flow time. Emerging data support the potential use of ECPR in selected cases with OHCA as part of a healthcare system where ECPR is part of a highly functioning system (ie, high-volume with trained teams and established coordination between systems of care). Although there are ethical challenges—in particular, considering individual vs. societal benefit and avoidance of futility—ongoing trials will determine optimal patient selection and management in the future, with the potential to transform outcomes in selected individuals.

| ISSUE | ACTION | NOTES |
|---|---|---|
| **Identification of underlying cause** | • Coronary angiography unless obvious non-cardiac cause<br>• CT-PA<br>• Comprehensive echocardiography<br>• Repeat ECGs | • Irrespective of age or presenting rhythm<br>• Will need appropriate phasing to ensure adequate PA opacification |
| **Circuit flow instability** | • Search for potential blood loss or ECMO-driven LV distension | • Cardiac tamponade, intra-abdominal and thoracic hemorrhage should be excluded |
| **Restoration of potentially perfusing rhythm** | • Refractory arrhythmia: consider further attempts of electrical cardioversion aiming to restore sinus rhythm as soon as possible | • If unsuccessful:<br>  o Consider potential causes (ie, coronary ischaemia)<br>  o Correct arterial blood gas abnormalities & all other potentially precipitating factors |
| **LV distension/no pulsatility** | • Consider LV venting | • Options:<br>  o IABP, direct LV vent, Impella, atrial septostomy |
| **Post-arrest pulmonary oedema** | • Exclude LV distension<br>• Ensure adequate PEEP | • Aiming to avoid hypocarbia |
| **Avoid hyperoxia** | • Carefully blend ECMO gas flow with air and oxygen mix targeting patient arterial oxygen saturation 92-97% | • Hyperoxia may be associated with worse neurological outcome, including in the ECPR population |
| **Targeted temperature management** | • Accurately achieved using heat exchanger<br>• Aim 33-36 for first 24h, then gradually rewarm to 37C | • Recommendations extrapolated from non-ECPR patient populations |
| **Limb ischemia** | • If not already done, insert distal perfusion cannula on side of femoral arterial cannulation | • Should be undertaken within 4h of cannulation but should not delay cardiac reperfusion/other urgent diagnostic imaging/interventions |
| **Brain structure/function** | • CT brain<br>• Neuro-care bundle implementation<br>• Neuroprognostication aligned with CPR practices | • Neuro-care bundles used in addition to standard post-CPR multimodality neuroprognostication[8] |
| **Ensuring adequate monitoring** | • Initiate cerebral and peripheral tissue NIRS | • Repeated measurement of surrogates of end-organ perfusion and repeated echocardiography may be needed in initial hours post-ECPR |

**Table 32-4.** CPR-specific early postarrest management (within hours).

| ISSUE | COMMENTS |
|---|---|
| Program development | • Should be part of an established ECMO programme<br>• Multidisciplinary & multiprofessional engagement mandatory<br>• Eligibility criteria should be clear and reproducible<br>• In-house ECPR protocols must be robust, and agreed through the hospital governance processes<br>• ECPR for OHCA provides a significant logistical obstacle: integrated prehospital protocols (including patient identification, timely transport with high-quality CPR) are key, and should be integrated into ongoing training and education processes |
| Training and education | • Regular individual, system and team-based simulation recommended |
| Quality Improvement | • Data monitoring, audit and quality improvement strategies should be embedded in the programme<br>• Quality of care & outcome metrics should be measured, reported and reviewed regularly<br>• Case reviews should be undertaken for every case |
| Governance | • Every ECPR programme should have a robust governance process<br>• Ideally every patient should be part of an ongoing clinical trial and/or registry to allow for benchmarking and optimise research opportunities |

**Table 32-5.** Key factors for ECPR program logistics.[5]

# References

1. Tsao CW, Aday AW, Almarzooq ZI, et al. Heart Disease and Stroke Statistics-2022 Update: A Report From the American Heart Association. Circulation 2022;145:e153–639.
2. Bartos JA, Grunau B, Carlson C, et al. Improved Survival with Extracorporeal Cardiopulmonary Resuscitation Despite Progressive Metabolic Derangement Associated with Prolonged Resuscitation. Circulation 2020:119.042173.
3. Mørk SR, Bøtker MT, Christensen S,. Survival and neurological outcome after out-of-hospital cardiac arrest treated with and without mechanical circulatory support. Resusc Plus 2022;10:100230.
4. Reynolds JC, Grunau BE, Rittenberger JC, et al. Association Between Duration of Resuscitation and Favorable Outcome After Out-of-Hospital Cardiac Arrest: Implications for Prolonging or Terminating Resuscitation. Circulation 2016;134:2084–94.
5. Richardson ASC, Tonna JE, Nanjayya V, et al. Extracorporeal Cardiopulmonary Resuscitation in Adults. Interim Guideline Consensus Statement From the Extracorporeal Life Support Organization. ASAIO J 2021;67:221–8.
6. Olasveengen TM, Semeraro F, Ristagno G, et al. European Resuscitation Council Guidelines 2021: Basic Life Support. Resuscitation 2021;161:98–114.
7. Wyckoff MH, Singletary EM, Soar J, et al. 2021 International Consensus on Cardiopulmonary Resuscitation and Emergency Cardiovascular Care Science With Treatment Recommendations: Summary From the Basic Life Support; Advanced Life Support; Neonatal Life Support; Education, Implementation, and Teams; First Aid Task Forces; and the COVID-19 Working Group. Resuscitation 2021;169:229–311.
8. Merchant RM, Topjian AA, Panchal AR, et al. Part 1: Executive Summary: 2020 American Heart Association Guidelines for Cardiopulmonary Resuscitation and Emergency Cardiovascular Care. Circulation 2020;142:S337–57.
9. Abrams D, MacLaren G, Lorusso R, et al. Extracorporeal cardiopulmonary resuscitation in adults: evidence and implications. Intensive Care Med 2022;48:1–15.
10. Andersen LW, Østergaard JN, Antonsen S, et al. The Danish in-hospital cardiac arrest registry (DANARREST). Clin Epidemiol 2019;11:397–402.
11. Yannopoulos D, Bartos J, Raveendran G, et al. Advanced reperfusion strategies for patients with out-of-hospital cardiac arrest and refractory ventricular fibrillation (ARREST): a phase 2, single centre, open-label, randomised controlled trial. Lancet (London, England) 2020;396:1807–16.
12. Belohlavek J, Smalcova J, Rob D, et al. Effect of Intra-arrest Transport, Extracorporeal Cardiopulmonary Resuscitation, and Immediate Invasive Assessment and Treatment on Functional Neurologic Outcome in Refractory Out-of-Hospital Cardiac Arrest: A Randomized Clinical Trial. JAMA 2022;327:737–47.
13. Bol ME, Suverein MM, Lorusso R, et al. Early initiation of extracorporeal life support in refractory out-of-hospital cardiac arrest: Design and rationale of the INCEPTION trial. Am Heart J 2019;210:58–68.
14. Tonna JE, Selzman CH, Girotra S, et al. Resuscitation Using ECPR During In-Hospital Cardiac Arrest (RESCUE-IHCA) Mortality Prediction Score and External Validation. JACC Cardiovasc Interv 2022;15:237–47.
15. Koen 'T Joncke, Nathanaël T, Philippe D. A systematic review of current ECPR protocols. A step towards standardisation. Resusc Plus 2020;3:100018.
16. Kawakami S, Tahara Y, Koga H, et al. The association between time to extracorporeal cardiopulmonary resuscitation and outcome in patients with out-of-hospital cardiac arrest. Eur Hear Journal Acute Cardiovasc Care 2022;11:279–89.
17. Chen Y-S, Lin J-W, Yu H-Y, et al. Cardiopulmonary resuscitation with assisted extracorporeal life-support versus conventional cardiopulmonary resuscitation in adults with in-hospital cardiac arrest: an observational study and propensity analysis. Lancet (London, England) 2008;372:554–61.
18. Kim SJ, Kim HJ, Lee HY, et al. Comparing extracorporeal cardiopulmonary resuscitation with conventional cardiopulmonary resuscitation: A meta-analysis. Resuscitation 2016;103:106–16.
19. Panchal AR, Bartos JA, Cabañas JG, et al. Part 3: adult basic and advanced life support: 2020 American Heart Association guidelines for cardiopulmonary resuscitation and emergency cardiovascular care. Circulation 2020;142:S366–468.
20. Soar J, Böttiger BW, Carli P, et al. European resuscitation council guidelines 2021: adult advanced life support. Resuscitation 2021;161:115–51.
21. Brooks SC, Anderson ML, Bruder E, et al. Part 6: alternative techniques and ancillary devices for cardiopulmonary resuscitation: 2015 American Heart Association guidelines update for cardiopulmonary resuscitation and emergency cardiovascular care. Circulation 2015;132:S436–43.
22. Soar J, Callaway CW, Aibiki M, et al. Part 4: advanced life support: 2015 international consensus on cardiopulmonary resuscitation and emergency cardiovascular care science with treatment recommendations. Resuscitation 2015;95:e71–120.
23. Bloch A, Schai N, Friess J-O, et al. ECPR in a tertiary care hospital: Presentation of challenges on

the basis of a real case. Trends Anaesth Crit Care 2018;21:27–32.

24. Tonna J, Selzman C, Bartos J, et al. Critical care management, hospital case volume, and survival after extracorporeal cardiopulmonary resuscitation. Circulation 2020;142:A117–A117.

25. MacLaren G, Masoumi A, Brodie D. ECPR for out-of-hospital cardiac arrest: more evidence is needed. Crit Care 2020;24:1–3.

26. Yannopoulos D, Bartos JA, Martin C, et al. Minnesota Resuscitation Consortium's Advanced Perfusion and Reperfusion Cardiac Life Support Strategy for Out-of-Hospital Refractory Ventricular Fibrillation. J Am Heart Assoc 2016;5.

27. Tonna JE, Johnson NJ, Greenwood J, et al. Practice characteristics of Emergency Department extracorporeal cardiopulmonary resuscitation (eCPR) programs in the United States: The current state of the art of Emergency Department extracorporeal membrane oxygenation (ED ECMO). Resuscitation 2016;107:38–46.

28. Bartos JA, Frascone RJ, Conterato M, et al. The Minnesota mobile extracorporeal cardiopulmonary resuscitation consortium for treatment of out-of-hospital refractory ventricular fibrillation: Program description, performance, and outcomes. EClinicalMedicine 2020:100632.

29. Koster RW, Beenen LF, van der Boom EB, et al. Safety of mechanical chest compression devices AutoPulse and LUCAS in cardiac arrest: a randomized clinical trial for non-inferiority. Eur Heart J 2017;38:3006–13.

30. Burkhoff D, Sayer G, Doshi D, et al. Hemodynamics of mechanical circulatory support. J Am Coll Cardiol 2015;66:2663–74.

31. Mortensen JD. Clinical sequelae from arterial needle puncture, cannulation, and incision. Circulation 1967;35:1118–23.

32. Seidenberg B, Hurwitt ES. Retrograde femoral (Seldinger) aortography: surgical complications in 26 cases. Ann Surg 1966;163:221.

33. Colvin MP, Curran JP, Jarvis D, et al. Femoral artery pressure monitoring. Use of the Seldinger technique. Anaesthesia 1977;32:451–5.

34. Kaufeld T, Beckmann E, Ius F, et al. Risk factors for critical limb ischemia in patients undergoing femoral cannulation for venoarterial extracorporeal membrane oxygenation: Is distal limb perfusion a mandatory approach? Perfusion 2019;34:453–9.

35. Ruggeri L, Franco A, Alba AC, et al. Coagulation derangements in patients with refractory cardiac arrest treated with extracorporeal cardiopulmonary resuscitation. J Cardiothorac Vasc Anesth 2019;33:1877–82.

36. Cartwright B, Bruce HM, Kershaw G, et al. Hemostasis, coagulation and thrombin in venoarterial and venovenous extracorporeal membrane oxygenation: the HECTIC study. Sci Rep 2021;11:1–10.

37. Richardson ASC, Schmidt M, et al. ECMO Cardio-Pulmonary Resuscitation (ECPR), trends in survival from an international multicentre cohort study over 12-years. Resuscitation 2017;112:34–40.

38. Taran S, Steel A, Healey A, et al. Organ donation in patients on extracorporeal membrane oxygenation: considerations for determination of death and withdrawal of life support. Can J Anesth Can d'anesthésie 2020;67:1035–43.

39. Tonna JE, Selzman CH, Mallin MP, et al. Development and implementation of a comprehensive, multidisciplinary emergency department extracorporeal membrane oxygenation program. Ann Emerg Med 2017;70:32–40.

40. Richardson AS, Tonna J, Nanjayya V, et al. Extracorporeal cardiopulmonary resuscitation in adults. Interim guideline consensus statement from the Extracorporeal Life Support Organization. ASAIO J 2021; 67:221-228.

# 33

## Complications, Followup, and Outcomes of Adults with Cardiac Failure

*Hannah Rando, Sung-Min Cho, Daniele Camboni, Michael Mazzeffi*

### Introduction

VA ECMO is used to support adults with cardiogenic shock from multiple etiologies including myocardial infarction, massive pulmonary embolism, drug overdose, poisoning, electrical storm, rejection after heart transplantation, and postcardiotomy shock following cardiopulmonary bypass (CBP). VA ECMO is also used for ECPR for patients with refractory cardiac arrest. Although venovenoarterial (VVA) ECMO is sometimes used in the management of adult patients with combined cardiac and respiratory failure, our principal focus will be on VA ECMO and its associated complications.

### Complications of VA ECMO for Cardiac Failure

Despite recent advances in ECMO care, the frequency of complications for VA ECMO remains high, with up to 60% of all VA ECMO patients experiencing an adverse event during their treatment.[1] Complications associated with ECMO cannulation itself are discussed in Chapter 4, but here we will use a system-based approach to discuss the most common major complications that occur during VA ECMO support.

### Neurologic

Neurologic complication represents one of the most severe complications for adult VA ECMO patients. In a cohort study performed by Hou et al. in 2021, approximately 21% of VA ECMO patients experienced a neurologic complication, including ischemic stroke, intracranial hemorrhage (ICH), differential hypoxemia (previously referred to as North South syndrome or Harlequin syndrome), or brain death.[2] The true incidence of neurologic complications is likely underestimated, however, because of the lack of standardized neuromonitoring and difficulty obtaining neuroimaging in critically ill VA ECMO patients. An autopsy study performed by Rastan et al. demonstrated a 30% rate of undiagnosed thromboembolic events, reinforcing discrepancies between clinical and postmortem neurologic injury.[3] A similar study performed by Cho et al. demonstrated acute brain injury in 68% of ECMO patients, with the most common acute brain injury being hypoxic-ischemic brain injury (44%) followed by ICH and ischemic infarct.[4]

For this reason, implementation of standardized neuromonitoring protocol has been suggested to improve neurologic outcomes. After instituting a standardized approach including neurologic examinations, transcranial

Doppler (TCD), electroencephalography (EEG), somatosensory evoked potentials (SSEPs),, and neuroimaging, Cho et al. demonstrated more frequent diagnosis of acute brain injury as well as a greater proportion of patients with favorable neurologic outcome at time of discharge.[5,6] Others have advocated for regular measurement of neuron-specific enolase levels, a serum biomarker that corresponds with neurologic outcome and mortality and a potential adjunct in determining ideal timing of neuroimaging, although ongoing hemolysis in ECMO may confound the interpretation.[7] Cerebral near-infrared spectroscopy (NIRS) has also shown promise in early detection of acute brain injury, with a demonstrated sensitivity of 86% and specificity of 55% in a prospective cohort study performed by Hunt et al.[8] Further research is needed to determine the optimal components and timing of neurologic monitoring for VA ECMO patients.

Hypoxic ischemic brain injury (HIBI) is a result of global cerebral ischemia caused by reduced cerebral blood flow or oxygen delivery. It represents one of the most common complications in VA ECMO patients and can be seen in up to 14-61% of cases.[9] In the majority of cardiac ECMO patients, HIBI occurs prior to cannulation due to hemodynamic instability. Early reversal of hypoxia and ischemia is the primary tenet of management. Other management strategies are similar to standard cardiac arrest management and include targeted temperature management, neurological monitoring, and management of neurologic sequelae such as seizures and cerebral edema.[9]

Another common neurologic complication noted in VA ECMO patients is ischemic stroke, which occurs in 4-7% of patients, and is most commonly from thromboembolism, highlighting the importance of adequate systemic anticoagulation and routine surveillance of ECMO circuit clot and intracardiac thrombus.[10] Unfortunately, intracranial hemorrhage (ICH) occurs at an only slightly lower frequency and has an extremely high mortality of 80-90% when it occurs. The clinician is therefore tasked with balancing the opposing risks of thromboembolism and hemorrhage when managing anticoagulation in a VA ECMO patient. ICH tends to occur earlier during the ECLS course, while ischemic strokes tend to occur later in the course of a VA ECMO run. Risk factors for ICH include low platelet count, female sex, and central cannulation, whereas ischemic stroke is more likely to occur in the setting of renal replacement therapy and ECMO circuit mechanical failure.[10,11]

Differential hypoxemia is a complication unique to peripheral VA ECMO. The phenomenon occurs when deoxygenated blood that is ejected antegrade from the heart mixes with well oxygenated blood that flows retrograde up the descending thoracic aorta, putting any organ perfused by the mixed or deoxygenated blood (ie, heart or brain) at risk for ischemia. The location of the mixing point depends on intrinsic cardiac function and its recovery against the amount of ECLS support provided. Patients that are especially susceptible to differential hypoxemia are those with recovered native cardiac function but persistent pulmonary insufficiency. Since the lungs are unable to perform effective gas exchange, deoxygenated blood returns to the left ventricle and is subsequently ejected into the aorta, where it mixes with blood that flows retrograde from the ECMO circuit. Differential hypoxemia is estimated to occur in approximately 9% of peripheral VA ECMO patients, and can manifest as coronary, cerebral, and/or upper extremity hypoxemia.[12] Diagnosis is typically made with arterial blood gases sampled from the right radial artery, as the innominate artery is the first to receive deoxygenated blood from the aortic arch. Management options include increasing ECMO blood flow, augmenting oxygenation of pulmonary blood flow by adjusting ventilator settings, converting to central cannulation, or placement of an additional cannula into the right internal jugular vein (V-VA ECMO configuration) to direct oxygenated blood into the right atrium.

## Pulmonary

While less commonly discussed, pulmonary pathology represents an important source of morbidity and mortality in adult VA ECMO patients. Patients are at risk for many of the same pulmonary complications as other critically ill patients, including pneumonia, pulmonary embolism, pulmonary edema, and pulmonary hemorrhage. Multifactorial respiratory failure commonly occurs in patients with critical illness myopathy or neuropathy, as the diaphragm begins to atrophy by the fourth day of mechanical ventilation support.[13] During VA ECMO support, there is significant risk for pulmonary embolism, due to the formation of thrombus on the venous cannula and deep venous thrombosis. The risk persists even after decannulation because of the frequent presence of post-decannulation deep venous thrombosis, estimated to occur in up to 30% of patients.[14] There is a paucity of data regarding management of venous thromboembolism in the adult cardiac ECMO population, but given the frailty of this patient population and the possibility of clinically occult disease, some advocate for routine screening with Doppler ultrasound after decannulation, or regular prescription of therapeutic anticoagulation for three months after decannulation.[14,15]

Pulmonary congestion is one of the most widely recognized sequelae of VA ECMO cannulation and is multifactorial. First, left ventricular dysfunction causes inadequate left ventricular ejection, particularly in the setting of increased afterload with retrograde blood flow in the aorta (peripheral VA ECMO). Increased left ventricular diastolic pressure leads to increased left atrial and ultimately increased pulmonary capillary pressure. Management strategies for pulmonary edema include increasing cardiac contractility and strategies aimed at reducing left heart pressures. These include use of inotropic agents, mechanical unloading with an intraaortic balloon pump (IABP), Impella, or catheter-mounted left ventricular assist device (LVAD), performing an atrial septostomy to reduce left atrial pressure, or surgical placement of a left ventricular vent via the right superior pulmonary vein.[16,17]

Pulmonary malperfusion can occur during VA ECMO because of decreased transpulmonary blood flow. In a porcine model, Vardi et al. demonstrated a significant reduction in pulmonary capillary blood flow as VA ECMO blood flow was increased.[18] This reduction, in conjunction with increased left atrial pressure, resulted in a decreased transpulmonary perfusion gradient and the potential for pulmonary malperfusion. Strategies to reduce lung ischemia during VA ECMO include reducing ECMO blood flow to maintain partial pulmonary perfusion or converting to VVA ECMO with a cannula in the jugular vein to provide oxygenated blood within the pulmonary arteries.[16]

The frequency of pulmonary complications in adult VA ECMO patients is not well described. The ELSO Registry does not provide data on complications such as pulmonary edema or embolism. There is some data on pulmonary hemorrhage, which frequently occurs as a consequence of pulmonary congestion, ischemia, thrombocytopenia, and systemic anticoagulation. Although seen more commonly in VV ECMO patients, pulmonary hemorrhage was described in 2.8% of VA ECMO patients in the 2017 ELSO Registry report.[19]

## Cardiac

During VA ECMO, blood flow from the arterial cannula generates supraphysiologic afterload, which can cause left ventricular distension, increased myocardial wall tension, and increased myocardial oxygen demand.

In patients with cardiogenic shock from left ventricular failure, elevated left ventricular end diastolic pressure results in progressive subendocardial ischemia and impaired myocardial recovery.[20] Furthermore, if left ventricular distension is left unattended, blood continues to accumulate under pressure until ventricular and systemic pressures equalize. This can result in severe pulmonary edema, intracardiac thrombus, and fatal pulmonary hemorrhage. For this reason, either use of a pulmonary artery catheter to monitor left sided filling pressures or routine and regular use of echocardiography to measure left ventricular distension is advised. Management of left ventricular distension consists of cardiac augmentation with inotropic agents, mechanical unloading of the left ventricle, or surgical vent placement. Mechanical unloading is often performed with an IABP, which simultaneously decreases afterload and enhances diastolic coronary blood flow, or an Impella, which offloads the left ventricle by aspirating blood from the ventricle and ejecting it into the aorta. Direct ventricular decompression can also be performed through a preexisting sternotomy or mini thoracotomy with surgical vent placement via the right upper pulmonary vein or left ventricular apex. Surgical vents utilize larger cannulae, thereby providing improved venous drainage and left ventricular unloading, but carry a higher risk of bleeding compared to minimally invasive strategies (Chapter 4).[21]

### Vascular

Access site vascular complications are estimated to occur in 20% of ECLS patients and include posterior vessel wall perforation, dissection, pseudoaneurysm, and thrombosis.[22,23] ECLS patients are also susceptible to large hematoma formation, even with relatively minor vascular injury because of systemic anticoagulation, thrombocytopenia, and coagulopathy that occurs during ECLS.

Many vascular complications can be managed conservatively, while others require open or endovascular repair. A study performed by Tanaka et al. in 2016 demonstrated a discharge rate of 18% in patients with vascular complications, compared to a 49% discharge rate in those without, highlighting the important impact that vascular complications can have on patient outcome.[24]

Lower extremity ischemia ipsilateral to the ECMO return cannula is another important vascular complication, although the rate of critical limb ischemia requiring surgical intervention is low (<2%) in experienced ECMO centers.[25] Lower extremity ischemia is caused by either thromboembolism or vessel occlusion from the cannula itself and presents with pallor or cool extremities. Other commonly described manifestations of limb ischemia such as pain and neurologic deficits may be difficult to identify due to patient sedation. In a pooled analysis of 1866 patients supported on VA ECMO, the authors reported lower limb ischemia in 17% of patients, with 10% developing compartment syndrome and 5% ultimately requiring lower extremity amputation.[26] Risk factors for limb ischemia include large cannula size, preexisting peripheral arterial disease, and multiple cannulation attempts.[27,28] If limb ischemia is not detected promptly, it can result in rhabdomyolysis, acute kidney injury, compartment syndrome, and potential limb loss. For this reason, the contemporary standard of care is to perform antegrade distal lower extremity perfusion. Additionally, regular monitoring of distal leg perfusion using near-infrared spectroscopy (NIRS) and/or Doppler ultrasound is recommended, although protocols vary by institution. Use of Doppler ultrasound may be deceptive as continuous ECMO flow may make distal pulses less pulsatile and therefore less detectable. NIRS monitoring can be advantageous in this setting as it monitors the difference between oxygenated and deoxygenated hemoglobin and does not require pulsatile blood flow. Patton-Rivera et al. recently demonstrated utility in comparison of NIRS in both cannulated and noncannulated extremities to differentiate between cannula-related obstruction and other sources of hypoperfusion (eg, high dose vasopressors).[29]

## Hematologic

Bleeding is the most common major complication that occurs during VA ECMO, reported in 30%-70% of patients.[30-32] Common locations of bleeding include the site of cannulation, oropharynx, upper and lower gastrointestinal tract, thorax, cranium, or retroperitoneum. Bleeding is in part related to systemic anticoagulation, but is likely multifactorial in nature. Other contributing factors include acquired von Willebrand syndrome, endothelial dysfunction from nonpulsatile blood flow, thrombocytopenia, platelet surface receptor shedding, abnormal platelet aggregation, increased tissue factor pathway inhibitor levels, and the trauma associated with CPR and invasive procedures.[23,33-36] The risk of bleeding is highest in the postcardiotomy population and commonly occurs at the surgical site.[37]

In an individual patient, bleeding risks must be balanced with thromboembolic risks. Although thromboembolic complications are less prevalent with the introduction of biocompatible ECMO circuit materials, they remain relatively common and can have devastating clinical consequences including ischemic stroke or limb ischemia, as previously described. Anticoagulation with unfractionated heparin remains the most widely used approach at this time, with a variety of coagulation assays available to assess anticoagulant effect. The optimal intensity of anticoagulation, as well as the potential for novel anticoagulant use remain under active clinical investigation, but currently anticoagulation strategies remain center and patient specific and best guided by

clinical judgement. Although some centers have moved towards using no anticoagulation during VA ECMO, this practice is not widespread and may be associated with a higher frequency of thrombosis (eg, circuit thrombosis rate up to 50%), with very limited clinical data available at present.[38]

## Renal

Acute renal failure is reported in up to 60% of VA ECMO patients, and is associated with increased mortality.[39] Up to 46% of patients require continuous renal replacement therapy (CRRT), which can be initiated by connecting the CRRT circuit into the ECMO circuit.[26] There are few studies (although no randomized controlled trials) comparing early versus late initiation of CRRT in ECLS patients, which demonstrate no difference in mortality.[40] Factors contributing to acute renal failure in ECLS patients include refractory hypotension prior to cannulation, hemolysis resulting in hemoglobinuria, microemboli to the renal vasculature, and kidney hypoperfusion secondary to renin angiotensin aldosterone system dysfunction.[23]

## Outcomes in Adult Cardiac ECMO Patients

### Survival Outcomes

Survival for VA ECMO patients is variable depending on treatment duration, ECMO indication, and multiple patient factors, such as preexisting comorbidities.[41] The ELSO Registry reports overall survival to decannulation of 59% in adult cardiac patients, with 44% surviving to hospital discharge.[42] The survival outcome is better in patients with decompensated congestive heart failure causing cardiogenic shock, with probability of survival of approximately 40-50%.[41,43] In a single-center observational cohort study, risk factors independently associated with higher mortality included severe liver or renal failure and female sex.[44] Similarly, in a retrospective cohort study of 3,846 patients using ELSO Registry data, Schmidt et al. found higher mortality in individuals with chronic renal failure and pre-ECMO organ failure, suggesting precannulation comorbidities play a significant role in outcomes.[41]

Survival for adult patients requiring ECPR is the lowest with only 25-35% of patients surviving to discharge (Chapter 32). Furthermore, acute brain injury is common in ECPR patients with only 40% of patients having a good functional outcome, even in high-volume ECLS centers.[45] Younger patients appear to have better neurologic outcomes with ECPR, as do those with shorter time from arrest to ECMO cannulation.[46,47] Postcardiotomy VA ECMO patients have similar survival to discharge outcomes of around 20-40%.[48,49] Retrospective observational studies have suggested risk factors for in-hospital mortality in this patient population included advanced age, diabetes, obesity, renal insufficiency, and high operative and postoperative lactate.[50,51]

### Long-term Outcomes and Followup

Long-term survival and quality of life outcomes are difficult to characterize for adult ECLS patients, as most longitudinal outcome studies are in neonatal or pediatric patients or are based on single-center experiences. A metaanalysis performed by Wilson-Smith et al. in 2019 sought to better characterize long-term outcomes for VA ECMO patients with cardiogenic shock. In a combined cohort of 17,515 patients, the survival rates at 1, 2, 3, and 5 years were 36.7%, 34.8%, 33.8%, and 29.9%, respectively, suggesting relatively stable survival expectations following hospital discharge.[52] Similar results have been shown in the postcardiotomy shock population. A metaanalysis performed by Meani et al. evaluated fifteen studies and included 2,852 patients supported on VA ECMO for postcardiotomy shock. When comparing reported in-hospital survival and one-year survival, differences ranged from 0% to 21%, suggesting relatively low long-term mortality in those who survive initial hospitalization.[49] The study was limited by the variability in followup time, and the authors noted that only six articles reported 5-year survival and only two reported 10-year survival.

Of equal importance is the long-term assessment of quality of life in VA ECMO patients. Several single-center studies have demonstrated lower Short-Form 36 (SF-36) or EuroQol (EG-5D) scores for patients supported on ECMO, suggesting persistent sequelae that can impact health-related quality of life, although it should be noted that these scores were more favorable than many other chronic health conditions such as congestive heart failure or chronic renal insufficiency.[44,53] These patients may therefore benefit from longer term psychosocial or physical rehabilitation targeted to their individual needs. Both posttraumatic stress disorder and anxiety disorders are relatively common after VA ECMO, occurring in up to 40% of patients.[54]

There are currently no formal recommendations for patient followup after VA ECMO decannulation, in part related to the deficit in research on long-term outcomes. Given the potential for late onset complications such as venous thromboembolism,[14,15] as well as the evidence of reduced quality of life after hospitalization, there may be a role for multidisciplinary ECLS clinics to optimize patient care after decannulation. Clinical trials would be of value in ascertaining the benefit of regular followup visits or imaging in the adult cardiac population.

### Conclusions

VA ECMO is used to support adult patients with refractory cardiogenic shock, ECPR for out-of-hospital and in-hospital cardiac arrest, and postcardiotomy shock characterized by an inability to wean from CPB. The outcomes in the adult cardiac population remain poor and patients are susceptible to irreversible neurologic, pulmonary, cardiovascular, and renal complications. Future research should be targeted towards identification of modifiable risk factors and development of targeted interventions to reduce ECLS-associated complications and improve functional outcomes.

# References

1. Lee SY, Jeon KH, Lee HJ, et al. Complications of veno-arterial extracorporeal membrane oxygenation for refractory cardiogenic shock or cardiac arrest. Int J Artif Organs. 2020;43(1):37-44.

2. Hou D, Wang H, Yang F, et al. Neurologic Complications in Adult Post-cardiotomy Cardiogenic Shock Patients Receiving Venoarterial Extracorporeal Membrane Oxygenation: A Cohort Study. Front Med (Lausanne). 2021 Aug;8:721774.

3. Rastan AJ, Lachmann N, Walther T, et al. Autopsy findings in patients on postcardiotomy extracorporeal membrane oxygenation (ECMO). Int J Artif Organs. 2006 Dec;29(12):1121-31.

4. Cho S, Geocadin RG, Caturegli G, et al. Understanding characteristics of acute brain injury in adult extracorporeal membrane oxygenation: An autopsy study. Critical Care Medicine. 2020;48(6):e532.

5. Cho S, Ziai W, Mayasi Y, et al. Noninvasive neurological monitoring in extracorporeal membrane oxygenation. ASAIO J. 2020;66(4):388-393.

6. Ong CS, Etchill E, Dong J, et al. Neuromonitoring detects brain injury in patients receiving extracorporeal membrane oxygenation support. The Journal of Thoracic and Cardiovascular Surgery. 2021.

7. Floerchinger B, Philipp A, Foltan M, et al. Neuron-specific enolase serum levels predict severe neuronal injury after extracorporeal life support in resuscitation. Eur J Cardiothorac Surg. 2014;45(3):496-501.

8. Hunt MF, Clark KT, Whitman G, et al. The use of cerebral NIRS monitoring to identify acute brain injury in patients with VA-ECMO. J Intensive Care Med. 2021;36(12):1403-1409.

9. Cho S, Farrokh S, Whitman G, et al. Neurocritical care for extracorporeal membrane oxygenation patients. Crit Care Med. 2019;47(12):1773-1781.

10. Le Guennec L, Cholet C, Huang F, et al. Ischemic and hemorrhagic brain injury during venoarterial-extracorporeal membrane oxygenation. Ann Intensive Care. 2018;8(1):129.

11. Cho S, Canner J, Chiarini G, et al. Modifiable risk factors and mortality from ischemic and hemorrhagic strokes in patients receiving venoarterial extracorporeal membrane oxygenation: Results from the extracorporeal life support organization registry. Crit Care Med. 2020;48(10):e897-e905.

12. Rupprecht L, Lunz D, Philipp A, et al. Pitfalls in percutaneous extracorporeal membrane oxygenation cannulation. Heart Lung Vessel. 2005;7:320–326.

13. Goligher EC, Dres M, Fan E, et al. Mechanical Ventilation-induced Diaphragm Atrophy Strongly Impacts Clinical Outcomes. Am J Respir Crit Care Med. 2018;197(2):204-213.

14. Vazquez ZGS, Sodha NR, Devers C, et al. Prevalence of deep vein thrombosis in patients supported with extracorporeal membrane oxygenation. ASAIO Journal 2021; (10):e169-e171.

15. Maestro-Benedicto A, Duran-Cambra A, Vila-Perales M, et al. Anticoagulation after VA-ECMO decannulation, providing new insights. European Heart Journal Acute Cardiovascular Care. 2021;10(Supplement_1):zuab020.168.

16. Roumy A, Liaudet L, Rusca M, et al. Pulmonary complications associated with veno-arterial extracorporeal membrane oxygenation: a comprehensive review. Crit Care. 2020;24:212.

17. Mlcek M, Meani P, Cotza M, et al. Atrial Septostomy for Left Ventricular Unloading During Extracorporeal Membrane Oxygenation for Cardiogenic Shock: Animal Model. JACC Cardiovasc Interv. 2021;14(24):2698-2707.

18. Vardi A, Jessen ME, Chao RY, et al. Effect of extracorporeal membrane oxygenation flow on pulmonary capillary blood flow. Crit Care Med. 1995;23(4):726–32.

19. ECLS registry report international summary. Extracorporeal Life Support Organization. 2017.

20. Cevasco M, Takayama H, Ando M, et al. Left ventricular distension and venting strategies for patients on venoarterial extracorporeal membrane oxygenation. J Thorac Dis. 2019;11(4):1676-1683.

21. Choi MS, Sung K, Cho YH. Clinical Pearls of Venoarterial Extracorporeal Membrane Oxygenation for Cardiogenic Shock. Korean Circ J. 2019;49(8):657-677.

22. Bisdas T, Beutel G, Warnecke G, et al. Vascular complications in patients undergoing femoral cannulation for extracorporeal membrane oxygenation support. Ann Thorac Surg. 2011 Aug;92(2):626-31.

23. Tsangaris A, Alexy T, Kalra R, et al. Overview of Veno-Arterial Extracorporeal Membrane Oxygenation (VA-ECMO) Support for the Management of Cardiogenic Shock. Front Cardiovasc Med. 2021;8:686558.

24. Tanaka D, Hirose H, Cavarocchi N, et al. The Impact of Vascular Complications on Survival of Patients on Venoarterial Extracorporeal Membrane Oxygenation. Ann Thorac Surg. 2016;101(5):1729-1734.

25. Pasrija C, Mazzeffi MA, Kon ZN. A percutaneous strategy for safe femoral venoarterial extracorporeal life support. J Thorac Cardiovasc Surg. 2017;153(2):370-371.

26. Cheng R, Hachamovitch R, Kittleson M, et al. Complications of extracorporeal membrane oxygenation for treatment of cardiogenic shock and cardiac arrest: a meta-analysis of 1,866 adult patients. Ann Thorac Surg. 2014;97(2):610-616.

27. Foley PJ, Morris RJ, Woo EY, et al. Limb ischemia during femoral cannulation for cardiopulmonary support. J Vasc Surg. 2010;52(4):850-853.

28. Lamb KM, DiMuzio PJ, Johnson A, et al. Arterial protocol including prophylactic distal perfusion catheter decreases limb ischemia complications in patients undergoing extracorporeal membrane oxygenation. J Vasc Surg. 2017;65(4):1074-1079.

29. Bonicolini E, Martucci G, Simons J, et al. Limb ischemia in peripheral veno-arterial extracorporeal membrane oxygenation: A narrative review of incidence, prevention, monitoring, and treatment. Critical care (London, England). 2019;23(1):266.

30. Mazzeffi MA, Tanaka K, Roberts A, et al. Bleeding, Thrombosis, and Transfusion With Two Heparin Anticoagulation Protocols in Venoarterial ECMO Patients. J Cardiothorac Vasc Anesth. 2019;33(5):1216-1220.

31. Olson SR, Murphree CR, Zonies D, et al. Thrombosis and Bleeding in Extracorporeal Membrane Oxygenation (ECMO) Without Anticoagulation: A Systematic Review. ASAIO J. 2021;67(3):290-296.

32. Raffa GM, Kowalewski M, Brodie D, et al. Meta-Analysis of Peripheral or Central Extracorporeal Membrane Oxygenation in Postcardiotomy and Non-Postcardiotomy Shock. Ann Thorac Surg. 2019;107(1):311-321.

33. Tauber H, Ott H, Streif W, et al. Extracorporeal membrane oxygenation induces short-term loss of high-molecular-weight von Willebrand factor multimers. Anesth Analg. 2015;120(4):730-736.

34. Jiritano F, Serraino GF, Ten Cate H, et al. Platelets and extra-corporeal membrane oxygenation in adult patients: a systematic review and meta-analysis. Intensive Care Med. 2020;46(6):1154-1169.

35. Mazzeffi M, Judd M, Rabin J, et al. Tissue Factor Pathway Inhibitor Levels During Veno-Arterial Extracorporeal Membrane Oxygenation in Adults. ASAIO J. 2021;67(8):878-883.

36. Chen Z, Koenig SC, Slaughter MS, et al. Quantitative Characterization of Shear-Induced Platelet Receptor Shedding: Glycoprotein Ibα, Glycoprotein VI, and Glycoprotein IIb/IIIa. ASAIO J. 2018;64(6):773-778.

37. Aubron C, DePuydt J, Belon F, et al. Predictive factors of bleeding events in adults undergoing extracorporeal membrane oxygenation. Ann Intensive Care. 2016;6(1):1-10. https://link.springer.com/article/10.1186/s13613-016-0196-7.

38. Fina D, Matteucci M, Jiritano F, et al. Extracorporeal membrane oxygenation without therapeutic anticoagulation in adults: A systematic review of the current literature. Int J Artif Organs. 2020;43(9):570-578.

39. Lee SW, Yu M, Lee H, et al. Risk factors for acute kidney injury and in-hospital mortality in patients receiving extracorporeal membrane oxygenation. PLOS ONE. 2015;10(10):e0140674.

40. Paek JH, Park S, Lee A, et al. Timing for initiation of sequential continuous renal replacement therapy in patients on extracorporeal membrane oxygenation. Kidney Res Clin Pract. 2018;37(3):239-247.

41. Schmidt M, Burrell A, Roberts L, et al. Predicting survival after ECMO for refractory cardiogenic shock: The survival after veno-arterial-ECMO (SAVE)-score. Eur Heart J. 2015;36(33):2246-2256.

42. ECLS international summary of statistics. Extracorporeal Life Support Organization Web site. https://www.elso.org/Registry/InternationalSummaryandReports/InternationalSummary.aspx. Updated 2021.

43. Rao P, Khalpey Z, Smith R, et al. Venoarterial extracorporeal membrane oxygenation for cardiogenic shock and cardiac arrest. Circulation: Heart Failure. 2018;11(9):e004905.

44. Combes A, Leprince P, Luyt C, et al. Outcomes and long-term quality-of-life of patients supported by extracorporeal membrane oxygenation for refractory cardiogenic shock. Crit Care Med. 2008;36(5).

45. Podell JE, Krause EM, Rector R, et al. Neurologic Outcomes After Extracorporeal Cardiopulmonary Resuscitation: Recent Experience at a Single High-Volume Center ASAIO J. 2022 Feb 1;68(2):247-254.

46. Zakhary B, Nanjayya VB, Sheldrake J, et al. Predictors of mortality after extracorporeal cardiopulmonary resuscitation. Crit Care Resusc. 2018;20(3):223-230.

47. Mazzeffi, M, Sanchez PG, Herr D, et al. Outcomes of extracorporeal cardiopulmonary resuscitation for refractory cardiac arrest in adult cardiac surgery patients. The Journal of thoracic and cardiovascular surgery. 2016;152(4):1133-1139.

48. F. Biancari, A. Perrotti, M. Dalen, M., et al. Meta-analysis of the outcome after postcardiotomy venoarterial extracorporeal membrane oxygenation in adult patients. J Cardiothorac Vasc Anesth. 32 (3) (2018), pp. 1175-1182.

49. Meani, P., Matteucci, M., Jiritano, F., et al. Long-term survival and major outcomes in post-cardiotomy extracorporeal membrane oxygenation for adult patients in cardiogenic shock. Annals of Cardiothoracic Surgery. 2019;8(1).

50. Hu RTC, Broad JD, Osawa EA, et al. 30-Day Outcomes Post Veno-Arterial Extra Corporeal Membrane Oxygenation (VA-ECMO) After Cardiac Surgery and Predictors of Survival. Heart Lung Circ. 2020;29(8):1217-1225.

51. Rastan AJ, Dege A, Mohr M, et al. Early and late outcomes of 517 consecutive adult patients treated with extracorporeal membrane oxygenation for refractory postcardiotomy cardiogenic shock. J Thorac Cardiovasc Surg. 2010;139(2):302-311.e1.

52. Wilson-Smith AR, Bogdanova Y, Roydhouse S, et al. Outcomes of venoarterial extracorporeal membrane oxygenation for refractory cardiogenic shock: systematic review and meta-analysis. Ann Cardiothorac Surg. 2019;8(1):1-8.

53. Camboni D, Philipp A, Rottenkolber V, et al. Long-term survival and quality of life after extracorporeal life support: A 10-year report. Eur J Cardiothorac Surg. 2017;52(2):241-247.

54. Kolle A, Irgens EC, Moi AL, et al. The Psychological and HRQoL related Aftermaths of Extra Corporeal Membrane Oxygenation Treatment: A Cross-Sectional Study. Intensive Crit Care Nurs. 2021;65:103058.

# 34

## Pregnancy

*Cara Agerstrand, Emily Naoum, Kollengode Ramanathan, Farah Siddiqui, Priya Nair*

## Introduction

The fundamental principles of ECLS management in pregnant patients are similar to nonpregnant patients; however, pregnancy introduces a level of complexity given the need to consider the health of both the patient and developing fetus. A thorough understanding of the physiologic changes and potential complications of pregnancy and demands of the fetus are required to optimize outcomes for both.

There is growing global clinical experience caring for this population, although evidence guiding management is limited.[1-3] Much of the early experience with peripartum ECLS was gained during the 2009 influenza A (H1N1) pandemic.[2-4] Since that time, ECLS has been used for a variety of cardiopulmonary indications, including for severe cases of COVID-19.[5-8] This chapter will review the physiologic changes of normal pregnancy and offer guidance for patient selection and management in this uniquely challenging population.

## Physiological Changes During Pregnancy

### Respiratory

Pregnancy-related changes in lung mechanics become apparent by the mid-second trimester. There is a slight decrease in total lung capacity and a marked decrease in functional residual capacity due to diaphragmatic elevation.[9-10] Spirometry is largely unchanged.[11] Late in pregnancy there is a 30% reduction in chest wall compliance with an associated decrease in total respiratory system compliance.[12,13]

Minute ventilation increases 50% during pregnancy due to a progesterone-mediated increase in tidal volume, which results in a respiratory alkalosis with a pH of 7.40-7.47, partial pressure of arterial carbon dioxide ($PaCO_2$) of 30-32 mmHg and a compensatory increase in bicarbonate excretion.[9] The relative depletion of buffering capacity renders the pregnant patient less adaptable to metabolic acidosis (eg, in the setting of sepsis). Oxygen consumption increases by 20% and $CO_2$ production by 60% at term, due to increased metabolism and fetal demands.[9]

### Cardiovascular

Cardiovascular changes begin early in the first trimester, with most plateauing by late second trimester. Cardiac output increases as much as 45% due to changes in stroke volume and heart rate, blood pressure decreases 5-10 mmHg and systemic vascular resistance (SVR) decreases 35-40%.[14] In the third trimester, mechanical compression of the vena cava may limit venous return and result in lower blood pressure and cardiac output, particularly while supine.[9,15] In that setting, uterine blood flow and transplacental gas exchange may be impaired.[16]

## Hematologic

Plasma volume increases by nearly 50% during pregnancy.[13,17] Despite a concomitant increase in red cell mass, this hemodilution results in a 25% decrease in hematocrit.[18] Pregnancy is a hypercoagulable state and carries a substantially increased risk of arterial and venous thromboembolism.[19] The risk of pelvic and left lower extremity thromboses are particularly increased due to vascular stasis from the gravid uterus.[19]

## Immunologic

Immunologic changes during pregnancy render the patient more susceptible to infection, particularly to organisms requiring a cell-mediated immune response, such as viruses, fungi, and mycobacteria.[20] Pregnancy also increases the risk of developing severe infection, as has been demonstrated with influenza and COVID-19, where there is higher likelihood of requiring invasive mechanical ventilation or ECLS compared to non-peripartum patients.[21,22]

## Etiology of Severe Cardiopulmonary Failure during Pregnancy

### Acute Respiratory Distress Syndrome

Pregnancy is associated with an increased incidence of the acute respiratory distress syndrome (ARDS), which occurs in 1 of 5000 deliveries.[23] ARDS is the most common indication for ECLS in the peripartum period.[1,2,7] Survival is similar to that in non-peripartum patients of child-bearing age, including in those requiring ECLS support.[3,10] The etiology of ARDS during

pregnancy may be due to conditions seen in nonpregnant patients (eg, bacterial pneumonia or gastric aspiration) or from pregnancy-specific conditions (eg, preeclampsia).

### Status Asthmaticus

Pregnancy may worsen underlying asthma due to alterations in lung mechanics and immunologic response, particularly in the late second and early third trimesters and in patients with poor baseline asthmatic control.[9,24] Asthma during pregnancy is associated with multiple comorbid conditions including preeclampsia, placenta abruption, placenta previa, obstetric hemorrhage and preterm delivery.[25]

### Cardiac Failure

Pregnancy-related cardiac failure can result from chronic conditions, including exacerbation of an existing cardiomyopathy, pulmonary arterial hypertension, or severe valvular disease. The risk of decompensation is highest in the third trimester and parturition, due to fluctuations in intrathoracic pressure and volume status. Following delivery, an abrupt increase in venous return and SVR places the patient at risk of fluid overload and pulmonary edema, as well.[17,26,27] Cardiac failure during pregnancy may also result from acute processes, such as arrhythmia, pulmonary embolism or peripartum cardiomyopathy, the last of which develops late in pregnancy or postpartum in patients without underlying cardiac disease.[7,28-30]

## ECLS Considerations during Pregnancy

The physiologic changes of pregnancy and the presence of the fetus necessitate certain special considerations for ECLS initiation and management beyond what is generally practiced in the care of a nonpregnant patient. Critically ill pregnant patients at risk of cardiac or pulmonary decompensation should receive early referral to an ECLS center with both maternal fetal medicine and neonatal intensive care capabilities.

### Indications for Therapy

The general approach to ECLS during pregnancy should be similar to that in nonpregnant patients. Pregnant patients with ARDS and status asthmaticus should be cannulated onto VV ECMO. In ARDS, gas exchange criteria for ECLS initiation should align with the Extracorporeal Membrane Oxygenation for Severe Acute Respiratory Distress Syndrome (EOLIA) trial, taking into account patient trajectory and fetal considerations.[31] ECLS is indicated when the patient is unable to achieve adequate, stable gas exchange despite optimized conventional management or for signs of fetal instability in a patient with borderline gas exchange. Status asthmaticus, refractory hypercapnic acidosis, barotrauma, hemodynamic instability, or fetal distress should prompt consideration of VV ECMO.[32-34]

VA ECMO should be considered in severe cardiac failure, including right heart failure from pulmonary arterial hypertension, when there are signs of deterioration in hemodynamics or systemic perfusion despite inotropic support, or in the setting of fetal instability.[27] VA ECMO has also been used successfully as ECPR in peripartum patients suffering cardiac arrest.[1,7]

### Contraindications

There are no pregnancy-specific contraindications to ECLS. In general, the relatively young patient age, absence of major comorbid conditions, and acuity of the disease processes favor the use of ECLS in appropriate circumstances. Although the risk of bleeding and thrombosis are increased during pregnancy, the potential benefit of ECLS outweighs these risks. Successful outcomes have been reported even in patients with massive obstetric hemorrhage and profound coagulopathies prior to ECMO cannulation, and neither should be considered contraindications to ECLS initiation in this specific population.[1,35]

### Mechanical Ventilation and Gas Exchange Targets

Pregnant patients with ARDS receiving ECLS should be managed with a lung rest approach to mechanical ventilation, with consideration of fetal demands.[36] Fetal oxygenation is dependent on several factors including uterine artery blood flow, uterine arterial oxygen content, hemoglobin level, and oxygen saturation. Therefore, impairment in gas exchange as well as hypotension, vasoconstriction, and uterine contractions can affect placental oxygen delivery.[9]

Pregnant patients receiving ECLS should maintain $PaO_2 \geq 70$ mmHg and $SaO_2 \geq 95\%$ to ensure adequate fetal oxygenation.[37,38] Adequate $PaO_2$ is also required to maintain fetal acid-base status. If patient hypoxemia occurs, the ECLS circuit should be preferentially used to augment systemic oxygenation. Positive end expiratory pressure should be applied with caution given the potential for decreased cardiac output and impairment in placental perfusion at elevated intrathoracic pressures.

Fetal $CO_2$ clearance is dependent on a transplacental gradient of 8-10 mmHg.[39] As baseline $PaCO_2$ is 30-32 mmHg during pregnancy, sweep should be titrated to maintain a mild respiratory alkalosis. Caution must be taken to avoid significant hypocapnia, which may result in fetal alkalosis, uterine artery constriction and leftward shift of the fetal oxygen dissociation curve resulting in fetal hypoxia.[37,39,40] Severe hypercapnia with a $PaCO_2 > 60$ mmHg should also be avoided, as rightward shift of the dissociation curve may limit oxygen binding to fetal hemoglobin.[37]

## Hemodynamic Targets

Strategies of cardiovascular support should be similar to those used in nonpregnant patients, including volume optimization and use of inotropes, vasopressors, and pulmonary vasodilators, as appropriate. A MAP ≥65 mmHg should be maintained and indicators of systemic hypoperfusion (including lactate, creatinine, transaminases, and urine output) should be monitored.[37] Hypertension during pregnancy predisposes to life-threatening complications, such as intracranial hemorrhage, and requires pharmacologic control.[41,42] Significant hypotension can result in reduced placental perfusion and fetal bradycardia, so drastic drops in blood pressure should be avoided. Administration of crystalloid can reduce the risk of fetal distress when using intravenous antihypertensive medications.[43]

## Cannulation Strategies

The augmented cardiac output of pregnancy often requires a high ECLS blood flow to maintain systemic oxygen delivery.[44] Pre-cannulation vascular ultrasound is recommended to facilitate selection of the largest cannula that can be safely accommodated in the vessel.

Both single-site and dual-site cannulation approaches to VV ECMO have been used in pregnancy.[1,5] In the third trimester, caval compression by the gravid uterus may limit drainage from the femoral venous cannula; however, left lateral positioning (15 degree tilt achieved with a wedge under the right hip) may alleviate this compression.[45] Inability to achieve adequate blood flow despite optimized patient positioning and judicious intravascular volume administration may require insertion of a second venous drainage cannula.

## Anticoagulation

Heparin and direct thrombin inhibitors can be administered using conventional targets.[46] A low-dose approach to anticoagulation similar to that of nonpregnant patients is recommended, with close monitoring of circuit function and evaluation for signs of systemic thrombosis, bleeding and DIC.[1,3,31]

## Pharmacology

Pharmacokinetics are complex during pregnancy, given the increased volume of distribution combined with decreased serum albumin concentrations and drug elimination.[47] Sequestration of lipophilic medications further complicates medication administration.[48]

The risk-benefit of all medications should be considered with input from specialists familiar with their risk profiles. Medications with the lowest risk of morbidity to both patient and fetus should be selected, although use of potentially fetotoxic medications may be required if suitable alternatives do not exist. When considering steroids, prednisolone has less placental transfer than dexamethasone. Prolonged use of both dexamethasone and betamethasone has been associated with childhood neurocognitive and neurosensory disorders.[49] Benzodiazepines and opiates may result in neonatal respiratory depression and withdrawal syndromes.

## Fetal Monitoring and Management

### Fetal Monitoring and Optimization

Patient stability is often reflected in fetal status. Fetal monitoring is routinely performed, but practices vary by institution, gestational age, neonatal resuscitative resources, and patient and family preference. A viability scan by transabdominal ultrasound can detect a fetal heartbeat from 12 weeks gestation. Daily fetal ultrasounds are routinely performed as the pregnancy progresses. Continuous fetal heart rate monitoring serves as a marker of adequate uteroplacental perfusion; however, appropriateness of use depends on the potential for respiratory and hemodynamic optimization and feasibility of intervention for acute fetal concerns (Table 34-1).[50]

Neonatal survival has been reported from 22 weeks, although survival is less likely in the presence of severe maternal illness. A course of antenatal steroids is recommended between 24-36 weeks gestation to promote fetal lung development and mitigate the risk of neonatal respiratory distress and intraventricular hemorrhage.[51,52] Magnesium sulphate infusion should be considered for deliveries less than 32 weeks because it has been shown to improve the infant's neurodevelopmental score.[52] In the third trimester, positioning the patient with a left lateral preference whenever possible may improve uterine artery blood flow and placental perfusion.[53]

## Timing of Delivery

The decision of whether to deliver the fetus is a major challenge when caring for an antenatal patient receiving ECLS (Figure 34-1). While ECLS is not an indication for delivery, its initiation should prompt a multidisciplinary risk assessment of continuing the pregnancy and the development of a delivery plan.[50] The Society for Maternal Fetal Medicine has supported the use of ECLS to facilitate *in utero* fetal development in patients with refractory hypoxemia due to COVID-19 at less than 32 weeks' gestation.[54]

Prolonging pregnancy is generally in the interest of the fetus; however, the principal consideration must be whether delivery will improve the patient's cardiopulmonary status. This should include an assessment of the burden of the fetoplacental unit on the patient's oxygen consumption because oxygen delivery to the placenta accounts for 10% of cardiac output (600-700 mL oxygen/min) at term, balanced

| MODE OF MONITORING | | USE | |
|---|---|---|---|
| Fetal Heartbeat | Scan/sonic aide/handheld Dopper | Fetal viability, can be used from 16-week gestation | Easy access to assess fetal life, absence of fetal heartbeat should be confirmed with scan |
| Fetal Growth Assessment | Ultrasound scan | Assess estimated fetal size, useful in predicting chronic placental disease. Useful to confirm placental location particularly placenta previa | Scans are also useful for additional information such as multiple pregnancy, polyhydramnios (increased liquor) that can increase diaphragmatic elevation |
| Umbilical and Fetal Dopplers | Ultrasound scan-continuous pulsed Doppler | Indication of chronic fetal hypoxia or acidemia | |
| CTG | Cardiotocograph used after 26 weeks | Used to predict acute fetal hypoxia or acidemia | A trained midwife or obstetrician required to interpret results |

**Table 34-1.** Mode of monitoring.

against the risk of deterioration that may result from delivery-related hemodynamic, immunologic, and hemorrhagic insults.[9]

Although the health of the patient is the primary indication for delivery, clinical deterioration in either the patient or fetus should prompt a multidisciplinary discussion regarding the risk-benefit calculus of delivery. This calculus will likely evolve as the pregnancy progresses and needs to be frequently revisited. Experienced members of the intensive care, cardiology, ECLS, obstetric, maternal fetal medicine, anesthesiology, neonatology, hematology, nursing, and pharmacy teams should be included in these multidisciplinary discussions, as appropriate.[55]

## Mode of Delivery

Planning for the mode of delivery is also crucial. Patient-specific factors, such as the etiology of cardiopulmonary failure, ECLS configuration and clinical stability should be considered when determining delivery mode. Successful outcomes have been reported with both cesarean and vaginal deliveries, though cesarean delivery is more common.[7] Vaginal birth by induction of labor is often challenging because oxygenation, blood pressure and pain may be more difficult to control, and it carries risk of intrapartum fetal hypoxia and acidosis.

When delivery is anticipated, the multidisciplinary delivery plan including

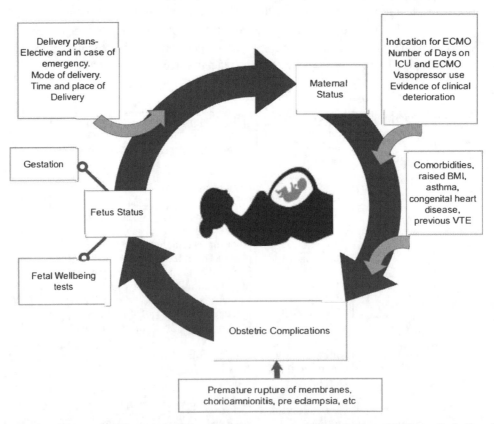

**Figure 34-1.** Illustrates important and dynamic factors to consider in timing of delivery, including the health and stability of the patient, the presence of obstetric complications and fetal gestational age and wellbeing. It also highlights the need to ensure a delivery plan is in place for any pregnant patient supported with ECMO. BMI=Body mass index, VTE=Venous thromboembolism.

anesthetic, hemodynamic, hematologic, ECLS, and neonatal management should be reviewed. Anticoagulation can be held, with close monitoring of circuit function. Equipment needed for emergent delivery as well as neonatal care should be readily accessible.[56]

## Pregnancy Complications

### Preeclampsia

Preeclampsia is an important diagnosis in the spectrum of hypertensive disorders of pregnancy, severe forms of which are associated with devastating complications including eclamptic seizures, intracranial hemorrhage, posterior reversible encephalopathy syndrome, ARDS, hepatic subcapsular hematoma and rupture, renal failure, and placental abruption. Hemolysis, elevated liver enzymes, and low platelets (HELLP) syndrome is considered a severe form of preeclampsia and is also associated with these complications.[41,42,57]

Suspicion of preeclampsia should arise in patients with hypertension or proteinuria. Preeclampsia with severe features (systolic blood pressure >160 mmHg, diastolic blood pressure >110 mmHg, thrombocytopenia, impaired liver function, renal insufficiency, pulmonary edema, cerebral or visual symptoms) warrants treatment with magnesium sulfate to reduce seizure risk. Of note, magnesium therapy is associated with pulmonary edema, neuromuscular weakness and uterine atony and requires monitoring to prevent supratherapeutic concentrations.[41,42]

### Placental Abruption

Abruption of the placental bed can result in severe hemorrhage, coagulopathy, and fetal death. Risk factors for abruption include hypertension, advanced maternal age, trauma, tobacco or cocaine use, and preterm, premature rupture of membranes. Even mild abruption may result in fetal compromise and spontaneous labor with the potential for miscarriage. Aggressive management of blood loss and treatment of coagulopathy is crucial, as is multidisciplinary planning regarding timing and mode of delivery.

### Amniotic Fluid Embolism

Amniotic fluid embolism (AFE) is a catastrophic complication of pregnancy that occurs during labor or immediately postpartum and results in a complex and profound inflammatory response characterized by pulmonary hypertension, myocardial depression, central nervous system injury, activation of the coagulation cascade, and ARDS.[58] AFE classically presents with hypoxemia, hypotension, and coagulopathy, possibly with hemorrhage and cardiac arrest. ECLS may improve the likelihood of neurologically intact survival in patients with AFE.[7]

### Fetal Demise

Patients with severe systemic illness have increased risk of fetal demise. A retained fetus predisposes to infection and DIC, therefore delivery should be considered. Vaginal delivery may be preferred in this scenario. If spontaneous labor does not develop, induction of labor may be required. Due to the risk of severe hemorrhage during parturition, cessation of anticoagulation should be considered and uterotonics readily available.

### Postpartum Hemorrhage

Postpartum hemorrhage may occur due to uterine atony, surgical incisions, cervical or vaginal lacerations, retained placenta or coagulopathy.[59,60] Uterotonics including oxytocin, carbetocin, methylergonovine, and prostaglandins should be considered. Cell salvage may be used in the setting of cesarean delivery, as well. Additional interventions include uterine compression sutures, uterine artery ligation or embolization, intrauterine balloon tamponade, and hysterectomy.[59] Vigilance should be maintained postpartum to monitor for late bleeding.

### *Sepsis*

Pneumonia, pyelonephritis, chorioamnionitis and endometritis are the most common causes of sepsis in the parturient.[61,62] Identifying sepsis during pregnancy can be challenging due to the physiologic changes of normal pregnancy, including increased heart rate, decreased blood pressure, and increased white blood cell concentration. Traditional screening tools for sepsis have limited sensitivity and specificity in pregnant patients and therefore early warning systems have been developed.[62,63] Early and appropriate antibiotic therapy is imperative to reduce mortality.

### ECLS Complications

ECLS-related complications are similar to those seen in non-peripartum patients. Bleeding is the most common complication, estimated in 20-50% of cases, with some recent studies suggesting comparable rates to non-peripartum patients.[7, 8, 27, 64, 65] Reassuringly, an analysis of over 250 cases of peripartum ECLS did not identify bleeding as a risk factor for mortality.[6] Given the hypercoagulability of pregnancy, there is concern regarding the risk of thrombotic events and DIC; however the extent of the issue is unclear.[7,8,27,65]

### Outcomes

Early referral to an ECLS center is recommended for all critically ill pregnant patients due to an estimated high number of preventable deaths.[66] Favorable outcomes have been reported when using ECLS for both respiratory and cardiac indications in an antenatal population.[1-3,7,64] Based on a systematic review of over 350 ECLS-supported peripartum patients, 81 of whom were pregnant while receiving ECLS, the median age was 29.5 years and median gestation was 24 weeks.[7] Roughly one-third of patients delivered on ECLS.[7] Survival outcomes are impacted by the underlying disease process, but are reported to be 70-80% for patients with both respiratory and cardiac indications for ECLS.[2,7] Excellent survival has also been reported with ECPR in this population, with improved outcomes compared to non-peripartum patients.[7,64] In cases of peripartum cardiomyopathy, one-tenth of survivors required bridge to ventricular assist devices or heart transplantation, with favorable hospital survival.[27] While outcomes in COVID-19 continue to evolve, ELSO Registry data of 100 peripartum patients suggests survival superior to a matched non-peripartum cohort.[8] Fetal survival in ECLS-supported pregnant patients is reported at 65-70%, though outcomes vary based on indication for ECLS and gestational age at cannulation.[1,2,7,67]

# References

1. Agerstrand C, Abrams D, Biscotti M, et al. Extracorporeal membrane oxygenation for cardiopulmonary failure during pregnancy and postpartum. Ann Thorac Surg. 2016;102(3):774-9.
2. Moore SA, Dietl CA, Coleman DM. Extracorporeal life support during pregnancy. J Thorac Cardiovasc Surg. 2016;151(4):1154-60.
3. Nair P, Davies AR, Beca J, et al. Extracorporeal membrane oxygenation for severe ARDS in pregnant and postpartum women during the 2009 H1N1 pandemic. Intensive Care Med. 2011;37(4):648-54.
4. Saad AF, Rahman M, Maybauer DM, et al. Extracorporeal membrane oxygenation in pregnant and postpartum women with H1N1-related acute respiratory distress syndrome: a systematic review and meta-analysis. Obstet Gynecol. 2016;127(2):241-7.
5. Barrantes JH, Ortoleva J, O'Neil ER, et al. Successful treatment of pregnant and postpartum women with severe COVID-19 associated acute respiratory distress syndrome with extracorporeal membrane oxygenation. ASAIO J. 2021;67(2):132-6.
6. Regan AK, Arah O, Fell DB, et al. SARS-CoV-2 infection during pregnancy and associated perinatal health outcomes: a national US cohort study. J Infect Dis. 2022 Mar 2;225(5):759-767.
7. Naoum EE, Chalupka A, Haft J, et al. Extracorporeal life support in pregnancy: a systematic review. J Am Heart Assoc. 2020;9(13):e016072.
8. O'Neil ER, Lin H, Shamshirsaz AA, et al. Pregnant and peripartum women with COVID-19 have high survival with extracorporeal membrane oxygenation: an Extracorporeal Life Support Organization registry analysis. Am J Respir Crit Care Med. 2022;205(2):248-50.
9. Chesnutt AN. Physiology of normal pregnancy. Crit Care Clin. 2004;20(4):609-15.
10. Mehta N, Chen K, Hardy E, et al. Respiratory disease in pregnancy. Best Pract Res Clin Obstet & Gynaecol. 2015;29(5):598-611.
11. Weinberger SE, Weiss ST, Cohen WR, et al. Pregnancy and the lung. Am Rev Respir Dis. 1980;121(3):559-81.
12. Marx GF, Murthy PK, Orkin LR. Static compliance before and after vaginal delivery. Br J Anaesth. 1970;42(12):1100-4.
13. Campbell LA, Klocke RA. Implications for the pregnant patient. Am J Resp Crit Care Med. 2001;163(5):1051-4.
14. Sanghavi M, Rutherford JD. Cardiovascular physiology of pregnancy. Circulation. 2014;130(12):1003-8.
15. Kerr MG, Scott DB, Samuel E. Studies of the inferior vena cava in late pregnancy. Br Med J. 1964;1(5382):522.4-33.
16. Massoth C, Chappell D, Kranke P, et al. Supine hypotensive syndrome of pregnancy: a review of current knowledge. Eur J Anaesthesiol. 2021;38:1-8.
17. Anjum H, Surani S. Pulmonary hypertension in pregnancy: a review. Medicina. 2021;57(3):259.
18. Chesley LC. Plasma and red cell volumes during pregnancy. Am J Obstet Gynecol. 1972;112(3):440-50.
19. James AH. Venous thromboembolism in pregnancy. Arterioscler Thromb Vasc Biol. 2009;29(3):326-31.
20. Abu-Raya B, Michalski C, Sadarangani M, et al. Maternal immunological adaptation during normal pregnancy. Front Immunol. 2020;11:575197.
21. Jamieson DJ, Rasmussen SA. An update on COVID-19 and pregnancy. Am J Obstet Gynecol. 2022;226(2):177-86.
22. Lapinsky SE. Critical illness as a result of influenza A/H1N1 infection in pregnancy. BMJ. 2010;340:c1235.
23. Pollock W, Rose L, Dennis CL. Pregnant and postpartum admissions to the intensive care unit: a systematic review. Intensive Care Med. 2010;36(9):1465-74.
24. Tamási L, Horváth I, Bohács A, et al. Asthma in pregnancy – immunological changes and clinical management. Respir Med. 2011;105(2):159-64.
25. Bonham CA, Patterson KC, Strek ME. Asthma outcomes and management during pregnancy. Chest. 2018;153(2):515-27.
26. Kiely DG, Condliffe R, Wilson VJ, et al. Pregnancy and pulmonary hypertension: a practical approach to management. Obstet Med. 2013;6(4):144-54.
27. Olson TL, O'Neil ER, Ramanathan K, et al. Extracorporeal membrane oxygenation in peripartum cardiomyopathy: a review of the ELSO registry. Int J Cardiol. 2020;311:71-6.
28. Sharma NS, Wille KM, Bellot SC, et al. Modern use of extracorporeal life support in pregnancy and postpartum. ASAIO J. 2015;61(1):110-4.
29. Sliwa K, Hilfiker-Kleiner D, Petrie MC, et al. Current state of knowledge on aetiology, diagnosis, management, and therapy of peripartum cardiomyopathy: a position statement from the Heart Failure Association of the European Society of Cardiology Working Group on peripartum cardiomyopathy. Eur J Heart Fail. 2010;12(8):767-78.
30. Davis MB, Arany Z, McNamara DM, et al. Peripartum cardiomyopathy: JACC state-of-the-art review. J Am Coll Cardiol. 2020;75(2):207-21.
31. Combes A, Hajage D, Capellier G, et al. Extracorporeal membrane oxygenation for severe acute respiratory distress syndrome. N Engl J Med. 2018;378(21):1965-75.

32. Bromberger BJ, Agerstrand C, Abrams D, et al. Extracorporeal carbon dioxide removal in the treatment of status asthmaticus. Crit Care Med. 2020;48(12):e1226-e31.

33. Clifford C, Mhatre M, Craigo S. Successful use of extracorporeal membrane oxygenation for status asthmaticus in a woman with a periviable pregnancy. Obstet Gynecol. 2018;132(4):1007-10.

34. Steinack C, Lenherr R, Hendra H, et al. The use of life-saving extracorporeal membrane oxygenation (ECMO) for pregnant woman with status asthmaticus. J Asthma. 2017;54(1):84-8.

35. Creel-Bulos C, Hassani B, Stentz MJ, et al. Extracorporeal membrane oxygenation for amniotic fluid embolism-induced cardiac arrest in the first trimester of pregnancy: a case report. Crit Care Explor. 2020;2(7):e0162.

36. Fan E, Gattinoni L, Combes A, et al. Venovenous extracorporeal membrane oxygenation for acute respiratory failure. Intensive Care Med. 2016;42(5):712-24.

37. Guntupalli KK, Karnad DR, Bandi V, et al. Critical illness in pregnancy: part II: common medical conditions complicating pregnancy and puerperium. Chest. 2015;148(5):1333-45.

38. Lapinsky SE. Acute respiratory failure in pregnancy. Obstet Med. 2015;8(3):126-32.

39. Omo-Aghoja L. Maternal and fetal acid-base chemistry: a major determinant of perinatal outcome. Ann Med Health Sci Res. 2014;4(1):8-17.

40. Levinson G, Shnider SM, DeLorimier AA, et al. Effects of maternal hyperventilation on uterine blood flow and fetal oxygenation and acid-base status. Anesthesiology. 1974;40(4):340-7.

41. Royal College of Obstetricians and Gynecologists. Hypertension in pregnancy: the management of hypertensive disorders during pregnancy. London, UK: RCOG Press. 2010 Aug.

42. ACOG practice bulletin, number 222: Gestational hypertension and preeclampsia. Obstet Gynecol. 2020;135(6):e237-e60.

43. Vigil-De Gracia P, Lasso M, Ruiz E, et al. Severe hypertension in pregnancy: hydralazine or labetalol: a randomized clinical trial. Eur J Obstet Gynecol Reprod Biol. 2006;128(1):157-62.

44. Schmidt M, Tachon G, Devilliers C, et al. Blood oxygenation and decarboxylation determinants during venovenous ECMO for respiratory failure in adults. Intensive Care Med. 2013;39(5):838-46.

45. Catanzarite V, Willms D, Wong D, et al. Acute respiratory distress syndrome in pregnancy and the puerperium: causes, courses, and outcomes. Obstet Gynecol. 2001;97(5 Pt 1):760-4.

46. Yarrington CD, Valente AM, Economy KE. Cardiovascular management in pregnancy. Circulation. 2015;132(14):1354-64.

47. Costantine M. Physiologic and pharmacokinetic changes in pregnancy. Front Pharmacol. 2014;5(65).

48. Shekar K, Fraser JF, Smith MT, et al. Pharmacokinetic changes in patients receiving extracorporeal membrane oxygenation. J Crit Care. 2012;27(6):741.e9-18.

49. Melamed N, Asztalos E, Murphy K, et al. Neurodevelopmental disorders among term infants exposed to antenatal corticosteroids during pregnancy: a population-based study. BMJ Open. 2019;9(9):e031197.

50. ACOG practice bulletin no. 211: critical care in pregnancy. Obstet Gynecol. 2019;133(5):e303-e19.

51. McGoldrick E, Stewart F, Parker R, et al. Antenatal corticosteroids for accelerating fetal lung maturation for women at risk of preterm birth. Cochrane Database Syst Rev. 2020;12(12):Cd004454.

52. Costantine MM, Weiner SJ. Effects of antenatal exposure to magnesium sulfate on neuroprotection and mortality in preterm infants: a meta-analysis. Obstet Gynecol. 2009;114(2 Pt 1):354-64.

53. Anderson NH, Gordon A, Li M, et al. Association of supine going-to-sleep position in late pregnancy with reduced birth weight: a secondary analysis of an individual participant data meta-analysis. JAMA Net Open. 2019;2(10):e1912614.

54. Halscott T, Vaught J, SMFM COVID-19 Task Force. Management considerations for pregnant patients with COVID-19. Society for Maternal Fetal Medicine. Feb 2, 2021. Available at:https://s3.amazonaws.com/cdn.smfm.org/media/2734/SMFM_COVID_Management_of_COVID_pos_preg_patients_2-2-21_(final).pdf. SfM-FMSMcfppwC-aJAf. Accessed Jan 31, 2022.

55. Aziz A, Ona S, Martinez RH, et al. Building an obstetric intensive care unit during the COVID-19 pandemic at a tertiary hospital and selected maternal-fetal and delivery considerations. Semin Perinatol. 2020;44(7):151298.

56. Combs CA, Einerson BD, Toner LE. Society for Maternal-Fetal Medicine special statement: surgical safety checklists for cesarean delivery. Am J Obstet Gynecol. 2021;225(5):B43-b9.

57. Guntupalli KK, Hall N, Karnad DR, et al. Critical illness in pregnancy: part I: an approach to a pregnant patient in the ICU and common obstetric disorders. Chest. 2015;148(4):1093-104.

58. Shamshirsaz AA, Clark SL. Amniotic fluid embolism. Obstet Gynecol Clin North Am. 2016;43(4):779-90.

59. ACOG Practice Bulletin No. 183: Postpartum Hemorrhage. Obstet Gynecol. 2017;130(4):e168-e86.

60. Merriam AA, Wright JD, Siddiq Z, et al. Risk for postpartum hemorrhage, transfusion, and

hemorrhage-related morbidity at low, moderate, and high volume hospitals. J Matern Fetal Neonatal Med. 2018;31(8):1025-34.

61. Acosta CD, Kurinczuk JJ, Lucas DN, et al. Severe maternal sepsis in the UK, 2011-2012: a national case-control study. PLoS Med. 2014;11(7):e1001672.

62. Bauer ME, Housey M, Bauer ST, et al. Risk factors, etiologies, and screening tools for sepsis in pregnant Women: a multicenter case-control study. Anesth Analg. 2019;129(6):1613-20.

63. Mhyre JM, D'Oria R, Hameed AB, et al. The maternal early warning criteria: a proposal from the national partnership for maternal safety. Obstet Gynecol. 2014;124(4):782-6.

64. Ramanathan K, Tan CS, Rycus P, et al. Extracorporeal membrane oxygenation in pregnancy: an analysis of the extracorporeal life support organization registry. Crit Care Med. 2020;48(5):696-703.

65. Taha B, Guglielminotti J, Li G, et al. Utilization and outcomes of extracorporeal membrane oxygenation in obstetric patients in the United States, 1999-2014: a retrospective cross-sectional study. Anesth Analg. 2022 Aug 1;135(2):268-276.

66. Freedman RL, Lucas DN. MBRRACE-UK: saving lives, improving mothers' care - implications for anaesthetists. Int J Obstet Anesth. 2015;24(2):161-73.

67. Zhang JJY, Ong JA, Syn NL, et al. Extracorporeal membrane oxygenation in pregnant and postpartum women: a systematic review and meta-regression analysis. J Intensive Care Med. 2021;36(2):220-8.

# 35

## Trauma and Environmental Injury

*Justyna Swol, Robert B. Laverty, Erik DeSoucy, Shingo Ichiba, Jeremy W. Cannon*

## Introduction

Unintentional injuries are the leading cause of death in the U.S. for ages ≤44, for which the mortality burden is far greater at younger ages.[1] Hemorrhagic shock is the leading cause of preventable mortality following trauma,[2,3] and, for those that survive the initial hemorrhagic insult, multiorgan failure further contributes to mortality in this population.[4,5] Respiratory failure is the most common type of organ failure seen in these patients and is also associated with the highest mortality.[6] Historically, acute respiratory distress syndrome (ARDS) occurs upwards of 30% of patients with severe traumatic brain injury and 5-10% of all severely injured patients, a figure which appears to be decreasing over time, likely due to advances in lung protective ventilation strategies and reduction in crystalloid based resuscitation.[7,8] ARDS is associated with mortality rates of 19-26% in patients following blunt and penetrating trauma, a figure which unfortunately has remained unchanged over the last few decades.[9-11]

The first ever clinical application of ECLS was in 1972 for an adult trauma patient following a motor vehicle crash, who sustained an aortic injury and developed respiratory failure after open repair. He was ultimately trialed on VA ECMO and survived to hospital discharge.[12]

Over the last 10 years, there has been a marked increase in ECLS use in trauma patients as shown in results from the ELSO Registry (Figure 35-1).[13] This chapter will provide an overview of indications and management of ECLS in adult and pediatric trauma patients. Military ECLS data is presented along with its application to the civilian setting, mass casualty events, blast lung injury, and burns. We also provide an overview of ECLS for environmental injuries such as hypothermia and Tsunami lung, an entity mechanistically similar to near drowning.

## Patient Selection

### Respiratory Failure

For patients with reversible injuries, ECLS can offer supplemental cardiopulmonary capacity in the early resuscitation phase for patients with specific injury patterns (eg, mainstem bronchial injury) and during treatment of secondary complications (eg, ARDS). Chest injuries cause many deaths every year and blunt thoracic trauma is an especially vexing mechanism of injury in severely injured trauma patients. The blunt force of the injury typically produces an underlying pulmonary contusion, decreased functional lung volume, shunt, and ventilation-perfusion mismatch leading to respiratory failure. Indications for the initiation of ECLS in trauma patients largely mirror those in other populations; respiratory failure is the most cited indication and initiation should be considered when patients meet criteria according to ELSO guidelines.[14] Pulmonary contusions, inhalation injuries, blast injury, direct tissue injury, and atelectasis can all lead to ARDS. In the setting of tracheal-bronchial tree disruption, profound hypoventilation may result, and ECLS cannulation is lifesaving, acting as a bridge to further reconstructive surgery.[15] VV ECMO is typically used in these patients.[10,13,16-20] Retrospective cohort studies have reported survival rates ranging from 44% to 87% in trauma patients.[20-27]

**Burns and Inhalation Injury**

Patients with severe burns develop a vasodilatory, hyperdynamic state secondary to activation of systemic inflammatory mediators from thermal dermal injury and require large amounts of initial fluid resuscitation. These patients are at high risk for pulmonary edema as well as pneumonitis and pneumonia due to inhalation injury, direct thermal airway injury, and sepsis. Respiratory failure is the major cause of mortality in burn injury. ECLS provides time for lung recovery in the setting of inhalation injury with or without cutaneous burns.[28,29] Early debridement is a tenant of modern burn care. However, these procedures may be performed while on ECLS, if necessary, with the expectation of significant blood product transfusion requirements. Increases in oxygen consumption and cardiac output can be difficult to overcome with VV ECMO due to failure to capture a high enough proportion of the venous return. Configuration change with an additional oxygenator may be helpful in this situation.[30] Scald burns show a tendency of higher survival than flame burns.[28,29] The survival rate for ECLS in burn patients ranges between 17%

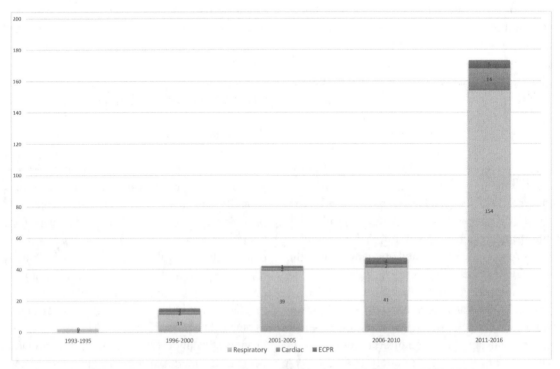

**Figure 35-1.** ECLS runs in trauma reported in the ELSO Registry 1993-2021.

and 66%[31] for adults and between 53% and 67% in children.[32] According to retrospective data from the ELSO Registry, overall survival to hospital discharge of 58 adult burn patients with severe ARDS was 43%. Multivariate logistic regression analysis identified acidosis (pH <7.16) and use of inotropic/vasopressors before ECLS as risk factors associated with increased risk of mortality. Non survivors had higher rates of renal replacement therapy utilization (70% vs. 36%, p=0.016).[18,33]

### *Blast Lung Injury*

Blast lung injury (BLI) is the result of exposure to the primary blast wave and the sudden increase in pressure associated with detonation of traditional explosive munitions or improvised explosive devices during combat or terrorist attacks. Primary BLI is defined as "radiological and clinical evidence of acute lung injury occurring within 12 hours of exposure and not due to secondary or tertiary injury."[34,35] Explosions produce high pressure energy waves and extreme heat, inducing direct lung injury. Blast survivors often also exhibit sequelae of the secondary and tertiary effects including penetrating and blunt trauma, hemorrhage, pneumothorax, and may develop multiorgan failure.[36] Blast lung injury can be rapidly fatal in up to 20% of patients.[34,35,37] Chest x-rays often show a 'butterfly' pattern in the initial stage (Figure 35-2)[36] which is characterized by diffuse alveolar edema secondary to the inflammatory-mediated capillary permeability, often beginning within the first 72 hours of injury, and lasting between 7 and 10 days.[38] Although published experience with BLI supported on ECLS is still very limited, early implementation of ECLS in battlefield hospitals has been shown to improve survival in combat injured patients.[38] Advances in ECLS technology have extended the use of this lifesaving device to resource-limited austere medical facilities to stabilize combat injured patients with severe respiratory failure unresponsive to lung protective ventilatory strategies.[27,39,40]

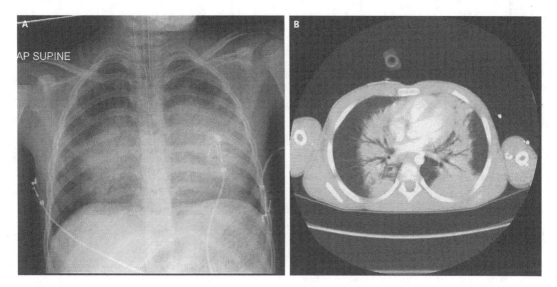

**Figure 35-2.** "Butterfly" pattern in the initial stage of blast lung injury when an improvised explosive device detonated very close to the 8 years old boy. With permission from Barnhard et al., NEJM 2013.[36]

## Cardiogenic Shock and Cardiac Arrest in Trauma

ECLS may also be used in the setting of cardiogenic shock or cardiac arrest, which is known to occur following traumatic injuries.[41,42] Indications for ECLS cannulation include myocardial contusion, cardiac arrest, and impairments in cardiac output unresponsive to conventional cardiopulmonary resuscitation and support. A recent review of the ELSO Registry reported survival to hospital discharge rates of 50% in trauma patients supported on ECLS following cardiac failure and 25% for those rescued with ECPR.[13] These patients are managed with a VA configuration to provide both gas exchange and perfusion support. Similarly, trauma patients who underwent a resuscitative thoracotomy and were then immediately cannulated for ECLS were shown to have survival rates of 48% and a trend towards improved mortality versus those who underwent resuscitative thoracotomy alone.[4] However, it is important to keep in mind that some of these patients may have had noncardiac causes for arrest such as tension pneumothorax or exsanguination. Work in this area is ongoing and includes clinical trials such as induced deep hypothermia after traumatic arrest to preserve brain function (ClinicalTrials.gov Identifier: NCT01042015). Population demographics can influence trauma epidemiology and associated risks of cardiovascular events leading to cardiogenic shock in need of ECLS support. Thus, aging individuals may suffer severe injury (eg, when driving) following myocardial infarction[44] and blunt thoracic trauma can cause acute myocardial infarction.[45] Thus, evaluation of underlying cardiac function and coronary perfusion is recommended.

## Bleeding and Hemorrhagic Shock

Patients who have severe but potentially survivable injuries treated may still succumb to the compounding effects of hypovolemic shock, hypoxemia, hypothermia, metabolic acidosis, and coagulopathy. However, trauma related bleeding conditions and coagulopathies have previously been considered contraindications for the use of ECLS. While ECLS is not a direct therapy for coagulopathy, when used without anticoagulation it can correct hypercarbia and hypoxemia, ameliorate metabolic acidosis, help to restore hemodynamic stability and correct hypothermia, thus addressing at least 2 of the components of the 'triad of death' and serving as a bridge to surgical or endovascular intervention for hemorrhage control.[41,46] Endovascular interventions such as thoracic aorta endovascular repair (TEVAR) and resuscitative endovascular balloon occlusion of the aorta (REBOA) are relatively new adjuncts in the management of the trauma patient and have reported improved mortality over their open alternatives.[47,48] In cases of distal malperfusion due to the aortic injury morphology or the need for aortic cross clamping during surgery, cannulation for ECLS has been reported to preserve distal aortic perfusion while awaiting definitive repair or when bypass is not available.[49,50]

## Special Considerations

The use of ECLS in patients with traumatic brain injuries (TBI) remains controversial due to the recommendation for anticoagulation and the risk of lethal intracerebral bleeding.[51] However, a prolonged (>5 days) anticoagulation-free ECLS course is possible.[52] In TBI patients, femoral-femoral cannulation for VV ECMO should be considered standard due to the risk of jugular venous outflow obstruction from internal jugular cannulation. A systematic review reported survival rates of 60%-93% in patients with TBI who were subsequently placed on ECLS.[7,53] These studies demonstrated a trend towards lower anticoagulation use in these patients and no deaths related to intracranial hemorrhage.[54]

Special consideration for ECLS should be given to patients with certain injuries that can make conventional management of ARDS difficult, such as those with spinal cord injuries which may preclude the use of head of bed elevation and proning.[14] Other unique populations are those with extremity injuries in whom consideration should be given to modifying ECLS cannulation approaches to avoid exacerbating ischemic limb injuries by obstructing arterial inflow or venous outflow.[16,55,56]

**Pediatric Patients**

ECLS in pediatric trauma patients has comparable survival to other ELSO cohorts undergoing ECLS for non-traumatic causes.[57] Drowning (38.7%) was the most common mechanism, followed by burns (21.1%), and thoracic trauma (17.8%). The majority of patients (62.3%) were male and on VA ECMO (54.5%) in a cohort of 573 patients with a median age of 4.82 years identified in the ELSO Registry. Complication rates were high (at 81.9%), with the most frequent types being cardiovascular, mechanical, and hemorrhagic. However, the incidence of complications (overall and by type) was similar to those reported in other ELSO cohorts. Overall survival was 55.3%; 74.3% for patients on VV ECMO compared to 41.7% for those on VA ECMO.[57]

**Special Considerations in Environmental Injury**

*Severe Accidental Hypothermia*

Severe accidental hypothermia, defined by a core temperature <28° C, is a special cause of cardiac arrest associated with significant morbidity and mortality but potentially good neurological outcomes.[58] A recent metaanalysis reported a mean survival rate of 46% and good neurologic outcome in 40% of patients requiring ECLS for accidental hypothermia.[59]

The Hypothermia Outcome Prediction after ECLS (HOPE) score, also available as an online calculator at www.hypothermiascore.org, was developed as a predictive algorithm to determine the survival probabilities of these patients.[60] Advocates called a cutoff of ≥10% predicted survival to use extracorporeal rewarming, generally performed via VA ECMO.[61]

Hypothermic patients with asystole may be rewarmed with ECLS until the inhibited myocardium resumes electrical activity (usually around 28-30° C), with shockable rhythm defibrillation being required to achieve the return of spontaneous circulation (ROSC). At core temperatures <30° C, ventricular fibrillation is often resistant to pharmacotherapy and defibrillation; however, it may be successful when ECLS provides adequate blood flow and a stable rate of rewarming.[61] After ROSC, normothermia (35-36° C) is recommended during the first 24 hours.[62] Rapid rewarming rates of about 4-5° C/hour are recommended until ROSC and adequate perfusion, followed by slower rewarming at 1-2° C/hour. After ROSC patients often develop severe coagulopathy and multiple organ failure, with cardiac and respiratory failure requiring further advanced organ support with ECLS beyond initial rewarming.[63] Normothermia, along with stabilized metabolic, hemodynamic, and pulmonary function are the requirements for ECLS weaning and decannulation.[61]

*Submersion and Nonfatal Drowning During Tsunami*

Drowning in a tsunami wave is considered to differ markedly from drowning in fresh or saltwater bodies. The landfall during a tsunami carries various objects along with it (eg, soil, sand, buildings, vehicles, dust/wastes, oil, etc.). Aspiration of these contaminants lead to severe lung damage called 'tsunami lung,' characterized by a combination of chemical induced pneumonitis and bacterial pneumonia affecting the entire lung.[64] Most victims will die of drowning. Those who survive transport to a medical facility should be closely monitored for progressive respiratory failure due to tsunami lung. Due to resource limitations during disaster and mass casualty events, case reports of tsunami lung managed with ECLS are sparse.

## Contraindications

Patient selection for ECLS support in trauma incorporates thoughtful consideration of the injury severity, prognosis and possibility for definitive therapy, the patient's age and comorbidities, severity of cardiopulmonary dysfunction, the physiology and state of other organs dysfunction (eg, brain, kidney, and liver), and resource availability.[13,19] Patients with confirmed or suspected nonsurvivable injuries should not be placed on ECLS, although the extracorporeal organ support has been utilized in some cases as a bridge to organ donation, although this may present additional ethical and legal hurdles (Chapter 45).

## Anticoagulation

A recent systematic review of trauma patients on ECLS showed that 86% received systemic anticoagulation, largely with unfractionated heparin.[65] Activated clotting time and activated partial thromboplastin time were the two most common laboratory assays used for monitoring, with therapeutic goals of 180-220 sec and 40-80 sec, respectively.[65] Viscoelastic testing thromboelastography (TEG) and rotational thromboelastometry (ROTEM) can also be used to monitor anticoagulation during ECLS.[66] The heparinase assay can be particularly useful uncovering underlying coagulopathy independent of heparin that can be addressed with targeted therapeutic interventions. Heparin-bonded circuits are also available and have been shown to decrease the need for systemic anticoagulation in trauma patients.[41] ECLS runs without anticoagulation for a limited time is possible while the primary injuries are being evaluated and treated.[52]

Furthermore, a combination of traumatic, hemodilution, and ECLS-induced coagulopathy may occur. When possible, correct preexisting coagulopathy, with general goals being an INR ≤1.5, platelet count ≥50 k, and fibrinogen ≥150 mg/dL. Patients who develop bleeding complications on ECLS should be evaluated promptly for need of surgical or procedural intervention. Consideration should be given to the cessation of systemic anticoagulation and initiation of aminocaproic acid or tranexamic acid, both of which have been shown to decrease rates of surgical site bleeding in pediatric patients on ECLS.[67,68]

## Surgery During ECLS

Trauma patients on ECLS may have a need for operative intervention during their hospitalization (Chapter 51). Hemostasis, however, remains challenging given all the aforementioned factors. It may also be difficult to define bleeding from operative sites after ECLS started vs. bleeding as a complication of surgery while already on ECLS. Retrospective reviews have suggested it is safe to perform required surgical procedures but with expected increased rates of postoperative bleeding complications.[69] Development of hemothoraces, pneumothoraces, or pleural effusions requiring tube thoracostomy is another known clinical sequela in these patients. These can typically be managed with a small-bore (14 Fr) pigtail catheter without the need for holding anticoagulation. Patients managed with ECLS for a protracted period of time will also commonly need conversion to tracheostomy during their stay.[70] Early tracheostomy during the first 10-14 days after intubation bridges to spontaneous breathing and weaning from mechanical ventilation[71] and can be safely performed in this population. Higher rates of bleeding may be seen when performed via a percutaneous technique.[72,73] Institutional protocols vary, but most hold anticoagulation 1-6 hours prior to the procedure.

## Complications

As alluded to, the most common complications seen in trauma patients on ECLS are bleeding and thrombosis, underscoring the need for meticulous anticoagulation management. A systematic review reported bleeding rates of 23%, most commonly from surgical sites followed by cannulation sites.[65] Furthermore, 19% of patients had a thrombotic complication, with femoral deep vein thrombosis reported as the most common followed by clotting of the oxygenator and/or circuit. Less commonly reported complications include abdominal compartment syndrome, cannula dislodgement, access site injury (acute limb ischemia), and need for fasciotomy.

## Outcomes and Survival

Retrospective cohort studies in trauma patients on ECLS for respiratory support have reported survival rates ranging from 44%-87%, several of which demonstrated a survival benefit when matched to controls treated with conventional ventilation management alone.[20-27] More recent retrospective reviews, however, have reported improved survival rates and show that the number of trauma facilities utilizing ECLS has been increasing over recent years to include use by the U.S. Department of Defense for severely injured civilian and military patients.[14,16]

## Conclusion

The decision to initiate ECLS in trauma patients is complex and should involve a multidisciplinary team. The strongest evidence remains for respiratory failure refractory to conventional ventilatory management, but emerging data supports use in the setting of severe thoracic trauma including blast injury, traumatic brain injuries, and burns. ECLS in the setting of traumatic arrest is an area of active, ongoing research. For trauma patients managed on ECLS, teams must balance the risk of bleeding and thrombotic complications in this patient population and closely monitor anticoagulation regimens.

## References

1. Heron M. Deaths: Leading Causes for 2019. Natl Vital Stat Rep. 2021;70(9):1-114.
2. Sauaia A, Moore FA, Moore EE, et al. Epidemiology of trauma deaths: a reassessment. J Trauma. 1995;38(2):185-93.
3. Cannon JW. Hemorrhagic Shock. N Engl J Med. 2018;378(4):370-9.
4. Trunkey DD. Trauma. Accidental and intentional injuries account for more years of life lost in the U.S. than cancer and heart disease. Among the prescribed remedies are improved preventive efforts, speedier surgery and further research. Sci Am. 1983;249(2):28-35.
5. Eastridge BJ, Holcomb JB, Shackelford S. Outcomes of traumatic hemorrhagic shock and the epidemiology of preventable death from injury. Transfusion. 2019;59(S2):1423-8.
6. Regel G, Grotz M, Weltner T, et al. Pattern of organ failure following severe trauma. World J Surg. 1996;20(4):422-9.
7. Bedeir K, Seethala R, Kelly E. Extracorporeal life support in trauma: Worth the risks? A systematic review of published series. J Trauma Acute Care Surg. 2017;82(2):400-6.
8. Aisiku IP, Yamal JM, Doshi P, et al. The incidence of ARDS and associated mortality in severe TBI using the Berlin definition. J Trauma Acute Care Surg. 2016;80(2):308-12.
9. Navarrete-Navarro P, Rodriguez A, Reynolds N, et al. Adult respiratory distress syndrome among blunt and penetrating trauma patients: demographics, mortality, and resource utilization over 8 years. J Crit Care. 2001;16(2):47-53.
10. Birkner DR, Halvachizadeh S, Pape HC, et al. Mortality of Adult Respiratory Distress Syndrome in Trauma Patients: A Systematic Review over a Period of Four Decades. World J Surg. 2020;44(7):2243-54.
11. Fahr M, Jones G, O'Neal H, et al. Acute Respiratory Distress Syndrome Incidence, But Not Mortality, Has Decreased Nationwide: A National Trauma Data Bank Study. Am Surg. 2017;83(4):323-31.
12. Hill JD, O'Brien TG, Murray JJ, et al. Prolonged extracorporeal oxygenation for acute post-traumatic respiratory failure (shock-lung syndrome). Use of the Bramson membrane lung. N Engl J Med. 1972;286(12):629-34.
13. Swol J, Brodie D, Napolitano L, et al. Indications and outcomes of extracorporeal life support in trauma patients. J Trauma Acute Care Surg. 2018;84(6):831-7.
14. Cannon JW, Gutsche JT, Brodie D. Optimal Strategies for Severe Acute Respiratory Distress Syndrome. Crit Care Clin. 2017;33(2):259-75.
15. Zhou R, Liu B, Lin K, et al. ECMO support for right main bronchial disruption in multiple trauma patient with brain injury--a case report and literature review. Perfusion. 2015;30(5):403-6.
16. Ainsworth CR, Dellavolpe J, Chung KK, et al. Revisiting extracorporeal membrane oxygenation for ARDS in burns: A case series and review of the literature. Burns. 2018;44(6):1433-8.
17. Burke CR, Chan T, Brogan TV, et al. Extracorporeal life support for victims of drowning. Resuscitation. 2016;104:19-23.
18. Burke CR, Chan T, McMullan DM. Extracorporeal Life Support Use in Adult Burn Patients. J Burn Care Res. 2017;38(3):174-8.
19. Swol J, Belohlavek J, Brodie D, et al. Extracorporeal life support in the emergency department: A narrative review for the emergency physician. Resuscitation. 2018;133:108-17.
20. Ull C, Schildhauer TA, Strauch JT, Swol J. Outcome measures of extracorporeal life support (ECLS) in trauma patients versus patients without trauma: a 7-year single-center retrospective cohort study. J Artif Organs. 2017;20(2):117-24.
21. Cordell-Smith JA, Roberts N, Peek GJ, et al. Traumatic lung injury treated by extracorporeal membrane oxygenation (ECMO). Injury. 2006;37(1):29-32.
22. Guirand DM, Okoye OT, Schmidt BS, et al. Venovenous extracorporeal life support improves survival in adult trauma patients with acute hypoxemic respiratory failure: a multicenter retrospective cohort study. J Trauma Acute Care Surg. 2014;76(5):1275-81.
23. Bosarge PL, Raff LA, McGwin G, et al. Early initiation of extracorporeal membrane oxygenation improves survival in adult trauma patients with severe adult respiratory distress syndrome. J Trauma Acute Care Surg. 2016;81(2):236-43.
24. Munoz J, Santa-Teresa P, Tomey MJ, et al. Extracorporeal membrane oxygenation (ECMO) in adults with acute respiratory distress syndrome (ARDS): A 6-year experience and case-control study. Heart Lung. 2017;46(2):100-5.
25. Ahmad SB, Menaker J, Kufera J, et al. Extracorporeal membrane oxygenation after traumatic injury. J Trauma Acute Care Surg. 2017;82(3):587-91.
26. Ahmed N, Kuo YH, Pratt A. Outcomes of Extracorporeal Membrane Oxygenation in Acute Respiratory Distress Syndrome Following Traumatic Injury: A Propensity-Matched Analysis. Crit Care Explor. 2021;3(5):e0421.
27. Piper LC, Nam JJ, Kuckelman JP, et al. A Case Report of Combat Blast Injury Requiring Combat Casualty Care, Far-Forward ECMO, Air Transport, and All Levels of Military Critical Care. Mil Med. 2021.

28. Asmussen S, Maybauer DM, Fraser JF, et al. Extracorporeal membrane oxygenation in burn and smoke inhalation injury. Burns. 2013;39(3):429-35.

29. Nelson J, Cairns B, Charles A. Early extracorporeal life support as rescue therapy for severe acute respiratory distress syndrome after inhalation injury. J Burn Care Res. 2009;30(6):1035-8.

30. Szentgyorgyi L, Shepherd C, Dunn KW, et al. Extracorporeal membrane oxygenation in severe respiratory failure resulting from burns and smoke inhalation injury. Burns. 2018;44(5):1091-9.

31. Hsu PS, Tsai YT, Lin CY, et al. Benefit of extracorporeal membrane oxygenation in major burns after stun grenade explosion: Experience from a single military medical center. Burns. 2017;43(3):674-80.

32. Watson JA, Englum BR, Kim J, et al. Extracorporeal life support use in pediatric trauma: a review of the National Trauma Data Bank. J Pediatr Surg. 2017;52(1):136-9.

33. Song H, Yuan Z, Peng Y, Luo G. Extracorporeal membrane oxygenation combined with continuous renal replacement therapy for the treatment of severe burns: current status and challenges. Burns & trauma. 2021;9:tkab017-tkab.

34. Mackenzie I, Tunnicliffe B, Clasper J, et al. What the Intensive Care Doctor Needs to Know about Blast-Related Lung Injury. Journal of the Intensive Care Society. 2013;14(4):303-12.

35. Mackenzie IM, Tunnicliffe B. Blast injuries to the lung: epidemiology and management. Philos Trans R Soc Lond B Biol Sci. 2011;366(1562):295-9.

36. Barnard E, Johnston A. Blast Lung. New England Journal of Medicine. 2013;368(11):1045.

37. Boutillier J, Deck C, Magnan P, et al. A critical literature review on primary blast thorax injury and their outcomes. J Trauma Acute Care Surg. 2016;81(2):371-9.

38. Mohamed MAT, Maraqa T, Bacchetta MD, et al. The Feasibility of Venovenous ECMO at Role-2 Facilities in Austere Military Environments. Mil Med. 2018;183(9-10):e644-e8.

39. Bein T, Zonies D, Philipp A, et al. Transportable extracorporeal lung support for rescue of severe respiratory failure in combat casualties. J Trauma Acute Care Surg. 2012;73(6):1450-6.

40. Read MD, Nam JJ, Biscotti M, et al. Evolution of the United States Military Extracorporeal Membrane Oxygenation Transport Team. Military Medicine. 2020;185(11-12):e2055-e60.

41. Arlt M, Philipp A, Voelkel S, et al. Extracorporeal membrane oxygenation in severe trauma patients with bleeding shock. Resuscitation. 2010;81(7):804-9.

42. Tisherman SA, Alam HB, Rhee PM, et al. Development of the emergency preservation and resuscitation for cardiac arrest from trauma clinical trial. J Trauma Acute Care Surg. 2017;83(5):803-9.

43. Owattanapanich N, Inaba K, Allen B, et al. Extracorporeal Membrane Oxygenation May Improve Outcomes After Resuscitative Thoracotomy: A National Trauma Data Bank Analysis. Am Surg. 2021 Dec;87(10):1565-1568.

44. Alkhouli M, Alqahtani F. Incidence and Outcomes of Acute Myocardial Infarction During Motor Vehicle Accident Related Hospitalizations. American Journal of Cardiology. 2019;123(5):725-8.

45. Kara H, Avcı A, Akinci M, et al. Blunt chest trauma as a cause of acute myocardial infarction. Acta Clin Belg. 2014;69(5):367-70.

46. Willers A, Swol J, Kowalewski M, et al. Extracorporeal Life Support in Hemorrhagic Conditions: A Systematic Review. ASAIO J. 2021;67(5):476-84.

47. Xenos ES, Abedi NN, Davenport DL, et al. Meta-analysis of endovascular vs open repair for traumatic descending thoracic aortic rupture. J Vasc Surg. 2008;48(5):1343-51.

48. Brenner M, Inaba K, Aiolfi A, et al. Resuscitative Endovascular Balloon Occlusion of the Aorta and Resuscitative Thoracotomy in Select Patients with Hemorrhagic Shock: Early Results from the American Association for the Surgery of Trauma's Aortic Occlusion in Resuscitation for Trauma and Acute Care Surgery Registry. J Am Coll Surg. 2018;226(5):730-40.

49. Wada D, Hayakawa K, Kanayama S, et al. A case of blunt thoracic aortic injury requiring ECMO for acute malperfusion before TEVAR. Scand J Trauma Resusc Emerg Med. 2017;25(1):110.

50. Huang SC, Chen YS, Wang SS, et al. Extracorporeal membrane oxygenation support during repair of traumatic aortic transection. Journal of the Formosan Medical Association = Taiwan yi zhi. 2005;104(9):677-80.

51. Muellenbach RM, Redel A, Kustermann J, et al. [Extracorporeal membrane oxygenation and severe traumatic brain injury. Is the ECMO-therapy in traumatic lung failure and severe traumatic brain injury really contraindicated?]. Anaesthesist. 2011;60(7):647-52.

52. Muellenbach RM, Kredel M, Kunze E, et al. Prolonged heparin-free extracorporeal membrane oxygenation in multiple injured acute respiratory distress syndrome patients with traumatic brain injury. J Trauma Acute Care Surg. 2012;72(5):1444-7.

53. Menut R, Larrieu N, Conil JM, et al. Use of ECMO (extracorporeal membrane oxygenation) in a traumatic brain injured patient with severe hypoxemia. Ann Fr Anesth Reanim. 2013;32(10):701-3.

54. Biscotti M, Gannon WD, Abrams D, et al. Extracorporeal membrane oxygenation use in

patients with traumatic brain injury. Perfusion. 2015;30(5):407-9.

55. Soussi S, Gallais P, Kachatryan L, et al. Extracorporeal membrane oxygenation in burn patients with refractory acute respiratory distress syndrome leads to 28 % 90-day survival. Intensive Care Med. 2016;42(11):1826-7.

56. Eldredge RS, Zhai Y, Cochran A. Effectiveness of ECMO for burn-related acute respiratory distress syndrome. Burns. 2019;45(2):317-21.

57. Behr CA, Strotmeyer SJ, Swol J, et al. Characteristics and outcomes of extracorporeal life support in pediatric trauma patients. J Trauma Acute Care Surg. 2020;89(4):631-5.

58. Dow J, Giesbrecht GG, Danzl DF, et al. Wilderness Medical Society Clinical Practice Guidelines for the Out-of-Hospital Evaluation and Treatment of Accidental Hypothermia: 2019 Update. Wilderness & Environmental Medicine. 2019;30(4):S47-S69.

59. Saczkowski RS, Brown DJA, Abu-Laban RB, et al. Prediction and risk stratification of survival in accidental hypothermia requiring extracorporeal life support: An individual patient data meta-analysis. Resuscitation. 2018;127:51-7.

60. Pasquier M, Hugli O, Paal P, et al. Hypothermia outcome prediction after extracorporeal life support for hypothermic cardiac arrest patients: The HOPE score. Resuscitation. 2018;126:58-64.

61. Swol J, Darocha T, Paal P, et al. Extracorporeal Life Support in Accidental Hypothermia with Cardiac Arrest-A Narrative Review. ASAIO J. 2021.

62. Carsten Lott AT, Anette Alfonzo, Alessandro Barelli, et al. European Resuscitation Council Guidelines for Cardiac arrest in special circumstances 2020. Resuscitation 2021;in press.

63. Kosinski S, Pasquier M, Podsiadlo P, et al. The role of extracorporeal life support in patients with hypothermic cardiac arrest. Resuscitation. 2019;134:157-8.

64. Inoue Y, Fujino Y, Onodera M, et al. Tsunami lung. J Anesth. 2012;26(2):246-9.

65. Wang C, Zhang L, Qin T, et al. Extracorporeal membrane oxygenation in trauma patients: a systematic review. World J Emerg Surg. 2020;15(1):51.

66. Panigada M, G EI, Brioni M, et al. Thromboelastography-based anticoagulation management during extracorporeal membrane oxygenation: a safety and feasibility pilot study. Ann Intensive Care. 2018;8(1):7.

67. Downard CD, Betit P, Chang RW, et al. Impact of AMICAR on hemorrhagic complications of ECMO: a ten-year review. J Pediatr Surg. 2003;38(8):1212-6.

68. van der Staak FH, de Haan AF, et al. Surgical repair of congenital diaphragmatic hernia during extracorporeal membrane oxygenation: hemorrhagic complications and the effect of tranexamic acid. J Pediatr Surg. 1997;32(4):594-9.

69. Ried M, Bein T, Philipp A, et al. Extracorporeal lung support in trauma patients with severe chest injury and acute lung failure: a 10-year institutional experience. Critical care. 2013;17(3):R110.

70. Swol J, Strauch JT, Schildhauer TA. Tracheostomy as a bridge to spontaneous breathing and awake-ECMO in non-transplant surgical patients. European Journal of Heart Failure. 2017;19:120-3.

71. Swol J, Shekar K, Protti A, et al. Extubate Before Venovenous Extracorporeal Membranous Oxygenation Decannulation or Decannulate While Remaining on the Ventilator? The EuroELSO 2019 Weaning Survey. ASAIO J. 2021;67(4):e86-e9.

72. Salna M, Tipograf Y, Liou P, et al. Tracheostomy Is Safe During Extracorporeal Membrane Oxygenation Support. ASAIO J. 2020;66(6):652-6.

73. Kelley KM, Galvagno SM, Wallis M, et al. Tracheostomy in Patients on Venovenous Extracorporeal Membrane Oxygenation: Is It Safe? Am Surg. 2021;87(8):1292-8.

# 36

## Septic Shock

*Graeme MacLaren, Nicolas Bréchot, Warwick Butt*

## Introduction

In adult patients, sepsis is defined as "life-threatening organ dysfunction caused by a dysregulated host response to infection," while septic shock is a "subset of sepsis in which underlying circulatory, cellular, and metabolic abnormalities are associated with a greater risk of mortality than sepsis alone."[1] In practical terms, adult septic shock is infection associated with: 1) persistent hypotension requiring vasopressors to maintain a mean arterial pressure ≥65 mmHg and 2) a serum lactate >2 mmol/L despite fluid resuscitation.[1] Known as Sepsis-3, these definitions were conceived, validated, and applied without consideration for children. While the general underlying principles may be applied to children, they have not been validated in large cohorts and have not yet been widely adopted in pediatric medicine.

Sepsis was historically regarded as a contraindication to ECLS. In the 1990s, however, a number of studies demonstrated that it could be potentially lifesaving in neonatal and pediatric septic shock,[2-5] a view strengthened by later reports involving larger numbers of patients.[6-9] ECLS for refractory septic shock in neonates is now regarded as a standard indication, with in-hospital survival rates of approximately 75-80%.[10,11] However, universal acceptance of ECLS for septic shock in older

patients has been limited by retrospective study designs, historically poor outcomes in some centers, lack of comparative evaluation of cannulation strategies, and perhaps by an underappreciation of the pathophysiological and hemodynamic responses to infection with changes in age. The most common hemodynamic pattern of septic shock in adult patients, distributive shock, is widely regarded as a contraindication to ECLS in the absence of other indications because of poor outcomes.[12]

Sepsis is associated with only one pulmonary pathophysiological response, acute respiratory distress syndrome (ARDS); but several hemodynamic responses, including dilation and failure of one or both ventricles, an increase in pulmonary vascular resistance, and a fall in systemic vascular resistance, all may exist in relative isolation or in combination.[10] ECLS can be used to support patients with sepsis and any combination of:

- ARDS
- Right heart failure
- Left heart failure, and/or
- Distributive shock.

This chapter will outline the indications and contraindications for ECLS in sepsis; review the hemodynamic responses to infection in patients of all ages and the implications these have for cannulation; discuss circuit management in sepsis; and summarize outcomes. The chapter will focus on the use of ECLS as mechanical circulatory support in refractory septic shock, which requires more detailed consideration than isolated respiratory failure from sepsis.

## Indications

Pneumonia or sepsis-induced ARDS usually presents without the need for mechanical circulatory support, in which case the indication for ECLS is similar to other causes of hypoxic respiratory failure (Chapters 8, 13, 23). Some of these patients may have hypotension caused by severe hypoxia, hypercapnia, pulmonary hypertension, and right heart dysfunction. However, these secondary cardiovascular effects usually improve substantially with venovenous (VV) ECMO, with its attendant benefits on oxygenation, acid-base balance, carbon dioxide, temperature, and intrathoracic pressure.

In neonatal and pediatric septic shock, the use of ECLS as mechanical circulatory support is regarded as a therapy of last resort, when refractory shock progresses despite all attempts at ventilatory strategies, fluid, pharmacological, and disease-modifying therapy, or when cardiac arrest has occurred. One study of 80 children receiving VA ECMO for refractory septic shock demonstrated that ECMO was associated with better outcomes only if the predicted risk of mortality was >50%.[9] The rapidity of shock progression and physiological decline is more important than the absolute amount of inotropic support, but in general, ECLS should be considered if a child:

- is receiving doses of >0.8-1 mcg/kg/min of epinephrine or its equivalent (ie, an inotrope score[13] >80-100)
- has had adequate fluid resuscitation and other appropriate pharmacological strategies[10,14]
- continues to deteriorate with rising lactate, acidosis, worsening hypotension or multiorgan dysfunction.

In adult septic shock, several observational series have demonstrated poor outcomes with the use of ECLS for distributive shock.[15-17] More recently, a study of 82 adult patients demonstrated that the use of VA ECMO in refractory sepsis-induced cardiogenic shock was associated with decreased mortality compared to 130 matched controls.[18] The indications for ECMO in this study were:

- hemodynamic compromise, defined as an inotrope score >75 or serum lactate >4 mmol/L
- severe myocardial dysfunction, defined as a cardiac index <3.0 L/m/m² or left ventricular ejection fraction (LVEF) <35%.

The speed at which ECLS can be initiated is institution-dependent and this must be borne in mind by clinicians seeking to try every possible less invasive strategy in patients with rapidly progressive shock.

## Contraindications

The standard contraindications apply in septic patients being considered for ECLS, such as preexisting severe neurological dysfunction or incurable malignancy. An additional consideration in sepsis is the oncology patient. These patients have been historically regarded as poor ECLS candidates, but contemporary outcomes are acceptable in many instances.[19-21] Neutropenic sepsis is not a contraindication to ECLS, but can be challenging because of other commonly associated problems, such as thrombocytopenia and fragile integument. Nonetheless, successful outcomes have been reported.[22]

The nature of the infecting organism should not be regarded as a major determinant of the appropriateness of ECLS, although some organisms, most notably *Bordetella pertussis* and disseminated herpes simplex virus in infants, are associated with poorer outcomes.[23,24]

**Cannulation strategies**

Cannulation is one of the most important management issues in ECLS for sepsis and must be individually tailored to the patient's circulatory and respiratory status (Chapter 4). An understanding of the pathophysiology of septic shock coupled with adequate hemodynamic information is important in planning an appropriate cannulation strategy.

For sepsis-induced isolated respiratory failure requiring ECLS, VV cannulation is preferred because it is associated with better outcomes. VV ECMO avoids the complications of VA ECMO such as systemic embolization, arterial trauma, and increased left ventricular afterload, while preserving pulmonary blood flow, pulsatile systemic flow, and oxygenation of blood in the systemic ventricle and thus the coronary arteries. VV ECMO is also preferred in those patients with ARDS that persists after resolution of shock, when the patient is ready to be weaned off mechanical circulatory support but not ready to cease extracorporeal gas exchange because of ongoing severe respiratory failure. In these instances, consideration should be given to changing to VV cannulation if it is anticipated that lung recovery will require more than 1-2 days of additional ECLS.

If ECLS is being considered primarily as mechanical circulatory support for refractory septic shock, then the patient's hemodynamic response to sepsis must first be established. Septic shock has three principle hemodynamic manifestations based on the most compromised part of the circulation: right heart failure, left heart failure with inadequate systemic oxygen delivery, or distributive shock with poor oxygen extraction.[10]

Right heart failure associated with persistent pulmonary hypertension of the newborn (PPHN) is the most frequent manifestation of septic shock in neonates. Right heart failure from a combination of sepsis-induced ventricular dysfunction and high positive-pressure ventilation can also be seen in older patients. After the neonatal period, septic children often suffer from isolated left ventricular failure with preserved vasomotor tone and impaired oxygen delivery. The age at which a child will alter their hemodynamic response from left heart failure ('cold' shock) to distributive shock ('warm' shock) is highly variable and cannot be reliably predicted from the child's age. However, by late adolescence and into adulthood, the most common hemodynamic response to sepsis is distributive shock. This is characterized by a reduction in ventricular function and vasomotor tone, an increase in heart rate, and often by a reduction in oxygen extraction at a cellular level. The categorization of shock requires a combination of clinical assessment; blood tests (eg, venous oximetry, lactate); echocardiography; and an assessment of cardiac output. It is best performed by an experienced critical care physician.[10]

Possible ECLS cannulation strategies become apparent once the hemodynamic pattern of shock has been identified (Table 36-1). Those with right heart failure and concomitant respiratory failure can be supported with VV ECMO if the shock is not particularly advanced, as the consequent reduction in intrathoracic pressure and optimization of oxygenation and carbon dioxide clearance may be sufficient to improve myocardial performance and peripheral circulation, especially in small children. Otherwise, peripheral VA ECMO or central ECMO can be used.

In pediatric left heart failure, peripheral or high flow central ECMO is appropriate. Serial echocardiograms should be performed to monitor left heart distension. If this is worsening, then steps should be taken to alleviate it before left atrial distension and hypertension lead to hemorrhagic pulmonary edema.[25] Increasing circuit flows may limit atrial distension. If this is unsuccessful, then options include, 1) percutaneous atrial septostomy, 2) mini-thoracotomy and insertion of a left atrial vent cannula via the left superior pulmonary vein, 3) submammary incision and insertion of an apical left ventricular cannula, or 4) a direct left atrial vent cannula can be inserted on central ECMO, ie, biatrial drainage (Chapter 4). If the femoral artery is used in older children or adults, then an additional perfusion cannula should be inserted to supply oxygenated blood to the affected leg to prevent limb ischemia.[26,27] An additional consideration in patients on peripheral VA ECMO is that coronary and cerebral arterial blood may be supplied by the left ventricle and not the ECMO circuit (ie, differential oxygenation). It is thus important that an appropriate amount of oxygen is provided by the ventilator and that a surrogate marker of coronary oxygenation (eg, right radial artery blood, near infrared spectroscopy, right hand pulse oximetry) is used to monitor for possible complications, such as differential hypoxemia. If there is decreased oxygen saturation in the right arm, then increasing peripheral VA flow (if possible) and thus decreasing flow through the pulmonary circulation may be sufficient to allow for adequate coronary and cerebral oxygenation. If not, then an additional venous drainage cannula may provide sufficient flow to avoid cerebral hypoxia, either as an additional drainage cannula to increase total circuit flow or as a return cannula to oxygenate blood as it traverses the pulmonary circulation. This last solution, venovenoarterial (VVA) ECMO, is

| CANNULATION STRATEGY | TYPICAL PATIENT | ADVANTAGES | DISADVANTAGES |
|---|---|---|---|
| Venovenous | Neonate | • No differential hypoxemia<br>• Rapid cannulation<br>• One cannula | • No direct circulatory support<br>• Inappropriate in advanced shock |
| Peripheral venoarterial (carotid) | Infant | • Direct circulatory support<br>• Rapid cannulation | • Limited flow rates |
| Peripheral venoarterial (femoral) | Young adult with septic cardiomyopathy | • Direct circulatory support<br>• Rapid cannulation | • Risk of differential hypoxemia<br>• Limb ischemia |
| Veno venoarterial | Adolescent or adult with severe combined circulatory and respiratory failure | • Corrects differential hypoxemia<br>• Proportion of respiratory and circulatory support easily adjusted to meet physiological needs | • Requires 3 cannulas<br>• Gate clamp on the return venous limb may increase the risk of hemolysis |
| Central (atrioaortic) | Child | • Highest possible flow rates<br>• No differential hypoxemia<br>• Associated with lower mortality in children[9,29] | • Requires cardiac surgical services<br>• Increased risks of local bleeding and mediastinitis |

**Table 36-1.** Basic ECMO cannulation strategies in septic shock.

technically challenging in small children but easily performed in adolescents and adults.[28]

### *Central Cannulation in Children*

Central cannulation is commonly used in most major pediatric and adult cardiac transplantation centers for other indications. With this technique, analogous to cardiopulmonary bypass, a cardiac surgeon performs a sternotomy and cannulates the right atrium directly. Venous blood is pumped through the circuit and returned through a cannula placed in the ascending aorta. The largest available cannulas should be placed to maximize laminar flow and minimize excessive suction pressure. The latter requires monitoring because hypovolemia or cannula obstruction will limit inflow and create an increase in suction, with resultant turbulent flow, microcavitation, and hemolysis. The pump inlet pressure should be measured at the connection between the atrial cannula and the inlet tubing and should be maintained between -20 mmHg and zero. If the pressure is consistently more negative than -20 mmHg, then it should be assumed that the pump revolutions have been set too high, the patient is hypovolemic, or the cannulae are kinked, obstructed, or too small. Suggested cannula sizes and estimated flow ranges are listed in Table 36-2. If possible, the skin should be sutured around the cannulas to reduce bleeding, and the defect between the sternal edges closed over with a silastic membrane sutured into place.

| PATIENT WEIGHT (kg) | ATRIAL CANNULA (Fr) | AORTIC CANNULA (Fr) | ANTICIPATED FLOWS (L/min) |
|---|---|---|---|
| <10 | 14-28 | 10-16 | 1-2 |
| 10-20 | 20-36 | 14-20 | 3-4 |
| 21-40 | 24-46 | 18-21 | 4-6 |
| 41-60 | 28-50 | 20-24 | 6-8 |
| >60 | 36-52 | 22-24 | 8-10 |

**Table 36-2.** Suggested cannula sizes for pediatric central ECMO.[8]

Possible benefits of this technique include:

- Achieving high flow rates, which may lead to faster resolution of shock
- Avoiding differential hypoxemia
- Complete cardiac and pulmonary support

Possible disadvantages include:

- Requires specialty cardiac surgical services
- Risk of mediastinitis
- Risk of local hemorrhage is greater than with percutaneous techniques

There is some evidence that high flow, central ECMO is associated with improved survival in pediatric septic shock. In one single center study of 45 children with refractory septic shock, 73% of patients who received central ECMO survived compared to 38% who received peripheral ECMO (p=0.05).[6] In a subsequent case series from the same center, 17 (74%) of 23 children supported with central cannulation for septic shock survived to hospital discharge, some of whom had suffered from distributive shock and recurrent cardiac arrest.[8] These patients received long-term followup. None of the survivors suffered from severe disability and the majority made a complete recovery. A more recent multicenter study demonstrated an association between the use of central ECMO and decreased mortality in children with septic shock when compared to peripheral cannulation (OR 0.31, 95%CI 0.1-0.98, p=0.05).[9] Another multicenter study found that high flow ECMO (>150 ml/kg/min) was associated with better survival than standard ECMO flows or no ECMO in refractory septic shock (82% vs. 43%, vs. 48%, respectively, p=0.03).[29]

### Management during ECMO

For patients with circulatory failure on VA ECMO, the goals of ECMO are the same as for other indications: restore organ blood flow and adequate tissue oxygenation while awaiting recovery, without causing further damage to the lungs or heart. The ECMO pump now becomes analogous to the heart. Instead of adjusting inotropes to enhance cardiac output, circuit flows 'replace' the cardiac output and thus must be titrated to provide adequate oxygen delivery. A term that is frequently used when referring to ECMO circuit flows is 'full flow' and is taken from the cardiac operating room. However, this term is misleading and should be abandoned in ICU. Analogous to the concept that no given cardiac output can ever be considered 'normal',[30] there is no circuit flow that can be regarded as 'full flow'. The term fails to take oxygen consumption into consideration and falsely implies that there is a universally applicable level above which no benefit would be seen from further increases in flow. Instead, circuit flows should be goal-directed, targeting rapid normalization of lactate, improvement in $SvO_2$ >65-70%, and restoration of age-appropriate mean arterial pressures. In sepsis, this may require very high flows (eg, >150-200 ml/kg/min in young children).[29] Appropriate monitoring of pump inlet pressures (see above) and regular measurement of plasma free hemoglobin should be used to detect excessive pump revolutions or cannula misplacement. Hemolysis is a serious complication, and every attempt should be made to prevent it. One study of 207 children on ECLS demonstrated that those patients with severe hemolysis (plasma free Hb >1 g/L) had a six-fold increased risk of death compared to those who did not.[31] Similar findings have been seen in adult patients.[32]

Inotropes can usually be weaned off or to minimal doses within a few hours of achieving adequate circuit flows. Vasoconstrictors may be necessary to maintain age-appropriate mean arterial pressure, but it is not unusual to see systemic hypertension ensue around this time, particularly with the high flows of central

ECMO, in which case short-acting vasodilators (eg, sodium nitroprusside) can be initiated to improve centrifugal pump flow and improve peripheral circulation. Ventilation should be reduced to lung-protective settings (eg, rate 5-10, peak inspiratory pressure <20 $cmH_2O$, PEEP 5-12, $FiO_2$ <0.5) unless on peripheral VA ECMO, in which case the $FiO_2$ and PEEP must still be set sufficiently high to preserve coronary oxygenation. If differential hypoxemia becomes apparent, then conversion to central or VVA ECMO may be appropriate, depending on the patient's age and local surgical expertise.[8,28]

The coagulation cascade is intricately involved in the process of inflammation and septic patients frequently have disseminated intravascular coagulation (DIC). Thrombus may form in parts of the ECMO circuit or patient while there is hemorrhage in other areas. DIC should be aggressively treated with blood products while heparin is titrated to activated clotting times (ACT), activated partial thromboplastin times (APTT), or anti-Xa levels. In septic children, the target ACT is generally 2 times normal unless bleeding is profuse, in which case the target may be temporarily lowered to 1.5 times normal until the bleeding slows or stops. Adequate blood product support with recombinant factor replacement, fresh frozen plasma (aiming INR <1.3-1.5), cryoprecipitate (aiming fibrinogen >2.0 g/L), and platelets (aiming >50-80 x $10^9$/L, depending on the patient's age) is standard. Coagulopathy should not be allowed to replace controlled pharmacological anticoagulation in circuit management.

Other measures such as effective empiric antibiotics and immediate treatment of any septic foci are vital. The pharmacokinetics of many antibiotics in patients receiving ECLS have been inadequately studied (Chapter 49). As failure to provide adequate and timely empiric antibiotics has been associated with substantial increases in mortality,[33,34] initial antibiotics should be given as early as possible, cover all likely pathogens, and be at the maximum dose recommended by standard formularies, especially those with a wide therapeutic index such as β-lactam antibiotics. Therapeutic drug monitoring should be used whenever possible.

## Outcomes

ECLS for neonatal sepsis is associated with in-hospital survival rates of approximately 75-80%.[11] In pediatric septic shock, historical experience suggested that the use of ECLS in older children was associated with survival to hospital discharge of 50% at best,[6,10] although this may have recently improved.[35] The use of high flow, central ECMO is associated with survival rates approaching 75%.[6,8]

The increasing use of ECLS for adult septic shock has demonstrated that peripheral ECMO for distributive shock is generally associated with poor outcomes.[12,15-17] However, in adult patients with refractory septic cardiomyopathy, ECLS may have an important role.[18,36,37] In one study of 212 adult patients with septic cardiomyopathy, 60% of patients supported on VA ECMO survived vs. 25% without ECMO (risk ratio for mortality 0.54, 95% CI 0.40-0.70, p<0.0001).[18]

## Conclusions

The use of ECLS for highly selected patients with refractory septic shock has increased in recent years, with the majority of patients of all ages surviving to discharge in experienced centers.[8,18,35,36] ECLS is generally required very early in the course of sepsis, usually before antibiotics have taken effect.[7] The optimal approach to cannulation should be individualized and varies with the age of the patient, the hemodynamic pattern of shock, and the experience of the center.[37]

## References

1. Singer M, Deutschman CS, Seymour CW, et al. The Third International Consensus definitions for sepsis and septic shock (Sepsis-3). JAMA 2016; 315:801-810.
2. McCune S, Short BL, Miller MK, et al. Extracorporeal membrane oxygenation therapy in neonates with septic shock. J Pediatr Surg 1990; 25:479-482.
3. Hocker JR, Simpson PM, Rabalais GP, et al. Extracorporeal membrane oxygenation and early-onset group B streptococcal sepsis. Pediatrics 1992; 89:1-4.
4. Beca J, Butt W. Extracorporeal membrane oxygenation for refractory septic shock in children. Pediatrics 1994; 93:726-729.
5. Goldman AP, Kerr SJ, Butt W, et al. Extracorporeal support for intractable cardiorespiratory failure due to meningococcal disease. Lancet 1997; 349:466-469.
6. MacLaren G, Butt W, Best D, et al. Extracorporeal membrane oxygenation for refractory septic shock in children: one institution's experience. Pediatr Crit Care Med 2007; 8:447-451.
7. Bartlett RH. Extracorporeal support for septic shock. Pediatr Crit Care Med 2007; 8:498-499.
8. MacLaren G, Butt W, Best D, et al. Central extracorporeal membrane oxygenation for refractory pediatric septic shock. Pediatr Crit Care Med 2011; 12:133-136.
9. Schlapbach LJ, Chiletti R, Straney L, et al. Defining benefit threshold for extracorporeal membrane oxygenation in children with sepsis – a binational multicenter cohort study. Crit Care. 2019 Dec 30;23(1):429.
10. Davis AL, Carcillo JA, Aneja RK, et al. American College of Critical Care Medicine clinical practice parameters for hemodynamic support of pediatric and neonatal septic shock. Crit Care Med 2017; 45:1061-1093.
11. Extracorporeal Life Support Organization (ELSO). ECLS registry report, International Summary. October 2021.
12. Schmidt M, Bréchot N, Combes A. Ten situations in which ECMO is unlikely to be successful. Intensive Care Med 2016; 42:750-752.
13. Wernovsky G, Wypij D, Jonas RA, et al. Postoperative course and hemodynamic profile after the arterial switch operation in neonates and infants. Circulation 1995; 92:2226-2235.
14. Weiss SL, Peters MJ, Alhazzani W, et al. Surviving sepsis campaign international guidelines for the management of septic shock and sepsis-associated organ dysfunction in children. Intensive Care Med 2020; 46(Suppl 1):10-67.
15. Huang CT, Tsai YJ, Tsai PR, Ko WJ. Extracorporeal membrane oxygenation resuscitation in adult patients with refractory septic shock. J Thorac Cardiovasc Surg 2013; 146:1041-6.
16. Park TK, Yang JH, Jeon K, et al. Extracorporeal membrane oxygenation for refractory septic shock in adults. Eur J Cardiothorac Surg 2015; 47:e68-74.
17. Cheng A, Sun HY, Lee CW, et al. Survival of septic adults compared with nonseptic adults receiving extracorporeal membrane oxygenation for cardiopulmonary failure: a propensity-matched analysis. J Crit Care 2013; 28:532.e1-10.
18. Bréchot N, Hajage D, Kimmoun A, et al. Venoarterial extracorporeal membrane oxygenation to rescue sepsis-induced cardiogenic shock: a retrospective, multicentre, international cohort study. Lancet 2020; 396:545-552.
19. Gow KW, Lao OB, Leong T, et al. Extracorporeal life support for adults with malignancy and respiratory or cardiac failure: The Extracorporeal Life Support experience. Am J Surg 2010; 199:669-675.
20. Gow KW, Heiss KF, Wulkan ML, et al. Extracorporeal lilfe support for support of children with malignancy and respiratory or cardiac failure: The extracorporeal life support experience. Crit Care Med 2009; 37:1308-1316.
21. Di Nardo M, Ahmad AH, Merli P, et al. Extracorporeal membrane oxygenation in children receiving haematopoietic cell transplantation and immune effector cell therapy: an international and multidisciplinary consensus statement. Lancet Child Adolesc Health 2022; 6:116-128.
22. Smith S, Butt W, Best D, et al. Long-term survival after extracorporeal life support in children with neutropenic sepsis. Intensive Care Med 2016; 42:942-943.
23. Prodhan P, Wilkes R, Ross A, et al. Neonatal herpes virus infection and extracorporeal life support. Pediatr Crit Care Med 2010; 11:599-602.
24. Domico M, Ridout D, MacLaren G, et al. Extracorporeal membrane oxygenation for pertussis: predictors of outcome including pulmonary hypertension and leukodepletion. Pediatr Crit Care Med 2018; 19:254-261.
25. Eastaugh LJ, Thiagarajan RR, Darst JR, et al. Percutaneous left atrial decompression in patients supported with extracorporeal membrane oxygenation for cardiac disease. Pediatr Crit Care Med 2015; 16:59-65.
26. Spurlock DJ, Toomasian JM, Romano MA, et al. A simple technique to prevent limb ischemia during venoarterial ECMO using the femoral artery: the posterior tibial approach. Perfusion 2012; 27:141-145.
27. Jia D, Yang IX, Ling RR, et al. Vascular complications of extracorporeal membrane oxygenation: A

systematic review and meta-analysis. Crit Care Med 2020; 48:e1269-e1277.

28. Vogel DJ, Murray J, Czapran AZ, et al. Veno-arterio-venous ECMO for septic cardiomyopathy: a single-centre experience. Perfusion 2018; 33:57-64.

29. Oberender F, Ganeshalingham A, Fortenberry JD, et al. Venoarterial extracorporeal membrane oxygenation versus conventional therapy in severe pediatric septic shock. Peditr Crit Care Med 2018; 19:965-972.

30. Pinsky MR. Hemodynamic evaluation and monitoring in the ICU. Chest 2007; 132:2020-2029.

31. Lou S, MacLaren G, Best D, Delzoppo C, et al. Hemolysis in pediatric patients receiving centrifugal-pump extracorporeal membrane oxygenation: prevalence, risk factors, and outcomes. Crit Care Med 2014; 42:1213-20.

32. Omar HR, Mirsaeidi M, Socias S, et al. Plasma free hemoglobin is an independent predictor of mortality among patients on extracorporeal membrane oxygenation support. PLoS One 2015; 10:e0124034.

33. Kumar A, Roberts D, Wood KE, et al. Duration of hypotension before initiation of effective antimicrobial therapy is the critical determinant of survival in human septic shock. Crit Care Med 2006; 34:1589-1596.

34. Kumar A, Ellis P, Arabi Y, et al. Initiation of inappropriate antimicrobial therapy results in fivefold reduction of survival in human septic shock. Chest 2009; 136:1237-48.

35. Melnikov G, Grabowski S, Broman LM. Extracorporeal membrane oxygenation for septic shock in children. ASAIO J 2022; 68:262-267.

36. Falk L, Hultman J, Broman LM. Extracorporeal membrane oxygenation for septic shock. Crit Care Med 2019; 47:1097-1105.

37. MacLaren G. In sepsis-induced heart failure, extracorporeal membrane oxygenation can provide support. Lancet 2020; 396:515-517.

# 37

## Poisoning

*Adam Blumenberg, Eleonore Valencia, Giles Peek, Amy Dzierba*

## Introduction

Poisoning is a prevalent cause of severe disease and death worldwide. The consequent cardiovascular and/or respiratory failure may be refractory to conventional supportive therapies and potentially lethal, in which case ECLS may be lifesaving. Specifically, the acuity of disease secondary to certain poisonings and the rapidity by which it progresses may limit the effect of antidotes and affect the body's natural metabolism of the toxin. Additionally, most toxic substances do not have a specific antidote and critical illness is treated with hemodynamic and ventilatory support until recovery or death. ECLS may be utilized as a bridge to native recovery or transplantation in select patients. Ongoing challenges to the use of ECLS in the setting of poisoning include cases in which the type of toxic substance(s) and disease-reversibility are indeterminate, as well as the optimal timing to cannulate or transfer to an ECMO-capable center.

## Epidemiology

According to 2019 data from the World Health Organization, the global mortality rate attributed to unintentional poisoning was 1.1 per 100,000 population, and Africa remains disproportionately afflicted.[1] Although the mortality rate has decreased by more than 25% over the past two decades, it is likely an underestimate, given the lack of infrastructure for accurate data collection in many countries.

The American Association of Poison Control Centers (AAPCC) comprised of 55 poison centers serving the United States, American Samoa, Federated States of Micronesia, Guam, Puerto Rico, and the US Virgin Islands, has reported a gradual decline in poisonings over time. The exposure rate was 6.3 per 1000 population in 2020 compared to 8.0 per 1000 population in 2000. Children ≤5 years predominated in exposure rates, but only comprised a minority of fatalities (1.3%), with most deaths occurring in persons aged 30 to 39 years. The vast majority of cases were unintentional, with intentional overdoses more associated with clinically significant and severe disease. Four percent of poisonings required critical care. The leading substances implicated in fatal cases included sedatives, hypnotics, antipsychotics, pharmaceutical and illegal opioid preparations, acetaminophen, alcohols, stimulants, and street drugs.[2]

There are important geographic differences in the patterns of poisoning among children and adults. In a multicenter, international pediatric study of acute poisoning presentations, unintentional ingestion of therapeutic drugs was most frequent in South America, North

America, Northern Europe, Southern Europe, and the Western Pacific. Unintentional ingestion of household products predominated in Western Europe and the Eastern Mediterranean.[3] Pesticides, commonly organophosphates, aluminum phosphide, and paraquat, continue to be the predominant toxins implicated in unintentional ingestions in rural Southern Asia, South-Eastern Asia, Africa, South America, and Central America; however, there are increasing reports of intentional ingestions in urban areas also.[4-6] Drugs, such as benzodiazepines, antidepressants, and prescription opioids, as well as illicit opioids, remain a prevalent source of poisoning in high-income countries and are becoming ubiquitous in low- and middle-income countries, too.[7-9]

**General Approach to the Poisoned Patient**

Toxic substances exert their effects on the human body through a variety of mechanisms. Many pharmaceuticals lose receptor specificity in toxic concentrations and may cause organ dysfunction beyond an extrapolated form of their therapeutic effect in a process known as toxicodynamics. For example, while aspirin is used therapeutically as a cyclooxygenase inhibitor, in toxic concentrations it is a mitochondrial poison. Certain drugs may have longer durations of action and different distribution patterns in the setting of toxic rather than therapeutic doses in a process known as toxicokinetics. For example, while therapeutic doses of loperamide do not reach the systemic circulation due to hepatic first-pass metabolism and P-glycoprotein efflux, in overdose these enzymes become saturated and loperamide may poison the heart and brain. Life-threatening effects of poisoning include hemodynamic collapse through cardiogenic shock, diffuse vasodilation, acute respiratory distress syndrome (ARDS), mitochondrial failure, altered mental status leading to loss of airway reflexes, status epilepticus, refractory ventricular dysrhythmias, and refractory cardiac arrest.

Direct cardiac toxins such as beta blockers and calcium channel blockers may cause acute cardiogenic shock and low cardiac output via bradydysrhythmias, negative inotropy, and decreased peripheral vascular resistance. Vasodilators such as calcium channel blockers may cause distributive shock as well as high output cardiac failure in which heart rate and cardiac output fail to compensate for low vascular resistance. Ion channel inhibitors, such as drugs with sodium or potassium channel inhibition, may cause cardiogenic shock and refractory ventricular dysrhythmias due to acquired channelopathy. Such drugs include class I antiarrhythmics, antiepileptic drugs, cocaine, antipsychotics, local anesthetics, and antidepressants.[10,11] Stimulant drugs such as methamphetamine, cocaine, ecstasy (3,4-Methylenedioxymethamphetamine) may induce acute cardiomyopathy due to catecholaminergic excess and subsequent demand ischemia.[12] Substances which inhibit mitochondrial function such as carbon monoxide, aluminum phosphide, cyanide, and azide may induce shock.[13,14] Toxins may induce respiratory failure due to direct tissue destruction from caustic agents such as hydrocarbons, lye, or phenol,[15] or due to pulmonary toxicity such as with bleomycin, amiodarone, or paraquat.[16,17] Respiratory failure may also occur secondary to pulmonary edema from stimulants or opioids and naloxone, or intoxication-related aspiration.[18-20]

Intentional ingestions during suicide attempts may involve multiple drugs and drug classes.[2] The exact doses and substances may be unknown because the ingestion history is often incomplete or unreliable. While some substances (such as acetaminophen, ethanol, salicylates, and lithium) are quantifiable at many regional hospitals in real time, most toxins cannot be reliably confirmed in a clinically relevant time frame. A multidrug overdose may include a potentially lethal quantity of one or more drugs as well as benign dose of other substances. Treatment should be based on the clinical syndrome as well as the likely toxin(s).

## First Line Treatment

Care for critically ill poisoned patients requires a multidisciplinary team and should be performed in consultation with a medical toxicologist. Many countries have poison centers available by phone any time of day, however only 47% of WHO member states have a poison center.[1] If available, local poison center contact information should be easily available in all healthcare environments. Most critically ill poisoned patients should be monitored and treated with supportive therapies in the ICU such as administration of intravenous fluids, optimization of electrolytes and metabolic derangements, and utilization of vasoactive medications. Respiratory failure may require endotracheal intubation and mechanical ventilation. Altered mental status may also require intubation if airway reflexes are impaired. Certain poison ingestions are amenable to gastrointestinal decontamination with activated charcoal, gastric lavage, or whole bowel irrigation, all of which have potential complications and are not indicated in most poisonings.[21,22] A flowchart proposing management is available in Figure 37-1.

Specific antidotes and targeted treatments have improved the prognosis for patients with certain toxicities. Opioid-induced respiratory failure may be reversed with naloxone and digoxin-induced cardiac failure with digoxin immune fab. Liver failure from acetaminophen may be prevented with n-acetyl cysteine (NAC), and renal failure from ethylene glycol may be prevented with fomepizole or ethanol. Certain poisons such as aspirin, lithium, and metformin may be removed via hemodialysis.[23-25]

Many toxic substances do not have an antidote, and sometimes conventional treatments fail. Mortality may reach 10-20% in the setting of cardiovascular failure and may reach 90% when hemodynamic impairment is refractory to standard treatment.[26,27]

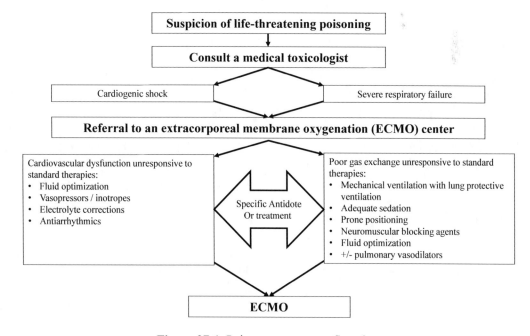

**Figure 37-1.** Poison management flowchart.

## Rationale for VA and VV ECMO in Poisoning

A general principle of most poisonings is that organ dysfunction is temporary because the human body can metabolize toxic substances. Over the course of hours to days, the kidneys excrete toxins, and the liver chemically modifies toxic to nontoxic substances. The duration of toxicity depends on the dose, the toxicokinetics of a given substance or combination of substances, and the function of the organ responsible for metabolizing it. Since hemodynamic and/or pulmonary dysfunction is typically transient, there is a strong rationale for using mechanical cardiopulmonary assistance in severely poisoned patients. ECLS provides stable perfusion and gas exchange through the time required to metabolize toxic substances from the body. Additionally, ECLS provides support when the therapy of the toxic substance may worsen hemodynamics.[28] For example, iron toxicity may cause shock but is optimally treated with the chelator deferoxamine which may exacerbate hypotension. Toxic alcohols and aspirin poisoning may require hemodialysis, which can only be performed on a hemodynamically stable patient.[29] There are reports of ECLS used to support patients receiving hemoperfusion,[30] plasma exchange,[31] plasmapheresis,[35] CytoSorb,[36] and other modalities (Chapter 42).

Antidotes exist for certain poisons such as digoxin immune fab for cardiac glycoside toxicity. Often, antidotes may take time to acquire, administer, or reach therapeutic effect. ECLS may provide support during periods of hemodynamic instability or ventricular dysrhythmias until the antidote takes effect.[28,37] Certain toxic substances may lead to permanent organ failure which is optimally treated with organ transplant. For example, lung destruction secondary to a caustic agent or paraquat may be supported by ECLS while awaiting organ availability.[38]

## Animal Studies

ECLS has been studied in three major animal models of drug poisoning. In a model of lidocaine poisoning in dogs consisting of a 30 mg/kg IV injection, 8 dogs received ECLS support over 90 minutes and were compared to 8 dogs treated conventionally (mechanical ventilation, vasopressors, cardioversion, and antiarrhythmics). All dogs in the ECLS group survived, compared to only two in the control group. Interestingly, ECLS-treated animals had a drug clearance comparable to normal individuals in this experiment.[39] In a model of cardiac arrest following desipramine infusion in dogs, ECLS also rescued all animals (6/6), while only 1/6 animals survived in the conventional treatment group.[40] Lastly, in a model of amitriptyline poisoning in which 20 swine were receiving 0.5 mg/kg/min amitriptyline until the blood pressure dropped below 30 mmHg for 1 min (near-lethal toxicity), ECLS rescued all animals (10/10), while 9/10 died in the conventional treatment group.[41]

## Human Studies

Despite an absence of randomized clinical trials for ECLS in acute poisoning, there is a strong pragmatic basis for its use. To date, ECLS has been used as a salvage therapy in patients presenting with cardiogenic shock or arrhythmia refractory to conventional treatment. There are no randomized controlled trials of ECLS in poisoned patients. The literature on the application of ECLS for human poisoning is limited to case reports, retrospective analyses of single and multicenter data, and systematic reviews. Specific criteria regarding patient selection, timing, indications and contraindications for individual poisonings remain elusive.[42]

The reported use of ECLS as salvage therapy for severe poisoning is low. Data from the AAPCC suggests that ECLS utilization is increasing, with a reported use of 0.007% in 2020.[2] In a more recent, longitudinal study of the AAPCC's National Poison Data System, Cole et al described an increasing use of ECLS from 2000 to 2018, in particular among adults, for a variety of both single- and multi-substance ingestions involving pharmaceuticals and non-pharmaceuticals. The rate of survival remained stable over time at 70%, with the highest mortality occurring in cases of hematologic and metabolic toxins. Interestingly, the authors reported higher ECLS utilization in urban regions of the United States.[43]

In 2009, Daubi et al. reported the outcomes of 17 patients supported with peripheral VA ECMO for acute poisoning.[44] Fifteen suffered from cardiotoxic intoxication including 11 with membrane stabilizing agents, combined with various antipsychotic drugs. All had severe myocardial dysfunction at the time of ECMO implantation, received high dose catecholamines, and suffered multiple organ failure. Seven received ECPR with a mean low-flow time of $101 \pm 55$ min. Time from admission to ECMO was $6.4 \pm 7$ hrs. Cannulation was performed in the operating room for 13 patients and at the bedside for 4. Fifteen patients were weaned from ECMO, and 13 (76%) were discharged alive without neurological sequelae. Mean ECMO duration was short ($4.5 \pm 2.4$ days), but a high rate of complications occurred: 6 episodes of limb ischemia and 2 episodes of cannulation site bleeding. The authors concluded that despite a high morbidity associated with the technique, VA ECMO could rescue patients with refractory myocardial dysfunction associated with drug poisoning.

In 2012, Masson et al. reported the outcomes of 62 patients with severe shock or persistent (>30 min) cardiac arrest after drug poisoning.[45] Fourteen patients underwent VA ECMO, whereas 48 were managed conventionally. Patients treated with or without ECMO at ICU admission were on high dose vasopressors and had comparable drug ingestion histories, Simplified Acute Physiology Score (SAPS II score) ($66 \pm 18$), Sequential Organ Failure Assessment (SOFA) score (median: 11 [IQR, 9-13]), Glasgow Coma Scale score (median: 3 [IQR, 3-11]), need for ventilator support (n=56) and extrarenal support (n=23). Survival rate was 86% in the ECMO group, compared to only 48% in patients who received conventional therapies and none of the patients with persistent cardiac arrest survived without ECMO support. In a multivariate analysis, adjusting for SAPS II and beta-blocker intoxication, ECMO support remained significantly associated with lower mortality (Adjusted Odds Ratio, 0.18; 95% CI, 0.03-0.96; p=0.04). Interestingly, none of the 6 ECMO-treated patients who were intoxicated with membrane stabilizing agents died, whereas death occurred in 15 of the 23 patients managed conventionally in this setting. In a sensitivity analysis of the 52 intoxicated patients who did not have cardiac arrest, ECMO remained associated with survival (OR for death 0.28; 95% CI 0.05-1.48, p=0.17), although the difference did not reach statistical significance. The mean time from admission to ECMO was short ($8 \pm 7$ hours), as well as ECMO duration ($6 \pm 2.9$ days).

In 2015, Wang et al. evaluated 10 cases of poisoning who received ECMO referred to the ToxIC registry out of 26,271 toxicologic exposure cases who were reported during the study period. The ToxIC registry is a practice-based, multicenter research and surveillance network with data on tens of thousands of toxic exposures.[29,46] Six patients were under 18 years old and 4 were adults. The toxins were carbon monoxide, a cyanogenic amine, methanol, psychiatric drugs, cardiovascular drugs, analgesics, antidiabetics, and sedative/hypnotics. Most patients developed hemodynamic instability, seizures, dysrhythmias, metabolic acidosis, and multiorgan failure. Other interventions included vasopressors, CPR (4), continuous renal replacement therapy (CRRT)

(5), bicarbonate (4), intravenous fat emulsion (2), and hemodialysis (1). ECMO was initiated on average 35 hours into their course and lasted an average of 170 hours, and 8/10 survived.

In 2019, Weiner et al. evaluated 104 cases of poisoning who received VA ECMO referred to the ELSO Registry out of 15,511 VA ECMO cases who were reported during the study period.[47,48] The median patient age was 34 years and 53.5% were male. The toxins were 47.2% cardiovascular drugs, 8.7% opioids, 3.8% cocaine, 3.8% antidepressants, with the remainder unknown or unspecified. Prior to initiation of VA ECMO, 92.4% received vasopressor infusion for hemodynamic support, 85.9% received two or more vasopressors, and 33.0% had a cardiac arrest prior to cannulation. The median duration of VA ECMO was 68 hours with an interquartile range of 48 to 113 hours, and 52.9% of the cases survived to discharge. Specific toxin, demographics, and nature of pre-ECMO support was similar in survivors and nonsurvivors, except that a greater proportion of nonsurvivors had placement of an intraaortic balloon pump. VA ECMO improved parameters reflecting hemodynamics (MAP, SBP, and DBP), acidosis (pH, bicarbonate), and oxygenation (pO2, SpO2, and SvO2). Nonsurvivors showed persistently low pH 24 hours after VA ECMO initiation compared to survivors. Ramanathan et al. also examined the ELSO database and found in 83 patients who received ECMO for poisoning an overall 41% survival rate and nearly 90% survival in patients who received VV ECMO for inhalational injuries or aspiration.[49]

In 2020, Cole et al. evaluated 407 cases (332 adults and 75 children) of poisoning who received ECLS referred to the National Poison Data System.[43] The National Poison Data System is a central database for the USA's 55 poison centers containing over 74 million case records.[50] The median patient age was 27 years with 47.5% female. A single substance was responsible for toxicity in 51.5% of cases

and the median was 3. Overall survival with ECLS was 70%, and patients with metabolic or hematologic poisoning (eg, carbon monoxide, aluminum phosphide) had a lower likelihood of survival than those poisoned by other substances (49% vs. 72%; p=0.004).

In 2021, Upchurch et al. systematically reviewed the English-language literature and analyzed 156 articles regarding poisoned patients who received ECMO. The authors recommended consideration of VA ECMO in absence of contraindications for all patients with acute poisoning and refractory cardiogenic shock or refractory cardiac arrest. The authors recommend VV ECMO in poisoning be considered by the same criteria as in nonpoisoned patients.[51,52] The authors noted that while there are no absolute contraindications to ECMO, it might be hypothetically ineffective in certain toxicities such as those that cause cellular respiratory failure or severe coagulopathy.

In 2022, DiNardo and colleagues reviewed the US experience of ECLS for poisoning in children as reported to the ELSO Registry between 2003 and 2019. Eighty-six children with a median age of 12.0 year were reported; 52.9% were female. The most commonly reported substance exposures were hydrocarbons (n=17; 19.8%), followed by chemical asphyxiants (n=14; 16.3%), neuroactive agents (n=14; 16.3%), opioid/analgesics (n=13;15.1%), and cardiovascular agents (n=12; 14.0%). 83.7% of the cases had a single substance poisoning. The intention of the exposure was unknown in 65.1%, self-harm in 20.9%, and 10.5% was unintentional. Overall survival was (65.1%). Most patients received VA ECMO. A bimodal distribution of ECMO support was observed among two age groups: less than or equal to 3 years (n=34) and 13–17 years (n=41). Hemodynamic and metabolic parameters improved for all patients with ECMO. Persistent systolic hypotension, acidemia/metabolic acidosis, and elevated $PaO_2$ after 24 hours of ECMO support were associated with mortality.

ECMO duration and PICU length of stay were significantly longer in survivors compared to nonsurvivors (139.5 vs. 70.5 hr; p=0.007 and 25.0 vs. 4.0 d; p=0.002, respectively).[53]

**Ethical Considerations**

Approximately a third of poisoning fatalities are due to intentional self-harm or suicide attempts.[54] The majority of patients who recover from these do not repeat suicide attempts.[55,56] The four ethical pillars of autonomy, beneficence, nonmaleficence, and justice are issues that must be addressed on an individual basis.[57] Honoring patient autonomy may be particularly challenging if the reason for critical illness is attempted suicide, however ECMO should not be withheld from a patient on the basis of suicidality or psychiatric illness.

**Technical Considerations and Potential Contraindications of ECLS in Poisoning**

There is no major difference in decision making in using ECLS for poisoning than in any other scenario. ECLS can be used to support respiratory, cardiac, or cardiorespiratory function for patients in whom the poison has depressed these organ systems so severely that conventional supportive measures are failing. The majority of patients will have a mixture of cardiac and respiratory insufficiency and will therefore be cannulated for VA ECMO support using the age-appropriate techniques discussed in Chapter 4. Patients with poisoning predominantly affecting the lungs, or example paraquat or diesel fuel aspiration, may be treated with VV ECMO as for any other type of ARDS. However, if electing to use VV support, clinicians should observe for evolving right ventricular (RV) dysfunction. If RV function is deteriorating, the patient may need to be switched to VVA support or to RV-PA cannulation. Another important consideration is potential reversibility, for instance a patient who has developed cerebral herniation related to acetaminophen (paracetamol) toxicity would not be an appropriate ECLS candidate. On the other hand, certain toxins may induce central nervous system depression that can mimic brain death lasting for days or weeks only to completely resolve; and clinicians should not conclude medical futility based on prolonged encephalopathy.[58]

Certain specific toxins and treatments may interact with ECLS circuits. Intravenous fat emulsion, which may be used to treat cardiotoxicity caused by calcium channel blockers and beta blockers, may interfere with ECLS by cracking stopcocks (23.8%), causing fat agglutination (26.2%), clogging the membrane lung (4.8%), and increasing blood clot formation in the circuits (4.8%).[59] Hydroxocobalamin, the preferred antidote for cyanide poisoning, is a bright red pigment and may activate blood leak alarms on hemodialysis machines.[60] Methylene Blue, the preferred treatment for acquired methemoglobinemia, may dye the fluid in the ECMO heat exchanger due to diffusion across the polyurethane heat exchange fibers.[61] Additionally, certain drugs such as midazolam, acetaminophen, lorazepam, fentanyl, and morphine have been shown to adsorb to the ECLS circuit (Chapter 49).[62,63] It is possible that other toxic substances and their pharmacological treatments may be absorbed by the ECLS circuit.

Some toxic substances may induce coagulopathy or hemolysis, which could potentially make ECLS less effective or more dangerous. Toxin-induced hemorrhagic disease may be exacerbated by central cannulation and by the anticoagulation needed for ECLS. Rattlesnake (Crotalidae) venom includes enzymes that digest cellular membranes and proteins, and may cause thrombocytopenia, fibrinolysis, and excessive bleeding.[64] Acute iron toxicity may cause disseminated intravascular coagulation and gastrointestinal hemorrhage.[65] Similarly, toxin-induced hemolysis such as in the setting of arsine gas poisoning may be exacerbated by mechanical circulatory support.

One peculiarity of ECLS support in poisoning is when the poison causes disruption to normal coupling of oxygen delivery and consumption and depresses oxygen consumption at a cellular level. In this situation, the clinician is faced with a patient on VA support who does not seem to be using enough oxygen. $SvO_2$ and NIRS may both be above 90% with flow of 100-120 ml/kg/min.[66] In this situation one should not be tempted to reduce flow, as it seems the patient is profoundly supply dependent. The resumption of normal metabolism is heralded by a reduction of $SvO_2$ and NIRS to normal levels. It is theoretically possible that poisoning with drugs which stimulate the metabolism (eg, salicylates and dinitrophenol) could create increased oxygen consumption. In this situation, it is recommended that ECMO flow be increased as much as necessary to reestablish a normal $DO_2$:$VO_2$ and obtain $SvO_2$ >65%. This may necessitate increasing VA flows to 200 ml/kg/min or even more, which may require insertion of additional venous drainage cannulas or even trans-thoracic cannulation.

Autoregulation of systemic vascular resistance may also be affected by poisons, for instance calcium channel blocker overdoses cause profound vasodilation, while amphetamines cause vasoconstriction. It may be necessary to manipulate the patient's SVR in these situations with vasopressors or vasodilators. These drugs should be titrated to optimize VA ECMO flow as discussed above, and the SVR adjusted to give an age-appropriate mean blood pressure. Complications of ECMO are no different from those seen with other indications, with the exception of complications related to the poisons themselves, such as limb ischemia caused by ergot-alkaloids as described by St. Anthony in 1676.[67]

**Conclusion**

ECLS can be used to successfully support adults and children following poisoning to allow bridge to recovery or transplantation. There is reasonable evidence from laboratory studies and case series that ECLS increases survival in patients who have failed conventional supportive care, particularly those in cardiac arrest. The lack of randomized controlled trials of ECLS vs. conventional care in poisoning should not deter clinicians from initiating ECLS when indicated. Specific treatment for the poisoning itself should be guided by advice from a toxicologist and a National Poisons Information service, if available.

# References

1. World Health Organization. Poison control and unintentional poisoning. Accessed January 8, 2022. https://www.who.int/data/gho/data/themes/topics/indicator-groups/poison-control-and-unintentional-poisoning.

2. Gummin DD, Mowry JB, Beuhler MC, et al. 2020 Annual Report of the American Association of Poison Control Centers' National Poison Data System (NPDS): 38th Annual Report. 2021;59(12):1282-1501.

3. Gonzalez-Urdiales P, Kuppermann N, Dalziel SR, et al. Pediatric Intentional Self-poisoning Evaluated in the Emergency Department: An International Study. Pediatr Emerg Care. 2021;37(12):e1631-e1636.

4. Boedeker W, Watts M, Clausing P, et al. The global distribution of acute unintentional pesticide poisoning: estimations based on a systematic review. BMC Public Heal 2020 201. 2020;20(1):1-19.

5. Mehrpour O, Akbari A, Jahani F, et al. Epidemiological and clinical profiles of acute poisoning in patients admitted to the intensive care unit in eastern Iran (2010 to 2017). BMC Emerg Med. 2018;18(1):1-9.

6. Senarathna L, Jayamanna SF, Kelly PJ, et al. Changing epidemiologic patterns of deliberate self poisoning in a rural district of Sri Lanka. BMC Public Health. 2012;12(1):1-8.

7. Martins SS, Sampson L, Cerdá M, et al. Worldwide Prevalence and Trends in Unintentional Drug Overdose: A Systematic Review of the Literature. Am J Public Health. 2015;105(11):e29-e49.

8. Lund C, Teige B, Drottning P, et al. A one-year observational study of all hospitalized and fatal acute poisonings in Oslo: epidemiology, intention and follow-up. BMC Public Health. 2012;12(1).

9. Clark D, Murray DB, Ray D. Epidemiology and Outcomes of Patients Admitted to Critical Care after Self-Poisoning: http://dx. 2011;12(4):268-273.

10. Derlet RW, Horowitz BZ. Cardiotoxic drugs. Emerg Med Clin North Am. 1995;13(4):771-791. Accessed January 8, 2022. https://www.unboundmedicine.com/medline/citation/7588189/Cardiotoxic_drugs_.

11. Mladěnka P, Applová L, Patočka J, et al. Comprehensive review of cardiovascular toxicity of drugs and related agents. Med Res Rev. 2018;38(4):1332.

12. Morrison LK, Kromm J, Gaudet J, et al. Rescue extracorporeal membrane oxygenation therapy in methamphetamine toxicity. CJEM. 2018;20(S2):S14-S19.

13. Geng S, Hao X, Xu H, et al. Cardiac injury after acute carbon monoxide poisoning and its clinical treatment scheme. Exp Ther Med. 2020;20(2):1098.

14. Gurjar M, Baronia AK, Azim A, et al. Managing aluminum phosphide poisonings. J Emergencies, Trauma Shock. 2011;4(3):378.

15. Gorguner M, Akgun M. Acute inhalation injury. Eurasian J Med. 2010;42(1):28-35. Accessed November 9, 2017. https://pubmed.ncbi.nlm.nih.gov/25610115/.

16. Shah A, Pasrija C, Kronfli A, et al. Veno-Venous Extracorporeal Membrane Oxygenation Use in the Treatment of Bleomycin Pulmonary Toxicity. Innovations (Phila). 2017;12(2):144-146.

17. Wolkove N, Baltzan M. Amiodarone pulmonary toxicity. Can Respir J. 2009;16(2):43.

18. Radke JB, Owen KP, Sutter ME, et al. The effects of opioids on the lung. Clin Rev Allergy Immunol. 2014;46(1):54-64.

19. Jiwa N, Sheth H, Silverman R. Naloxone-Induced Non-Cardiogenic Pulmonary Edema: A Case Report. Drug Saf - Case Reports. 2018;5(1).

20. Tseng W, Sutter ME, Albertson TE. Stimulants and the lung : review of literature. Clin Rev Allergy Immunol. 2014;46(1):82-100.

21. Seger D. Position paper: Single-dose activated charcoal. Clin Toxicol. 2005;43(2):61-87.

22. Cooper GM. A randomized clinical trial of activated charcoal for the routine management of oral drug overdose. Qjm. 2005;98(9):655-660.

23. Juurlink DN, Gosselin S, Kielstein JT, et al. Extracorporeal Treatment for Salicylate Poisoning: Systematic Review and Recommendations From the EXTRIP Workgroup. Ann Emerg Med. 2015;66(2):165-181.

24. Decker BS, Goldfarb DS, Dargan PI, et al. Extracorporeal Treatment for Lithium Poisoning: Systematic Review and Recommendations from the EXTRIP Workgroup. Clin J Am Soc Nephrol. 2015;10(5):875-887.

25. Calello DP, Liu KD, Wiegand TJ, et al. Extracorporeal Treatment for Metformin Poisoning: Systematic Review and Recommendations From the Extracorporeal Treatments in Poisoning Workgroup. Crit Care Med. 2015;43(8):1716-1730.

26. Köppel C, Oberdisse U, Heinemeyer G. Clinical Course and Outcome in Class IC Antiarrhythmic Overdose 2008;28(4):433-444.

27. Perez A, Paredes VL, Rea TD. Critical drug overdoses and emergency medical services: Where should we put our efforts? [2] (multiple letters). Acad Emerg Med. 2004;11(12):1369.

28. Upchurch C, Blumenberg A, Brodie D, et al. Extracorporeal membrane oxygenation use in poisoning: a narrative review with clinical recommendations. Clin Toxicol. 2021; 59:877-887.

29. Wang GS, Levitan R, Wiegand TJ, et al. Extracorporeal Membrane Oxygenation (ECMO) for Severe

Toxicological Exposures: Review of the Toxicology Investigators Consortium (ToxIC). J Med Toxicol. 2016;12(1):95-99.

30. Ferrari F, Carletti A, Peroni N, et al. Brief Report: A Case of Tramadol Overdose: Extracorporeal Life Support and Hemoperfusion as Life-Saving Treatment. Blood Purif. 2020;49(4):509-512.

31. Kolcz J, Pietrzyk J, Januszewska K, et al. Extracorporeal life support in severe propranolol and verapamil intoxication. J Intensive Care Med. 2007;22(6):381-385.

32. Ishigami S, Hase S, Nakashima H, et al. Intravenous chlorhexidine gluconate causing acute respiratory distress syndrome. J Toxicol Clin Toxicol. 2001;39(1):77-80.

33. Sato H, Kyan R, Uemura S, et al. Usefulness of venoarterial extracorporeal membranous oxygenation for fatal cibenzoline succinate poisoning. Acute Med Surg. 2020;7(1).

34. Ramanathan K, Mohanty B, Tang S, et al. Extracorporeal therapy for amlodipine poisoning. J Artif Organs. 2020;23(2):183-186.

35. Koschny R, Lutz M, Seckinger J, et al. Extracorporeal life support and plasmapheresis in a case of severe polyintoxication. J Emerg Med. 2014;47(5):527-531.

36. Schroeder I, Zoller M, Angstwurm M, et al. Venlafaxine intoxication with development of takotsubo cardiomyopathy: successful use of extracorporeal life support, intravenous lipid emulsion and CytoSorb®. Int J Artif Organs. 2017;40(7):358-360.

37. Thooft A, Goubella A, Fagnoul D, et al. Combination of veno-arterial extracorporeal membrane oxygenation and hypothermia for out-of-hospital cardiac arrest due to Taxus intoxication. CJEM. 2014;16(6):504-507.

38. Tang X, Sun B, He H, et al. Successful extracorporeal membrane oxygenation therapy as a bridge to sequential bilateral lung transplantation for a patient after severe paraquat poisoning. Clin Toxicol (Phila). 2015;53(9):908-913.

39. Freedman MD, Gal J, Freed CR. Extracorporeal pump assistance--novel treatment for acute lidocaine poisoning. Eur J Clin Pharmacol. 1982;22(2):129-135.

40. Martin TK, RL M, EA M, SM S. Extracorporeal life support vs thumper after lethal desipramine OD [abstract]. Vet Hum Toxicol. 1990;32:349.

41. Larkin GL, Graeber GM, Hollingsed MJ. Experimental amitriptyline poisoning: treatment of severe cardiovascular toxicity with cardiopulmonary bypass. Ann Emerg Med. 1994;23(3):480-486.

42. Mycyk M. Extracorporeal Membrane Oxygenation Shows Promise for Treatment of Poisoning Some of the Time: The Challenge to Do Better by Aiming Higher. Crit Care Med. 2020;48(8):e985.

43. Cole JB, Olives TD, Ulici A, et al. Extracorporeal Membrane Oxygenation for Poisonings Reported to U.S. Poison Centers from 2000 to 2018: An Analysis of the National Poison Data System. Crit Care Med. 2020;48(8):1111-1119.

44. Daubin C, Lehoux P, Ivascau C, et al. Extracorporeal life support in severe drug intoxication: a retrospective cohort study of seventeen cases. Crit Care. 2009;13(4):R138.

45. Masson R, Colas V, Parienti JJ, et al. A comparison of survival with and without extracorporeal life support treatment for severe poisoning due to drug intoxication. Resuscitation. 2012;83(11):1413-1417.

46. Wax PM, Kleinschmidt KC, Brent J, Investigators ATCR. The Toxicology Investigators Consortium (ToxIC) Registry. J Med Toxicol. 2011;7(4):259-265.

47. Lorusso R, Alexander P, Rycus P, et al. The Extracorporeal Life Support Organization Registry: update and perspectives. Ann Cardiothorac Surg. 2019;8(1):93-98.

48. Weiner L, Mazzeffi MA, Hines EQ, et al. Clinical utility of venoarterial-extracorporeal membrane oxygenation (VA-ECMO) in patients with drug-induced cardiogenic shock: a retrospective study of the Extracorporeal Life Support Organizations' ECMO case registry. Clin Toxicol (Phila). 2020;58(7):705-710.

49. Ramanathan K, Tan CS, Rycus P, et al. Extracorporeal membrane oxygenation for poisoning in adult patients: outcomes and predictors of mortality. Intensive Care Med. 2017;43(10):1538-1539.

50. Carpenter JE, Chang AS, Bronstein AC, et al. Identifying incidents of public health significance using the national poison data system, 2013-2018. Am J Public Health. 2020;110(10):1528-1531.

51. Combes A, Price S, Slutsky AS, et al. Temporary circulatory support for cardiogenic shock. Lancet. 2020;396(10245):199-212.

52. Ranieri VM, Rubenfeld GD, Thompson BT, et al. Acute respiratory distress syndrome: the Berlin Definition. JAMA. 2012;307(23):2526-2533.

53. Di Nardo M, Alunni Fegatelli D, Marano M, et al. Use of Extracorporeal Membrane Oxygenation in Acutely Poisoned Pediatric Patients in United States: A Retrospective Analysis of the Extracorporeal Life Support Registry From 2003 to 2019. Crit Care Med. 2022 Apr 1;50(4):655-664.

54. Hoppe-Roberts J, Lloyd L, Chyka P. Poisoning mortality in the United States: comparison of national mortality statistics and poison control center reports. Ann Emerg Med. 2000;35(5):440-448.

55. Groholt B, Ekeberg Ø. Prognosis after adolescent suicide attempt: mental health, psychiatric treatment, and suicide attempts in a nine-year follow-up study. Suicide Life Threat Behav. 2009;39(2):125-136.

56. Reid WH. Prognosis after suicide attempt: standard of care and the consequences of not meeting it. J Psychiatr Pract. 2009;15(2):141-144.

57. Eckman PM, Katz JN, El Banayosy A, et al. Veno-Arterial Extracorporeal Membrane Oxygenation for Cardiogenic Shock: An Introduction for the Busy Clinician. Circulation. 2019;140(24):2019-2037.

58. Murphy L, Wolfer H, Hendrickson RG. Toxicologic Confounders of Brain Death Determination: A Narrative Review. Neurocrit Care. 2021;34(3):1072-1089.

59. Lee HMD, Archer JRH, Dargan PI, et al. What are the adverse effects associated with the combined use of intravenous lipid emulsion and extracorporeal membrane oxygenation in the poisoned patient? Clin Toxicol (Phila). 2015;53(3):145-150.

60. Datar P, Sidhu JS, Virk J, et al. A Case of Hydroxocobalamin-Induced False Blood Leak Alarm on Dialysis Machine. J Investig Med High Impact Case Reports. 2019;7:2324709619883466.

61. Wieruszewski PM, Nabzdyk CG, Bowman HM, et al. Refractory Hypotension During ECMO: Words of Caution When Using Methylene Blue. J Cardiothorac Vasc Anesth. 2022 Feb;36(2):631-632.

62. Harthan AA, Buckley KW, Heger ML, et al. Medication adsorption into contemporary extracorporeal membrane oxygenator circuits. J Pediatr Pharmacol Ther. 2014;19(4):288-295.

63. Wildschut ED, Ahsman MJ, Allegaert K, et al. Determinants of drug absorption in different ECMO circuits. Intensive Care Med. 2010;36(12):2109-2116.

64. Slagboom J, Kool J, Harrison RA, et al. Haemotoxic snake venoms: their functional activity, impact on snakebite victims and pharmaceutical promise. Br J Haematol. 2017;177(6):947-959.

65. Robotham JL, Lietman PS. Acute Iron Poisoning: A Review. Am J Dis Child. 1980;134(9):875-879.

66. Lehoux J, Hena Z, McCabe M, et al. Aluminium phosphide poisoning resulting in cardiac arrest, successful treatment with Extracorporeal Cardiopulmonary resuscitation (ECPR): a case report. Perfus (United Kingdom). 2018;33(7):597-598.

67. Henry LG, Blackwood JS, Conley JE, et al. Ergotism. Arch Surg. 1975;110(8):929-932.

# 38

## Elderly Patients

*Roberto Lorusso, Koji Takeda, Shinichiro Ohshimo, Mariusz Kowalewski, Anna Mara Scandroglio, Giovanni Landoni, Yih-Sharng Chen*

## Introduction

Venoarterial ECMO represents a compelling treatment modality and is increasingly used in adults with refractory cardiogenic shock (CS).[1-6] According to ELSO Registry data, a dramatic increase in the number of ECLS cases among elderly (>70 years old) patients has been seen over the last 2 decades, with a rise of 280% between the years 2005-2010 and 2011-2015,[7] an increase nearly 50% greater in the elderly than in their younger counterparts. More sophisticated VA ECMO technology, more clinical confidence in implantation and postoperative management, as well as inclusion in resuscitation protocols (ie, ECPR), have been associated with broadening of ECMO indications. Consequently, VA ECMO has now become an important and potentially valid solution for patients previously not considered candidates for temporary mechanical circulatory support (MCS), to permit and promote organ recovery or to facilitate transition to more advanced and durable therapies. At the same time, VA ECMO is resource-intensive and often burdened by a complicated postimplantation course, which is particularly true in elderly patients. In most elderly patients, the general objective of VA ECMO is as a 'bridge to recovery' because more advanced approaches such as heart transplantation or durable left ventricular assist devices (LVAD) implantation are either contraindicated or considered futile.

## Epidemiology and Trends in the Use of ECLS in the Elderly

Temporary mechanical circulatory support and ECLS use for patients with acute circulatory or respiratory failure has dramatically increased in the past decades. In the United States, an estimated 11,887 patients received temporary MCS for circulatory failure between 2004 and 2011.[1] The rise of percutaneous device use was particularly remarkable, with an increase of 1511%, whereas rates of in-hospital mortality have been stable or decreased over time. In Germany, 45,647 patients were treated with ECLS from 2007 to 2018.[2] Of those, the number of VV ECMO cases increased by 236% from 825 in 2007 to 2,768 in 2018. Hospital mortality declined from 70.1% in 2008 to 53.9% in 2018. ECLS use for respiratory failure has been paralleled by an increase in the use of VA ECMO for cardiogenic shock in the United States.[3] According to the 2021 ELSO Registry report, there were 75,735 adult ECLS runs in the world and included in the registry.[4]

Population ageing is a global phenomenon. In 2019, there were 703 million persons aged 65 years or over in the global population. This number is projected to double to 1.5 billion in 2050.[5] As the general population grows older, the number of elderly patients at risk of acute circulatory or respiratory failure further increases. For example, the incidence of cardiogenic shock complicating acute myocardial infarction (AMI) in patients over the age of 75 had increased nearly by 5% within 7 years in the United States.[6] The rapid growth and positive outcomes of temporary MCS or ECLS use in acute circulatory and respiratory failure has resulted in a reduced treatment threshold to apply these therapies to elderly patients, although increasing age is a widely reported risk factor and is associated with increased mortality.[8] In the National Inpatient Sample analysis, patients over 65 years old accounted for 39.6% of patients on temporary MCS from 2004 to 2007 in the U.S. From 2008-2011, this age group grew to represent 47.2%.[1] In the German registry, the largest increase of VA ECMO use was observed in the 75 to 80 year-old age groups from 2007 to 2018.[2] In the analysis of Impella (Abiomed, Danvers, MA) use for the treatment of patients with AMI at U.S. centers between 2009-2016, there were 4164 patients (29.8%) over 70 years old. Of those, 1108 patients (26.6%) were over 80.[7] A recent ELSO Registry analysis from 1992 to 2015 found that patients over 70 years old accounted for 13.6% of patients on VA ECMO for cardiogenic shock. From 1993-1998 to 2011-2015, this age group grew from 7.6% to 14.8%. The mean age of this cohort was 75.3 +/- 4.5 years, and 63.9% were male. ECLS was more frequently used for postcardiotomy shock in the elderly cohort.[9]

Thus, there is a world-wide trend of liberal utilization of temporary MCS and ECLS over time. This chapter highlights the indication, management, and outcomes of ECLS and temporary MCS in the elderly.

## Circulatory Support

Previous reports comparing elderly versus younger patients undergoing VA ECMO for CS showed that in-hospital mortality was significantly higher in the former group.[8] The reports on outcomes across elderly populations undergoing VA ECMO therapy vary in terms of mortality rates.[7-27] Reasons for the observed divergent rates in these reports are multifactorial, including 1) different age thresholds to define "elderly"; 2) different etiologies of CS; 3) combining VA and VV ECMO patients; 4) diverse risk profiles and different indications for ECMO. In addition, the vast majority of previous studies are single-center experiences, often subject to selection bias. Besides, results in elderly patients may be less likely to be published for various reasons, including higher mortality, reluctance to share poor results, and reports often being limited to uncontrolled case series. Nevertheless, some reports are available. One recent report from the ELSO Registry[7] demonstrated that the total number of elderly patients increased each year (from 7% to 15%) within the frames of the registry (Figure 38-1).

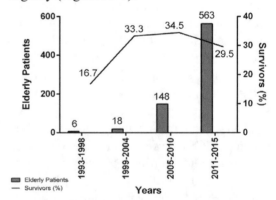

**Figure 38-1.** The in-hospital survival rates of elderly patients (≥70 years of age) submitted to VA ECMO for cardiogenic shock and enrolled in the ELSO Registry collected as of June 2015. A slight decline in survival rate was seen during the last year-group but was not statistically significant. (Used with permission from Lorusso R, et al.)[16]

One important finding of this report was that overall outcomes were not necessarily unacceptable. Patient selection most likely plays a critical role in the chance of achieving favorable results.

Another recent study,[23] again using ELSO Registry data and including 2,644 patients over 70 years old, was the first on this scale to address the trends of application, outcomes, and mortality predictors in elderly populations undergoing VA ECMO for cardiogenic shock. Besides showing a trend in the increase of VA ECMO use among the elderly for CS, it demonstrated that a significant proportion of patients underwent VA ECMO for postcardiotomy CS. Overall in-hospital mortality in this challenging setting was 68.3%, with the highest crude mortality observed in the 75-79 year old subgroup (70.1%). Interestingly, when observing age-adjusted outcomes, even the most advanced age group (ie, ≥ 80 years old) had in-hospital mortality rates which did not necessarily contraindicate the use of ECMO.

## Postcardiotomy and Non-postcardiotomy Shock

Elderly patients have particular characteristics with regard to indications for ECMO. The most frequent condition for VA ECMO implantation appears to be non-postcardiotomy CS, in contrast to what has already been shown in several other studies.[16-18] Figure 38-2 lists the indications and associated mortality. Regardless of age, several settings exist such as myocarditis, posttranscatheter aortic valve replacement (TAVR) CS, and acute coronary syndromes (ACS), where survival rates can be relatively favorable. Conversely, sepsis and decompensated heart failure in octogenarians supported with VA ECMO have dismal prognoses.

The situation is even more complex when the postcardiotomy setting is considered. While this population at baseline generally have relatively robust general health in order to undergo major elective heart surgery, postcardiotomy shock as

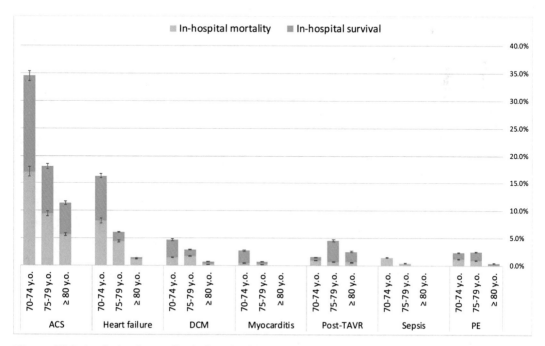

**Figure 38-2.** Analysis of mortality indices in elderly patients according to indication for VA ECMO in non postcardiotomy cardiogenic shock. (Reproduced with modifications from Kowalewski M et al.)[23]

an indication for VA ECMO is less common in older patients compared to younger subjects.[7] It may be explained, in part, by the fact that VA ECMO for postcardiotomy indications has been recently associated with poor results.[6] It is, however, more likely because of pre-ECMO comorbidities, the impact of preoperative cardiac illnesses and complicated surgical procedures, together with intraoperative features (eg, cannulation strategy[19]) as well as the type of complications more frequently observed such as bleeding and stroke.[6] Figure 38-3 depicts mortality in the postcardiotomy population, taking into account the division by age groups and type of surgery performed.

## Respiratory Support

According to ELSO Registry data,[28] annual VV ECMO usage has continued to rapidly increase since 2009, reaching 18,000 cases/year in 2020. With advancing age, the thorax becomes stiffer and the strength of the respiratory muscles decreases. During exercise, pulmonary arterial pressure increases with age. Reduced ciliary motility delays the clearance of pathogenic microorganisms in the airway. The $PaO_2$ also gradually decreases with age, while the pH and $PaCO_2$ do not significantly change. In this way, respiratory control, thoracic movement, and gas exchange capacity all decline with age.

Since VV ECMO is essentially a supportive therapy, it is not indicated when the lungs are affected by an irreversible process. However, the latest ELSO guidelines[29] do not define a clear age threshold for VV ECMO, although older age is a relative contraindication. Age has been widely known as a risk factor for the development of ARDS. However, the pathophysiological mechanisms underlying the increased risk and severity of ARDS in the elderly have not been well understood. Patients with ARDS often have multiple risk

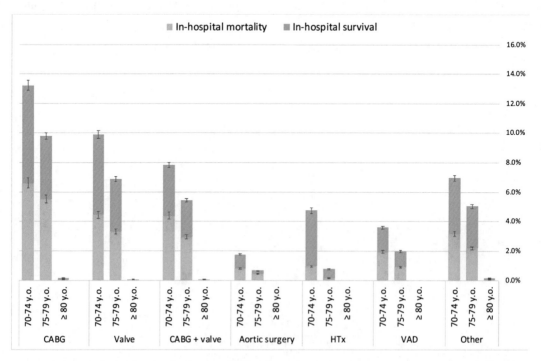

**Figure 38-3.** Analysis of mortality indices in elderly patients according to indication for V-A ECMO in postcardiotomy cardiogenic shock. (Reproduced with modifications from Kowalewski M et al.)[23]

factors and comorbidities, some of which may be influenced by age itself. Therefore, it is difficult to completely separate the effects of age and comorbidity on ECMO outcomes. Data on the use of ECMO in the elderly are limited and are generally from retrospective studies. Available data suggest that older age alone is not a contraindication to ECMO, but rather its use should be determined on a case-by-case basis.[30]

In earlier eras of ECLS, advanced age was considered a relative contraindication. For example, the pivotal CESAR trial only included patients below 65 years of age.[31] While the EOLIA trial did not have any specific upper age limit, the mean age of the participants was 52 years old.[32] A review of ELSO Registry data from 1990 to 2013 by Mendiratta et al. identified a total of 368 patients over the age of 65 receiving ECLS for respiratory failure.[30] In-hospital survival was 41%, lower than that of all other adults (55%), although selection bias may have been an issue. The authors also noted that over two thirds of cases were performed after 2010.

A multicenter study in South Korea from 2014 to 2015 reported 51 cases in patients older than 65 years from a total of 209 VV ECMO patients.[35] Survival was around 30% in elderly patients, and almost twice that in patients younger than 50 years of age.

The COVID-19 pandemic caused a new surge in ECMO research, with many series published from centers around the world. The mean age of patients treated with ECMO in ELSO Registry publications was 50 years of age, in line with that of previous series.[34] However, experience varied considerably between countries. In Germany, for example, a nationwide cohort analysis of 3875 VV ECMO runs between January 2020 and November 2021 included 924 patients over 65 years of age.[2] The study reported an overall survival rate of 34%, substantially lower than previous reports of ECMO for ARDS in Germany before the pandemic. As only 18% of elderly patients were

discharged alive, the authors recommended against initiation of ECMO in these patients. The experience from Japan was rather different: while only 35 ECMO runs were reported among 4695 in-hospital elderly patients, half of them survived to hospital discharge.[35]

## Predicting Outcomes in the Elderly

Various scoring systems have been suggested to predict the survival of patients with VV ECMO and VA ECMO (Table 38-1). The PRESERVE score was developed to predict 6-month survival after ECMO in patients with severe ARDS.[36] The RESP[37] and Roch[38] scores were developed to predict survival at discharge. The PRESET score was developed to predict ICU survival,[39] while the ECMOnet score was developed to predict in-hospital survival in patients with severe influenza A(H1N1) influenza.[40] A VV ECMO mortality score was developed to predict overall mortality.[41] Three of these scoring systems included age as a risk factor: PRESERVE score (3 points for age >55, 2 points for age 45-55, 0 points for age <45), RESP score (-3 points for age $\geq$60, -2 points for age 50-59, 0 points for age $\leq$49), and Roch score (1 point for age $\geq$45, 0 points for age <45). The remaining 3 scores did not include age. Furthermore, these scoring systems only predicted an increase in mortality and did not suggest that age alone was a contraindication to ECMO. These scoring systems include other variables such as obesity, immunosuppression, other organ dysfunction (SOFA score, platelets, total bilirubin, creatinine, mean blood pressure, central nervous system impairment), ventilatory and hospitalization days before starting ECMO, ventilator settings (PEEP, plateau pressure, peak inspiratory pressure), arterial blood gas analysis (pH, $PaCO_2$), use of supine position and muscle relaxants, primary disease of ARDS, circulatory failure (lactate levels), anemia, and many other factors. This suggests that older age alone does not determine poor outcomes following VV

ECMO, but rather that multiple other factors are involved. Scoring systems are also available for VA ECMO and include REMEMBER and SAVE scores. The Survival after VA ECMO (SAVE) Score[42] predicts survival in adult patients after ECMO for refractory CS. While patients receiving CPR during cannulation were not included in the derivation of the SAVE Score and, therefore, the score may not apply to these patients, age over 63 years was associated with a 50% increase in mortality compared to 18-38 year olds, regardless of other comorbidities. The (pRedicting mortality in patients undergoing venoarterial Extracorporeal MEMBrane oxygenation after coronary artEry bypass gRafting) REMEMBER[43] score was created with six pre-ECMO parameters: older age, left main coronary artery disease, inotrope score >75, CK-MB >130 IU/L, serum creatinine >150 umol/L, and platelet count <100 × 109/L, but was limited to patients undergoing isolated coronary surgery.

What needs to be addressed in future research is a risk stratification tool and a scoring system for both circulatory (postcardiotomy and non-postcardiotomy) and respiratory support which combines the predictive abilities of available scoring systems but is validated among a wider group of patients, rather than being limited to single indications.[44]

## Complications and Discontinuation of Therapy

A limited number of studies have specifically evaluated complications occurring in elderly patients using VV ECMO. However, following similar studies in VA ECMO,[45] it is clear that hemorrhagic, renal, mechanical, metabolic, neurological, and infectious complications are also more common in elderly patients with VV ECMO. The risk of these complications is particularly high because the duration of VV ECMO is longer than that of VA ECMO. It is important for physicians to promptly recognize these complications and appropriately treat them. Although older age is associated with a higher risk of complications, there is no established threshold above which ECMO is futile.[46]

| ECMO | VV ECMO | | | | | |
|---|---|---|---|---|---|---|
| Scoring system | PRESERVE | ECMOnet | RESP | Roch-Score | VV ECMO mortality | PRESET |
| Publication year | 2013 | 2013 | 2014 | 2014 | 2016 | 2017 |
| Age included in the score | Yes | No | Yes | Yes | No | No |
| Other variables considered | BMI, immunocompromised status, prone positioning, days MV, sepsis-related organ failure, plateau pressure and PEEP. | bilirubin value, MAP, HCT, preECMO hospital length of stay and sCr levels | immunocompromised status, days of MV, diagnosis, central nervous system dysfunction, acute associated non-pulmonary infection, NMB or NO use, bicarbonate infusion, cardiac arrest, PaCO2, and PIP | SOFA score, and a diagnosis of influenza pneumonia | immunocompromised status, duration of mechanical ventilation and SOFA score | Admission pH, MAP, lactate, platelet concentrations, and pre-ECMO hospital stay |

| ECMO | VA ECMO | | | |
|---|---|---|---|---|
| Scoring system | SAVE | ENCOURAGE | PREDICT VA-ECMO | REMEMBER |
| Publication year | 2015 | 2016 | 2018 | 2019 |
| Age included in the score | Yes | Yes | No | Yes |
| Other variables considered | CKD, ventilation prior to ECMO initiation, pre-ECMO organ failures, pre-ECMO cardiac arrest, CHD, pulse pressure, weight, acute myocarditis, heart transplant, VT or VF, blood pressure, bicarbonate level | female sex, body mass index >25 kg/m(2), Glasgow coma score <6, creatinine >150 µmol/L, lactate (<2, 2-8, or >8 mmol/L), and prothrombin activity <50%. | lactate, pH and standard bicarbonate concentration | left main coronary artery disease, inotropic score > 75, CK-MB > 130 IU/L, serum creatinine > 150 umol/L, and platelet count < 100 × 109/L. |

BMI=body mass index; MAP=mean arterial pressure; NMB=neuromuscular blockade; NO=nitric oxide; PaCO₂=partial pressure of arterial carbon dioxide; PEEP=positive end-expiratory pressure; PIP=peak inspiratory pressure; SOFA=sequential organ failure assessment.

**Table 38-1.** Comparison of scoring systems for predicting outcomes of VV and VA ECMO.

## Conclusions

Although advanced age is associated with limited success rates following ECLS, age alone is not directly related to an ominous prognosis. Rather, the comorbidities and frailty that are linked with age further drive poor outcomes. It may be that careful patient selection may ultimately provide some elderly patients with results comparable to their younger counterparts.

## References

1. Stretch R, Sauer CM, Yuh DD, et al. National trends in the utilization of short-term mechanical circulatory support: Incidence, outcomes, and cost analysis. J Am Coll Cardiol. 2014;64:1407-1415.
2. Friedrichson B, Mutlak H, Zacharowski K, et al. Insight into ECMO, mortality and ARDS: a nationwide analysis of 45,647 ECMO runs. Crit Care. 2021 Jan 28;25(1):38.
3. McCarthy FH, McDermott KM, Kini V, et al. Trends in u.S. Extracorporeal membrane oxygenation use and outcomes: 2002-2012. Semin Thorac Cardiovasc Surg. 2015;27:81-88.
4. ELSO registry report: https://www.elso.org/Portals/0/Files/Reports/2021_April/International%20Report%20April_page1.pdf.
5. United Nations Department of Economic Affairs. World Population Ageing 2019: Highlights (2019).
6. Kolte D, Khera S, Aronow WS, et al. Trends in incidence, management, and outcomes of cardiogenic shock complicating ST-elevation myocardial infarction in the United States. J Am Heart Assoc. 2014 Jan 13;3(1):e000590.
7. O'Neill WW, Grines C, Schreiber T, et al. Analysis of outcomes for 15,259 US patients with acute myocardial infarction cardiogenic shock (AMICS) supported with the Impella device. Am Heart J 2018 Aug;202:33-38.
8. Biancari F, Perrotti A, Ruggieri VG, et al. Five-year survival after post-cardiotomy veno-arterial extracorporeal membrane oxygenation. Eur Heart J Acute Cardiovasc Care. 2021 Aug 24;10(6):595-601.
9. Lorusso R, Gelsomino S, Parise O, et al. Venoarterial extracorporeal membrane oxygenation for refractory cardiogenic shock in elderly patients: Trends in application and outcome from the extracorporeal life support organization (elso) registry. Ann Thorac Surg. 2017;104:62-69.
10. Bellumkonda L, Gul B, Masri SC. Evolving concepts in diagnosis and management of cardiogenic shock. Am J Cardiol. 2018;122:1104-111.
11. Stretch R, Sauer CM, Yuh DD, et al. National trends in the utilization of short-term mechanical circulatory support: Incidence, outcomes, and cost analysis. J Am Coll Cardiol. 2014;64:1407-1415.
12. McCarthy FH, McDermott KM, Kini V, et al. Trends in U.S. Extracorporeal membrane oxygenation use and outcomes: 2002-2012. Semin Thorac Cardiovasc Surg. 2015;27:81-88.
13. Sauer CM, Yuh DD, Bonde P. Extracorporeal membrane oxygenation use has increased by 433% in adults in the united states from 2006 to 2011. ASAIO J. 2015;61:31-36.
14. Maxwell BG, Powers AJ, Sheikh AY, et al. Resource use trends in extracorporeal membrane oxygenation in adults: An analysis of the nationwide inpatient sample 1998-2009. J Thorac Cardiovasc Surg. 2014;148:416-421 e411.
15. Whitman GJ. Extracorporeal membrane oxygenation for the treatment of postcardiotomy shock. J Thorac Cardiovasc Surg. 2017;153:95-101.
16. Lorusso R, Gelsomino S, Parise O, et al. Venoarterial extracorporeal membrane oxygenation for refractory cardiogenic shock in elderly patients: Trends in application and outcome from the extracorporeal life support organization (elso) registry. Ann Thorac Surg. 2017;104:62-69.
17. Lee SN, Jo MS, Yoo KD. Impact of age on extracorporeal membrane oxygenation survival of patients with cardiac failure. Clin Interv Aging. 2017;12:1347-1353.
18. Yeh TC, Chang HH, Ger LP, et al. Clinical risk factors of extracorporeal membrane oxygenation support in older adults. PLoS One. 2018;13:e0195445.
19. Saito S, Nakatani T, Kobayashi J, et al. Is extracorporeal life support contraindicated in elderly patients? Ann Thorac Surg. 2007;83:140-145.
20. Wang L, Yang F, Wang X, et al. Predicting mortality in patients undergoing va-ecmo after coronary artery bypass grafting: The remember score. Crit Care. 2019;23:11.
21. Baek MS, Chung CR, Kim HJ, et al. Age is major factor for predicting survival in patients with acute respiratory failure on extracorporeal membrane oxygenation: A korean multicenter study. J Thorac Dis. 2018;10:1406-1417.
22. Strom JB, Zhao Y, Shen C, et al. National trends, predictors of use, and in-hospital outcomes in mechanical circulatory support for cardiogenic shock. EuroIntervention. 2018;13:e2152-e2159.
23. Kowalewski M, Zieliński K, Maria Raffa G, et al. Mortality Predictors in Elderly Patients With Cardiogenic Shock on Venoarterial Extracorporeal Life Support. Analysis From the Extracorporeal Life Support Organization Registry. Crit Care Med. 2021 Jan 1;49(1):7-18.
24. Pontailler M, Demondion P, Lebreton G, et al. Experience with Extracorporeal Life Support for Cardiogenic Shock in the Older Population more than 70 Years of Age. ASAIO J. 2017;63:279-284.
25. Sertic F, Diagne D, Rame E, et al. Short-term outcomes and predictors of in-hospital mortality with the use of veno-arterial extracorporeal membrane oxygenation in elderly patients with refractory cardiogenic shock. J Cardiovasc Surg (Torino). 2019 Oct;60(5):636-638.
26. Salna M, Takeda K, Kurlansky P, et al. The influence of advanced age on venous-arterial extracorporeal

membrane oxygenation outcomes. Eur J Cardiothorac Surg. 2018;53:1151-1157.

27. Kowalewski M, Zieliński K, Brodie D, et al. Venoarterial Extracorporeal Membrane Oxygenation for Postcardiotomy Shock-Analysis of the Extracorporeal Life Support Organization Registry. Crit Care Med. 2021 Jul 1;49(7):1107-1117.

28. ECLS Registry Report & International Summary of Statistics. URL: https//www.elso.org/Registry/InternationalSummary.aspx (31.12.2021 accessed).

29. Tonna JE, Abrams D, Brodie D, et al. Management of Adult Patients Supported with Venovenous Extracorporeal Membrane Oxygenation (VV ECMO): Guideline from the Extracorporeal Life Support Organization (ELSO). ASAIO J 2021;67:601–10.

30. Mendiratta P, Tang X, Collins RT, et al. Extracorporeal membrane oxygenation for respiratory failure in the elderly: a review of the Extracorporeal Life Support Organization registry. ASAIO J 2014;60:385–90.

31. Peek GJ, Mugford M, Tiruvoipati R, et al. Efficacy and economic assessment of conventional ventilatory support versus extracorporeal membrane oxygenation for severe adult respiratory failure (CESAR): a multicentre randomised controlled trial. Lancet 2009;374:1351-63.

32. Combes A, Hajage D, Capellier G, et al. Extracorporeal Membrane Oxygenation for Severe Acute Respiratory Distress Syndrome. N Engl J Med 2018;378:1965-1975.

33. Baek MS, Chung CR, Kim HJ, et al. Age is major factor for predicting survival in patients with acute respiratory failure on extracorporeal membrane oxygenation: a Korean multicenter study. J Thorac Dis 2018;10:1406-1417.

34. Barbaro RP, MacLaren G, Boonstra PS, et al. Extracorporeal Life Support Organization. Extracorporeal membrane oxygenation for COVID-19: evolving outcomes from the international Extracorporeal Life Support Organization Registry. Lancet 2021;398:1230-1238.

35. Asai Y, Nomoto H, Hayakawa K, et al. Comorbidities as Risk Factors for Severe Disease in Hospitalized Elderly COVID-19 Patients by Different Age-Groups in Japan. Gerontology 2022; 7:1-11.

36. Schmidt M, Zogheib E, Rozé H, et al. The PRESERVE mortality risk score and analysis of long-term outcomes after extracorporeal membrane oxygenation for severe acute respiratory distress syndrome. Intensive Care Med 2013;39:1704–13.

37. Schmidt M, Bailey M, Sheldrake J, et al. Predicting survival after extracorporeal membrane oxygenation for severe acute respiratory failure. The Respiratory Extracorporeal Membrane Oxygenation Survival Prediction (RESP) score. Am J Respir Crit Care Med 2014;189:1374–82.

38. Roch A, Hraiech S, Masson E, et al. Outcome of acute respiratory distress syndrome patients treated with extracorporeal membrane oxygenation and brought to a referral center. Intensive Care Med 2014;40:74–83.

39. Hilder M, Herbstreit F, Adamzik M, et al. Comparison of mortality prediction models in acute respiratory distress syndrome undergoing extracorporeal membrane oxygenation and development of a novel prediction score: the PREdiction of Survival on ECMO Therapy-Score (PRESET-Score). Crit Care 2017;21:301.

40. Pappalardo F, Pieri M, Greco T, et al. Predicting mortality risk in patients undergoing venovenous ECMO for ARDS due to influenza A (H1N1) pneumonia: the ECMOnet score. Intensive Care Med 2013;39:275–81.

41. Cheng YT, Wu MY, Chang YS, et al. Developing a simple preinterventional score to predict hospital mortality in adult venovenous extracorporeal membrane oxygenation: A pilot study. Medicine (Baltimore) 2016;95:e4380.

42. Schmidt M, Burrell A, Roberts L, et al. Predicting survival after ECMO for refractory cardiogenic shock: the survival after veno-arterial-ECMO (SAVE)-score. Eur Heart J. 2015 Sep 1;36(33):2246-56.

43. Wang L, Yang F, Wang X, et al. Predicting mortality in patients undergoing VA-ECMO after coronary artery bypass grafting: the REMEMBER score. Crit Care. 2019 Jan 11;23(1):11.

44. Maca J, Matousek V, Bursa F, et al. Extracorporeal membrane oxygenation survival: External validation of current predictive scoring systems focusing on influenza A etiology. Artif Organs 2021;45:881–92.

45. Kowalewski M, Zieliński K, Maria Raffa G, et al. Mortality Predictors in Elderly Patients with Cardiogenic Shock on Venoarterial Extracorporeal Life Support. Analysis from the Extracorporeal Life Support Organization Registry*. Crit Care Med 2021;49:1107–17.

46. ELSO Guidelines for Cardiopulmonary Extracorporeal Life Support Extracorporeal Life Support Organization, Version 1.4 August 2017. Ann Arbor, MI, USA. www.elso.org.

# Malignancy and Immunodeficiency

*Matteo Di Nardo, R. Scott Stephens, Jonathan C. Yeung, Peter Schellongowski, Matthieu Schmidt, Melania M. Bembea*

## Introduction

Concerns over whether ECLS should be offered to immunocompromised patients have led to many controversial and thought-provoking discussions in the last decade. The lack of specific criteria and uncertain prognosis for ECLS use in this subset of patients renders ECLS candidacy more challenging. This chapter provides current insights and, where possible, new data on ECLS candidacy in patients with solid and blood cell tumors, patients receiving hematopoietic stem cell transplantation (HSCT), and those with autoimmune diseases or Human Immunodeficiency Virus (HIV).

## ECLS Support in Pediatric and Adult Patients with Solid Organ and Blood Cancer

Pediatric and adult cancer patients account for approximately 15%-40% of all intensive care unit (ICU) admissions.[1,2] Though historically dismal,[3] outcomes for critically ill cancer patients have improved in recent years, and current ICU and hospital survival stands at over 50%.[4-8] Furthermore, substantial evidence suggests that many adult ICU survivors regain a favorable quality of life and tolerate continued, and potentially curative, anticancer therapies. At the same time, novel and highly effective anticancer therapies, including immune checkpoint inhibitors (ICI) and immune effector cells, carry the risk of significant toxicity, including fulminant cardiopulmonary failure, but with the potential for long-term control or cure of the malignancy.[9] This is particularly important because long-term survival after critical illness is defined by the prognosis of the underlying malignant disease, and may not differ from cancer patients who were never admitted to the ICU.[1,2] Thus, a uniform reluctance to admit to provide advanced critical care support to patients with cancer can no longer be justified.[6]

### *ECLS Utilization in Patients with Malignancy*

Conventional criteria for ECLS candidacy have focused on otherwise healthy patients with respiratory and/or cardiac failure. In many cases, these criteria have excluded patients with active malignancy.[10] However, over the last decade, ECLS use has increased in pediatric and adult patients with malignancy.[11-17] This may be due to a combination of increased use of ECLS in complicated patient populations and improved cancer-specific survival rates.

Data on ECLS outcomes in patients with malignancies are limited, and predominantly include single-center studies and case series. There are a few exceptions, and these larger studies may be the most informative with regards to outcomes. In 2010, an analysis of the ELSO Registry reported an overall hospital survival rate of 32% in 72 adult patients with malignancy undergoing ECLS support.[12] Respiratory failure was the most common reason for ECLS. There was no difference in survival according to type of malignancy (solid vs. hematologic), but patients with respiratory failure had worse outcomes than patients with cardiac failure. Specific to pediatric patients, a review of children from the ELSO Registry from 1994-2007 by Gow et al. included 107 patients with oncologic disease (HSCT patients were excluded), with 35% survival to discharge.[18] More recently, an abstract by Armijo-Garcia et al. reported 178 ECLS patients with malignancy (also excluding HSCT patients) from 2008-2012, with a 48% survival to discharge, despite similar complication rates compared to those reported previously. Hematologic or solid malignancy did not impact survival.[19] Recently, Bridges et al. reported a multicenter cohort of children with cancer who were supported with VV ECMO for respiratory failure.[11] Analysis of this cohort of 21 patients demonstrated 38% pediatric ICU survival. Type of cancer (hematologic vs. solid tumor) was not associated with survival. In these patients, survival was not different for those placed on ECLS within one month of diagnosis as compared to being more remote from diagnosis.

To add to this evidence, larger series reporting outcomes of immunocompromised patients supported with ECLS are also informative. Schmidt et al. reported a 30% six-month survival rate in 203 immunocompromised patients with ARDS.[20] Hematologic malignancy patients had significantly worse outcomes than other immunocompromised patients. Older age, thrombocytopenia, hypercapnia, and higher driving pressures were all associated with mortality, while recent-onset immunosuppression was associated with a lower risk of mortality. More recently, a series

of 118 immunocompromised patients supported with ECLS for respiratory failure reported a 34% hospital survival rate and a 25 % six-month survival rate.[21] However, hematologic malignancy patients had particularly poor outcomes (0% six-month survival).

### Indications, Contraindications, and Specific Considerations

There are no definitive indications and contraindications for ECLS support in patients with malignancy. Thus, the decision whether ECLS deployment is appropriate should be informed by specific status details of the patient's malignant disease and chance of survival, whether cancer-specific treatment has commenced, the likelihood of successful treatment, the time frame in which treatment might take effect, secondary organ involvement (eg, kidney, liver, etc.), and whether the critical illness is potentially reversible.[22] During this complex decisionmaking, it is worth noting that 5-year survival for many cancers is similar to or better than that for other conditions for which ECLS support is common (eg, bridge to lung transplant, extracorporeal cardiopulmonary resuscitation).[23,24] Thus, survival-to-hospital discharge may not be the most important outcome to be evaluated in the clinical decisionmaking surrounding ECLS candidacy, but rather 'good long-term survival', "which includes adequate neurological, psychological and functional recovery coupled to an acceptable quality of life."[24] In addition, predicted survival is continuously changing with the advent of novel anticancer therapies with high efficacy. Thus, since standardized criteria for ECLS candidacy do not currently exist in cancer patients, ECLS should be evaluated on a case-by-case basis searching for interdisciplinary consensus between the ECLS, oncology, and palliative care teams, the patient (when feasible), and family.

Additional specific considerations regarding ECLS in patients with malignancies include the risks of bleeding and infections while on ECLS. Many cancer patients are thrombocytopenic due to the underlying malignancy or to chemotherapy-induced myelosuppression. Thrombocytopenia may preclude the use of anticoagulation while on ECLS if platelet counts cannot be adequately maintained with transfusions. Infection is a major risk in immunocompromised cancer patients, and may either be the cause for requiring ECLS support (eg, pneumonia leading to ARDS) or can develop while on ECLS. In patients who are severely immunocompromised, infections are the most common cause of respiratory failure and septic shock. Evaluation of the patient's immune status is crucial in these circumstances. Since ECLS is not a therapy, physicians should carefully evaluate patients' immune status before considering ECLS. Some infections, in fact, can be cured only when immune reconstitution has recovered. Thus, ECLS should be considered with extreme caution in patients with refractory neutropenia or thrombocytopenia.

Of note, ECLS should not be the reason to postpone or withhold chemotherapy.[25-27] For example, in the case of a patient with life-threatening mediastinal mass, reduction in tumor burden with urgent chemotherapy may rapidly improve the patient's condition.[28] However, when chemotherapy is given, attention to the changes in pharmacokinetics during ECLS should be considered.[29]

**ECLS in Patients with Massive Mediastinal Masses**

The induction of anesthesia for patients with massive anterior mediastinal masses (lymphomas, germ cell tumors, lymphoblastic leukemias, etc.) for diagnostic or therapeutic reasons is challenging and may require the use of ECLS.[30-34] These masses are slow growing and may result in significant mass effect on the airway and cardiovascular structures which are compensated by the awake patient, for example, with avoidance of the supine position and tension of the airway muscles to maintain patency. Upon induction, these mechanisms are lost, potentially leading to rapid loss of airway, compression of great vessels, and cardiovascular collapse. The change from atmospheric pressure ventilation to positive-pressure ventilation and the arterio- and venodilation caused by anesthetic agents may additionally promote cardiovascular collapse following induction. Clinically, high-risk patients can be identified by the inability to lie supine. Consequently, diagnostic biopsies should be performed awake wherever possible.

Assessment of the patient should include the aforementioned clinical exam, cross-sectional imaging, and echocardiography. High-risk patients potentially requiring ECLS may include ones with superior vena cava syndrome, pulmonary artery compression, tracheal or bronchial compression >50% (particularly of the distal trachea/carina where an endotracheal tube cannot be easily passed), and/or cardiac compression. Pediatric patients are at high risk even when tracheal compression is <50%. In these circumstances, consideration should be given for an ECLS circuit to be kept primed in the operating theater with femoral access sheaths prepared with local anesthesia.[28] After that, awake fiberoptic intubation can be attempted to secure the airway. If intubation fails or the patient develops peri arrest symptoms, the patient should be immediately repositioned upright to reestablish awake physiology. Awake ECLS should then be initiated as a bridge for temporary cardiopulmonary stabilization for induction of anesthesia and surgery. If the patient arrests despite best attempts, ECLS via the existing groin sheaths should be undertaken, but the surgical team should not focus solely on this modality for rescue. Cannulation can often take >5 minutes, by which time neurological compromise may already have occurred. Simultaneous rapid sternotomy to relieve the intrathoracic pressure should be considered to maximize outcomes in this difficult situation.

## ECLS in Patients Undergoing HSCT

In the last decade, survival of critically ill patients admitted to ICU and receiving allogeneic or autologous HSCT has increased, particularly in children.[35-39] In light of these results, a renewed interested in ECLS has grown, especially in pediatric patients receiving HSCT, based on recent data showing improved survival compared with previous years.[40-46] Allogeneic stem cell transplantation has been generally considered an absolute contraindication for ECLS because of poor survival.[47,48] In contrast, ECLS in patients receiving autologous stem cell transplantation appeared to show better outcomes, even although few cases were reported.[13,49,50] Recent data in pediatrics show that there is no difference in term of ECLS survival between patients receiving autologous vs. allogeneic HSCT[46]; however, it is well known that both are associated with different transplant-related mortality, which is lower in autologous (<5%) than in allogeneic HSCT (up to 10-20%).[51,52] Pooled data from European adult centers showed very poor outcomes in allogeneic stem cell transplanted patients who received ECLS, with a survival ranging from 10 to 20% and the only survivors were admitted long after engraftment (>100 days).[48] Recovery of immune reconstitution is essential to face infectious causes of respiratory or cardiac failure. In the first three months after engraftment, immune reconstitution is still impaired and this may explain the poor outcomes reported in adults, especially when particular types of HSCT are used (eg, T-B depleted or haploidentical HSCT). For these reasons, many adult centers currently consider allogeneic HSCT as an absolute contraindication for ECLS. A different perspective is viewed in pediatric

patients receiving allogeneic HSCT, where the use of adopted immunotherapies (eg, donor third-party cytotoxic lymphocytes) showed effective treatment of bacterial, viral, and fungal pathogens when immune reconstitution is still impaired, even during ECLS.[53]

Currently, ECLS candidacy and management of HSCT patient receiving ECLS for respiratory and/or cardiac failure is based on retrospective studies, case series and case reports; however, there is general consensus that ECLS could be considered in children receiving HSCT for nonmalignant disease or with malignancies at low risk of recurrence with a reasonable disease-free survival.[53] ECLS candidacy in adult patients receiving HSCT is still controversial and should be evaluated on a case-by-case basis and with an interdisciplinary team.

### Technical Considerations on ECLS Candidacy

ECLS candidacy in HSCT patients includes evaluation of the underlying disease treated with HSCT (eg, hematologic disease [benign vs. malignant], inborn errors of metabolism, or immune deficiency), the current critical illness requiring ECLS and its potential reversibility in a reasonable amount of time, the organ reserve prior to ECLS, and the refractoriness of thrombocytopenia.[53] Other valuable details supporting the decisionmaking are the type of conditioning regimen used (myeloablative vs. nonmyeloablative) before HSCT, the type of HSCT (autologous vs. allogeneic), the graft source (peripheral blood, bone marrow, umbilical cord blood) and its manipulation, as well as the human leukocyte antigen (HLA)-matching.

### Use of ECLS to Manage Respiratory Failure after HSCT

Acute respiratory failure and cardiac failure due to septic shock are the most common causes of ICU admission after HSCT. Acute respiratory failure may be due to infectious or noninfectious causes and etiology has an important impact on outcomes. Pulmonary infections before neutrophil engraftment are often difficult to manage without the support of the innate and the adaptive immune responses.[54,55] When pulmonary infections occur after neutrophil engraftment, bacterial infections are more successfully treated than viral and fungal infections, which remain challenging because of the absence of functional lymphocytes. However, early detection of infections and specific adoptive immunotherapies (virus specific T-cells and third-party T-cells directed to viral and fungal pathogens) may allow for effective treatment when immune reconstitution is still impaired.[56.] Therefore, ECLS may be considered after neutrophil engraftment when the likelihood of recovery of the critical illness is high in a reasonable period of time (2-3 weeks) with the use of these advanced treatments.[53]

Noninfectious causes of acute lung injury after HSCT are related to the process of immune recovery. Early diagnosis of these diseases and appropriate therapy can avoid the use of ECLS and its related risks (bleeding, infection, etc.).[57] Idiopathic pneumonia syndrome (IPS) is a group of lung diseases characterized by noninfectious involvement of the lung after HSCT, which may affect the pulmonary parenchyma, the vascular endothelium, or the airway epithelium. Recent data obtained in both adults and children show that IPS has a good clinical response to steroids and tumor necrosis factor-alpha inhibition. Refractory IPS may benefit from ECLS.[58,59] Diffuse alveolar hemorrhage (DAH) is another form of IPS that was historically regarded as an absolute contraindication to ECLS. Systemic glucocorticoids are considered the mainstay of therapy; however, there is a high variability in dosing and duration of therapy. Recent pediatric data have shown successful outcomes with the use of ECLS to manage patients unresponsive

to maximal medical treatment.[60,61] Bronchiolitis obliterans represents a late complication of HSCT and occurs almost exclusively in allogeneic recipients with chronic GVHD. ECLS can be used in bronchiolitis obliterans as a bridge to lung transplantation in patients who remain in remission of their primary disease and who have not developed secondary malignancies and/or have active chronic GVHD.[62,63] Currently, there is insufficient data to recommend the use of ECLS to manage respiratory and/or cardiac failure in patients with sinusoidal obstruction syndrome or transplant associated thrombotic microangiopathy. Decision regarding ECLS candidacy in patients with these complications should be made with caution and on a case-by-case basis.[53]

### Use of ECLS to Manage Heart Failure after HSCT

Congestive heart failure can be a complication of HSCT, especially in patients receiving autologous transplantation. Potentially cardiotoxic exposures unique to HSCT include myeloablative conditioning with high-dose chemotherapy (alkylators, anthracyclines, antimetabolites, antimicrotubules, and antibodies) and total body irradiation.[64,65] Viral myocarditis can be a fatal complication after HSCT due to the impaired immune reconstitution. Antiviral treatments, adoptive immunotherapies with virus specific T-cells and immunoglobulin supplementations may be of help to improve cardiac function, while immunosuppressive therapies may of help in virus-negative myocarditis.[66]

### Anticoagulation Management in Patients Receiving HSCT

Tailored anticoagulation management balancing the risks of bleeding and thrombosis is essential in HSCT patients receiving ECLS. In HSCT patients supported with ECLS, we recommend maintaining the platelet count higher than 40.000/µL.[53] We also suggest to maintain fibrinogen levels higher than 200 mg/dL and antithrombin activity between 80-100% with plasma-derived concentrate.[53] In patients at high risk of bleeding, some centers reported positive data with the use of ECLS without any anticoagulation. This was achieved using high blood flow (eg, 2 L/min for VA ECMO and 3-3.5 L/min for VV ECMO).[67-69] However, data are lacking in this population. Notably, in refractory bleeding, thrombocytopenia and acquired von Willebrand syndrome should be considered.[70]

### ECLS in Adult Patients with HIV

Pulmonary infections and respiratory failure are the most common causes of ICU admission in HIV patients. Although the frequency of ICU admission has decreased since the use of Highly Active Antiretroviral Therapy (HAART), several cohorts have described the use of ECLS in patients with HIV and respiratory failure.[71] In a retrospective multicenter study including 203 immunocompromised patients on ECLS, 6-month survival was 24% in patients with HIV. Besides, a low pre-ECLS platelet count was an independent predictor of mortality.[72] These results were recently confirmed in 126 patients with HIV from the ELSO Registry.[71] Overall survival to discharge was 36%. Respiratory ECLS was the primary indication (78%) with 39% survival, while cardiac and ECPR indications accounted for 16% and 6% of patients, with survival rates of 30% and 12.5%, respectively.

### *Pneumocystis jirovecii Pneumonia*

The main cause for ECLS in immuno-compromised HIV-positive patients is *Pneumocystis jirovecii* Pneumonia (PJP). Capatos et al. reported an aggressive approach to the management and cannulation of HIV patients with severe respiratory failure within three institutions in South Africa.[73] Survival to discharge among their 22 HIV-positive patients was 68%, and 60% in those with PJP. However, these apparently good outcomes, approaching those reported for bacterial or viral ARDS,[74,75] has been tempered by more recent studies.[71] In summary, the survival rate of patients with HIV-related ARDS treated with ECLS appears lower than those reported in the CESAR[74] or the EOLIA[75] trials.

### ECLS in Autoimmune Disease

Patients with autoimmune diseases may present with acute respiratory failure or cardiovascular failure due to different etiological categories: exacerbation of the underlying disease or complications thereof, including bleeding, pulmonary embolism, infections, macrophage activation syndrome, or complications of the treatment, such as infections, toxicity, and myocarditis.[76-78] The experience with ECLS in adult patients with autoimmune diseases is limited to mostly smaller case series or single case reports.[79,80] Therefore, ECLS candidacy and management still remains an interdisciplinary and individualized process. Furthermore, in some patients, the diagnosis of an autoimmune disease is only made during ECLS. In these situations, ECLS may serve as bridge to recovery or as a bridge to lung transplantation.

In general, the prognosis of acute respiratory failure in immunosuppressed patients with unidentified etiology is poor.[81] Besides infectious complications, diffuse alveolar hemorrhage (DAH) has been the most common reason for acute respiratory failure necessitating VV ECMO in autoimmune disease.[79] Successful treatment of DAH with VV ECMO has been reported in patients with lupus erythematosus, polymyositis, anti-MDA5 dermatomyositis, polyarteritis nodosa, Wegener´s granulomatosis, microscopic polyangiitis, antiphospholipid syndrome, as well as secondary vasculitis (eg, immune-mediated vasculitis to medication).[79,82-84] Earlier reports stated that systemic anticoagulation was administered to most patients despite DAH.[85] However, it is unclear if this remains necessary with the latest generation devices, improved biocompatibility, as well as heparin-coated cannulas and lines. Survival rates of VV ECMO treated patients with DAH have been as high as 90% in some patient series.[86] However, recent reports also emphasize the high risk of bleeding, including central nervous systemic bleeding.[84] VA ECMO has been used successfully in cases of lupus-associated myocarditis with refractory cardiogenic shock, eosinophilic granulomatosis with polyangiitis, Takayasu arteritis and rheumatoid arthritis,[87] as well as in patients with catastrophic antiphospholipid syndrome accompanied by fulminant pulmonary embolism.[88] In the largest case series of patients with autoimmune disease treated with ECLS, a total of 90 patients were treated with either VV ECMO for respiratory failure (53%), or VA ECMO for cardiovascular failure (47%).[80] The combined hospital survival rate was 49% but survival was higher in patients with vasculitis. Of note, the respective survival rates for VV and VA ECMO patients matched the general outcomes of the ELSO Registry.[80]

The use of ECLS to manage pediatric autoimmune disease is relatively rare and limited to brief reports.[89-94] A recent analysis of the ELSO Registry reported that the use of ECLS in children with immune-mediated disorders has progressively increased in the last decade, with survival rates to hospital discharge of 50%.[89] Of note, survival decreased over time and differed between respiratory and cardiac cases, the latter being more successful. Respiratory comorbidities (eg, pulmonary haemorrhage, pulmonary infections) are the most critical complications of autoimmune diseases and may be successfully supported with ECLS. Patients with juvenile idiopathic arthritis, dermatomyositis, and hemophagocytic lymphohistiocytosis (HLH) had the worst prognosis.[89] Currently, the use of ECLS to manage HLH remains controversial because of poor outcomes[27,90,91,95,96] and should be evaluated on a case-by-case basis.

In conclusion, patients with refractory acute respiratory and/or cardiac failure complicating autoimmune diseases represent a poorly studied and complex population. ECLS candidacy requires an interdisciplinary and individualized evaluation while aggressive therapy for the primary disorder is promptly instituted.

## References

1.  Soares M, Bozza FA, Azevedo LC, et al. Effects of Organizational Characteristics on Outcomes and Resource Use in Patients With Cancer Admitted to Intensive Care Units. J Clin Oncol. 2016;34(27):3315-3324.
2.  Wösten-van Asperen RM, van Gestel JPJ, van Grotel M, et al. PICU mortality of children with cancer admitted to pediatric intensive care unit a systematic review and meta-analysis. Crit Rev Oncol Hematol. 2019;142:153-163.
3.  Mokart D, Pastores SM, Darmon M. Has survival increased in cancer patients admitted to the ICU? Yes. Intensive Care Med. 2014;40(10):1570-1572.
4.  Vincent F, Soares M, Mokart D, et al. In-hospital and day-120 survival of critically ill solid cancer patients after discharge of the intensive care units: results of a retrospective multicenter study-A Groupe de recherche respiratoire en reanimation en Onco-Hematologie (Grrr-OH) study. Ann Intensive Care. 2018;8(1):40.
5.  Georges Q, Azoulay E, Mokart D, et al. Influence of neutropenia on mortality of critically ill cancer patients: results of a meta-analysis on individual data. Crit Care. 2018;22(1):326.
6.  Azoulay E, Mokart D, Pene F, et al. Outcomes of critically ill patients with hematologic malignancies: prospective multicenter data from France and Belgium--a groupe de recherche respiratoire en reanimation onco-hematologique study. J Clin Oncol. 2013;31(22):2810-2818.
7.  Darmon M, Bourmaud A, Georges Q, et al. Changes in critically ill cancer patients' short-term outcome over the last decades: results of systematic review with meta-analysis on individual data. Intensive Care Med. 2019;45(7):977-987.
8.  Ali AM, Sayed HA, Mohammed MM. The Outcome of Critically Ill Pediatric Cancer Patients Admitted to the Pediatric Intensive Care Unit in a Tertiary University Oncology Center in a Developing Country: A 5-Year Experience. J Pediatr Hematol Oncol. 2016;38(5):355-359.
9.  Riveiro-Barciela M, Trallero-Araguás E, Martínez-Valle F. Toxicities from immunotherapy: From clinical trials to real-world clinical practice. Med Clin (Barc). 2020;155(12):541-547.
10. Combes A, Hajage D, Capellier G, et al. Extracorporeal Membrane Oxygenation for Severe Acute Respiratory Distress Syndrome. N Engl J Med. 2018;378(21):1965-1975.
11. Bridges BC, Kilbaugh TJ, Barbaro RP, et al. Veno-Venous Extracorporeal Membrane Oxygenation for Children With Cancer or Hematopoietic Cell Transplant: A Ten Center Cohort. ASAIO J. 2021;67(8):923-929.
12. Gow KW, Lao OB, Leong T, Fortenberry JD. Extracorporeal life support for adults with malignancy and respiratory or cardiac failure: The Extracorporeal Life Support experience. Am J Surg. 2010;199(5):669-675.
13. Pravin RR, Huang BX, Sultana R, et al. Mortality Trends of Oncology and Hematopoietic Stem Cell Transplant Patients Supported on Extracorporeal Membrane Oxygenation: A Systematic Review and Meta-Analysis. J Intensive Care Med. 2022 Apr;37(4):555-564.
14. Potratz JC, Guddorf S, Ahlmann M, et al. Extracorporeal Membrane Oxygenation in Children With Cancer or Hematopoietic Cell Transplantation: Single-Center Experience in 20 Consecutive Patients. Front Oncol. 2021;11:664928.
15. Ranta S, Kalzén H, Nilsson A, et al. Extracorporeal Membrane Oxygenation Support in Children With Hematologic Malignancies in Sweden. J Pediatr Hematol Oncol. 2021;43(2):e272-e275.
16. Kebudi R, Oflaz Sozmen B, Bahar M, et al. Prolonged extracorporeal membrane oxygenation in pediatric leukemia with severe acute respiratory distress syndrome and persistent fungemia. Pediatr Blood Cancer. 2021;68(6):e28966.
17. Alexander PMA, Thiagarajan RR. Pediatric oncology-The final frontier for extracorporeal membrane oxygenation in children? Pediatr Blood Cancer. 2020;67(10):e28521.
18. Gow KW, Heiss KF, Wulkan ML, et al. Extracorporeal life support for support of children with malignancy and respiratory or cardiac failure: The extracorporeal life support experience. Crit Care Med. 2009;37(4):1308-1316.
19. Armijo-Garcia V FC, Carrillo S, Gelfond J, Meyer AD, et al. Outcome of extracorporeal life support for children with malignancy: A report from the Extracorporeal Life Support Organization (ELSO) registry. In. Proceedings of the 24th Annual ELSO Meeting Program 2012; Philadelphia, PA.
20. Schmidt M, Schellongowski P, Patroniti N, et al. Six-month Outcome of Immunocompromised Severe ARDS Patients Rescued by ECMO. An International Multicenter Retrospective Study. Am J Respir Crit Care Med. 2018 May 15;197(10):1297-1307.
21. Na SJ, Park SH, Hong SB, et al. Clinical outcomes of immunocompromised patients on extracorporeal membrane oxygenation support for severe acute respiratory failure. Eur J Cardiothorac Surg. 2020;57(4):788-795.
22. Reddy DRS, Botz GH. Triage and Prognostication of Cancer Patients Admitted to the Intensive Care Unit. Crit Care Clin. 2021;37(1):1-18.

23. Inci I, Ehrsam JP, Van Raemdonck D, et al. Extracorporeal life support as a bridge to pulmonary retransplantation: prognostic factors for survival in a multicentre cohort analysis. Eur J Cardiothorac Surg. 2022 Jan 24;61(2):405-412.

24. MacLaren G. When to initiate ECMO with low likelihood of success. Crit Care. 2018;22(1):217.

25. Rotz SJ, Almeida FA, Koyfman S, et al. Continuous infusion chemotherapy, radiotherapy, and FDG-PET are feasible during extracorporeal membrane oxygenation. Pediatr Blood Cancer. 2020;67(9):e28429.

26. Sekandarzad A, Udi J, Waller CF, et al. Extracorporeal Membrane Oxygenation Support as a Bridge to Recovery during Chemotherapy in a Young Patient with Metastatic Choriocarcinoma and Severe Acute Respiratory Distress Syndrome. Oncol Res Treat. 2020;43(10):559-564.

27. Weyand AC, Barbaro RP, Walkovich KJ, et al. Adjustments to pharmacologic therapies for hemophagocytic lymphohistiocytosis while on extracorporeal support. Pediatr Blood Cancer. 2021;68(6):e29007.

28. Leow L, Sampath HK, Yong KJ, et al. Rescue extracorporeal membrane oxygenation for massive anterior mediastinal masses. J Artif Organs. 2021;24(4):450-457.

29. Shekar K, Fraser JF, Smith MT, et al. Pharmacokinetic changes in patients receiving extracorporeal membrane oxygenation. J Crit Care. 2012;27(6):741 e749-718.

30. Ramanathan K, Leow L, Mithiran H. ECMO and adult mediastinal masses. Indian J Thorac Cardiovasc Surg. 2021;37(Suppl 2):338-343.

31. Potere B, Boulos R, Awad H, et al. The Role of Extracorporeal Membrane Oxygenation in the Anesthetic Management of Superior Vena Cava Syndrome: Is it Time to Use a Scoring System? J Cardiothorac Vasc Anesth. 2022 Jun;36(6):1777-1787.

32. Worku B, DeBois W, Sobol I, et al. Extracorporeal Membrane Oxygenation as a Bridge through Chemotherapy in B-Cell Lymphoma. J Extra Corpor Technol. 2015;47(1):52-54.

33. Song P, Josten NJ, Cheng AM. Posterior Mediastinal Mass Resection Requiring Venoarterial and Venovenous Extracorporeal Membrane Oxygenation Support. J Cardiothorac Vasc Anesth. 2022 Apr;36(4):1127-1131.

34. Brenn BR, Reddy SK, Van Arendonk KJ, et al. Perioperative management of an anterior mediastinal teratoma in an infant: one more tool in the toolbox. BMJ Case Rep. 2018 Nov 1;2018:bcr2018227022.

35. Aspesberro F, Guthrie KA, Woolfrey AE, et al. Outcome of pediatric hematopoietic stem cell transplant recipients requiring mechanical ventilation. J Intensive Care Med. 2014;29(1):31-37.

36. Huynh TN, Weigt SS, Belperio JA, et al. Outcome and prognostic indicators of patients with hematopoietic stem cell transplants admitted to the intensive care unit. J Transplant. 2009;2009:917294.

37. Gournay V, Dumas G, Lavillegrand JR, et al. Outcome of allogeneic hematopoietic stem cell transplant recipients admitted to the intensive care unit with a focus on haploidentical graft and sequential conditioning regimen: results of a retrospective study. Ann Hematol. 2021;100(11):2787-2797.

38. Mokart D, Granata A, Crocchiolo R, et al. Allogeneic hematopoietic stem cell transplantation after reduced intensity conditioning regimen: Outcomes of patients admitted to intensive care unit. J Crit Care. 2015;30(5):1107-1113.

39. Afessa B, Azoulay E. Critical care of the hematopoietic stem cell transplant recipient. Crit Care Clin. 2010;26(1):133-150.

40. Gow KW, Wulkan ML, Heiss KF, et al. Extracorporeal membrane oxygenation for support of children after hematopoietic stem cell transplantation: the Extracorporeal Life Support Organization experience. J Pediatr Surg. 2006;41(4):662-667.

41. Di Nardo M, Locatelli F, Palmer K, et al. Extracorporeal membrane oxygenation in pediatric recipients of hematopoietic stem cell transplantation: an updated analysis of the Extracorporeal Life Support Organization experience. Intensive Care Med. 2014;40(5):754-756.

42. Maue DK, Hobson MJ, Friedman ML, et al. Outcomes of pediatric oncology and hematopoietic cell transplant patients receiving extracorporeal membrane oxygenation. Perfusion. 2019;34(7):598-604.

43. Steppan DA, Coleman RD, Viamonte HK, et al. Outcomes of pediatric patients with oncologic disease or following hematopoietic stem cell transplant supported on extracorporeal membrane oxygenation: The PEDECOR experience. Pediatr Blood Cancer. 2020;67(10):e28403.

44. Coleman RD, Goldman J, Moffett B, et al. Extracorporeal Membrane Oxygenation Mortality in High-Risk Populations: An Analysis of the Pediatric Health Information System Database. ASAIO J. 2020;66(3):327-331.

45. Bridges BC, Kilbaugh TJ, Barbaro RP, et al. Veno-Venous Extracorporeal Membrane Oxygenation for Children With Cancer or Hematopoietic Cell Transplant: A Ten Center Cohort. ASAIO J. 2021 Aug 1;67(8):923-929.

46. Olson TL, O'Neil ER, Kurtz KJ, et al. Improving Outcomes for Children Requiring Extracorporeal Membrane Oxygenation Therapy Following Hematopoietic Stem Cell Transplantation. Crit Care Med. 2021 Apr 1;49(4):e381-e393.

47. Schmidt M, Bréchot N, Combes A. Ten situations in which ECMO is unlikely to be successful. Intensive Care Med. 2016;42(5):750-752.

48. Wohlfarth P, Beutel G, Lebiedz P, et al. Characteristics and Outcome of Patients After Allogeneic Hematopoietic Stem Cell Transplantation Treated With Extracorporeal Membrane Oxygenation for Acute Respiratory Distress Syndrome. Crit Care Med. 2017;45(5):e500-e507.

49. Wolfson RK, Kahana MD, Nachman JB, et al. Extracorporeal membrane oxygenation after stem cell transplant: clinical decision-making in the absence of evidence. Pediatr Crit Care Med. 2005;6(2):200-203.

50. Williams FZ, Vats A, Cash T, et al. Successful Use of Extracorporeal Life Support in a Hematopoietic Stem Cell Transplant Patient with Neuroblastoma. J Extra Corpor Technol. 2018;50(1):61-64.

51. Holmqvist AS, Chen Y, Wu J, et al. Assessment of Late Mortality Risk After Allogeneic Blood or Marrow Transplantation Performed in Childhood. JAMA Oncol. 2018;4(12):e182453.

52. Yen HJ, Eissa HM, Bhatt NS, et al. Patient-reported outcomes in survivors of childhood hematologic malignancies with hematopoietic stem cell transplant. Blood. 2020;135(21):1847-1858.

53. Di Nardo M, Ahmad AH, Merli P, et al. Extracorporeal membrane oxygenation in children receiving haematopoietic cell transplantation and immune effector cell therapy: an international and multidisciplinary consensus statement. Lancet Child Adolesc Health. Lancet Child Adolesc Health 2022; 6:116-128.

54. Di Nardo M, Locatelli F, Di Florio F, et al. Extracorporeal membrane oxygenation as a bridge to allogeneic T-cell depleted hematopoietic stem cell transplantation in infants with severe combined immune deficiency: is it feasible? Intensive Care Med. 2014;40(10):1600-1601.

55. Hsiao LT, Chung FP, Chiou TJ, et al. The limitations of extracorporeal membrane oxygenation as a bridge to allogeneic hematopoietic stem cell transplantation. Intensive Care Med. 2014;40(12):1971-1972.

56. Di Nardo M, Li Pira G, Amodeo A, et al. Adoptive immunotherapy with antigen-specific T cells during extracorporeal membrane oxygenation (ECMO) for adenovirus-related respiratory failure in a child given haploidentical stem cell transplantation. Pediatr Blood Cancer. 2014;61(2):376-379.

57. Chima RS, Abulebda K, Jodele S. Advances in critical care of the pediatric hematopoietic stem cell transplant patient. Pediatr Clin North Am. 2013;60(3):689-707.

58. Liao WI, Tsai SH, Chiu SK. Successful use of extracorporeal membrane oxygenation in a hematopoietic stem cell transplant patient with idiopathic pneumonia syndrome. Respir Care. 2013;58(2):e6-10.

59. Koinuma T, Nunomiya S, Wada M, et al. Concurrent treatment with a tumor necrosis factor-alpha inhibitor and veno-venous extracorporeal membrane oxygenation in a post-hematopoietic stem cell transplant patient with idiopathic pneumonia syndrome: a case report. J Intensive Care. 2014;2(1):48.

60. Morris SH, Haight AE, Kamat P, et al. Successful use of extracorporeal life support in a hematopoietic stem cell transplant patient with diffuse alveolar hemorrhage. Pediatr Crit Care Med. 2010;11(1):e4-7.

61. Fan K, Hurley C, McNeil MJ, et al. Case Report: Management Approach and Use of Extracorporeal Membrane Oxygenation for Diffuse Alveolar Hemorrhage After Pediatric Hematopoietic Cell Transplant. Front Pediatr. 2020;8:587601.

62. Cheng GS, Edelman JD, Madtes DK, et al. Outcomes of lung transplantation after allogeneic hematopoietic stem cell transplantation. Biol Blood Marrow Transplant. 2014;20(8):1169-1175.

63. Jung S, Yoon HM, Yoon J, et al. The association of lung function changes with outcomes in children with bronchiolitis obliterans syndrome after hematopoietic stem cell transplantation. Pediatr Pulmonol. 2021;56(10):3332-3341.

64. Dandoy CE, Jodele S, Paff Z, et al. Team-based approach to identify cardiac toxicity in critically ill hematopoietic stem cell transplant recipients. Pediatr Blood Cancer. 2017;64(10).

65. Meserve EE, Lehmann LE, Perez-Atayde AR, et al. Cyclophosphamide-associated cardiotoxicity in a child after stem cell transplantation for β-thalassemia major: case report and review of the literature. Pediatr Dev Pathol. 2014;17(1):50-54.

66. Sumi M, Kitahara M, Shishido T, et al. Myocarditis with Advanced Atrioventricular Block after Allogeneic Stem Cell Transplantation: A Case Report and Literature Review. Intern Med. 2020;59(1):113-118.

67. Kurihara C, Walter JM, Karim A, et al. Feasibility of Venovenous Extracorporeal Membrane Oxygenation Without Systemic Anticoagulation. Ann Thorac Surg. 2020;110(4):1209-1215.

68. Wood KL, Ayers B, Gosev I, et al. Venoarterial-Extracorporeal Membrane Oxygenation Without Routine Systemic Anticoagulation Decreases Adverse Events. Ann Thorac Surg. 2020;109(5):1458-1466.

69. Fina D, Matteucci M, Jiritano F, et al. Extracorporeal membrane oxygenation without systemic anticoagulation: a case-series in challenging conditions. J Thorac Dis. 2020;12(5):2113-2119.

70. Kalbhenn J, Schmidt R, Nakamura L, et al. Early diagnosis of acquired von Willebrand Syndrome (AVWS) is elementary for clinical practice in patients

treated with ECMO therapy. J Atheroscler Thromb. 2015;22(3):265-271.

71. Brogan TV, Thiagarajan RR, Lorusso R, et al. The use of extracorporeal membrane oxygenation in human immunodeficiency virus-positive patients: a review of a multicenter database. Perfusion. 2020;35(8):772-777.

72. Schmidt M, Schellongowski P, Patroniti N, et al. Six-Month Outcome of Immunocompromised Patients with Severe Acute Respiratory Distress Syndrome Rescued by Extracorporeal Membrane Oxygenation. An International Multicenter Retrospective Study. Am J Respir Crit Care Med. 2018;197(10):1297-1307.

73. Capatos G, Burke CR, Ogino MT, et al. Venovenous extracorporeal life support in patients with HIV infection and Pneumocystis jirovecii pneumonia. Perfusion. 2018;33(6):433-437.

74. Peek GJ, Mugford M, Tiruvoipati R, et al. Efficacy and economic assessment of conventional ventilatory support versus extracorporeal membrane oxygenation for severe adult respiratory failure (CESAR): a multicentre randomised controlled trial. Lancet. 2009;374(9698):1351-1363.

75. Combes A, Hajage D, Capellier G, et al. Extracorporeal Membrane Oxygenation for Severe Acute Respiratory Distress Syndrome. N Engl J Med. 2018;378(21):1965-1975.

76. Restrepo-Escobar M, N AR, Hernández-Zapata LJ, Velásquez M, et al. Factors associated with infection amongst paediatric patients with systemic lupus erythematosus treated in the intensive care unit. Lupus. 2019;28(9):1141-1147.

77. Zamir G, Haviv-Yadid Y, Sharif K, et al. Mortality of patients with systemic lupus erythematosus admitted to the intensive care unit - A retrospective single-center study. Best Pract Res Clin Rheumatol. 2018;32(5):701-709.

78. Pineton de Chambrun M, Larcher R, Pène F, et al. CAPS criteria fail to identify most severely-ill thrombotic antiphospholipid syndrome patients requiring intensive care unit admission. J Autoimmun. 2019;103:102292.

79. Rodríguez RCS, Flores-Umanzor E, Cepas-Guillen PL, et al. Extracorporeal membrane oxygenation in cardiopulmonary disease of rheumatic conditions: A systematic review. Med Clin (Barc). 2020;155(10):454-458.

80. Bay P, Lebreton G, Mathian A, et al. Outcomes of severe systemic rheumatic disease patients requiring extracorporeal membrane oxygenation. Ann Intensive Care. 2021;11(1):29.

81. Demoule A, Antonelli M, Schellongowski P, et al. Respiratory Mechanics and Outcomes in Immunocompromised Patients With ARDS: A Secondary Analysis of the EFRAIM Study. Chest. 2020;158(5):1947-1957.

82. Yin K, March RJ, Hoopes CW, et al. Extracorporeal membrane oxygenation in the management of granulomatosis with polyangiitis. J Card Surg. 2021;36(2):743-747.

83. Delvino P, Monti S, Balduzzi S, et al. The role of extra-corporeal membrane oxygenation (ECMO) in the treatment of diffuse alveolar haemorrhage secondary to ANCA-associated vasculitis: report of two cases and review of the literature. Rheumatol Int. 2019;39(2):367-375.

84. Seeliger B, Stahl K, Schenk H, et al. Extracorporeal Membrane Oxygenation for Severe ARDS Due to Immune Diffuse Alveolar Hemorrhage: A Retrospective Observational Study. Chest. 2020;157(3):744-747.

85. Abrams D, Agerstrand CL, Biscotti M, Burkart KM, et al. Extracorporeal membrane oxygenation in the management of diffuse alveolar hemorrhage. ASAIO J. 2015;61(2):216-218.

86. Reddy HG, Maynes EJ, Saxena A, et al. Utilization of extracorporeal life support for diffuse alveolar damage and diffuse alveolar hemorrhage: A systematic review. Artif Organs. 2021;45(6):559-568.

87. Battisha A, Sawalha K, Altibi AM, et al. Cardiogenic shock in autoimmune rheumatologic diseases: an insight on etiologies, management, and treatment outcomes. Heart Fail Rev. 2022;27(1):93-101.

88. Repéssé X, Freund Y, Mathian A, et al. Successful extracorporeal membrane oxygenation for refractory cardiogenic shock due to the catastrophic antiphospholipid syndrome. Ann Intern Med. 2010;153(7):487-488.

89. Barreto JA, Mehta A, Thiagarajan RR, et al. The Use of Extracorporeal Life Support in Children With Immune-Mediated Diseases. Pediatr Crit Care Med. 2022;23(1):e60-e65.

90. Saites VA, Hadler R, Gutsche JT, et al. Extracorporeal Membrane Oxygenation for Hemophagocytic Lymphohistiocytosis. Am J Case Rep. 2016;17:686-689.

91. Cheng A, Williams F, Fortenberry J, et al. Use of Extracorporeal Support in Hemophagocytic Lymphohistiocytosis Secondary to Ehrlichiosis. Pediatrics. 2016;138(4).

92. Zulian F, Martinez Toledo MM, Amigoni A, et al. Successful use of extracorporeal membrane oxygenation for severe interstitial lung disease in a child with dermatomyositis. Intensive Care Med. 2007;33(9):1663-1666.

93. Patel JJ, Lipchik RJ. Systemic lupus-induced diffuse alveolar hemorrhage treated with extracorporeal membrane oxygenation: a case report and review of the literature. J Intensive Care Med. 2014;29(2):104-109.

94. Kolovos NS, Schuerer DJ, Moler FW, et al. Extracorporal life support for pulmonary hemorrhage in children: a case series. Crit Care Med. 2002;30(3):577-580.

95. Cashen K, Chu RL, Klein J, et al. Extracorporeal membrane oxygenation outcomes in children with hemophagocytic lymphohistiocytosis. Perfusion. 2017;32(2):151-156.

96. von Bahr Greenwood T, Holzgraefe B, Chiang SCC, et al. Clinical and laboratory signs of haemophagocytic lymphohistiocytosis associated with pandemic influenza A (H1N1) infection in patients needing extracorporeal membrane oxygenation: A retrospective observational study. Eur J Anaesthesiol. 2021;38(7):692-701.

# 40

## Lung Transplantation

*Marcelo Cypel, Christian Bermudez, Amy E. Hackmann*

Lung transplant remains an effective therapeutic option for endstage lung disease. With continued efforts to refine operative technique, patient selection, and optimization of postoperative care, both the short- and long-term survival for lung transplant has been gradually improving.

The use of ECLS plays a major role to support during transplant procedures, as well as before and after transplantation. Lung transplant centers must be very familiar with this technology in order to properly care for this patient population. Significant improvements in ECLS associated technologies, as well as a better understanding of ECMO physiology, have led to less morbidity and a more liberal use of this support modality. In 2020, nearly 7% of lung transplants were supported on ECMO preoperatively.[1] In this chapter we will discuss the use of ECLS as a bridge to lung transplantation, as an intraoperative strategy, and finally for posttransplant support.

## ECLS as Bridge to Lung Transplantation

As their pulmonary disease progresses, listed patients awaiting lung transplant may deteriorate and require mechanical support for their failing lungs. These support strategies include extracorporeal membrane oxygenation and $CO_2$ removal technologies

to supplement or entirely replace pulmonary function. Furthermore, some patients require hemodynamic support for the right ventricle, or more rarely develop biventricular failure. The principal goals of these bridging strategies are to restore acceptable physiology, avoid end-organ injury, and maintain or improve functional capacity and physical conditioning while awaiting transplantation.

### Hypoxemia and/or Hypercapnia

VV ECMO is the preferred option for bridging patients with isolated hypoxemia and/or hypercapnia in the absence of hemodynamic instability or significant right ventricular dysfunction. This can be typical of cystic fibrosis (hypercapnia) or pulmonary fibrosis (hypoxia) patients. In this population, VV ECMO provides superior results compared to VA ECMO, especially by providing better central oxygenation and decreased risks of ECMO-related complications. In patients with VV ECMO as a bridge to lung transplantation, periodic evaluation of right ventricular function should be performed. In cases where hemodynamic support is needed, conversion to OxyRVAD or VVA ECMO support should be considered depending on center experience, urgency of the situation, and patient size characteristics. Peripheral VA ECMO alone is not sufficient to restore oxygenation with normal LV function in these patients, while antegrade flow provided by central cannulation strategies is acceptable.

In select circumstances where hypercapnic respiratory failure is the predominant issue, extracorporeal $CO_2$ removal ($ECCO_2R$) can effectively be used as a bridging strategy.[2]

The theoretical advantages over ECMO in this select population is the need for only single-site, relatively small-bore, upper body access. Continuous evaluation of progressive hypoxia should be evaluated to guide if and when alternative bridging strategies such as full ECMO are required. In addition, $ECCO_2R$ can be associated with higher bleeding complications given the need for higher anticoagulation with low flow in these circuits, as well as increased shear stress on blood cells at low flow.

To facilitate ambulation and physiotherapy, single site dual lumen cannulas (i.e., Crescent, Medtronic or Avalon Elite, Getinge) are preferred at some centers for patients bridged on VV ECMO to transplantation. However, in larger patients with significant lung function impairment, these cannulas can often provide insufficient flow to fully support oxygenation.

Some patients may be better served with a conventional 2 cannula VV ECMO approach, such as when cannulation is very urgent or the expected requisite flows are higher than those which single site cannulas can provide. This is a very effective mode of support and, with careful planning, full ambulation even with femoral venous cannulas has been demonstrated to be safe and effective.[3] Thus, femoral venous cannulation is not a contraindication for ambulation.

### Right Ventricular Failure

Patients listed for lung transplantation with pulmonary hypertension should be considered for bridge with mechanical support when clinical signs of right heart failure are evident,

such as need for inotropes, poor mixed venous saturation, and early signs of kidney and liver dysfunction.

Patients developing severe right-sided heart failure require comprehensive care, including treatment of factors causing or contributing to heart failure, fluid management, and strategies to improve cardiac function. MCS should be initiated when the clinical course suggests that significant right heart failure is present and associated with imminent secondary organ dysfunction despite optimized medical therapy.[4]

The most common MCS approach for patients with pulmonary hypertension is VA ECMO. VA ECMO placed under local anesthesia via the femoral vessels is well tolerated and safe. However, femoral VA ECMO limits mobilization and is associated with risks of ischemic limb complications if support is required for several weeks. Thus, many centers have preferred the use of central VA ECMO, either via cannulation of the axillary artery, innominate artery, or ascending aorta.[5,6] Some recent reports with the use of central VA ECMO via minianterior right thoracotomy in the 3rd intercostal space have shown promising results, both in terms of durability and patient mobilization.[7] A few centers use pulmonary artery-left atrium pumpless interventional Lung Assist Device (iLA, Novalung, Xenios). In this mode, the device is placed in parallel with pulmonary circulation. Due to its very low resistance, it provides an excellent means of decompressing the right ventricle. In a previous report, over 80% of patients were successfully bridged with this approach.[4] Although a very useful strategy, this device is not available in all jurisdictions. The use of right ventricular assist devices is generally not recommended in patients with PAH awaiting lung transplantation due to the high risk of pulmonary hemorrhage. However, some evidence may suggest that this technique can be useful when an OxyRVAD is kept at low flow in patients with chronic lung disease or post COVID-19 ARDS complicated with secondary pulmonary hypertension as a bridge to transplant.[8] Some patients with PAH and large atrial septal defect may be bridged with VV ECMO.[9]

### *Sepsis*

Patients bridged with ECMO may develop significant pulmonary sepsis leading to secondary organ dysfunction. Especially in patients with cystic fibrosis and bronchiectasis on mechanical ventilation, secretions tend to accumulate with multidrug-resistant organisms and uncontrolled sepsis can develop despite broad antibiotic coverage. In 2016, Cypel and colleagues performed bilateral pneumonectomies (to remove the source of sepsis) in conjunction with central VA ECMO and PA-LA Novalung (biventricular support).[10] A successful bilateral lung transplant was performed six days later. Barac and colleagues repeated this approach, albeit with a slight modification (a shunt between the left pulmonary artery and left pulmonary vein was used).[11] Again, a successful double lung transplant was performed less than a week after the pneumonectomies. Given the small experience to date with this approach, it should be considered only in exceptional situations and in centers with large experience both in mechanical support and lung transplantation.

### *Bridge to Lung Transplant in Patients with Acute Lung Injuries*

Very selected patients with ARDS, including influenza- and COVID-19-related ARDS supported with ECMO, can be considered for transplantation in the absence of any signs of lung recovery. As we gain experience in this setting, the conditions to consider a patient for transplantation may include: Age less than 65 years old, absence of second-organ dysfunction (possibly excluding acute renal failure), absence of signs of lung recovery despite prolonged

ECMO support, evidence of lung fibrosis or bullous destruction on CT, ability to consent for transplantation, participation in physiotherapy, and meets all other standard criteria for lung transplantation (including social support).[12,13] The decision of how long to wait for recovery prior to transplantation remains under investigation. More data is accumulating to better inform such decisions.

Recent data from the scientific registry of transplant recipients (SRTR) in the United States reported 118 COVID-19 ARDS patients who underwent lung transplantation. The 30- and 90-day mortality was 1.7 and 3.4%, respectively.[14] Importantly, given the prolonged hospital stay of many of these patients, their recovery may be lengthy as well.

### *Patient Management*

For patients bridged with ECMO to lung transplantation, several aspects of management require focused attention. First, as patients are often on support for a prolonged time, ICU care focused on increasing rehabilitation efforts and supporting adequate nutrition during this catabolic state are important. Also, to limit immunologic challenges posttransplant, transfusions should be limited. Lastly, care of the patient should focus on avoiding multiorgan dysfunction to improve transplant candidacy and long-term outcomes.

### Intraoperative Mechanical Support

The use of mechanical support devices provides several advantages in routine lung transplantation. These include hemodynamic stability; facilitating dissection of the pulmonary hilum; and allowing for protective reperfusion and ventilation. Some of these advantages are somewhat diminished by risks such as a higher rate of intraoperative blood transfusion, reoperations, activation of proinflammatory cytokines, and a higher rate of non-pulmonary complications. However, there is now evidence that most of these disadvantages are mostly associated with the use of cardiopulmonary bypass rather than ECMO. Indications for the use of mechanical support during the lung transplant operation is shown in Table 40-1.

One of the most beneficial effects of VA ECMO during lung transplantation is graft protection against reperfusion injury. When performing a sequential bilateral lung transplantation without MCS, the first implanted graft is exposed to the full cardiac output, a situation which can augment ischemia-related damage, and can lead to the 'first lung syndrome.' The positive effect of controlled reperfusion on primary graft function achieved through a routine VA ECMO strategy has been recently highlighted.[15] Of note, ECMO flows should target about 50-70% of patient cardiac output so that continuous perfusion of the newly implanted lung is achieved. To that end, maintaining adequate patient volume status is critical, and the surgical team, anesthesia team, and perfusionist should communicate to achieve this goal.

### VA ECMO vs. Full Cardiopulmonary Bypass

While for many years the traditional intraoperative support system during lung transplant has been CPB, VA ECMO has become the preferred mode for intraoperative support in lung transplantation at certain centers.

VA ECMO has demonstrated several advantages related to patient outcomes when compared to CPB. This includes decreased rates of bleeding complications, neurologic complications, reoperations, primary graft dysfunction, and renal dysfunction.[16-20] Thus, CPB is currently mostly reserved for transplant procedures where concomitant cardiac surgical procedures are also required. It can also be used in cases where the technical complexity or difficult exposure requires complete decompression of the cardiac structures to allow better conduct of the operation. The bypass circuit may be modified in order to switch quickly from VA ECMO to cardiopulmonary bypass, if needed.

### VA ECMO vs. VV ECMO

The preferred mode of MCS during lung transplantation is VA ECMO. As explained above, VA ECMO diverts blood flow from the pulmonary circulation, protecting the new graft. In addition, it provides hemodynamic support during manipulation of the mediastinum. Although VA ECMO may have potential benefits over CPB, it is important to consider that this is a closed system with constant suction pressure and requires careful attention to prevent venous injuries that can lead to air entrainment in the circuit. The two limbs of the VV ECMO circuit can be joined with a Y connector to use as the venous drainage on VA ECMO (ie, VV-A cannulation).

| RECIPIENT RELATED | DONOR RELATED |
|---|---|
| Primary pulmonary hypertension | High risk donor: Long ischemic time, edema, others |
| Secondary pulmonary hypertension (IPF) | Lobar transplant |
| Secondary pulmonary hypertension (IPF) | |
| Patient with ischemic heart disease | |
| Hypoxemia or high PAP after contra-lateral pneumonectomy; needing FiO$_2$ >70% or PAP >50 mmHg | |
| Bleeding from PA or LA | |
| Small chest | |
| Pediatric transplant | |
| Airway difficulties | |

**Table 40-1.** Indications for mechanical support during lung transplant operations.

Some patients that are bridged to transplant on VV ECMO can stay on that mode of support during the operation if they maintain hemodynamic stability and do not have significant pulmonary hypertension. This is typically the case in cystic fibrosis and emphysema patients.[21]

### *Central vs. Peripheral ECMO*

Both the use of central and peripheral ECMO have been successfully reported to support patients during lung transplant operations. However, most centers prefer central cannulation due to ease of access and ability to provide full support.

### *Anticoagulation*

Most centers run intraoperative ECMO on low ACT targets. Generally, patients receive 60 IU/kg of heparin to bring the ACT above 200-250 seconds for cannulation. Subsequent ACTs are maintained between 160-180 seconds during the procedure. Some recent reports have described the intraoperative use of ECMO without therapeutic anticoagulation for patients with high risk of bleeding.[22] Using a circuit without anticoagulation should only be considered in select circumstances, such as patients bridged to retransplantation where the risk of bleeding is significantly higher.

### ECMO for Patient Support after Lung Transplantation

Maintaining ECMO support after lung transplant provides several advantages during the early postoperative period. It secures immediate respiratory and possibly hemodynamic stability. It allows progressive initiation of reverse cardiac remodeling in pulmonary hypertension patients. Furthermore, it avoids deterioration of dysfunctional donor lungs which may need emergent secondary ECMO for severe graft failure. On the other hand, it carries additional risks of bleeding because of anticoagulation and coagulopathy, vascular access complications, infection, venous and/or arterial thrombosis, and pulmonary embolism because of cannulation.

There are currently two main situations when MCS is utilized at the end of lung transplant: 1) Severe Primary Graft Dysfunction (PGD) reflected by hypoxemia, hypercapnia, and secondary high pulmonary artery pressures and 2) The patient is at high risk for severe primary graft dysfunction—such as significant intraoperative transfusion requirements or prolonged donor ischemic times—and 'prophylactic' MCS prolongation aims to improve the early postoperative phase.

VV ECMO has been preferred over VA ECMO for recipients with severe PGD. While the resolution of PGD may take longer with VV ECMO compared to VA due to absence of protective flow, the rate of complications may be significantly less.[23-25] By correcting hypoxemia and acidosis, VV ECMO can improve pulmonary artery pressures and improve right ventricular performance even in patients with some early hemodynamic compromise.[23]

However, patients with PGD and severe hemodynamic compromise may require peripheral or central VA ECMO. In this situation, it is critically important to use partial flows to ensure aortic flow pulsatility. This pulsatility is needed to avoid stasis in the pulmonary circulation and allow for proper graft perfusion and to prevent thrombosis of the right ventricle or pulmonary circulation. In the case of postoperative VA ECMO support, more infrequently seen but clinically important nonetheless, is the possibility of pulmonary vein thrombosis, reinforcing the importance of maintaining some pulsatility and initiation of anticoagulation when postoperative bleeding has decreased.

Peripheral cannulation has been increasingly used in cases of VV and VA support for postoperative PGD or hemodynamic instability. Preoperative planning may be needed to have adequate vascular access available in high-risk cases that can be difficult to obtain late during the procedure. Placing a second right internal jugular vein access or switching the Swan Ganz catheter to the left internal jugular vein can be considered for this purpose. Peripheral cannulation may also allow complete chest closure in certain cases and may be associated with less risk of bleeding.

**Conclusion**

The role of ECLS in lung transplantation has been increasing in recent years, especially as patients undergoing lung transplant become sicker at presentation. Patients can be supported with ECLS in all phases of lung transplant care. Understanding both the strengths and the limitations of different modalities and strategies is crucial to ongoing success.

# References

1. Chambers, D.C., et al., The International Thoracic Organ Transplant Registry of the International Society for Heart and Lung Transplantation: Thirty-eighth adult lung transplantation report - 2021; Focus on recipient characteristics. J Heart Lung Transplant, 2021. 40(10): p. 1060-1072.

2. Hakim, A.H., et al., Contemporary Outcomes of Extracorporeal Membrane Oxygenation Used as Bridge to Lung Transplantation. Ann Thorac Surg, 2018. 106(1): p. 192-198.

3. Abrams D, et al. Early Mobilization during Extracorporeal Membrane Oxygenation for Cardiopulmonary Failure in Adults: Factors Associated with Intensity of Treatment Ann Am Thorac Soc 2022 Jan;19(1):90-98.

4. de Perrot, M., et al., Impact of extracorporeal life support on outcome in patients with idiopathic pulmonary arterial hypertension awaiting lung transplantation. J Heart Lung Transplant, 2011. 30(9): p. 997-1002.

5. Biscotti, M., et al., Extracorporeal membrane oxygenation with subclavian artery cannulation in awake patients with pulmonary hypertension. ASAIO J, 2014. 60(6): p. 748-50.

6. Chicotka, S , et al. The "Central Sport Model": Extracorporeal Membrane Oxygenation Using the Innominate Artery for Smaller Patients as Bridge to Lung Transplantation. ASAIO J. 2017 Jul/Aug;63(4):e39-e44.

7. Downey, P., et al., Ambulatory central veno-arterial extracorporeal membrane oxygenation in lung transplant candidates. J Heart Lung Transplant, 2019. 38(12): p. 1317-1319.

8. Sinha, N., et al., ProtekDuo as a bridge to lung transplant and heart-lung transplant. Clin Transplant, 2021. 35(5): p. e14273.

9. Kon, Z.N., et al., Venovenous Extracorporeal Membrane Oxygenation With Atrial Septostomy as a Bridge to Lung Transplantation. Ann Thorac Surg, 2016. 101(3): p. 1166-9.

10. Cypel, M., et al., Bilateral pneumonectomy to treat uncontrolled sepsis in a patient awaiting lung transplantation. J Thorac Cardiovasc Surg, 2017. 153(4): p. e67-e69.

11. Barac, Y.D., et al., Bilateral pneumonectomy with veno-arterial extracorporeal membrane oxygenation as a bridge to lung transplant. J Heart Lung Transplant, 2019. 38(11): p. 1231-1232.

12. Cypel, M., S. Keshavjee, When to consider lung transplantation for COVID-19. Lancet Respir Med, 2020. 8(10): p. 944-946.

13. Bharat, A., et al., Early outcomes after lung transplantation for severe COVID-19: a series of the first consecutive cases from four countries. Lancet Respir Med, 2021. 9(5): p. 487-497.

14. Roach, A., et al., Lung Transplantation for Covid-19-Related Respiratory Failure in the United States. New Engl J Med 2022; 386:1187-1188.

15. Hoetzenecker, K., et al., Bilateral lung transplantation on intraoperative extracorporeal membrane oxygenator: An observational study. J Thorac Cardiovasc Surg, 2020. 160(1): p. 320-327 e1.

16. Machuca, T.N., et al., Outcomes of intraoperative extracorporeal membrane oxygenation versus cardiopulmonary bypass for lung transplantation. J Thorac Cardiovasc Surg, 2015. 149(4): p. 1152-7.

17. Bermudez, C.A., et al., Outcomes of intraoperative venoarterial extracorporeal membrane oxygenation versus cardiopulmonary bypass during lung transplantation. Ann Thorac Surg, 2014. 98(6): p. 1936-42; discussion 1942-3.

18. Ius, F., et al., Lung transplantation on cardiopulmonary support: venoarterial extracorporeal membrane oxygenation outperformed cardiopulmonary bypass. J Thorac Cardiovasc Surg, 2012. 144(6): p. 1510-6.

19. Biscotti, M., et al., Comparison of extracorporeal membrane oxygenation versus cardiopulmonary bypass for lung transplantation. J Thorac Cardiovasc Surg, 2014. 148(5): p. 2410-5.

20. Loor, G., et al., Effect of mode of intraoperative support on primary graft dysfunction after lung transplant. J Thorac Cardiovasc Surg, 2022. Feb 4:S0022-5223(22)00119-2.

21. Hashimoto, K., et al., Intraoperative extracorporeal support during lung transplantation in patients bridged with venovenous extracorporeal membrane oxygenation. J Heart Lung Transplant, 2018. 37(12): p. 1418-1424.

22. Bharat, A., M.M. DeCamp, Veno-arterial extracorporeal membrane oxygenation without therapeutic anticoagulation for intra-operative cardiopulmonary support during lung transplantation. J Thorac Dis, 2017. 9(7): p. E629-E631.

23. Hartwig, M.G., et al., Improved survival but marginal allograft function in patients treated with extracorporeal membrane oxygenation after lung transplantation. Ann Thorac Surg, 2012. 93(2): p. 366-71.

24. Dahlberg, P.S., et al., Medium-term results of extracorporeal membrane oxygenation for severe acute lung injury after lung transplantation. J Heart Lung Transplant, 2004. 23(8): p. 979-84.

25. Harano, T., et al., Extracorporeal Membrane Oxygenation for Primary Graft Dysfunction After Lung Transplantation. ASAIO J, 2021. 67(9): p. 1071-1078.

# 41

## Heart Transplantation

*Jonathan H. Smith, Yves d'Udekem, Jonathan Haft, Peta M.A. Alexander*

### Context Outcomes of Heart Transplantation in Adults and Children

ECLS has been used as a bridge to heart transplantation for patients with heart failure not responsive to medical therapies. This has become more common in adults in the USA since the changes in the Organ Procurement and Transplantation Network/United Network for Organ Sharing (OPTN/UNOS) criteria in 2018.[1] Technical aspects of ECLS for heart transplantation are common to ECLS in general and are discussed in Chapters 4, 6, and 51. Matters related to children are further delineated in Chapters 17-20 and to adult patients in Chapters 27-29 and 31. Bridging strategies and pretransplant management are discussed in Chapter 20 for children and Chapter 30 for adult patients. This chapter will discuss the use of ECLS in the treatment of primary graft dysfunction (PGD) after heart transplantation and the use of ECLS when late failure of the graft occurs.

Primary graft dysfunction/failure (PGD) refers to poor function of the transplanted heart after weaning from cardiopulmonary bypass and has been defined by Kobashigawa (Table 41-1).[2] Only the most severe cases will require ECLS.

The pathology in failed grafts[3] is a combination of ischemic changes +/- vascular thrombosis. It is not possible to know whether thrombosis or necrosis occurs pre or postimplantation. Other mechanisms of damage to dysfunctional donor hearts may be catecholamine excess during brain death or prolonged ischemic time.[4] Secondary graft dysfunction refers to graft failure where a surgical, anatomical, or immunological factor is clearly implicated (eg, acute rejection, myocardial ischemia, pulmonary hypertension, vasoplegia).

Adult heart transplantation has a one-year survival of 84-86% and a five-year survival (conditional on survival at 1 year) of 86%. The principal causes of early death are PGD and acute rejection.[5] Primary graft dysfunction is

| DONOR RISK FACTORS | RECIPIENT RISK FACTORS | PROCEDURAL FACTORS |
|---|---|---|
| Age | Age | Ischemic time |
| Cause of death | Weight | Donor recipient sex |
| Trauma | Mechanical support | mismatch |
| Cardiac dysfunction | Congenital heart disease | Weight mismatch |
| Inotropic support | Reoperations | Noncardiac organ |
| Comorbidities | Comorbidities, renal or | donation |
| Cardiac arrest downtime | liver dysfunction | Procurement team |
| Drug abuse | LVAD explant | experience |
| Left ventricular | Ventilator dependent | Center volume |
| hypertrophy | Multiorgan transplant | Cardioplegic solution |
| Valvular disease | Allosensitization | Increased blood |
| Hormone treatment | High PVR | transfusion |
| Wall motion | Infection | Emergency or elective |
| abnormalities | Retransplant | transplant |
| Sepsis | | |
| Marginal donor | | |
| allocation | | |
| Troponin trend | | |
| Hypernatraemia | | |

**Table 41-1.** Risk factors for primary graft dysfunction after Kobashigawa.[2]

the early complication of heart transplantation, occurring in 10-22% of adult heart transplant recipients.[6-8] Early graft failure caused the deaths of 3.6% of adult recipients in the registry report by Lund.[9] The mortality of primary graft dysfunction treated with ECLS is between 25-53% of the patients affected. In adults, factors that are implicated are donor age, recipient diabetes mellitus, pretransplant mechanical support, duration of operation, and the donor ischemic time.[10-12]

Pediatric heart transplantation has a one-year survival of 90% and a five-year survival (conditional on survival at 1 year) of 90%. In pediatric transplantation, the incidence of PGD of a severity to require ECLS is 5-17%. PGD is associated with 25-46% mortality in published series.[13-15] Predisposing factors are younger age, preoperative ECLS, longer ischemic time, higher serum bilirubin and congenital heart disease.[2]

The categories 'high risk recipient' and 'marginal donor' are occasionally used and give a poorly calibrated but sensible indication of risk that is related to the donor diagnosis, duration of ischemic time, condition of the recipient, and state of preservation of the donor organ.[16,17] Unit experience and good coordination of the transplant organ retrieval will help. The use of hearts from DCD donors is becoming more common,[18] as is the use of ex vivo perfusion.[19] The latter can reduce the ischemic time, which may reduce PGD (Chapter 45).

## The Transplant Operation

The operation is the consequence of lengthy assessment and consent procedures. Coordination with the donor center, likely cross clamp time, presence of VAD or ECLS pretransplant, difficulty of dissection, and other precautions required should all be discussed at the presurgical meeting. Surgical process is dissection, institution of cardiopulmonary bypass, cardiectomy, graft implantation, followed by reperfusion and separation from cardiopulmonary bypass.

## Assessment of Cardiac Function

During and after weaning from cardiopulmonary bypass, assessment of donor cardiac function is done by visual inspection, TEE (or epicardial echo in smaller patients), near infrared spectroscopy, and hemodynamic measurements including pulmonary artery pressures and thermodilution cardiac output. Laboratory adjuncts include arterial blood lactate, base deficit, and mixed venous saturation, which can provide additional information about perfusion adequacy.

Patients commonly require low dose inotrope and vasoconstrictor requirements, but those who remain hemodynamically unstable (CVP >15, SBP <90 mmHg, MAP<70, PCWP >20 mmHg, and CI <2.0) despite one or two attempts to separate from bypass with a need for high dose inotropes should be considered for additional circulatory support (Table 41-2). Pulmonary artery hypertension may be present, so many centres routinely use selective pulmonary vasodilators such as inhaled nitric oxide or inhaled epoprostenol to support right heart function in the early post-operative period.[20] In adults, an intraaortic balloon pump

| PGD LEFT VENTRICLE (PGD-LV) | Mild PGD LV one of the criteria must be met | 1. LV Ejection fraction <40% 2. RAP >15 mmHg or PCWP >20 and CI <2 L/min/m² on low dose inotropes for more than one hour |
| | Moderate PGD-LV must have one criterion from **A** and one from **B** | **A** 1. LV Ejection fraction <40% 2. RAP >15 mmHg or PCWP >20 and CI <2 L/min/m² with hypotension <70 mmHg for more than one hour |
| | | **B** 1. On high dose inotropes, score >10 2. Newly placed IABP independent of inotropes |
| | Severe PGD-LV | Dependence on single or biventricular support more than an IABP including ECMO |
| PGD RIGHT VENTRICLE (PGD-RV) | Diagnosis requires both 1 and 2, or 3 alone | 1. RAP >15 mmHg, PCWP <15 and CI <2 L/min/m² 2. TPG <15 mmHg and PA systolic pressure <50 mmHg 3. Need for RVAD |

**Table 41-2.** Classification of Primary Graft Dysfunction (PGD), after Kobashigawa.[2]

(IABP) may be considered for further therapy for impaired left ventricular dysfunction[21]; however, in the case of refractory graft failure, early ECLS provides greater systemic blood flow and is easily placed in the operating room. If femoral ECLS cannulation was to be used, a femoral IABP may obstruct ECLS flow and increase the risk for peripheral vascular complications.[12,22,23] In the case of a known marginal donor or increased risk factors such as a prolonged ischemic time, ECLS may be instituted prophylactically to ensure adequate perfusion in the early post-operative period.

In pediatric practice, similar methods of assessment are used.[24] Patients with good function, low filling pressures and low lactates will not require ECLS. However, donor heart performance can be idiosyncratic and unpredictable. Assessment depends on the clinical data available and team experience. While poor function is often evident at the time of implantation, it may deteriorate in the hours after admission to the ICU. Should the heart appear suboptimal from the start, for instance when a 'marginal donor' is used as part of a strategy to deal with the waiting list, the use of ECLS may be deployed electively.[25]

### Threshold for ECLS in Primary Graft Failure

Numerous risk factors have been identified[2] and two risk scores have been reported.[11,26] Early studies of PGD were limited by variable definitions used by different centres. The ISHLT consensus guidelines of 2014 standardized the diagnosis, enabling more consistent reporting. In recipients who have several of the acknowledged risk factors for PGD, many centers now have a low threshold for the implementation of early support with ECLS. The diagnosis is almost always clinical once anatomical or surgical problems are excluded.

### *Timing*

Diagnosis of PGD must be made within 24 hours of transplant and exclude secondary causes such as bleeding, technical issues, and hyperacute rejection. In pediatric practice, there are more marked size discrepancies between donor and recipient hearts,[27] a similar relationship between ischemic time and hypotension after transplantation, but a higher chance of pulmonary hypertension complicating the procedure.[20]

The current consensus is that earlier ECLS initiation is better. Many prefer to cannulate to ECLS in the operating theater rather than in the ICU with a patient with borderline hemodynamics and graft function.

### Aims of Support

The goal of ECLS after heart transplantation is to allow for the allograft to rest and recover while maintaining adequate organ perfusion. Hemodynamics should be closely monitored, and cardiac recovery frequently assessed with echocardiography. Neurologic, renal, hepatic, pulmonary, and other end organ perfusion should be maintained, and appropriate replacement therapy used when indicated. In the immediate postoperative period, one can run without heparin until hemostasis is assured; this strategy requires ready availability of another circuit in case of circuit thrombosis, particularly in children. After restarting anticoagulation, the team should monitor for cerebrovascular events and gastrointestinal hemorrhage. If acute rejection is suspected, endomyocardial biopsies should be obtained via right heart catheterization and immunosuppression augmented as indicated.

### Left Heart Decompression

In addition to the venting techniques discussed in Chapter 4 and 51, there is an opportunity for the surgeon to create an ASD in the graft during implantation or leave an existing atrial communication. This may help avoid the need for a vent.

## Coagulation Management

Standard techniques are used (Chapters 18, 28, and 51).

## Assessing Recovery

Recovery usually occurs between 2-5 days after implantation.[28] Evidence of recovery includes return of pulsatility in the presence of adequate, but not excessive, inotrope use. If the overall condition of the patient allows, elective reduction in flow and echo assessment with RV filling should follow.[29] If propitious, weaning continues and the patient can then be 'clamped off' ECLS prior to decannulation (Chapters 19 and 29). Decannulation takes place in the operating theater. The chest is left open for 24 hours or more and closed later.[30]

## Immunosuppression

Local immunosuppression protocols should be managed while the patients are supported on ECLS, including early intravenous steroids, and combination therapy. The volume of distribution of the ECLS circuit and potential for adsorption to the circuit components may complicate dosing of immunosuppressants, so levels (tacrolimus, mycophenolate derivatives) or cell counts (thymoglobulin–CD3) must be monitored to ensure therapeutic dosing.

## Outcome

Most of the early deaths after heart transplantation in adults and children are due to failure to recover from PGD, multiorgan failure (which is often a consequence of PGD), and some with brain injury which is a consequence of the cardiovascular failure from PGD. Early complications are graft failure, acute rejection, infection, and multiorgan failure.[5] In pediatrics, postoperative ECLS support also increases the risk of stroke.[31] Vasoplegia occurs in 16% of the adult group.[32] Primary graft dysfunction is associated with increased costs and higher mortality.[33]

Successful weaning of ECLS has been reported in 60-100% of PGD patients and 30-day or survival-to-discharge has been reported between 46-100%.[12,34] In children who require ECLS after transplantation, survival typically reaches 50-60%[15,24] If a patient survives the early period, ECLS-treated PGD is not associated with decreased survival at 1 or 5 years.[13,14]

The choice for mechanical assist device for severe PGD is understudied. Taghavi found similar survival between patients supported with RVAD or ECLS in isolated right-sided dysfunction, but overall graft recovery was improved in the ECLS-treated patients.[35] PGD has also been successfully managed with short-term paracorporeal VAD, although a direct comparison with ECLS was not made.[36]

## Failure to Recover Donor Heart

Should the graft not recover, then a critical assessment of the donor heart with echocardiography, CT, and cardiac catheterization may be required. A biopsy to assess the degree of rejection can be performed on ECLS. If rejection is discovered, immunosuppression is augmented. A discussion on the likelihood and feasibility of successful medium-term support to recovery or re-transplantation should then take place.[37,38]

## ECLS for Late Graft Failure after Heart Transplantation

Patients who suffer graft failure beyond the first 48 hours of heart transplant can be supported with ECLS. This 'late graft failure' usually occurs due to acute cellular mediated rejection or chronic allograft vasculopathy. When indicated, ECLS should be considered soon after presentation to provide support during periods of augmentation of immunosuppression. Kittleson showed improved outcomes when ECLS was used as preemptive therapy as opposed to an element of cardiopulmonary resuscitation. Survival to discharge was 79% in the former group, although only 26% were alive at one year.[39,40]

ECLS deployed to support augmentation of immunosuppression may be effective and allow assessment of recovery, VAD, or retransplantation. The last of these is less likely to be successful within one year of the initial transplant, and is a risk factor for early death in 6-17 year old patients.[41]

**Conclusion**

Primary graft failure is a life-threatening complication of heart transplantation and requires careful evaluation. Once surgical and immunological factors have been excluded, management should be to support cardiac function to recovery while minimizing complications. Early initiation of VA ECMO in the operating room is an effective therapy that will improve the early outcome of this disorder. The complications are those of cardiac ECMO, although attention to dosing of immunosuppression is required. Recovery of cardiac function can be expected within 7 days.

Late graft failure has different and more intractable causes. A recipient who presents with this who is not in a peri-arrest condition may benefit from short-term support to maintain life, investigate the cause, and augment immunosuppression. Subsequent therapy will need thoughtful discussion and suitability for retransplantation may depend on the cause of deterioration.

# References

1. Reich H, Ramzy D, Moriguchi J et al. Acceptable Post–Heart Transplant Outcomes Support Temporary MCS Prioritization in the New OPTN UNOS Heart Allocation Policy. Transplantation Proceedings. 2021;53:353-357.

2. Kobashigawa J, Zuckermann A, Macdonald P et al. Report from a consensus conference on primary graft dysfunction after cardiac transplantation. The Journal of heart and lung transplantation : the official publication of the International Society for Heart Transplantation. 2014;33:327-340.

3. Benck L, Manzoor D, Kransdorf EP, et al. Pathological Assessment of Primary Graft Dysfunction Does Not Suggest a Prominent Role for an Adaptive Immune Response. Circulation. 2020;142:A15646-A15646.

4. Banner NR, Thomas HL, Curnow E et al. The importance of cold and warm cardiac ischemia for survival after heart transplantation. Transplantation. 2008;86:542-547.

5. Vanderlaan RD, Manlhiot C, Edwards LB, et al. Risk factors for specific causes of death following pediatric heart transplant: An analysis of the registry of the International Society of Heart and Lung Transplantation. Pediatric Transplantation. 2015;19:896-905.

6. Carmena MDGC, Bueno MG, Almenar L et al. Primary graft failure after heart transplantation: characteristics in a contemporary cohort and performance of the RADIAL risk score. The Journal of Heart and Lung Transplantation. 2013;32:1187-1195.

7. Lim JH, Hwang HY, Yeom SY, et al. Percutaneous extracorporeal membrane oxygenation for graft dysfunction after heart transplantation. Korean J Thorac Cardiovasc Surg. 2014;47:100-105.

8. Seguchi O, Fujita T, Murata Y et al. Incidence, etiology, and outcome of primary graft dysfunction in adult heart transplant recipients: a single-center experience in Japan. Heart Vessels. 2016; 31:555-562.

9. Lund LH, Edwards LB, Kucheryavaya AY et al. The Registry of the International Society for Heart and Lung Transplantation: Thirty-second Official Adult Heart Transplantation Report-2015; Focus Theme: Early Graft Failure. The Journal of heart and lung transplantation: the official publication of the International Society for Heart Transplantation. 2015;34:1244.

10. Truby LK, Takeda K, Topkara VK et al. Risk of severe primary graft dysfunction in patients bridged to heart transplantation with continuous-flow left ventricular assist devices. The Journal of Heart and Lung Transplantation. 2018;37:1433-1442.

11. Avtaar Singh SS, DAS DE S, Rushton S, et al. PREDICTA: A Model to Predict Primary Graft Dysfunction After Adult Heart Transplantation in the United Kingdom. J Card Fail. 2019;25:971-977.

12. DeRoo SC, Takayama H, Nemeth S et al. Extracorporeal membrane oxygenation for primary graft dysfunction after heart transplant. J Thorac Cardiovasc Surg. 2019;158:1576-1584.e3.

13. Godown J, Bearl DW, Thurm C et al. Extracorporeal membrane oxygenation use in the first 24 hours following pediatric heart transplantation: Incidence, risk factors, and outcomes. Pediatr Transplant. 2019;23:e13414.

14. Profita EL, Gauvreau K, Rycus P, et al. Incidence, predictors, and outcomes after severe primary graft dysfunction in pediatric heart transplant recipients. 2019;38:601-608.

15. Nair AG, Sleeper LA, Smoot LB et al. Extracorporeal Membrane Oxygenation Support After Heart Transplantation in Children—Outcomes of a Single Center Cohort. Pediatric Critical Care Medicine. 2020;21:332-339.

16. Ross HJ, Law Y, Book WM et al. Transplantation and mechanical circulatory support in congenital heart disease: a scientific statement from the American Heart Association. Circulation. 2016;133:802-820.

17. O'Connor MJ, Glatz AC, Rossano JW et al. Cumulative effect of preoperative risk factors on mortality after pediatric heart transplantation. The Annals of Thoracic Surgery. 2018;106:561-566.

18. Messer SJ, Axell RG, Colah S et al. Functional assessment and transplantation of the donor heart after circulatory death. J Heart Lung Transplant. 2016;35:1443-1452.

19. Sponga S, Benedetti G, de Manna ND et al. Heart transplant outcomes in patients with mechanical circulatory support: cold storage versus normothermic perfusion organ preservation. Interact Cardiovasc Thorac Surg. 2021;32:476-482.

20. Hoskote A, Carter C, Rees P, et al. Acute right ventricular failure after pediatric cardiac transplant: predictors and long-term outcome in current era of transplantation medicine. The Journal of thoracic and cardiovascular surgery. 2010;139:146-153.

21. Loforte A, Murana G, Cefarelli M et al. Role of Intra-Aortic Balloon Pump and Extracorporeal Membrane Oxygenation in Early Graft Failure After Cardiac Transplantation. Artificial Organs. 2016;40:E136-E145.

22. Listijono DR, Watson A, Pye R et al. Usefulness of extracorporeal membrane oxygenation for early cardiac allograft dysfunction. The Journal of Heart and Lung Transplantation. 2011;30:783-789.

23. Entwistle JWC. Commentary: The evolving management of primary graft dysfunction in heart transplantation. The Journal of Thoracic and Cardiovascular Surgery. 2019;158:1587-1588.

24. Su JA, Kelly RB, Grogan T, et al. Extracorporeal membrane oxygenation support after pediatric orthotopic heart transplantation. 2015;19:68-75.

25. Kirk R, Griselli M, Smith J, et al. Elective extracorporeal membrane oxygenation bridge to recovery in otherwise" unusable" donor hearts for children: Preliminary outcomes. The Journal of Heart and Lung Transplantation. 2013;32:839-840.

26. Segovia J, Cosío MD, Barceló JM et al. RADIAL: a novel primary graft failure risk score in heart transplantation. J Heart Lung Transplant. 2011;30:644-651.

27. Huang J, Trinkaus K, Huddleston CB, et al. Risk factors for primary graft failure after pediatric cardiac transplantation: importance of recipient and donor characteristics. J Heart Lung Transplant. 2004;23:716-722.

28. Fiser SM, Tribble CG, Kaza AK et al. When to discontinue extracorporeal membrane oxygenation for postcardiotomy support. The Annals of thoracic surgery. 2001;71:210-214.

29. Aissaoui N, Luyt CE, Leprince P et al. Predictors of successful extracorporeal membrane oxygenation (ECLS) weaning after assistance for refractory cardiogenic shock. Intensive Care Med. 2011;37:1738-1745.

30. Simmonds J, Dominguez T, Longman J et al. Predictors and Outcome of Extracorporeal Life Support After Pediatric Heart Transplantation. The Annals of Thoracic Surgery. 2015;99:2166-2172.

31. Morgan CT, Manlhiot C, McCrindle BW, et al. Outcome, incidence and risk factors for stroke after pediatric heart transplantation: An analysis of the International Society for Heart and Lung Transplantation Registry. The Journal of Heart and Lung Transplantation. 2016;35:597-602.

32. Truby LK, Takeda K, Farr M et al. Incidence and Impact of On-Cardiopulmonary Bypass Vasoplegia During Heart Transplantation. ASAIO J. 2018;64:43-51.

33. Quader M, Hawkins RB, Mehaffey JH et al. Primary graft dysfunction after heart transplantation: Outcomes and resource utilization. J Card Surg. 2019;34:1519-1525.

34. Lima EB, Cunha CR, Barzilai VS et al. Experience of ECLS in primary graft dysfunction after orthotopic heart transplantation. Arq Bras Cardiol. 2015;105:285-291.

35. Taghavi S, Zuckermann A, Ankersmit J et al. Extracorporeal membrane oxygenation is superior to right ventricular assist device for acute right ventricular failure after heart transplantation. Ann Thorac Surg. 2004;78:1644-1649.

36. Thomas HL, Dronavalli VB, Parameshwar J, et al. Incidence and outcome of Levitronix CentriMag support as rescue therapy for early cardiac allograft failure: a United Kingdom national study. Eur J Cardiothorac Surg. 2011;40:1348-1354.

37. Kanter KR, Vincent RN, Berg AM, et al. Cardiac retransplantation in children. The Annals of thoracic surgery. 2004;78:644-649.

38. Mahle WT. Cardiac retransplantation in children. Pediatric transplantation. 2008;12:274-280.

39. Kittleson MM, Patel JK, Moriguchi JD et al. Heart transplant recipients supported with extracorporeal membrane oxygenation: outcomes from a single-center experience. 2011;30:1250-1256.

40. Perri G, Hasan A, Cassidy J et al. Extracorporeal life support after paediatric heart transplantation. European Journal of Cardio-Thoracic Surgery. 2012ezs115.

41. Dipchand AI, Edwards LB, Kucheryavaya AY et al. The registry of the International Society for Heart and Lung Transplantation: seventeenth official pediatric heart transplantation report--2014; focus theme: retransplantation. 2014;33:985-995.

# 42

## Extracorporeal Elimination

*Brian C. Bridges, Katja M. Gist, Alexander Supady, Christoph Benk, Leen Vercaemst, Thomas Müller, David S. Cooper, Matthew L. Paden*

## Introduction

As the volume and complexity of patients receiving cardiac and/or respiratory support with ECLS increases, so does the use of additional extracorporeal organ support. For the patient supported with traditional extracorporeal membrane oxygenation, other extracorporeal organ support therapies can be used in line with the ECLS circuit. The ECLS circuit can serve as a platform in which other extracorporeal organ support therapies can be added. In this chapter, we will outline the other forms of extracorporeal organ support and elimination therapies that can be used in conjunction with ECLS.

## Kidney Replacement Therapy During ECLS

### Acute Kidney Injury and Fluid Overload

Acute kidney injury (AKI) is common in patients supported with ECLS and is associated with significant morbidity and mortality in both single and multicenter studies across the age spectrum.[1-3] The incidence of AKI in ECLS is highly variable, ranging from 40-85%, with approximately 40-45% requiring kidney replacement therapy (KRT, also known as renal replacement therapy, RRT).[1-4] The Kidney Disease: Improving Global Outcomes (KDIGO) consensus definition, and the neonatal (age

<28 days) modification are used to diagnose AKI based on changes in serum creatinine or urine output.[5,6] ELSO defines AKI by serum creatinine or need for dialysis.[7] A summary of the KDIGO and ELSO AKI definitions are included in Table 42-1.

Pathologic fluid overload (FO) is also highly prevalent in patients supported with ECLS.[8-11] FO often precedes initiation of ECLS, and unfortunately, many patients continue to accumulate additional fluid while on ECLS.[11,12] Like AKI, FO is also associated with increased morbidity and mortality.[3,8,10,11] In fact, fluid homeostasis and AKI are interrelated, and the effects of pathologic FO and AKI appear to synergistically worsen outcomes.[12,13] The threshold of pathologic FO is unknown.

| KDIGO DEFINITION | | |
|---|---|---|
| | Serum Creatinine | Urine Output |
| Stage 1 | 1.5-1.9x baseline OR ≥0.3mg/dL (≥26.5 µmol/l) increase | <0.5ml/kg/h for 6-12 hours |
| Stage 2 | 2.0-2.9x baseline | <0.5ml/kg/h for ≥12 hours |
| Stage 3 | 3.0x baseline OR ≥4mg/dL (≥353.6 µmol/l) OR Initiation of RRT OR In patients < 18 years, decrease in eGFR to <35ml/min/1.73m² | <0.3ml/kg/g for ≥24 hours OR Anuria for ≥12 hours |
| ELSO DEFINITION (Serum Creatinine) | | |
| > 1.5 mg/dL >3 mg/dL Dialysis | | |

**Table 42-1.** Acute Kidney Injury Definitions by KDIGO and ELSO. (Neonatal modification not included.)

However, most studies have used a cutoff of 10% and evaluated its impact on outcomes prior to ECLS initiation, peak during ECLS, and at ECLS termination.[6,9,12]

### Kidney Replacement Therapy and ECLS

KRT is an important tool used for the management of AKI and FO for patients supported with ECLS. A recent international survey disseminated by the Kidney Interventions During Membrane Oxygenation (KIDMO) group demonstrated that among 60 centers, 85% of respondents used KRT for the prevention or treatment of FO. Just under 50% of respondents indicated that KRT was used for AKI and/or electrolyte derangements.[14] Multiple KRT modalities exist, and the mode of clearance can be modified based on center practices, type of filter, patient need, or the desired effect (ultrafiltration, diffusion, convection, or both). The KRT modalities, advantages, and disadvantages are summarized in Table 42-2.

| MODALITY | DESCRIPTION/INDICATION | ADVANTAGES | DISADVANTAGES |
|---|---|---|---|
| Continuous Kidney Replacement Therapy (CKRT)* | SCUF: Removes excessive fluid from the blood via ultrafiltration | • No dialysate or replacement fluid needed<br>• Can be performed with an in-line filter or an external device<br>• Cheaper than other forms of CKRT | • Use of an in-line filter results in decreased fluid removal precision |
| | CVVH: Removes large volumes of fluid via convection; replacement fluid is added | • Removal of large molecules<br>• Precise control of fluid balance with an external device (integrated or in parallel) | • Patient immobilization<br>• Expensive |
| | CVVHD: Removal of fluid mainly by diffusion using dialysate | • Removal of small to medium sized molecules<br>• Precise control of fluid balance with an external device (integrated or in parallel) | |
| | CVVHDF: Both convection and diffusion are used and requires an external device | • Removal of a range of molecule sizes | |
| Sustained low efficiency dialysis (SLED)** | Conventional IHD machines are used to provide extended duration KRT (8-12 hours) in critically ill patients with hemodynamic instability | • Potentially lower costs<br>• Can be performed without anticoagulation<br>• Removal of small and mid-sized molecules | • Unfamiliarity<br>• Unclear effects on drug pharmacokinetics<br>• Hypophosphatemia |
| Intermittent hemodialysis (IHD) | A separate device that is either integrated into the ECLS circuit or applied through separate vascular access. | • Lower cost than CKRT<br>• Patient mobilization between sessions | • More rapid fluid removal may result in ECLS circuit issues and hemodynamic issues<br>• Disequilibrium syndrome<br>• Requires special nursing expertise |

*CVVH and CVVHD can be performed with an in-line filter by adding IV pumps for replacement fluid and/or dialysate. **Sustained low efficiency dialysis also referred to as prolonged intermittent renal replacement therapy (PIRRT).
Abbreviations: SCUF=slow continuous ultrafiltration, CVVH=continuous venovenous hemofiltration, CVVHD=continuous venovenous hemodialysis, CVVHDF=continuous venovenous hemodiafiltration.

**Table 42-2.** Description of kidney replacement therapy modalities.

KRT can be performed using an in-line filter or an external device. The use of an in-line filter is a common practice in some neonatal and pediatric ECLS centers. An in-line filter is typically placed after the pump and before the oxygenator to trap air and clots. The positive pressure from the pump drives the blood through the filter and it is returned to the ECLS circuit before the oxygenator. Slow continuous ultrafiltration (SCUF) is the most common modality used with this setup. However, continuous venovenous hemofiltration (CVVH) and continuous venovenous hemodialysis (CVVHD) can be delivered by adding replacement fluid or dialysis fluid respectively using standard infusion pumps. With this modality, ultrafiltration is regulated by connecting a standard infusion device to the effluent port of the hemofilter. There are several advantages to using an in-line hemofilter, including low cost, smaller priming volume, and the ability to generate large ultrafiltration volumes. Unfortunately, there are also several important disadvantages. Fluid removal precision is decreased, amounting to differences as much as 800 ml/day.[15] There is also limited solute clearance and the requirement for an external infusion device to control ultrafiltration and delivery of replacement fluid. These hemofilters are often not designed for high pressure systems and the volume delivery of the infusion pump is often limited to 1 liter/hour, and thus convective and diffusive clearance is less than with conventional membranes. Finally, flow rates are limited by either a stopcock or flow restrictor, both of which generate flow turbulence that can trigger hemolysis and thrombus formation.

An external device can either be connected to the ECLS circuit or placed in parallel through separate venous access points. In this parallel setup, no manipulation of the ECLS circuit is needed and the dose and modality can be adjusted based on center specific protocols and patient needs. The major disadvantages of

this methodology include the need for separate venous access points—which in small pediatric patients may be challenging, if not impossible.

Many centers use a KRT device in conjunction with the ECLS circuit. The inflow line of the KRT device is placed after the pump, either before or after the oxygenator to avoid air entrapment, and the return line is placed postpump and preoxygenator to avoid sending air or clot to the patient (Figure 42-1). Because the access pressures of the KRT device are usually negative, attention should be paid to the set pressure limits of both the ECLS circuit and KRT device.

Unfortunately, there are no consensus statements on what constitutes the best timing for KRT initiation. Furthermore, the theoretical benefits of early initiation for rapid resolution of FO have been refuted by several trials evaluating an early vs. late start KRT strategy in critically ill adults not supported by ECLS.[16-18] Paek and colleagues evaluated the timing of KRT initiation in patients supported by ECLS. Early initiation was defined as <72 hours after ECLS initiation. They found no difference in mortality between the early and late KRT groups.[19] Based on the existing data, one should consider KRT when the host response alone is maladaptive

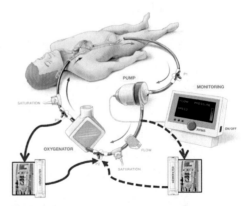

**Figure 42-1.** Extracorporeal life support circuit with CKRT device integration. The access portion of the CKRT device is connected after the oxygenator or before the oxygenator and after the pump. The return line is post pump and before the oxygenator.

in processes such as electrolyte homeostasis, managing azotemia in the setting of bleeding and neurologic impairment, or when there is inadequate native urine output. Indeed, KRT may also be necessary when proper nutrition cannot be delivered.[20,21] The 21st Acute Disease Quality Initiative (ADQI) group concluded that there was insufficient evidence for the preemptive use of KRT in patients treated with ECLS, and its use should be based on absolute and relative indications in critically ill patients.[22]

### Outcomes and Recovery of Renal Function

Severe AKI, AKI requiring KRT, and FO in ECLS supported patients are associated with mortality in both children and adults.[1,4,23] A recent metaanalysis demonstrated a pooled adjusted odds of mortality in adult patients requiring KRT on ECLS of 3.3,[1] although there seems to be an era effect, with a 20% reduction in the most recent 5 years (2015-2020).[1,23] Similarly, the adjusted odds of mortality in a metaanalysis of pediatric patients requiring KRT and ECLS was 3.6-fold greater than patients with no AKI.[4] In a subanalysis of the KIDMO database including only pediatric ECLS patients who received KRT, FO was reduced at KRT discontinuation among survivors. FO at both KRT initiation and discontinuation were associated with increased ECLS duration and a 10-20% increased adjusted odds of mortality.[9]

Among adults, the risk of subsequent major adverse kidney events (MAKE) at one year after AKI are significant,[24,25] in addition to notable decrements in glomerular filtration rate.[25] Recovery of kidney function was observed in 96% of children receiving ECLS and KRT from a single center.[26] Additional longitudinal studies are needed to assess the impact of severe AKI or FO needing KRT on both survival and chronic kidney disease (CKD). Zwiers et al. reported on the incidence of CKD and hypertension among a cohort of neonates treated with ECLS. The median followup duration was 8.2 years, and 32% had at least one sign of CKD and/or hypertension. Severe AKI was associated with 4-times greater odds of signs of CKD or hypertension.[27]

### Therapeutic Plasma Exchange During ECLS

Therapeutic plasma exchange (TPE) is an extracorporeal procedure that removes plasma from other blood components and replaces it with 5% albumin and/or fresh frozen plasma. TPE has the benefit of removing proinflammatory mediators, cytokines, antibodies, pathogenic autoantibodies, pro- and anticoagulant proteins, immunoglobins, and toxic macromolecules.[28-32] TPE is performed using a centrifugal based system or with a highly permeable membrane. These allow for the separation of plasma from the cellular elements contained within the blood. With centrifugation, the system extracts the

| | CENTRIFUGE | MEMBRANE |
|---|---|---|
| Mechanism | Centrifugal force | Capillary membrane filter |
| Plasma extraction (%) | 80 | 30 |
| Anticoagulation | Citrate | Heparin or bivalirudin |
| Separation | Specific gravity | Molecular size |
| Blood volume in the circuit (mL) | 180 | 125 |
| Molecular weight cutoff (kD) | N/A | 3000 |
| Fluid replacement | Albumin and/or fresh frozen plasma | Albumin and/or fresh frozen plasma |

**Table 42-3.** Comparison of centrifugation and membrane therapeutic plasma exchange. (Adapted from Williams and colleagues.[65])

whole blood, adds anticoagulant, separates the blood components, collects specific components, and returns the uncollected components back to the patient. With this method, blood components are separated based on specific gravity (density) rather than molecular size. With membrane filtration, plasma is separated from the blood by a plasma filter membrane or a protein solution postfilter. Blood components are separated based on molecular size using convection. The replacement fluid, in conjunction with the patient's blood and cellular components are then returned to the patient. A comparison of centrifugation and membrane plasma exchange is included in Table 42-3. Single or multiple TPE sessions lasting 3-4 hours can be performed in isolation or in tandem with other extracorporeal therapies including ECLS and/or CKRT. The amount of plasma exchanged with each treatment course can vary and is typically 1-2 times the total plasma volume.

The American Society for Apheresis (ASFA) recently updated the guidelines for the use of TPE and encompasses a broad array of conditions graded by level of evidence.[33] Overall, there is a paucity of data on the use of TPE with ECLS. Technically, performing TPE concurrently with ECLS is done in a similar fashion to CKRT (Figure 42-2). In fact, the TPE

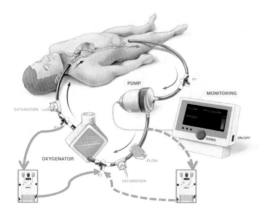

**Figure 42-2.** Extracorporeal life support circuit with therapeutic plasma exchange device integration.

device can be connected to the ECLS circuit with CKRT without interrupting the flow of the ECLS circuit. TPE can also be performed using a separate access point. In a recent study of TPE performed in patients on ECLS, there was relatively good tolerance, with hypocalcemia being the most common complication.[34]

TPE in tandem with ECLS is most reported in patients with septic shock and multisystem organ failure. ASFA has categorized this as a class III recommendation (optimum role of TPE is not established and decision making should be individualized) and Grade 2B recommendation (weak recommendation, moderate quality of evidence).[33] TPE is thought to improve organ function in sepsis by removing inflammatory mediators and replenishing anticoagulant proteins, with an improvement in mortality in a retrospective study of pediatric patients with thrombocytopenia associated multiple organ failure (TAMOF).[35] The first randomized controlled trial by Kawai and colleagues demonstrated a reduction in the risk of death and fewer organ failures for children and adults treated with TPE versus conventional therapy.[36] Unfortunately, prospective studies evaluating the use of TPE in children and adults have been largely conflicting,[37-40] and a large systematic review and metaanalysis concluded that there was insufficient evidence to recommend TPE as an adjunctive therapy for patients with septic shock.[41]

TPE is a standard treatment for thrombotic thrombocytopenic purpura (TTP), a condition that results in severe thrombocytopenia, microangiopathic hemolytic anemia, and neurologic abnormalities. TAMOF is thought to be a unique sepsis phenotype in which there is a microangiopathy like TTP, with platelet consumption and organ failure secondary to microvascular thromboses.[36-42] TPE is beneficial in TTP because it results in the repletion of ADAMTS13 and removal of thrombogenic von Willebrand factor multimers. Nguyen and colleagues performed a randomized controlled trial in children with TAMOF, and found that no patients who received TPE died, while 80% who were randomized to standard sepsis management died.[39] In ECLS-supported patients with critical cardiac disease and TAMOF, TPE use was associated with recovery from organ failure.[42]

**Therapeutic Cytapheresis**

Therapeutic cytapheresis refers to the removal of the cellular components of blood. Red blood cell exchange, in which a patient's native red blood cells are removed and replaced with donor red blood cells, is commonly performed in patients with complications of sickle cell disease such as neurologic changes from stroke or acute chest syndrome. The removal of white blood cells, or leukocytapheresis, has been used to reduce the hyperviscosity and symptoms of severely elevated white blood cell counts observed with acute leukemia. Guidelines and the available evidence for the use of therapeutic cytapheresis are available from the ASFA.[43]

One of the most reported indications for cytapheresis for patients supported with ECLS is therapeutic leukocytapheresis for infants with severe pertussis. Infants with severe pertussis can suffer from hypoxia, pulmonary hypertension, and cardiovascular failure that is refractory to conventional therapy. Historically, infants requiring ECLS for pertussis have had a high mortality rate. There is evidence that the refractory hypoxia and pulmonary hypertension in severe pertussis is mediated by the hyperleukocytosis that is associated with the disease, and that the degree of hyperleukocytosis is independently associated with increased mortality.[44,45] In postmortem exams of infants with fatal pertussis, there is evidence of leukocyte thrombi in the pulmonary vasculature.[46,47] There have been attempts to attenuate the hyperleukocytosis associated with severe pertussis with the hopes of improving the outcomes of these critically ill children.

In 2006, Grzeszczak et al. described the use of leukocytapheresis in a 5-week-old patient requiring support with ECLS for pertussis. In this case report, leukocytapheresis was temporally associated with a normalization of the white blood cell count, cardiopulmonary stability, and eventual survival to hospital discharge.[48]

In a single-center review of 19 critically ill infants with severe pertussis, patients treated after the institution of a leukodepletion strategy had a mortality of 10% compared to a historic mortality of 44% before the use of leukodepletion.[49] A retrospective, multicenter study of infants requiring ECLS for severe pertussis demonstrated an overall survival of 28%. Younger age, lower $PaO_2/FiO_2$ ratio, the need of vasoactive infusions, pulmonary hypertension, and decreased time from intubation to cannulation onto ECLS were associated with increased mortality. A multivariate analysis demonstrated that infants treated with leukocytapheresis during ECLS support for pertussis had increased survival to hospital discharge.[50]

**Hemoadsorption Therapies**

In recent decades, extracorporeal hemo-adsorption has been suggested as an adjunctive treatment option for different clinical conditions, particularly for patients in severe inflammatory states. So far, the evidence for a clinical benefit from the use of hemoadsorption devices is scarce and no study has shown a survival benefit.[51] Hemoadsorption devices have to be incorporated in extracorporeal blood circuits; therefore, their use in combination with ECLS is feasible.[52,53]

***Technical Aspects and Implementation in ECLS Circuits***

When CKRT is already in place in the ECLS circuit, the adsorber can be incorporated in series with the hemofilter in line with the CKRT circuit (Figure 42-3). If no CKRT device is used in conjunction with ECLS, the hemoadsorption circuit should be connected to ports with a positive pressure difference between the inlet and outlet ports, enabling the recommended forward blood flow through the device (Figure 42-4). It is important to note that the return port in this configuration is situated in a negative pressure zone with centrifugal pumps, and this can lead to disastrous air emboli upon accidental disconnection.

### *Clinical Evidence for the Use of Hemoadsorption in Combination with ECLS*

The removal of endotoxin, inflammatory cytokines, or other harmful substances directly from the patient's blood may be a sound rationale for the use of hemoadsorption; but to date, there is only limited data demonstrating a clinical benefit when used in combination with ECLS.[53] Case reports and single-center case series of patients supported with hemoadsorption in combination with ECLS suggest a benefit of this treatment for patients with severe respiratory failure, sepsis, and cardiovascular failure.[54-57] However, studies comparing patients treated with hemoadsorption to a control group have not confirmed a significant treatment effect with respect to a reduction of inflammatory parameters or clinical improvement.[58-60] In a retrospective observational study, a negative effect of hemoadsorption on patient survival after cardiac arrest was suggested.[61] Similarly, in randomized controlled trials assessing the effect of hemoadsorption in combination with ECLS or cardiopulmonary bypass during cardiac surgery, no conclusive evidence for a benefit of hemoadsorption could be found.[58,62-66] A randomized trial in patients with severe COVID-19 supported with venovenous ECLS even showed a survival disadvantage for patients treated for the first 72 hours after initiation of ECLS with the CytoSorb adsorber.[67,68]

Taken together, there may be a sound pathophysiological rationale for the combined use of hemoadsorption and ECLS and its technical application is feasible and seemingly safe. However, current evidence does not support its routine clinical use. Without a proven benefit in rigorously conducted clinical trials, the routine use of hemoadsorption in patients supported with ECLS cannot be recommended.

### Extracorporeal Liver Support

Extracorporeal liver support has been used in patients with acute and acute-on-chronic liver failure as both a bridge to recovery and bridge to

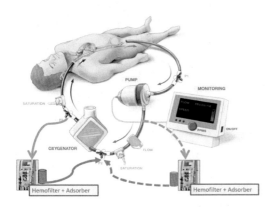

**Figure 42-3.** Adsorption filter in parallel to the ECLS circuit and in series with the CKRT circuit.

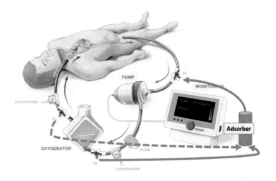

**Figure 42-4.** Adsorption filter circuit in parallel to the ECLS circuit with filter flow determined by pressure gradient.

transplant. Extracorporeal liver support includes single-pass albumin dialysis (SPAD), molecular adsorbent recirculating system (MARS®), Prometheus® fractionated plasma separation and adsorption system, and high-volume plasma exchange. SPAD can be performed with a commercially available continuous kidney replacement therapy device. With SPAD, blood flows through a hemofilter countercurrent to a dialysate solution containing albumin to remove protein bound molecules that are not typically removed by standard kidney support therapy. As the used albumin solution is discarded, this process requires a large volume of albumin and incurs considerable cost.[69] With the MARS system, blood also flows through a hemofilter with a countercurrent dialysate fluid with albumin to remove protein bound solutes. The spent albumin solution then undergoes dialysis to remove water soluble toxins and then passes through an anion exchanger resin adsorber and a charcoal absorber. The replenished albumin solution is then reused and recycled through the primary circuit. The Prometheus system filters albumin from the patient's blood, and the albumin enriched plasma is passed through a resin adsorber column and an anion exchanger adsorber column to remove protein bound toxins. After passing through the two adsorber columns, the replenished albumin solution passes through the primary circuit for the removal of water-soluble molecules using a hemofilter and conventional dialysis.[69-70] High volume plasma exchange, as described in a previous section, has been used in both pediatric and adult acute liver failure. In some centers, therapeutic plasma exchange is used in tandem with continuous kidney replacement therapy to remove both protein bound and water soluble toxins and to treat fluid overload in patients with acute liver failure.[71,72]

There are a few reports on the use of extracorporeal liver support in conjunction with traditional ECLS. A case series of adult ECLS patients with severe hyperbilirubinemia who were supported with MARS had a survival of 40% compared to historic controls that had no survivors with severe hyperbilirubinemia.[73] In a retrospective, single center study of adult ECLS patients with acute liver failure, patients supported with ECLS and MARS therapy had an ECLS survival of 64% vs. an ECLS survival of only 21% in the standard medical care group (p=0.02). There was a trend in improved 30-day mortality in the ECLS patients supported with MARS, 43% vs. 14% in the ECLS with standard care group, but this difference was not statistically significant.[74]

**Conclusion**

The use of additional organ support therapies in conjunction with traditional ECLS will continue to increase as the number and acuity of patients placed on ECLS support while awaiting recovery of native organ function or bridge to organ transplant increase. There is still a great deal of work needed to determine the best timing, technique, and application of these forms of extracorporeal organ support and elimination therapies.

# References

1. Thongprayoon C, Cheungpasitporn W, Lertjitbanjong P, et al. Incidence and Impact of Acute Kidney Injury in Patients Receiving Extracorporeal Membrane Oxygenation: A Meta-Analysis. J Clin Med. 2019;8(7).

2. Delmas C, Zapetskaia T, Conil JM, et al. 3-month prognostic impact of severe acute renal failure under veno-venous ECMO support: Importance of time of onset. Journal of critical care. 2018;44:63-71.

3. Fleming GM, Sahay R, Zappitelli M, et al. The Incidence of Acute Kidney Injury and Its Effect on Neonatal and Pediatric Extracorporeal Membrane Oxygenation Outcomes: A Multicenter Report From the Kidney Intervention During Extracorporeal Membrane Oxygenation Study Group. Pediatr Crit Care Med. 2016;17(12):1157-1169.

4. Hansrivijit P, Lertjitbanjong P, Thongprayoon C, et al. Acute Kidney Injury in Pediatric Patients on Extracorporeal Membrane Oxygenation: A Systematic Review and Meta-analysis. Medicines (Basel). 2019;6(4).

5. Kellum JA, Lameire N, Group KAGW. Diagnosis, evaluation, and management of acute kidney injury: a KDIGO summary (Part 1). Critical care. 2013;17(1):204.

6. Selewski DT, Charlton JR, Jetton JG, et al. Neonatal Acute Kidney Injury. Pediatrics. 2015;136(2):e463-473.

7. Codes for Extracorporeal Life Support (ECLS) Complications. https://www.elso.org/Registry/SupportDocuments/ECLSComplicationsCode.aspx. Accessed December 31, 2021.

8. Schmidt M, Bailey M, Kelly J, et al. Impact of fluid balance on outcome of adult patients treated with extracorporeal membrane oxygenation. Inten care Med. 2014;40(9):1256-1266.

9. Gorga SM, Sahay RD, Askenazi DJ, et al. Fluid overload and fluid removal in pediatric patients on extracorporeal membrane oxygenation requiring continuous renal replacement therapy: a multicenter retrospective cohort study. Pediatric nephrology. 2020;35(5):871-882.

10. Dado DN, Ainsworth CR, Thomas SB, et al. Outcomes among Patients Treated with Renal Replacement Therapy during Extracorporeal Membrane Oxygenation: A Single-Center Retrospective Study. Blood purification. 2020;49(3):341-347.

11. Selewski DT, Askenazi DJ, Bridges BC, et al. The Impact of Fluid Overload on Outcomes in Children Treated With Extracorporeal Membrane Oxygenation: A Multicenter Retrospective Cohort Study. Pedia Crit Care Med :. 2017;18(12):1126-1135.

12. Gist KM, Misfeldt A, Sahay RD, et al. Acute Kidney Injury and Fluid Overload in Pediatric Extracorporeal Cardio-Pulmonary Resuscitation: A Multicenter Retrospective Cohort Study. ASAIO J. 2021.

13. Gist KM, Selewski DT, Brinton J, et al. Assessment of the Independent and Synergistic Effects of Fluid Overload and Acute Kidney Injury on Outcomes of Critically Ill Children. Pedia Crit Care Med. 2020;21(2):170-177.

14. Gorga SM, Lima L, Askenazi DJ, et al. Fluid Balance Management Informs Renal Replacement Therapy Use During Pediatric Extracorporeal Membrane Oxygenation: A Survey Report From the Kidney Intervention During Extracorporeal Membrane Oxygenation Group. ASAIO J. 2022;68(3):407-412.

15. Sucosky P, Dasi LP, Paden ML, et al. Assessment of Current Continuous Hemofiltration Systems and Development of a Novel Accurate Fluid Management System for Use in Extracorporeal Membrane Oxygenation. J Med Devices. 2008;2(3).

16. Barbar SD, Clere-Jehl R, Bourredjem A, et al. Timing of Renal-Replacement Therapy in Patients with Acute Kidney Injury and Sepsis. New Engl J Med. 2018;379(15):1431-1442.

17. Gaudry S, Hajage D, Schortgen F, et al. Initiation Strategies for Renal-Replacement Therapy in the Intensive Care Unit. New Engl J Med. 2016;375(2):122-133.

18. Investigators S-A, Canadian Critical Care Trials G, Australian, et al. Timing of Initiation of Renal-Replacement Therapy in Acute Kidney Injury. New Engl J Med. 2020;383(3):240-251.

19. Paek JH, Park S, Lee A, et al. Timing for initiation of sequential continuous renal replacement therapy in patients on extracorporeal membrane oxygenation. Kidney Res Clin Pract. 2018;37(3):239-247.

20. Murphy HJ, Cahill JB, Twombley KE, et al. Implementing a practice change: early initiation of continuous renal replacement therapy during neonatal extracorporeal life support standardizes care and improves short-term outcomes. J Artif Organs. 2018;21(1):76-85.

21. Murphy HJ, Finch CW, Taylor SN. Neonatal Extracorporeal Life Support: A Review of Nutrition Considerations. Nutr Clin Pract. 2018;33(5):625-632.

22. Joannidis M, Forni LG, Klein SJ, et al. Lung-kidney interactions in critically ill patients: consensus report of the Acute Disease Quality Initiative (ADQI) 21 Workgroup. Intensive care medicine. 2020;46(4):654-672.

23. Mitra S, Ling RR, Tan CS, et al. Concurrent Use of Renal Replacement Therapy during Extracorporeal Membrane Oxygenation Support: A Systematic Review and Meta-Analysis. J Clin Med. 2021;10(2).

24. Coresh J, Turin TC, Matsushita K, et al. Decline in estimated glomerular filtration rate and subsequent

risk of end-stage renal disease and mortality. JAMA. 2014;311(24):2518-2531.

25. Vinclair C, De Montmollin E, Sonneville R, et al. Factors associated with major adverse kidney events in patients who underwent veno-arterial extracorporeal membrane oxygenation. Annals of intensive care. 2020;10(1):44.

26. Paden ML, Warshaw BL, Heard ML, et al. Recovery of renal function and survival after continuous renal replacement therapy during extracorporeal membrane oxygenation. Pediatr Crit Care Med. 2011;12(2):153-158.

27. Zwiers AJ, H IJ, van Rosmalen J, et al. CKD and hypertension during long-term follow-up in children and adolescents previously treated with extracorporeal membrane oxygenation. Clin J Amer Society Nephrology : CJASN. 2014;9(12):2070-2078.

28. Belousova T, Tong Y, Bai Y, et al. Utilization of therapeutic plasma exchange for hyperbilirubinemia in a premature newborn on extracorporeal membrane oxygenation. J Clin Apher. 2019;34(5):615-622.

29. Canter MO, Daniels J, Bridges BC. Adjunctive Therapies During Extracorporeal Membrane Oxygenation to Enhance Multiple Organ Support in Critically Ill Children. Front Pediatr. 2018;6:78.

30. Cheng CW, Hendrickson JE, Tormey CA, et al. Therapeutic Plasma Exchange and Its Impact on Drug Levels: An ACLPS Critical Review. American Journal of Clinical Pathology. 2017;148(3):190-198.

31. Eyre M, Hacohen Y, Barton C, et al. Therapeutic plasma exchange in paediatric neurology: a critical review and proposed treatment algorithm. Dev Med Child Neurol. 2018;60(8):765-779.

32. Kassif Lerner R, Pollak U. The use of therapeutic plasma exchange for pediatric patients supported on extracorporeal membranous oxygenator therapy: A narrative review. Perfusion. 2022 Mar;37(2):113-122.

33. Schwartz J, Padmanabhan A, Aqui N, et al. Guidelines on the Use of Therapeutic Apheresis in Clinical Practice-Evidence-Based Approach from the Writing Committee of the American Society for Apheresis: The Seventh Special Issue. J Clin Apher. 2016;31(3):149-162.

34. Dyer M, Neal MD, Rollins-Raval MA, et al. Simultaneous extracorporeal membrane oxygenation and therapeutic plasma exchange procedures are tolerable in both pediatric and adult patients. Transfusion. 2014;54(4):1158-1165.

35. Sevketoglu E, Yildizdas D, Horoz OO, et al. Use of therapeutic plasma exchange in children with thrombocytopenia-associated multiple organ failure in the Turkish thrombocytopenia-associated multiple organ failure network. Pediatr Crit Care Med. 2014;15(8):e354-359.

36. Kawai Y, Cornell TT, Cooley EG, et al. Therapeutic plasma exchange may improve hemodynamics and organ failure among children with sepsis-induced multiple organ dysfunction syndrome receiving extracorporeal life support. Pediatr Crit Care Med. 2015;16(4):366-374.

37. Busund R, Koukline V, Utrobin U, et al. Plasmapheresis in severe sepsis and septic shock: a prospective, randomised, controlled trial. Intensive Care Med. 2002;28(10):1434-1439.

38. Long EJ, Taylor A, Delzoppo C, et al. A randomised controlled trial of plasma filtration in severe paediatric sepsis. Critical care and resuscitation : journal of the Australasian Academy of Critical Care Medicine. 2013;15(3):198-204.

39. Nguyen TC, Han YY, Kiss JE, et al. Intensive plasma exchange increases a disintegrin and metalloprotease with thrombospondin motifs-13 activity and reverses organ dysfunction in children with thrombocytopenia-associated multiple organ failure. Crit Care Med. 2008;36(10):2878-2887.

40. Reeves JH, Butt WW, Shann F, et al. Continuous plasmafiltration in sepsis syndrome. Plasmafiltration in Sepsis Study Group. Crit Care Med. 1999;27(10):2096-2104.

41. Rimmer E, Houston BL, Kumar A, et al. The efficacy and safety of plasma exchange in patients with sepsis and septic shock: a systematic review and meta-analysis. Crit Care. 2014;18(6):699.

42. Chong M, Lopez-Magallon AJ, Saenz L, et al. Use of Therapeutic Plasma Exchange during Extracorporeal Life Support in Critically Ill Cardiac Children with Thrombocytopenia-Associated Multi-Organ Failure. Front Pediatr. 2017;5:254.

43. Padmanabhan A, Connelly-Smith L, Aqui N, et al. Guidelines on the Use of Therapeutic Apheresis in Clinical Practice - Evidence-Based Approach from the Writing Committee of the American Society for Apheresis: The Eighth Special Issue. J Clin Apher. 2019;34(3):171-354.

44. Pierce C, Klein N, Peters M. Is leukocytosis a predictor of mortality in severe pertussis infection? Intensive Care Med. 2000;26(10):1512-1514.

45. Mikelova LK, Halperin SA, Scheifele D, et al. Predictors of death in infants hospitalized with pertussis: a case-control study of 16 pertussis deaths in Canada. J Pediatr. 2003;143(5):576-581.

46. Williams GD, Numa A, Sokol J, et al. ECLS in pertussis: does it have a role? Intensive Care Med. 1998;24(10):1089-1092.

47. Paddock CD, Sanden GN, Cherry JD, et al. Pathology and pathogenesis of fatal Bordetella pertussis infection in infants. Clin Infect Dis. 2008;47(3):328-338.

48. Grzeszczak MJ, Churchwell KB, Edwards KM, et al. Leukopheresis therapy for severe infantile pertussis with myocardial and pulmonary failure. Pediatr Crit Care Med. 2006;7(6):580-582.

49. Rowlands HE, Goldman AP, Harrington K, et al. Impact of rapid leukodepletion on the outcome of severe clinical pertussis in young infants. Pediatrics. 2010;126(4):e816-827.

50. Domico M, Ridout D, MacLaren G, et al. Extracorporeal Membrane Oxygenation for Pertussis: Predictors of Outcome Including Pulmonary Hypertension and Leukodepletion. Pediatr Crit Care Med. 2018;19(3):254-261.

51. Supady A, Brodie D, Wengenmayer T. Extracorporeal haemoadsorption: does the evidence support its routine use in critical care? Lancet Respir Med. 2022;10(3):307-312.

52. Bonavia A, Groff A, Karamchandani K, et al. Clinical Utility of Extracorporeal Cytokine Hemoadsorption Therapy: A Literature Review. Blood Purif. 2018;46(4):337-349.

53. Napp LC, Ziegeler S, Kindgen-Milles D. Rationale of Hemoadsorption during Extracorporeal Membrane Oxygenation Support. Blood Purif. 2019;48(3):203-214.

54. Bruenger F, Kizner L, Weile J, et al. First successful combination of ECMO with cytokine removal therapy in cardiogenic septic shock: a case report. Int J Artif Organs. 2015;38(2):113-116.

55. Calabro MG, Febres D, Recca G, et al. Blood Purification With CytoSorb in Critically Ill Patients: Single-Center Preliminary Experience. Artif Organs. 2019;43(2):189-194.

56. Kogelmann K, Scheller M, Druner M, et al. Use of hemoadsorption in sepsis-associated ECMO-dependent severe ARDS: A case series. J Intensive Care Soc. 2020;21(2):183-190.

57. Träger K, Schütz C, Fischer G, et al. Cytokine Reduction in the Setting of an ARDS-Associated Inflammatory Response with Multiple Organ Failure. Case Rep Crit Care. 2016;2016:9852073.

58. Rieder M, Zahn T, Benk C, et al. Cytokine adsorption in a patient with severe coronavirus disease 2019 related acute respiratory distress syndrome requiring extracorporeal membrane oxygenation therapy: A case report. Artif Organs. 2021;45(2):191-194.

59. Scharf C, Schroeder I, Paal M, et al. Can the cytokine adsorber CytoSorb(®) help to mitigate cytokine storm and reduce mortality in critically ill patients? A propensity score matching analysis. Ann Intensive Care. 2021;11(1):115.

60. Supady A, Zahn T, Rieder M, et al. Effect of Cytokine Adsorption on Survival and Circulatory Stabilization in Patients Receiving Extracorporeal Cardiopulmonary Resuscitation. ASAIO J. 2022;68(1):64-72.

61. Akin M, Garcheva V, Sieweke JT, et al. Early use of hemoadsorption in patients after out-of hospital cardiac arrest - a matched pair analysis. PLoS One. 2020;15(11):e0241709.

62. Bernardi MH, Rinoesl H, Dragosits K, et al. Effect of hemoadsorption during cardiopulmonary bypass surgery - a blinded, randomized, controlled pilot study using a novel adsorbent. Crit Care. 2016;20:96.

63. Bernardi MH, Rinoesl H, Ristl R, et al. Hemoadsorption does not Have Influence on Hemolysis During Cardiopulmonary Bypass. ASAIO J. 2019;65(7):738-743.

64. Garau I, Marz A, Sehner S, et al. Hemadsorption during cardiopulmonary bypass reduces interleukin 8 and tumor necrosis factor alpha serum levels in cardiac surgery: a randomized controlled trial. Minerva Anestesiol. 2019;85(7):715-723.

65. Poli EC, Alberio L, Bauer-Doerries A, et al. Cytokine clearance with CytoSorb(R) during cardiac surgery: a pilot randomized controlled trial. Crit Care. 2019;23(1):108.

66. Taleska Stupica G, Sostaric M, Bozhinovska M, et al. Extracorporeal Hemadsorption versus Glucocorticoids during Cardiopulmonary Bypass: A Prospective, Randomized, Controlled Trial. Cardiovasc Ther. 2020;2020:7834173.

67. Supady A. Cytokine adsorption and ECMO in patients with COVID-19 - Author's reply. Lancet Respir Med. 20219(8):e72-e74.

68. Supady A, Weber E, Rieder M, et al. Cytokine adsorption in patients with severe COVID-19 pneumonia requiring extracorporeal membrane oxygenation (CYCOV): a single centre, open-label, randomised, controlled trial. Lancet Respir Med. 2021;9(7):755-762.

69. Rademacher S, Oppert M, Jorres A. Artificial extracorporeal liver support therapy in patients with severe liver failure. Expert Rev Gastroenterol Hepatol. 2011;5(5):591-599.

70. Jain V, Dhawan A. Extracorporeal Liver Support Systems in Paediatric Liver Failure. J Pediatr Gastroenterol Nutr. 2017;64(6):855-863.

71. Akcan Arikan A, Srivaths P, Himes RW, et al. Hybrid Extracorporeal Therapies as a Bridge to Pediatric Liver Transplantation. Pediatr Crit Care Med. 2018;19(7):e342-e349.

72. Zoica BS, Deep A. Extracorporeal renal and liver support in pediatric acute liver failure. Pediatr Nephrol. 2021;36(5):1119-1128.

73. Peek GJ, Killer HM, Sosnowski MA, et al. Modular extracorporeal life support for multiorgan failure patients. Liver. 2002;22 Suppl 2:69-71.

74. Sparks BE, Cavarocchi NC, Hirose H. Extracorporeal membrane oxygenation with multiple-organ failure: Can molecular adsorbent recirculating system therapy improve survival? J Heart Lung Transplant. 2017;36(1):71-76.

# 43

## Extracorporeal Carbon Dioxide Removal

*Matthew E. Cove, Christian Karagiannidis, Elena Spinelli, Darryl Abrams, Antonio Pesenti*

## Introduction

Over the past 50 years, extracorporeal carbon dioxide removal ($ECCO_2R$) has developed in parallel to ECMO. Although the therapies overlap and share similar equipment, the primary aim of $ECCO_2R$ is carbon dioxide ($CO_2$) removal alone; whereas, ECMO aims to provide both oxygen delivery and $CO_2$ removal. From the earliest animal experiments in the 1970s, $ECCO_2R$ has been recognized as a tool for uncoupling pulmonary $CO_2$ elimination from oxygenation.[1] Its earliest clinical applications were the support of low-frequency ventilation in patients with ARDS,[2,3] but perhaps the true potential of $ECCO_2R$ was only recognized in the early 2000s,[4,5] when lower tidal volume ventilation was firmly established as a lifesaving intervention in ARDS[6] and the principles of ventilation-induced lung injury (VILI) were more completely understood.[7]

Recent technological advances have led to the development of a variety of $ECCO_2R$ devices. These have been used in an attempt to help a range of patients with respiratory failure, including the support of ultra-low tidal volumes in ARDS,[8-11] expedited ventilator weaning in patients with chronic obstructive pulmonary disease (COPD),[12,13] and as an alternative to invasive mechanical ventilation (IMV) in patients with exacerbations of chronic pulmonary diseases,[14,15] providing a bridge to recovery (BTR) or a bridge to transplantation (BTT).[16] This chapter focuses on the principles of $ECCO_2R$ compared to ECMO and highlights the current clinical evidence and procedures for its use in patients with respiratory failure.

## $ECCO_2R$ Compared to ECMO

The primary aim of $ECCO_2R$ is the direct removal of $CO_2$ from blood; whereas, that of ECMO is both oxygen delivery and $CO_2$ removal. Since both therapies involve gas exchange, the basic components are similar, principally a blood pump and membrane lung. The latter is typically constructed using gas permeable, liquid impermeable, hollow fibers, but important differences between $CO_2$ and oxygen transport in blood affords greater flexibility in the design of $ECCO_2R$ circuit components. Oxygen is poorly soluble and transported bound to hemoglobin; whereas, $CO_2$ is transported mostly in the form of soluble bicarbonate. Constraints imposed by hemoglobin saturation kinetics result in ECMO requiring much higher blood flow rates than $ECCO_2R$.

The implication of hemoglobin saturation kinetics is that blood cannot carry significantly more oxygen when hemoglobin oxygen saturation reaches 100%. Further increases in partial pressure of oxygen ($PaO_2$) are possible, but they contribute little to total oxygen content because solubility is so poor.[17] As a result, each liter of venous blood can only carry an extra 40-60 mL/L of oxygen, assuming normal hemoglobin (15 g/dL) and mixed venous saturation.[4,18] This principle determines the normal range for cardiac output. An average resting 75 kg adult consumes approximately 250 mL of oxygen per minute (3.3–3.5 ml/kg/min[19-21]) and, given the oxygen-carrying capacity of venous blood, they need a blood flow of 4 to 6 L/min to meet this demand.[22] To achieve the therapeutic goal of oxygen delivery, ECMO requires similar blood flow rates.

Compared to oxygen, each liter of blood carries substantially more $CO_2$, albeit mostly in the form of bicarbonate. Metabolically produced $CO_2$ diffuses into red blood cells, where it reacts with water yielding bicarbonate ($HCO_3^-$) and hydrogen ions ($H^+$), a slow reaction accelerated by carbonic anhydrase. The formation of bicarbonate and hydrogen ions is favored because deoxygenated hemoglobin has a high affinity for binding hydrogen ions. This has the effect of lowering the relative concentration of hydrogen ions and, by Le Chatelier's principle, shifts the reaction equilibrium towards the production of more hydrogen ions and bicarbonate.

The process is reversed when blood passes through the lungs. Oxygenated hemoglobin loses its affinity for hydrogen ions, raising the concentration of free hydrogen ions and causing bicarbonate to be converted back into $CO_2$, facilitating pulmonary elimination. These interactions are known as the Haldane effect,[23] which is simply the more familiar Bohr effect viewed from the aspect of $CO_2$ transport physiology.[24] The ability of increased hydrogen ion concentration to release $CO_2$ from bicarbonate has been exploited experimentally to improve $ECCO_2R$ efficiency. Electrodialysis and acidic compounds have been used to elevate the hydrogen ion concentration in blood passing through the membrane lung, increasing the amount of $CO_2$ removed.[25-27]

Under normal circumstances, about 80% of $CO_2$ is transported bound as bicarbonate,[28] and venous blood with a pH of 7.37 and $PaCO_2$ of 46 mmHg contains approximately 26 mmol/L of bicarbonate,[28] the equivalent of nearly 600 ml of $CO_2$.[29] Since an average 75 kg adult at rest produces about 250 ml of $CO_2$ every minute, each half litre of blood contains more $CO_2$ than that produced metabolically each minute. This means $ECCO_2R$ can be achieved at much lower blood flow rates than ECMO. Current devices aim to provide $ECCO_2R$ with rates between 250 mL and 1500 mL/min, depending on the technical circumstances.

## Current ECCO$_2$R Strategies

In general, $ECCO_2R$ systems may be grouped into pumpless and pump-driven systems. Pumpless systems rely on the arteriovenous (AV) pressure gradient to generate circuit flow. AV $ECCO_2R$ systems usually operate passively at blood flow rates of 1-1.5 L/min, depending on cannula size, and may remove 50-60% of total $CO_2$.[30] Effective operation of these devices requires a preserved cardiac output and the absence of shock, frequently precluding their use in critically ill patients.

Pump-driven systems are more commonly used. Some devices are derived from renal replacement therapy units and driven by roller pumps, whereas others are derived from high-flow ECMO circuits and therefore driven by rotational, mostly centrifugal, blood pumps. The efficacy of $ECCO_2R$ systems depends mainly on the blood flow rate and secondarily on the sweep gas flow and membrane lung surface area.[31-34] Very low blood flow rates of 250 mL/min, such as those currently used in continuous renal replacement therapy, have only a minor impact on $CO_2$ removal, removing about 40-60 mL of $CO_2$ per minute.[35] Blood flow rates around 500 mL/min remove between

60 and 80 ml of $CO_2$ per minute, which can be nearly doubled by increasing the flow rate to 1000 mL/min, achieving $CO_2$ removal rates around 150 mL/min. Sweep gas flow has a weaker impact on $CO_2$ removal.[33] In daily clinical practice, sweep gas flow should be carefully titrated to avoid large arterial $CO_2$ differences within a short time.

It is important that the surface area of membrane lungs used in $ECCO_2R$ systems is matched to the flow range, to avoid clotting risk from long blood passing times in membrane lungs with large surface areas. Very low surface areas of 0.4 $m^2$ should be used for blood flow rates of 500 mL/min or less, whereas surface areas of 0.8 $m^2$ or more are suitable for blood flow rates above 500 mL/min.[31]

Many pump-driven $ECCO_2R$ systems rely on rotational pumps designed for the high blood flow rates used in ECMO, but this creates technical challenges. Reducing the blood flow rate with rotary pumps designed for higher flow rates changes the flow characteristics considerably, dramatically increasing recirculation and shear stress, which amplifies hemolysis and bleeding complications.[36,37] Of note, hemolysis is one of the major complications shown to worsen clinical outcomes and is independently associated with mortality.[38,39] Recent studies have demonstrated significant bleeding complications in patients with acute exacerbation of COPD supported with $ECCO_2R$.[38,40,41] Similar observations were reported in neonatal and pediatric patients.[42]

Although cannula size and design have less often been a focus of interest, recent simulations show that current cannulas have regions of static flow conditions at lower blood flow rates, potentially leading to more clotting.[43] Overall, the use of lower blood rates may allow for smaller cannulas and more options in the choice of pump compared to ECMO, but simply providing $ECCO_2R$ with components designed for higher ECMO flows is likely to increase complications.

## Clinical Considerations for $ECCO_2R$

In general, $ECCO_2R$ has been used to support two broad groups of patients, those with respiratory failure from ARDS and those with exacerbations of chronic lung diseases, such as asthma, COPD, and pulmonary fibrosis. In all these patients, the goal of $ECCO_2R$ is to reduce the intensity, facilitate the removal of, or provide an alternative to IMV.

### *Acute Respiratory Distress Syndrome (ARDS)*

$ECCO_2R$ is a potential strategy to facilitate very low tidal volume ventilation in moderate forms of ARDS, so-called ultra-lung-protective ventilation.[44] Lung protective ventilation, defined as targeting tidal volumes of 6 ml/kg predicted body weight (PBW) or less, and plateau airway pressures less than or equal to 30 $cmH_2O$, has been demonstrated to improve survival in ARDS and is the current standard of care.[6] However, animal and human studies suggest there may be additional protection when targeting even lower tidal volumes and airway pressures by further reducing VILI,[8,9,45,46] especially in patients with higher respiratory system elastance,[47,48] but the ability to implement these ultra-lung-protective ventilation strategies is limited by hypercapnia and acidosis.[49] $ECCO_2R$ provides a means to mitigate the development of hypercapnia and acidosis, thereby facilitating the application of ultra-lung-protective ventilation.[50]

Despite the pathophysiological rationale and encouraging preliminary data,[2,8,9,51-54] the largest randomized controlled trial to date, the pRotective vEntilation With Veno-venouS Lung assisT in Respiratory Failure (REST) study, did not demonstrate decreased mortality in patients receiving lower tidal volumes supported by $ECCO_2R$, and actually showed fewer ventilator-free days, compared to those receiving conventional low tidal volume ventilation (6 ml/kg PBW).[11] This may be partly because the reduction in tidal volume in $ECCO_2R$-supported patients was smaller than planned (4-4.5 ml/kg compared to the target of ≤3 ml/kg) and was achieved at the price of higher respiratory rates, greater hypercapnia and respiratory acidosis, as well as longer use of neuromuscular blocking agents and mandatory modes of ventilation, perhaps reflecting the low efficiency of the $ECCO_2R$ device used. In particular, overlooking the respiratory rate ignores the fact that it is an important determinant of mechanical power, and thus increases the risk of VILI.[55] Experimental studies have shown that reducing the respiratory rate improves lung protection in ARDS.[56,57] The negative results may also have been affected by the fact that patients were enrolled based on the level of hypoxemia alone ($PaO_2$ to $FiO_2$ ratio ≤150 mmHg), without necessarily meeting criteria for ARDS.[11] While using oxygenation criteria alone is pragmatic for a large randomized controlled trial, prognostically enriches the population, and helps with generalizability if the trial were positive, it also means it cannot be certain all patients enrolled would necessarily benefit from the lower tidal volumes supported by $ECCO_2R$.

The REST trial highlights the invasive nature of $ECCO_2R$ therapy and, in relatively unselected patients with acute hypoxemic respiratory failure, that the risks related to anticoagulation and cannula placement may exceed any potential benefits. The use of $ECCO_2R$ in ARDS still requires further investigation: assessing the risks of VILI and hypercapnia, determining the most effective targets for ultra-lung protective ventilation, and identifying the patients most likely to derive benefit.[58]

### Exacerbations of Chronic Lung Disease

$ECCO_2R$ may be considered in intubated patients with acute-on-chronic lung disease when hypercapnia and respiratory acidosis persist despite the use of IMV, or it may be applied as an alternative to IMV with the aim of avoiding endotracheal intubation and ventilator-associated complications.

During acute exacerbations of COPD, patients receiving IMV can experience worsening dynamic hyperinflation; ventilation/perfusion mismatch; and increased $CO_2$ production, all of which contribute to the development of severe respiratory acidosis. $ECCO_2R$ can disrupt this vicious cycle by reducing the amount of $CO_2$ that needs to be cleared through the native lungs, facilitating a reduction in tidal volume and set respiratory rate, in turn allowing for a more prolonged expiratory time. Several case series have demonstrated the ability of $ECCO_2R$ to correct severe acute respiratory acidosis[12,13,41,59,60] and facilitate extubation.[12,60] In some circumstances, early implementation of $ECCO_2R$ in nonintubated patients has been found to decrease the work of breathing and correct respiratory acidosis, preventing the failure of noninvasive respiratory support and thus avoiding the inherent risks of IMV altogether.[13,38,41,61,62]

Despite a good physiological rationale, the potential benefits of minimizing IMV in COPD patients are not straightforward. Matched studies with historical controls have reported conflicting results both in terms of decreased need for intubation and mortality rates.[41,62] Furthermore, the incidence of $ECCO_2R$-related complications varies in these patients and has been reported to be as high as 44%.[38] Successful application of $ECCO_2R$ in COPD patients will depend on identifying optimal timing of initiation, patient selection, and technical considerations (eg, cannula size selection, minimization of device-related complications).

A less frequent indication for $ECCO_2R$ therapy is severe, refractory status asthmaticus,[63] to specifically prevent the deleterious consequences of IMV on lung hyperinflation and hemodynamic stability. Currently, the data for such use is limited to observational studies.[64-67] Similarly, exacerbations or progression of chronic lung diseases in patients awaiting lung transplantation may benefit from initiation of $ECCO_2R$ when the goal is avoidance of intubation and IMV, which may otherwise compromise transplant candidacy. Small retrospective studies have reported successful use of $ECCO_2R$ as a bridge to transplant in experienced centers.[68,69]

**Initiating and Managing $ECCO_2R$**

$ECCO_2R$ is a tool that can help clinicians modify ventilation support to mitigate the harmful effects of IMV, ultimately reducing VILI. Successful $ECCO_2R$ therapy, therefore, demands careful attention to ventilator management (or avoidance of IMV altogether), as well as management of the $ECCO_2R$ circuit itself.

*Physiological Targets and Ventilator Management*

In patients with ARDS, the greatest contributor to morbidity and mortality is believed to be from VILI,[70] and therefore greater emphasis should be placed on reducing the factors contributing to VILI (eg, excess lung stress, strain, and shear forces) by applying ultra-lung-protective ventilation.[71] Most $ECCO_2R$ trials have targeted tidal volumes of 3 to 4 ml/kg PBW with a corresponding decrease in plateau airway pressures, while maintaining or reducing respiratory rates below pre-$ECCO_2R$ settings.[8,9,11,50,71] In the absence of prospective randomized data that definitively defines optimal ventilator settings during $ECCO_2R$, it may be reasonable to apply the ventilator parameters used in the ECMO arm of the EOLIA trial, in other words, plateau airway pressure $\leq 24$ $cmH_2O$ and PEEP $\geq 10$ $cmH_2O$, corresponding to a driving pressure $\leq 14$ $cmH_2O$ and tidal volumes well below 6 ml/kg PBW.[72] Using $ECCO_2R$ to achieve similar settings in ARDS patients has been shown to reduce

inflammatory markers associated with VILI.[8] Respiratory rates ranged between 10 and 30 breaths per minute in the EOLIA trial but, given the potential contribution of respiratory rate to VILI,[55,73] it may be reasonable to target the lowest rate feasible.[71] Of note, the application of these ventilator settings, in combination with $ECCO_2R$, may worsen underlying hypoxemia through a variety of proposed mechanisms, potentially necessitating the use of a higher $FiO_2$.[71,74]

In obstructive airway diseases, there may be a greater emphasis on and rationale for removal of IMV, owing to the contribution of positive pressure ventilation to dynamic hyperinflation and increases in intrinsic PEEP (ie, autoPEEP), along with the fact that dyspnea and increased respiratory drive may persist despite the ability to achieve adequate pH and arterial partial pressure of carbon dioxide ($PaCO_2$) with IMV alone. Endotracheal extubation may have additional advantages in this patient population, including avoidance of ventilator-associated pneumonia and VILI, more effective delivery of inhaled medications and enteral nutrition, and a greater likelihood of success with early mobilization.[12,75,76] The same rationale may be applied to patients with endstage lung disease receiving $ECCO_2R$ as a bridge to transplantation, given the importance of avoiding ventilator complications and maximizing pretransplant physical conditioning.[16]

The ability to either minimize ventilator settings or remove IMV altogether will depend on the ability of $ECCO_2R$ to maintain pH and $PaCO_2$ within acceptable ranges, which will vary by a given device's efficiency at carbon dioxide removal. Notably, in the SUPERNOVA pilot trial, devices with relatively higher extracorporeal blood flow rates (eg, 0.8-1.0 L/min) were more successful at facilitating ultra-lung protective ventilation targets than a device set to lower blood flow rates (eg, 0.3-0.5 L/min).[10,50]

In most circumstances, and without a significant concomitant metabolic acidosis, the sweep gas flow rate should be adjusted to achieve a near-normal pH. In the subset of patients receiving $ECCO_2R$ who have chronic hypercapnia with a compensatory metabolic alkalosis and who may be candidates for lung transplantation, the sweep gas flow rate should be adjusted to achieve a slightly alkalemic pH (eg, 7.41-7.45) to allow for a gradual reversal of the alkalosis in anticipation of improved ventilatory capacity and native gas exchange after transplantation. It is important to note, however, that intracranial hemorrhage (ICH) during ECLS has been associated with a rapid decrease in $PaCO_2$ post-ECLS initiation,[77] highlighting the importance of achieving a gradual correction of $PaCO_2$ over several hours rather than an abrupt decrease at the time of cannulation.

### Anticoagulation Strategy

Thrombotic risk within the circuit generally increases as extracorporeal blood flow rates decrease. This may be particularly true with current $ECCO_2R$ technology, which tends to couple low blood flow rates with a relatively high extracorporeal membrane surface area. The use of low levels of systemic anticoagulation (as has increasingly been adopted for ECMO management[75,78]) increases the thrombotic risk even further. The existing literature reports varying rates of circuit thrombosis at blood flow rates less than 1 L/min when activated partial thromboplastin times of ~1.5 to 2 times baseline are targeted.[11,13,41] If, in fact, $ECCO_2R$ is associated with higher rates of thrombosis than ECMO, it might necessitate higher anticoagulation targets to mitigate that sequela and the concomitant bleeding risk would then have to be taken into consideration when assessing the risk-benefit profile of $ECCO_2R$. Ultimately, more data is needed to determine the optimal level of anticoagulation for $ECCO_2R$, which will depend, in part, on the blood flow used.

Additionally, it is important to consider that currently available circuit pumps are generally designed for optimal performance at >4 L/min of blood flow, with lower blood flows (eg, <2 L/min) associated with higher rates of hemolysis and recirculation within the pump, greater loss of high molecular weight von Willebrand factor multimers, decreased platelet aggregation, increased platelet destruction, and prolonged clotting times in various ex vivo, in vitro, and computational models.[36,37,79]

### Management Considerations in the Event of Circuit Failure

In the event of circuit failure, the management of patients should rely on conventional management of hypercapnia while the circuit malfunction is corrected. In endotracheally intubated patients, minute ventilation should be increased as needed. In nonendotracheally intubated patients, noninvasive positive-pressure ventilation should be considered. If noninvasive ventilatory support is insufficient, endotracheal intubation and IMV should be initiated.

### Weaning ECCO₂R

In patients receiving $ECCO_2R$ as BTR, assessments of readiness to wean should be undertaken as the acute process is resolving. In patients receiving IMV, the sweep gas flow rate may be reduced in order to maintain normal pH, while ventilator settings are liberalized within the limits of lung-protective ventilation as native lung function improves (eg, 6 ml/kg PBW, plateau airway pressure ≤30 cm $H_2O$). In patients who are breathing without the assistance of the ventilator, the sweep gas flow rate may be incrementally lowered with corresponding assessments of both the patient's respiratory status and pH by arterial blood gas to ensure adequate spontaneous ventilation without excess work of breathing. In patients with acute exacerbations of COPD or status asthmaticus, there should be close monitoring for dynamic hyperinflation or increased work of breathing as $ECCO_2R$ is weaned.

## Conclusions

$ECCO_2R$ has the potential to support a range of patients with respiratory failure. While current clinical indications include status asthmaticus and BTT, questions remain over appropriate patient selection, optimal timing of therapy, and the right balance between the level of invasiveness of the $ECCO_2R$ strategy and efficiency of $CO_2$ removal, particularly for ARDS and acute exacerbations of COPD. Until there are clearer answers to these questions, $ECCO_2R$ should be used cautiously and, where possible, only in studies designed to answer such questions.

# References

1. Kolobow T, Gattinoni L, Tomlinson TA, et al. Control of Breathing Using an Extracorporeal Membrane Lung. Anesthesiology. 1977;46(2):138–41.
2. Gattinoni L, Agostoni A, Pesenti A, et al. Treatment of acute respiratory failure with low-frequency positive-pressure ventilation and extracorporeal removal of CO2. The Lancet. 1980 Aug 9;2(8189):292–4.
3. Morris AH, Wallace CJ, Menlove RL, et al. Randomized clinical trial of pressure-controlled inverse ratio ventilation and extracorporeal CO2 removal for adult respiratory distress syndrome. American Journal of Respiratory and Critical Care Medicine. 1994;149(2):295–305.
4. Cove ME, MacLaren G, Federspiel WJ, et al. Bench to bedside review: Extracorporeal carbon dioxide removal, past present and future. Critical care (London, England). 2012;16(5):232.
5. Pesenti A, Patroniti N, Fumagalli R. Carbon dioxide dialysis will save the lung. Critical Care Medicine. 2010 Oct;38(10 Suppl):S549-54.
6. Network TARDS. Ventilation with lower tidal volumes as compared with traditional tidal volumes for acute lung injury and the acute respiratory distress syndrome. The Acute Respiratory Distress Syndrome Network. New England Journal of Medicine. 2000 May 4;342(18):1301–8.
7. Tremblay LN, Slutsky AS. Ventilator-induced lung injury: from the bench to the bedside. Intensive Care Medicine. 2006 Jan;32(1):24–33.
8. Terragni PP, Sorbo LD, Mascia L, et al. Tidal volume lower than 6 ml/kg enhances lung protection: role of extracorporeal carbon dioxide removal. Anesthesiology. 2009 Oct;111(4):826–35.
9. Bein T, Weber-Carstens S, Goldmann A, et al. Lower tidal volume strategy (≈3 ml/kg) combined with extracorporeal CO2 removal versus "conventional" protective ventilation (6 ml/kg) in severe ARDS: the prospective randomized Xtravent-study. Intensive Care Medicine. 2013 May;39(5):847–56.
10. Combes A, Tonetti T, Fanelli V, et al. Efficacy and safety of lower versus higher CO2 extraction devices to allow ultraprotective ventilation: secondary analysis of the SUPERNOVA study. Thorax. 2019;74(12):1179.
11. McNamee JJ, Gillies MA, Barrett NA, et al. Effect of Lower Tidal Volume Ventilation Facilitated by Extracorporeal Carbon Dioxide Removal vs Standard Care Ventilation on 90-Day Mortality in Patients With Acute Hypoxemic Respiratory Failure. JAMA 2021;326(11):1013–23.
12. Abrams DC, Brenner K, Burkart KM, et al. Pilot study of extracorporeal carbon dioxide removal to facilitate extubation and ambulation in exacerbations of chronic obstructive pulmonary disease. Annals of the American Thoracic Society. 2013 Aug;10(4):307–14.
13. Burki NK, Mani RK, Herth FJF, et al. A novel extracorporeal CO(2) removal system: results of a pilot study of hypercapnic respiratory failure in patients with COPD. Chest. 2013 Mar;143(3):678–86.
14. Tiruvoipati R, Buscher H, Winearls J, et al. Early experience of a new extracorporeal carbon dioxide removal device for acute hypercapnic respiratory failure. Critical care and resuscitation : journal of the Australasian Academy of Critical Care Medicine. 2016 Dec;18(4):261–9.
15. Vianello A, Arcaro G, Paladini L, et al. Successful management of acute respiratory failure in an Idiopathic Pulmonary Fibrosis patient using an extracorporeal carbon dioxide removal system. Sarcoidosis Vasc Diffuse Lung Dis Official J Wasog World Assoc Sarcoidosis Other Granulomatous Disord. 2016;33(2):186–90.
16. Abrams D, Brodie D, Arcasoy SM. Extracorporeal Life Support in Lung Transplantation. Clin Chest Med. 2017;38(4):655–66.
17. Pittman RN. Regulation of Tissue Oxygenation. San Rafael (CA): Morgan & Claypool Life Sciences; 2011. Chapter 4, Oxygen Transport.
18. Dunn J-O, Mythen M, Grocott M. Physiology of oxygen transport. Bja Educ. 2016;16(10):341–8.
19. Ainsworth RE, Haskell WL, Leona HS, et al. Compendium of Physical Activities: classification of energy costs of human physical activities. Medicine Sci Sports Exerc. 1993;25(1):71.
20. Ainsworth BE, Haskell WL, Whitt MC, et al. Compendium of Physical Activities: an update of activity codes and MET intensities. Medicine Sci Sports Exerc. 2000;32(9):S498–516.
21. Part a: Executive Summary. Nutr Rev [Internet]. 2009;67(2):114–20. Available from: https://doi.org/10.1111/j.1753-4887.2008.00136.x.
22. Wolff CB. Normal cardiac output, oxygen delivery and oxygen extraction. Adv Exp Med Biol. 2008;599:169–82.
23. Christiansen J, Douglas CG, Haldane JS. The absorption and dissociation of carbon dioxide by human blood. J Physiology. 1914;48(4):244–71.
24. Siggaard-Andersen O, Garby L. The Bohr Effect and the Haldane Effect. Scand J Clin Laboratory Investigation. 2009;31(1):1–8.
25. Zanella A, Castagna L, Salerno D, et al. Respiratory Electrodialysis. A Novel, Highly Efficient Extracorporeal CO2 Removal Technique. American Journal of Respiratory and Critical Care Medicine. 2015 Sep 15;192(6):719–26.
26. Scaravilli V, Kreyer S, Linden K, et al. Enhanced Extracorporeal CO2 Removal by Regional Blood Acidification: Effect of Infusion of Three

Metabolizable Acids. ASAIO journal (American Society for Artificial Internal Organs : 1992). 2015 Sep;61(5):533–9.

27. Arazawa DT, Kimmel JD, Finn MC, et al. Acidic sweep gas with carbonic anhydrase coated hollow fiber membranes synergistically accelerates CO2 removal from blood. Acta biomaterialia. 2015 Oct;25:143–9.

28. Geers C, Gros G. Carbon dioxide transport and carbonic anhydrase in blood and muscle. Physiological reviews. 2000 Apr;80(2):681–715.

29. Cove ME, Vu LH, Ring T, Federspiel WJ, et al. Respiratory Dialysis—A Novel Low Bicarbonate Dialysate to Provide Extracorporeal CO2 Removal. Crit Care Med 2020;48(7):e592-e598.

30. Muller T, Lubnow M, Philipp A, et al. Extracorporeal pumpless interventional lung assist in clinical practice: determinants of efficacy. Eur Respir J. 2008;33(3):551–8.

31. Karagiannidis C, Strassmann S, Brodie D, et al. Impact of membrane lung surface area and blood flow on extracorporeal CO2 removal during severe respiratory acidosis. Intensive Care Medicine Experimental. 2017 Dec;5(1):34.

32. Karagiannidis C, Kampe KA, Sipmann FS, et al. Veno-venous extracorporeal CO2 removal for the treatment of severe respiratory acidosis: pathophysiological and technical considerations. Crit Care. 2014;18(3):R124.

33. Strassmann S, Merten M, Schäfer S, et al. Impact of sweep gas flow on extracorporeal CO2 removal (ECCO2R). Intensive Care Medicine Exp. 2019;7(1):17.

34. Karagiannidis C, Hesselmann F, Fan E. Physiological and Technical Considerations of Extracorporeal CO2 Removal. Crit Care. 2019;23(1):75.

35. Godet T, Combes A, Zogheib E, et al. Novel carbon dioxide removal device driven by a renal-replacement system without hemofilter: an experimental approach and validation. Critical Care. 2014;18(Suppl 1):P316.

36. Schöps M, Groß-Hardt SH, et al. Hemolysis at low blood flow rates: in-vitro and in-silico evaluation of a centrifugal blood pump. J Transl Med. 2021;19(1):2.

37. Gross-Hardt S, Hesselmann F, Arens J, et al. Low-flow assessment of current ECMO/ECCO2R rotary blood pumps and the potential effect on hemocompatibility. Crit Care. 2019;23(1):348.

38. Braune S, Sieweke A, Brettner F, et al. The feasibility and safety of extracorporeal carbon dioxide removal to avoid intubation in patients with COPD unresponsive to noninvasive ventilation for acute hypercapnic respiratory failure (ECLAIR study): multicentre case-control study. Intensive Care Medicine. 2016 Sep;42(9):1437–44.

39. Sklar MC, Beloncle F, Katsios CM, et al. Extracorporeal carbon dioxide removal in patients with chronic obstructive pulmonary disease: a systematic review. Intens Care Med. 2015;41(10):1752–62.

40. Karagiannidis C, Strassmann S, Schwarz S, et al. Control of respiratory drive by extracorporeal CO2 removal in acute exacerbation of COPD breathing on non-invasive NAVA. Critical Care Lond Engl. 2019;23(1):135.

41. Sorbo LD, Pisani L, Filippini C, et al. Extracorporeal Co2 removal in hypercapnic patients at risk of noninvasive ventilation failure: a matched cohort study with historical control. Critical Care Medicine. 2015 Jan;43(1):120–7.

42. Okochi S, Cheung EW, Barton S, et al. An Analysis of Risk Factors for Hemolysis in Children on Extracorporeal Membrane Oxygenation. Pediatric Critical Care Medicine J Soc Critical Care Medicine World Fed Pediatric Intensive Critical Care Soc. 2018;19(11):1059–66.

43. Vatani A, Liao S, Burrell AJC, et al. Improved Drainage Cannula Design to Reduce Thrombosis in Veno-Arterial Extracorporeal Membrane Oxygenation. Asaio J Am Soc Artif Intern Organs 1992. 2022;68(2):205–13.

44. Abrams D, Agerstrand C, Beitler JR, et al. Risks and Benefits of Ultra-Lung-Protective Invasive Mechanical Ventilation Strategies with a Focus on Extracorporeal Support. Am J Resp Crit Care. 2022.

45. Frank JA, Gutierrez JA, Jones KD, et al. Low tidal volume reduces epithelial and endothelial injury in acid-injured rat lungs. American Journal of Respiratory and Critical Care Medicine. 2002 Jan 15;165(2):242–9.

46. Hager DN, Krishnan JA, Hayden DL, Brower RG, Network ACT. Tidal volume reduction in patients with acute lung injury when plateau pressures are not high. American Journal of Respiratory and Critical Care Medicine. 2005 Nov 15;172(10):1241–5.

47. Goligher EC, Costa ELV, Yarnell CJ, et al. Effect of Lowering V t on Mortality in Acute Respiratory Distress Syndrome Varies with Respiratory System Elastance. Am J Resp Crit Care. 2021;203(11):1378–85.

48. Goligher EC, Combes A, Brodie D, et al. Determinants of the effect of extracorporeal carbon dioxide removal in the SUPERNOVA trial: implications for trial design. Intens Care Med. 2019;45(9):1219–30.

49. Richard JC, Marque S, Gros A, et al. Feasibility and safety of ultra-low tidal volume ventilation without extracorporeal circulation in moderately severe and severe ARDS patients. Intens Care Med. 2019;45(11):1590–8.

50. Combes A, Fanelli V, Pham T, Ranieri VM, investigators ES of ICMTG and the "Strategy of

U-P lung ventilation with ECR for N-O moderate to severe A (SUPERNOVA). Feasibility and safety of extracorporeal CO2 removal to enhance protective ventilation in acute respiratory distress syndrome: the SUPERNOVA study. Intensive Care Medicine. 2019 May;45(5):592–600.

51. Gattinoni L, Kolobow T, Agostoni A, et al. Clinical application of low frequency positive pressure ventilation with extracorporeal CO2 removal (LFPPV-ECCO2R) in treatment of adult respiratory distress syndrome (ARDS). Int J Artif Organs. 1979;2(6):282–3.

52. Gattinoni L, Kolobow T, Damia G, et al. Extracorporeal carbon dioxide removal (ECCO2R): a new form of respiratory assistance. Int J Artif Organs. 1979;2(4):183–5.

53. Gattinoni L, Pesenti A, Caspani ML, et al. The role of total static lung compliance in the management of severe ARDS unresponsive to conventional treatment. Intens Care Med. 1984;10(3):121–6.

54. Gattinoni L, Pesenti A, Mascheroni D, et al. Low-frequency positive-pressure ventilation with extracorporeal CO2 removal in severe acute respiratory failure. . 1986 Aug 15;256(7):881–6.

55. Gattinoni L, Tonetti T, Cressoni M, et al. Ventilator-related causes of lung injury: the mechanical power. Intens Care Med. 2016;42(10):1567–75.

56. Grasso S, Stripoli T, Mazzone P, et al. Low Respiratory Rate Plus Minimally Invasive Extracorporeal Co2 Removal Decreases Systemic and Pulmonary Inflammatory Mediators in Experimental Acute Respiratory Distress Syndrome&ast; Crit Care Med. 2014;42(6):e451–60.

57. Araos J, Alegria L, Garcia P, et al. Near-Apneic Ventilation Decreases Lung Injury and Fibroproliferation in an Acute Respiratory Distress Syndrome Model with Extracorporeal Membrane Oxygenation. Am J Resp Crit Care. 2018;199(5):603–12.

58. Goligher EC, Amato MBP, Slutsky AS. Applying Precision Medicine to Trial Design Using Physiology. Extracorporeal CO2Removal for Acute Respiratory Distress Syndrome. American Journal of Respiratory and Critical Care Medicine. 2017 Sep 1;196(5):558–68.

59. Abrams D, Roncon-Albuquerque R, Brodie D. What's new in extracorporeal carbon dioxide removal for COPD? Intens Care Med. 2015;41(5):906–8.

60. Roncon-Albuquerque R, Carona G, Neves A, et al. Venovenous extracorporeal CO2 removal for early extubation in COPD exacerbations requiring invasive mechanical ventilation. Intens Care Med. 2014;40(12):1969–70.

61. Kluge S, Braune SA, Engel M, et al. Avoiding invasive mechanical ventilation by extracorporeal carbon dioxide removal in patients failing noninvasive ventilation. Intens Care Med. 2012;38(10):1632–9.

62. Braune S, Burchardi H, Engel M, et al. The use of extracorporeal carbon dioxide removal to avoid intubation in patients failing non-invasive ventilation – a cost analysis. Bmc Anesthesiol. 2015;15(1):160.

63. Yeo HJ, Kim D, Jeon D, et al. Extracorporeal membrane oxygenation for life-threatening asthma refractory to mechanical ventilation: analysis of the Extracorporeal Life Support Organization registry. Crit Care. 2017;21(1):297.

64. Mikkelsen ME, Woo YJ, Sager JS, et al. Outcomes Using Extracorporeal Life Support for Adult Respiratory Failure due to Status Asthmaticus. Asaio J. 2009;55(1):47–52.

65. Brenner K, Abrams DC, Agerstrand CL, et al. Extracorporeal carbon dioxide removal for refractory status asthmaticus: experience in distinct exacerbation phenotypes. Perfusion. 2013 Dec 20;29(1):26–8.

66. Lascio GD, Prifti E, Messai E, et al. Extracorporeal membrane oxygenation support for life-threatening acute severe status asthmaticus. Perfusion. 2017;32(2):157–63.

67. Bromberger BJ, Agerstrand C, Abrams D, et al. Extracorporeal Carbon Dioxide Removal in the Treatment of Status Asthmaticus. Crit Care Med. 2020;Publish Ahead of Print.

68. Schellongowski P, Riss K, Staudinger T, et al. Extracorporeal CO2 removal as bridge to lung transplantation in life-threatening hypercapnia. Transplant Int. 2015;28(3):297–304.

69. Collaud S, Benden C, Ganter C, et al. Extracorporeal Life Support as Bridge to Lung Retransplantation: A Multicenter Pooled Data Analysis. Ann Thorac Surg. 2016;102(5):1680–6.

70. Slutsky AS, Ranieri VM. Ventilator-Induced Lung Injury. New England Journal of Medicine. 2013 Nov 28;369(22):2126–36.

71. Abrams D, Schmidt M, Pham T, et al. Mechanical Ventilation for Acute Respiratory Distress Syndrome during Extracorporeal Life Support. Research and Practice. Am J Resp Crit Care. 2019;201(5):514–25.

72. Combes A, Hajage D, Capellier G, et al. Extracorporeal Membrane Oxygenation for Severe Acute Respiratory Distress Syndrome. New England Journal of Medicine. 2018 May 24;378(21):1965–75.

73. Costa ELV, Slutsky AS, Brochard LJ, et al. Ventilatory Variables and Mechanical Power in Patients with Acute Respiratory Distress Syndrome. Am J Resp Crit Care. 2021;204(3):303–11.

74. Gattinoni L. Ultra-protective ventilation and hypoxemia. Crit Care. 2016;20(1):130.

75. Brodie D, Slutsky AS, Combes A. Extracorporeal Life Support for Adults with Respiratory Failure and Related Indications: A Review. . 2019;322(6):557–68.

76. Abrams D, Madahar P, Eckhardt CM, et al. Early Mobilization during ECMO for Cardiopulmonary Failure in Adults: Factors Associated with Intensity of Treatment. Ann Am Thorac Soc. 2022 Jan;19(1):90-98.
77. Luyt C-E, Bréchot N, Demondion P, et al. Brain injury during venovenous extracorporeal membrane oxygenation. Intens Care Med. 2016;42(5):897–907.
78. Agerstrand CL, Burkart KM, Abrams DC, et al. Blood Conservation in Extracorporeal Membrane Oxygenation for Acute Respiratory Distress Syndrome. Ann Thorac Surg. 2015;99(2):590–5.
79. Ki KK, Passmore MR, Chan CHH, et al. Low flow rate alters haemostatic parameters in an ex-vivo extracorporeal membrane oxygenation circuit. Intensive Care Medicine Exp. 2019;7(1):51.

# 44

## Other Mechanical Circulatory Support

*Federico Pappalardo, Roberto Lorusso, Ravi R. Thiagarajan, Timothy Maul, Alain Combes*

### Introduction

In this chapter, we will discuss the use of Mechanical Circulatory Support (MCS) other than ECMO in both adults and children. This will include the use of the Impella, Intra-Aortic Balloon Pump, Implantable and Paracorporeal Ventricular Assist Devices (VAD), and the Total Artificial Heart (TAH). We will also consider using these devices in conjunction with ECMO and also with an oxygenator in the VAD circuit.

### Impella

The Impella pump (Abiomed Inc., Danvers, MA) is a catheter mounted, constant speed, axial flow pump. The Impella is a family of products, which can generally be split into two categories: pumps intended for the heart's left side (Impella 2.5, CP, 5.0, LD, and 5.5), and for the right side (Impella RP) (Figure 44-1). Impella effectively volume unloads the LV and increases forward flow, reducing myocardial oxygen consumption, and reducing pulmonary capillary wedge pressure. The right side Impella RP pump has its inlet located in the inferior vena cava at the level of the diaphragm, and crosses two valves to propel blood into the outlet within the pulmonary trunk, bypassing the right ventricle. The intravascular Impella pumps are driven by a miniature motor, which is located at the tip of a catheter shaft and is actively purged with a glucose solution. The nitinol-reinforced

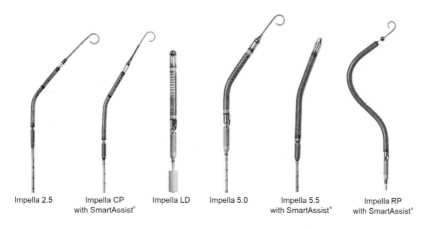

Impella 2.5   Impella CP   Impella LD   Impella 5.0   Impella 5.5   Impella RP
              with SmartAssist®                       with SmartAssist®   with SmartAssist®

**Figure 44-1.** Impella Family.

thin wall cannula spans across the valve(s), connecting the pump inlet and outlet.

The main differences between the left side Impella types are the maximum blood flow rate they can deliver and their overall size; the larger pumps can deliver more flow, with the tradeoff of insertion site bore size. Therefore, pump selection should be made at baseline according to the expected flow required by the clinical conditions. Impella 2.5 and CP—with 12 Fr and 14 Fr cannula and motor sizes, and 9 Fr catheter size—can deliver ~2.5 L/min and ~3.7 L/min of mean flow, respectively, and are intended for percutaneous femoral insertion. They are both approved for up to 4 days of use in the United States and 5 days in Europe. The larger Impella pumps are capable of delivering full cardiac support and maximum LV unloading and are surgically inserted via the axillary artery or ascending aorta, which allows the patient to ambulate while on support. The Impella 5.5 has been significantly downsized as compared to its Impella 5.0/LD and can accomplish a higher blood flow rate, with peak flows around 6 L/min (Figure 44-2). Preliminary clinical experience with the Impella 5.5 appears favorable.[1]

One randomized study and some retrospective and registry studies have evaluated the outcomes of cardiogenic shock patients treated with Impella devices. The SHOCK (IMPRESS) trial included 48 STEMI patients randomized to receive Impella CP or IABP. Day 30 and 6-month mortality were similar (50% vs. 46% and 50% vs. 50%, p=0·92) for Impella and IABP patients, respectively, while more bleeding events occurred in the Impella group.[2] More recently, a retrospective study matched 237 AMI patients who received Impella support for AMI-induced cardiogenic shock with 237 patients from the IABP-SHOCK II trial. There was no significant difference in 30-day all-cause mortality (48·5% vs. 46·4%, p=0·64). Severe or life-threatening bleeding (8·5% vs. 3·0%, p<0·01) and peripheral vascular complications (9·8% vs. 3·8%, p=0·01) were more frequent in the Impella group.[3] In the Premier Healthcare Database including 4782 patients undergoing PCI at 432 hospitals, Impella use was associated with more adverse events and higher costs.[4] After propensity score adjustment, and accounting for clustering of patients by hospitals, Impella use was associated with death (odds ratio, 1·24 (95% CI, 1·13-1·36); bleeding (odds ratio, 1·10 (95% CI, 1·00-1·21) and stroke (odds ratio, 1·34 (95% CI, 1·18-1·53). Similarly, among 1680 propensity-matched pairs of

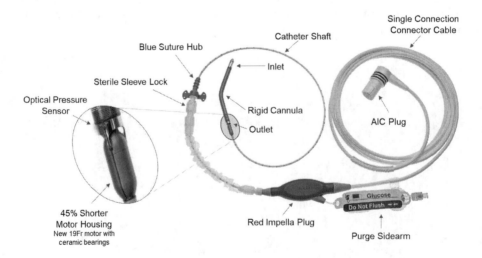

**Figure 44-2.** Impella 5.5.

AMI cardiogenic shock patients who received Impella or IABP in the CathPCI and the Chest Pain-MI registries, the use of the intravascular microaxial left-ventricular assist device was associated with higher mortality (45% vs. 34%; absolute risk difference, 11%, 95% CI, 8%-14%; p<0·001) and higher risk of in-hospital major bleeding (31% vs. 16%; absolute risk difference, 15%, 95% CI, 13%-18%; p<0·001).[5] These associations were consistent regardless of whether patients received a device before or after PCI. A large, randomized trial comparing the Impella CP with conventional treatment in 360 AMI cardiogenic shock patients is ongoing (NCT01633502).

The Impella RP, intended for percutaneous support and unloading of the right heart, has a preformed cannula shape for insertion via the femoral vein. With a 22 Fr cannula, 21 Fr motor and 11 Fr catheter, the Impella RP is able to deliver ~4 L/min of mean blood flow. It is approved for 14 days in the United States and Europe.

## Combining Impella and ECMO (ECpella)

Simultaneous use of ECMO and Impella is possible and can vary in type and motivation. Most notably, patients supported by VA ECMO may require Impella implantation to unload the LV. In the setting of severe LV dysfunction, the increased afterload of VA ECMO can lead to increases in LV cavity pressure and to pulmonary venous hypertension with subsequent pulmonary edema. There is also heightened myocardial wall stress due to increased LV end diastolic pressure, which contributes to ischemia, decreased $O_2$ delivery to heart muscle, and ventricular arrhythmias, all of which hinder cardiac recovery. Furthermore, inadequate unloading of the LV, in association with stasis, can lead to thrombus formation within the heart chambers and pulmonary circulation. This complication is a major determinant of poor outcome, limiting options for recovery, heart transplantation, or transition to long-term VAD systems. Traditional management strategies for LV decompression (commonly referred to as venting) include several surgical techniques, unique cannulation strategies such as LAVA (VA ECMO with LA drainage), or the IABP (Chapter 4). These methods may not effectively volume unload and decompress the left ventricle. Active unloading of the LV with Impella CP or Impella 5.5 while on VA ECMO, referred to as ECpella (sometimes also called ECMella or ImpECMO), is an attractive percutaneous option because it not only decompresses the ventricle but also augments forward flow. It actively volume unloads the LV, increases microcirculation, and rests the heart while on VA ECMO support. ECpella also provides an attractive option to wean the extracorporeal circuit as soon as practical, and to leave the patient solely on Impella support.[6-9]

In an international, multicenter cohort study of 686 patients with cardiogenic shock treated with VA ECMO, use of left ventricular unloading with Impella was associated with lower mortality, especially if the pump was inserted very early after ECMO initiation. However, the 'ECpella' strategy was also associated with higher risks of complications, such as severe bleeding or interventions because of access site–related ischemia.[8]

Patients supported with Impella alone may require subsequent ECMO implantation, particularly if the chosen Impella device is not able to provide adequate flow for the patient's clinical conditions. If the LV remains dilated with Impella only, adding ECMO at an early enough stage can significantly support recovery because full unloading by a small Impella is only achievable if part of the cardiac output is taken by the VA ECMO circuit. Similarly, early weaning from the ECMO is desirable to reduce complication rates.[9]

| AUTHOR[ref] | SETTING | PATIENT/ANI-MAL/MODEL | STUDY DESIGN | EFFECTS/OUTCOMES |
|---|---|---|---|---|
| *Positive Effects* | | | | |
| *Meani*[1] | Postcardiotomy and ECPR | 10 | Retrospective | IABP was effective in 8/10 patients to allow reopening of the aortic valve which was protractedly closed during peripheral VA ECMO |
| *Chen*[2] | Postcardiotomy shock | 60 | Single-center, Retrospective | Better short-term outcome – Better long-term outcome in patient after heart transplant |
| *Brechot*[3] | All etiologies | 259 (104 with IABP) | Single-center, Retrospective Propensity Matching | Lower rate of pulmonary edema and more days off mechanical ventilation |
| *Kida*[4] | Cardiogenic shock, all etiologies | 519 (459 with IABP) | Registry | VA ECMO+IABP significantly associated with reduced risk of short-term mortality |
| *Li*[5] | All etiologies (29 studies) | 4576 | Systematic Review Meta-analysis | VA ECMO+IABP associated with decreased in-hospital mortality – No difference in relation to complications |
| *Chen*[6] | Postcardiotomy | 152 | Single-centre, Retrospective | Concurrent ECMO and IABP application had better short-term survival and reduced peripheral perfusion complications |
| *Char*[7] | All etiologies | 283 (68 pts with IABP and 72 ECMO+Impella) | Single-centre, Retrospective | Association ECMO+IABP reduced morbidity and mortality at hospital discharge and at 180 days |
| *Vallabhajosyula*[8] | All etiologies | 4653 | Systematic Review Meta-analysis | ECMO + IABP has 18.5% lower mortality than ECMO alone in AMI pts, whereas no influence in overall cardiogenic shock etiologies |
| *Gass*[9] | All etiologies | 135 | Single-centre, Retrospective | Prior IABP use independent predictor of reduced in-hospital mortality, stroke and vascular injury |
| *Neutral Effects* | | | | |
| *Huang*[10] | Postcardiotomy cardiogenic shock | 2251 | Systematic Review Meta-analysis | VA ECMO+IABP did not Improve either weaning nor survival |
| *Wuang*[11] | All etiologies (12 Observational studies) | 3704 | Review Meta-analysis | Improved Weaning rate, but no effect on in-hospital mortality |
| *Wang*[12] | Cardiogenic Shock, all etiologies (3 Studies) | | Systematic Review | Improved Weaning rate, but no effect on in-hospital mortality |
| *Cheng*[13] | Cardiogenic Shock, all etiologies (16 Studies) | 1517 | Systemic Review | No difference on in-hospital survival |
| *Lin*[14] | All etiologies | 529 (302 ECMO+IABP) | Single-centre, Retrospective Propensity Matching | ECMO+IABP did not improve in-hospital outcome |
| *Experimental Models* | | | | |
| *Belohlavek*[15] | Prolonged cardiac arrest (comparing ECMO alone, femoro-femoral or femoro-subclavian) versus ECMO + IABP | 11 pigs | Animal study | VA ECMO+IABP reduced coronary perfusion |
| *Reymond*[16] | Silicon mock circulation | Phantom model | In-vitro study | VA ECMO+IABP improved coronary flow (more pronounced at lower rate, decreased with more severe heart failure) |

IABP=intra-aortic balloon pump; ECMO=extracorporeal membrane oxygenation; pts=patients; All etiologies include cardiogenic shock and cardiac arrest patients.

**Table 44-1.** Clinical evidence of the effects of associated intraaortic balloon counterpulsation with venoarterial extracorporeal membrane oxygenation.

## Combining IABP and VA ECMO

The use of VA ECMO and IABP is the subject of much practice variation between centers because the actual impact of such a mechanical support device over left ventricular unloading and outcome is not fully elucidated yet. There are a few specific aspects which characterize the dual device action. The first one is directly connected to the effects of the IABP on the circulation, whereby the IABP enhances LV ejection (and therefore unloading) by reducing aortic systolic blood pressure. This combination of severely reduced LV contractility and the presence of peripheral VA ECMO may easily lead to protracted closure of the aortic valve, preventing the aortic valve from opening. By inserting an IABP, the aortic valve may start to reopen in all heart beats.[10]

The second aspect is the timing of insertion of IABP in ECMO patients. Concomitant application of VA ECMO and IABP may be associated with better outcomes then late insertion of IABP.[11]

The beneficial effects of IABP in reducing LV end diastolic pressure and thereby pulmonary capillary pressure has been highlighted by Brechot and colleagues, who showed reduced rate of pulmonary edema in patients with the combination of ECMO and IABP.[12] Kida and colleagues, in a study analyzing more than 500 VA ECMO patients supported after acute myocardial infarction, found that combined ECLS-IABP was associated with a reduced risk of 30-day mortality.[13] Other studies, either single-center or systematic review and metaanalyses, have shown beneficial effects of IABP in VA ECMO patients (Table 44-1). The largest study published to date from the ELSO Registry confirmed the improved outcomes of patients receiving LV mechanical unloading. In this study, IABP was associated with similar mortality and lower rates of renal injury and medical and surgical site bleeding than the Impella.[6] However, neutral effects of IABP in VA ECMO have also been described, underlining the need for dedicated prospective, randomized studies in this respect (Table 44-1).

## Escalation and De-escalation of MCS

Outcomes may be improved with either simultaneous or consecutive combinations of MCS devices, with correct timing and indications for implantation, escalation, and de-escalation, customized for each patient and clinical scenario. Previous studies demonstrated a temporal relationship between the early use of percutaneous MCS and improved clinical outcomes in cardiogenic shock patients.[14-16]

## Escalation

### *Criteria and Timing*

As the dynamics of myocardial dysfunction are extremely complex in cardiogenic shock due to the interplay between primary and secondary myocardial dysfunction, and eventually the occurrence of right ventricular failure, clinical assessment and judgment should trigger the need for escalation of mechanical circulatory support and selection of the most appropriate configuration (eg, ECMO and IABP, ECPella, ECMO and ProtekDuo, BiPella, Impella, VAD). Aortic regurgitation should be addressed at this stage.

Reasons for Escalation:

- Persistence of shock,
- Pulmonary edema,
- Right ventricular failure,
- Vasoactive Inotrope Score (VIS) >20[17]
- Inability to wean from inotropes.

**Possible Uni- or Biventricular Escalation**

Multiparametric evaluation is fundamental to make the correct diagnosis of persistent cardiogenic shock isolated to the left (systemic) ventricle or related to both ventricles, and consequently to select the appropriate timing and MCS escalation strategy (Figures 44-3 and 44-4).

*__Univentricular dysfunction__* (isolated LV dysfunction with preserved right ventricular contractility) allows elective MCS escalation (a few to 24 hours). Usually, first line MCS in patients with poor LV function and SCAI stage C is femoral percutaneous devices (either Impella CP or VA ECMO). In cases of more profound cardiogenic shock (SCAI stage D or E), VA ECMO or transition from femoral percutaneous to an upper body approach with a more powerful pump (Impella 5.0/5.5) is advised.

Advantages of the Impella 5.0/5.5 vs. VA ECMO, which remains a reasonable option in this context, are the following:

- Impella 5.0/5.5 provides full cardiac support, even in the absence of residual LV function.
- Axillary Impella 5.0/5.5 may be associated with lower vascular complication rates than VA ECMO[18,19]
- The longer duration of support allows time to evaluate myocardial recovery and, if not present, Impella 5.0/5.5 represents a valuable bridge-to-decision device towards long-term therapies such as LVAD implantation or heart transplant (Chapter 30).

*__Biventricular dysfunction__* with concomitant right heart failure development requires urgent decision-making and MCS escalation.

The precise diagnosis of the underlying cause of RV failure is fundamental for undertaking the correct escalation strategy. RV failure should

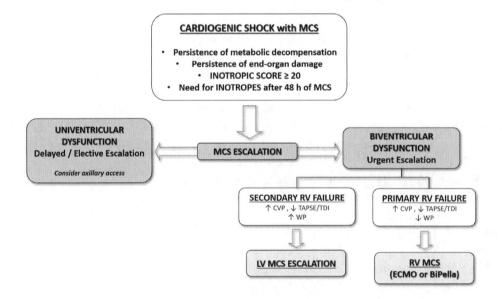

RV: Right Ventricular; LV: Left Ventricular CVP: Central Venous Pressure; WP: Wedge Pressure

**Figure 44-3.** MCS Escalation.

be detected both with hemodynamic and echocardiographic monitoring, eg, increased central venous pressure (>16 mmHg), reduced RV function on echocardiography (eg, Tricuspid Annulus Peak Systolic Excursion and tissue doppler S' wave), and/or invasive parameters (eg, low PAPi <1.8 or high RAP/PAOP ratio >0.6). First, the most common differential diagnoses of RV failure have to be ruled out: primary lung problems (eg, pneumothorax, pleural effusion, atelectasis), pulmonary embolism, right ventricular outflow obstruction, tamponade, LV pump displacement or suction, and persistence of metabolic decompensation (acidosis, hypercapnia). Second, in order to select the best MCS escalation strategy, correct classification of the underlying cause is important:

*Secondary RV failure* is characterized by increased LV filling pressure and requires LV MCS escalation with upgrade of LV unloading by increasing pump flow or with a more powerful pump (see univentricular dysfunction).

*Primary RV failure* presents normal LV filling pressure values and requires escalation with direct RV MCS support. Biventricular MCS strategies are VA ECMO support, addition of an RVAD with ProtekDuo®, or BiPELLA.[20]

***Ventricular Dysfunction in Single Ventricle Congenital Heart Disease.*** Patients with univentricular hearts who have undergone palliation by means of the Norwood and Fontan pathways are presenting with heart failure in increasing numbers. They may present at any stage in the palliation and at any age. Patients with cavopulmonary connections (Glenn and Fontan Circulations) often have elevated venous pressures with accompanying cirrhosis, renal impairment, and protein losing enteropathy. Presentation is usually subacute, resembling the time course of isolated left ventricular failure described above. MCS is challenging and strategies to support these patients are still evolving. Further information can be found below and in Chapters 4, 20, 31, and 41.

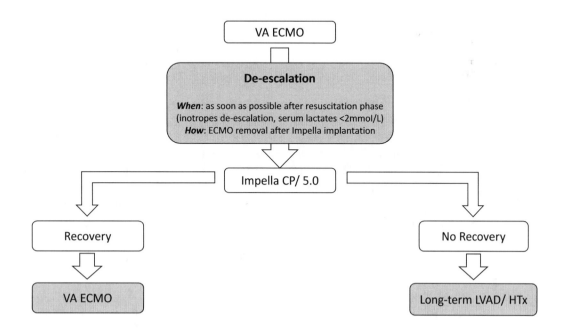

**Figure 44-4.** MCS De-escalation.

## De-escalation

VA ECMO is still considered the standard MCS in patients with profound cardiogenic shock (INTERMACS / SCAI E patients) or refractory cardiac arrest (ECPR). VA ECMO is a reasonable rescue therapy in refractory cardiogenic shock patients, although it is associated with substantial complication rates. Weaning may be successful in up to 60% of patients surviving the acute phase of cardiogenic shock. However, some of these patients may require long-term VAD support or heart transplantation, due to the lack of myocardial recovery. When a bridge to LVAD implantation is discussed, switching VA ECMO for Impella 5.0/5.5 represents a potentially valuable bridge-to-decision to test RV function. In the case of severe RV failure, two Centrimag intrathoracic devices (for RV and LV support) may be used for midterm (6-8 weeks) support in patients who are not immediate candidates for VAD or heart transplant surgery. Using the Impella 5.0/5.5 via axillary surgical access has also been proposed by some authors as a strategy for MCS de-escalation after VA ECMO.

## Total Artificial Heart

Two orthotopic artificial hearts have been developed. They have unique advantages over other machines because they solve problems of persistent ventricular arrhythmias, RV failure, or severe heart valve diseases. The CARMAT TAH (C-TAH) is a biventricular, pulsatile, electrically powered, hydraulically actuated flow pump with all components embodied in a single device, mimicking the natural heart implanted in the pericardial sac. Its most original feature is the use of bioprosthetic materials, similar to those used for bioprosthetic heart valves to reduce the need for anticoagulation. The SynCardia Temporary CardioWest Total Artificial is a biventricular, pneumatic, pulsatile pump that totally replaces the native ventricles.

Over 1,000 implantations have been performed worldwide over the last 4 decades and the recent development of a smaller driving console may allow greater patient mobility and eventually discharge from the hospital.

## TandemHeart

The TandemHeart is a percutaneous VAD consisting of an extracorporeal centrifugal continuous flow pump that drains blood from the left atrium and then pumps it into the femoral artery at a flow rate of up to 4 L/min. The left atrial catheter is usually inserted via the femoral vein into the right atrium and then across the atrial septum into the left atrium. The TandemHeart increases cardiac output and mean arterial pressure and decreases cardiac filling pressures by venting the left atrium. This effect may be partially offset by the increased LV afterload due to retrograde blood flow up the aorta toward the aortic root. The TandemHeart was associated with significant improvements in hemodynamic and metabolic outcomes when compared to IABP in two small, randomized trials. However, survival was not improved, and there were more complications in patients treated with the TandemHeart.[20-22]

## Specific Pediatric Considerations

While ECLS modalities such as VA ECMO are frequently utilized in pediatric patients for cardiorespiratory failure because of their ease of deployment, they may not be the optimal strategy for recovery or bridge to transplantation. Considerations for patients in isolated cardiac failure such as extended duration, LV decompression, mobilization/ rehabilitation, and blood product sensitization may make other forms of MCS a superior option. Many patients find themselves in a bridge-to-bridge, bridge-to-transplantation, or bridge-to-decision situation that warrants a change from VA ECMO to more durable MCS such as VAD

(Chapter 20). Indeed, short VA ECMO runs prior to VAD implantation have been demonstrated to be useful in some circumstances.[24] The decision to utilize a VAD or ECMO in pediatric heart failure is multifactorial and fluid (Figure 44-5). The underlying cardiac dysfunction plays an important role in decisionmaking. Historically, cardiomyopathy has been the main diagnosis requiring MCS in pediatrics, but congenital heart disease has increasingly been seen as an indication for MCS.[24-26] Because pediatric patients have considerable variation in size, MCS strategies vary accordingly from paracorporeal to implantable devices. For the purposes of this chapter, we will describe utilization in terms of modality (paracorporeal or implantable) and category (continuous or pulsatile).

### *Paracorporeal Continuous*

Paracorporeal continuous MCS devices include centrifugal pumps that are frequently utilized for ECMO, but without an oxygenator.[27] Cannulation strategies include standard ECMO cannulas or specific paracorporeal MCS cannulas directly connected to the atrium or ventricle (left or right) and artery (pulmonary or aorta), which are tunneled through the skin to facilitate sternal closure. Percutaneous insertion for right ventricular support is possible for larger children ($>1.2m^2$ BSA), who are comparable in size to small adults. Paracorporeal continuous MCS has been reported to offer three times longer support duration and improved survival over traditional ECMO. Nonetheless, VA ECMO has been successfully used to bridge patients to cardiac transplantation even after many months of support.[28]

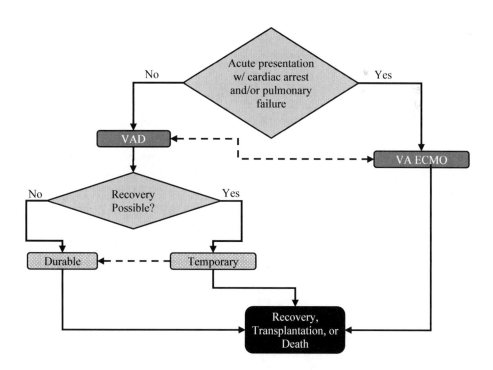

**Figure 44-5.** Pediatric Heart Failure Decision Tree: VAD or VA ECMO.

### Paracorporeal Pulsatile

Paracorporeal pulsatile MCS devices have experienced the longest history in pediatrics. From adult devices employed in larger pediatric patients to specifically designed pediatric devices that can range down to patients under 3 kg, these devices have demonstrated superior outcomes to ECMO when they are able to be placed electively.[24] Currently, the Berlin Heart GMBh Excor is the only commercially available device. Pulsatile VADs in the paracorporeal setting are pneumatically driven devices with blood-filled polymer sacs enclosed in hard external housings. Filling and emptying of the blood sac are controlled through vacuum-assisted refilling and applied pneumatic pressure, respectively. The pneumatic system controls the timing of systole and diastole and can adjust the applied vacuum or pressure to compensate for changes in preload and afterload. One-way valves (polymeric trileaflet) positioned at the entrance and exit of the blood sac create unidirectional flow through the device and are key areas of concern for thrombus formation.[29,30] A mobile air compressor provides the necessary pneumatic power, which has seen significant reduction in size from washing machine sized devices without battery backup in the 1990s to suitcase-sized systems with more than 5 hours of battery life today. Specific cannulas designed to interface with these devices are used and are tunneled through the skin to permit sternal closure. These cannulas are also suitable for long term transthoracic ECMO and paracorporeal continuous flow VAD use and are becoming increasingly popular (Chapter 4).

### Implantable Continuous

The continued miniaturization of adult implantable continuous flow VADs has afforded some adolescent children the ability to navigate transplant wait-list times and rehabilitate. Some may even receive care at home, although outpatient VAD care still carries the potential for serious life-threatening complications.[31-33] These devices are typically centrifugal or axial flow pumps that directly connect to the ventricle and have an outflow graft that is sewn to the corresponding artery. The main body of the VAD remains in the pericardial space, and only a small driveline that conveys power and control to the VAD exits the skin. The driveline is an important source for infection, which can be highly resistant to treatment. The future hope of fully implantable pumps without a driveline (wireless connectivity) will potentially negate this risk, leading to a major positive improvement in patient experience. Current implantable continuous flow VADs are intended to support patients with a BSA >1.2 m². While reported adult outcomes have been excellent, published pediatric experience is limited, with recent FDA approval occurring in December 2020, and no currently approved status for children in Europe.[32, 34]

### VAD + Oxygenator (OxyVAD)

One of the advantages of paracorporeal MCS in pediatric patients is that those who develop pulmonary failure secondary to cardiac failure can take advantage of hybrid ECMO approaches by adding oxygenators into these paracorporeal VAD systems. The addition of an oxygenator to a paracorporeal VAD is a relatively straightforward process, essentially splicing tubing, and connectors at the VAD outlet to interpose an oxygenator. The published experience with OxyVAD configurations demonstrates both frequent use and reasonably good short-term outcomes.[35-41] The PEDIMACS registry of pediatric VADs reported only 7% of their patients had prior ECMO runs, but this nearly doubled to 13% having respiratory failure within 3 months of implantation.[42] Overall outcomes were positive, with only 5 patients (19%) expiring on support or within 1 month of decannulation, which is better than the 54% mortality reported in the ELSO Registry for pediatric cardiac ECMO.[43] However, in certain contexts, there may be no actual benefit conferred to the patient by utilizing OxyVAD configurations compared to multiple combined modalities.[41]

There are many reasons for adding an oxygenator to a paracorporeal VAD rather than initiating separate ECMO support, or instituting ECMO in the place of the VAD. These include avoiding additional surgical procedures to minimize short-term procedural risks, as well as long-term complications including access vessel thrombosis and infection while avoiding simultaneous management of two complex mechanical circulatory support systems. Important factors to consider prior to initiating OxyVAD include patient age and size, disease process, anticoagulation requirements, and the capabilities and comfort of the center in managing infrequently used, nontraditional systems. Smaller patients (<10 kg) have a higher incidence of pulmonary and biventricular failure, requiring multiple modalities in their bridge-to-transplantation process compared to their larger counterparts.[42,44] These patients also require smaller devices with lower margins for error that are not well equipped for overcoming high resistances. Primary respiratory failure (viral or pulmonary edema) can easily be managed with a OxyVAD configuration, while bacterial sepsis involving multiorgan dysfunction and cardiovascular instability will benefit from the control and vascular access afforded by conversion to VA ECMO.[40] Anticoagulation on a OxyVAD patient is primarily dependent upon left- or right-sided support and mirrors that provided to similar ECMO patients due to the additional surface area of the oxygenator. The experience of the entire medical management team from physicians to nurses, perfusionists, and respiratory therapists is a significant factor to consider. Teams that are comfortable with the day-to-day management of ECMO patients are likely to be successful with OxyVAD configurations because personnel are well equipped to troubleshoot technical issues with each of the specific devices and are more equipped to recognize and respond to emergencies.

**Outcomes**

Successful bridge to transplantation or explantation to recovery (81% at 1 year) with a VAD is dependent on multiple factors, including device classification, underlying patient conditions, and the transplant landscape. Implantable continuous VADs offer superior survival outcomes, followed by pulsatile paracorporeal, and worst in those supported on short-term paracorporeal continuous pumps (reflecting high-risk patient substrate).[24,45] Infants, weight <20 kg (even higher if <5 kg), INTERMACS 1 classification, congenital heart disease, and biventricular VAD support are among the high-risk factors for mortality.[24-26,45,46] Right ventricular failure after primary durable LVAD implantation is associated with adverse outcomes,[47] and the need for right ventricular assist device (RVAD) or delayed implantation increases risk for death on-device (hazard ratio 6.9, >3 months), which makes early intervention with temporary/durable RVAD support and prioritization towards a higher waitlist status necessary.[47] Finally, regional differences in transplantation availability can also prove challenging, with children waiting longer in Europe (early transplant rates of 35% at 6 months) compared to the US (50% at 6 months).[25]

## References

1.  Bernhardt A., Potapov E., Schibilsky D, et al. First in man evaluation of a novel circulatory support device: Early experience with the Impella 5.5 after CE mark approval in Germany. J Heart Lung Transplant 2021 Aug;40(8):850-855.
2.  Ouweneel DM, Eriksen E, Sjauw KD, et al. Percutaneous Mechanical Circulatory Support Versus Intra-Aortic Balloon Pump in Cardiogenic Shock After Acute Myocardial Infarction. J Am Coll Cardiol 2017; 69(3): 278-87.
3.  Schrage B, Ibrahim K, Loehn T, et al. Impella Support for Acute Myocardial Infarction Complicated by Cardiogenic Shock. Circulation 2019; 139(10): 1249-58.
4.  Amin AP, Spertus JA, Curtis JP, et al. The Evolving Landscape of Impella Use in the United States Among Patients Undergoing Percutaneous Coronary Intervention with Mechanical Circulatory Support. Circulation 2020; 141(4): 273-84.
5.  Dhruva SS, Ross JS, Mortazavi BJ, et al. Association of Use of an Intravascular Microaxial Left Ventricular Assist Device vs Intra-aortic Balloon Pump with In-Hospital Mortality and Major Bleeding Among Patients With Acute Myocardial Infarction Complicated by Cardiogenic Shock. JAMA 2020; 323:734-745.
6.  Grandin E, Nunez J, Willar B, et al. Mechanical left ventricular unloading in patients undergoing venoarterial extracorporeal membrane oxygenation. J Am Coll Card 2022; 79:1239-1250.
7.  Pappalardo F, Schulte C, Pieri M, et al. Concomitant implantation of Impella® on top of veno-arterial extracorporeal membrane oxygenation may improve survival of patients with cardiogenic shock. Eur J Heart Fail. 2017 Mar;19(3):404-412.
8.  Schrage B, Becher PM, Bernhardt A, et al. Left Ventricular Unloading Is Associated With Lower Mortality in Patients With Cardiogenic Shock Treated With Venoarterial Extracorporeal Membrane Oxygenation: Results From an International, Multicenter Cohort Study. Circulation. 2020 Dec;142(22):2095-2106.
9.  Bertoldi LF, Pappalardo F, Lubos E, et al. Bridging INTERMACS 1 patients from VA-ECMO to LVAD via Impella 5.0: De-escalate and ambulate. J Crit Care. 2020; 57:259-263.
10. Meani P, Delnoij T, Raffa GM, et al. Protracted aortic valve closure during peripheral veno-arterial extracorporeal life support: is intra-aortic pump an effective solution? Perfusion 2019;34:35-41.
11. Chen K, Hou J, Tang H, Hu S. Concurrent implantation of intra-aortic balloon pump and extracorporeal membrane oxygenation improved survival of patients with postcardiotomy cardiogenic shock. Artif Organs 2019;43:142-9.
12. Brechot N, Demondion P, Santi F, et al. Intra-aortic balloon pump protects against hydrostatic pulmonary edema during peripheral veno-arterial extracorporeal membrane oxygenation. Eur Heart J Acute Cardiovasc Care 2018;7:62-69.
13. Kida H, Sotomi Y, Hikoso S, et al. Prognostic significance of intra-aortic balloon pumping support in patients with acute myocardial infarction and veno-arterial extracorporeal membrane oxygenation thrapy. J Cardiol 2022; 79:179-85.
14. Basir MB, Schreiber TL, Grines CL, et al. Effect of early initiation of mechanical circulatory support on survival in cardiogenic shock. Am J Cardiol 2017; 119:845-851.
15. Pieri M, Sorrentino T, Oppizzi M, et al. The role of different mechanical circulatory support devices and their timing of implantation on myocardial damage and mid-term recovery in acute myocardial infarction related cardiogenic shock. J Interv Cardiol. 2018; 31:717–724.
16. Tongers J, Sieweke JT, Kühn C, et al. Early escalation of mechanical circulatory support stabilizes and potentially rescues patients in refractory cardiogenic shock. Circ Heart Fail. 2020; 13:e005853.
17. Na SJ, Chung CR, Cho YH, et al. Vasoactive Inotropic Score as a Predictor of Mortality in Adult Patients With Cardiogenic Shock: Medical Therapy Versus ECMO. Rev Esp Cardiol (Engl Ed). 2019; 72(1):40-47.
18. Karami M, den Uil CA, Ouweneel DM, et al. Mechanical circulatory support in cardiogenic shock from acute myocardial infarction: Impella CP/5.0 versus ECMO. Eur Heart J Acute Cardiovasc Care. 2020 Mar; 9(2):164-172.
19. Bertoglio L, Katsarou M, Scandroglio M, et al. Surgical transaxillary placement of the Impella 5.0 ventricular assist device. J Card Surg. 2019; 34(2):92-98.
20. Ruhparwar A, Zubarevich A, Osswald A, et al. ECPELLA 2.0—Minimally invasive biventricular groin-free full mechanical circulatory support with Impella 5.0/5.5 pump and ProtekDuo cannula as a bridge-to-bridge concept: A first-in-man method description. J Card Surg. 2020; 35:195–199.
21. Burkhoff D, Cohen H, Brunckhorst C, O'Neill WW. A randomized multicenter clinical study to evaluate the safety and efficacy of the TandemHeart percutaneous ventricular assist device versus conventional therapy with intraaortic balloon pumping for treatment of cardiogenic shock. Am Heart J 2006; 152(3): 469.e1-8.
22. Thiele H, Sick P, Boudriot E, et al. Randomized comparison of intra-aortic balloon support with a

percutaneous left ventricular assist device in patients with revascularized acute myocardial infarction complicated by cardiogenic shock. Eur Heart J 2005; 26(13): 1276-83.

23. Interagency Registry for Mechanically Assisted Circulatory Support. Appendix A - adverse event definitions. UAB School of Medicine. https://www.uab.edu/medicine/intermacs/intermacs-documents.

24. Morales DLS, Adachi I, Peng DM, et al. Fourth Annual Pediatric Interagency Registry for Mechanical Circulatory Support (Pedimacs) Report. Ann Thorac Surg. 2020;110(6):1819-1831.

25. de By T, Antonides CFJ, Schweiger M, et al. The European Registry for Patients with Mechanical Circulatory Support (EUROMACS): second EUROMACS Paediatric (Paedi-EUROMACS) report. Eur J Cardiothorac Surg. 2020;57(6):1038-1050.

26. Peng DM, Koehl DA, Cantor RS, et al. Outcomes of children with congenital heart disease implanted with ventricular assist devices: An analysis of the Pediatric Interagency Registry for Mechanical Circulatory Support (Pedimacs). J Heart Lung Transplant. 2019;38(4):420-430.

27. Yarlagadda VV, Maeda K, Zhang Y, et al. Temporary Circulatory Support in U.S. Children Awaiting Heart Transplantation. J Am Coll Cardiol. 2017;70(18):2250-2260.

28. Shanefield, S., Knewitz D, Philip J, et al. Support with extracorporeal membrane oxygenation for over 1 year duration as a bridge to cardiac transplantation: A case report and review of the literature. Cardiol Young, 2021; 31(9): 1495-1497.29.

29. Wagner WR, Johnson PC, Kormos RL, Griffith BP. Evaluation of bioprosthetic valve-associated thrombus in ventricular assist device patients. Circulation. 1993;88(5 Pt 1):2023-2029.

30. Maeda K, Almond C, Hollander SA, et al. Characteristics of deposits and pump exchange in the Berlin Heart EXCOR ventricular assist device: Experience with 67 cases. Pediatr Transplant. 2018;22(4):e13181.

31. Burki S, Adachi I. Pediatric ventricular assist devices: current challenges and future prospects. Vasc Health Risk Manag. 2017;13:177-185.

32. Hoskote A, Stiller B, Thiagarajan RR. What's new in mechanical support strategies for the intensivist in children with severe cardiac failure. Intensive Care Med. 2021; 47(10):1152-1155.

33. Pokrajac N, Cantwell LM, Murray JM, Dykes JC. Characteristics and Outcomes of Pediatric Patients With a Ventricular Assist Device Presenting to the Emergency Department. Pediatr Emerg Care. 2022. Feb 1;38(2):e924-e928.

34. O'Connor MJ, Lorts A, Davies RR, et al. Early experience with the HeartMate 3 continuous-flow ventricular assist device in pediatric patients and patients with congenital heart disease: A multicenter registry analysis. J Heart Lung Transplant. 2020; 39(6):573-579.

35. Betit P, Matte GS, Howe R, et al. The addition of a membrane oxygenator to a ventricular assist device in a patient with acute respiratory distress syndrome. J Extra Corpor Technol. 2011; 43(4):264-266.

36. Garcia-Guereta L, Cabo J, de la Oliva P, et al. Ventricular assist device application with the intermediate use of a membrane oxygenator as a bridge to pediatric heart transplantation. J Heart Lung Transplant. 2009; 28(7):740-742.

37. Monge MC, Kulat BT, Eltayeb O, et al. Novel Modifications of a Ventricular Assist Device for Infants and Children. Ann Thorac Surg. 2016; 102(1):147-153.

38. Monge MC, Kulat BT, Eltayeb O, et al. Successful Bridge-to-Transplant of Functionally Univentricular Patients With a Modified Continuous-Flow Ventricular Assist Device. Artif Organs. 2017; 41(1):25-31.

39. Zaccagni HJ, Timpa JG, O'Meara LC, Alten JA. Long-term membrane oxygenator use to support an infant with acute respiratory distress syndrome on biventricular assist device. Interact Cardiovasc Thorac Surg. 2013; 17(1):196-198.

40. Conway J, Al-Aklabi M, Granoski D, et al. Supporting pediatric patients with short-term continuous-flow devices. J Heart Lung Transplant. 2016; 35(5):603-609.

41. De Rita F, Hasan A, Haynes S, et al. Outcome of mechanical cardiac support in children using more than one modality as a bridge to heart transplantation. Eur J Cardiothorac Surg. 2015; 48(6):917-922.

42. Rossano JW, Lorts A, VanderPluym CJ, et al. Outcomes of pediatric patients supported with continuous-flow ventricular assist devices: A report from the Pediatric Interagency Registry for Mechanical Circulatory Support (PediMACS). J Heart Lung Transplant. 2016; 35(5):585-590.

43. ECLS Registry : Live online query Extracorporeal Life Support Organization; June 10th 2022.

44. Mansfield RT, Lin KY, Zaoutis T, et al. The Use of Pediatric Ventricular Assist Devices in Children's Hospitals From 2000 to 2010: Morbidity, Mortality, and Hospital Charges. Pediatr Crit Care Med. 2015;16(6):522-528.

45. VanderPluym CJ, Cantor RS, Machado D, et al. Utilization and Outcomes of Children Treated with Direct Thrombin Inhibitors on Paracorporeal Ventricular Assist Device Support. ASAIO J. 2020;66(8):939-945.

46. Miera O, Morales DLS, Thul J, Amodeo A, Menon AK, Humpl T. Improvement of survival in low-weight children on the Berlin Heart EXCOR ventricular

assist device supportdagger. Eur J Cardiothorac Surg. 2019;55(5):913-919.

47. Simpson KE, Kirklin JK, Cantor RS, et al. Right heart failure with left ventricular assist device implantation in children: An analysis of the Pedimacs registry database. J Heart Lung Transplant. 2020; 39(3):231-240.

# 45

## Extracorporeal Therapy to Facilitate Organ Donation

*Alvaro Rojas-Pena, Peter S. MacDonald, Ina Jochmans, David Paredes-Zapata, Robert H. Bartlett*

### Introduction

Over the last 10 years, the use of ECMO and the number of ELSO registered ECMO centers have increased significantly worldwide. Currently, there are more than 700 ELSO registered centers and more than 17,500 ECMO cases per year are being reported.[1] This rapid increase in the acceptance of the technology, greater clinical expertise, patient selection, and more ECMO healthcare providers are key factors in the rapid growth of ECMO in all areas of clinical practice where cardiac and/or respiratory support are needed, and this snowball effect is no different in organ procurement and transplantation.

In 2006, the Institute of Medicine (IOM) published a report titled "Organ Donation; Opportunities for Action."[2] The IOM recommendation was to increase the pool of donated organs by successfully recovering and transplanting organs donated after circulatory death (DCD). The report estimated that 22,000 additional donors could be candidates for DCD after uncontrolled cardiac arrest (uDCD). The IOM recommended expansion of the population of potential donors via the implementation of initiatives to increase DCD donation, and research on organ quality and enhanced organ function. Since this report, organ procurement organizations (OPOs) have joined forces to maximize DCD donation in the U.S. and these joint efforts have shown excellent results. In 2021, there were 41,354 organ transplants and 13,861 deceased donors in the U.S., a historical record high as reported by the United Network for Organ Sharing (UNOS). In addition, UNOS reported a total of 4,187 DCD donors in 2021, an increase of 29.9% compared to 2020, as well as a steady increase in DCD donation over the last 10 years.[3] However, despite record highs in total number of transplants performed and total number of deceased donors in 2021, the lack of organs suitable for transplantation continues to be a major problem in transplantation. Based on Organ Procurement and Transplantation Network (OPTN) data as of June 1, 2022, there were 116,447 patients on the organ transplantation list.

ECMO provides normal tissue perfusion in the absence of cardiac activity and has the potential to improve organ quality when initiated following cessation of circulation and declaration of death in DCD donors. The use of ECMO in DCD donation is referred to as Normothermic Regional Perfusion (NRP). A few centers worldwide have over 15 years of experience with ECMO-assisted organ donation of abdominal organs (liver, kidney, and pancreas).[4-10] Recently, the technology has been adapted to include recovery of thoracic organs (hearts and lungs).[11-16] This chapter summarizes the principles of organ donation, discusses the importance of understanding the physiology of brain death and presents the experience with the use of ECMO-assisted organ donation. ECMO support for organ donation has been applied in 3 different clinical settings as described in Table 45-1.

## Understanding Deceased Organ Donation

A guiding principle of vital organ donation is the dead donor rule (DDR), which is an ethical principle rather than a legal doctrine.[18] A vital organ cannot be removed until the donor is determined to be dead according to medical standards and legal criteria and removing a vital organ cannot cause the death of the donor. Even autonomous choice cannot override the DDR: patients who do not meet the criteria for death cannot donate vital organs (eg, heart, whole liver), no matter how fervent their desire to be a donor. In the United States, the Uniform Determination of

Death Act (UDDA) states, "An individual who has sustained either: 1) irreversible cessation of circulatory and respiratory functions; or 2) irreversible cessation of all functions of the entire brain, including the brain stem, is dead. A determination of death must be made in accordance with accepted medical standards."[19]

In deceased organ donation, two pathways can lead to the diagnosis of death: diagnosis of death based on neurological criteria—donation after brain death (DBD) also called donation after neurologic determination of death (NDD). In this summary we will refer to these donors as DBD and diagnosis of death based on circulatory criteria—donation after circulatory death (DCD).

## Donation after Brain Death (DBD)

Isolated brain death causes apnea that results in cardiac arrest in minutes. If apnea is prevented by mechanical ventilation, vital organ function gradually progresses from

| DONOR TYPE* | MAASTRICHT CATEGORY | DESCRIPTION | COUNTRIES WITH SUCCESSFUL DCD PROTOCOLS |
|---|---|---|---|
| Uncontrolled DCD (uDCD) | Maastricht Type I and II | Individuals that suffer cardiac arrest and are declared dead because the treating team determines that they cannot be resuscitated. | Australia, Belgium, Czech Republic, France, Israel, Italy, Latvia, Lithuania, Netherlands, Poland, Portugal, Russia, Spain, Switzerland, UK |
| | Maastricht Type IV | Brain dead donors that either suffer cardiac arrest prior to organ recovery and follow the DCD organ recovery pathway. | N/A |
| Controlled DCD (cDCD) | Maastricht Type III | Deaths that occur following planned WLST (mechanical and pharmacological) support. | Australia, Austria, Belgium, Canada, China, Czech Republic, France, Ireland, Italy, Netherlands, New Zealand, Norway, Spain, Switzerland, Sweden, UK, USA |
| DBD or NDD | N/A | A patient who becomes brain dead while ECMO support was started as a resuscitative effort. | China, France, Italy, Taiwan, USA |

*Modified from the Non-heart Beating Donors Maastricht Categories.[17]
DBD=donation after brain death; DCD=Donors after circulatory death; NDD=Neurologic death donors; WLST=Withdrawal of life sustaining treatment; N/A=Not applicable

**Table 45-1.** Clinical scenarios for ECMO support assisted organ donation.

normal to failure in a reproducible, identifiable, and relentless fashion.[20,21] Transplanting organs from brain dead donors into recipients with organ failure became a reality after the publication of the Harvard criteria for brain death in 1968.[22] The window for recovering organs for transplantation is only as long as the period between brain death and organ failure— approximately 48 hours. Understanding the pathophysiology of brain death is the background for procuring organs from brain dead subjects for transplantation.

After brain death (with mechanical ventilation) and after the "Cushing response" of hypertension and bradycardia, vital organ function remains normal for 6-12 hours. The first manifestation of organ malfunction is loss of distal tubular function in the kidney, resulting in profound diuresis (diabetes insipidus). This is from a lack of antidiuretic hormone secretion from the brain. Untreated, diabetes insipidus leads to hypovolemia and organ failure from hypovolemic shock. When diabetes insipidus is prevented by administration of vasopressin (antidiuretic hormone), blood volume is maintained, and vital organ function continues for another 12-24 hours. The next manifestation of organ failure is loss of systemic vasomotor tone, resulting in vasodilation, relative hypovolemia, and hypotension. The physiologic picture resembles anaphylaxis. Untreated, this phenomenon results in cardiac arrest from hypovolemic shock within a few hours. This vascular collapse can be treated with systemic alpha-adrenergic agents and infusion of fluids. But after about 6 hours of this treatment (24-48 hours from brain death), increasing dosages of pressors are required to maintain blood pressure, and generalized capillary leakage begins, resulting in generalized edema. Continuous infusion of fluid is required to maintain the blood volume, and those organs that malfunction while edematous begin to fail. Pulmonary edema results in lung dysfunction. Cardiac edema results in a loss of diastolic compliance and decreased cardiac output. Intestinal edema results in profuse diarrhea. Eventually a combination of hypoxemia, hypercarbia, acidosis, and low cardiac output results in cardiac arrest. In some ways, this multiple organ failure syndrome resembles an accelerated version of the loss of other hormones secreted by the brain (adrenocorticotropic hormone, thyroid stimulating hormone, and vasopressin). But administration of these hormones in large doses (or administration of secondary hormones like thyroid hormone and adrenal cortical steroids) has only a slight delaying effect on the multiple organ failure syndrome.

## Donation after Circulatory Death (DCD)

When death is pronounced based on the absence of circulation, vital organs are exposed to severe hypoxia at normothermic temperatures. Nevertheless, under certain conditions, organ donation can take place. Kootstra et al. described four categories of DCD donors[17] that are still in use today, albeit with some modifications (Table 45-1). We now refer to uncontrolled (uDCD) and controlled (cDCD) DCD donation, where "uncontrolled" refers to the fact that the circulatory arrest is unexpected and unanticipated, as is the case in a failed resuscitation or a potential DBD donor who suddenly suffers a cardiac arrest. On the other hand, in cDCD the circulatory arrest is expected and anticipated. Indeed, when the treating team of a patient on life sustaining treatment has decided, in agreement with the family, that further treatment is futile and life sustaining treatment will be withdrawn, the pathway of cDCD donation can be started. In this case, the withdrawal of life sustaining treatment (WLST) takes place in a scheduled fashion with the organ procurement teams standing by. Like DBD donation, a DCD program requires rigorous adherence to legal and ethical protocols.

In comparison to DBD donation, DCD donation is associated with a lower yield of transplantable organs and higher rates of posttransplant complications which may increase morbidity and mortality. Livers suffer an increased risk of ischemic biliary complications and primary nonfunction, while kidneys are at higher risk of primary nonfunction or delayed graft function.[23-25] The reason is that the organs begin to sustain warm ischemic (WI) injury when the circulation stops. Nevertheless, once organ function of a DCD organ has recovered, the long-term outcomes are good and comparable to those after DBD donation.[26-28] To decrease the risk of these ischemia-related posttransplant complications, well-established DCD donation protocols can include in situ organ preservation (ECMO-assisted organ donation, or Normothermic Regional Perfusion (NRP), and/or ex-situ resuscitation, evaluation, and repair of organs post-procurement by isolated organ perfusion. Both cDCD and uDCD offer great potential for tissue donation. The success of a DCD program requires the establishment of protocols that include national ethical, professional, and legal frameworks to address both public and professional concerns with all aspects of the DCD pathway.[29]

## Donation of Abdominal Organs from DCD

### Methods for DCD Organ Recovery

Rapid Recovery (RR, conventional) technique for procuring abdominal DCD organs: Rapid recovery (RR) instituted after declaration of death is the standard procedure for DCD organ retrieval in many centers. After cessation of circulation, a 'stand-off' or "no-touch" period is respected to ensure that circulation does not recover spontaneously (cardiac autoresuscitation). Although this period is 5 minutes in most countries and centers, it can vary between 3 and 20 minutes.

After this 'stand-off' period, and in the absence of spontaneous recovery of circulation, the patient is declared dead and organ procurement can start. In RR, a rapid sterno laparotomy is performed, the infrarenal aorta is cannulated and after the descending aorta is clamped (usually above the diaphragm), cold preservation solution is flushed through the aortic cannula. The peritoneal cavity is filled with slush ice for topical cooling. In parallel, heart and lungs can also be procured (see section, 'Donation of cardiac grafts from cDCD'). When the cold-flush is finished, liver, pancreas, and kidneys are removed, flushed on the back table, and stored until transplantation. Another technique of rapid recovery, historically used in uDCD but now mostly abandoned, includes cannulation of the femoral artery for immediate cold perfusion of the body before opening the abdomen.

ECMO-assisted DCD donation or Normothermic Regional Perfusion (Figure 45-1): Normothermic Regional Perfusion (NRP) was first used in 1989 by Spanish transplant surgeons using a percutaneously placed regional perfusion cardiopulmonary bypass circuit.[30]

NRP involves placement of femoral arterial and venous cannula either percutaneously or via cut down, or placement of the arterial and venous cannulas directly in the aorta and vena cava or in the iliac vessels.[31] Depending on the clinical scenario and local practice, the cannula may be placed prior to, or following, declaration of death.[31] The circuit consists of, at a minimum, a centrifugal pump and an oxygenator. A heat exchanger may or may not be included in the circuit. If included, circulation is normothermic (37° C). If not included, ECMO occurs at ambient room temperature (~30° C).[9] Historically, hypothermic temperatures (<20° C) were also used, but this practice has not been reported after 2005.[25] The entire system is about the size of a hemodialysis unit and can be transported on a wheeled cart. A proximal aortic occlusion balloon is inserted into the thoracic aorta to enable selective perfusion of the abdominal organs, or the descending aorta is clamped (usually above the diaphragm). This improves the efficiency of the ECMO circuit by limiting the circulating volume and it avoids re-establishing perfusion to the brain. Typically, ECMO target flow is >50 mL/kg/min (2–3 L/min).[31]

### NRP Compared to RR

There are several logistical and physiologic hurdles to the utilization of organs from DCD. The chief physiologic barrier is warm ischemia. The rational to reestablish the flow of oxygenated blood after the declaration of death using ECMO is the reversal of anaerobic metabolism by replenishing mitochondrial stores of adenosine triphosphate (ATP) creating an ischemic-preconditioning environment;[32-34] and the facilitation of the assessment of organ function and viability after reperfusion.[25,31]

### Outcomes of Abdominal Organs Transplanted after NRP

A recent systematic review and metaanalyses showed that transplantation of uDCD livers and kidneys after NRP is associated with inferior graft and patient survival relative to DBD.[25] Some kidney registry analyses suggest NRP

decreases primary nonfunction and delayed graft function rates compared to RR in uDCD. No studies comparing NRP with RR in uDCD for the liver are reported, reflecting a hesitancy to transplant uDCD livers without some form of perfusion (in situ or ex situ).[25] While transplantation of uDCD liver and kidneys after NRP should not necessarily be avoided altogether, these organs should be used with caution, weighing risks of continued waiting against risks of utilising uDCD grafts, even with NRP.[25]

In cDCD, there is currently no evidence that NRP reduces risks of primary nonfunction or mortality after liver transplantation compared to RR, although metaanalyses suggest NRP leads to a significant reduction in overall biliary complications (eg, ischemic cholangiopathy by 75%, anastomotic strictures by 65%) compared to RR.[25]

In kidney transplantation, variable rates or primary nonfunction and delayed graft function are described. A direct comparison with RR in DCD suggests reduced delayed graft function with NRP.[35] There is no evidence that the risk of DGF after NRP is different compared to that in DBD kidney transplantation, while it is well-known that RR leads to higher DGF rates compared to DBD. Kidney graft survival rates with NRP appear good, but variable definitions

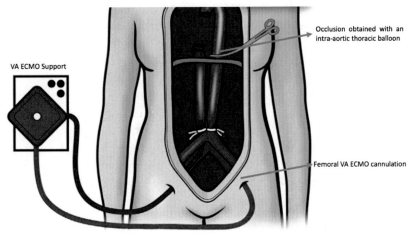

**Figure 45-1.** Schematic of Normothermic Regional Perfusion (NPR).

are used. Pancreas transplantation after NRP is feasible and safe, but large series have not been reported.[9, 24]

## Donation of Cardiac Grafts from cDCD

DCD is rapidly emerging as an important pathway to heart transplantation from adult deceased donors with the potential to increase total heart transplant activity by more than 20%.[36] Following the first report of successful distant retrieval and transplantation of three adult DCD hearts in 2014,[37] adult DCD heart transplant programs have commenced in the UK, Europe, Australia, and North America.[13,15,38] Recently, a preliminary report of the US multicenter DCD heart trial demonstrated improved 2-year survival of recipients of hearts from DCD donors compared to recipients of hearts from DBD donors.[38] While upper age limits for acceptance of DCD donors for heart transplantation vary between centers, in general the upper age limit has been lower than for DBD donors (typically restricted to those <50 years). This is due in part to the more limited ability to screen the DCD donor for preexisting heart disease and due to the concern regarding the susceptibility of the heart from the older donor to the obligatory period of warm ischemia that is intrinsic to the DCD pathway. An echocardiogram demonstrating normal biventricular and valve function prior to WLST is the major requirement.

### *Assessing Functional Warm Ischemia During Withdrawal of Life Support*

Preclinical studies suggest that provided the functional warm ischemia time (fWIT) is less than 30 minutes, the heart of the DCD donor is fully recoverable and transplantable.[39,40] However, whereas progression to circulatory death in these preclinical models is rapid and predictable, the time course of progression to circulatory arrest in human DCD donors is more variable.[41] In addition, although there is agreement that a sustained fall in systolic blood pressure below normal marks the onset of fWIT following WLST, there is ongoing debate as to what level of systolic blood pressure should be used, 90 or 50 mmHg.[41] In the US DCD Heart Trial, warm ischemic time was defined as time from when mean systolic blood pressure (SBP) was <50 mmHg or peripheral saturation <70% to aortic crossclamp and administration of cold cardioplegia in the donor.[38] Recently, Sanchez-Camara and colleagues from Spain performed serial endomyocardial biopsies in noncardiac human donors who underwent a DCD withdrawal protocol.[42] They reported that biomarkers of calcium homeostasis, mitochondrial function, and cellular viability remained unchanged up to the time of circulatory arrest and only began to become compromised 10 minutes after circulatory arrest.[42] These findings strongly suggest that the asystolic warm ischemic time (aWIT) (defined as the period between circulatory arrest and either administration of preservation flush solution or restoration of the circulation in situ discussed in the next section) is the critical interval in determining the extent of myocardial ischemic injury during WLST. The major clinical implication of this finding is that the location of WLST (ICU vs. anesthesia bay vs. operating table) is the major modifiable determinant of the duration of aWIT. In a systematic review of liver transplantation from DCD donors, Cao et al. reported that posttransplant survival was better and ischemic cholangiopathy was less when WLST occurred in the operating room compared with WLST in the ICU.[43] Similarly, an increase in the aWIT has been reported to be an independent predictor of primary nonfunction and graft failure after kidney transplantation from DCD donors.[44]

### Cardiac Graft Retrieval Protocols

Jurisdictional variations regarding the diagnosis of circulatory death and the interventions that are permitted before and after death have influenced the development of specific retrieval protocols (Table 45-2).[45]

Antemortem interventions including administration of heparin[43,46] and placement of guidewires or perfusion cannulas prior to WLST[15,47] reduce the risk of postmortem thrombosis and shorten the fWIT respectively but are not allowed in some jurisdictions. Where this is possible, death is only declared after the 'stand-off' period (time until a clinical status of death is reached). The mandated 'stand-off' time between circulatory arrest and commencement of retrieval surgery varies from 2 to 20 minutes and obviously has a major impact on fWIT. Finally, there is variation regarding what postmortem interventions are permitted, specifically re-establishment of the circulation in situ, which is prohibited in some jurisdictions. In jurisdictions that do not permit re-establishment of the circulation after death, direct procurement of the DCD heart followed by normothermic machine perfusion has been

| | ST VINCENT'S (Aus)[12] | PAPWORTH (UK)[13,14] | LIEGE (Belgium)[15,47] | VANDERBILT[16] |
|---|---|---|---|---|
| **Donor age group** | Adult < 55 years | Adult < 55 years | Adult and pediatric | Adult < 35 years |
| **Location of WLST** | ICU / Anesthesia bay | ICU or Anesthesia bay | Operating room | Not stated |
| **Ante-mortem interventions** | None | None | Heparin | Heparin |
| | | | Perfusion cannulas | |
| | | | TEE + Swan-Ganz | |
| **Sedation (Comfort care)** | Variable | Variable | Sevoflurane | Variable |
| **Death** | Circulatory arrest: 2–5 min | Circulatory arrest: >5 min | Arterial BP < 30 mmHg Circulatory arrest: > 5 min | Circulatory arrest: 2–5 min |
| **fWIT** | <30 min after SBP < 90mmHg | <30 min after SBP < 50 mmHg | Not Stated* | <35 min after SBP < 50mmHg |
| **Post-mortem interventions** | Cold flush (direct procurement) | NRP OR Cold flush | NRP | NRP |
| **Graft retrieval** | DP-NMP | DP-NMP, NRP-NMP for distant retrieval | NRP-SCS (co-located, or interhospital transfer) | NRP-SCS for distant retrieval |
| | | NRP-SCS (co-location) | | |

*Expected fWIT <30min; DP-NMP=Direct procurement followed by normothermic machine perfusion; fWIT=Functional warm ischemic time; ICU=Intensive care unit; NRP=Normothermic regional perfusion NRP-NMP=Normothermic regional perfusion followed by normothermic machine perfusion; NRP-SCS=Normothermic regional perfusion followed by static cold storage; SBP=Systolic blood pressure; TEE=Transesophageal echocardiogram; WLST=Withdrawal of life sustaining treatment.

**Table 45-2.** Current published DCD retrieval protocols for retrieval of the adult DCD heart highlighting variability between centers due to regional differences in legislation (adapted from Crespo-Leiro et al.[45])

the technique that has allowed successful transplantation of DCD hearts (Figure 45-2).[48,49]

In jurisdictions that permit reestablishment of the circulation after death, thoracoabdominal normothermic regional perfusion after isolation of the cerebral circulation has allowed resuscitation and functional assessment of the DCD heart in situ prior to retrieval and transplantation (Figure 45-2).[13,15,16,47] The procurement techniques are outlined below.

Direct procurement followed by ex situ normothermic machine perfusion: Following sternotomy, blood is rapidly drained from the right atrium via a large bore cannula into a collection bag containing heparin. More recently, tirofiban has been added to the collection bag to prevent platelet activation.[50] This blood is used to prime the ex situ perfusion circuit. Cold preservation solution is then administered, terminating the fWIT. The heart is excised and connected to the normothermic machine perfusion device (OCS, TransMedics, MA, USA), after which ex situ normothermic perfusion is commenced. Cardiac viability is assessed from a combination of perfusion and

metabolic parameters including myocardial lactate extraction.[41, 48]

In situ thoracoabdominal normothermic regional perfusion followed by machine perfusion or static cold storage: Following sternotomy and crossclamping of the head and neck vessels (sometimes in combination with either open or active drainage) to prevent recirculation to the brain, thoracoabdominal normothermic regional perfusion using ECMO is instituted.[13,51] The fWIT ends with the resumption of circulation with oxygenated blood via the ECMO circuit. Following a period of ECMO perfusion, the heart is weaned from support and its function assessed in situ. The Papworth group initially transported the DCD heart using the Transmedics OCS; however, they and more recently others have reported successful transport of DCD hearts using static cold storage.[14-16,46]

Whether one technique is better than the other remains to be adequately studied. If in situ reanimation followed by static cold storage demonstrates noninferior outcomes to direct procurement with ex situ normothermic

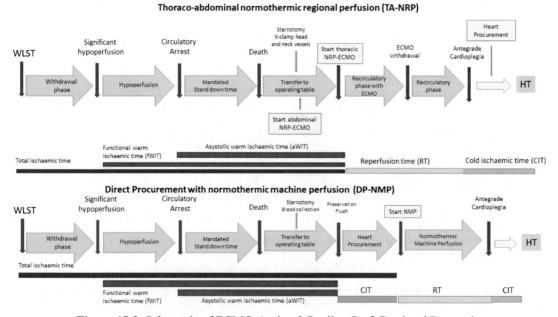

**Figure 45-2.** Schematic of ECMO-Assisted Cardiac Graft Retrieval Protocols.

perfusion, it may be preferred in jurisdictions that permit thoracoabdominal normothermic regional perfusion due to the ability to study the reanimated heart in situ and lower cost since the transport machine will not be required.

## Ethical and Legal Considerations in NRP DCD Donation

The processes of death determination and subsequent organ recovery should be guided by established protocols and uphold ethical and legal requirements. A recent Consensus Statement, drafted by a working group of the European Society of Organ Transplantation, details the minimal ethical, logistical, and technical requirements that form the foundation of a safe and effective NRP program.[31] As NRP is an integral part of DCD procedures, DCD ethical considerations apply, keeping in mind that compliance with national, professional, and institutional guidelines is essential and may further direct ethical discussions.[31,52-55]

It is fundamental that NRP procedures are in accordance with the DDR. As such, the definition of circulatory arrest and determination of death should be performed according to medical, professional, and national standards.[31,56-58] From an ethical viewpoint, the definition of death in DCD settings is generally accepted as the permanent rather than the irreversible cessation of circulation.[59-65] 'Permanent' means that no efforts are made to restart circulation and autoresuscitation is no longer possible. This point is commonly accepted to be achieved after 5 minutes of continuous apnea, circulatory loss, and unresponsiveness, but in some countries, legislation requires a longer observational period.[63]

In NRP-settings, 'permanent' has an additional dimension, since NRP restores circulation to a limited vascular region.[51] Brain reperfusion would negate permanence, and any NRP technique needs to ensure brain reperfusion does not occur.[66-68] Technical adaptations to the NRP procedure have been proposed,[51] but the debate on if and how to safeguard the criterion of cessation of circulation continues.[69] Transparent protocols, in accordance with the latest standards in medical care, are needed.[31]

## ECMO-assisted DBD Organ Donation

In addition to maintaining circulation after cardiac cessation in DCD, ECMO can also be used to support brain dead donors that have severe cardiac or pulmonary dysfunction, including cardiopulmonary arrest that occurs before the team is assembled to recover organs.[6] While this is an unusual indication for ECMO, it may allow organs to be recovered in a setting where recovery of viable organs would have been otherwise impossible. In this situation, the aortic occlusion balloon can be omitted to speed up placing the donor on ECMO since there is no need to avoid blood flow to the coronary and carotid arteries. In this case, it is important to note the following:

ECMO effect on drug pharmacokinetics:[70] Patients on ECMO have an increased volume of distribution, decreased drug metabolism, and decreased excretion secondary to multiorgan failure, which affects agents such as sedatives and neuromuscular blockers (Chapter 49). These factors may lead to residual drug effects and potential confounding if insufficient time or interventions (eg, dialysis) are provided for clearance. Therefore, extra time and the therapeutic drug monitoring may be required to exclude drug effects prior to determination of death in patients on ECMO. In addition, the use of antagonizing agents becomes an alternative when time is limited, or drug assays are not available. In case of a potential drug effect, any ancillary test must be performed in addition to clinical examination.

Apnea test on ECMO for brain death determination: ECMO rapidly and efficiently clears $CO_2$. Therefore, ECMO settings need to be modified to ensure adequate increase of $CO_2$ while maintaining normoxemia. This is achieved by decreasing the sweep gas flow to the membrane lung (ML); however, at very low flows hypoxemia and hypercapnia may occur without significant acidemia if the pH is normalized early in the process. In addition, patients on VA ECMO require special attention to the location of arterial blood gas sampling, since not all vascular sites necessarily reflect cerebral blood composition. The following interventions need to be considered to successfully perform an apnea test on ECMO:

- Collect baseline blood gases from both peripheral cannula and post-ML,
- Observe patient respiratory efforts (lower chest and abdomen) because any respiratory efforts preclude neurologic death,
- Set ML sweep gas $FsO_2$ to 1.0,
- Adjust ECMO blood flow to ensure $SpO_2$ >92% during apnea testing,
- Reduce sweep gas to 0.5-1 L/min to induce hypercapnia (adding 5% $CO_2$ may be required),
- Disconnect patient from the ventilator,
- After 5 min, obtain blood gases to ensure that $CO_2$ is rising and modify sweep gas flow or $CO_2$ concentration as needed,
- Repeat blood gases every 5-10 minutes until thresholds have been met ($PaCO_2$ >60 mmHg, rise in $PaCO_2$ >20 mmHg, pH <7.28),
- Once the apnea test is completed, return to baseline ECMO parameters.

**When Patients on ECMO Become Donors**

Finally, it is important to note that some patients on ECMO can become DBD or DCD donors. As mentioned previously, following specific protocols to maintain the legal and ethical definition of death is critical. If the ECMO patient meets DBD criteria after following the steps for the definition of death described above, it is our experience that ECMO

support continues in a classical way throughout the donor surgery. When the retrieval team is ready, cold organ flushing is started via the existent ECMO arterial cannula. If the ECMO patient meets criteria for DCD, then ECMO supports must be stopped during WLST to assure determination of circulatory death as previously described. Once death is determined, several approaches have been used: 1) a sterno laparotomy is performed and the descending aorta is clamped above the diaphragm followed by flushing of the abdominal organs via the ECMO cannulas; 2) placement of an intravascular balloon (thoracic aorta) via the femoral artery cannula or the femoral artery to avoid cerebral perfusion, then restarting ECMO during NRP until organ procurement, aiming to minimize fWIT; 3) a sternotomy or sterno laparotomy with clamping of the thoracic aorta is an alternative means before starting NRP.

# References

1.  https://www.elso.org/Registry/ InternationalSummaryandReports/ InternationalSummary.aspx Accessed: May 15th, 2022.
2.  (IOM) IOM. Organ Donation: Opportunities for Action. 2006 ed. Washington, D.C: The National Academies Press; 2006.
3.  2021 Annual Report of the U.S. Organ Procurement and Transplantation Network and the Scientific Registry of Transplant Recipients: Transplant Data 1994-2021. Department of Health and Human Services, Health Resources and Services Administration, Healthcare Systems Bureau, Division of Transplantation, Rockville, MD; United Network for Organ Sharing, Richmond, VA; University Renal Research and Education Association, Ann Arbor, MI.
4.  Valero R, Cabrer C, Oppenheimer F, et al. Normothermic recirculation reduces primary graft dysfunction of kidneys obtained from non-heart-beating donors. Transpl Int. 2000;13(4):303-10.
5.  Lee JH, Hong SY, Oh CK, et ak. Kidney transplantation from a donor following cardiac death supported with extracorporeal membrane oxygenation. J Korean Med Sci. 2012 Feb;27(2):115-9.
6.  Gravel MT, Arenas JD, Chenault R 2nd, et al. Kidney transplantation from organ donors following cardiopulmonary death using extracorporeal membrane oxygenation support. Ann Transplant. 2004;9(1):57-8.
7.  Rudich SM, Arenas JD, Magee JC, et al. Extracorporeal support of the non-heart-beating organ donor. Transplantation. 2002 Jan 15;73(1):158-9.
8.  Magliocca JF, Magee JC, Rowe SA, et al. Extracorporeal support for organ donation after cardiac death effectively expands the donor pool. J Trauma. 2005 Jun;58(6):1095-101; discussion 1101-2.
9.  Rojas-Peña A, Sall LE, Gravel MT, et al. Donation after circulatory determination of death: the university of michigan experience with extracorporeal support. Transplantation. 2014 Aug 15;98(3):328-34.
10. Ortega-Deballon I, Hornby L, Shemie SD. Protocols for uncontrolled donation after circulatory death: a systematic review of international guidelines, practices and transplant outcomes. Crit Care. 2015 Jun 24;19(1):268.
11. Scheuer SE, Jansz PC, Macdonald PS. Heart transplantation following donation after circulatory death: Expanding the donor pool. J Heart Lung Transplant. 2021 Sep;40(9):882-889. Epub 2021 Apr 8.
12. Chew HC, Iyer A, Connellan M, et al. Outcomes of Donation After Circulatory Death Heart Transplantation in Australia. J Am Coll Cardiol. 2019 Apr 2;73(12):1447-1459.
13. Messer SJ, Axell RG, Colah S, et al. Functional assessment and transplantation of the donor heart after circulatory death. J Heart Lung Transplant. 2016 Dec;35(12):1443-1452. Epub 2016 Jul 16.
14. Messer S, Page A, Colah S, et al. Human heart transplantation from donation after circulatory-determined death donors using normothermic regional perfusion and cold storage. J Heart Lung Transplant. 2018 Jul;37(7):865-869.
15. Tchana-Sato V, Ledoux D, Detry O, et al. Successful clinical transplantation of hearts donated after circulatory death using normothermic regional perfusion. J Heart Lung Transplant. 2019 Jun;38(6):593-598.
16. Hoffman JRH, McMaster WG, Rali AS, et al. Early US experience with cardiac donation after circulatory death (DCD) using normothermic regional perfusion. J Heart Lung Transplant. 2021 Nov;40(11):1408-1418. Epub 2021 Jul 10.
17. Kootstra G, Daemen JH, Oomen AP. Categories of non-heart-beating donors. Transplant Proc. 1995 Oct;27(5):2893-4.
18. Truog RD, Miller FG. The dead donor rule and organ transplantation. N Engl J Med. 2008 Aug 14;359(7):674-5.
19. National Conference of Commissioners on Uniform State Laws. Amendments to Uniform Brain Death Act, Uniform Determination of Death Act. [Chicago] :[The Conference], 1980.
20. Bartlett RH. Vitalin: the rationale for a hypothetical hormone. J Am Coll Surg. 2004 Aug;199(2):286-92.
21. Novitzky D, Cooper DK, Reichart B. Hemodynamic and metabolic responses to hormonal therapy in brain-dead potential organ donors. Transplantation. 1987 Jun;43(6):852-4.
22. A definition of irreversible coma. Report of the Ad Hoc Committee of the Harvard Medical School to Examine the Definition of Brain Death. JAMA. 1968 Aug 5;205(6):337-40.
23. Sung RS, Galloway J, Tuttle-Newhall JE, et al. Organ donation and utilization in the United States, 1997-2006. Am J Transplant. 2008 Apr;8(4 Pt 2):922-34.
24. Merion RM, Pelletier SJ, Goodrich N, et al. Donation after cardiac death as a strategy to increase deceased donor liver availability. Ann Surg. 2006 Oct;244(4):555-62.
25. De Beule J, Vandendriessche K, Pengel LHM, et al. A systematic review and meta-analyses of regional perfusion in donation after circulatory death solid organ transplantation. Transpl Int. 2021 Nov;34(11):2046-2060. Epub 2021 Oct 19.
26. Foss S, Nordheim E, Sørensen DW, et al. First Scandinavian Protocol for Controlled Donation After

Circulatory Death Using Normothermic Regional Perfusion. Transplant Direct. 2018 Jun 13;4(7):e366.

27. Summers DM, Watson CJ, Pettigrew GJ, et al. Kidney donation after circulatory death (DCD): state of the art. Kidney Int. 2015 Aug;88(2):241-9. Epub 2015 Mar 18.

28. Tang JX, Na N, Li JJ, et al. Outcomes of Controlled Donation After Cardiac Death Compared With Donation After Brain Death in Liver Transplantation: A Systematic Review and Meta-analysis. Transplant Proc. 2018 Jan-Feb;50(1):33-41.

29. Smith M, Dominguez-Gil B, Greer DM, et al. Organ donation after circulatory death: current status and future potential. Intensive Care Med. 2019 Mar;45(3):310-321. Epub 2019 Feb 6.

30. Sánchez-Fructuoso AI, Prats D, Torrente J, et al. Renal transplantation from non-heart beating donors: a promising alternative to enlarge the donor pool. J Am Soc Nephrol. 2000 Feb;11(2):350-358.

31. Jochmans I, Hessheimer AJ, Neyrinck AP, et al. Consensus statement on normothermic regional perfusion in donation after circulatory death: Report from the European Society for Organ Transplantation's Transplant Learning Journey. Transpl Int. 2021 Nov;34(11):2019-2030.

32. Amador A, Grande L, Martí J, et al. Ischemic pre-conditioning in deceased donor liver transplantation: a prospective randomized clinical trial. Am J Transplant. 2007 Sep;7(9):2180-9.

33. Net M, Valero R, Almenara R, et al. The effect of normothermic recirculation is mediated by ischemic preconditioning in NHBD liver transplantation. Am J Transplant. 2005 Oct;5(10):2385-92.

34. García-Valdecasas JC, Tabet J, Valero R, et al. Liver conditioning after cardiac arrest: the use of normothermic recirculation in an experimental animal model. Transpl Int. 1998;11(6):424-32.

35. Padilla M, Coll E, Fernández-Pérez C, et al. Improved short-term outcomes of kidney transplants in controlled donation after the circulatory determination of death with the use of normothermic regional perfusion. Am J Transplant. 2021 Nov;21(11):3618-3628.

36. Suarez-Pierre A, Iguidbashian J, Stuart C, et al. Appraisal of Donation After Circulatory Death: How Far Could We Expand the Heart Donor Pool? Ann Thorac Surg. 2022 Feb 17:S0003-4975(22)00197-7.

37. Dhital KK, Iyer A, Connellan M, et al. Adult heart transplantation with distant procurement and ex-vivo preservation of donor hearts after circulatory death: a case series. Lancet. 2015 Jun 27;385(9987):2585-91.

38. J.N. Schroder, A. Shah, V. Pretorius, et al. Expanding Heart Transplants from Donors After Circulatory Death (DCD) - Results of the First Randomized Controlled Trial Using the Organ Care System (OCS™) Heart - (OCS DCD Heart Trial). The Journal of Heart and Lung Transplantation 2022;41(4):Supplement Page S72. SSN 1053-2498.

39. Iyer A, Gao L, Doyle A, et al. Increasing the tolerance of DCD hearts to warm ischemia by pharmacological postconditioning. Am J Transplant. 2014 Aug;14(8):1744-52.

40. White CW, Lillico R, Sandha J, et al. Physiologic Changes in the Heart Following Cessation of Mechanical Ventilation in a Porcine Model of Donation After Circulatory Death: Implications for Cardiac Transplantation. Am J Transplant. 2016 Mar;16(3):783-93.

41. Scheuer SE, Jansz PC, Macdonald PS. Heart transplantation following donation after circulatory death: Expanding the donor pool. J Heart Lung Transplant. 2021 Sep;40(9):882-889.

42. Sánchez-Cámara S, Asensio-López MC, Royo-Villanova M, et al. Critical warm ischemia time point for cardiac donation after circulatory death. Am J Transplant. 2022 May;22(5):1321-1328.

43. Cao Y, Shahrestani S, Chew HC, et al. Donation After Circulatory Death for Liver Transplantation: A Meta-Analysis on the Location of Life Support Withdrawal Affecting Outcomes. Transplantation. 2016 Jul;100(7):1513-24.

44. Heylen L, Jochmans I, Samuel U, et al. The duration of asystolic ischemia determines the risk of graft failure after circulatory-dead donor kidney transplantation: A Eurotransplant cohort study. Am J Transplant. 2018 Apr;18(4):881-889.

45. Crespo-Leiro MG, Costanzo MR, et al. Heart transplantation: focus on donor recovery strategies, left ventricular assist devices, and novel therapies. Eur Heart J. 2022 Jun 14;43(23):2237-2246.

46. Gao L, Doyle A, Villanueva J, et al. Enhanced functional recovery of the heart donated after circulatory death determination with antemortem heparin. J Heart Lung Transplant. 2020 Jun;39(6):607-609.

47. Vandendriessche K, Tchana-Sato V, Ledoux D, et al. Transplantation of donor hearts after circulatory death using normothermic regional perfusion and cold storage preservation. Eur J Cardiothorac Surg. 2021 Oct 22;60(4):813-819.

48. Chew HC, Iyer A, Connellan M, et a. Outcomes of Donation After Circulatory Death Heart Transplantation in Australia. J Am Coll Cardiol. 2019 Apr 2;73(12):1447-1459.

49. Messer S, Cernic S, Page A, et al. A 5-year single-center early experience of heart transplantation from donation after circulatory-determined death donors. J Heart Lung Transplant. 2020 Dec;39(12):1463-1475.

50. Scheuer SE, Soto C, Joseph J, et al. Platelet activation after withdrawal of life support in donation after

circulatory death donors. J Heart Lung Transplant. 2020;39(12):1494-6.

51. Manara A, Shemie SD, Large S, et al. Maintaining the permanence principle for death during in situ normothermic regional perfusion for donation after circulatory death organ recovery: A United Kingdom and Canadian proposal. Am J Transplant. 2020 Aug;20(8):2017-2025.

52. Domínguez-Gil B, Ascher N, Capron AM, et al. Expanding controlled donation after the circulatory determination of death: statement from an international collaborative. Intensive Care Med. 2021 Mar;47(3):265-281.

53. Haase B, Bos M, Boffa C, et al. Ethical, legal, and societal issues and recommendations for controlled and uncontrolled DCD. Transpl Int. 2016 Jul;29(7):771-9. Epub 2016 Jan 13.

54. Saemann L, Karck M, Korkmaz-Icöz S, et al. Ethical Decision Diagrams on Donation After Cardiocirculatory Death Heart Transplantation Considering Organ Preservation Techniques. Transplant Direct. 2020 Oct 19;6(11):e617.

55. Jericho BG. Organ Donation After Circulatory Death: Ethical Issues and International Practices. Anesth Analg. 2019 Feb;128(2):280-285.

56. Dhanani S, Hornby L, Ward R, Shemie S. Variability in the determination of death after cardiac arrest: a review of guidelines and statements. J Intensive Care Med. 2012 Jul-Aug;27(4):238-52.

57. Othman MH, Dutta A, Kondziella D. Public opinion and legislations related to brain death, circulatory death and organ donation. J Neurol Sci. 2020 Jun 15;413:116800.

58. Shemie SD. Clarifying the paradigm for the ethics of donation and transplantation: was 'dead' really so clear before organ donation? Philos Ethics Humanit Med. 2007 Aug 24;2:18.

59. McGee A, Gardiner D. Permanence can be Defended. Bioethics. 2017 Mar;31(3):220-230. Epub 2016 Dec 28.

60. White FJ 3rd. Controversy in the Determination of Death: The Definition and Moment of Death. Linacre Q. 2019 Nov;86(4):366-380.

61. Bernat JL. Conceptual Issues in DCDD Donor Death Determination. Hastings Cent Rep. 2018 Nov;48 Suppl 4:S26-S28.

62. Bos MA. Ethical and legal issues in non-heart-beating organ donation. Transplant Proc. 2005 Mar;37(2):574-6.

63. Dhanani S, Hornby L, van Beinum A, et al. Resumption of Cardiac Activity after Withdrawal of Life-Sustaining Measures. N Engl J Med. 2021 Jan 28;384(4):345-352. PMID: 33503343.

64. Gardiner D, Shemie S, Manara A, Opdam H. International perspective on the diagnosis of death. Br J Anaesth. 2012 Jan;108 Suppl 1:i14-28.

65. Dalle Ave AL, Gardiner D, Shaw DM. Cardio-pulmonary resuscitation of brain-dead organ donors: a literature review and suggestions for practice. Transpl Int. 2016 Jan;29(1):12-9.

66. Shapey IM, Summers A, Augustine T, et al. Systematic review to assess the possibility of return of cerebral and cardiac activity after normothermic regional perfusion for donors after circulatory death. Br J Surg. 2019 Feb;106(3):174-180.

67. Bernat JL, Capron AM, Bleck TP, et al. The circulatory-respiratory determination of death in organ donation. Crit Care Med. 2010 Mar;38(3):963-70.

68. Perez-Villares JM, Rubio JJ, Del Río F, et al. Validation of a new proposal to avoid donor resuscitation in controlled donation after circulatory death with normothermic regional perfusion. Resuscitation. 2017 Aug;117:46-49.

69. Entwistle JW, Drake DH, Fenton KN, et al. Normothermic regional perfusion: Ethical issues in thoracic organ donation. J Thorac Cardiovasc Surg. 2022 Jul;164(1):147-154.

70. Ha MA, Sieg AC. Evaluation of altered drug pharmacokinetics in critically ill adults receiving extracorporeal membrane oxygenation. Pharmacotherapy 2017; 37: 221-35.

# 46

## Transport

*David Zonies, Cara Agerstrand, Erin August, Mackenzie R. Cook, Bernadette S. Elliott, Ahmed Labib, Demetris Yannopoulos*

### History

Transport of patients supported with ECLS dates to the 1970s when Dr. Robert Bartlett and colleagues described the interhospital transport of two pediatric patients.[1] In the decades that followed, both ground and air transport of ECLS-supported patients has been utilized by select centers globally, with the bulk of early experience originating from several medical centers in the United States, Sweden, France, Germany, and Taiwan.[2-11] Neonates, pediatric, and adult patients receiving ECLS for both respiratory and cardiac support have been successfully transported, with survival outcomes comparable to the ELSO Registry and patients not requiring interinstitutional ECLS transport.[4,8,9,12,13]

As ECLS has become increasingly incorporated into management strategies for patients with severe cardiopulmonary failure and ECLS equipment has become more compact, lightweight, and mobile, the number of centers conducting ECLS transport has increased. The influenza A (H1N1) pandemic of 2009 and the coronavirus disease 2019 (COVID-19) pandemic have further promoted the expansion of ECLS transport, with the establishment of regional and national referral networks and the goal of increasing access to

ECLS and improving outcomes for the most critically ill patients.[13-15]

### Outcomes of Transport

Transport of critically ill patients on multiorgan support presents unique challenges and can be associated with morbidity and mortality. To address this issue, professional organizations, including ELSO, have issued specific guidance for transportation of the critically ill patient.[16] A dedicated transport team utilizing specialized equipment improves quality of transport of extremely sick patients with cardiorespiratory failure.[17,18] Outcomes of transport on ECLS can be described in terms of safety and efficacy. Several single-center reports spanning the last two decades suggest transport on ECLS is safe and feasible.[4,7]

Recent multicenter systematic reviews offer the advantage of large sample size, varying transport platforms, team composition, and cannulation protocols while still demonstrating infrequent complications and very rare transport-associated fatalities. Javidfar demonstrated a "safe mobile ECLS culture" after reviewing 110 mobile ECLS missions during the peak of COVID-19.[19] Good clinical outcomes after transport have been widely described. Interestingly, outcome is occasionally better in those patients who have ECLS implantation at a referring facility, often perceived to be a less familiar and potentially less equipped environment.[20,21]

**Transport System Models of Care**

Patients who are cannulated at a referral hospital by the ECLS transport team and subsequently returned to the ECLS center are referred to as a primary transport. Patients who are successfully placed on ECLS at an outside hospital and then transferred by a transport team are referred to secondary ECLS transport. In addition to traditional primary and secondary ECLS transport, patients with ECLS may be transported between hospitals (interhospital) or within the same center for therapeutic and/or diagnostic purposes (intrahospital). The overriding priority at all times is patient and medical personnel safety. Whatever the indication, distance or duration of transport, the same principles and preparation must be followed. Logistics of transportation can be categorized under the following: equipment (essential and optional), manpower, and platform.

The most common indication for transporting a patient supported with ECLS is the need to move a patient from a center that does not provide ECLS, or which does not have the means to provide care beyond initiation of ECLS to an established ECLS center. Mobile ECLS services available 24/7 are needed to provide effective logistics and reliable infrastructure for patient safety.[22] ELSO has assisted in providing foundations and resources to ECLS transport centers, as well as centers looking for ECLS support by means of ELSO transport guidelines and the ELSO website member directory.

Transport mode, team composition, required life support devices, and patient weight can all limit patient movement options. A larger team can be transported by ground because it is the least restrictive. Flight options will be limited by space and weight, with rotor wing being the most restrictive. It is critical for the team to understand these limitations when decisions are made. Current ELSO transport guidelines recommend ground transport up to 400km (250-300 miles), rotor wing for distances up to 650km (300-400 miles), and fixed wing for further distances. It is also important to remember that with fixed wing transport, additional ground transport will be required.

The most established transport system is one that uses a hub (the ECLS center) and spoke hospital model. The hub ECLS center is typically a quaternary cardiopulmonary care center. Spoke hospitals can widely vary depending on the resources available. Care agreements for receiving patients after ECLS has been removed are in many cases necessary due to the ICU bed constraints in most large centers. Those agreements need to be in place for smooth operations and collaboration to be successful.

**Transport Team Composition**

ECLS transport team composition is based on various factors, including whether patients are initially placed on support by the team (primary transport), already on support (secondary transport), and overall team expertise. Safety is the key to a successful transport, whether the ECLS center has a hospital-based team, partnership with a transport service, or uses a third party. Common team compositions include any of the following: surgeon, intensivist, operating room nurse, operating room technician, perfusionist, ECLS specialist (RN), respiratory therapist, and ICU RN. Space and weight restrictions on aircraft or an ambulance will influence these options. The minimum required personnel include a cannulator with ECLS experience (eg, surgeon/intensivist) and ECLS specialist (eg, ECLS trained nurse or respiratory therapist). If using a third party, it is recommended to verify a cannulating physician's credentials and privileges. In the United States, this may

```
┌─────────────────────────────────────┐
│  ☐  Referral intake form completed   │
│                                      │
│  ☐  Criteria met to accept (2 physi- │
│     cian agreement)                  │
│                                      │
│  ☐  Activation declared and commu-   │
│     nicated to referring and transfer│
│                                      │
│  ☐  Ground/Flight Service activated  │
│                                      │
│  ☐  Equipment checklist verified     │
│                                      │
│  ☐  Emergency Privileges obtained    │
│     at referring facility (sent emer-│
│     gency packet)                    │
│                                      │
│  ☐  Pre-arrival equipment/supplies   │
│     sent to referring                │
│                                      │
│  ☐  Patient re-assessed and deter-   │
│     mined to remain candidate?       │
│                                      │
│  ☐  Patient devices secured prior to │
│     transport                        │
│                                      │
│  ☐  Leave ECMO documentation         │
│     with families                    │
│                                      │
│  ☐  Obtain family contact informa-   │
│     tion for updates                 │
│                                      │
│  ☐  Notify receiving facility of     │
│     estimated arrival time and any   │
│     special equipment needs          │
└─────────────────────────────────────┘
```

**Figure 46-1.** Example transport team checklist.

vary based on the state you are in or look to transport from.

Team members may be exchanged or omitted based on partnerships with EMS/flight teams who have flight RNs and paramedics as required for modality safety standards of all crew members on board. In many cases, the flight team (nurse/paramedic) complements the ECLS team and can manage the ventilator and infusion pumps, permitting the ECLS team to focus on ECLS specific tasks.[23] In a high-stakes environment, procedural checklists, team pauses (eg, "time-outs") are essential to ensure high quality care (Figure 46-1). It is highly recommended to be as regimented as possible when mobile.[3,24]

## Indications and Contraindications for Mobile Transport

The utilization of a mobile ECLS team to facilitate initiation of ECLS for patients in need can be broadly implemented within healthcare systems that have shared care agreements and established collaborations. Once communications are established between the referring center, the ECLS center and the accepting ECLS critical care physician, a decision of whether a patient needs to be transferred for ECLS cannulation at the accepting facility or a team needs to be dispatched to initiate ECLS support followed by transport needs to be made. For those decisions to be made efficiently, institutional and interprofessional trust needs to be established in order to optimize care and outcomes for individual patients.

The main variable for the decision and timing to transfer a patient with or without ECLS support is their overall severity of illness and prediction of clinical deterioration with high risk of death without ECLS. Along with clinical indications, transport complexities such as mode (air vs. ground), weather, traffic and team expertise are equally important.

The decision whether to send a team to cannulate or not depends on the indications. In general, pulmonary ECLS support for most causes can be initiated after transporting the patient to the receiving ECLS center. These patients are partially supported with ventilatory strategies that allow for some period with adequate support. The same is true for patients that are slowly progressing with cardiopulmonary failure needing ECLS support if they are identified early. Patients with severe cardiogenic shock and cardiac arrest are in general supported first with ECLS and subsequently transferred due to the unpredictability of their clinical course. In those patients, death can be imminent with complex arrhythmias and circulatory and respiratory collapse that cannot be effectively treated enroute with standard less invasive therapies.

When selecting patients for mobile ECLS, the most common contraindications are those discussed elsewhere in this book for ECLS support. Clinical contraindications may be evident prior to transport dispatch, and it is also possible that between the time of dispatch and team arrival at the referring hospital, there is sufficient clinical change such that ECLS support is no longer appropriate. The ECLS transport team must possess sufficient expertise to recognize this clinical change and communicate compassionately and effectively with the referring team and the patient's family. An important consideration in mobile ECLS support is that some patients, if they were physically located at the receiving institution, would not require ECLS support but are too unstable for transport to the receiving facility without ECLS.[25,26]

The decision to activate a mobile ECLS team should also include the physical and human resources of the receiving institution. These patients can be incredibly resource-intensive and lack of available resources to care for them is an increasingly common problem in the COVID-19 era.[27] Physical and human resource contraindications may be partially mitigated with proactive sharing of regional resources among a number of ECLS capable centers.[28,29]

An additional contraindication that must be considered in mobile ECLS is the availability of a safe transport solution. While often not directly the purview of the clinical team, close coordination with transport logistics and an understanding of available transport options is essential. The pilots, drivers, transport nurses, and technicians represent equal stakeholders who may risk violation of duty hours, crew rest, and expertise in particular airframes that can accommodate the patient. A close relationship with the logistical partner of the ECLS transport team can help predict and mitigate these barriers and it behooves the mobile ECLS team to recall that safety in the air and on the road should always be the team's primary concern.

**Mobile Transport Equipment**

Equipment should be standardized with few optional aspects only based on specific limitations. For example, a nonessential item may be excluded based on the particular case, weight restrictions, distance, and team composition. Minimal requirements include a pump, circuit power cables, cannulas, and ancillary supplies required for ECLS cannulation and emergencies (Figure 46-2a,b). Assuming the flight service supplies standard ACLS equipment, devices including a monitor, defibrillator, ventilator, infusion pumps, portable ultrasound, circuit device warmer, near-infrared spectroscopy or alternate perfusion monitoring may not be required from the ECLS team. Redundancy should be carefully considered for essential items to prevent transport failures and mitigate emergencies in the event of malfunction.

Most transports will occur with a local EMS agency (air or ground). Initial and ongoing cross training is essential for a highly reliable team. For flight operations, most services require annual flight safety updates. This also gives a good opportunity for the ECLS team to become more comfortable with equipment and resource locations. Specifically, teams should become familiar with vehicle configuration, power and oxygen capacities, and weight limitations for aircraft. Ground vehicles often provide larger working areas and team comfort, at the cost

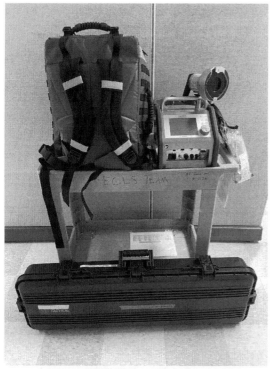

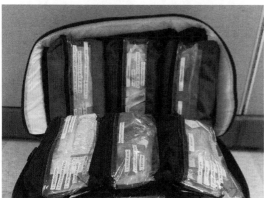

**Figure 46-2.** a) ECMO transport equipment. Backpack with supplies, cannula carrying case, ECMO pump, and ECMO circuit; b) Multicompartment ECMO backpack for transport.

of time in transit. Aircraft afford faster travel, but at the cost of space and weight capabilities. Fixed wing transport incurs additional loading and unloading risks, as well as additional patient movements.

**Team Training**

Team training and provider education for a successful mobile ECLS program should be designed around avoiding common complications, preparing for known challenges, and creating a team capable of managing unforeseen events (Chapter 54). Building a mobile capability into an established ECLS program that provides in situ ECLS support allows the nascent transport program to draw upon significant institutional experience.[28] If possible, this is the preferred approach rather than creating a de novo transport program.

While there are no established standards for mobile ECLS team composition, in order to meet these challenges, the mobile ECLS team members should be among the most experienced in the group.[7,30,31] Experience with cannulation and initiation as well as clinical management and troubleshooting gained at the bedside in the home institution is invaluable when on a mobile ECLS run. Specific credentialing may be considered for physicians to provide mobile ECLS care.

A standardized approach to mobile ECLS eases the cognitive load upon transport team members. Development and implementation of institutional checklists and clinical practice guidelines is advisable. The ELSO guidelines on safe ECLS transport include examples of checklists to be run prior to departure for transport to and from the referring hospital.[25]

When training the team, it is important to consider that cannulation will frequently occur at the bedside in the referring ICU with limited or no access to fluoroscopy. A dual-site cannulation approach for VV ECMO, with sonographic confirmation of guidewire positioning and cannula position supported by plain radiography may be the most versatile, and therefore preferred, strategy.[3,22,28,32,33] Cross training of nurses and ECLS specialists to assist with cannulation may also allow for smaller transport teams, potentially improving

response time and extending the practical range for mobile ECLS retrieval.

Particularly when growing a transport program, institutional and individual experience with mobile ECLS can be rapidly expanded by bringing extra team members on transports as observers.[28] It is advisable to only add members

### Patient Information Form (ECMO Referral)

- Patient location (Hospital, City, State, Unit/Bed #):

- Requesting provider:

- Call back phone number:

- Is family aware of potential for ECMO? Yes/No (circle one)

- Consent/assent obtained, by whom?

- Admission diagnosis:

- Mode of ECMO Support:

- Brief patient history (working diagnosis, past medical history, reason for ECMO, etc.):
_____
_____
_____

| |
|---|
| Date/Time: |
| Patient Name: |
| Patient Health Number: |
| DOB: |
| Admission date: |

| |
|---|
| Flu positive? Yes/No (circle one) |
| Viral panel: |
| COVID-19? Yes/No (circle one) |

Current and admission weight:
Height:
Chronic renal failure? Yes/No (circle one)
Dialysis? Yes/No (circle one)
Acute renal failure? Yes/No (circle one)
Active bleeding? Yes/No (circle one)          If yes, where?
Requiring transfusion Yes/No (circle one)
Current continuous medications:
Current neurological status:

| |
|---|
| Cardiac arrest this admission? Yes/No (circle one) |
| Trauma? Yes/No (circle one) |
| Surgery/type/date: |

**Latest laboratory results**

| | | | |
|---|---|---|---|
| WBC: | Na: | ALT: | INR: |
| HGB: | K: | AST: | PT: |
| Platelets: | Urea | Total bilirubin: | APTT: |
| Fibrinogen: | Creatinine: | Albumin: | Glucose: |
| Lactate: | $HCO_3$: | LDH: | Pregnancy test: |
| Procalcitonin: | Blood type: | *(please have 2 units PRBC available.)* | |

**Latest ABG**
pH:
$pCO_2$:
$pO_2$:
Base excess:

**Chest X-Ray**
Findings:

| Latest Vitals | Ventilator settings | I/O status |
|---|---|---|
| HR: | Date of intubation: | Last 24 hours |
| ABP: | Mode: | |
| Resp: | $FiO_2$: | Since admission: |
| $SpO_2$: | PEEP: | |
| Temp: | When was the $FiO_2$ last < 60%? | Nutrition: |

**ECHO**
Ejection fraction:
Aortic Valve status:          Mitral Valve status:          Pericardial effusion? Yes/No (circle one)
CT Head:          CT Chest/Abdomen:

ELSO Clinical Intake Form: ECMO Referral for Transport

**Figure 46-3.** ECMO referral intake form.

with prior ECLS experience to the mobile team, to allow them to build upon baseline knowledge and skills as they adapt to the challenged of mobile ECLS. Routine case reviews should be undertaken by the whole mobile ECLS group (regardless of the presence or absence of complications) to accelerate knowledge acquisition, spur process improvement, support team learning, and speed the onboarding of new members.[28,34]

High fidelity simulations with group debriefs likely have a similarly important role in building, maintaining, and expanding an effective mobile ECLS team. Well-constructed high fidelity simulation events will help experienced and new team members develop, test, and implement the behaviors and skills necessary to respond to the challenges of an ECLS transport.[28,34-38] In a high functioning system, complications and challenges identified during debriefings can be added into the high-fidelity simulation events to improve future team performance.

**Transport Considerations**

Receiving referrals should be a streamlined process for efficiency with standardized criteria and intake data collected for decision making of acceptance or declination for candidate patients (Figure 46-3). Gathering candidate information from more than one source of the referring team can save valuable hours of travel to a patient who is not a candidate for ECLS but was accepted without a comprehensive understanding of status and comorbidities. The type of support should be determined from the outset so all key stakeholders participate in the referral (eg, VA ECMO may require a shock team or cardiac surgeon; VV ECMO may require an intensivist). Best practice includes a detailed discussion on a recorded transfer center phone line whether the patient is accepted or declined. Multifactorial considerations are made for each accepted transport, to include

resource allocation, physiologic status, unit census, facility, and team capacity. The decision of acceptance or declination often requires concurrence of two or more providers to ensure patient selection consistency. Once a patient is accepted, best practice also includes sending the referral center a document outlining expectations and necessary standard equipment that should be available at bedside prior to the team's arrival (Figure 46-4). This document can include the availability of consenting persons for transport, the team responsible for obtaining consent and contact persons for questions or issues incurred as the transport team is advancing. Most important for providers is the need for emergency privileges. This is usually requested through an on-call administrator with delegated authority of the hospital medical executive board or the chief medical officer. If the team is crossing state or provincial lines, specific state licensure may be required for both providers and nurses.

Next, the transport team will communicate with the transport service to verify mode of transport based on availability and projected timeline. This should also be communicated to the referring center with as much lead time as possible. Another best practice is to have basic reading material available to be left with family or medical decision makers to understand what ECLS entails. This literature is helpful as the family will process the information on varied timelines.

Once the patient is assessed at the bedside, updates are provided by the referring team, and the decision is finalized to proceed with ECLS, consent should be obtained. Transport team members will perform the duties within their roles to ensure cannulation equipment is prepared and the circuit is primed and ready for initiation. Cannulation should not be performed until all emergency equipment and cannulation equipment are prepared and readily available. Postcannulation care should include securement of all tubes and lines for movement, transfer to the transport gurney or sled, transition of all monitors, ventilator, and infusions to the transport team equipment with reassessment of patient status throughout (Figure 46-5).

Prior to departure, the team should permit the family to see the patient if possible. The receiving team should be notified and updated with patient status and estimated time of arrival. Documentation of the cannulation and transport status throughout should maintain facility requirements for post procedure patients and unstable critical care patients until settled in the ICU (Figure 46-6).

**ECMO TRANSPORT**

Thank you for your patient referral and the opportunity to serve your patient's needs.

**What to expect:**

Our team will initiate ECMO at the patient bedside. Cannulas are inserted percutaneously via Seldinger technique. For veno-venous (VV) ECMO, we will use a femoral vein and an internal jugular vein or the bilateral femoral veins. For veno-arterial (VA) ECMO, we will transition the patient to our ECMO circuit.

Once ECMO is initiated, support will be titrated to the patient's pulmonary and cardiac needs. Once stable on ECMO, we will begin preparation for transport back to OHSU. However, if there are complications or ongoing instability, we may remain at your facility for a few hours before departing.

**Please address the following tasks to expedite ECMO initiation.**

**Administrative:**
☐ Consent: Have the patient's legal surrogate present or available by phone for consent.
Ensure the patient's family knows that their loved one is being considered for ECMO and that our team will reach out to them for consent. We will provide an overview of ECMO including a discussion regarding risks and benefits.
☐ Emergency Credentialing: Provide our physician with contact information and email of credentialing office, administrator on call, or chief medical officer to request emergency privileges. We will send a privilege packet over for review and approval.
☐ Medical Records: Have patient chart and medical records available (including H&P and most recent notes, labs, and imaging).

**Patient Preparation:**
☐ Reverse coagulopathy ensuring hemoglobin >7.0 g/dL, platelets > 100K, and INR < 2.0.
☐ Ensure an arterial line is in place.
☐ Place and verify central lines for medications if not already in place.
☐ Current labs available:
      ☐ Current Type and Screen
      ☐ CBC
      ☐ Coagulation panel
      ☐ ABG

**ICU Preparation:**
☐ Clear room of non-essential equipment.
☐ Clear a space behind the head of the patient placing the ventilator and all pumps to one side.
☐ Have ultrasound machine and two bedside tables in the room.
☐ Have one bedside table outside the room.
☐ Have crash cart with defibrillator outside the room.
☐ Have a norepinephrine infusion available.
☐ Have one liter crystalloid bolus primed and in a pressure bag inside room
☐ Four units of PRBC/FFP *prepared and ready*, but do not need to have at bedside.

**Personnel:**
☐ Please have someone to meet the ECMO team on arrival and escort them to the patient.

We will bring personnel and equipment to place the ECMO cannulas and operate the pump. We will rely on your facility for bedside nursing, respiratory therapy, radiology, and other support.

*Referring Checklist ECMO, Rev. Dec, 2021*

**Figure 46-4.** Prearrival checklist provided to referring institution.

The ECLS team should communicate their needs with the transporting crew to plug equipment into either an ambulance or aircraft power supply. This assures that power requirements are met, and fire risk is minimized. Power inverters or transformers on ground or air transport in the USA are usually supplied to convert current from 115V/400 Hz to 60 Hz standard power. Specific to air medical transport, ECLS equipment and monitors should be verified to be compliant via airworthiness certification. This provides a measure of safety for both the aircrew, team, and patient. The ECLS team must verify that equipment does not generate radio interference with any aircraft navigation or communication systems. Finally, power requirements must be verified, especially as some peripheral ECLS equipment can draw significant power (eg, high amperage heater-cooler devices). Having a datasheet with all equipment listing power requirements (voltage and amperage) readily available will assist the transport team.

Oxygen capacity is a critical issue during ECLS transport. In most cases, sufficient oxygen supply is available from on-board medical aircraft or ambulances. However, one must be prepared for unexpected delays (eg, patient, weather, etc.) and have an understanding of oxygen consumption and cylinder capacity for both the ECLS circuit and ventilator. Simple calculators are available on-line to make such calculations once the team knows the types of oxygen cylinders, transport time estimation, and flow rates. It is imperative to verify that cylinders are fully charged with enough capacity for 150-200% requirements.[39] If the transport crosses international borders, ensure that the correct electrical and gas adapters are carried.

## Special Physiologic Concerns during Transport

Transport transitions add additional risk to the ECLS patient. Transfer between the facility and ambulance, ambulance to ambulance, and ambulance to aircraft puts patients at risk of hypothermia, especially in colder climes and in small children. Hypothermia can lead to coagulopathy and may be associated with worse clinical outcomes. Significant effort should be made to assure both external (blankets) and central warming (heating bath) adjuncts when available for adults, children, and neonates.

Additional stressors of flight exist during ascent and descent. The team should be aware of the effects of acceleration and deceleration during critical moments of flight which may contribute to temporary venous insufficiency to the circuit and pump. As previously mentioned, the risk of hypothermia increases with increased altitude and should be closely monitored. Similarly, during long distance transport, insensible fluid losses increase due to lower humidity and partial gas pressure at altitude. Similarly, based on Boyle's law, gas volume will

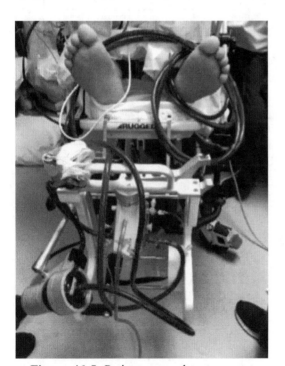

**Figure 46-5.** Patient secured to transport stretcher with ECMO pump. Tubing should be long enough to maneuver around the patient.

expand at altitude so gas filled spaces should be decompressed for safety. This includes gastric decompression if not already completed. Although Dalton's law stipulates a more hypoxic environment with increasing altitude, it is negligible for patients on ECLS support at typical 5000-8000' cabin altitude pressure.

## Mobile ECLS Complications

The technical, hemorrhagic, thrombotic, and infectious complications associated with ECLS cannulation and long-term support do not appear to be significantly different in patients who have ECLS initiated prior to or after transport and are addressed elsewhere

| ECMO INITIATION/TRANSPORT RECORD | | | | | | | | | |
|---|---|---|---|---|---|---|---|---|---|
| **DATE** | | | | | PATIENT STICKER | | | | |
| **ECMO MD** | | Name | | | | | | | |
| **ECMO RN** | | OHSU MRN | | | | | | | |
| **LF RN** | | DOB | | | | | | | |
| **Referring** | | VA ECMO | ☐ | | | | | | |
| | | VV ECMO | ☐ | | Sex: | Age: | Height: | Wt: | |
| Times | | Console Name | | | Allergies: | | | | |
| Referring Arrival | | Drainage Cannula | | | Diagnosis | | | | |
| Procedure Start | | Insertion Location | | | Pt. History | | | | |
| ECMO Initiation | | Size | | | | | | | |
| Procedure End | | Return Cannula | | | | | | | |
| Transport Start | | Insertion Location | | | | | | | |
| OHSU Arrival | | Size | | | | | | | |

**ELSO Required Data**

| | | | | | | | | |
|---|---|---|---|---|---|---|---|---|
| Pre-ECMO (circle): | CRRT/HD | inhaled epo | nitric oxide | proned (# hrs_____) | | plasmapheresis | | |
| Pre-ECMO (circle): | alprostadil | bicarb (IV) | epoprostenol (SQ) | NMB > 6 hrs | sildenafil | systemic steroids | THAM | |
| Vasoactive Meds: | epi | norepi | vaso | milrinone dobutamine | other: | | | |
| Pre-ECMO VS: | SBP: | DBP: | MAP: | SvO2: | INTUBATION: date/time: | | Pre-ECMO BVM? Y / N | |

| Pre-ECMO ABG (closest to ECMO start time) | | | | | | | Pre-ECMO Vent Settings *MAP is Mean Airway Pressure, PIP is Peak Insp. Pressure | | | |
|---|---|---|---|---|---|---|---|---|---|---|
| Time | pH | CO2 | pO2 | HCO3 | O2 sat | Lactate | Rate | FiO$_2$ | PEEP | MAP/PIP |
| | | | | | | | | | | |

| ABG/VBG: | | | | | | | Ventilator Settings | | | |
|---|---|---|---|---|---|---|---|---|---|---|
| Time | pH | CO2 | pO2 | HCO3 | O2 sat | Lactate | Rate | FiO$_2$ | PEEP | Other Notes: (PC/MAP/PIP) |
| | | | | | | | | | | |
| | | | | | | | | | | |
| | | | | | | | | | | |

| TIME | FLOW L/MIN | RPM | SGF/FsO2 | P$_{VEN}$ | P$_{ART}$/Delta P | HGB/HCT | SvO2/ Tven | BP/MAP | SpO$_2$ | NOTES |
|---|---|---|---|---|---|---|---|---|---|---|
| | | | | | | | | | | |
| | | | | | | | | | | |
| | | | | | | | | | | |
| | | | | | | | | | | |
| | | | | | | | | | | |
| | | | | | | | | | | |
| | | | | | | | | | | |
| SIGNATURE | | | | | | | | | | |

**Figure 46-6.** Transport medical record documentation.

in this book (Chapters 6,7,12,16,22,26,33). Nonetheless, there are specific mobile ECLS related complications that warrant discussion, both because they can be prepared for and because at least one complication may be seen in up to a quarter of all transports.[22,24]

Death during ECLS transport is very rare and mobile ECLS deaths appear to be primarily related to cannulation complications and underlying patient illness, rather than transport specific etiologies. The most common transport specific complication is actually not ECLS related but rather sudden ventilator failure or airway dislodgement.[24,40] Pump specific complications are uncommon but can be catastrophic if not managed acutely. This includes loss of blood flow, air entrainment, oxygenator thrombosis, and access site insufficiency.[24,32] A higher rate of pump related complications have been reported with fixed-wing transport, likely related to the additional loading and unloading from ambulance to aircraft that is usually required. Pump and ventilator complications during transport warrant specific attention during team preparation, debriefing, and training due to their common occurrence en route, the challenges associated with responding to these issues under cramped and adverse circumstances, difficulties with team communication, and the potentially significant patient impact.

**Special Circumstances**

The COVID-19 pandemic has highlighted additional challenges in ECLS transport, including the need for an adaptive approach to ECLS utilization during surge conditions and health system stress (Chapters 53,57,59). Pandemic related resource constraints may affect ICU bed capacity, the availability of ECLS equipment, as well as the number of trained personnel. Development of centralized networks within healthcare systems, as well as regionally and nationally, has been employed to optimize resource utilization and increase access to ECLS when demand vastly overwhelms capacity.

Components of such strategies may include an assessment of local, regional, and national ECLS capacity, including ICU beds, ECLS circuits, disposable equipment, the alignment of ECLS referral and eligibility criteria at varying levels of surge conditions, the creation of centralized communications and referral hubs, coordination of interhospital transport, and dissemination of information to hospitals, public health, and governmental entities. Such systems, ideally in place before surge or crisis conditions are reached, may more effectively and equitably allocate limited ECLS resources.

The safety of the ECLS transport team must be considered, as well. COVID-19 adapted ambulances, with the driver's compartment completely separated from the patient compartment and incorporation of high efficiency particulate air filters with external exhaust systems have been used to mitigate viral transmission in the confined space of the ambulance.[41] Viral and bacterial filters may be placed on all mechanical ventilators during patient transport. ECLS transport teams should have protocols in place for the donning and doffing of personal protective equipment, as well as for minimizing contamination of the ECLS supply bag. A transport route (between the ambulance and intensive care unit) should be selected to minimize potential exposure to others.

# References

1. Bartlett RH, Gazzaniga AB, Fong SW, et al Extracorporeal membrane oxygenator support for cardiopulmonary failure. Experience in 28 cases. J Thorac Cardiovasc Surg. Mar 1977;73(3):375-86.
2. Cornish JD, Carter JM, Gerstmann DR, et al. Extracorporeal membrane oxygenation as a means of stabilizing and transporting high risk neonates. ASAIO Trans. Oct-Dec 1991;37(4):564-8.
3. Foley DS, Pranikoff T, Younger JG, et al. A review of 100 patients transported on extracorporeal life support. ASAIO journal (American Society for Artificial Internal Organs : 1992). Nov-Dec 2002;48(6):612-9.
4. Bryner B, Cooley E, Copenhaver W, et al. Two decades' experience with interfacility transport on extracorporeal membrane oxygenation. Ann Thorac Surg. Oct 2014;98(4):1363-70.
5. Coppola CP, Tyree M, Larry K, et al. A 22-year experience in global transport extracorporeal membrane oxygenation. J Pediatr Surg. Jan 2008;43(1):46-52; discussion 52.
6. Clement KC, Fiser RT, Fiser WP, et al. Single-institution experience with interhospital extracorporeal membrane oxygenation transport: A descriptive study. Pediatr Crit Care Med. Jul 2010;11(4):509-13.
7. Biscotti M, Agerstrand C, Abrams D, et al. One Hundred Transports on Extracorporeal Support to an Extracorporeal Membrane Oxygenation Center. Ann Thorac Surg. Jul 2015;100(1):34-9; discussion 39-40.
8. Fletcher-Sandersjöö A, Frenckner B, Broman M. A Single-Center Experience of 900 Interhospital Transports on Extracorporeal Membrane Oxygenation. The Annals of Thoracic Surgery. 2019/01/01/ 2019;107(1):119-127.
9. Beurtheret S, Mordant P, Paoletti X, et al. Emergency circulatory support in refractory cardiogenic shock patients in remote institutions: a pilot study (the cardiac-RESCUE program). Eur Heart J. Jan 2013;34(2):112-20.
10. Roch A, Hraiech S, Masson E, et al. Outcome of acute respiratory distress syndrome patients treated with extracorporeal membrane oxygenation and brought to a referral center. Intensive Care Med. Jan 2014;40(1):74-83.
11. Huang SC, Chen YS, Chi NH, et al. Out-of-center extracorporeal membrane oxygenation for adult cardiogenic shock patients. Artificial organs. Jan 2006;30(1):24-8.
12. Salna M, Chicotka S, Biscotti M, 3rd, et al. Morbid obesity is not a contraindication to transport on extracorporeal support. Eur J Cardiothorac Surg. Apr 1 2018;53(4):793-798.
13. Patroniti N, Zangrillo A, Pappalardo F, et al. The Italian ECMO network experience during the 2009 influenza A(H1N1) pandemic: preparation for severe respiratory emergency outbreaks. Intensive Care Medicine. 2011/07/06 2011;37(9):1447.
14. Lebreton G, Schmidt M, Ponnaiah M, et al. Extracorporeal membrane oxygenation network organisation and clinical outcomes during the COVID-19 pandemic in Greater Paris, France: a multicentre cohort study. Lancet Respir Med. 2021;9(8):851-862.
15. Diaz RA, Graf J, Zambrano JM, et al. Extracorporeal Membrane Oxygenation for COVID-19-associated Severe Acute Respiratory Distress Syndrome in Chile: A Nationwide Incidence and Cohort Study. Am J Respir Crit Care Med. Jul 1 2021;204(1):34-43.
16. Dirnberger D, Fiser RT, Harvey C, et al. Guidelines for ECMO Transport. Jan 1, 2022, 2021. Accessed Jan 1, 2021.
17. Gebremichael M, Borg U, Habashi NM, et al. Interhospital transport of the extremely ill patient: the mobile intensive care unit. Crit Care Med. Jan 2000;28(1):79-85.
18. Wiegersma JS, Droogh JM, Zijlstra JG, et al. Quality of interhospital transport of the critically ill: impact of a Mobile Intensive Care Unit with a specialized retrieval team. Crit Care. 2011;15(1):R75.
19. Javidfar J, Brodie D, Takayama H, et al. Safe transport of critically ill adult patients on extracorporeal membrane oxygenation support to a regional extracorporeal membrane oxygenation center. ASAIO journal (American Society for Artificial Internal Organs : 1992). Sep-Oct 2011;57(5):421-5.
20. Fleissner F, Mogaldea A, Martens A, et al. ECLS supported transport of ICU patients: does out-of-house implantation impact survival? J Cardiothorac Surg. Jun 2 2021;16(1):158.
21. Lee H, Sung K, Suh GY, et al. Outcomes of transported and in-house patients on extracorporeal life support: a propensity score-matching study. European journal of cardio-thoracic surgery : official journal of the European Association for Cardio-thoracic Surgery. Feb 1 2020;57(2):317-324.
22. Broman LM, Holzgraefe B, Palmer K, et al. The Stockholm experience: interhospital transports on extracorporeal membrane oxygenation. Crit Care. Jul 9 2015;19:278.
23. Labib A, August E, Agerstrand C, et al. Extracorporeal Life Support Organization Guideline for Transport and Retrieval of Adult and Pediatric Patients with ECMO Support. ASAIO journal (American Society for Artificial Internal Organs : 1992). Apr 1 2022;68(4):447-455.
24. Fletcher-Sandersjoo A, Frenckner B, Broman M. A Single-Center Experience of 900 Interhospital

Transports on Extracorporeal Membrane Oxygenation. The Annals of thoracic surgery. Jan 2019;107(1):119-127.

25. Dirnberger D, Fiser R, Harvey C, et al. Extracorporeal Life Support Organization: Guidlines for ECMO Transport. Accessed January 10, 2022. https://www.elso.org/Resources/Guidelines.aspx.

26. Forrest P, Ratchford J, Burns B, et al. Retrieval of critically ill adults using extracorporeal membrane oxygenation: an Australian experience. Intensive Care Med. May 2011;37(5):824-30.

27. Peek GJ, Mugford M, Tiruvoipati R, et al. Efficacy and economic assessment of conventional ventilatory support versus extracorporeal membrane oxygenation for severe adult respiratory failure (CESAR): a multicentre randomised controlled trial. Lancet. Oct 2009;374(9698):1351-63.

28. Odish MF, Yi C, Chicotka S, et al. Implementation and Outcomes of a Mobile Extracorporeal Membrane Oxygenation Program in the United States During the Coronavirus Disease 2019 Pandemic. J Cardiothorac Vasc Anesth. Oct 2021;35(10):2869-2874.

29. Odish M, Yi C, Eigner J, et al. The Southern California Extracorporeal Membrane Oxygenation Consortium During the Coronavirus Disease 2019 Pandemic. Disaster Med Public Health Prep. Jun 8 2021:1-8.

30. Vaja R, Chauhan I, Joshi V, et al. Five-year experience with mobile adult extracorporeal membrane oxygenation in a tertiary referral center. J Crit Care. Dec 2015;30(6):1195-8.

31. Bellingan G, Olivier T, Batson S, et al. Comparison of a specialist retrieval team with current United Kingdom practice for the transport of critically ill patients. Intensive Care Med. Jun 2000;26(6):740-4.

32. Burrell AJC, Pilcher DV, Pellegrino VA, et al. Retrieval of Adult Patients on Extracorporeal Membrane Oxygenation by an Intensive Care Physician Model. Artificial organs. Mar 2018;42(3):254-262.

33. Ranney DN, Bonadonna D, Yerokun BA, et al. Extracorporeal Membrane Oxygenation and Interfacility Transfer: A Regional Referral Experience. The Annals of thoracic surgery. Nov 2017;104(5):1471-1478.

34. ELSO Guidelines for Training and Continuing Education of ECMO Specialists. Updated 2010. Accessed January 11, 2022.

35. Sin SWC, Ng PY, Ngai WCW, et al. Simulation training for crises during venoarterial extracorporeal membrane oxygenation. J Thorac Dis. May 2019;11(5):2144-2152.

36. Burkhart HM, Riley JB, Lynch JJ, et al. Simulation-based postcardiotomy extracorporeal membrane oxygenation crisis training for thoracic surgery residents. The Annals of thoracic surgery. Mar 2013;95(3):901-6.

37. Zakhary BM, Kam LM, Kaufman BS, et al. The Utility of High-Fidelity Simulation for Training Critical Care Fellows in the Management of Extracorporeal Membrane Oxygenation Emergencies: A Randomized Controlled Trial. Crit Care Med. Aug 2017;45(8):1367-1373.

38. Riley JB, Searles BE, Darling EM, et al. The Effectiveness of Three Different Curricular Models to Teach Fundamental ECMO Specialist Skills to Entry Level Perfusionists. J Extra Corpor Technol. Dec 2021;53(4):245-250.

39. Oxygen Cylindar Calculator. World Federation of Societies of Anesthesiologists. Accessed June 1 2022, 2022. https://opencriticalcare.org/oxygen-cylinder-duration-calculator.

40. Mendes PV, de Albuquerque Gallo C, Besen B, et al. Transportation of patients on extracorporeal membrane oxygenation: a tertiary medical center experience and systematic review of the literature. Ann Intensive Care. Dec 2017;7(1):14.

41. Agerstrand C, Dubois R, Takeda K, et al. Extracorporeal Membrane Oxygenation for Coronavirus Disease 2019: Crisis Standards of Care. ASAIO journal (American Society for Artificial Internal Organs : 1992). Mar 1 2021;67(3):245-2.

# 47

## Physiotherapy and Mobilization

*Jessica B. Cornman, Chris L. Wells, Daniel L. Herr, Marcelo Cypel, Marta Cucchi,*
*Matthieu Schmidt, Jordi Riera, Carol L. Hodgson*

## Introduction

Patients requiring ECLS for severe acute respiratory and cardiac failure are frequently managed with deep sedation and neuromuscular blockers, particularly in the first few days after initiation.[1] In the case of acute respiratory failure, particular attention is given to applying a protective lung ventilation strategy which may include prone positioning.[2,3] As a result of the severity of the illness, and the requirement for sedation and paralysis, patients managed on ECLS often have long periods of immobility and bedrest.

The combination of critical illness and prolonged immobility have been identified as key factors in poor functional recovery in ICU survivors. In a multicenter cohort study of 222 survivors of acute lung injury, muscle strength and physical function were measured over two years after the onset of the acute lung injury.[4] Duration of bedrest during the critical illness was the only factor associated with the development of prolonged neuromuscular weakness.[4] Prolonged immobility has been associated with physical and cognitive deficits that may persist for up to 5 years after the ICU stay.[5]

Intensive Care unit acquired weakness (ICUAW) has been defined as neuromuscular weakness that is usually symmetrical, predominantly affects the proximal limbs and respiratory muscles, develops during critically illness, and has no other explanation aside from the critical illness itself.[6] A number of risk factors have been identified for development of ICUAW and can be divided into preadmission risk factors and factors related to the ICU stay.[6] Pre-ICU risk factors include age, the type and number of comorbidities, frailty and the level of independence prior to admission.[6] Risk factors that may be related to the ICU admission, and commonly seen in patients managed on ECLS, include hyperglycemia, sepsis and inflammation, severity of illness, prolonged duration of mechanical ventilation, and prolonged immobility or duration of bed rest.[6]

Early rehabilitation in ICU is one strategy to mitigate the development of ICUAW and improve muscle strength and physical function.[7] The timing of early rehabilitation in ICU varies considerably in the literature.[7] The rationale for starting rehabilitation early is based on the rapid physiological deterioration in muscle structure and function observed within the first few days of an ICU admission.[8]

Early rehabilitation in the ICU has been shown to be safe and feasible in general ICU populations.[7,9] In a systematic review and metaanalysis of safety of rehabilitation in the ICU that included over 7,500 patients and

22,000 rehabilitation sessions, the incidence of any potential safety events was low (2.6%), and very rare (0.6%) for events that required additional care requirements.[9] A number of guidelines have been published recommending the implementation of early rehabilitation in ICU.[10] Factors that have been identified that facilitate a culture that prioritizes early rehabilitation are leadership including a mobility champion, and adequate resources and training.[11]

In pilot studies and phase II clinical trials, patients who receive early rehabilitation in ICU have demonstrated improved rates of independent functioning at hospital discharge,[12] improved muscle strength,[7] earlier liberation from mechanical ventilation, reduced rates of delirium, shorter length of stay in ICU and hospital,[12] and more days alive and out of hospital at 6 months.[7]

In summary, while early rehabilitation in general ICU populations has increased, the use of ECLS is often associated with periods of very prolonged immobility and bedrest. This is as a result of deep sedation, respiratory or hemodynamic instability, anticoagulation and bleeding, cannula position, and fear of kinking or dislodging the cannulas.[13] Current literature shows that in most centers, standard care includes minimal active rehabilitation during ECLS.

**Awake ECLS**

The term Awake Extracorporeal Life Support (ECLS) was first coined in the study by Fuehner et al. published in 2012.[14] The patients treated with this strategy were described as awake and liberated from mechanical ventilation, which led to proactive involvement in physical therapy (PT). Therefore, the milestone of this strategy is embedded in the concept of a patient being extubated and cognitively alert.[15-31] Initially, the respiratory status eligible to commence an awake strategy is defined

as "spontaneous breathing." The elasticity of this concept evolved since the early days of ECLS and has allowed for a wider inclusion of different practices: patients are considered involved in an awake ECLS strategy, despite being still supported with invasive mechanical ventilation through an endotracheal tube or a tracheostomy. This concept allowed for a shift in prioritizing the focus in the awake ECLS approach away from extubation towards the cognitive state of the patient, which has further promoted early rehabilitation to restore function. The use of a sedation scale to assess the patient's level of alertness or agitation may optimize the weaning of sedation. The Richmond Agitation Sedation Scale (RASS),[13,20,21,32,33] the Riker Sedation Agitation Scale (SAS),[34] and the Ramsay Sedation Scale[26] are the most common assessment tools reportedly used to assess awake status.

A third element particular to the awake ECLS strategy is early rehabilitation and mobilization. The aim is to achieve ambulatory status to maintain and improve patients' motor function and nerve function.[35-40] In patients bridging to transplant (BTT), ambulatory status has been associated with a reduction of secondary complications and an improved overall success of the procedure, including survival.[15,41,42] As such, ambulation during ECLS in patients who are BTT is widely supported to improve outcome.[27,29,43-46]

There is increasing literature that supports the benefit of ICU rehabilitation for patients receiving ECLS. In a small, multicenter, pilot randomized trial, Hodgson et al reported a higher level of functional independence at hospital discharge for those survivors who participated in early mobilization and rehabilitation when compared to patients receiving standard care.[6] Participation with physical therapy was associated with higher level of function and activity tolerance to either be discharged home (24%) or to acute rehabilitation centers (69%).[32] However, as this was a small pilot trial, these results are preliminary and need to be considered hypothesis generating. There are no large, randomized trials to confirm the safety and benefit of early rehabilitation of patients during ECMO. Further trials are in currently in progress (ClinicalTrials.gov Identifier: NCT05003609).

In a retrospective cohort study in Toronto in 2017, after controlling for clinical baseline and severity of illness, it was reported that patients receiving physical therapy while receiving ECLS had 42% lower ICU mortality than those who did not receive therapy.[34] Similarly, in a small retrospective study of patients cannulated in the right internal jugular vein with VV ECMO, Boling et al reported a greater survival rate at time of hospital discharge for patients who achieved ambulatory status (12/18, 67%) when compared to all ECMO patients (45%).[15] In a systematic review including over 300 patients, rehabilitation during ECLS was associated with a decrease in duration of mechanical ventilation, ICU days and cost.[47] Finally, Bain et al., in a retrospective study in 2016 that compared hospital cost for patients who achieved ambulation status while on ECLS vs. a nonambulatory group, found there was a 22% reduction in total hospital costs and 73% reduction in post-transplant ICU cost in the ambulatory ECLS group.[48]

## Barriers to Early Mobilization

In a recent scoping review of early rehabilitation of patients during ECLS, facilitators and barriers were identified in 69 and 29 studies, respectively.[13] The most common facilitators were upper body cannulation, weaning sedation, and having a multidisciplinary team with expertise in ECLS management. The most common barriers to early rehabilitation during ECLS were the use of heavy sedation and medical instability.[13]

Other barriers to early mobilization in patients receiving ECLS for ARDS include the concerns of patient-self-induced lung injury (P-SILI). ARDS patients usually have a high respiratory drive, even with values of $PaO_2$ and $PaCO_2$ normalized by the ECLS system.[49,50] This is due to the stimulation of lung mechanoreceptors by the inflammation itself, leading to an intense and profound inspiration that may further damage the alveoli and other structures due to a huge increase in transpulmonary pressure. During the first phases of ECLS support (24-72 hours), the lung injury induced by the ventilator must be minimized and P-SILI must be avoided. In later phases, sedatives and neuromuscular blockers should be titrated down and withdrawn. In this phase, the intensity of breathing should be monitored, for example by esophageal pressure monitoring.[51] Some centers use low doses of neuromuscular blockers to minimize the transpulmonary switch.[52] Studies with animal models are currently exploring ways of blocking the neural networks.[53]

## Initiation of Early Rehabilitation and Mobility

Table 47-1 provides an example of a checklist for rehabilitation and mobilization of patients during ECLS. Rehabilitation begins with a thorough review of the electronic medical record with a focus on understanding the underlying medical condition leading to the need for ECLS support, the hospital course including ECLS, mechanical ventilation support, vasoactive and ionotropic infusions, level of sedation, nutritional status, and laboratory findings. The therapist is looking for stable hemodynamics without increasing doses of medications or changes in arterial blood gases, and stable ventilatory settings if present, especially $FiO_2$ and PEEP levels. The therapist should verify with the critical care team that the cannulas are correctly positioned and are secured with no frank bleeding. Nursing staff should review the flow at rest and with basic procedures (such as repositioning in bed and washing). Finally, the therapist should verify the level of sedation and the presence of any neuromuscular blockers. If the patient is moderately or heavily sedated (eg, the RASS is less than -2), the critical care team should discuss if the sedation can be lightened so the patient can actively participate in rehabilitation.[32,54]

The patient supported on ECLS who is orally intubated should be able to participate in active rehabilitation and mobilization. In general, patients who are orally intubated may be more anxious and uncomfortable and will require reassurance from the healthcare team and they may require anxiolytics before mobilization. If the patient is undergoing a weaning trial on the ventilator, rehabilitation may be hindered if weaning is occurring concurrently due to increased oxygen consumption. Sufficient ventilatory support needs to be maintained to allow functional progression without increasing the risk of cardiorespiratory compromise and undo stress and anxiety to the patient. In this case, the healthcare team need to discuss and

| Pre-Rehabilitation Planning | · Identify potential candidates for rehabilitation early<br>· Confirm candidates for rehabilitation amongst the medical, nursing and physiotherapy staff, including the ECMO specialists<br>· Organize additional staff as required<br>· Coordinate a time for rehabilitation with all staff<br>· Confirm parameters for the ECMO Fresh Gas Flow (FGF) and blood flow with the ECMO specialist<br>· Discuss roles during rehabilitation and an agreed back-up plan or escalation pathway during the rehabilitation session if required<br>· Discuss the rehabilitation plan with the patient to ensure treatment goals are agreed<br>· Ensure all equipment required for an emergency is at the bedside (e.g. 4 clamps)<br>· Prepare the ventilator for portable operation if required<br>· Check cannulae are secured and stable<br>· Check the ETT / tracheostomy is secure and suction prior to mobilisation to ensure integrity of the tube |
|---|---|
| Considerations During Rehabilitation | · Notify the consultant immediately prior to the rehabilitation session<br>· Do not commence rehabilitation unless the consultant and medical team are available to assist if required<br>· Confirm each staff members role during the rehabilitation session immediately prior to commencing<br>· Confirm with the patient that they are ready to participate and continue to assess throughout the rehabilitation session<br>· Assess the cannulae stability regularly, including during and after every position change<br>· Assess the patient physiology continuously during the session<br>· Titrate FGF and blood flow as needed |
| Post-Rehabilitation Checklist | · Check the patients' vitals to confirm stability – contact the primary team immediately if they are not stable<br>· Reassess the patient (eg, pain, level of exertion, SOB, tolerance of the rehab session)<br>· Confirm the cannulae position is unchanged and that they are secure, including checking the cannulae length<br>· Return the oxygen gas line to the wall as appropriate<br>· ECMO specialist to check ECMO FGF and blood flow and return to pre-rehabilitation settings if it is safe to do so<br>· The senior physiotherapist documents the rehabilitation session, including the rehabilitation dose (distance, time, highest mobility level), the response to rehabilitation, symptoms, vital signs, and number of staff required<br>· ECMO nurse documents any changes to ECMO settings |

**Table 47-1.** Checklist for early rehabilitation of patients during ECMO.

decide prioritization of the ventilator weaning schedule and the rehabilitation plan.

Active mobilization comes with risks and benefits that the therapist needs to consider when planning each session. With every session, the therapist should complete an assessment of cognitive function, delirium, the ability to follow commands, and engage the patient in the therapy process. The therapist should try to assess anxiety that may become a barrier to active mobilization. Techniques such as breathing control or slower mobility progression may reduce anxiety. The therapist should complete a neuromuscular assessment to determine if the patient is safe to perform functional tasks. The use of the ASIA (American Spinal Injury Association) impairment scale is a standard objective tool that may be used to complete these serial assessments and

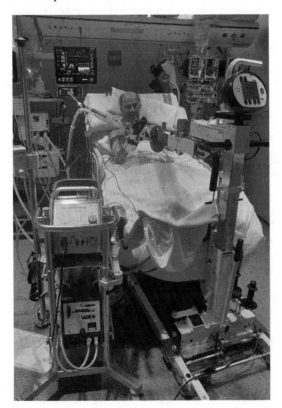

**Figure 47-1.** Bed level activity with supported on ECMO. Printed with patient permission from University of Maryland Medical System.

detect neuromuscular changes, particularly in the presence of femoral cannulation.[55] Hip flexion to at least 90 degrees to assess ECLS flows should also be assessed for patients with femoral cannulation prior to transferring to a seated position.

The patient may begin with bed-level activities (Figure 47-1) and progress according to tolerance and participation, based on interdisciplinary team discussion and collaboration (Table 47-2). Prior to initiation of out-of-bed mobility, the goals of the session should be discussed and agreed upon by the multidisciplinary team. Once the team has agreed on a rehabilitation plan, it should be discussed with the patient and family to ensure their understanding, engagement, and consent prior to initiation of mobility.

Advancing a patient to initiate gait training and safe ambulation (Figure 47-2 and 47-3) requires a coordinated effort of the healthcare team and should be decided with input from the medical staff responsible for the patient's management. Once agreed by the healthcare team, it is recommended that gait training be initially directed by the physical therapist so a comprehensive neuromuscular assessment can be completed to assure patient safety. Once it is determined the patient is safe to ambulate with less than minimal assistance, and demonstrates no significant gait deviation, nursing can also contribute to ambulating the patient if trained in safe patient handling techniques. The therapist should gather a sufficient number of staff members and clearly assign roles. Each team member should communicate any issues to the therapist who is overseeing the ambulation session. It is vital that the ECLS specialist support the cannulas, monitor flows, and maintain a distance between patient and the ECLS device to avoid tension on the cannulas. The team should plan for and be prepared to address any adverse event during ambulation (eg, having a chair nearby if required and emergency equipment in case of cannula dislodgement or bleeding). Finally, at the conclusion of any ambulation, the cannula sites should be inspected to detect and address migration or bleeding (Table 47-1).

## Complications during Mobilization

Reported complications during ECMO mobilization are generally uncommon and can be categorized into major and minor. Efforts should be made to prevent and manage these complications.[13] Major complications are events that require an emergent response and could cause serious harm or death to the patient. These ECLS-specific complications include accidental decannulation, cannula fracture, significant cannula migration, severe bleeding from insertion site, cannula kinking that can lead to interruptions to blood flow with cardiorespiratory instability, and ECLS machine malfunction or circuit failure (Chapter 7).[13] Other major complications that may occur (and are not specific to ECLS) include cardiac arrest, stroke, pulmonary emboli, cardiac arrythmias, and falls. Minor complications are events that do not require an emergent response and the

| FUNCTIONAL LEVELS | BED DEPENDENT | CHAIR DEPENDENT | AMBULATORY |
|---|---|---|---|
| Definitions | · General strength in primary functional muscles group <3/5<br>· ≥ moderate assistance with bed mobility and supine to sit transfers<br>· ≥ static sitting balance<br>· < 20 minutes of activity tolerance | · General strength in primary muscle groups 3/5 to 4/5<br>· < moderate assistance with bed mobility and supine to sit transfers<br>· < minimal assistance with sitting and standing balance<br>· ≤ Minimal assistance for sit to stand<br>· 20 to 30 minutes of activity tolerance | · General strength in primary muscle groups ≥ 4/5<br>· < minimal assistance with bed mobility and supine to sit transfers<br>· ≤ close contact with sitting balance<br>· ≤ minimal assistance with sit to stand transfers<br>· ≤ contact guard with standing balance<br>· ≤ minimal assistance with gait training<br>· 30 – 40 minutes of activity tolerance |
| Functional Progression Training | · Bed mobility<br>· Sitting balance training<br>· Sitting tolerance<br>· Pretransfer training (sit-to stand and lateral transfers, sit pivot)<br>Pediatric:<br>· bed level play skills<br>· ring sitting in bed<br>· lift transfer parent or caregivers lap | · Bed mobility<br>· Advanced sitting balance<br>· Sit-to-stand or lateral transfers<br>· Standing balance<br>· Pre-gait training<br>Pediatric:<br>· sitting play either on mat or bench<br>· standing and cruising<br>· utilization of ride-on toy<br>· gait training in gait trainer | · Sit-to-stand transfers<br>· Advanced standing balance<br>· Gait training<br>Pediatric:<br>· gait with or without push toy<br>· riding adaptive bike/trike<br>· utilization of active video games |
| Muscle strength: low repetitions, high resistance, 2–3 sets, short recovery time | Closed kinetic exercises: leg press; terminal knee extension; hip abduction and extension; dorsiflexors; scapular depression; latissimus dorsi, triceps, trunk, and extremity PNF; hand putty | Modified sit-to-stand transfers, modified step-ups, reverse SLR, continue with closed kinetic exercises for previous level, add shoulder flexion and abduction | Continue with closed kinetic chain exercises and advance previous exercises. Add squats, step-ups, deltoids, and biceps exercises |
| Muscle endurance: 30–90 s of high intensity interval training, 3–5 intervals, active recovery | · Rhythmic stabilization in supine or side-lying position<br>· PRE: Leg press, reverse SLR, Shoulder extension and triceps<br>· Restorator for UE and LE ** | · Rhythmic stabilization in sitting<br>· Progress PRE<br>· Modified sit-to-stand transfer.<br>· Restorator for UE and LE** | · Rhythmic stabilization in standing<br>· PRE Squats and step-ups, modified military press-ups and triceps<br>· Marching in place<br>· Restorator for UE and LE** |
| ROM/ Joint Integrity | · General ROM of extremities, trunk, scapular, pelvis, dorsiflexion and hamstring muscle extensibility<br>· manage any joint contracture | · Trunk, spine, scapular, pelvis mobility<br>· Continue with extensibility exercises<br>· Joint mobilization management | · Continue and advance previous level |
| Aerobic, continuous work for 6 min | · Restorator for UE and LE** | · Restorator for UE and LE** | · Restorator for UE and LE**<br>· Ambulation |
| Pulmonary | · Airway clearance<br>· Breath control exercises<br>· Ventilatory strategies<br>· Breathing pattern facilitation<br>· Inspiratory muscle training | · Continue and advance previous section | · Continue and advance previous section |

SLR=straight leg raise; UE=upper extremity; LE=lower extremity; ROM=range of motion; PRE=progressive resistive exercise.
**Will be dependent on cannulation sites. Monitor cannulation sites closely for bleeding and cannulation security.

**Table 47-2.** Activity progression while supported on ECMO.[81]

patient is not at immediate risk of injury or death, and may resolve with discontinuation of, or modification to, the mobilization activity. These include minor cannula migration (not requiring repositioning), minor bleeding at insertion sites that ceases spontaneously or with manual pressure, interruptions in blood flow without cardiorespiratory instability, transient desaturation, minor arrythmias, or hypotension.[13]

## Multidisciplinary Team Approach

It is important to acknowledge that early rehabilitation combined with an Awake ECLS strategy is time- and labor-intense for the team implementing mobilization and ensuring cannula and patient safety.[56] This approach requires both a culture of multidisciplinary

collaboration and institutional resource investment, which will allow sustainability.[57]

Investing in specific and consistent rehabilitation and mobilization training for the multidisciplinary team is deemed pivotal for the practice to be successful.[29,32] It will better identify barriers and optimize timing, dosage, and safety concerns. Regular meetings with multidisciplinary team members is considered important to screen patients for suitability to mobilize during ECLS.[58]

Introducing active mobilization for patients during ECLS increases the workload and complexity of care for the nursing staff. With other healthcare team members, the nursing team must assess and determine suitability for mobilization. The introduction of a standardized screening tool allows more homogenous assessment among multidisciplinary team members (Table 47-1).[32]

The multidisciplinary team is responsible for monitoring the patient during mobilization, including the ECLS cannula site(s) and bleeding, neurological changes, ECLS flows,

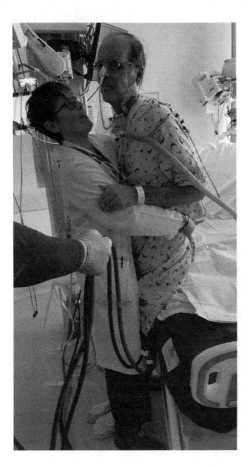

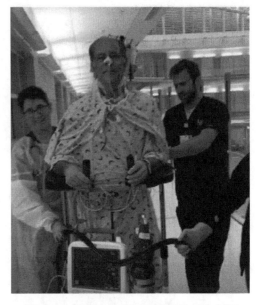

**Figure 47-2 a(left), b(right).** Mobility progression while supported on VA ECMO. Printed with patient permission from University of Maryland Medical System.

hemodynamic stability, respiratory stability, and the response to mobilization. Each organization, however, has a responsibility to identify the number and type of healthcare professionals required to safely monitor the ECLS circuit and the patient during rehabilitation.[59]

The members of the healthcare team needed to perform rehabilitation and mobilization with patients on ECLS is variable and depends upon the complexity of the patient and the number of lines, tubes and devices in use, organizational protocols, and legal requirements in different countries. It is important that the ECLS team discusses local guidelines for staffing of rehabilitation activities, including the number of staff required, the types of professions involved, the role of each profession, the education and training requirements, as this will maximize safety and efficiency of the rehabilitation service.

After completing the preintervention screening (Table 47-1), therapeutic exercises in bed or in a chair should be able to be completed with one therapist. During routine positioning of ECLS patients, two or three staff may be needed, based on medical and cannula stability. For active mobilization, the multidisciplinary team must include at least one specialized ECLS

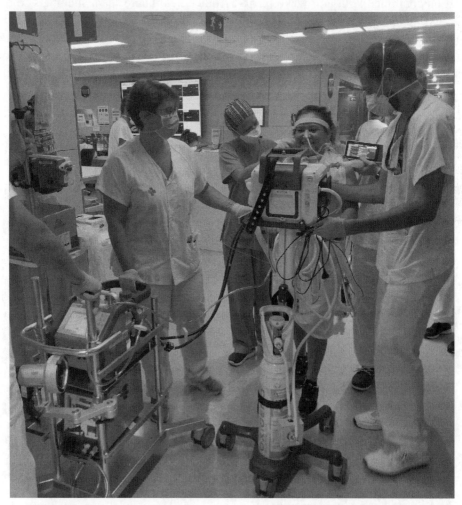

**Figure 47-3.** Ambulation while supported on ECMO. Printed with patient permission from University of Maryland Medical System.

staff member present to monitor the cannula, the circuit and adjust settings as required (such as sweep gas flow rates and increased oxygen demand).[44]

## Outcome Measures to Objectively Document Rehabilitation Progress and Potential

It is important to objectively document the functional status in a systematic manner to track progress and alert the team when there is functional regression. A core set of outcome measures to utilize in the evaluation of patients on ECLS has been published, including outcome measures for complications during ECLS, mortality and the level of recovery at 6-months.[60]

The Function Status Scale ICU[61] and the ICU Mobility Scale[62] are valid and reliable tools to track basic function and level of mobility in critically ill patients. For the measurement of muscle strength, the Medical Research Council Sum Score (MRC-SS) is the most common measure and weakness on this scale has been associated with increased mechanical ventilation days, ICU length of stay, and mortality in the general adult ICU population.[63-65] It is more challenging to assess muscle endurance in this population depending on the cannulation sites. There are 3 accepted sit-to-stand tests (5 times, 30 or 60 second tests) but caution needs to be taken if the patient is femorally cannulated. The use of an upper limb ergometer can be used to document muscle endurance in the cases of femoral cannulation if there are concerns with site bleeding or pain. To document functional status, the Activity Measure for Post-Acute Care (AM PAC) Basic Mobility and Activities of Daily Living are easy to complete and are useful in tracking progress and assisting in discharge recommendations.[66,67] The AM PAC Cognition, MOCA, or SLUMs can be used to objectively document the cognitive status of patients on ECLS support.[68,69]

Finally, to assess activity tolerance upon recovery, the core outcome set for ECLS recommends using the modified Rankin scale, the EQ5D and the Instrumental Activities of Daily Living (IADL) at 6-months after ECMO initiation.[60] In addition, the 6 MWT or an ergometer test can be objectively used.[70]

## Prone Positioning

To date, prone positioning (PP) is one of the most effective treatments for severe ARDS.[71] By homogenizing lung-aeration distribution,[72] lung ventilation, lung perfusion, and ventilation/perfusion ratio,[73] PP can enhance lung protection, while improving oxygenation and reducing mortality.[71] Besides, PP homogenizes the distribution of transpulmonary pressure, thereby mitigating the ventilator-induced lung-injury risk attributable to alveolar overstretching and cyclic atelectasis.[74]

Theoretically, the combination of PP with VV ECMO is promising because it could further enhance lung protection. However, its use is recent and mainly reported by experienced ECLS centers.[75-77] For instance, only 10% and 15% of patients were prone positioned during ECLS in the EOLIA trial[1] and the LIFEGARDS study,[2] respectively. More recently, several studies have suggested benefits when these two therapies are combined. In a retrospective, single-center study over 8 years including 298 VV ECMO treated adults with severe ARDS and 64 patients proned during ECMO, a propensity-score–matched analysis compared patients with PP during ECMO and those without.[78] Although both groups had similar ECMO durations, PP-ECMO patients' 90-day probability of being weaned off ECMO and alive was higher (0.75 vs. 0.54, p=0.03) and 90-day mortality was lower (20% vs. 42%, p<0.01) than for no-PP-ECMO patients. This 22% lower ICU mortality was close to that reported for the PROSEVA trial.[71] Similarly, Guervilly et al and Giani et al reported lower mortality rates when PP was added to

ECLS for retrospective case-series,[75,76] whereas only shorter ECLS durations were reported in another study.[79] Recently, a metaanalysis that included 13 studies with a combined population of 1836 patients, highlighted that the use of prone positioning in ARDS patients receiving VV ECMO was associated with a significant improvement in 28-day survival (74% vs. 58%, p<0.001). Survival was also improved at 60-days, 90-days, ICU and hospital discharge. However, the duration of mechanical ventilation was increased in VV ECMO patients with PP.[80]

Some studies have tried to identify which patients are more likely to respond to PP on ECMO because of the fear of life-threatening complications and uncertainty regarding PP benefits. An improvement in the static compliance may define a PP-responder during ECLS. Pre-PP quantitative lung computed tomography analysis showed that, despite similar dorsal lung-tissue distributions, patients with increased static compliance post-PP had lower percentages of nonaerated or poorly aerated lung tissue in ventral and medial–ventral regions.[81] However, if there is benefit to PP on ECLS, the best time to initiate this procedure and the optimal duration of PP is unknown.

Ongoing randomized controlled trials should help to answer that question.

Absolute or relative contraindications for PP on ECMO are listed in Table 47-3. To prevent potential complications associated with the procedure (eg, cannula dislodgement or suddenly decreased extracorporeal blood flow) (Table 47-4), the procedure should be protocolized and the healthcare team should have been trained ideally with simulation programs. Interestingly, ECLS-related complication rates were very low and frequently similar to the group of patients who were not placed in PP, when performed in experienced ECLS centers.[1,75] Notably, rare accidental extubation or decannulation occurred during the PP procedure, supporting its safety when performed by well-trained staff.

After carefully securing the ECLS cannula, checking the position of the tip of the femoral drainage cannula into the right atrium, and applying thin hydrocolloid dressing for pressure ulcer prevention, at least six experienced staff will be needed for the procedure. ICU lines and drains that are instead above the waist should be positioned towards the head of the bed and lines and tubes below the waist are positioned

| ABSOLUTE CONTRAINDICATIONS | HIGH RISK RELATIVE CONTRAINDICATIONS | OTHER RELATIVE CONTRAINDICATIONS |
|---|---|---|
| • Suspected raised intracranial pressure<br>• Spinal instability | • Recent sternotomy<br>• Facial surgery<br>• Severe hemodynamic instability | • Open abdomen<br>• Pregnancy<br>• Multiple trauma with unstable fractures |

**Table 47-3.** Absolute and relative contraindication for proning during ECMO.

| SEVERE COMPLICATIONS | LESS SEVERE COMPLICATIONS |
|---|---|
| • Transient desaturation<br>• Lower ECMO flow<br>• Hemodynamic instability<br>• Accidental extubation<br>• Accidental decannulation<br>• Central line displacement | • Pressure ulcers<br>• Vomiting<br>• Increases in need for sedation ± paralysis<br>• Nerve damage<br>• Bleeding from ECMO cannula sites |

**Table 47-4.** Potential complications of prone positioning during ECMO.

towards the foot of the bed. EKG leads should be repositioned to avoid the patient lying on them. Prior to turning the range of motion of the cervical spine and shoulders should be cleared to identify any necessary positional alterations that will be necessary to avoid musculoskeletal or neurological injuries. One person at the head will hold the endotracheal tube and the jugular cannula; another person at the feet will guide the procedure while holding the cannulas and avoiding any tension, and two persons will stand on each side of the bed to perform the double sheets technique for turning. Mechanical lifts can be used to assist staff in proning, especially with large patients, and can lead to using fewer staff if the team is well trained in the use of lifts. A transverse positioning device can be placed under the pelvis and the chest to limit intraabdominal pressure, which could reduce the ECMO flow. As in the PROSEVA trial, PP duration on ECMO should be maintained for at least 16 hours even if the optimal duration on ECMO is unknown.

# References

1. Combes A, Hajage D, Capellier G, et al. Extracorporeal Membrane Oxygenation for Severe Acute Respiratory Distress Syndrome. N Engl J Med. 2018;378(21):1965-1975.

2. Schmidt M, Pham T, Arcadipane A, et al. Mechanical Ventilation Management during Extracorporeal Membrane Oxygenation for Acute Respiratory Distress Syndrome. An International Multicenter Prospective Cohort. Am J Respir Crit Care Med. 2019;200(8):1002-1012.

3. Serpa Neto A, Schmidt M, Azevedo LCP, et al. Associations between ventilator settings during extracorporeal membrane oxygenation for refractory hypoxemia and outcome in patients with acute respiratory distress syndrome: a pooled individual patient data analysis : Mechanical ventilation during ECMO. Intensive Care Med. 2016;42(11):1672-1684.

4. Fan E, Dowdy DW, Colantuoni E, et al. Physical complications in acute lung injury survivors: a two-year longitudinal prospective study. Crit Care Med. 2014;42(4):849-859.

5. Herridge MS, Tansey CM, Matté A, et al. Functional disability 5 years after acute respiratory distress syndrome. N Engl J Med. 2011;364(14):1293-1304.

6. Hodgson CL, Tipping CJ. Physiotherapy management of intensive care unit-acquired weakness. J Physiother. 2017;63(1):4-10.

7. Tipping CJ, Harrold M, Holland A, Romero L, Nisbet T, Hodgson CL. The effects of active mobilisation and rehabilitation in ICU on mortality and function: a systematic review. Intensive Care Med. 2017;43(2):171-183.

8. Puthucheary ZA, Rawal J, McPhail M, et al. Acute skeletal muscle wasting in critical illness. JAMA. 2013;310(15):1591-1600.

9. Nydahl P, Sricharoenchai T, Chandra S, et al. Safety of Patient Mobilization and Rehabilitation in the Intensive Care Unit. Systematic Review with Meta-Analysis. Ann Am Thorac Soc. 2017;14(5):766-777.

10. Lang JK, Paykel MS, Haines KJ, Hodgson CL. Clinical Practice Guidelines for Early Mobilization in the ICU: A Systematic Review. Crit Care Med. 2020;48(11):e1121-e1128.

11. Cuthbertson BH, Goddard SL, Lorencatto F, et al. Barriers and Facilitators to Early Rehabilitation in the ICU: A Theory Driven Delphi Study. Crit Care Med. 2020;48(12):e1171-e1178.

12. Schweickert WD, Pohlman MC, Pohlman AS, et al. Early physical and occupational therapy in mechanically ventilated, critically ill patients: a randomised controlled trial. Lancet Lond Engl. 2009;373(9678):1874-1882.

13. Hayes K, Hodgson CL, Webb MJ, Romero L, Holland AE. Rehabilitation of adult patients on extracorporeal membrane oxygenation: A scoping review. Aust Crit Care Off J Confed Aust Crit Care Nurses. Published online October 25, 2021:S1036-7314(21)00136-3.

14. Fuehner T, Kuehn C, Hadem J, et al. Extracorporeal Membrane Oxygenation in Awake Patients as Bridge to Lung Transplantation. Am J Respir Crit Care Med. 2012;185(7):763-768.

15. Boling B, Dennis DR, Tribble TA, Rajagopalan N, Hoopes CW. Safety of Nurse-Led Ambulation for Patients on Venovenous Extracorporeal Membrane Oxygenation. Prog Transplant Aliso Viejo Calif. 2016;26(2):112-116.

16. Hoopes CW, Kukreja J, Golden J, Davenport DL, Diaz-Guzman E, Zwischenberger JB. Extracorporeal membrane oxygenation as a bridge to pulmonary transplantation. J Thorac Cardiovasc Surg. 2013;145(3):862-867; discussion 867-868.

17. Youn T, Kim D, Park TK, et al. Clinical Outcomes of Early Extubation Strategy in Patients Undergoing Extracorporeal Membrane Oxygenation as a Bridge to Heart Transplantation. J Korean Med Sci. 2020;35(42):e346.

18. Xia J, Gu S, Li M, et al. Spontaneous breathing in patients with severe acute respiratory distress syndrome receiving prolonged extracorporeal membrane oxygenation. BMC Pulm Med. 2019;19(1):237.

19. Deng L, Xia Q, Chi C, Hu G. Awake veno-arterial extracorporeal membrane oxygenation in patients with perioperative period acute heart failure in cardiac surgery. J Thorac Dis. 2020;12(5):2179-2187.

20. Ellouze O, Lamirel J, Perrot J, et al. Extubation of patients undergoing extracorporeal life support. A retrospective study. Perfusion. 2019;34(1):50-57.

21. Bataillard A, Hebrard A, Gaide-Chevronnay L, et al. Extubation in patients undergoing extracorporeal life support. Int J Artif Organs. 2017;40(12):696-700.

22. Pasrija C, Mackowick KM, Raithel M, et al. Ambulation With Femoral Arterial Cannulation Can Be Safely Performed on Venoarterial Extracorporeal Membrane Oxygenation. Ann Thorac Surg. 2019;107(5):1389-1394.

23. Sommer W, Marsch G, Kaufeld T, et al. Cardiac Awake Extracorporeal Life Support—Bridge to Decision? Artif Organs. 2015;39(5):400-408.

24. Tipograf Y, Salna M, Minko E, et al. Outcomes of Extracorporeal Membrane Oxygenation as a Bridge to Lung Transplantation. Ann Thorac Surg. 2019;107(5):1456-1463.

25. Downey P, Ragalie W, Gudzenko V, Ardehali A. Ambulatory central veno-arterial extracorporeal membrane oxygenation in lung transplant candidates. J Heart Lung Transplant. 2019;38(12):1317-1319.

26. Yeo HJ, Cho WH, Kim D. Awake extracorporeal membrane oxygenation in patients with severe postoperative acute respiratory distress syndrome. J Thorac Dis. 2016;8(1):37-42.

27. Benazzo A, Schwarz S, Frommlet F, et al. Twenty-year experience with extracorporeal life support as bridge to lung transplantation. J Thorac Cardiovasc Surg. 2019;157(6):2515-2525.e10.

28. Taniguchi H, Ogawa F, Honzawa H, et al. Veno-venous extracorporeal membrane oxygenation for severe pneumonia: COVID-19 case in Japan. Acute Med Surg. 2020;7(1):e509.

29. Hakim AH, Ahmad U, McCurry KR, et al. Contemporary Outcomes of Extracorporeal Membrane Oxygenation Used as Bridge to Lung Transplantation. Ann Thorac Surg. 2018;106(1):192-198.

30. Magunia H, Guerrero AM, Keller M, et al. Extubation and Noninvasive Ventilation of Patients Supported by Extracorporeal Life Support for Cardiogenic Shock: A Single-Center Retrospective Observational Cohort Study. J Intensive Care Med. 2021;36(7):783-792.

31. Crotti S, Bottino N, Spinelli E. Spontaneous breathing during veno-venous extracorporeal membrane oxygenation. J Thorac Dis. 2018;10(Suppl 5):S661-S669.

32. Wells CL, Forrester J, Vogel J, Rector R, Tabatabai A, Herr D. Safety and Feasibility of Early Physical Therapy for Patients on Extracorporeal Membrane Oxygenator: University of Maryland Medical Center Experience. Crit Care Med. 2018;46(1):53-59.

33. Braune S, Bojes P, Mecklenburg A, et al. Feasibility, safety, and resource utilisation of active mobilisation of patients on extracorporeal life support: a prospective observational study. Ann Intensive Care. 2020;10(1):161.

34. Munshi L, Kobayashi T, DeBacker J, et al. Intensive Care Physiotherapy during Extracorporeal Membrane Oxygenation for Acute Respiratory Distress Syndrome. Ann Am Thorac Soc. 2017;14(2):246-253.

35. Keshavamurthy S, Bazan V, Tribble TA, Baz MA, Zwischenberger JB. Ambulatory extracorporeal membrane oxygenation (ECMO) as a bridge to lung transplantation. Indian J Thorac Cardiovasc Surg. Published online September 1, 2021:1-14.

36. Garcia JP, Kon ZN, Evans C, et al. Ambulatory veno-venous extracorporeal membrane oxygenation: innovation and pitfalls. J Thorac Cardiovasc Surg. 2011;142(4):755-761.

37. Hayes D, Kukreja J, Tobias JD, Ballard HO, Hoopes CW. Ambulatory venovenous extracorporeal respiratory support as a bridge for cystic fibrosis patients to emergent lung transplantation. J Cyst Fibros Off J Eur Cyst Fibros Soc. 2012;11(1):40-45.

38. Rahimi RA, Skrzat J, Reddy DRS, et al. Physical Rehabilitation of Patients in the Intensive Care Unit Requiring Extracorporeal Membrane Oxygenation: A Small Case Series. Phys Ther. 2013;93(2):248-255.

39. Rehder KJ, Turner DA, Hartwig MG, et al. Active rehabilitation during extracorporeal membrane oxygenation as a bridge to lung transplantation. Respir Care. 2013;58(8):1291-1298.

40. Turner DA, Cheifetz IM, Rehder KJ, et al. Active rehabilitation and physical therapy during extracorporeal membrane oxygenation while awaiting lung transplantation: A practical approach*. Crit Care Med. 2011;39(12):2593-2598.

41. Lehr CJ, Zaas DW, Cheifetz IM, Turner DA. Ambulatory Extracorporeal Membrane Oxygenation as a Bridge to Lung Transplantation. CHEST. 2015;147(5):1213-1218.

42. Spinelli E, Protti A. Get Fit for Lung Transplant With Ambulatory Extracorporeal Membrane Oxygenation! Respir Care. 2016;61(1):117-118.

43. Yanagida R, Seethamraju H, Davenport DL, Tribble TA, Zwischenberger JB, Hoopes CW. Bridging to lung transplantation with double-lumen venovenous extracorporeal membrane oxygenation. Int J Artif Organs. 2019;42(11):621-627.

44. Abrams D, Javidfar J, Farrand E, et al. Early mobilization of patients receiving extracorporeal membrane oxygenation: a retrospective cohort study. Crit Care Lond Engl. 2014;18(1):R38.

45. Mohite PN, Kaul S, Sabashnikov A, et al. Extracorporeal life support in patients with refractory cardiogenic shock: keep them awake. Interact Cardiovasc Thorac Surg. 2015;20(6):755-760.

46. Langer T, Santini A, Bottino N, et al. "Awake" extracorporeal membrane oxygenation (ECMO): pathophysiology, technical considerations, and clinical pioneering. Crit Care Lond Engl. 2016;20(1):150.

47. Ferreira D da C, Marcolino MAZ, Macagnan FE, Plentz RDM, Kessler A. Safety and potential benefits of physical therapy in adult patients on extracorporeal membrane oxygenation support: a systematic review. Rev Bras Ter Intensiva. 2019;31(2):227-239.

48. Bain JC, Turner DA, Rehder KJ, et al. Economic Outcomes of Extracorporeal Membrane Oxygenation With and Without Ambulation as a Bridge to Lung Transplantation. Respir Care. 2016;61(1):1-7.

49. Spinelli E, Mauri T, Beitler JR, Pesenti A, Brodie D. Respiratory drive in the acute respiratory distress syndrome: pathophysiology, monitoring, and therapeutic interventions. Intensive Care Med. 2020;46(4):606-618.

50. Jonkman AH, de Vries HJ, Heunks LMA. Physiology of the Respiratory Drive in ICU Patients: Implications for Diagnosis and Treatment. Crit Care Lond Engl. 2020;24(1):104.

51. Telias I, Spadaro S. Techniques to monitor respiratory drive and inspiratory effort. Curr Opin Crit Care. 2020;26(1):3-10.

52. Doorduin J, Nollet JL, Roesthuis LH, et al. Partial Neuromuscular Blockade during Partial Ventilatory Support in Sedated Patients with High Tidal Volumes. Am J Respir Crit Care Med. 2017;195(8):1033-1042.

53. Brander L, Moerer O, Hedenstierna G, et al. Neural control of ventilation prevents both over-distension and de-recruitment of experimentally injured lungs. Respir Physiol Neurobiol. 2017;237:57-67.

54. Patrick K, Adams A. Mobilization of Patients Receiving Extracorporeal Membrane Oxygenation Before Lung Transplant. Crit Care Nurse. 2021;41(4):39-45.

55. Kalsi-Ryan S. International Standards for Neurological Classification of Spinal Cord Injury (ISNCSCI) *. In: Vaccaro AR, Fisher CG, Wilson JR, eds. 50 Landmark Papers. 1st ed. CRC Press; 2018:83-86.

56. Haji JY, Mehra S, Doraiswamy P. Awake ECMO and mobilizing patients on ECMO. Indian J Thorac Cardiovasc Surg. Published online January 18, 2021:1-10.

57. Hoopes C. Ambulatory Extracorporeal Membrane Oxygenation. Oper Tech Thorac Cardiovasc Surg. 2014;19(2):129-137.

58. Bonizzoli M, Lazzeri C, Drago A, et al. Effects of a physiotherapic program in patients on veno-venous extracorporeal membrane oxygenation: an 8-year single-center experience. Minerva Anestesiol. 2019;85(9):989-994.

59. Botsch A, Protain E, Smith AR, Szilagyi R. Nursing Implications in the ECMO Patient. IntechOpen; 2019.

60. Hodgson CL, Fulcher B, Mariajoseph FP, et al. A Core Outcome Set for Research in Patients on Extracorporeal Membrane Oxygenation. Crit Care Med. 2021;49(12):e1252-e1254.

61. Huang M, Chan KS, Zanni JM, et al. Functional Status Score for the Intensive Care Unit (FSS-ICU): An International Clinimetric Analysis of Validity, Responsiveness, and Minimal Important Difference. Crit Care Med. 2016;44(12):e1155-e1164.

62. Hodgson C, Needham D, Haines K, et al. Feasibility and inter-rater reliability of the ICU Mobility Scale. Heart Lung J Crit Care. 2014;43(1):19-24.

63. Vanhorebeek I, Latronico N, Van den Berghe G. ICU-acquired weakness. Intensive Care Med. 2020;46(4):637-653.

64. De Jonghe B, Cook D, Griffith L, et al. Adaptation to the Intensive Care Environment (ATICE): development and validation of a new sedation assessment instrument. Crit Care Med. 2003;31(9):2344-2354.

65. Society of Critical Care Medicine | SCCM. Accessed January 19, 2022. https://sccm.org/Home.

66. Jette DU, Stilphen M, Ranganathan VK, Passek SD, Frost FS, Jette AM. AM-PAC "6-Clicks" functional assessment scores predict acute care hospital discharge destination. Phys Ther. 2014;94(9):1252-1261.

67. Hoyer EH, Young DL, Klein LM, et al. Toward a Common Language for Measuring Patient Mobility in the Hospital: Reliability and Construct Validity of Interprofessional Mobility Measures. Phys Ther. 2018;98(2):133-142.

68. Koski L. Validity and applications of the Montreal cognitive assessment for the assessment of vascular cognitive impairment. Cerebrovasc Dis Basel Switz. 2013;36(1):6-18.

69. SLU Mental Status Exam. Accessed January 18, 2022. https://www.slu.edu/medicine/internal-medicine/geriatric-medicine/aging-successfully/assessment-tools/mental-status-exam.php.

70. ACSMs Guidelines for Exercise Testing and Prescription. ACSM_CMS. Accessed January 18, 2022. https://www.acsm.org/education-resources/books/guidelines-exercise-testing-prescription.

71. Guérin C, Reignier J, Richard JC, et al. Prone positioning in severe acute respiratory distress syndrome. N Engl J Med. 2013;368(23):2159-2168.

72. Gattinoni L, Pelosi P, Vitale G, Pesenti A, D'Andrea L, Mascheroni D. Body position changes redistribute lung computed-tomographic density in patients with acute respiratory failure. Anesthesiology. 1991;74(1):15-23.

73. Richter T, Bellani G, Scott Harris R, et al. Effect of prone position on regional shunt, aeration, and perfusion in experimental acute lung injury. Am J Respir Crit Care Med. 2005;172(4):480-487.

74. Mutoh T, Guest RJ, Lamm WJ, Albert RK. Prone position alters the effect of volume overload on regional pleural pressures and improves hypoxemia in pigs in vivo. Am Rev Respir Dis. 1992;146(2):300-306.

75. Guervilly C, Prud'homme E, Pauly V, et al. Prone positioning and extracorporeal membrane oxygenation for severe acute respiratory distress syndrome: time for a randomized trial? Intensive Care Med. 2019;45(7):1040-1042.

76. Giani M, Martucci G, Madotto F, et al. Prone Positioning during Venovenous Extracorporeal Membrane Oxygenation in Acute Respiratory Distress Syndrome. A Multicenter Cohort Study and Propensity-matched Analysis. Ann Am Thorac Soc. 2021;18(3):495-501.

77. Kimmoun A, Roche S, Bridey C, et al. Prolonged prone positioning under VV-ECMO is safe and improves oxygenation and respiratory compliance. Ann Intensive Care. 2015;5(1):35.

78. Petit M, Fetita C, Gaudemer A, et al. Prone-positioning for severe acute respiratory distress syndrome requiring extracorporeal membrane oxygenation. Crit Care Med 2022; 50:264-274.

79. Rilinger J, Zotzmann V, Bemtgen X, et al. Prone positioning in severe ARDS requiring extracorporeal membrane oxygenation. Crit Care Lond Engl. 2020;24(1):397.

80. Papazian L, Schmidt M, Hajage D, et al. Effect of prone positioning on survival in adult patients receiving venovenous extracorporeal membrane oxygenation for acute respiratory distress syndrome: a systematic review and meta-analysis. Intensive Care Med. Published online January 17, 2022.

81. Petit M, Fetita C, Gaudemer A, et al. Prone-Positioning for Severe Acute Respiratory Distress Syndrome Requiring Extracorporeal Membrane Oxygenation. Crit Care Med. Published online July 14, 2021.

# 48

## Bedside Ultrasound

*Ghislaine Douflé, Erik Su, Ravi R. Thiagarajan, Dirk W. Donker, Eddy Fan*

In recent years, bedside ultrasound (US) has gained wide acceptance within critical care. Bedside US is particularly advantageous for comprehensive imaging on ECLS, as it is readily available, low risk, and avoids a labor-intensive intrahospital transport. This chapter will focus on US modalities, presenting specific aspects pertaining to ECLS.

### Pre-ECLS

The role of echocardiography pre-ECLS is essential to confirm indication and choice of configuration. Comprehensive echocardiography should be performed to document any cardiovascular abnormalities, including for patients with respiratory failure needing VV ECMO.[1] Indeed, patients with severe hypoxemia due to left-sided valvular disease or severe left ventricular (LV) dysfunction may require a different management strategy.

In severe right ventricular (RV) dysfunction, signs of chronicity should be identified as these patients may require VA or VVA ECMO.[2] Alternatively, patients with acute RV failure due to ARDS often stabilize once on VV ECMO but may develop differential hypoxemia if placed on peripheral VA ECMO, and may need to be switched to VV or VVA ECMO.[3-8]

Patients requiring circulatory support need a thorough assessment of cardiac function (ie, biventricular morphology and function, presence of intracardiac thrombus). Contraindications (eg, severe aortic regurgitation, aortic dissection) or pathologies requiring surgical interventions (eg, papillary muscle, interventricular septal rupture) must be diagnosed before proceeding to cannulation. The presence and consequences of a pericardial effusion should be evaluated precannulation. Right atrial anatomy (eg, presence of a prominent Eustachian valve, Chiari network, or atrial septal defect), presence of RA or RV thrombi, position of pacemaker leads, and patency of the superior and inferior vena cava (SVC and IVC) should also be assessed precannulation (Figures 48-1 and 48-2).[9]

### ECLS Procedural Guidance

#### *Ultrasound-guided Vascular Access*

A thorough examination of the peripheral vessels around the expected puncture point is crucial to exclude occlusive thrombi or stenosis.[10-13] The size of the vessel will determine the cannula size that can be safely inserted (Fr = 3 x narrowest vascular diameter in mm). A small gap of a few Fr is recommended for

**Figures: All figures are at the end of this chapter.**

ease of insertion and patient safety. Realtime ultrasound-guided vascular puncture is recommended for faster access and minimizes the risk of vascular complications.

### Echocardiography Guidance for ECLS

Both transthoracic and transesophageal echocardiography (TTE and TEE) can be used to guide cannulation. In mechanically ventilated adult patients, visualization of the guidewires is enhanced on TEE compared to TTE.[14,15] Adequate echocardiography training is mandatory to safely guide ECMO cannulation, as both wires and cannula can generate significant scattering and artifacts, and rapid switching between views is needed.[14] Once vascular access is obtained, guidewires can be advanced under realtime echo guidance. The TTE views needed are the subcostal views of the IVC and descending aorta for VA ECMO.[16] The subcostal RV inflow outflow (RVIO) and the parasternal RV inflow (RVI) may better visualize the wires in the RA. On TEE, the key views are the midesophageal (ME) bicaval and IVC views, and the descending aorta for VA ECMO.[17]

### VV ECMO

*Two cannulation sites.* Both wires should ideally be in both vena cava so that they do not inadvertently abut against any cardiac chambers (Figure 48-3 and 48-4). Careful monitoring of the wires during sequential vascular dilations is needed, as wires may coil in the heart, cross the interatrial septum, or enter a subhepatic vein (Figure 48-5).[9,18,19] Wires looped in the RA or RV may lead to dysrhythmias and increase the risk of cardiac perforation (Figures 48-6 and 48-7).[20] The final position of the cannula should maximize drainage while avoiding clinically relevant recirculation. Several factors affect the amount of recirculation, such as configuration, distance between cannulas, direction of the reinjection jet, and location of the main draining point within multistage cannulas.[21,22] The position of the drainage cannula needs to account for potential loss in lung volume that may occur with a lung rest strategy once the patient is on ECLS. This may cause the diaphragm to shift upward and change the cannula position within the IVC and in relation to the cardiac chambers.[23] Therefore, the drainage cannula may be placed within the RA and its position reassessed after ventilatory adjustment (Figure 48-8). The reinfusion cannula may not always be visualized in the SVC but should be a few centimeters above the SVC/RA junction (Figure 48-9). For femorofemoral V-V ECMO, the drainage cannula may be placed within the RA and the single stage reinfusion cannula mid RA. This allows adequate flows and minimal recirculation as long as a sufficient distance is maintained between the proximal drainage hole and the tip of the reinjection cannula.[24]

*Single site cannulation.* Dual-lumen bicaval cannulas (DLBC) and RA-PA cannulas can be placed under echo guidance.[25-30] Constant monitoring of the wire is of the utmost importance during dilations and insertion of the cannula. For DLBC, the wire should be far into the IVC beyond the takeoff of the hepatic veins and should remain straight when inserting the cannula.[31,32] Alternating between the ME bicaval and IVC views is required. The IVC-RA junction may be challenging to visualize on TEE; switching between TEE and TTE subcostal views may provide a better visualization of the cannula in the IVC. The reinjection jet should be in the RA and directed towards the tricuspid valve. For RA-PA cannulation, one needs to see the wire up to the PA and carefully follow the cannula over the wire.[33,34] It may be challenging to image the whole cannula at once but the RVIO allows visualization of the cannula's progression through the RA, RV, and main PA. The cannula tip should be 2 to 3 cm above the pulmonary valve but should not be selective in the PA branches. This can be ascertained from the ME RVIO, ME view of the pulmonary valve, and the PA upper esophageal view (Figure 48-10).

## *VA ECMO*

Similar principles apply for the insertion of the drainage cannula as on VV ECMO. As recirculation is not a concern on VA ECMO, the drainage cannula can be advanced across the RA and within the SVC. The arterial wire should be seen in the aorta. The reinfusion cannula is usually not seen on echocardiography but may be seen on a pelvic ultrasound in the femoral or iliac artery. One should check for the absence of aortic dissection post cannulation.[35]

For all cannulations, the absence of a new pericardial or pleural effusion should be ascertained postprocedure, and the size of a preexisting effusion must be reassessed.

## Monitoring on ECLS

### *Echocardiographic Monitoring on VV ECMO*

Echocardiography plays an integral role in managing patients supported with VV ECMO.[6,36] TTE views provide adequate echogenicity in most cases, especially when tidal volumes are minimal.[37] In addition to monitoring cardiac function (more specifically RV function), echocardiography is helpful to troubleshoot persistent hypoxemia and inadequate flows that cannot be explained by circuit failure. Even if the initial position was deemed adequate, cannula position should be reassessed with echocardiography in case of lower flows, as x-rays are not as sensitive to locate the cannula position relative to the cardiac chambers.[38,39] Echocardiography allows discrimination between hypovolemia, cannula malposition, and thrombus formation. If needed, cannula repositioning should be done under echo guidance. In case of hypoxemia,

echocardiography can help diagnose insufficient ECMO flows in proportion to the patient's cardiac output. Ultrasound dilution technique combined with echocardiography can also help quantify the recirculation fraction.[35,40] Moreover, colour Doppler is helpful in visualizing the reinjection flow direction of DLBC on the TTE RVI, RVIO, and subcostal views. On TEE, the ME bicaval, modified bicaval, and proximal IVC views are best to assess flow direction of DLBC. Loss in lung volumes may change the relative position of the cannula within the RA and cause the reinjection flow to become intrahepatic, thus causing inefficient oxygenation and elevation of liver enzymes (Figure 48-11a and 48-11b).[15] On VV ECMO, impaired venous return due to pericardial tamponade will have the same hemodynamic consequences as without ECMO. However, pulsus paradoxus and its echocardiographic equivalent (transmitral and transtricuspid respiratory variations) may be missing in case of minimal tidal volumes. RA compression may not always be evident as the ECMO flow may be initially maintained.

### *Echocardiographic Monitoring on VA ECMO*

Echocardiographic assessment is indispensable throughout the course of VA ECMO. Frequent evaluation of biventricular geometry and function and valvular pathologies (mitral and aortic regurgitation) are necessary to ensure adequate ventricular unloading while maintaining sufficient circulatory support and organ perfusion. Complex interactions between ventricular preload and afterload make it challenging to accurately measure intrinsic ventricular contractility; all parameters should be interpreted with caution and reported with the ECMO flows at the time of assessment. Increased LV afterload due to ECMO flows (especially retrograde aortic flows with femoral VA ECMO) can lead to LV overdistention, increased ventricular filling pressure, and pulmonary edema. A transient decrease in LV systolic function in infants or "cardiac stun" on VA ECMO is well described in the literature.[41] Daily echocardiographic assessment paired with perfusion parameters allows optimization of ECMO and inotropic support while monitoring for signs of recovery or lack thereof. When LV contractility is severely impaired, opening of the aortic valve may be limited or absent despite lower ECMO flows and inotropic support. This further increases LV distension and can lead to thrombi formation in the aortic root and ventricles, with the possibility of complete thrombosis of either ventricular cavity (Figure 48-12).[14] Adequate opening of the aortic valve at different ECMO flows can be monitored with echocardiography. Consistent loss of pulsatility and a significant amount of spontaneous echo contrast, despite inotropic support and adequate fluid loading, may prompt insertion of a venting device.[42-46] The diagnosis of tamponade is even more challenging on VA ECMO, as organ perfusion and hemodynamics may be initially maintained. Additionally, the RV may be underfilled and collapsed from the ECMO drainage alone. Loss of pulsatility may occur, while drops in flows may be delayed, especially for loculated effusions. Serial echocardiography may be needed to monitor the evolution and size of the effusion.

### Lung Ultrasound (Lung US)

Lung US can be used to assess for presence of pleural effusions, pneumothoraces, and assess lung aeration. Caution should be used when diagnosing a pneumothorax on ECMO with ultraprotective ventilation. Even in the absence of pneumothorax, lung sliding may not be observed due to complete lung collapse while a lung pulse will still be present. In two pilot studies monitoring patients with lung US, lung US scores (LUS) did not differ between survivors and non survivors at the time of ECMO initiation. Improvement of LUS was observed in patients who improved and could be decannulated from VV ECMO, while persistently high LUS portended a poor prognosis.[47,48] Others described the potential use of LUS as a surrogate for lung compliance.[49]

### Neuromonitoring with Transcranial Doppler (TCD)

It is important to recognize that continuous flow confounds traditional measurements of pulsatility on VA ECMO and is well described in the pediatric literature. Arteriospasm may be masked in situations where the heart is contributing little to cerebral blood flow, but some series indicate that an increase in pulsatility index, not otherwise associated with improved cardiac function, may indicate an acute neurological injury and remains an area for investigation.[50,51] The first 3-5 days after cannulation have been identified as the highest risk for intracranial hemorrhage in infants.[52] This has supported the concept of using daily screening with head US during the first week of ECMO support, as mentioned in recent ELSO guidelines.[53,54] Yet, concerns exist regarding the sensitivity of US. In one autopsy and imaging study, 19 of 74 patients had neurologic or MR imaging sequela despite a normal head US.[55,56] Reports of TCD use in adults on ECMO have largely been descriptions of feasibility. As in children, overall pulsatility is diminished by the proportion of cardiac output captured by the continuous flow on VA ECMO.[57,58] Considerations for use of TCD in brain death evaluation have been discussed: in cases of pulsatile blood flow, there is agreement that oscillating arterial flow, absence of diastolic flow with short systolic spikes, and absence of flow, in comparison to a previously documented flow on TCD performed by the same operator, are consistent with brain death.[59] The absence of flow is potentially problematic on VA ECMO in case of poor cardiac ejection, as continuous cerebral blood flow may be difficult to detect.[60,61]

## Weaning

On VV ECMO, hypoxemia and hypercapnia may worsen RV function during weaning of VV ECMO, but there is, to our knowledge, no study focusing on RV function in this setting.

Weaning from VA ECMO is an intricate process requiring integration of clinical and echocardiographic parameters.[62] Attempts at liberating from VA ECMO should be made as soon as possible to avoid complications from prolonged ECMO support. Evaluation of cardiac size and function with a stepwise reduction in ECMO flows (as low as 1 L/min in adult patients) provides invaluable information to guide the timing of separation from ECMO. Parameters described to assess readiness for liberation include biventricular function as measured with LV ejection fraction (EF) 20-25%, tissue Doppler S' at the mitral annulus $\geq6$ cm/s, LVOT velocity time integral $\geq10$ cm, and ventricular interdependence.[63,64] 2D strain values were not different between weaned and non-weaned patients.[65] As RV failure portends a worse prognosis, it is crucial to specifically evaluate RV function.[66] A 3D RVEF above 24% has been shown to be the best parameter to predict successful liberation from VA ECMO, while RV strain, RV fractional area of change, and central venous pressure were independently associated with RVEF.[67] Ventricular interdependence has also been described as a predictor of successful decannulation.[68] Unless the ECMO circuit is clamped, assessing true RV intrinsic contractility may be difficult since the RV is not fully loaded, even at low flows. To minimize the risk of circuit clotting, some authors have suggested using an arteriovenous bridge or pump controlled retrograde trial off.[69-71] More recently, indices assessing RV coupling to the pulmonary circulation (tricuspid annular S' velocity/right ventricular systolic pressure (RVSP), tricuspid annular plane systolic excursion (TAPSE)/RVSP, RV free wall lateral strain/RVSP with cut-off values of $\geq0.33$,

0.45, 0.45, respectively) performed better at predicting successful weaning than previously described parameters, even at moderate flows.[72]

## Post-ECLS Care

The incidence of cannula-related thrombosis after ECLS is a frequent complication despite adequate anticoagulation, with an incidence ranging from 18.1% to 100% (the latter incidence was from a small cohort of patients supported with VV ECMO for COVID-19 ARDS), thus warranting systematic vascular imaging of previous cannulation sites.[73-76]

## Specific Neonatal and Pediatric Considerations

Unique considerations regarding US in neonates and children on ECMO exist by virtue of cannulation strategy, patient size, and body composition. Understanding the particularities of US for neonates and children is paramount for diagnostic accuracy and appropriate management. Smaller face size of probes promotes mobility and may help small structures appear larger on screens, while larger probes are needed for children approaching adult body habitus. Children, particularly neonates, demonstrate higher water content and bone immaturity, which facilitate ultrasound transmission.[77] Conversely, it may be difficult to locate a window in small children covered with dressings. Modified and foreshortened views may be the only views available.

In patients with congenital diaphragmatic hernia (CDH), diaphragm position, lung inflation, and abnormal cardiac position may complicate interpretation of cannula position. Cannula position can change in patients with right sided CDH and after CDH surgical intervention.

With right carotid artery return cannulas, optimal placement should be at the junction of the right brachiocephalic artery (BCA)

and the ascending aorta (Figure 48-13). A cannula protruding in the aorta can direct more proportional flow towards the aortic root, thereby reducing aortic valve opening, impeding decompression of the left ventricle, and increasing left atrial pressure. A cannula placed higher in the BCA or carotid artery is feasible but becomes a concern for increased risk of dislodgement. For neonates, one may also consider obtaining ductal views of a patent ductus arteriosus (PDA) to determine directionality of flow and the contribution of right-to-left shunting through the PDA as a source for systemic desaturation on VA ECMO.[78,79]

**Conclusion**

The use of bedside ultrasound is an integral part of the management of patients on ECLS. From indication and initiation to weaning, it is an indispensable tool that allows rapid assessment of patients on ECLS. Physicians managing ECLS patients should be familiar with specificities of ultrasound on ECLS to accurately assess and interpret ultrasonographic findings.

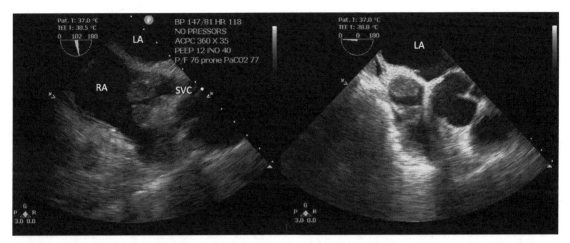

**Figure 48-1.** TEE ME bicaval views showing two right atrial thrombi at the SVC and RA junction. Decision was made to proceed with Femorofemoral V-V ECMO cannulation to avoid dislodging the thrombi during cannulation.

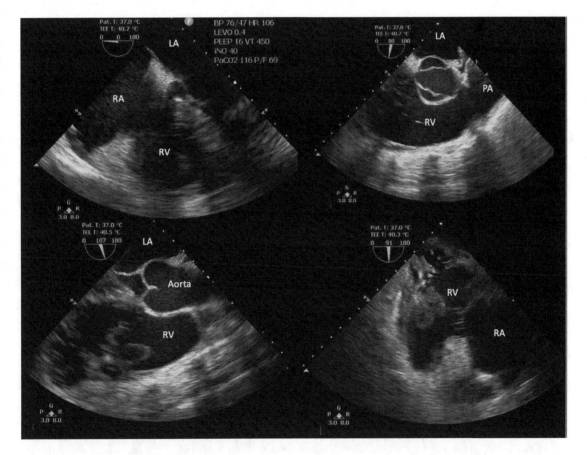

**Figure 48-2.** TEE ME four chamber view focused on the RV (top left). A RV thrombus is seen within the RV. ME RVIO view showing part of the RV clot (top right). Modified ME RV view showing the multilobular clot attached to the subvalvular apparatus of the tricuspid valve (bottom Left). Transgastric RVI view showing the clot (bottom right).

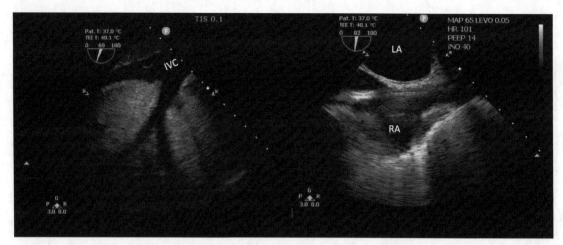

**Figure 48-3.** TEE. View at the esophageal and gastric junction showing the IVC with the femoral wire being advanced (left). ME bicaval view showing both wires across the RA and both vena cavae (right).

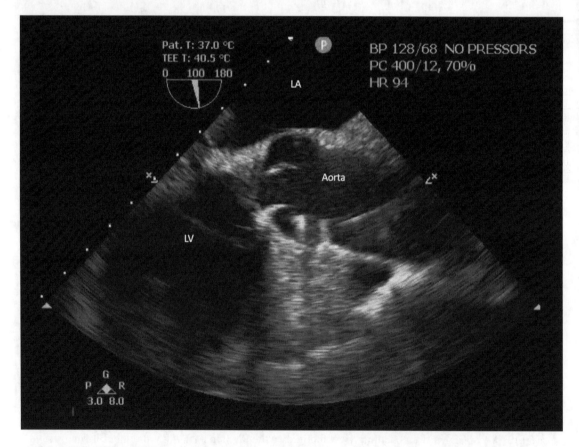

**Figure 48-4.** TEE ME view of the ascending aorta with a guidewire inadvertently inserted in the ascending aorta after transfixing the internal jugular vein. The guidewire was removed, and a new venipuncture was performed.

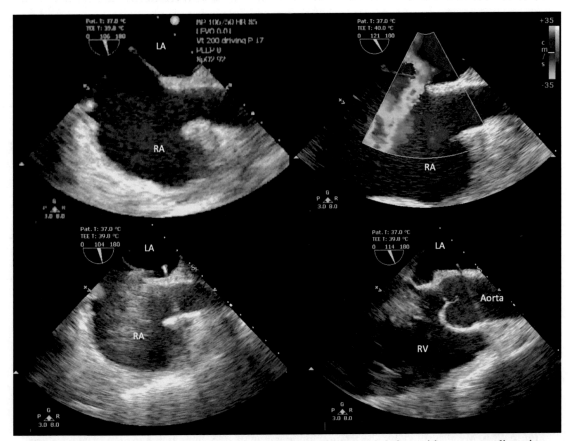

**Figure 48-5.** ME bicaval view depicting a secundum atrial septal defect with corresponding view with colour flow Doppler added showing a left to right shunt (top). ME long axis view showing the guide wire crossing the atrial septal defect and ending in the LA (bottom left). ME long axis view with the guidewire in the LA (bottom right).

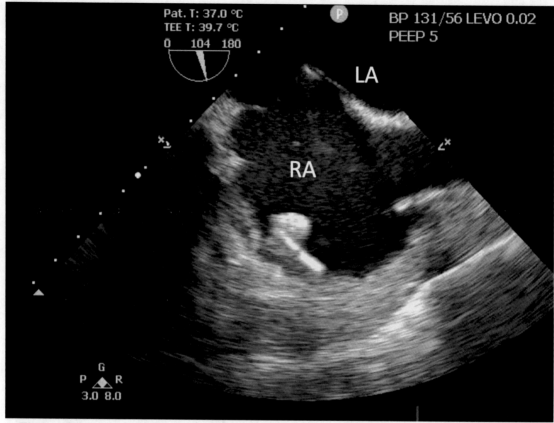

**Figure 48-6.** ME bicaval view. The femoral guidewire is seen looping within the RA. The wire was repositioned in the SVC before insertion of the cannula.

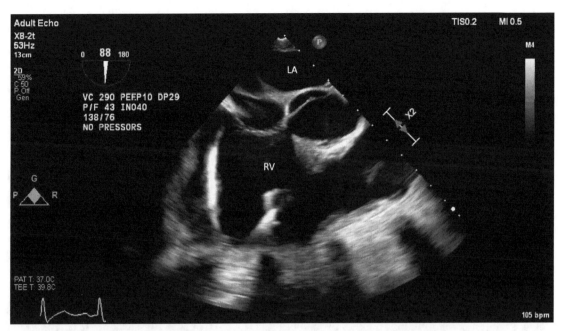

**Figure 48-7.** Modified ME view of the RV. A guidewire is seen looping in the RV.

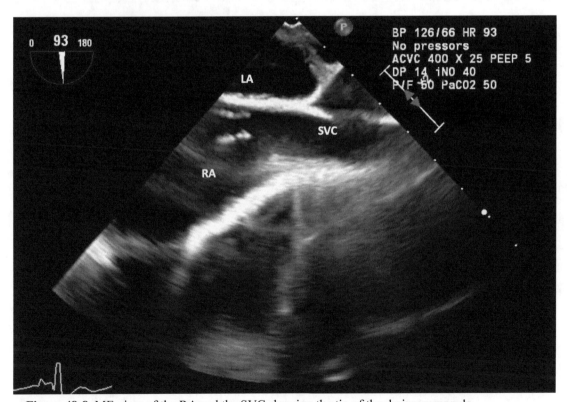

**Figure 48-8.** ME view of the RA and the SVC showing the tip of the drainage cannula.

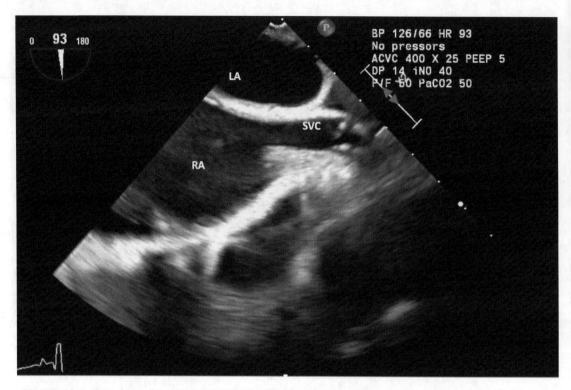

**Figure 48-9.** ME view of the RA and the SVC showing the tip of the reinjection cannula.

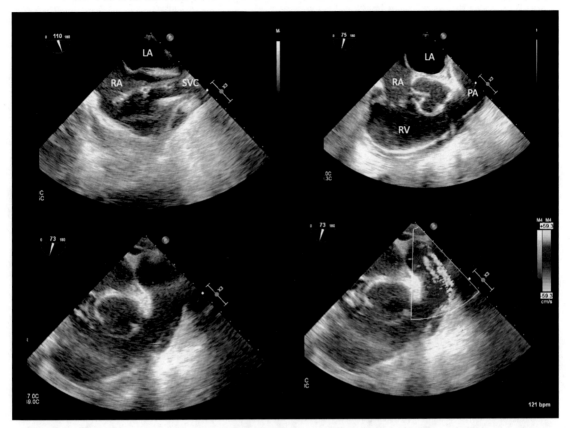

**Figure 48-10.** TEE ME views showing a RA-PA cannula. The drainage holes can be seen in the RA (top left). The cannula itself is seen lying along the wall of the RV (top right), with the tip of the cannula 2 to 3 cm above the pulmonary valve (bottom left). Cannula with reinjection flow seen with colour flow Doppler (bottom right).

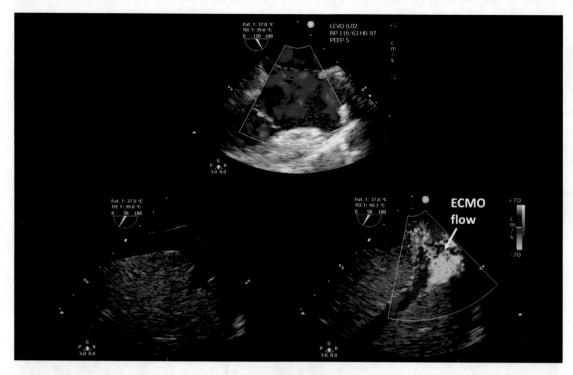

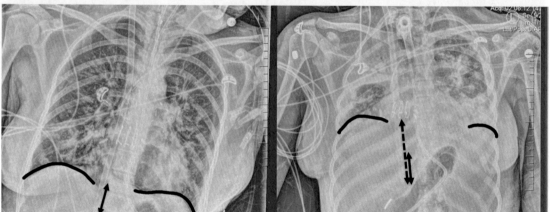

**Figure 48-11a(top), b(bottom).** TEE views ME modified bicaval of a patient with a dual lumen bicaval cannula. The jet was initially directed towards the tricuspid valve. However, a few days later, without any significant change in the cannula position the patient remained hypoxemic. A repeat TEE showed that the reinjection flow was predominantly reinjected in the hepatic veins. The comparison of the two-chest x-ray showed a significant loss in lung volumes and subsequent elevation of the diaphragm. The relative position of the reinjection hole in relation to the cardiac chambers changed causing the reinjection flow to be reinjected within the liver instead of in the RA. The cannula was withdrawn under TEE guidance until the reinjection was seen in the RA.

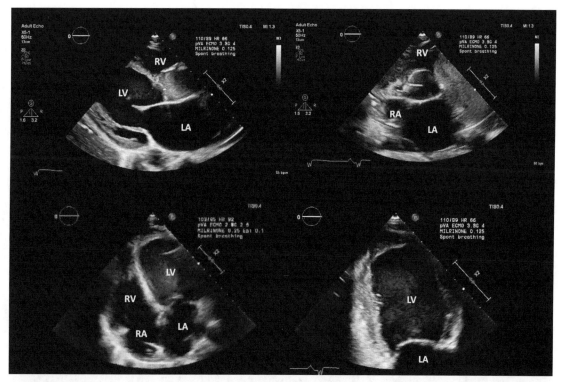

**Figure 48-12.** TTE views of a patient on peripheral VA ECMO for dilated cardiomyopathy. Parasternal view showing no opening of the aortic valve and significant spontaneous echo contrast in the aortic root (top left). Parasternal short axis of the aortic valve of the same patient with spontaneous contrast in the RV, PA and in the aortic root (top right). Apical four chamber view with LV thrombus and spontaneous echo contrast (bottom left). Apical two chamber view focused on the LV with the apical thrombus (bottom right).

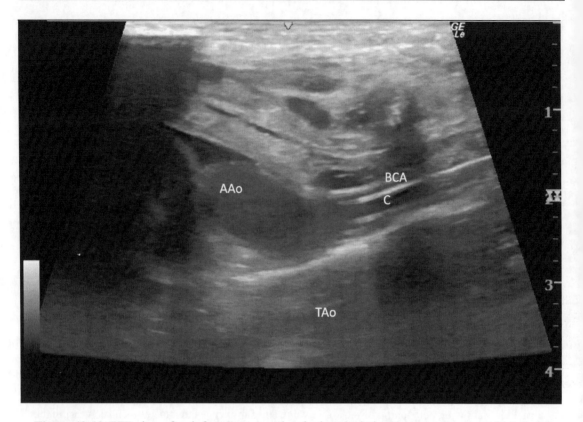

**Figure 48-13.** TTE view of an infant: Parasternal arch view depicting the ascending aorta (AAo), the brachiocephalic artery (BCA) containing a correctly positioned aortic return cannula (C). The transverse aortic arch (TAo) is also depicted with a bright artifact crossing the arch horizontally between the ascending and transverse aortic arch.

# References

1. Lang RM, Badano LP, Mor-Avi V, et al. Recommendations for cardiac chamber quantification by echocardiography in adults: an update from the American Society of Echocardiography and the European Association of Cardiovascular Imaging. J Am Soc Echocardiogr. Jan 2015;28(1):1-39 e14.
2. Rudski LG, Lai WW, Afilalo J, et al. Guidelines for the echocardiographic assessment of the right heart in adults: a report from the American Society of Echocardiography endorsed by the European Association of Echocardiography, a registered branch of the European Society of Cardiology, and the Canadian Society of Echocardiography. J Am Soc Echocardiogr. Jul 2010;23(7):685-713; quiz 786-8.
3. Hoetzenecker K, Donahoe L, Yeung JC, et al. Extracorporeal life support as a bridge to lung transplantation-experience of a high-volume transplant center. J Thorac Cardiovasc Surg. Mar 2018;155(3):1316-1328 e1.
4. Douflé G, Ferguson ND. Monitoring during extracorporeal membrane oxygenation. Curr Opin Crit Care. Apr 8 2016.
5. Lazzeri C, Bonizzoli M, Cianchi G, et al. Right ventricular dysfunction and Pre Implantation Vasopressors in Refractory ARDS Supported by V-V-ECMO. Heart Lung Circ. 2018;27(12):1483-1488.
6. Reis Miranda D, van Thiel R, Brodie D, Bakker J. Right ventricular unloading after initiation of venovenous extracorporeal membrane oxygenation. Am J Respir Crit Care Med. Feb 1 2015;191(3):346-8.
7. Bunge JJH, Caliskan K, Gommers D, et al. Right ventricular dysfunction during acute respiratory distress syndrome and veno-venous extracorporeal membrane oxygenation. J Thorac Dis. Mar 2018;10(Suppl 5):S674-S682.
8. Goursaud S, Valette X, Dupeyrat J, et al. Ultraprotective ventilation allowed by extracorporeal CO2 removal improves the right ventricular function in acute respiratory distress syndrome patients: a quasi-experimental pilot study. Ann Intensive Care. Jan 7 2021;11(1):3.
9. Giraud R, Banfi C, Bendjelid K. Echocardiography should be mandatory in ECMO venous cannula placement. Eur Heart J Cardiovasc Imaging. 2018;19(12):1429-1430.
10. Lamperti M, Bodenham AR, Pittiruti M, et al. International evidence-based recommendations on ultrasound-guided vascular access. Intensive Care Med. Jul 2012;38(7):1105-17.
11. Randolph AG, Cook DJ, Gonzales CA, et al. Ultrasound guidance for placement of central venous catheters: A meta-analysis of the literature. Crit Care Med. 1996;24(12):2053-2058.
12. Hind D, Calvert N, McWilliams R, et al. Ultrasonic locating devices for central venous cannulation: meta-analysis. BMJ. Aug 16 2003;327(7411):361.
13. Silverberg MJ, Kory P. Intensive care ultrasound: II. Central vascular access and venous diagnostic ultrasound. Ann Am Thorac Soc. Oct 2013;10(5):549-56.
14. Donker DW, Meuwese CL, Braithwaite SA, et al. Echocardiography in extracorporeal life support: A key player in procedural guidance, tailoring and monitoring. Perfusion. May 2018;33(1_suppl):31-41.
15. Douflé G, Roscoe A, Billia F, et al. Echocardiography for adult patients supported with extracorporeal membrane oxygenation. Crit Care. 2015;19:326.
16. Mitchell C, Rahko PS, Blauwet LA, et al. Guidelines for Performing a Comprehensive Transthoracic Echocardiographic Examination in Adults: Recommendations from the American Society of Echocardiography. J Am Soc Echocardiogr. Jan 2019;32(1):1-64.
17. Hahn RT, Abraham T, Adams MS, et al. Guidelines for performing a comprehensive transesophageal echocardiographic examination: recommendations from the American Society of Echocardiography and the Society of Cardiovascular Anesthesiologists. J Am Soc Echocardiogr. Sep 2013;26(9):921-64.
18. Navas-Blanco JR, Williams DV. Images in Anesthesiology: Inadvertent Extracorporeal Membrane Oxygenation Cannulation across a Patent Foramen Ovale. Anesthesiology. 2019;130(2):309-310.
19. Serck N, Lheureux O, Creteur J, et al. Hepatic vein cannulation during veno-arterial extracorporeal membrane oxygenation. Intensive Care Med. 2018;44(9):1571-1572.
20. Salazar PA, Blitzer D, Dolejs SC, et al. Echocardiographic Guidance During Neonatal and Pediatric Jugular Cannulation for ECMO. J Surg Res. Dec 2018;232:517-523.
21. Abrams D, Bacchetta M, Brodie D. Recirculation in venovenous extracorporeal membrane oxygenation. ASAIO J. Mar-Apr 2015;61(2):115-21.
22. Lindholm JA. Cannulation for veno-venous extracorporeal membrane oxygenation. J Thorac Dis. Mar 2018;10(Suppl 5):S606-S612.
23. Riccabona M, Dacar D, Zobel G, et al. Sonographically guided cannula positioning for extracorporeal membrane oxygenation. Pediatr Radiol. 1995;25(8):643-5.
24. The Alfred ICU. ECMO.icu. Accessed December 15th 2021, https://ecmo.icu/procedures-percutaneous-ecmo-cannulation/.
25. Dolch ME, Frey L, Buerkle MA, et al. Transesophageal echocardiography-guided technique for extracorporeal membrane oxygenation dual-lumen catheter placement. Case Reports. ASAIO J. Jul-Aug 2011;57(4):341-3.

26. Chimot L, Marque S, Gros A, et al. Avalon(c) bicaval dual-lumen cannula for venovenous extracorporeal membrane oxygenation: survey of cannula use in France. ASAIO J. Mar-Apr 2013;59(2):157-61.

27. Griffee M, Zimmerman J, McKellar S, et al. Echocardiography-Guided Dual-Lumen Venovenous Extracorporeal Membrane Oxygenation Cannula Placement in the ICU-A Retrospective Review. J Cardiothorac Vasc Anesth. 2020;34(3):698-705.

28. Trimlett RH, Cordingley JJ, Griffiths MJ, et al. A modified technique for insertion of dual lumen bicaval cannulae for venovenous extracorporeal membrane oxygenation. Intensive Care Med. Jun 2011;37(6):1036-7.

29. Hemamalini P, Dutta P, Attawar S. Transesophageal Echocardiography Compared to Fluoroscopy for Avalon Bicaval Dual-Lumen Cannula Positioning for Venovenous ECMO. Ann Card Anaesth. Jul-Sep 2020;23(3):283-287.

30. Moscatelli A, Febbo F, Buratti S, et al. Intensivists Performed Percutaneous Bicaval Double-Lumen Echo-Guided Extracorporeal Membrane Oxygenation Cannulation at Bedside in Newborns and Children: A Retrospective Analysis. Pediatr Crit Care Med. Jun 2019;20(6):551-559.

31. Rubino A, Vuylsteke A, Jenkins DP, et al. Direct complications of the Avalon bicaval dual-lumen cannula in respiratory extracorporeal membrane oxygenation (ECMO): Single-center experience. Int J Artif Organs. Oct 2014;37(10):741-7.

32. Hirose H, Yamane K, Marhefka G, et al. Right ventricular rupture and tamponade caused by malposition of the Avalon cannula for venovenous extracorporeal membrane oxygenation. J Cardiothorac Surg. 2012;7:36.

33. Hill GED, Traudt RJ, Durham LA, et al. Successful Treatment of Refractory Status Asthmaticus Accompanied by Right Ventricular Dysfunction Using a Protek Duo Tandem Heart Device. J Cardiothorac Vasc Anesth. 2019;33(11):3085-3089.

34. Cain MT, Smith NJ, Barash M, et al. Extracorporeal Membrane Oxygenation with Right Ventricular Assist Device for COVID-19 ARDS. J Surg Res. Mar 18 2021;264:81-89.

35. Clements D, Primmer J, Ryman P, et al. Measurements of recirculation during neonatal veno-venous extracorporeal membrane oxygenation: clinical application of the ultrasound dilution technique. J Extra Corpor Technol. Sep 2008;40(3):184-7.

36. Lazzeri C, Bonizzoli M, Cianchi G, et al. Right Ventricular Hypertrophy in Refractory Acute Respiratory Distress Syndrome Treated With Venovenous Extracorporeal Membrane Oxygenation Support. J Cardiothorac Vasc Anesth. Jun 2020;34(6):1441-1445.

37. Viau-Lapointe J, Douflé G. Transthoracic View of Extracorporeal Membrane Oxygenation Cannulae. Am J Resp Crit Care Med. 2019;199(10):e39-e40.

38. Thomas TH, Price R, Ramaciotti C, et al. Echocardiography, not chest radiography, for evaluation of cannula placement during pediatric extracorporeal membrane oxygenation. Pediatr Crit Care Med. Jan 2009;10(1):56-9.

39. Pawlowski TW, Stoller JZ, Rintoul NE, et al. Point-of-care ultrasound for the evaluation of venous cannula position in neonatal extracorporeal membrane oxygenation. J Perinatol. Jul 2021;41(7):1645-1650.

40. Korver EP, Ganushchak YM, Simons AP, et al. Quantification of recirculation as an adjuvant to transthoracic echocardiography for optimization of dual-lumen extracorporeal life support. Intensive Care Med. May 2012;38(5):906-9.

41. Dickson ME, Hirthler MA, Simoni J, et al. Stunned myocardium during extracorporeal membrane oxygenation. Am J Surg. Dec 1990;160(6):644-6.

42. Unai S, Nguyen M-L, Tanaka D, et al. Clinical Significance of Spontaneous Echo Contrast on Extracorporeal Membrane Oxygenation. Ann Thorac Surg. 2017;103(3):773-778.

43. Hireche-Chikaoui H, Grubler MR, Bloch A, et al. Nonejecting Hearts on Femoral Veno-Arterial Extracorporeal Membrane Oxygenation: Aortic Root Blood Stasis and Thrombus Formation-A Case Series and Review of the Literature. Crit Care Med. 2018;46(5):e459-e464.

44. Soleimani B, Pae WE. Management of left ventricular distension during peripheral extracorporeal membrane oxygenation for cardiogenic shock. Perfusion. Jul 2012;27(4):326-31.

45. Meani P, Gelsomino S, Natour E, et al. Modalities and Effects of Left Ventricle Unloading on Extracorporeal Life support: a Review of the Current Literature. Eur J Heart Fail. May 2017;19 Suppl 2:84-91.

46. Avalli L, Maggioni E, Sangalli F, et al. Percutaneous left-heart decompression during extracorporeal membrane oxygenation: an alternative to surgical and transseptal venting in adult patients. ASAIO J. Jan-Feb 2011;57(1):38-40.

47. Mongodi S, Pozzi M, Orlando A, et al. Lung ultrasound for daily monitoring of ARDS patients on extracorporeal membrane oxygenation: preliminary experience. Intensive Care Med. Jan 2018;44(1):123-124.

48. Lu X, Arbelot C, Schreiber A, et al. Ultrasound Assessment of Lung Aeration in Subjects Supported by Venovenous Extracorporeal Membrane Oxygenation. Respir Care. Dec 2019;64(12):1478-1487.

49. Ntoumenopoulos G, Buscher H, Scott S. Lung ultrasound score as an indicator of dynamic lung compliance during veno-venous extra-corpo-

real membrane oxygenation. Int J Artif Organs. Mar 2021;44(3):194-198.

50. O'Brien NF, Buttram SDW, Maa T, et al. Cerebrovascular Physiology During Pediatric Extracorporeal Membrane Oxygenation: A Multicenter Study Using Transcranial Doppler Ultrasonography. Pediatr Crit Care Med. Feb 2019;20(2):178-186.

51. Rilinger JF, Smith CM, deRegnier RAO, et al. Transcranial Doppler Identification of Neurologic Injury during Pediatric Extracorporeal Membrane Oxygenation Therapy. J Stroke Cerebrovasc Dis. Oct 2017;26(10):2336-2345.

52. Theodorou CM, Guenther TM, Honeychurch KL, et al. Utility of Routine Head Ultrasounds in Infants on Extracorporeal Life Support: When is it Safe to Stop Scanning? ASAIO J. Dec 22 2021.

53. Wild KT, Rintoul N, Kattan J, et al. Extracorporeal Life Support Organization (ELSO): Guidelines for Neonatal Respiratory Failure. ASAIO J. May 2020;66(5):463-470.

54. Maratta C, Potera RM, van Leeuwen G, et al. Extracorporeal Life Support Organization (ELSO): 2020 Pediatric Respiratory ELSO Guideline. ASAIO J. Sep/Oct 2020;66(9):975-979.

55. McCutcheon KC, Wise L, Lewis K, et al. The utility of cranial ultrasound as a screening tool for neonatal ECMO. J Perinat Med. Feb 25 2020;48(2):173-178.

56. Lazar EL, Abramson SJ, Weinstein S, et al. Neuroimaging of brain injury in neonates treated with extracorporeal membrane oxygenation: lessons learned from serial examinations. J Pediatr Surg. Feb 1994;29(2):186-90.

57. Kavi T, Esch M, Rinsky B, et al. Transcranial Doppler Changes in Patients Treated with Extracorporeal Membrane Oxygenation. J Stroke Cerebrovasc Dis. Dec 2016;25(12):2882-2885.

58. Salna M, Ikegami H, Willey JZ, et al. Transcranial Doppler is an effective method in assessing cerebral blood flow patterns during peripheral venoarterial extracorporeal membrane oxygenation. J Card Surg. Jun 2019;34(6):447-452.

59. Marinoni M, Cianchi G, Trapani S, et al. Retrospective Analysis of Transcranial Doppler Patterns in Veno-Arterial Extracorporeal Membrane Oxygenation Patients: Feasibility of Cerebral Circulatory Arrest Diagnosis. ASAIO J. Mar/Apr 2018;64(2):175-182.

60. Cestari M, Gobatto ALN, Hoshino M. Role and Limitations of Transcranial Doppler and Brain Death of Patients on Veno-Arterial Extracorporeal Membrane Oxygenation. ASAIO J. Jul/Aug 2018;64(4):e78.

61. Berthoud V, Ellouze O, Constandache T, et al. Transcranial Doppler Waveform Patterns in Nonpulsatile Blood Flow Under Venoarterial Extracorporeal Membrane Oxygenation for Brain Death Diagnosis. ASAIO J. Apr 2020;66(4):e64.

62. Brahmbhatt DH, Daly AL, Luk AC, et al. Liberation From Venoarterial Extracorporeal Membrane Oxygenation: A Review. Circ Heart Fail. Jul 2021;14(7):e007679.

63. Aissaoui N, Luyt CE, Leprince P, et al. Predictors of successful extracorporeal membrane oxygenation (ECMO) weaning after assistance for refractory cardiogenic shock. Clinical Trial. Intensive Care Med. Nov 2011;37(11):1738-45.

64. Punn R, Axelrod DM, Sherman-Levine S, et al. Predictors of mortality in pediatric patients on venoarterial extracorporeal membrane oxygenation. Pediatr Crit Care Med. Nov 2014;15(9):870-7.

65. Aissaoui N, Guerot E, Combes A, et al. Two-dimensional strain rate and Doppler tissue myocardial velocities: analysis by echocardiography of hemodynamic and functional changes of the failed left ventricle during different degrees of extracorporeal life support. Clinical Trial. J Am Soc Echocardiogr. Jun 2012;25(6):632-40.

66. Pappalardo F, Pieri M, Arnaez Corada B, et al. Timing and Strategy for Weaning From Venoarterial ECMO are Complex Issues. J Cardiothorac Vasc Anesth. Dec 12 2014.

67. Huang K-C, Lin L-Y, Chen Y-S, et al. Three-Dimensional Echocardiography-Derived Right Ventricular Ejection Fraction Correlates with Success of Decannulation and Prognosis in Patients Stabilized by Venoarterial Extracorporeal Life Support. J Am Soc Echocardiogr. 2018;31(2):169-179.

68. Aissaoui N, Caudron J, Leprince P, et al. Right-left ventricular interdependence: a promising predictor of successful extracorporeal membrane oxygenation (ECMO) weaning after assistance for refractory cardiogenic shock. Intensive Care Med. 2017;43(4):592-594.

69. Westrope C, Harvey C, Robinson S, et al. Pump controlled retrograde trial off from V-A-ECMO. ASAIO J. Sep-Oct 2013;59(5):517-9.

70. Babar ZU, Sharma AS, Ganushchak YM, et al. An arterio-venous bridge for gradual weaning from adult veno-arterial extracorporeal life support. Perfusion. Nov 2015;30(8):683-8.

71. Ling L, Chan KM. Weaning adult patients with cardiogenic shock on veno-arterial extracorporeal membrane oxygenation by pump-controlled retrograde trial off. Perfusion. Jul 2018;33(5):339-345.

72. Kim D, Park Y, Choi KH, et al. Prognostic Implication of RV Coupling to Pulmonary Circulation for Successful Weaning From Extracorporeal Membrane Oxygenation. JACC Cardiovasc Imaging. Aug 2021;14(8):1523-1531.

73. Cooper E, Burns J, Retter A, et al. Prevalence of Venous Thrombosis Following Venovenous Extracorporeal Membrane Oxygenation in Patients

With Severe Respiratory Failure. Crit Care Med. Dec 2015;43(12):e581-4.

74. Fisser C, Reichenbacher C, Muller T, et al. Incidence and Risk Factors for Cannula-Related Venous Thrombosis After Venovenous Extracorporeal Membrane Oxygenation in Adult Patients With Acute Respiratory Failure. Crit Care Med. Apr 2019;47(4):e332-e339.

75. Parzy G, Daviet F, Persico N, et al. Prevalence and Risk Factors for Thrombotic Complications Following Venovenous Extracorporeal Membrane Oxygenation: A CT Scan Study. Crit Care Med. Feb 2020;48(2):192-199.

76. Parzy G, Daviet F, Puech B, et al. Venous Thromboembolism Events Following Venovenous Extracorporeal Membrane Oxygenation for Severe Acute Respiratory Syndrome Coronavirus 2 Based on CT Scans. Crit Care Med. Oct 2020;48(10):e971-e975.

77. Su E, Dalesio N, Pustavoitau A. Point-of-care ultrasound in pediatric anesthesiology and critical care medicine. Can J Anaesth. Apr 2018;65(4):485-498.

78. Tanke R, Daniels O, Van Heyst A, et al. The influence of ductal left-to-right shunting during extracorporeal membrane oxygenation. J Pediatr Surg. Aug 2002;37(8):1165-8.

79. Miller LE, Stoller JZ, Fraga MV. Point-of-care ultrasound in the neonatal ICU. Curr Opin Pediatr. Apr 2020;32(2):216-227.

# 49

## Pharmacology

*Christa Jefferis Kirk, Mohd Hafiz Abdul-Aziz, Jason A. Roberts, Eleonore Valencia, Kevin Watt, Graeme MacLaren, Kiran Shekar*

### Introduction

Safe and effective pharmacotherapy during ECLS requires an understanding of multiple interdependent factors that impact the pharmacokinetics (PK) and pharmacodynamics (PD) of a given drug or combination of drugs. Critical illness influences drug absorption, distribution, metabolism, and elimination via alterations in total body water and plasma proteins, inadequate tissue perfusion, and impaired end organ function. ECLS further compounds these pharmacokinetic alterations through drug adsorption to ECLS circuitry, a larger volume of distribution (Vd), and decreased clearance (CL), all of which challenge the use of standard medication dosing and may necessitate individualization. Moreover, ECLS technology continues to evolve and experiences among different centers and populations vary, which may decrease the applicability of available literature. Therefore, to avoid life-threatening treatment failure or toxicity, it is essential to understand and monitor the dynamic interactions between critically ill patients, drug physiochemistry, and the ECLS circuit.[1]

### Pharmacokinetics and Pharmacodynamics in ECLS

Attaining a therapeutic drug concentration is dependent on medication-specific bioavailability, Vd, and clearance. Bioavailability is the amount of functional drug at its site of action and is affected by drug administration, distribution, and metabolism. Vd is the theoretical volume needed to dilute a drug to its effective serum concentration and is determined by the physiochemical properties of drugs including protein binding, lipophilicity, and distribution into tissues. Drugs that are hydrophilic have a lower Vd, and their concentrations are primarily influenced by changes in volume status. Highly lipophilic medications have better tissue penetration, resulting in lower plasma concentrations and increased Vd. Medications that are highly protein bound to plasma proteins (eg, albumin) will predominantly remain in the intravascular space and have higher Vd based on free serum drug concentrations.[2,3] Medication clearance is mainly dependent on kidney and liver function. Therefore, changes to Vd or clearance may impact the expected half-life of a drug, the basis for determination of both dose and frequency of administration.[4]

## Physiological Influences on Pharmacokinetics and Pharmacodynamics

Developmental changes in total body water, fat stores, plasma proteins, and metabolic enzymes during maturation create age-dependent PK and PD.[4,5] Neonates and children have higher body water, lower fat stores, and immature enzymatic and drug transport function compared to adults, which impacts drug bioavailability and Vd. Therefore, extrapolation of neonatal and pediatric data regarding pharmacology during ECLS to adults, and vice versa, should be undertaken with caution or not at all.[5,6]

Patients on ECLS may have substantial shifts in the distribution of intravascular and extravascular volume due to excess total body water, injury to the vascular endothelium, deranged concentrations of plasma proteins, or end-organ dysfunction. The therapeutic effect of a hydrophilic drug may be lessened in a patient with intravascular volume overload but may be more pronounced in patients with depleted intravascular volume. Critical illness-associated catabolism, common in cases of sepsis or trauma, decreases plasma proteins, which increases the level of unbound drug and risks toxic effects from highly protein-bound drugs. Bioavailability can be affected by decreased absorption of enterally administered medications in critically ill patients with delayed gastric emptying or ileus. Finally, metabolism and elimination are usually dependent on hepatic and renal function, while the biliary tract, feces, lungs, and other proteolytic mechanisms contribute less. Therefore, standard dosing of a given medication may result in treatment failure or toxicity in patients who have altered hepatic metabolism or renal clearance. Importantly, these pathologies rarely occur in isolation and can be additive, and therefore must be considered for safe and effective drug administration during critical illness.[4,6,7]

Figure 49-1 highlights the pharmacokinetic alterations in critically ill patients that create a delicate balance between treatment failure and adverse reactions related to drug toxicity. Medications must be vigilantly monitored and adjusted in critically ill patients to ensure safe and efficacious therapy.[1,6,7,8]

## Circuit Influences on Pharmacokinetics and Pharmacodynamics

The ECLS circuit impacts PK and PD via hemodilution and drug sequestration (Figure 49-1).[8] Hemodilution predominantly results from the additive effect of circuit volume to a patient's native circulating volume and can have a significant impact on Vd. The extent of hemodilution is dependent upon a patient's size in relation to the circuit; therefore, an infant will experience greater hemodilution than an adult. Hemodilution and the resultant alterations in Vd can also result from blood product and intravenous volume administration, fluid retention, extravascular fluid redistribution, and decreased plasma protein concentrations.[7]

Drug sequestration is a phenomenon in which a drug is adsorbed to or absorbed or deactivated by the ECLS circuit and can lead to decreased bioavailability and higher Vd.[6,7,8] The degree of sequestration is dependent on multiple factors, including the chemical properties of a given drug, administered colloids (eg, blood prime, albumin), and the materials and surface areas of the ECLS circuit and membrane lung.[9,10,11] ECLS materials, often made of plastic and/or silicone, react with certain drugs and comprise a large surface area, leading to decreased bioavailability of drugs as they become sequestered.[8,9,11,12] Highly lipophilic and protein bound medications are prone to sequestration because of their affinity for circuit materials and colloids.[6,7] A recent PK study of antimicrobials during ECLS showed that highly protein bound drugs have greater circuit sequestration with resultant decreases in Vd.[13] A saturation point may exist after which liberation of a sequestered drug back into the circulation may occur; however, this concept has not been well studied.[7] Finally, drug sequestration has been demonstrated to have a temporal association, with greater sequestration occurring in newly primed circuits and decreased sequestration in older circuits.[9] This is important to consider when a circuit change is indicated after medication therapies have been established.

### *Medication-Specific Influences on Pharmacokinetics and Pharmacodynamics*

The chemical properties of drugs can impact the degree to which hemodilution and sequestration occur. In general, medications with low Vd are considered to be hydrophilic and, therefore, will be more impacted by changes in volume status.[14] On the other hand, medications that are highly protein bound or distributed into the tissues have larger Vd and will thus be more affected by changes in plasma protein concentration and circuit sequestration.[14] This is particularly important to understand in the case of medications for which therapeutic drug monitoring is unavailable.

Log P values measure the partition or octanol-water coefficient between hydrophilic and lipophilic properties of a specific chemical. Higher log P values are associated with increased lipophilicity, which may indicate a higher likelihood of binding to circuit components or distribution into adipose tissue.[15] Wildschut and colleagues correlated log P values to medication recovery for seven commonly used medications in ECLS. Those with higher log P values were less likely to be recovered post-oxygenator, suggesting that

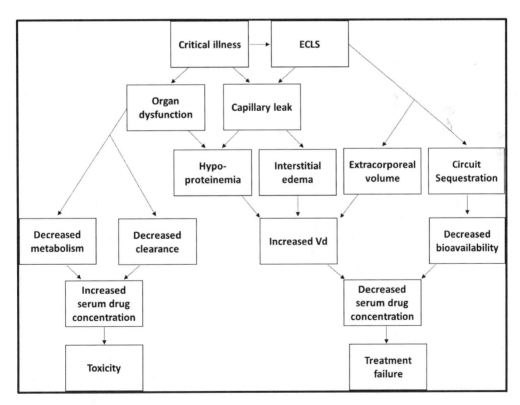

**Figure 49-1.** Risks associated with altered PK during critical illness and ECLS. Assumes intravenous administration and standard dosing.

medications with higher partition coefficients have higher affinities for circuit surfaces.[16,17] In 2015, the ASAP ECMO (Antibiotic, Sedative and Analgesic Pharmacokinetics during Extracorporeal Membrane Oxygenation) Study consortium reported similar results for both lipophilic and highly protein bound medications suggesting that, in addition to having higher Vd, they also bind to the circuit, substantially decreasing bioavailability.[13]

ECLS components, patient-specific clinical factors, and the physicochemical properties of medications have dynamic interdependent effects on drug PK and PD. Although much of the available literature may be limited to ex vivo studies, case series, and ECLS registry data, clinical applicability of these data can be expanded when discussed in conjunction with PK properties.

## Practical Guidance for Medication Dosing in ECLS

The continuously changing physiology of critically ill patients limits dosing standardization and necessitates vigilant monitoring and adjustment in medication management. The ASAP ECMO Study group has highlighted the primacy of PK and its impact on medication management during ECLS to decrease morbidity and mortality.[13] In the absence of clinically applicable empiric data, PK parameters can be used to develop an individualized dosing regimen that can be continuously updated based on patient, circuit, and medication-specific variables. It is imperative when making decisions about medication dosing to strongly weigh benefit more so than manageable risk. Aggressive dosing with close surveillance for the emergence of adverse drug reactions (ADRs) should direct medication management strategies. Once a decision is made on initial dosing, therapeutic drug monitoring, when available, can be used to tailor and adjust medication regimens to

ensure appropriate serum concentrations, while avoiding toxicity.

## *Using Pharmacokinetics and Pharmacodynamics for Medication Dosing*

The impact of altered Vd in patients requiring ECLS cannot be underestimated. Hydrophilic drugs have lower Vd and will be significantly affected by frequent volume shifts during ECLS. Therefore, increased loading doses and/or more frequent administration should be considered for patients with hypervolemia to achieve therapeutic concentrations more rapidly. For many drugs, as protein binding and lipophilicity increase, higher doses are needed due to changes in plasma protein concentrations or sequestration into the circuit. Very lipophilic medications or those that are significantly protein bound should be avoided, if possible, to prevent prolonged underdosing. If unavoidable, significantly higher, and more frequent dosing may be required at initiation and after circuit changes to decrease sequestration effects. Lastly, the presence of renal or hepatic dysfunction may also affect medication clearance. Table 49-1 suggests strategies for medication dosing based on PK properties.

## *Therapeutic Drug Monitoring*

Therapeutic drug monitoring (TDM) is the practice of measuring serum concentrations of drugs at a designated time and adjusting doses as needed to attain maximally effective concentrations.[18] It is particularly useful in managing medications that have a narrow therapeutic window, increased risk of toxicity, or require specific serum concentrations to achieve a desired outcome. The challenges in dosing medications during ECLS can be navigated with TDM when available. Well-documented TDM strategies include those associated with vancomycin, aminoglycosides, and immunosuppressive therapy, which may lead to use of alternative dosing strategies including more frequent administration, higher dosing, or prolonged infusions.[4,19,20,21] However, expanding technology has allowed for the use of TDM for other medications, including a variety of antimicrobials and antifungals. In a position paper about the use of TDM in critically ill patients, multiple international infectious disease experts established the need for practical TDM, including readily available laboratory services to improve outcomes in pediatric and adult patients. They provided guidance for how to use TDM to monitor a wide variety of antimicrobials, antifungals, and antiviral agents.[22] Providers should work with their laboratory and pharmacy colleagues to develop TDM protocols for critical medications used during ECLS

## Pharmacokinetic and Pharmacodynamic Modeling

More recently, researchers have been investigating the use of PK-PD modeling-based algorithms to better predict initial antimicrobial dosing within the context of individual variables.[5,13,19] Building on fundamental population PK-PD principles, these studies use

| Protein Binding | X Log P | Volume of Distribution (L/kg) | Risk | Dosing Strategy<br>Recommend close monitoring for ADEs when using higher dosing or increased frequency<br>Use TDM if concerns for therapeutic failure or toxicity at any time during treatment |
|---|---|---|---|---|
| **Low (<30%)** | <1 | <1 | Low | ECLS-specific dose adjustment not needed |
| | | | Moderate to High in neonates and infants | In neonates and infants Vd can be significantly increased by the ECLS volume - increasing risk of underdosing - consider higher doses or increased frequency |
| | 1-2 | 1-5 | Low to moderate | |
| | >2 | >5 | Moderate | Consider higher doses or increased frequency when appropriate |
| **Moderate (30-60%)** | <1 | <1 | Low to moderate | ECLS-specific dose adjustment not needed |
| | | | Moderate to High in neonates and infants | In neonates and infants Vd can be significantly increased by the ECLS volume - increasing risk of underdosing - consider higher doses or increased frequency |
| | 1-2 | 1-5 | Moderate | Consider higher doses or increased frequency when appropriate |
| | >2 | >5 | Moderate to High | Use higher loading and/or maintenance doses and/or increased frequency when appropriate |
| **High (>60%)** | <1 | <1 | Moderate<br>Moderate to High in neonates and infants* | Consider higher doses or increased frequency when appropriate |
| | 1-2 | 1-5 | Moderate to High | Use higher loading and/or maintenance doses and/or increased frequency when appropriate |
| | >2 | >5 | High | Avoid combinations if possible. If required – use higher loading doses and/or maintenance doses and increased frequency if appropriate. Follow medication levels if available. |

X log P=experimental octanol-water coefficient of medication as a measure of lipophilicity; ADE=adverse drug event; TDM=therapeutic drug monitoring

**Table 49-1.** Therapeutic implications of pharmacokinetic changes during ECLS.[7,14]

mathematical models to predict the likelihood of attaining therapeutic drug levels for patients on ECLS.[5,13,23] As more studies become available, ECLS dosing guidelines can be formulated to assist clinicians in choosing appropriate medication therapy. Advancements in the availability and understanding of population-specific PK-PD modeling and practical TDM have the potential to significantly improve both empiric and targeted drug regimens for patients requiring ECLS.

### Antimicrobial Therapy

The most prevalent types of infections in ECLS patients are bloodstream infections, lower respiratory tract infections, and urinary tract infections.[24] The Surviving Sepsis Campaign recommends the use of broad-spectrum antibiotics in the initial management of patients with sepsis and septic shock.[25] However, once the pathogen(s) are identified and their susceptibilities become available, empiric antimicrobials should be deescalated to more narrow spectrum agents to promote therapeutic appropriateness and reduce costs.[26] It is imperative to have rapid microbiological and susceptibility testing available to guide the choice of antimicrobial agent and ensure sufficient dosing.

The recent surge of multidrug resistant organisms (MDRO) combined with diminishing antibiotic development has highlighted the need to optimize the use of existing antimicrobials.[27] This becomes even more important in critically ill patients as pathogens isolated in the ICU are commonly less susceptible to standard antimicrobials.[28, 29] ECLS patients are at even more significant risk for MDRO infections as they often require a higher number and longer duration of invasive devices.

### *Pharmacokinetic and Pharmacodynamic Dosing Considerations*

Therapeutic antimicrobial effect is strongly associated with attainment of PK and PD targets specific to the underlying infection and chosen medication.[30] In preclinical studies, antimicrobial dosing based on PK-PD principles has been shown to minimize the risk of emergence of resistance by avoiding ineffective antibiotic exposure.[30,31]

In initiating broad spectrum empiric therapy, understanding drug physiochemistry is key to predicting the degree of drug loss to the ECLS circuit. Recently, multicenter prospective, open label PK studies in adults have developed PK-PD models to estimate appropriate empiric dosing of broad-spectrum antibiotics. Their findings highlight the need to use alternative dosing strategies such as prolonged infusions of piperacillin-tazobactam, loading doses of vancomycin, and lower doses of cefepime during ECLS with dosing adjustments for body mass index (BMI) and estimated creatinine clearance.[32,33,34,35] Table 49-2 lists the physiochemical properties and PK for common antimicrobials and antifungals used during ECLS and provides recommendations for empiric therapy and monitoring.

### Sedation and Analgesia

ECLS is invasive in nature and for this reason necessitates both sedation and analgesia which involves choosing and managing the correct drug to ensure patient safety and comfort. In targeting a set level of sedation, the choice of agent should keep the desired physiological endpoint in mind while understanding the interplay of PK-PD in a critically ill patient on ECLS.[36,37] Most commonly, an opioid will be used to address analgesia in combination with a sedative agent. There can be synergism from the combination of these agents; thus, dose-dependent side effects of any one agent

| Antimicrobial or antimicrobial class | Physicochemical properties | Pharmacokinetic implications | Dosing and management Recommendation |
|---|---|---|---|
| Aminoglycosides | Hydrophilic<br><br>Low to moderate protein binding | Minimal sequestration<br><br>Low Vd<br><br>Altered Cl | Adjust individual agents based on PK per Table 49-1<br><br>Utilize TDM guided dosing |
| Beta-lactams | Relatively hydrophilic<br><br>Variable protein binding | Relatively hydrophilic<br><br>Moderate to higher Vd<br><br>Altered clearance | Higher doses and more frequent or prolonged infusion may be considered for altered PK<br><br>Adjust individual agents based on PK per Table 49-1<br><br>Adjust per clearance<br><br>Utilize TDM if available |
| Carbapenems | Relatively hydrophilic<br><br>Variable protein binding | Relatively hydrophilic<br><br>Low Vd | Higher doses and more frequent or prolonged infusion may be considered for altered PK<br><br>Adjust individual agents based on PK per Table 49-1<br><br>Adjust per renal function<br><br>Utilize TDM if available |
| Fluoroquinolones | Lipophilic<br><br>Moderate protein binding | Increased sequestration<br><br>Higher Vd<br><br>Altered Cl | Higher or more frequent doses may be needed *initially* to overcome sequestration<br><br>Adjust individual agents based on PK per Table 49-1<br>Utilize TDM if available |
| Caspofungin<br>Micafungin | Low lipophilicity<br><br>Highly protein-bound | Moderate sequestration<br><br>Higher Vd | Higher loading doses may be needed to overcome Vd<br><br>Adjust individual agents based on PK per Table 49-1<br>Utilize TDM if available |
| Vancomycin | Hydrophilic<br><br>Moderate to high protein binding | Minimal sequestration<br><br>Higher Vd<br><br>Altered Cl | Higher loading doses may be needed to overcome Vd<br><br>Adjust individual agents based on PK per Table 49-1<br><br>Utilize TDM guided dosing |
| Voriconazole | High lipophilicity<br><br>Moderate protein-binding | High sequestration<br><br>Higher Vd | Significantly higher initial loading and daily doses<br><br>Utilize TDM if available |

Vd=volume of distribution; Cl=clearance; TDM=therapeutic drug monitoring
aMinimal sequestration characterized by logP <1 and protein binding less than 30%; moderate sequestration determined by logP between 1 and 2 and protein binding between 30-60%; high sequestration determined by logP >2 and protein binding greater than 60%.
*Arbitrary cut-off points for degree of sequestration and protein binding

**Table 49-2.** Summary of dosing recommendations for relevant antimicrobials.[14]

can be minimized while achieving a similar endpoint. The role of PK-PD in choosing the most appropriate agent will be further discussed in the agent-specific review section.

### Pharmacokinetic Dosing Considerations: Analgesics

Opioids are indispensable analgesics used in intensive care and, except for methadone, are generally pharmacodynamically similar. In international surveys, fentanyl remains one of the most popular agents used for analgesia in ECLS, followed by hydromorphone and morphine.[38,39] Fentanyl is a highly lipophilic opioid and has been shown to have a mean drug loss of 97% into an ex vivo ECLS circuit at 24 hours and clinically requires dose escalation over time.[19,38,39] The demonstration of ex vivo circuit drug loss and the ongoing need for dose escalation has not curbed the usage of this opioid across institutions. Proponents have described the advantage of inactive metabolites as a reason for the drug's choice, especially in patients with renal dysfunction.

Morphine is another commonly used opioid that, unlike fentanyl, appears to be minimally sequestrated in ex vivo models, with less than 1% drug loss at 24 hours.[8,40] However, morphine was similarly shown to require dose escalation over time which correlated with decreasing plasma concentrations.[37] Despite this phenomenon, based on the limited clinical data, it has been suggested as a superior alternative to fentanyl, due to its better PK profile in ECLS.[38,39]

Hydromorphone is a synthetic opioid that has low lipophilicity and protein binding. In a recent retrospective review of 52 adult ECLS patients, the use of hydromorphone resulted in lower sedation usage over 48 hours as compared to fentanyl.[42] There were many limitations to this study; however, clinically, when comparing the PK-PD parameters of both medications, hydromorphone is less likely to require

dosage escalation over time due to limited risk of interaction with the circuit or underlying physiology.

Enteral methadone has been used as an adjunctive opioid in ECLS. With its long duration of action, it has been shown to temper escalation of other agents and may have a role in reducing withdrawal symptoms.[43] It is important to note that methadone is very highly protein bound and may not be an ideal agent in patients who are experiencing ongoing protein losses or dramatic protein shifts.

### Pharmacokinetic Dosing Considerations: Sedatives

Sedatives are widely used in combination with analgesics to maintain patient comfort and safety during ECLS. Midazolam, a commonly used benzodiazepine in the ICU for sedation, has been shown to be significantly sequestrated in ex-vivo models, with only 13% drug recovery at 24 hours.[8] Clinically, there has been one retrospective study demonstrating the need for significantly higher doses of midazolam or equivalents in ECLS patients.[44] Another group showed comparatively decreased daily dose requirements without dose escalation but this was in combination with high-dose fentanyl for analgesia.[45] However, it can be anticipated from expected PK changes on ECLS that higher loading and maintenance doses should be considered.[14]

Propofol is a highly lipophilic and significantly protein-bound sedative that is significantly sequestered within the ECLS circuit and even theorized to undergo oxidative breakdown.[46] In an ex vivo model of a whole-blood primed ECLS circuit, 70% of propofol drug concentration diminished within the first 30 minutes of the experiment, and after 5 hours, only 11% of the initial concentration remained.[47] Based on these limited data, it appears that higher doses of propofol may be required over time for optimal sedation.[14] Moreover, maximal doses need to be further defined in this population due to the risk of propofol-related infusion syndrome with prolonged infusions.

Dexmedetomidine has gained popularity in the ICU for its absence of respiratory depression, potential reduction of delirium, and unique sedation profile characterized by anxiolysis and analgesia.[48] Consistent with its high lipophilicity and protein binding, much of the drug is lost through circuit adsorption.[49] Higher infusion rates or bolus doses may be required especially at ECLS initiation and circuit change.

Ketamine is pharmacodynamically distinct from other sedatives and is often used as an adjunctive agent in ECLS [50] An initial retrospective study showed a sedative-sparing effect with concurrent decrease in vasopressor requirements; however, this was not seen in a subsequent randomized controlled trial.[51] Of note, the protocols in this study were not tailored to ketamine's unique PD.[50,51] It is recommended to use the lowest effective infusion doses to avoid the adverse psychomimetic phenomena commonly associated with ketamine.

## Other Medications

Many cardiovascular medications are titrated to effect, making dosing in ECLS patients significantly less challenging than other classes of drugs. However, some medications may need higher loading doses and more aggressive rates of infusion based on PK-PD parameters. For example, larger doses of both alprostadil and sildenafil—both commonly used in neonates with congenital heart disease—are needed in patients on ECLS likely due to their larger Vd.[52,53]

The antiarrhythmics amiodarone, esmolol, lidocaine, and procainamide may require higher bolus doses and rates of infusion to achieve their desired effect due to increased protein binding and lipophilicity.[54,55] Amiodarone is extremely lipophilic (log P=7.6) and significantly protein bound (99%), dramatically increasing Vd. Not surprisingly, an ex vivo study of three different circuit priming fluids showed that amiodarone is extensively sequestered into the circuit (~70-80%).[56] Use of infusion rates as high as 25 mcg/kg/min have been reported.[55]

Anticonvulsant medications may also be affected by the ECLS circuit. Case reports have shown up to 15-35% losses of fosphenytoin into circuits while phenobarbital levels may be subtherapeutic with traditional dosing as well.[57,58] Larger loading and maintenance doses will be required to achieve therapeutic levels. Standard doses of levetiracetam have been shown to be effective in adults, even with the addition of CRRT.[59] Due to the high risk of subtherapeutic dosing, it is prudent to preferentially use medications with readily available TDM.

## Conclusion

Medication dosing during ECLS requires multidisciplinary cooperation to design efficacious treatment plans with vigilant monitoring and adjustment. Advances in TDM and expansion of PK-PD modeling in ECLS populations may lead to better and more accurate initial dosing in the future. Until then, the team can use known drug-specific PK and PD interactions with patient and circuit factors to estimate empiric dosing and continuously tailor therapy based on clinical assessment, TDM, and ongoing surveillance for ADRs.

# References

1.  Roberts JA. Pharmacokinetic issues for antibiotics in the critically ill patient. Crit Care Med. 2009;37(3):840-51.
2.  Schmidt S, Gonzalez D, Derendorf H. Significance of protein binding in pharmacokinetics and pharmacodynamics. J Pharm Sci. 2010;99(3):1107-1122.
3.  Ahsman M. Determinants of pharmacokinetic variability during extracorporeal membrane oxygenation [PhD Thesis]. Rotterdam, The Netherlands: Erasmus University Rotterdam; 2010.
4.  Fernandez E, Perez R, Hernandez A, et al. Factors and mechanisms for pharmacokinetic differences between pediatric population and adults. Pharmaceutics. 2011; 3:53-72.
5.  Gijsen M, Vlasselaers D, Spriet I, et al. Pharmacokinetics of antibiotics in pediatric intensive care: fostering variability to attain precision medicine. Antibiotics. 2021; 10:1182-1218.
6.  Hahn J, Choi JH, Chang MJ. Pharmacokinetic changes of antibiotic, antiviral, antituberculosis, and antifungal agents during extracorporeal membrane oxygenation in critically ill adult patients. J Clin Pharm Ther. 2017;42:661-71.
7.  Ha MA, Sieg AC. Evaluation of altered drug pharmacokinetics in critically ill adults receiving extracorporeal membrane oxygenation. Pharmacotherapy. 2017;37(2):221-235.
8.  Shekar K, Roberts JA, Mcdonald CI, et al. Sequestration of drugs in the circuit may lead to therapeutic failure during extracorporeal membrane oxygenation. Crit Care. 2012;16(5):R194.
9.  Mehta NM, Halwick DR, Dodson BL, et al. Potential drug sequestration during extracorporeal membrane oxygenation: results from an ex vivo experiment. Intensive Care Med. 2007;33(6):1018-1024.
10. Spriet I, Annaert P, Meersseman P, et al. Pharmacokinetics of caspofungin and voriconazole in critically ill patients during extracorporeal membrane oxygenation. J Antimicrob Chemother. 2009;63(4):767-70.
11. Preston TJ, Ratliff TM, Gomez D, et al. Modified surface coatings and their effect on drug adsorption within the extracorporeal life support circuit. J Extra Corpor Technol. 2010;42(3):199-202.
12. Preston TJ, Hodge AB, Riley JB, et al. In vitro drug adsorption and plasma free hemoglobin levels associated with hollow fiber oxygenators in the extracorporeal life support (ECLS) circuit. J Extra Corpor Technol. 2007;39(4):234-237.
13. Shekar K, Roberts JA, Welch S, et al. ASAP ECMO: Antibiotic, Sedative and Analgesic Pharmacokinetics during Extracorporeal Membrane Oxygenation: a multi-centre study to optimise drug therapy during ECMO. BMC Anesthesiol. 2012;12:29.
14. Cheng V, Abdul-Aziz MH, Roberts JA, et al. Optimising drug dosing in patients receiving extracorporeal membrane oxygenation. J Thorac Dis. 2018;10(Suppl 5):S629-S641.
15. Rosenbaum S. Basic Pharmacokinetics and Pharmacodynamics: An Integrated Textbook and Computer Simulations. Hoboken, NJ: John Wiley & Sons; 2011.
16. Wildschut ED, Ahsman MJ, Allegaert K, et al. Determinants of drug absorption in different ECMO circuits. Intensive Care Med. 2010;36(12):2109-2116.
17. Wildschut ED, de Hoog M, Ahsman MJ, et al. Plasma concentrations of oseltamivir and oseltamivir carboxylate in critically ill children on extracorporeal membrane oxygenation support. PLoS One. 2010;5(6):e10938.
18. Kang JS, Lee MH. Overview of therapeutic drug monitoring. Korean J Intern Med. 2009;24(1):1-10.
19. Bouglé A, Dujardin O, Lepère V, et al. PHARMECMO: Therapeutic drug monitoring and adequacy of current dosing regimens of antibiotics in patients on Extracorporeal Life Support. Anaesth Crit Care Pain Med. 2019;38(5):493-497.
20. Roberts JA, Paul SK, Akova M, et al. DALI: defining antibiotic levels in intensive care unit patients: are current β-lactam antibiotic doses sufficient for critically ill patients? Clin Infect Dis. 2014;58(8):1072-1083.
21. Kuhn D, Metz C, Seiler F, et al. Antibiotic therapeutic drug monitoring in intensive care patients treated with different modalities of extracorporeal membrane oxygenation (ECMO) and renal replacement therapy: a prospective, observational, single-center study. Crit Care. 2020;24:664-75.
22. Abdul-Aziz MH, Alffenaar JWC, Bassetti M, et al. Antimicrobial therapeutic drug monitoring in critically ill adult patients: a position paper. Int Care Med. 2020; 46:1127-1153.
23. Raffaeli G, Pokorna P, Allegaert K, et al. Drug disposition and pharmacotherapy in neonatal ECMO: from fragmented data to integrated knowledge. Front Pediatr. 2019;7:360.
24. Biffi S, Di Bella S, Scaravilli V, et al. Infections during extracorporeal membrane oxygenation: epidemiology, risk factors, pathogenesis and prevention. Int J Antimicrob Agents. 2017;50(1):9-16.
25. Rhodes A, Evans LE, Alhazzani W, et al. Surviving Sepsis Campaign: International Guidelines for Management of Sepsis and Septic Shock: 2016. Intensive Care Med. 2017;43(3):304-377.
26. Garnacho-Montero J, Gutiérrez-Pizarraya A, Escoresca-Ortega A, et al. De-escalation of empirical therapy is associated with lower mortality in patients

with severe sepsis and septic shock. Intensive Care Med. 2014;40(1):32-40.

27. Abdul-Aziz MH, Lipman J, Mouton JW, et al. Applying pharmacokinetic/pharmacodynamic principles in critically ill patients: optimizing efficacy and reducing resistance development. Semin Respir Crit Care Med. 2015;36(1):136-153.

28. Zhanel GG, DeCorby M, Laing N, et al. Antimicrobial-resistant pathogens in intensive care units in Canada: results of the Canadian National Intensive Care Unit (CAN-ICU) study, 2005-2006. Antimicrob Agents Chemother. 2008;52(4):1430-1437.

29. Rhomberg PR, Fritsche TR, Sader HS, et al. Antimicrobial susceptibility pattern comparisons among intensive care unit and general ward Gram-negative isolates from the Meropenem Yearly Susceptibility Test Information Collection Program (USA). Diagn Microbiol Infect Dis. 2006;56(1):57-62.

30. Abdul-Aziz MH, Lipman J, Mouton JW, et al. Applying pharmacokinetic/pharmacodynamic principles in critically ill patients: optimizing efficacy and reducing resistance development. Semin Respir Crit Care Med. 2015;36(1):136-153.

31. Roberts JA, Kruger P, Paterson DL, et al. Antibiotic resistance--what's dosing got to do with it?. Crit Care Med. 2008;36(8):2433-2440.

32. Cheng V, Abdul-Aziz MH, Burrows F, et al. Population pharmacokinetics of piperacillin and tazobactam in critically ill patients receiving extracorporeal membrane oxygenation: an ASAP ECMO Study. Antimicrob Agents Chemother. 2021;65(11):e0143821.

33. Cheng V, Abdul-Aziz MH, Burrows F, et al. Population pharmacokinetics of vancomycin in critically ill adult patients receiving extracorporeal membrane oxygenation (an ASAP ECMO Study). Antimicrob Agents Chemother. 2022;66(1):e0137721.

34. Cheng V, Abdul-Aziz MH, Burrows F, et al. Population pharmacokinetics of cefepime in critically ill patients receiving extracorporeal membrane oxygenation (an ASAP ECMO study). Int J Antimicrob Agents. 2021;58(6):106466.

35. Tang Girdwood S, Dong M, Tang P, et al. Population pharmacokinetic modeling of total and free ceftriaxone in critically ill children and young adults and Monte Carlo simulations support twice daily dosing for target attainment. Antimicrob Agents Chemother. 2022;66(1):e0142721.

36. Cheng V, Abdul-Aziz MH, Roberts JA, et al. Overcoming barriers to optimal drug dosing during ECMO in critically ill adult patients. Expert Opin Drug Metab Toxicol. 2019;15(2):103-112.

37. Roberts JA, Taccone FS, Lipman J. Understanding PK/PD. Intensive Care Med. 2016;42(11):1797-1800.

38. Marhong JD, DeBacker J, Viau-Lapointe J, et al. Sedation and mobilization during venovenous extracorporeal membrane oxygenation for acute respiratory failure: an international survey. Crit Care Med. 2017;45(11):1893–1899.

39. Dzierba AL, Abrams D, Madahar P, et al. Current practice and perceptions regarding pain, agitation and delirium management in patients receiving venovenous extracorporeal membrane oxygenation. J Crit Care. 2019;53:98-106.

40. Sun HY, Ko WJ, Tsai PR, et al. Infections occurring during extracorporeal membrane oxygenation use in adult patients. J Thorac Cardiovasc Surg. 2010;140(5):1125-32.e2.

41. Shekar K, Roberts JA, Mullany DV, et al. Increased sedation requirements in patients receiving extracorporeal membrane oxygenation for respiratory and cardiorespiratory failure. Anaesth Intensive Care. 2012;40(4):648-655.

42. Martin NJ, Peitz GJ, Olsen KM, et al. Hydromorphone compared to fentanyl in patients receiving extracorporeal membrane oxygenation. ASAIO J. 2021;67(4):443-448.

43. Dzierba AL, Abrams D, Brodie D. Medicating patients during extracorporeal membrane oxygenation: the evidence is building. Crit Care. 2017;21(1):66.

44. Nigoghossian CD, Dzierba AL, Etheridge J, et al. Effect of Extracorporeal Membrane Oxygenation Use on Sedative Requirements in Patients with Severe Acute Respiratory Distress Syndrome. Pharmacotherapy. 2016;36(6):607-616.

45. DeGrado JR, Hohlfelder B, Ritchie BM, et al. Evaluation of sedatives, analgesics, and neuromuscular blocking agents in adults receiving extracorporeal membrane oxygenation. J Crit Care. 2017;37:1-6.

46. Lemaitre F, Hasni N, Leprince P, et al. Propofol, midazolam, vancomycin and cyclosporine therapeutic drug monitoring in extracorporeal membrane oxygenation circuits primed with whole human blood. Crit Care. 2015;19(1):40.

47. Shekar K, Roberts JA, Mcdonald CI, et al. Protein-bound drugs are prone to sequestration in the extracorporeal membrane oxygenation circuit: results from an ex vivo study. Crit Care. 2015;19(1):164.

48. Patel M, Altshuler D, Lewis TC, et al. Sedation Requirements in Patients on Venovenous or Venoarterial Extracorporeal Membrane Oxygenation. Ann Pharmacother. 2020;54(2):122-130.

49. Nasr VG, Meserve J, Pereira LM, et al. Sedative and Analgesic Drug Sequestration After a Single Bolus Injection in an Ex Vivo Extracorporeal Membrane Oxygenation Infant Circuit. ASAIO J. 2019;65(2):187-191.

50. Tellor B, Shin N, Graetz TJ, et al. Ketamine infusion for patients receiving extracorporeal membrane oxygenation support: a case series. F1000Res. 2015;4:16.

51. Dzierba AL, Brodie D, Bacchetta M, et al. Ketamine use in sedation management in patients receiving extracorporeal membrane oxygenation. Intensive Care Med. 2016;42(11):1822-1823.

52. Ahsman MJ, Witjes BC, Wildschut ED, et al. Sildenafil exposure in neonates with pulmonary hypertension after administration via a nasogastric tube. Arch Dis Child Fetal Neonatal Ed. 2010;95(2):F109-F114.

53. Stone DM, Frattarelli DA, Karthikeyan S, et al. Altered prostaglandin E1 dosage during extracorporeal membrane oxygenation in a newborn with ductal-dependent congenital heart disease. Pediatr Cardiol. 2006;27(3):360-363.

54. Robinson B, Eshaghpour E, Ewing S, et al. Hypertrophic obstructive cardiomyopathy in an infant of a diabetic mother: support by extracorporeal membrane oxygenation and treatment with beta-adrenergic blockade and increased intravenous fluid administration. ASAIO J. 1998;44(6):845-847.

55. Kendrick JG, Macready JJ, Kissoon N. Amiodarone treatment of junctional ectopic tachycardia in a neonate receiving extracorporeal membrane oxygenation. Ann Pharmacother. 2006;40(10):1872-1875.

56. McDaniel CG, Honeycutt CC, Watt KM. Amiodarone Extraction by the Extracorporeal Membrane Oxygenation Circuit. J Extra Corpor Technol. 2021;53(1):68-74.

57. Dillman NO, Messinger MM, Dinh KN, et al. Evaluation of the Effects of Extracorporeal Membrane Oxygenation on Antiepileptic Drug Serum Concentrations in Pediatric Patients. J Pediatr Pharmacol Ther. 2017;22(5):352-357.

58. Thibault C, Massey SL, Abend NS, et al. Population pharmacokinetics of phenobarbital in neonates and infants on extracorporeal membrane oxygenation and the influence of concomitant renal replacement therapy. J Clin Pharmacol. 2021;61(3):378-387.

59. Nei SD, Wittwer ED, Kashani KB, et al. Levetiracetam pharmacokinetics in a patient receiving continuous venovenous hemofiltration and venoarterial extracorporeal membrane oxygenation. Pharmacotherapy. 2015;35(8):e127-e130.

# 50

## Anesthesia

*Jonathan Hastie, Madelyn Kahana, Susana Cruz Beltran, Nicholas Moore, Viviane G. Nasr*

## Introduction

As increasing numbers of adults and children are supported with ECLS, anesthesiologists will be called upon to provide care for those patients who require an intervention. Anesthesiologists are expected to have a breadth and depth of understanding of pharmacology and physiology while caring for patients supported with ECLS.

### Anesthetic Pharmacology and Physiology

Pharmacology in the ECLS patient is discussed in Chapter 49. This section focuses on anesthetic medications and physiologic principles specific to the anesthetic care of patients supported with ECLS.

### *Pharmacology of Intravenous Agents*

Medication levels may vary unpredictably during ECLS therapy. This unpredictability is due to complex interaction of mechanical and patient factors, disease-specific pathophysiology, and medications.[1] Mechanisms by which pharmacokinetics may be altered include an increased volume of distribution, sequestration of the therapeutic agent in the different components of the circuit, and reduction in elimination.[1] Moreover, pharmacokinetics may change throughout the time when a patient is supported with ECLS.[2] Failure to consider alterations in pharmacology may lead to therapeutic failure or medication toxicity.[3]

Significant alterations in propofol, midazolam, fentanyl, and morphine plasma levels have been reported when ECLS is initiated in both in vivo and ex vivo models.[4,5] Reductions in concentration may require a significant increase in the administered dose to achieve therapeutic plasma levels of active medications and their metabolites. These increased requirements may persist for the duration of ECLS support.[4] While maintaining the patient's comfort and relieving anxiety are important for intensive care, ensuring adequate sedation becomes paramount in the context of potentially noxious surgical and interventional stimulus.

An agent's physical properties determine the way the ECLS circuit may alter the pharmacokinetics. Sequestration in the ECLS circuit is thought to be significant for lipophilic medications and those that are highly protein-bound, while hemodilution with an increased circulating volume is relevant for hydrophilic medications.[1] Propofol, a protein-bound and highly lipophilic medication is also sequestered in the ECLS circuit. In vitro studies have demonstrated propofol concentrations between 20% and 32% of predicted in the simulated ECLS patient.[6] For sequestered medications, the tubing may act as a reservoir, and slowly release the medication once the infusion is discontinued.[1] Medications typically considered "short-acting" may thus have a prolonged duration of effect.

Precise understanding of the pharmacokinetics of intravenous anesthetics is limited by the variability of patient and ECLS circuit factors, as well as heterogeneity of research. The anesthesiologist should consider the likelihood of increased volume of distribution, sequestration of medications, and reduced elimination. Practically, this means bolus doses in general may need to be increased (particularly for hydrophilic medications), infusion rates will likely be substantially higher than those in the non-ECLS patient, and the duration of effect of infusions may be prolonged after cessation of the medication (Table 50-1).

### Pharmacology of Anesthetic Vapors

Volatile agents commonly used in anesthesia care are associated with two main concerns: the variability of anesthetic uptake in severely diseased lungs and the impact of oxygenator design on the potential for elimination of anesthetic vapors via the ECLS membrane.

Unlike the CPB circuit, which uses a microporous membrane oxygenator that is constructed from polypropylene and is permeable to anesthetic vapors,[7] modern ECLS circuits use diffusion membranes made from polymethylpentene.[8] The diffusion membrane presents a physical barrier between gases and blood to minimize plasma leakage over time, and postoxygenator gas analysis has shown minimal uptake of volatile agents.[9] As such, ECLS circuits using polymethylpentene diffusion oxygenators do not include vaporizers to administer volatile agents, nor do they significantly eliminate volatile agents. The administration of an inhalational anesthetic for a patient supported with ECLS would thus require the use of either an anesthesia machine or a vapor-conserving device used for high fresh-gas flow use of ICU ventilators.[10,11]

The nature of a patient's pathophysiology should be considered. A patient supported with high flow VV ECMO for severely diseased lungs may have inadequate uptake of inhaled volatile agents to achieve satisfactory blood concentrations, and hence intravenous medications are required. However, a patient requiring a lower level of support and with adequate lung function may have sufficient gas exchange, allowing the use of a volatile agent.

In addition to consideration of gas exchange in the patient's lungs, the circulation itself should be considered in deciding whether to

| ANESTHESIA MEDICATION | CONSIDERATIONS |
|---|---|
| Propofol | Lipophilic. Sequestration in ECLS circuit. Higher doses commonly needed for therapeutic effect. Risk of propofol infusion syndrome when used in ICU; may safely be used in short-term anesthetic care. |
| Midazolam | Lipophilic. Sequestration in ECLS circuit. Higher doses commonly needed for therapeutic effect. Prolonged effect after cessation of infusion. |
| Fentanyl | Lipophilic. Sequestration in ECLS circuit. Higher doses commonly needed for therapeutic effect. Prolonged effect after cessation of infusion. |
| Morphine | Hydrophilic. Increased volume of distribution. |
| Neuromuscular blockade | Increased volume of distribution. |
| Dexmedetomidine | Commonly used as adjunct sedation in the ICU. |

**Table 50-1.** Pharmacokinetic considerations of anesthetic medications in the patients supported with ECLS.

use volatile agents in anesthetic care. In a patient supported with VA ECMO with femoral venous and arterial cannulation with relatively preserved cardiac function, the upper body circulation receives blood primarily from the native cardiac ejection. If volatile agents are used, the brain may therefore receive blood with adequate concentrations. The lower body may primarily receive blood reinfused from the ECLS circuit, whose diffusion membrane oxygenator should have no significant effect on volatile agents.

Patients with minimal cardiac ejection, from either depressed cardiac function or relatively high flow VA ECMO support, are expected to have minimal pulmonary blood flow and would therefore be poor candidates to be anesthetized with volatile agents. Patients supported with more complicated configurations, such as VVA ECMO, likewise may be more reliably anesthetized with intravenous agents.

### Respiratory Physiology and ECLS

This section highlights a few salient points regarding respiratory physiology for the anesthesiologist caring for the ECMO patient.

VV ECMO is predominantly used for impaired gas exchange, or occasionally to allow healing of bronchopleural fistulas.[12,13] Understanding that the aim of ECLS is to aid lung function is key to planning ventilation strategies. Furthermore, when clinical situations change, adjustments to either ECLS or to patient gas exchange can compensate for the changes.

The effectiveness of ECLS gas exchange can be assessed in multiple ways including arterial blood gas analysis, pulse oximetry, and tissue saturation. The location from which an arterial blood gas is drawn will affect its interpretation. Pre- and postoxygenator blood gas analysis will demonstrate the effect of the ECMO membrane gas exchange. Pulse oximetry and tissue saturation monitoring using near infrared spectroscopy may also be used, particularly when there is concern for differential hypoxemia during femoral VA ECMO, for example.

The anesthesiologist should assess the patient's current support and recent trajectory over the last 24-48 hours. A comprehensive assessment of the patient's condition depends on discussion with the intensive care clinical team. Ventilator and ECLS settings should be noted (Table 50-2). As a starting point, an anesthesiologist may aim to maintain similar mechanical ventilation settings periprocedurally, though they may be modified as the clinical situation changes.

Based on patient and procedure factors, appropriate plans for monitoring oxygenation and ventilation should be made (Table 50-3). Most modern anesthesia machines can replicate the ICU ventilator settings, but institution-specific knowledge and planning are crucial. Additional options include using a transport ICU ventilator or changing the location of the procedure, if feasible.

During a procedure, acidosis may develop from poor perfusion, sepsis, or other reasons.

| VENTILATOR | ECMO |
|---|---|
| Mode of ventilation | Cannulation strategy |
| Tidal volume | Pump speed |
| Respiratory rate | Blood flow rate |
| Inspiratory time | $FsO_2$ |
| $FiO_2$ | Sweep gas flow rate |
| Positive end-expiratory pressure | |

**Table 50-2.** Respiratory assessment of the ECMO patient.

While the underlying reason for the acidosis is addressed, temporizing measures may be undertaken. To increase $CO_2$ clearance, increasing the sweep gas flow rate may be more effective and be associated with less risk of lung injury than increasing the patient's minute ventilation on the ventilator. Administration of a metabolic buffer may be appropriate at other times to temporarily mitigate acidosis.

Lastly, transport to and from the procedural area (when the procedure is not performed in the ICU) merits special concern for planning respiratory care. This is discussed at length in Chapter 46.

### Cardiac Physiology and ECLS

The anesthesiologist should have a thorough understanding of cardiac physiology in patients supported with ECLS. This is discussed at length in Chapters 27 and 28. Important points are reviewed here.

In patients supported with VV ECMO, an underfilled heart may benefit from fluid resuscitation or transfusion. Evidence of pulmonary congestion may prompt the initiation of an inotrope or fluid removal with diuresis or ultrafiltration. In other instances, the physiologic effects of impaired gas exchange may have hemodynamic effects which are amplified in the periprocedural setting. Hypoxemia can lead to an increase in sympathetic tone, or a decrease in myocardial performance. Acute hypercarbia will produce acidosis, which likewise can increase sympathetic tone when mild, or may lead to vasodilation and a decrease in myocardial function when more significant. The effect of vasoactive mediations may be attenuated in an acidotic milieu. Correcting the acidosis may improve responsiveness.

Central venous pressure (CVP) monitoring may be useful, but also misleading in certain situations. A cannula with a venous return near the CVP port may lead to erroneous measurements. Measured SVC pressure may not correlate with right atrial pressure. Regardless, the CVP *trend* during a procedure is likely a meaningful measurement.

Another potential hemodynamic effect of VV ECMO is the delayed effect time of a bolus of intravenous medication, as some or most of the delivered dose may be bypassed through the ECMO circuit before returning to the patient's right atrium. The magnitude of this effect will be a function of the proportion of venous return that is drained, the location of medication administration and venous drainage catheters, and the length of the ECMO circuit. Accounting for a delay in effect should prompt caution in repeating doses when managing hemodynamic instability.

| PROCEDURE | EXPLANATION |
|---|---|
| Coronary artery bypass grafting | Insufflation of leg for saphenous vein harvest leads to absorption of $CO_2$ and increased minute ventilation needs. |
| Laparoscopy | Abdominal insufflation leads to absorption of $CO_2$ and increased minute ventilation needs. |
| Thoracoscopy | Insufflation of the chest may lead to absorption of $CO_2$. One-lung ventilation decreases ability to clear $CO_2$. |
| Bronchoscopy | Airway procedures may be associated with apnea or decreased ability to ventilate. |
| Laryngoscopy | Decreased intraprocedure ventilation |

**Table 50-3.** Procedures with special considerations regarding ventilation.

The magnitude of the hemodynamic effect of VA ECMO depends on many factors, including patient size, native cardiac function, volume status, ECMO cannulation strategy, and ECMO pump speed. Understanding of the patient's circulatory state requires realtime monitoring of electrocardiogram (ECG) and arterial blood pressure tracing. CVP and pulmonary artery (PA) catheter monitoring may provide supplementary information.

Arterial pulsatility in the patient with VA ECMO will typically reflect native cardiac output. The pulse pressure, in combination with assessment of mean arterial pressure (MAP) and CVP further characterizes the patient's cardiac output. If a PA catheter is present, this can yield information in at least two important ways. One is that a mixed venous oxygen saturation can be used to calculate the cardiac output by the Fick Principle.[14] This calculated cardiac output reflects the global balance of oxygen supply and demand of the tissues. By subtracting the measured ECMO flow, the clinician may estimate the native cardiac output. Second, a PA catheter may be helpful in cases in which it is critical to maintain circulation across the lungs, such as a patient who has undergone mechanical mitral valve replacement or a lung transplant recipient at risk for pulmonary vein thrombosis at the site of anastomosis.

For surgical procedures, VA ECMO support may lead to improved intraoperative hemodynamics and better tolerance for changes associated with the procedure, such as surgical traction or compression of vital organs. For this reason, VA ECMO may be the preferred mode of intraoperative support for patients with marginal cardiac function undergoing lung transplantation.[15,16] However, the anesthesiologist should watch for surgical changes that can impair ECMO support itself. Changes in patient position, such as Trendelenburg or reverse Trendelenburg position, can affect cannula position or may impair venous drainage. Lateral positioning

may have similar effects. Abdominal or intrathoracic insufflation may impair venous drainage. Intraprocedure hemorrhage leading to hypovolemia will reduce the ability of ECLS to provide support. The degree of impairment of ECLS flow support may vary in a *nonlinear* fashion with volume status.

Preoperatively, the anesthetist should assess the hemodynamic impact of the ECLS circuit on the patient and observe for changes. The magnitude of negative pressure in the drainage cannula is reflective of cannula position relative to the vein, and a change can suggest a change in position or a change in circulating volume. Likewise, chatter of the drainage limb of the circuit or a drop in pump flow are consistent with decreased circulating volume. Some situations may require liberal fluid resuscitation or transfusion, while others benefit from a restrictive strategy. Adjustment in pump settings or change in vasopressor dose may be appropriate in which a restrictive strategy is used. As with all clinically significant decisions, changes in ECLS support are typically made in collaboration with the primary team managing the ECLS circuit.

## Developing and Implementing an Anesthesia Plan

This section highlights the practical aspects of managing patients supported with ECLS and undergoing a surgical procedure.

### *Patient Assessment*

Patients supported with ECLS may have a variety of airway support, including endotracheal tubes, tracheostomy tubes, high-flow nasal cannula oxygen, or noninvasive positive-pressure ventilation (NPPV). For patients without invasive airways, a standard airway assessment should be made.[17] For those with invasive airway equipment, the anesthesiologist should assess position, ease of insertion, stability, and duration.

As outlined in the Respiratory Physiology and ECLS section above, ventilator settings should be noted (Table 50-2). The anesthesiologist should address feasibility and appropriateness of mimicking these settings during transport and in the procedural area. Coordination with the respiratory therapist may allow use of the ICU ventilator on battery power to facilitate stability during transport.

Inhaled therapies, such as bronchodilators and pulmonary vasodilators, should be reviewed. Maintaining continuous inhaled therapies (eg, nitric oxide or epoprostenol) requires collaboration with a respiratory therapist. Vasoactive support, including continuous infusions and intermittently dosed medications must also be reviewed.

The patient's analgesic and sedative requirements to achieve the current status and anticipated surgical or interventional stimulation should be reviewed. The sedative dosages are a function of both pharmacodynamic tolerance and pharmacokinetic factors, such as sequestration.

Lastly, additional invasive therapies bear special relevance particularly for transport and anesthetic planning. The presence of IABP or intravascular heart assist pumps may require additional personnel to assist with transport and arrangement. Confirmation of correct positioning, or diagnosing malpositioning with imaging may be desirable, depending on the context and planned procedure.

### Procedural Considerations in the ECLS Patient

A multitude of procedures have been reported in patients supported with ECLS (Chapter 51). Despite the breadth of procedural considerations, common anesthetic considerations are reviewed below.

First, procedure location will have several implications, including whether the patient will be transported from the ICU and the need for an elevator. The location of the procedure also will determine proximity to resources, including pharmacy, laboratory services, blood bank, and support staff. Qualified clinicians to assist with unexpected events may be readily available in the operating room environment, somewhat less available in catheterization labs or endoscopy suites, and significantly less available in other remote locations.

Second, positioning of the ECLS patient for procedures should be considered. Supine position is ideal for managing patients supported with ECLS. However, the anesthetist should anticipate the effect of the patient's position (lateral or other) on cannula position, flow, and hemodynamics.

Third, the anticipated degree of noxious stimulation should be assessed and will be discussed further in the next section.

Fourth, hemodynamic and respiratory effects of the procedure are anticipated. These may result from pressure on or displacement of vital organs, induced arrhythmias, or insufflation of the chest or abdomen. Expected blood loss and fluid shifts should be considered. Certain procedures, such as lung transplantation in an ECLS patient with cystic fibrosis with chronic infection, may provoke a significant inflammatory response with vasodilation.

Lastly, additional routine considerations may include airway issues, equipment availability, use of fluoroscopy, or fire risk.

### Special Considerations for General Anesthesia

As described above, the patient's physiology and the ECLS strategy have implications on the anesthetic plan. Despite the limitations of volatile anesthetic agents, their use may have benefit in delivering general anesthesia in a patient who otherwise has tolerance or who requires large doses of intravenous medications owing to volume of distribution and sequestration. The anesthesiologist should ensure that therapeutic levels of the volatile anesthetic reach the cerebral circulation. Monitoring of the depth of anesthesia must be performed using end-tidal monitoring, and processed EEG monitoring, when available, in patients who receive neuromuscular blockade.

In addition to patient factors, the use of a volatile anesthetic may be challenging due to the limited availability of an anesthetic machine in remote locations, or the lack of scavenging systems to prevent contamination of the workspace with exhaled gases.

### *Special Considerations for Monitored Anesthesia Care*

If Monitored Anesthesia Care (MAC) is planned for the ECLS patient, sedation can be accomplished using opioids, sedative hypnotic agents such as propofol and benzodiazepines, sedatives such as dexmedetomidine, and nonopioid adjuvant medications. The pharmacokinetic principles described in the first part of this chapter remain relevant when considering dosing strategy and response. The anesthesiologist should consider the need and possibility to urgently convert to general anesthesia. These considerations include changes in position that will be required, airway management, and notification of additional team members.

### *Special Considerations for Regional Anesthesia*

Regional anesthesia may be considered in patients supported with ECLS. Specific considerations include:

1. The **location** of the procedure and patient **position** when performing the regional block.
2. The **coagulation** status of the patient. A patient with significant coagulopathy or

need for continuation of anticoagulant medications may be ineligible for neuraxial blockade, although a peripheral nerve block may be an option, particularly if there is perceived benefit in avoiding a general anesthetic.
3. The ability of and need for the patient to **cooperate** during the regional blockade.
4. The ability to develop a **contingency plan** in case the regional anesthetic fails.

These considerations together can create widely divergent scenarios relating to the appropriateness of a regional anesthetic. A patient who needs a toe amputation, who has normal coagulation, who can remain in the supine position, and who is cooperative and able to tolerate general anesthesia if needed may be a reasonable candidate for a regional anesthetic, such as ankle block or sciatic nerve block in the popliteal fossa. By contrast, a coagulopathic, noncooperative patient would not be eligible for an epidural.

### *Special Considerations for Care of the Pediatric or Neonatal Patient*

ECLS has been used in the pediatric population for nearly fifty years, and prior to the 2009 H1N1 pandemic, pediatric respiratory failure was the predominant context in which ECLS was used.[18,19] In current practice, however, ECLS in the neonatal and pediatric populations is used for respiratory support, cardiac support (bridging to mechanical circulatory support device, organ recovery, or cardiac transplantation), ECPR, and as preemptive support during anticipated times of hemodynamic instability during high-risk procedures[20-22] In these cases the pediatric anesthesiologist may care for these patients.

The anesthesiologist should consider that ECLS circuit design and configuration for neonates and pediatric patients accounts for their size and metabolism. Oxygen delivery for neonates in respiratory failure is approximately 6 ml/kg/min,[23] for pediatric patients 4-5 ml/kg/min,[24] while for adults 300 ml/m²/min, or approximately 3 ml/kg/min.[25] In VA ECMO, flow rates for neonates are 100-150 ml/kg/min and 70-100 ml/kg/min for pediatric patients.[26]

As previously discussed, the alterations in pharmacokinetics in the patient supported with ECLS are typically characterized by a larger volume of distribution and prolonged elimination, with a return to baseline after decannulation. However, some studies have suggested that some factors such as younger age, thoracic cannulation, and prolonged use of muscle relaxants are associated with an increased dosage requirement of benzodiazepines and opioids to achieve therapeutic effect.[27]

Pediatric cannulation strategy is based on the size of the patient. Small children are best cannulated via the neck vessels. The exact size, age, and weight for femoral arterial cannulation varies between operators and institutions (Chapter 4).[28]

Bleeding and thrombosis are of particular concern in pediatric patients supported with ECLS.[29,30] Anticoagulation with unfractionated heparin infusion is the most common clinical approach, and the clinician should recognize that heparin effect varies with age and depends on adequate antithrombin (AT) levels. Some institutions have adopted the use of direct thrombin inhibitors, which function independently of AT.[31] Transfusion strategies are typically institution-specific. For pediatric ECLS patients, phlebotomy for lab assessments contributes to transfusion requirements and should be done judiciously.[32] In general, the following parameters are targeted: INR <2, fibrinogen >100-150 mg/dL, and platelet >80,000-100,000.[32]

Vascular access in the critically ill pediatric patient is a common challenge, and patients supported with ECLS are no different. Continuous renal replacement therapy may be provided via the ECLS circuit.[33] Adequate vascular access is of particular importance in anesthesia care when rapid fluid shifts and procedural blood loss require prompt resuscitation. In some cases, the ECLS circuit may be the most efficient, reliable, and accessible access for administration of emergency medications and volume resuscitation. The anesthetist should be familiar with institutional practice and experience in these cases.

Other common principles of pediatric anesthetic care remain relevant for the pediatric ECLS patient, including fluid management and heat conservation. Optimal care delivery is provided by an anesthesiologist with expertise in pediatric anesthesiology and well versed in advanced cardiac and respiratory support.

### Team-Based Care

Teamwork among the multidisciplinary team is essential for best patient care. The anesthesiologist's role is prominent during transport care before and after the surgical procedure, while maintaining hemodynamic stability throughout the procedure, and while managing times of unexpected instability. Coordinating the team for transport of the ECLS patient involves confirming appropriate designation of team members to transport roles, ensuring adequate preparation has been made, and facilitating a team that is responsive to each of its members' concerns (Chapter 46). The use of checklists may facilitate that comprehensive safety measures are in place.

When unexpected instability occurs during a procedure, the anesthesiologist will have first-hand knowledge of the patient's cardiopulmonary status and can alert the team accordingly. Close communication between the anesthesiologist and the team member managing the ECLS circuit will ensure notification and shared understanding. Likewise, the proceduralist and the anesthesiologist will coordinate their management, with mutual updating about anticipated changes.

At times, anesthesia care for ECLS patients will be delivered in off-site locations which were not designed for large pieces of equipment and large teams. The anesthesiologist should be in tune to the space in which a procedure is performed and anticipate issues that may arise. These may include maximizing the ergonomics—and hence safety—of the workspace; minimizing exposure of the team to ionizing radiation; assessing the need and availability of gas outlets, suction, and scavenging systems; and confirming the adequacy of electrical sources and placement of power cords.

## Conclusion

Anesthesia care is commonly done in a variety of settings for ECLS patients, for cannulation, decannulation, cannula adjustment, and other invasive procedures. These procedures may be performed in the ICU, the operating room suites, the catheterization laboratory, or other remote locations. Specific challenges include the pharmacology of anesthetic agents and their interaction with the ECLS circuit, the critical illness of the patient, and the interactions of anesthetics and the procedure on the patient's cardiac and respiratory physiology. Patient safety and optimal care can be provided by an anesthesiologist with an in-depth understanding of these principles who thoughtfully constructs an anesthetic plan and exercises team leadership.

# References

1. Shekar K, Fraser JF, Smith MT, et al. Pharmacokinetic changes in patients receiving extracorporeal membrane oxygenation. J Crit Care. 2012;27(6):741 e749-718.

2. Mulla H, McCormack P, Lawson G, et al. Pharmacokinetics of midazolam in neonates undergoing extracorporeal membrane oxygenation. Anesthesiology. 2003;99(2):275-282.

3. Shekar K, Roberts JA, Smith MT, et al. The ECMO PK Project: an incremental research approach to advance understanding of the pharmacokinetic alterations and improve patient outcomes during extracorporeal membrane oxygenation. BMC Anesthesiol. 2013;13:7.

4. Shekar K, Roberts JA, Ghassabian S, et al. Sedation during extracorporeal membrane oxygenation-why more is less. Anaesth Intensive Care. 2012;40(6):1067-1069.

5. Nasr VG, Meserve J, Pereira LM, et al. Sedative and Analgesic Drug Sequestration After a Single Bolus Injection in an Ex Vivo Extracorporeal Membrane Oxygenation Infant Circuit. ASAIO J. 2019;65(2):187-191.

6. Hammaren E, Rosenberg PH, Hynynen M. Coating of extracorporeal circuit with heparin does not prevent sequestration of propofol in vitro. Br J Anaesth. 1999;82(1):38-40.

7. Hickey S, Gaylor JD, Kenny GN. In vitro uptake and elimination of isoflurane by different membrane oxygenators. J Cardiothorac Vasc Anesth. 1996;10(3):352-355.

8. Betit P. Technical Advances in the Field of ECMO. Respir Care. 2018;63(9):1162-1173.

9. Philipp A, Wiesenack C, Behr R, et al. High risk of intraoperative awareness during cardiopulmonary bypass with isoflurane administration via diffusion membrane oxygenators. Perfusion. 2002;17(3):175-178.

10. Kermad A, Speltz J, Danziger G, et al. Comparison of isoflurane and propofol sedation in critically ill COVID-19 patients-a retrospective chart review. J Anesth. 2021;35(5):625-632.

11. Scherer C, Kupka D, Stocker TJ, et al. Isoflurane Sedation in Patients Undergoing Venoarterial Extracorporeal Membrane Oxygenation Treatment for Cardiogenic Shock-An Observational Propensity-Matched Study. Crit Care Explor. 2020;2(3):e0086.

12. Grant AA, Lineen EB, Klima A, et al. Refractory traumatic bronchopleural fistula: Is extracorporeal membrane oxygenation the new gold standard? J Card Surg. 2020;35(1):242-245.

13. Daoud O, Augustin P, Mordant P, et al. Extracorporeal membrane oxygenation in 5 patients with bronchial fistula with severe acute lung injury. Ann Thorac Surg. 2011;92(1):327-330.

14. Lim H. The physiology of extracorporeal membrane oxygenation: The Fick principle. Perfusion. 2021:2676591211055971.

15. Hayanga JWA, Chan EG, Musgrove K, et al. Extracorporeal Membrane Oxygenation in the Perioperative Care of the Lung Transplant Patient. Semin Cardiothorac Vasc Anesth. 2020;24(1):45-53.

16. Ius F, Tudorache I, Warnecke G. Extracorporeal support, during and after lung transplantation: the history of an idea. J Thorac Dis. 2018;10(8):5131-5148.

17. El-Ganzouri AR, McCarthy RJ, Tuman KJ, et al. Preoperative Airway Assessment: Predictive Value of a Multivariate Risk Index. Anesthesia & Analgesia. 1996;82(6):1197-1204.

18. Awad JA, Matte J, Brassard A. Prolonged extracorporeal respiration with a membrane gas exchanger. J Thorac Cardiovasc Surg. 1973;66(1):40-51.

19. Bartlett RH, Gazzaniga AB, Jefferies MR, et al. Extracorporeal membrane oxygenation (ECMO) cardiopulmonary support in infancy. Trans Am Soc Artif Intern Organs. 1976;22:80-93.

20. ELSO. International Report. Available at https://www.elso.org/Portals/0/Files/Reports/2021_April/International%20Report%20April_page1.pdf. Accessed January 26, 2021.

21. Lasa JJ, Rogers RS, Localio R, et al. Extracorporeal Cardiopulmonary Resuscitation (E-CPR) During Pediatric In-Hospital Cardiopulmonary Arrest Is Associated With Improved Survival to Discharge: A Report from the American Heart Association's Get With The Guidelines-Resuscitation (GWTG-R) Registry. Circulation. 2016;133(2):165-176.

22. Monaco F, Belletti A, Bove T, et al. Extracorporeal Membrane Oxygenation: Beyond Cardiac Surgery and Intensive Care Unit: Unconventional Uses and Future Perspectives. J Cardiothorac Vasc Anesth. 2018;32(4):1955-1970.

23. Wild KT, Rintoul N, Kattan J, et al. Extracorporeal Life Support Organization (ELSO): Guidelines for Neonatal Respiratory Failure. ASAIO J. 2020;66(5):463-470.

24. Maratta C, Potera RM, van Leeuwen G, et al. Extracorporeal Life Support Organization (ELSO): 2020 Pediatric Respiratory ELSO Guideline. ASAIO J. 2020;66(9):975-979.

25. Tonna JE, Abrams D, Brodie D, et al. Management of Adult Patients Supported with Venovenous Extracorporeal Membrane Oxygenation (VV ECMO): Guideline from the Extracorporeal Life Support Organization (ELSO). ASAIO J. 2021;67(6):601-610.

26. Brown G, Moynihan KM, Deatrick KB, et al. Extracorporeal Life Support Organization (ELSO): Guidelines for Pediatric Cardiac Failure. ASAIO J. 2021;67(5):463-475.

27. Anton-Martin P, Modem V, Taylor D, et al. A retrospective study of sedation and analgesic requirements of pediatric patients on extracorporeal membrane oxygenation (ECMO) from a single-center experience. Perfusion. 2017;32(3):183-191.

28. Garcia AV, Jeyaraju M, Ladd MR, et al. Survey of the American Pediatric Surgical Association on cannulation practices in pediatric ECMO. J Pediatr Surg. 2018;53(9):1843-1848.

29. Dalton HJ, Reeder R, Garcia-Filion P, et al. Factors Associated with Bleeding and Thrombosis in Children Receiving Extracorporeal Membrane Oxygenation. Am J Respir Crit Care Med. 2017;196(6):762-771.

30. Werho DK, Pasquali SK, Yu S, et al. Hemorrhagic complications in pediatric cardiac patients on extracorporeal membrane oxygenation: an analysis of the Extracorporeal Life Support Organization Registry. Pediatr Crit Care Med. 2015;16(3):276-288.

31. Sanfilippo F, Asmussen S, Maybauer DM, et al. Bivalirudin for Alternative Anticoagulation in Extracorporeal Membrane Oxygenation: A Systematic Review. J Intensive Care Med. 2017;32(5):312-319.

32. Zaleski KL, Nasr VG. ECMO Primer for the Pediatric Anesthesiologist. Int Anesthesiol Clin. 2019;57(4):72-83.

33. Santiago MJ, Sanchez A, Lopez-Herce J, et al. The use of continuous renal replacement therapy in series with extracorporeal membrane oxygenation. Kidney Int. 2009;76(12):1289-1292.

# 51

## Procedures During Extracorporeal Life Support

*Peter P. Roeleveld, Giles J. Peek, Stefan Fischer, Ali Akil, Theo Kofidis, Amy E. Hackmann, D. Michael McMullan*

## Introduction

The evolution of ECLS circuitry and management techniques over the last 50 years has enabled complex procedures and operations to be performed safely on ECLS patients. We no longer need to deny patients the chance of ECLS support based solely on their need for an operation. Nevertheless, surgical and interventional procedures on ECLS carry risks of life-threatening bleeding which should not be underestimated. This chapter addresses the basic principles and decisionmaking framework for successful procedures on ECLS and then provides an overview of such procedures.

In 1992, Atkinson et al. found that 14% of pediatric ECLS patients received surgical procedures (excluding cannulation and decannulation).[1] Noncardiac surgical procedures are performed in 20 to 50% of adult ECLS patients.[2,3] Most commonly, procedures included general surgical procedures (predominantly abdominal exploration, bowel resection, or fasciotomy), vascular procedures (control of vascular hemorrhage), and thoracic procedures (tracheostomy, lung biopsy, exploratory thoracotomy, lobectomy).[2] High mortality rates occurred in patients who received noncardiac procedures (NCP) on ECLS, with a trend to worse survival than when NCP were not performed. Other documented procedures included open cholecystectomy, craniotomy with hematoma evacuation, pericardial window, and urologic procedures.[3]

Prolonged experience with surgical interventions in children on ECLS indicates that such procedures are technically feasible with the best results achieved when the patient undergoes rapid post-procedural decannulation.[4] Nagaraj et al. described 48 procedures in 37 neonates on ECLS and concluded that cardiac defects, diaphragmatic hernia, lobar emphysema, and other conditions can be safely corrected. However, hemorrhagic and thoracic complications, and multiple surgical interventions were associated with significantly higher mortality.[1,4] In a retrospective single-center study in children, approximately one in seven children required surgical intervention during ECLS, of whom almost 90% developed a complication, resulting in a 50% mortality rate.[5] Data demonstrate that few procedures are prohibitive to intervention providing that the proceduralists are sufficiently experienced and take the necessary precautions because of the increased risk of mortality.

## Decision Threshold – Three Questions

The first question that the proceduralist must ask is, "can the procedure be avoided?" This question is more useful than, "is the procedure necessary?" because it focuses attention on the consequences for the patient if the procedure were not performed. An example of this could be a child on VV ECMO for a left sided pneumonia with a large left hemothorax that has been slowly growing for the last week. A chest drain or thoracotomy would carry a risk of bleeding, but without the procedure the child is unlikely to inflate the pneumonic lung sufficiently to separate from ECLS. A caveat to this question is, "does this procedure achieve the therapeutic aim with the least risk to the patient?"

The second question is, "when is the best time to perform the procedure?" In the above case the procedure can be planned semielectively with an ideal team and operating environment. In contrast, a tension hemothorax that impedes venous drainage requires emergency drainage. Some procedures can be deferred until after decannulation (eg, grafting a burn or repairing a fractured bone). This question balances the need for the procedure against the need to ensure optimal operating conditions by transfusing clotting factors and platelets, altering heparin infusions and administrating antifibrinolytics.

The third question is, "am I the right person to perform this procedure?" Stirling Moss, the famous British racing driver of the 1950s and 60s, had a rule that he would never drive at more than 80% of his capacity so that he always had some driving ability in reserve to cope with unforeseen circumstances. The operator should therefore ensure that the proposed procedure falls well within their competency. In general terms, for more complex procedures, the best operator should be called upon within the timeframe allowable in Question 2.

**General Principals**

*Preparation and Communication*

A thorough preoperative briefing should address equipment requirements, proposed procedures, areas of responsibility and authority, and potential complications with their solutions, preferably by using a checklist. The specific questions of antibiotic prophylaxis, anticoagulant management, and the preparation of a primed standby circuit should also be covered. There should always be someone present who is thoroughly knowledgeable with regards to the hemodynamic consequences and limitations of the ECLS.

*Avoid Air in the Circuit*

Venting the left atrium, right atrium, manipulating stopcocks and cannula bungs can entrain air into the circuit. In addition, cardiac catheterization can allow air to enter around the hemostatic sheath after catheter introduction if the venous pressure is low and the pump RPM is creating significant suction. Therefore, all precautions should be taken to avoid the entrainment of air.

*Obtain Absolute Hemostasis*

With many procedures, residual bleeding often persists but usually settles quickly. When operating on ECLS patients, one should strenuously attempt to ensure total hemostasis including aggressive packing, draining, and sometimes closing the cavity or wound to achieve tamponade or leaving it open to facilitate exploration. Bleeding from irritation around a tracheostomy can be easily controlled by removing the tracheostomy, intubating the patient orally and packing the tracheostomy wound. Usually, in several days, the oral tube can be removed, and the tracheostomy tube replaced.

**General Measures**

Specific protocols for performing procedures during ECLS can increase safety and decrease complications. These procedures can be interventional, surgical, diagnostic, therapeutic, or any combination of these. Specific procedures require unique approaches.

### Anticoagulation

Antifibrinolytics (aminocaproic acid, aprotinin, and tranexamic acid) reduce bleeding complications.[5,6,7] Aminocaproic acid significantly reduced the rate of surgical site bleeding in 298 pediatric ECLS patients undergoing surgical procedures but was associated with increased numbers of circuit changes[6] (100 mg/kg bolus followed by 30 mg/kg/hr for 72 hrs). No difference in thrombotic complications (CNS infarct or major vessel thrombosis) occurred. Tranexamic acid significantly reduced bleeding at the surgical site in neonates undergoing congenital diaphragmatic hernia repair while on ECLS.[7] Aprotinin has effectively been used in the past but is no longer easily available.

Routine ECLS anticoagulation protocols may need to be temporarily altered to reduce the risk of procedural bleeding. Discontinuation of heparin or direct thrombin inhibitor administration may be appropriate for some high-risk procedures. Furthermore, pharmacologic agents (eg, protamine) and blood components (plasma complexes, platelets) may be required to more rapidly optimize the coagulation state of ECLS patients undergoing those procedures associated with an increased risk of life-threatening complications (eg, neurosurgical procedures). Careful consideration must be given to the potential increased risk of circuit thrombosis and thromboembolism versus reduced risk of procedural bleeding.

### ECLS Management

Alterations in clotting and bleeding precipitated by procedures or by manipulating anticoagulation can impact ECLS effectiveness. Prior to procedures, it may be necessary to prepare to support the patient with conventional measures, such as ventilation, inotropes, and/or blood products in case of inadequate ECLS support. For some patients on VA ECMO, it may be appropriate to cool the patient either to 32° C or even to 18° C to provide neuroprotection during the procedure if ECLS must be discontinued and the patient is not felt to be capable of sustaining circulation with adequate gas exchange for a sufficient period.

### Patient Transport

Members of the ECLS team should be notified prior to transporting patients for procedures. Support from the multidisciplinary team should immediately be available in case of accidental decannulation or other mechanical complications during transport (Chapter 46). A backup ECLS circuit should remain available during transport and the procedure.

### ECLS Circuit Related Procedures

When changing the ECLS circuit, or its parts, interruption of cardiopulmonary support should be as brief as possible. Some centers have devised ways to replace ECLS without interrupting support by implanting a parallel circuit.[8] Others simply go 'as quickly as possible' while temporarily increasing standard intensive care support, such as ventilation and/or inotropes, if necessary. Training for these events can decrease the likelihood of complications (Chapter 54).

Revision of ECLS cannulas can be necessary to improve positioning, upgrade size, or remove cannula related clots. Migration of cannulas can also occur during ECLS, potentially compromising flow or causing injury to surrounding tissue, including the right ventricle, right atrium, or inferior vena cava. Therefore, malposition of the cannula should be corrected expeditiously using fluoroscopy, echocardiography, and/or guidewires.[9]

## Diagnostic Procedures

### Radiologic Procedures

Ultrasound, roentgenograms, and computed tomography (CT) are standard diagnostic procedures for patients on ECLS. Ultrasound studies and most plain radiographs can be performed safely at the bedside. Other radiological investigations, including CT scans, require careful attention during transfer to safely complete the studies. In a study of pediatric ECLS patients who underwent CT, clinically significant findings leading to changes in patient management were identified in the majority of patients who were not progressing after 7-18 days on respiratory ECLS. When interpreting CT angiography, one should consider that VA ECMO changes filling and blood flow of the cardiac chambers and pulmonary vessels as well as altering the path of the injected contrast.[10-12] Although experimental MRI has been performed in an ECMO animal model,[13] wire-enforced cannulas could not be used and no commercially available MRI certified ECLS system currently exists.

### Transesophageal Echo

Transesophageal echocardiography (TEE) has become an important diagnostic tool in ECLS management.[14] In VAD and respiratory ECLS patients, TEE can determine appropriate cannula placement, especially dual-lumen VV ECMO cannulas (Chapter 48).[15] In cardiac ECLS patients, TEE can diagnose (residual) cardiac defects or pericardial effusion, evaluate ventricular function, determine the need for left atrial decompression, facilitate bedside atrial septostomy or interatrial stenting, and guide weaning.[16,17] Systemic anticoagulation is not a contraindication for TEE. Contraindications and complications in ECLS patient are similar to those in non-ECLS patients. Although TEE is considered safe, even in neonates, and complications occur rarely, the benefit-risk ratio should be examined in each case.

### Bronchoscopy

In patients on VV or VA ECMO, flexible bronchoscopy, bronchoalveolar lavage (BAL) and bronchial washings have been found to be safe and effective in both adults and children.[18,19] Indications include central airway obstruction, persistent atelectasis, secretion clearance, evaluation of suspected pulmonary infection with BAL, or foreign body aspiration.[19,20] It is not usually necessary to adjust anticoagulation. Spontaneously resolving blood-tinged secretions occurred after approximately 20-30% of flexible bronchoscopies. It is not yet clear if bronchoscopy should be performed routinely or only based on clinical suspicion of need. A pragmatic approach of routine early bronchoscopy which can be repeated as required is an effective approach.

### Cardiac Catheterization

Residual anatomic lesions have a strong negative influence on survival among postcardiac surgical ECLS patients. When echocardiography does not definitely exclude or diagnose residual lesions in these patients, cardiac catheterization can provide insight into adequacy of the surgical repair and hemodynamics.[21] Also, cardiac catheterization improves outcomes in ECPR patients.[22] Other indications include assessment of coronary anatomy; endomyocardial biopsy; electrophysiologic studies; arrhythmia ablation; transcatheter patent ductus arteriosus (PDA), atrial septal defect (ASD) or ventricular septal defect (VSD) closure; and left heart decompression.[23-26]

Early cardiac catheterization has been shown to reduce ECLS duration and increase survival in children who fail an initial attempt at separation from ECLS without a clear reason for failure identified by echocardiography.[27] In a retrospective study, no major complications occurred in 28 cardiac catheter studies in 22 children on ECLS.[28] Booth et al. studied 60 cardiac catheterizations on ECLS. Complications included two myocardial perforations (3%), one during atrial stenting for LV decompression, and the other was presumed to be through the left ventricular free wall.[29] Both patients received pericardial drains. In both studies, management was adjusted based on cardiac catheterization data in approximately 80%.[28,28] Callahan et al. described 36 pediatric patients undergoing a total of 40 cardiac catheter studies. They noted no complications related to patient transport, one nonvascular complication (hypotension), and five vascular complications (compartment syndrome, limb edema, oozing from cannulation site, temporary pulse loss, venous thrombus). Survival to discharge was 72%. Unexpected diagnostic information was found in more than half (52%) of catheterizations.[30]

Tachyarrhythmias in children on ECLS have been safely managed with ablation. Silva et al. described 39 patients, median age 5.5 months, on MCS because of tachyarrhythmias. The majority could be treated with antiarrhythmic medication. Thirteen patients (33%) underwent successful ablation without complications related to MCS or anticoagulation.[24] In adults with tachycardia-induced cardiomyopathy, ablation of the aberrant rhythm focus has also been safe and successfully described for atrial and ventricular tachycardias.[31-33]

Vascular access for catheterization in ECLS patients can prove challenging, especially in small children or in adult patients cannulated through the femoral vessels. The use of ultrasound-guided percutaneous puncture of femoral vessels is advocated.[28] Sometimes, surgical cutdown is necessary. Access for the cardiac catheter can be afforded through an accessory limb connected to the arterial cannula, terminated with a hemostatic valve.[34-36] This may be the best solution because it avoids

the risks of inserting and removing additional catheters during ECLS. It is also possible to puncture the ECMO cannula itself to insert the catheter access (Chapter 4). While this approach is not recommended for long-term support, it is a useful conduit for percutaneous vessel closure devices on decannulation.

## *Endoscopy*

Gastrointestinal (GI) bleeding occurs in 3% to 6% of patients receiving ECLS.[37] It may require transfusions and diagnostic or therapeutic interventions such as gastroduodenoscopy and/or colonoscopy. Endoscopic electrocautery can safely help control GI bleeding.

## **General Surgical Procedures**

### *Vascular Access*

The insertion of central venous lines and arterial catheters can be challenging in the ECLS patient due to the increased risk of bleeding and the presence of edema. Catheter insertion should be performed by experienced caregivers. Surgical cutdowns may be a safer or necessary option in some circumstances but carry a higher risk of ongoing bleeding.

### *Thoracotomy Drains*

Pneumothorax and hemothorax occur in up to 10% of patients on ECLS.[38,39] Placing a chest tube carries a significant risk of bleeding complications.[40] A recent analysis of the Kids Inpatient Database (KID) demonstrated that chest drain placement did not affect survival rates.[41] The assessment of the necessity for a chest tube or whether a patient can be decannulated without the drain may prove difficult. Jackson et al. proposed that, in children on ECLS, indications for chest tube placement include situations in which pleural collections compromise pump flow or oxygenation, indicating tension physiology, or when they preclude weaning from ECLS.[41] When instilled via thoracostomy tube, the fibrinolytic agent tissue plasminogen activator has been used to effectively break-up and evacuate complex loculated intrapleural fluid collections without the need for additional thoracostomy or thoracotomy in some children.[42] Small pleural collections that are unlikely to compromise lung function can be expectantly managed while on ECLS.

### Tracheostomy

Placement of a tracheostomy can be helpful during prolonged ECLS support by enabling spontaneous breathing, minimizing sedation, vasopressor and inotropic requirement, encouraging physiotherapy and ambulation, and reducing time on ECLS.[43,44] Bedside percutaneous and open tracheostomies in adult ECLS patients have repeatedly been shown to be safe if heparin is withheld 1-4 hours pre and postprocedure.[45-47] Bleeding complications are minor, but which approach incurs less bleeding remains uncertain.[45,48] With careful optimization of coagulation management, complication rates of tracheostomies can be low and comparable to those of other critically ill patients when performed by experienced operator.[47,49]

Experience with tracheostomy in children on ECLS is more limited.[45] Agar et al. described 11 pediatric patients (median age 69.5 months) who underwent tracheostomy. Ten received tracheostomy for prolonged respiratory support and 1 to manage tracheal stenosis with no complications.[50] Schwartz et al. described 9 patients (7-25 years old) who underwent bedside tracheostomies while on ECLS with temporary cessation of anticoagulation. Only three patients had superficial bleeding and sedation could be weaned in all patients, enabling them to participate in rehabilitation.[51] A 2022 ELSO Registry study showed that tracheostomies in children were uncommon

(2.6% of 3685 children) and surgical site bleeding was reported in 26%.[52]

### Cesarean Section

ECLS is increasingly being used during pregnancy (Chapter 34). Successful cesarean section during ECLS has been increasingly reported prior to and during the COVID-19 pandemic.[53-59] In two reports, periprocedural heparin administration was discontinued for several hours and standard (Pfannenstiel) cesarean section was performed without bleeding or thromboembolic complications.[58,59] Two additional reports described the use of ECLS immediately prior to emergency cesarean section to facilitate anesthetic safety and to maintain adequate circulation in women with peripartum cardiomyopathy.[56,57] Park et al. used fluoroscopy-assisted insertion of a guidewire during cannulation of the inferior vena cava (IVC) because of concerns of IVC injury compressed by the gravid uterus. After cannulation, no heparin was started, and an uneventful emergency cesarean section was performed. Anticoagulation was started 3 days after delivery.[57]

### Miscellaneous

Other infrequent general surgical procedures in ECLS patients include reports of liver transplantation,[60] gastrorrhaphy,[61] and debridement of soft tissue infections.[62]

## Trauma and Burn Patients

### Trauma

ECLS can be effective in trauma patients with severe cardiopulmonary failure. Survival in trauma patients who receive ECLS is similar to that observed in nontrauma ECLS populations.[63] In a 2015 ELSO Registry study of 85 patients with blunt thoracic trauma, 12 patients (14.1%) underwent invasive procedures on ECLS, including cranial, thoracic, abdominal, or vascular operations, thoracostomy tube placements, and tracheostomy placements (Chapter 35).[64] Hemorrhagic complications occurred in one-third of patients, including surgical site bleeding (14%), cannula site bleeding (19%), and hemolysis or disseminated intravascular coagulation (8%). Subjects with injuries at high risk for hemorrhage or who underwent invasive procedures were not more likely to have a hemorrhagic complication.[64] Strategies to decrease the risk of bleeding include withholding anticoagulation therapy temporarily or, if possible, postponing the procedure until after separation from ECLS.

In chest trauma patients with airway disruption, ECLS can be used to guarantee gas exchange during repair of the airway.[65] Data from the ELSO Registry indicates that ECLS survival in adult burn victims is similar to that observed in non-burn patient populations treated with ECLS.[66] Chou et al. describe two burn patients with ARDS who underwent several escharotomies on ECLS. By maintaining ACTs under 140 seconds, keeping platelets above $100 \times 10^9$, and infusing desmopressin, they encountered no hemorrhagic complications.[67]

### Abdominal Surgery

Laparotomy for bowel resection, abscess removal, relief of abdominal compartment syndrome, or placement of peritoneal drainage catheters can be necessary procedures in patients during ECLS support.[68] An ELSO Registry study of 196 pediatric patients, who underwent a laparotomy while on ECMO, showed that surgical site bleeding was not associated with mortality.[69]

Abdominal compartment syndrome (ACS) can cause abdominal ischemia, limit venous return, and impair the ability to maintain adequate ECLS flows. ACS, defined by progressive intraabdominal distension and intraabdominal pressures >15 mmHg in children and >20 mmHg in adults, has many different causes.[69] ACS can be alleviated by decompressive laparotomy or, when significant ascites is present, by placing a drainage catheter.[70] Although ACS is a rare condition (2-10%) in adult ECLS patients, its presence may be associated with considerable mortality. The necessity of abdominal packing, because of severe bleeding, seems to be a risk factor for increased mortality.[68,71] As a possible noninvasive alternative to decompressive laparotomy, total water-assisted colonoscopy to alleviate ACS was successfully described by Martucci et al. in three adult patients on VV ECMO.[72]

In children with ACS on ECLS, successful placement of a peritoneal dialysis catheter has been described in small case series, using periprocedural aminocaproic acid.[73] Drainage of ascites led to improvement in hemodynamics and oxygenation. Rollins et al. performed decompressive laparotomies without complications, via midline incision from the xiphoid process to the pubis, using electrocautery in 7 pediatric patients that significantly improved venous return and oxygen delivery.[74] Furthermore, leaving the abdomen open after decompressive laparotomy while on ECLS is not contraindicated.[75]

Other forms of compartment syndromes include limb and orbital compartment syndrome, an extremely rare condition.[76,77] In retrospective studies, limb compartment syndrome requiring fasciotomy occurred in 7%-20% of patients with femoral artery cannulation.[78,79]

### Neurosurgery

Evacuation of intracranial blood or clots can be necessary in trauma patients. Friesenecker et al. described an adult trauma patient who developed a massive intracerebral hemorrhage on VA ECMO. Anticoagulation was adjusted to achieve ACTs of 150 seconds. He underwent successful craniotomy without bleeding complications and survived with a GCS of 11.[80] Craniotomy or craniectomy can also be performed in children supported with ECLS, but extreme precaution must be taken regarding anticoagulation.[81,82]

With increased use of mechanical circulatory support (MCS) as a bridge to transplantation or as destination therapy, patients presenting with neurological complications resulting from MCS are becoming more frequent. Limited knowledge exists regarding decisive treatment, patient selection, management of anticoagulation, and early estimation of prognosis. Krenzlin et al. described discouraging results in 11 adults and one child on ECLS requiring craniotomy for life-threatening intraparenchymal hemorrhage, of whom 75% experienced recurrence despite correction of coagulation abnormalities. Nine patients (75%) died in hospital, two survived in a vegetative state, and one survived with severe disability.[83] Wilson et al. described 36 of 330 adult LVAD patients who suffered ICH.[84] With suspension of anticoagulation, no device failures were seen. Intraparenchymal hemorrhage had the worst outcome with 59% 30-day mortality. Traumatic subarachnoid hemorrhages did not lead to any deaths at 30 days while traumatic subdural hemorrhages had 13% mortality at 30 days. Five of their patients with intraparenchymal hemorrhage underwent a neurosurgical intervention and 4 died. No patient with an initial GCS <11 survived beyond 30 days.[84] The poor outcome of craniotomy for intraparenchymal hemorrhage in ECLS patients has been described in other smaller reports in adults and children.[85] Evacuation of subdural hematomas carries better prognosis with survival and minimal neurological deficits.[84-86]

Death is related primarily to progression of intracranial hemorrhage and not to thrombotic complications.[84] No specific anticoagulation guidelines exist for this patient population and decisions should be based on patient and device specifics.[86] In general, anticoagulation

and antiplatelet therapy should be immediately reversed upon diagnosis of ICH in LVAD patients. Withholding aspirin for 1 week and warfarin for 10 days reduces the risk of hemorrhage expansion or rebleeding while minimizing the risk of thromboembolic events and pump failure for adults supported with LVAD.[84]

## Specific Surgical Procedures in Respiratory ECMO

### *Thoracotomy*

Pleural effusions or empyema may need to be drained using chest drains. Furthermore, pulmonary abscesses, cysts, bullae, or necrotic tissue may develop, requiring surgical intervention. Ideally, thoracotomy is postponed until after decannulation.[87] Nonetheless, occasionally it cannot be avoided, such as removal of a septic focus or to fully expand the lung despite the risk of bleeding. Bressman et al. reported bilateral thoracotomies in patients undergoing pulmonary resection due to complications of pneumonia. The authors withheld heparin for 24 hours and reported no complications.[88]

### *Lung Biopsy*

Lung biopsy can diagnose lung pathologies in ECLS patients of all ages and can help guide therapy or decisions to withdraw treatment. Lung biopsy may be indicated in neonates who show no signs of improvement after 10-14 days on respiratory ECLS. Open lung biopsy can be safely performed in the ICU or in the operating suite without major complications.[89] Most centers do not use antifibrinolytics, adjust ACT levels to 160-180 seconds, maintain platelets $>100-150 \times 10^9$, and fibrinogen $>2$ g/l prior to interventions with a significant risk of bleeding. No studies report on bronchoscopic transbronchial lung biopsy in pediatric ECLS patients, probably because of concerns of bleeding. Air leaks rarely occur after biopsy, probably due to low thoracopulmonary compliance, low tidal volumes, and low ventilating pressures in patients supported with ECLS.

In 9 adult ECLS patients with ARDS on VV ECMO, transbronchial biopsy was shown to be safe. However, patients did require a median of 3.4 units of packed red blood cells because of bleeding, despite the fact that 50% were not on systemic anticoagulation during the procedure.[90]

### *Congenital Diaphragmatic Hernia*

Repair of congenital diaphragmatic hernia can safely be performed on patients supported with ECLS.[91] The ideal timing of surgery has been the focus of debate for many years (Chapter 11). Most centers use antifibrinolytics for 24-72 hours to control postoperative bleeding.[91]

### ECLS for Procedural Support in Thoracic Surgery

ECLS may also be used to support gas exchange during thoracic surgical procedures. For some high-risk patients, this can be decisive in making their lesion operable ECLS may allow extensive resection, airway reconstruction, or enable protective lung ventilation during surgery. It is essential to understand the pathophysiology of the underlying disease and of the different ECLS modes, as well as the variety of cannulation options to adequately apply the different escalation and de-escalation strategies in accordance with the clinical situation (Table 51-1).[92]

### *Establishment of Technical Operability*

ECLS may allow complete resection of locally advanced tumors, especially if ventilation or perfusion of both lungs must be completely interrupted, or if surgery involving the heart and great vessels is planned.[93-96]

ECLS has possible advantages over the use of cardiopulmonary bypass (CPB) to facilitate such resections. CPB requires full anticoagulation with high dose heparin and consequently there is an increased risk of bleeding. There can also be a risk of tumor cell spread via blood aspirated from the surgical field using CPB suction, which is returned to the patient through the open reservoir system.[97] Using intraoperative VA ECMO to perform complex tracheobronchial or extensive pulmonary resections of locally advanced tumors[98] prevents potential tumor cell spreading due to the closed circulatory system.

For extended lung and airway resections with airway interventions in hemodynamically stable patients, high-flow VV ECMO is preferred and may be sufficient. In addition to the necessary interruption of ventilation during tracheal or carinal resection,[94,95] this ECLS mode has also been shown to be effective for lung resection in patients with previous contralateral pneumonectomy,[93,99-101] sleeve pneumonectomy,[102,103] and esophageal surgery,[104] showing the efficacy and safety of VV ECMO compared to the more invasive VA approach. Up to 40 minutes of intraoperative apnea has been reported.[101] Heparin-free ECLS

| HOW TO PERFORM LUNG SURGERY ON ECMO |
| --- |
| Increase ECLS flow to maximal possible |
| Disconnect the ventilator and deflate both the lungs |
| Perform the surgery |
| Maintain $SaO_2$ >75% and age-appropriate blood pressure |
| Hand bag ventilation with 100% $FiO_2$ for a few breaths can be used if the patient desaturates |
| Decortication is easier with the lung ventilated rather than collapsed |

**Table 51-1.** Technique for lung surgery on ECLS.

has also been reported to support tracheal stenting.[105]

### Establishment of Functional Operability

Patients with lung cancer and compromised lung function are often excluded from surgery due to functional limitations. In such cases, VV ECMO serves as a useful tool to establish functional operability. The successful use of bicaval high-flow VV ECMO for extensive tumor resections in patients with preoperatively impaired pulmonary function has been reported.[101,106]

Also, patients with compromised lung function due to lung emphysema and chronic obstructive pulmonary disease (COPD) are often declared to be inoperable. Single-site low-flow VV ECMO intraoperatively increases patient safety and allows functional operability during single lung ventilation, thereby avoiding hypercapnia-associated hemodynamic instability and allowing for protective lung ventilation. This experience was recently reported in COPD patients undergoing lung volume reduction surgery (LVRS), who presented with preoperative hypercapnia.[107]

However, ECLS offers safety not only intraoperatively but also in the initial postoperative course, especially in patients with impaired lung function requiring noninvasive ventilation. In addition, awake ECLS may possibly also be helpful during weaning from ventilation and supports respiratory therapy in those functionally compromised patients.[108,109] Airway and lung surgery can be safely facilitated by ECLS, often electively during lung transplantation or pneumonectomy (Chapter 40).[110-112]

## Specific Surgical Procedures in Cardiac ECMO

### Sternotomy/thoracotomy

Blood clots can fill the pericardial or pleural space impairing venous return or pump flow, especially in ECLS patients with central cannulation. Clot evacuation may prove necessary in these patients. In neonates with shunt-dependent circulation, clotting or obstruction of the systemic-pulmonary shunt may lead to acute hypoxia or loss of systemic circulation, sometimes requiring MCS. Revision of the shunt can be safely performed on VA or VV ECMO or after conversion to bypass, leading to improved outcomes.[113,114]

### Unloading the Left Ventricle (LV Venting)

When the left ventricle (LV) fails to eject, it can become overdistended during ECLS, resulting in acute pulmonary venous congestion and edema, or inadequate myocardial recovery. Treatment is decompression of the LV. Elective LV decompression may reduce the duration of ECLS[115,97] and can be done surgically by cannulating the left atrium or a pulmonary vein, percutaneously by atrial septal stenting or balloon atrial septostomy,[25,116-118] or via the transdiaphragmatic route into the LV apex.[119] In adults and children, echocardiographically-guided percutaneous blade and balloon atrial septostomy can be performed safely at the bedside.[120-122] Barbone et al. described introducing a pigtail catheter into the femoral artery and advancing it through the aortic valve into the LV under TEE guidance in 4 adult patients.[123] Ruprecht et al. have reviewed cardiac decompression during ECLS.[106,124] A small left lateral thoracotomy can be made and the LV apex can be cannulated directly for LV decompression.

## *Intracardiac Operations*

The removal of intracardiac clots, infective endocarditis,[125] or surgery for residual lesions usually requires transfer to CPB in the operating room (see Table 51-2).

## Conclusion

Few procedures in the lexicon of the surgeon and interventionist cannot be performed safely on ECLS with good preparation.

| HOW TO PERFORM CARDIAC SURGERY ON ECLS | |
| --- | --- |
| Use the ECLS circuit for support | The ECLS circuit is used to maintain oxygen delivery and circulatory support whilst the surgery is performed. |
| Use the ECLS circuit for DHCA | Simple procedures such as repair of obstructed total anomalous pulmonary venous drainage can be carried out by cooling on V-A ECMO to around 18° C. Cardioplegia is given by hand syringe and the operation can be carried out. Care must be taken to prevent distention of the heart during cooling and rewarming, sometimes some slow cardiac massage is helpful. Use of a cell saver is essential. |
| Convert to CPB | • Cool patient to 32° C while opening the chest on ECLS<br>• Give 3mg/Kg Heparin and allow to circulate, check ACT >500 sec.<br>• Clamp ECLS circuit, connect CPB circuit to ECLS cannulas, or additional cannulas if necessary. Go on CPB<br>• Connect ends of ECLS circuit together and recirculate, turn the sweep off. Flash sweep for a few seconds if blood becomes deoxygenated. Check ACT, blood gas periodically.<br>• Perform the surgery.<br>• If patient will not come off CPB, then reconnect to the same ECLS circuit if it is clean. If it was due to be changed, prime a new one.<br>• If the patient does come off CPB, their passivated ECLS circuit can be kept on standby for 6-12 hours. |

**Table 51-2.** CPB: cardiopulmonary bypass. DHCA: deep hypothermic circulatory arrest. Two examples for using the ECLS circuit for support: a) A patient on VV ECMO can have their Blalock-Thomas-Taussig shunt revised on ECLS. Vascular clamps are applied to the shunt and pulmonary artery to control blood loss. A cell saver can be useful. b) A patient on VA ECMO can have their coronary arteries grafted using off-pump coronary artery bypass graft equipment and techniques.

# References

1. Atkinson JB, Kitagawa H, Humphries B. Major surgical intervention during extracorporeal membrane oxygenation. Journal of Pediatric Surgery. 1992;27(9):1197-1198.

2. Taghavi S, Jayarajan SN, Mangi AA, et al. Examining noncardiac surgical procedures in patients on extracorporeal membrane oxygenation. In: ASAIO Journal. Vol 61. Lippincott Williams and Wilkins; 2015:520-525.

3. Chestovich PJ. Surgical procedures for patients receiving mechanical cardiac support. American Surgeon. 2011;77(10):1314-1317.

4. Nagaraj HS, Mitchell KA, Fallat ME, et al. Surgical complications and procedures in neonates on extracorporeal membrane oxygenation. Journal of Pediatric Surgery. 1992;27(8):1106-1110.

5. Kersten CM, Hermelijn SM, Wijnen RMH, et al. Surgery in Neonatal and Pediatric ECMO Patients Other Than Congenital Diaphragmatic Hernia Repair: A 10-Year Experience. Frontiers in Pediatrics. 2021;9.

6. Downard CD, Betit P, Chang RW, et al. Impact of Amicar on hemorrhagic complications of ECMO: a ten-year review. Journal of Pediatric Surgery. 2003;38(8):1212-1216.

7. van der Staak FHJ, de Haan AFJ, Geven WB, et al. Surgical repair of congenital diaphragmatic hernia during extracorporeal membrane oxygenation: Hemorrhagic complications and the effect of tranexamic acid. Journal of Pediatric Surgery. 1997;32(4):594-599.

8. Rubin S, Ali AN, Pages ON, et al. How to replace an extracorporeal life support without interruption of the cardiopulmonary assistance. Interactive CardioVascular and Thoracic Surgery. 2009;9(2):311-313.

9. Tanaka D, Pitcher HT, Cavarocchi N, et al. Migrated Avalon Veno-Venous Extracorporeal Membrane Oxygenation Cannula: How to Adjust Without Interruption of Flow. Journal of Cardiac Surgery. 2015;30(11):865-868.

10. Goodwin SJ, Randle E, Iguchi A, et al. Chest computed tomography in children undergoing extra-corporeal membrane oxygenation: A 9-year single-centre experience. Pediatric Radiology. 2014;44(6):750-760.

11. Hayes D, Tobias JD, Galantowicz M, et al. Video Fluoroscopy Swallow Study and Nutritional Support During Ambulatory Venovenous Extracorporeal Membrane Oxygenation as a Bridge to Lung Transplantation. World Journal for Pediatric and Congenital Heart Surgery. 2014;5(1):91-93.

12. Al-Ogaili Z, Foulner D, Passage J, et al. CT pulmonary angiography during veno-arterial extracorporeal membrane oxygenation in an adult. Journal of Medical Imaging and Radiation Oncology. 2013;57(3):345-347.

13. Lidegran MK, Frenckner BP, Mosskin M, et al. MRI of the Brain and Thorax during Extracorporeal Membrane Oxygenation: Preliminary Report from a Pig Model. ASAIO Journal. 2006;52(1):104-109.

14. Meers JB, Nanda NC, Watts TE, et al. Utility of transesophageal echocardiography to assess real time left atrial pressure changes and dynamic mitral regurgitation following placement of transseptal multistage venous cannula for systemic venous drainage and indirect left ventricular venting in venoarterial extracorporeal membrane oxygenation. Echocardiography. 2021;38(3):493-499.

15. Dolch ME, Frey L, Buerkle MA, et al. Transesophageal Echocardiography-Guided Technique for Extracorporeal Membrane Oxygenation Dual-Lumen Catheter Placement. ASAIO Journal. 2011;57(4):341-343.

16. Cavarocchi NC, Pitcher HT, Yang Q, et al. Weaning of extracorporeal membrane oxygenation using continuous hemodynamic transesophageal echocardiography. The Journal of Thoracic and Cardiovascular Surgery. 2013;146(6):1474-1479.

17. Johnston TA, Jaggers J, McGovern JJ, et al. Bedside transseptal balloon dilation atrial septostomy for decompression of the left heart during extracorporeal membrane oxygenation. Catheterization and Cardiovascular Interventions. 1999;46(2):197-199.

18. Kamat PP, Popler J, Davis J, et al. Use of flexible bronchoscopy in pediatric patients receiving extracorporeal membrane oxygenation (ECMO) support. Pediatric Pulmonology. 2011;46(11):1108-1113.

19. Baqais K, Mahoney M, Tobler K, Hui A, Noseworthy M. Pediatric Sand Aspiration Managed Using Bronchoscopy and Extracorporeal Membrane Oxygenation. Canadian Respiratory Journal. 2015;22(5):261-262.

20. Lin J, Frye L. The intersection of bronchoscopy and extracorporeal membrane oxygenation. Journal of Thoracic Disease. 2021;13(8):5176-5182.

21. Soynov IA, Kornilov IA, Kulyabin YY, et al. Residual Lesion Diagnostics in Pediatric Postcardiotomy Extracorporeal Membrane Oxygenation and Its Outcomes. World Journal for Pediatric and Congenital Heart Surgery. 2021;12(5):605-613.

22. Alsoufi B, Awan A, Manlhiot C, et al. Results of rapid-response extracorporeal cardiopulmonary resuscitation in children with refractory cardiac arrest following cardiac surgery. European Journal of Cardio-Thoracic Surgery. 2014;45(2):268-275.

23. Brown KL, Shekerdemian LS, Penny DJ. Transcatheter closure of a patent arterial duct in a patient on veno-

arterial extracorporeal membrane oxygenation. Intensive Care Medicine. 2002;28(4):501-503.

24. Silva JNA, Erickson CC, Carter CD, et al. Management of Pediatric Tachyarrhythmias on Mechanical Support. Circulation: Arrhythmia and Electrophysiology. 2014;7(4):658-663.

25. Alkhouli M, Narins CR, Lehoux J, et al. Percutaneous Decompression of the Left Ventricle in Cardiogenic Shock Patients on Venoarterial Extracorporeal Membrane Oxygenation. Journal of Cardiac Surgery. 2016;31(3):177-182.

26. Kommineni M, Lang RM, Russo MJ, et al. Percutaneous transcatheter closure of infarct related ventricular septal defects assisted with portable miniaturized extracorporeal membrane oxygenation: A case series. Cardiovascular Revascularization Medicine. 2013;14(4):241-245.

27. Burke CR, Chan T, Rubio AE, et al. Early Cardiac Catheterization Leads to Shortened Pediatric Extracorporeal Membrane Oxygenation Run Duration. Journal of Interventional Cardiology. 2017;30(2):170-176.

28. Panda BR, Alphonso N, Govindasamy M, et al. Cardiac Catheter Procedures During Extracorporeal Life Support: A Risk-Benefit Analysis. World J Pediatr Congenit Heart Surg. 2014 Jan 1;5(1):31-7.

29. Booth KL, Roth SJ, Perry SB, et al. Cardiac Catheterization of Patients Supported by Extracorporeal Membrane Oxygenation. J Am Coll Cardiol. 2002 Nov 6;40(9):1681-6.

30. Callahan R, Trucco SM, Wearden PD, et al. Outcomes of Pediatric Patients Undergoing Cardiac Catheterization While on Extracorporeal Membrane Oxygenation. Pediatric Cardiology. 2015;36(3):625-632.

31. Scherrer V, Lasgi C, Hariri S, et al. Radiofrequency Ablation under Extracorporeal Membrane Oxygenation for Atrial Tachycardia in Postpartum. Journal of Cardiac Surgery. 2012;27(5):647-649.

32. Cheruvu C, Walker B, Kuchar D, et al. Successful Ablation of Incessant AV Reentrant Tachycardia in a Patient on Extracorporeal Membrane Oxygenation. Heart, Lung and Circulation. 2014;23(1):e12-e15.

33. Rizkallah J, Shen S, Tischenko A, et al. Successful Ablation of Idiopathic Left Ventricular Tachycardia in an Adult Patient During Extracorporeal Membrane Oxygenation Treatment. Canadian Journal of Cardiology. 2013;29(12):1741.e17-1741.e19.

34. Endemann DH, Philipp A, Hengstenberg C, et al. A simple method of vascular access to perform emergency coronary angiography in patients with veno-arterial extracorporeal membrane oxygenation. Intensive Care Medicine. 2011;37(12):2046-2049.

35. Ucer E, Fredersdorf S, Jungbauer C, et al. A unique access for the ablation catheter to treat electrical storm in a patient with extracorporeal life support. Europace. 2014;16(2):299-302.

36. Thuys C, MacLaren G, d'Udekem Y, et al. Vascular Access for Pediatric Coronary Angiography on Extracorporeal Membrane Oxygenation. World Journal for Pediatric and Congenital Heart Surgery. 2015;6(1):126-129.

37. Brogan T v., Thiagarajan RR, Rycus PT, et al. Extracorporeal membrane oxygenation in adults with severe respiratory failure: a multi-center database. Intensive Care Medicine. 2009;35(12):2105-2114.

38. Zwischenberger JB, Cilley RE, Hirschl RB, et al. Life-threatening intrathoracic complications during treatment with extracorporeal membrane oxygenation. Journal of Pediatric Surgery. 1988;23(7):599-604.

39. Gross GW, Dougherty CH. Pleural hemorrhage in neonates on extracorporeal membrane oxygenation and after repair of congenital diaphragmatic hernia: imaging findings. American Journal of Roentgenology. 1995;164(4):951-955.

40. Jackson HT, Longshore S, Feldman J, et al. Chest tube placement in children during extracorporeal membrane oxygenation (ECMO). Journal of Pediatric Surgery. 2014;49(1):51-54.

41. Tashiro J, Perez EA, Lasko DS, et al. Post-ECMO chest tube placement: A propensity score-matched survival analysis. Journal of Pediatric Surgery. 2015;50(5):793-797.

42. Witt CE, Mesher AL, Hermsen JL, et al. Intrapleural Fibrinolysis During Pediatric Extracorporeal Life Support. World Journal for Pediatric and Congenital Heart Surgery. 2015;6(1):123-125.

43. DiChiacchio L, Boulos FM, Brigante F, et al. Early tracheostomy after initiation of venovenous extracorporeal membrane oxygenation is associated with decreased duration of extracorporeal membrane oxygenation support. Perfusion. 2020;35(6):509-514.

44. Grewal J, Sutt AL, Cornmell G, et al. Safety and Putative Benefits of Tracheostomy Tube Placement in Patients on Extracorporeal Membrane Oxygenation: A Single-Center Experience. Journal of Intensive Care Medicine. 2020;35(11):1153-1161.

45. Kelley KM, Galvagno SM, Wallis M, et al. Tracheostomy in Patients on Venovenous Extracorporeal Membrane Oxygenation: Is It Safe? The American Surgeon. 2021;87(8):1292-1298.

46. Smith MC, Evans PT, Prendergast KM, et al. Surgical outcomes and complications of bedside tracheostomy in the ICU for patients on ECMO. Perfusion. 2022;37(1):26-30.

47. Braune S, Kienast S, Hadem J, et al. Safety of percutaneous dilatational tracheostomy in patients on extracorporeal lung support. Intensive Care Medicine. 2013;39(10):1792-1799.

48. Salas De Armas IA, Dinh K, Akkanti B, et al. Tracheostomy While on Extracorporeal Membrane Oxygenation: A Comparison of Percutaneous and Open Procedures. J Extra Corpor Technol. 2020 Dec;52(4):266-271.

49. Schmidt M, Fisser C, Martucci G, et al. Tracheostomy management in patients with severe acute respiratory distress syndrome receiving extracorporeal membrane oxygenation: an International Multicenter Retrospective Study. Critical Care. 2021;25(1):238.

50. Agar NJM, Berkowitz RG. Airway Complications of Pediatric Extracorporeal Membrane Oxygenation. Annals of Otology, Rhinology & Laryngology. 2011;120(6):353-357.

51. Schwartz SP, Bonadonna D, Hartwig MG, et al. Bedside Tracheostomy on Pediatric ICU Subjects Supported by Extracorporeal Membrane Oxygenation. Respiratory Care. 2017;62(11):1447-1455.

52. Kohne JG, MacLaren G, Rider E, et al. Tracheostomy Practices and Outcomes in Children During Respiratory Extracorporeal Membrane Oxygenation. Pediatric Critical Care Medicine. 2022;23(4):268-276.

53. Douglass KM, Strobel KM, Richley M, et al. Maternal-Neonatal Dyad Outcomes of Maternal COVID-19 Requiring Extracorporeal Membrane Support: A Case Series. Am J Perinatol. 2021 Jan;38(1):82-87.

54. Quintero A, Vinck EE, Perez LE, et al. Extra-corporeal membrane oxygenation and emergency C-section for a pregnant COVID-19 positive patient. Perfusion. Perfusion. 2021 Oct 7:2676591211049769.

55. Gevaert S, van Belleghem Y, Bouchez S, et al. Acute and Critically Ill Peripartum Cardiomyopathy and "bridge to" Therapeutic Options: A Single Center Experience with Intra-Aortic Balloon Pump, Extra Corporeal Membrane Oxygenation and Continuous-Flow Left Ventricular Assist Devices. Vol 15.; 2011.

56. Kim HY, Jeon HJ, Yun JH, et al. Anesthetic experience using extracorporeal membrane oxygenation for cesarean section in the patient with peripartum cardiomyopathy-a case report. Korean J Anesthesiol. 2014;66:392-397.

57. Park SH, Chin JY, Choi MS, et al. Extracorporeal membrane oxygenation saved a mother and her son from fulminant peripartum cardiomyopathy. Journal of Obstetrics and Gynaecology Research. 2014;40(7):1940-1943.

58. Panarello G, D'Ancona G, Capitanio G, Occhipinti G, Attardo G, Bertani A, Arcadipane A. Cesarean section during ECMO support. Minerva Anestesiol. 2011 Jun;77(6):654-7.

59. Łysenko L, Urszula Zaleska-Dorobisz, Radosław Blok, et al. A successful cesarean section in a pregnant woman with A (H1N1) influenza requiring ECMO support. Kardiochirurgia i Torakochirurgia Polska. 2014;11(2).

60. Landsman IS, Karsanac CJ. Pediatric Liver Retransplantation on an Extracorporeal Membrane Oxygenation-Dependent Child. Anesthesia & Analgesia. 2010;111(5):1275-1278.

61. Howell CG, Hatley RM, Davis JB, et al. Successful gastrorrhaphy on ECMO. Journal of Pediatric Surgery. 1988;23(12):1161-1162.

62. Firstenberg MS, Abel E, Blais D, et al. The Use of Extracorporeal Membrane Oxygenation in Severe Necrotizing Soft Tissue Infections Complicated by Septic Shock. Am Surg. 2010 Nov;76(11):1287-9.

63. Burke CR, Crown A, Chan T, et al. Extracorporeal life support is safe in trauma patients. Injury. 2017;48(1):121-126.

64. Jacobs J v., Hooft NM, Robinson BR, et al. The use of extracorporeal membrane oxygenation in blunt thoracic trauma. Journal of Trauma and Acute Care Surgery. 2015;79(6):1049-1054.

65. Ballouhey Q, Fesseau R, Benouaich V, et al. Benefits of extracorporeal membrane oxygenation for major blunt tracheobronchial trauma in the paediatric age group. Eur J Cardiothorac Surg. 2013 Apr;43(4):864-5.

66. Burke CR, Chan T, McMullan DM. Extracorporeal Life Support Use in Adult Burn Patients. Journal of Burn Care & Research. 2017;38(3):174-178.

67. Chou NK, Chen YS, Ko WJ, et al. Application of Extracorporeal Membrane Oxygenation in Adult Burn Patients. Artificial Organs. 2001;25(8):622-626.

68. Schulz SA, Schaefer S, Richards DC, et al. The Need for Emergency Laparotomy With Open Abdomen Therapy in the Course of ECMO—A Retrospective Analysis of Course and Outcome. Front Surg. 2020 Sep 4;7:63.

69. Barry WE, Castle SL, Golden J, et al. Laparotomy complications on extracorporeal life support: Surgical site bleeding does not increase mortality. Journal of Pediatric Surgery. 2019;54(9):1736-1739.

70. Beck R, Halberthal M, Zonis Z, et al. Abdominal compartment syndrome in children. Pediatric Critical Care Medicine. 2001;2(1):51-56.

71. Glowka TR, Schewe JC, Muenster S, et al. Decompressive laparotomy for the treatment of the abdominal compartment syndrome during extracorporeal membrane oxygenation support. Journal of Critical Care. 2018;47:274-279.

72. Martucci G, Amata M, di Francesco F, et al. Management of intra-abdominal hypertension during ECMO: Total water-assisted colonoscopy as a step-up minimally invasive treatment, and a literature review. Endoscopy International Open. 2021;09(06):E848-E852.

73. Prodhan P, Imamura M, Garcia X, et al. Abdominal Compartment Syndrome in Newborns and Children Supported on Extracorporeal Membrane Oxygenation. ASAIO Journal. 2012;58(2):143-147.

74. Rollins MD, Deamorim-Filho J, et al. Decompressive laparotomy for abdominal compartment syndrome in children on ECMO: Effect on Support and Survival. Journal of Pediatric Surgery. 2013;48(7):1509-1513.

75. Brown J, Warnock B, Turk E, et al. Open abdomen during extracorporeal membrane oxygenation is a safe and effective treatment for abdominal compartment syndrome. J Pediatr Surg. 2021 Dec 1:S0022-3468(21)00793-4.

76. Yeo JH, Sung KH, Chung CY, et al. Acute compartment syndrome after extracorporeal membrane oxygenation. Journal of Orthopaedic Science. 2015;20(2):444-448.

77. Brodt J, Gologorsky D, Walter S, et al. Orbital Compartment Syndrome Following Extracorporeal Support. Journal of Cardiac Surgery. 2013;28(5):522-524.

78. Avalli L, Maggioni E, Sangalli F, et al. Percutaneous Left-Heart Decompression During Extracorporeal Membrane Oxygenation: An Alternative to Surgical and Transeptal Venting in Adult Patients. ASAIO Journal. 2011;57(1):38-40.

79. Yau P, Xia Y, Shariff S, et al. Factors Associated with Ipsilateral Limb Ischemia in Patients Undergoing Femoral Cannulation Extracorporeal Membrane Oxygenation. Annals of Vascular Surgery. 2019;54:60-65.

80. Friesenecker BE, Peer R, Rieder J, et al. Case Report Craniotomy during ECMO in a severely traumatized patient. Acta Neurochir (Wien). 2005 Sep;147(9):993-6; discussion 996.

81. Anton-Martin P, Braga B, Megison S, et al. Craniectomy and Traumatic Brain Injury in Children on Extracorporeal Membrane Oxygenation Support. Pediatric Emergency Care. 2018;34(11):e204-e210.

82. Mendoza-Palomar N, Melendo-Pérez S, Balcells J, et al. Influenza-Associated Disseminated Aspergillosis in a 9-Year-Old Girl Requiring ECMO Support. 2021 Sep 5;7(9):726.

83. Krenzlin H, Rosenthal C, Wolf S, et al. Surgical treatment of intraparenchymal hemorrhage during mechanical circulatory support for heart-failure-a single-centre experience. Acta Neurochir (Wien). 2014 Sep;156(9):1729-34.

84. Wilson TJ, Stetler WR Jr, Al-Holou WN, et al. Management of intracranial hemorrhage in patients with left ventricular assist devices. J Neurosurg. 2013;118:1063-1068.

85. Niebler RA, Lew M, Zangwill SD, et al. Thoughts and Progress Incidence and Outcome of Pediatric Patients With Intracranial Hemorrhage While Supported on Ventricular Assist Devices. Artif Organs. 2014 Jan;38(1):73-8.

86. Mayer RR HS, Reddy GD, Morales DL, et al. Neurosurgical complications of left ventricular assist devices in children. J Neurosurg Pediatrics. 2012;10:370-375.

87. Marasco SF, Preovolos A, Lim K, et al. Thoracotomy in adults while on ECMO is associated with uncontrollable bleeding. Perfusion. 2007;22:23-26.

88. Krueger K, Schmutz A, Zieger B, et al. Venovenous Extracorporeal Membrane Oxygenation With Prophylactic Subcutaneous Anticoagulation Only: An Observational Study in More Than 60 Patients. Heart Lung Vessel. 2015;7(4):330-331.

89. Houmes RJ, ten Kate CA, Wildschut ED, et al. Risk and relevance of open lung biopsy in pediatric ECMO patients: the Dutch experience. Journal of Pediatric Surgery. 2017;52(3):405-409.

90. Lipps KM, Bharat A, Walter JM. Lung Biopsy in Patients with Acute Respiratory Distress Syndrome Supported on Extracorporeal Membrane Oxygenation: A 2 Year Experience. ASAIO Journal. 2019;65(8):e92-e94.

91. Keijzer R, Wilschut DE, Houmes RJ, et al. Congenital diaphragmatic hernia: To repair on or off extracorporeal membrane oxygenation? Journal of Pediatric Surgery. 2012;47(4):631-636.

92. Akil A, Bölükbas S, Wiebe K. Extracorporeal Membrane Oxygenation in Thoracic Surgery:Establishing Functional and Technical Operability. Zentralbl Chir . 2019;1:78-85.

93. Rosskopfova P, Yannis Perentes J, Ris HB, et al. Extracorporeal support for pulmonary resection: current indications and results. World J Surg Oncol. 2016 Feb 2;14:25.

94. Hong Y, Jo KW, Lyu J, et al. Use of venovenous extracorporeal membrane oxygenation in central airway obstruction to facilitate interventions leading to definitive airway security. Journal of Critical Care. 2013;28(5):669-674.

95. Ko M, dos Santos PR, MacHuca TN, et al. Use of single-cannula venous-venous extracorporeal life support in the management of life-threatening airway obstruction. Annals of Thoracic Surgery. 2015;99(3):e63-e65.

96. de Perrot M, Fadel E, Mussot S, et al. Resection of locally advanced (T4) non-small cell lung cancer with cardiopulmonary bypass. Annals of Thoracic Surgery. 2005;79(5):1691-1696.

97. Pinto CA, Marcella S, August DA, et al. Cardiopulmonary bypass has a modest association with cancer progression: a retrospective cohort study. BMC Cancer. BMC Cancer. 2013 Nov 3;13:519.

98. Lang G, Ghanim B, Hötzenecker K, et al. Extracorporeal membrane oxygenation support for complex tracheo-

bronchial procedures. Eur J Cardiothorac Surg. 2015 Feb;47(2):250-5; discussion 256.

99. Keeyapaj W, Alfirevic A. Carinal resection using an airway exchange catheter-assisted venovenous ECMO technique. Can J Anaesth. 2012;59:1075-1076.

100. Wan Kim C, Hyung Kim D, Soo Son B, et al. Patients and Methods The Feasibility of Extracorporeal Membrane Oxygenation in the Variant Airway Problems. Ann Thorac Cardiovasc Surgery. 2015;21:517-522.

101. Redwan B, Ziegeler S, Freermann S, et al. Intraoperative veno-venous extracorporeal lung support in thoracic surgery: a single-centre experience. Interactive CardioVascular and Thoracic Surgery 766–772. 2015;21:766-772.

102. Kondo T, Sagawa M, Sato M. Left Sleeve Pneumonectomy Performed Through a Clamshell Incisionwith Extracorporeal Membrane Oxygenation for BronchogenicCarcinoma: Report of Two Cases. Surg Today . 1999;29:807-810.

103. Kodama K, Higashiyama M, Yokouchi. [Use of percutaneous cardiopulmonary support (PCPS) for extended surgery in patients with T4 tumor].. Kyobu Geka. 2000;53:721-725.

104. Schiff JH, K€ J, Teschner J, et al. Veno-venous extracorporeal membrane oxygenation (ECMO) support during anaesthesia for oesophagectomy. Anaesthesia. 2013;68:527-530.

105. Fina D, Matteucci M, Jiritano F. Extracorporeal membrane oxygenation without systemic anticoagulation: a case-series in challenging conditions. J Thorac Dis. 2020;12(5):2113-2119.

106. Redwan B, Ziegeler S, Dickgreber N, et al. Metastasectomy in a lung graft using high-flow venovenous extracorporeal lung support in a patient after single lung transplantation. Journal of Thoracic and Cardiovascular Surgery. 2015;150(5):e79-e81.

107. Akil A, Ziegeler S, Reichelt J, et al. Veno-Venous Extracorporeal Lung Support as a Bridge to or Through Lung Volume Reduction Surgery in Patients with Severe Hypercapnia. ASAIO Journal. 2020;66(8):952-959.

108. Li X, He H, Sun B. Veno-venous extracorporeal membrane oxygenation support during lung volume reduction surgery for a severe respiratory failure patient with emphysema. J Thorac Dis. 2016;8:240-243.

109. Langer T, Santini A, Bottino N, et al. "Awake" extracorporeal membrane oxygenation (ECMO): pathophysiology, technical considerations, and clinical pioneering. Published online 2016.

110. Ius F, Kuehn C, Tudorache I, et al. Lung transplantation on cardiopulmonary support: Venoarterial extracorporeal membrane oxygenation outperformed

cardiopulmonary bypass. Journal of Thoracic and Cardiovascular Surgery. 2012;144(6):1510-1516.

111. Redwan B, Ziegeler S, Freermann S, et al. Intraoperative veno-venous extracorporeal lung support in thoracic surgery: a single-centre experience. Interactive Cardiovasc Thorac Surg. 2015 Dec;21(6):766-72.

112. Liston DE, Richards MJ. Venoarterial extracorporeal membrane oxygenation (VA ECMO) to facilitate combined pneumonectomy and tracheoesophageal fistula repair. Journal of Cardiothoracic and Vascular Anesthesia. 2014;28(4):1021-1023.

113. Allan CK, Thiagarajan RR, del Nido PJ, et al. Indication for initiation of mechanical circulatory support impacts survival of infants with shunted single-ventricle circulation supported with extracorporeal membrane oxygenation. Journal of Thoracic and Cardiovascular Surgery. 2007;133(3):660-667.

114. Miyashita T, Hayashi Y, Ohnishi Y, et al. Anesthesia for an infant with hypoplastic left heart syndrome undergoing reconstruction of a systemic pulmonary shunt under extracorporeal membrane oxygenation. J Cardiothorac Vasc Anesth. 1998;12(4):497-498.

115. Hacking DF, Best D, Brizard CP, et al. Elective Decompression of the Left Ventricle in Pediatric Patients May Reduce the Duration of Venoarterial Extracorporeal Membrane Oxygenation. Artificial Organs. 2015;39(4):319-326.

116. Keenan JE, Schechter MA, Bonadonna DK, et al. Early Experience with a Novel Cannulation Strategy for Left Ventricular Decompression during Nonpostcardiotomy Venoarterial ECMO. ASAIO Journal. 2016;62(3):e30-e34.

117. Eastaugh LJ, Thiagarajan RR, Darst JR, et al. Percutaneous Left Atrial Decompression in Patients Supported With Extracorporeal Membrane Oxygenation for Cardiac Disease*. Pediatric Critical Care Medicine. 2015;16(1):59-65.

118. Hong TH, Byun JH, Lee HM, et al. Initial Experience of Transaortic Catheter Venting in Patients with Venoarterial Extracorporeal Membrane Oxygenation for Cardiogenic Shock. ASAIO Journal. 2016;62(2):117-122.

119. Eudailey KW, Yi SY, Mongero LB, et al. Case Report Trans-diaphragmatic left ventricular venting during peripheral venous-arterial extracorporeal membrane oxygenation Case Report. Perfusion. 2015;30(8):701-703.

120. O'Connor TA, Downing GJ, Ewing LL, et al. Echocardiographically guided balloon atrial septostomy during extracorporeal membrane oxygenation (ECMO). Pediatric Cardiology. 1993;14(3):167-168.

121. Seib PM, Faulkner SC, Erickson CC, et al. Blade and balloon atrial septostomy for left heart decompression

in patients with severe ventricular dysfunction on extracorporeal membrane oxygenation. Catheterization and Cardiovascular Interventions. 1999;46(2):179-186.

122. Dahdouh Z, Roule V, Lognoné T, et al. Atrial septostomy in cardiogenic shock related to H1N1 infection. Acute Cardiac Care. 2013;15(1):7-9.

123. Barbone A, Malvindi PG, Ferrara P, et al. Proposal for bail-out procedures-Assisted circulation Left ventricle unloading by percutaneous pigtail during extracorporeal membrane oxygenation. Interactive CardioVascular and Thoracic Surgery. 2011;13:293-295.

124. Rupprecht L, Flörchinger B, Schopka S, et al. Cardiac Decompression on Extracorporeal Life Support. ASAIO Journal. 2013;59(6):547-553.

125. Noyes AM, Ramu B, Parker MW, et al. Extracorporeal Membrane Oxygenation as a Bridgeto Surgery for Infective Endocarditis Complicated by Aorto-Atrial Fistula and Cardiopulmonary Collapse. Tex Heart Inst J. 2015 Oct 1;42(5):471-3.

# 52

## Starting a New Program

*Ahmed Rabie, Alyaa Elhazmi, Elizabeth A. Moore, D. Michael McMullan, Jumana Yusuf Haji, Eva M. Marwali, Neil Orford, Simon Finney, Daniel Brodie, Graeme MacLaren, Mohamed Azzam, Mark T. Ogino*

### Introduction

The increase in ECLS use since 2009 was associated with a concomitant rise in the number of ECLS centers.[1] Starting new ECLS programs may be less of a challenge than in the past because of the increased awareness of educational opportunities, expanding literature on the use of ECLS, accessibility to educational resources, and the availability of ELSO guidelines.[2,3] This chapter will discuss establishing a new ECLS program, including the needed infrastructure, engagement, launch, and maintenance plan. While an ECLS program can impact hospital revenue, the program's organizational structure, services, patients, and clinical provider relationships may be viewed within a business framework (Figure 52-1). When approached this way, ECLS program leaders may evaluate opportunities to improve efficiency, safety, and effectiveness early in establishing a program. Furthermore, consideration may be given to interrelated critical elements of a program when considering subsequent changes to a program, such as adding transport ECLS, ECPR, or the use of ECLS for mechanical cardiac support in a comprehensive heart failure management strategy. We will utilize the five phases of the project management framework developed by the Project Management Institution (PMI)[4,5]

with modifications tailored to the nature of the program, then describe the Plan, Do, Check, Act, and cycle (PDCA) to fit ECLS program maintenance and sustainability for any proposed area of program progression.[6,7]

### Phases to start a new ECLS program:

Five phases of project management will guide the successful launch of a new ECLS program. These phases are initiation, planning, execution, auditing, and development (Figure 52-1).[7]

### Phase 1: Initiation phase

This phase will define the scope and goals of an ECLS service, survey available resources, identify stakeholders and program leads, confirm the institutional commitment, and develop an ECLS program charter.

#### 1. Define scope and goals of ECLS service

The scope of ECLS services in a center must clearly state and align with the hospital's range of services, the population served, and available services elsewhere in the region. Some forms of ECLS require more resources and specialty services than others to provide comprehensive care. For example, cardiac

ECMO as mechanical circulatory support (MCS) may be more challenging to implement and maintain than respiratory ECMO due to the increased resources required, including cardiac surgery, cardiac catheterization laboratories, and cardiac critical care facilities.[8] It is essential to consider the type of ECLS needed to fit the available resources and institutional goals. To assess the needs of the target population, the leadership can leverage market data to understand local dynamics and opportunities. Additionally, a historical review of patient admissions and ECLS inclusion criteria can provide insight into the theoretical volumes a center could support.

## 2. Surveying the available resources and the potential program needs

ECLS is a resource-intensive service, both financially and in terms of staffing requirements. Therefore, it is vital to understand current institutional resources and ensure the commitment of hospital leadership to starting a new ECLS program. Required resources include initial investments in purchasing equipment and consumables, team training, and recruitment. There must also be a firm commitment to the ongoing needs of the program concerning training and education, service maintenance, adequately designed and staffed ICUs, and the availability and readiness of non-ICU services such as other interventional services, surgery, laboratory, and blood bank capabilities.

## 3. Identify stakeholders and program leads

More than many other advanced therapies, the safe and effective provision of ECLS relies on a multidisciplinary approach to patient management. Consequently, a multidisciplinary Steering Committee directs well-organized and highly functioning ECLS programs. This committee will play an important role in program development, policy development, strategic planning, and education. The ECLS steering committee's size and structure should reflect the local hospital environment's unique

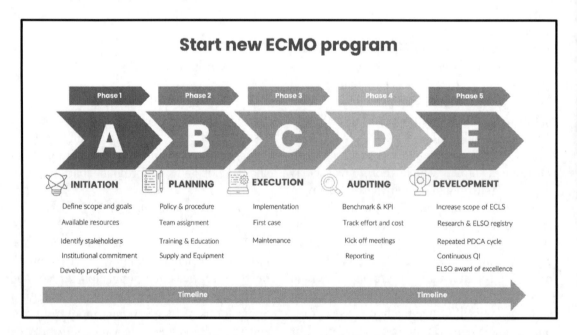

**Figure 52-1.** Five phases of a new project management developed by the Project Management Institute (PMI).

clinical setting and needs. The ECLS steering committee becomes the governing body responsible for developing policy, establishing care pathways and guidelines, overseeing provider credentialing, establishing educational goals and expectations, and engaging in routine safety and quality improvement activities. The success of a program is highly dependent on how well these activities are performed and whether consensus is achieved among critical stakeholders and the groups they represent.

It is necessary to identify a motivated and knowledgeable ECLS program director responsible for broad oversight of the program and serves as the program's champion. Ideally, the program director is an experienced ECLS provider. However, when identifying a leader with robust clinical experience is not feasible (eg, a new ECLS program in resource-limited environments), the program director should have completed an ELSO-endorsed or equivalent training program. Ultimately, the director is responsible for liaising between the multiple services and care teams involved in ECLS patients and represents the ECLS program to hospital clinical and administrative leadership. Finally, the hospital organizational leaders should clearly define the ECLS reporting structure. The ECLS program director should meet regularly with the hospital corporate leaders who have oversight of the program.[10]

Identifying a talented leader to fill the ECMO Coordinator/Manager role is equally crucial to a program's success. As the ECMO Coordinator, it is desirable to have someone experienced in ECLS. They will work with the program director in a partnered leadership model, running daily operations, budgeting, equipment management, staff deployment, and education.

### 4. Administration and institutional commitment

It is essential to ensure institutional commitment when starting a new ECLS program. A successful program requires support from the highest levels of leadership within an organization. It will need a strategic plan aligned with the hospital's mission and strategic plan.[11]

### 5. Develop ECLS program charter

The ECLS program director and Steering Committee should develop the ECLS program charter early in establishing a program. The charter should include the entire process of planning and assigning the subcommittee to achieve tasks either of clinical or operational importance. There should be clear timelines, objectives, deliverables, and outcomes. Many charter templates are available online.[12]

### Phase 2: Planning Phase

This phase will include a preset plan during the program charter's initiation.

### 1. Policies and procedures

The ECLS Steering Committee should create a task force to establish policies and procedures related to ECLS candidate selection and exclusion. The task force is responsible for a comprehensive review of the literature and drafting policies and procedures consistent with ELSO Guidelines.[13] The policies and procedures are drafted to provide ECLS clinicians with clear expectations for clinical and administrative responsibilities and explicit expectations for escalation. For example, ECLS centers will need to develop a process to ensure skills retention, a minimum number of annual pump hours, regular opportunities for high-fidelity didactic training, hands-on refresher courses, and periodic recertification. The Steering Committee will evaluate and approve these documents before initiating clinical ECLS activities. Once adopted, policies and procedures serve as the road map for operational activities and clinical management.

## 2. Team composition and assignment

A dedicated and well-trained multidisciplinary ECLS team is the key to success. Recruiting new team members to supervise and train bedside staff may be necessary.[14]

a. **ECLS cannulating physicians** may be anesthesiologists, intensivists, general surgeons, cardiothoracic surgeons, vascular surgeons, cardiologists, emergency medicine physicians, or other specialists, depending on the human resources available and the program's unique needs. Cardiac and pediatric surgeons typically perform pediatric and neonatal cannulations. Intensive care specialists perform percutaneous ECLS cannulation in children at some centers. In centers that utilize nonsurgeon providers for cannulation, the ECLS team must develop a reliable strategy for timely surgical backup assistance. The Steering Committee should review cannulation competence on an ongoing basis as part of a robust quality assurance program. The program director and an experienced surgeon can regularly provide direct, hands-on assistance to evaluate clinical competence and provide experienced-based education for ECLS team members.[15]

b. **ECLS physicians** are ECMO-trained physicians who provide medical expertise for cannulated patients. In addition, the ECLS physicians have the required practical knowledge and technical skills for troubleshooting and circuit interventions

c. **ECLS specialists** are clinical care providers with specialized knowledge and training in managing ECLS equipment and patients. ECLS specialists typically perform direct bedside care of ECLS patients for the duration of extracorporeal support. ECLS specialist staffing models may vary according to the available personnel and specific clinical needs.[16,17] Clinical perfusionists, ICU nurses, respiratory therapists, and physicians may undergo thorough training to become ECLS specialists. Many centers utilize a multiprovider model of care, especially for neonatal and pediatric ECMO. The ECLS specialist is primarily responsible for ECLS equipment, and a nurse is primarily responsible for the patient. In such a model, it is advantageous for the care team members to undergo some degree of crosstraining to leverage the individual's unique strengths in a complementary manner. A single provider of care model has been adopted as an accepted standard as integrated ECLS equipment became available. In this model of care, the nurse ECLS specialist provides comprehensive nursing care for the patient and manages the ECLS circuit, with or without backup support from a perfusionist.

d. **ECLS coordinator** is typically an ECMO specialist. They supervise and train technical staff, maintain equipment, and collect patient data. In addition, research, Key Performance Indicators (KPIs), outcome measures, and ELSO Registry participation require data collection as a required responsibility of the position.

## 3. Training and education

Proper training and education are essential for the success of a program. Therefore, centers should develop a program-specific approach to education, maintenance, knowledge dissemination, skill acquisition, and competency verification.

The program director, ECLS coordinator, and Steering Committee should develop an ECLS education program following the ELSO "Guidelines for Training and Continuing Education of ECMO Specialists" and "Guidelines for ECMO Centers," and the ELSO Specialist Training Manual.[14] ELSO training guidelines recommend an ECLS training course that runs for up to one week and includes 24-36 hours of didactic teaching and 8–16 hours of 'hands-on' training.[18] ECMO centers may perform 'hands-on' ECLS education in various settings, such as a training room, wet lab, animal laboratory, or simulation facility (Chapter 54). Educators incorporating high-fidelity simulation can enhance learning by providing immediate feedback, allowing repetitive practice, increasing difficulty with attaining skills, addressing various learner strategies, and permitting clinical variation in learner responses.[17] ELSO also provides educational conferences hosted by established ECLS institutions and several professional organizations.

The ELSO guidelines recommend that these training sessions are available to all ECLS clinicians at least every six months, with a recommendation for annual institutional recertification.

### 4. Supply and equipment

ECLS equipment should be evaluated and selected by members of the Steering Committee or appropriately knowledgeable delegates. The equipment inventory acquired should be based on the target or expected number of ECLS patients per year and the median duration of ECLS run according to the type of support. Clinical ECLS volume varies significantly by geographic region, proximity to other ECLS centers, patient demographics, and hospital mission. A minimum of two ECLS devices are required to start a program. The second device is the backup system available in the event of catastrophic equipment failure. It is essential to liaise with local equipment distributors to establish protocols for replacing and exchanging devices and consumables.[18]

## Phase 3: Execution Phase

### 1. Implementation

The Steering Committee must set a realistic timeline for implementing and developing an ECLS clinical service during the planning process, with a launch date that avoids additional risks associated with a lack of readiness. Ideally, a program should begin with low-complexity ECLS patients to minimize complications, maximize the likelihood of survival, and provide essential opportunities for staff education. In addition, early success raises the morale of the care team. Finally, it incentivizes hospital leadership to continue its support for the program.

### 2. First case

Another critical early guiding principle is that a new ECLS center should not endeavor to provide the full scope of ECLS. Initially, patients with favorable ELSO Registry outcome data are optimal candidates. Early successful outcomes allow confidence to develop among the team members. As the program matures, the Steering Committee may introduce increasingly complex forms of ECLS, including ECPR, interhospital ECLS transport, and bridge to organ transplantation. The evolution of the ECLS program will require additional resources, medical and surgical expertise, and staffing.

### 3. Maintenance

The sustainability of an ECLS program is related to quality, efficiency, and patient outcomes. Therefore, ongoing training, education, and competency assessment are critical to maintaining an ECLS program.

ECLS centers should develop center-specific continuous education and training guidelines, including didactic, hands-on simulation training, water drills, and proctored bedside training. The ECMO director and ECMO Coordinator are responsible for developing an ongoing schedule to evaluate ECLS clinical competency for all ECMO clinicians. Assessments include written tests of clinical knowledge and simulation lab-based psychomotor assessments of clinical judgment and decision-making; for example, patient and circuit troubleshooting, crisis management, team communication, and day-to-day and emergency scenario ECLS tasks. Observing ECLS care providers during actual patient situations provides invaluable information about competency and mastery of the clinician's skills. The program's total of ECMO-patient days will impact the time frame for ECLS specialists to acquire the skills, competence, and confidence to safely and independently care for ECLS patients.

Appropriate data collection and analysis resources will support a new center's philosophy of transparency and data sharing within the ECLS community. In addition, maintaining ELSO membership and up-to-date reporting to the ELSO registry provides the clinical benchmarks for the next phase of program development and auditing.

**Phase 4: Auditing Phase**

*1. Benchmark and key performance indicators*

A realistic estimate of patient outcomes and comparing clinical results against benchmark data provides administrators with a reasonable indicator of resource needs. The semiannual ELSO Registry reports contain center-specific data. It provides a complete analysis of center data that guides monitoring the center KPIs and outcomes. The Registry aggregates data from similar reporting centers, allowing comparative benchmarking analysis and enabling continuous benchmarking of a center's results and comparing its data locally or internationally.[1]

*2. Tracking effort and cost*

Monitoring the actual program performance against the planned implementation timeline is a continuous process via establishing an internal database, regular data collection, and analysis. Sets of performance indicators should monitor the adherence to program structure, process, and outcome, identify deficiencies, deviations from protocol, and opportunities for improvement.

*3. 'Kick-off' meetings*

Official meetings should be held regularly, depending on the center's volume, to discuss available analytic data. The administrative leaders may use meeting minutes to review the program's progress and performance and outline recommendations for improvement and implementation of a plan.

**Phase 5: Development Phase**

This phase is essential for programmatic success by leveraging a continuous quality improvement paradigm. Programs should evaluate and update goals at the predetermined timeline established in the initial charter. There are always opportunities for improvement in each program. These may include but are not limited to privileging, credentials, advanced training, competency assessment, evaluation of center volume (as determined by the needs of the community), increased scope of ECLS coverage, patient selection, and integration of clinical research.

In the development phase, a team may consider expanding the scope of service to include additional ECLS services, such as respiratory, circulatory, ECPR, or ECLS transportation, as well as expanding the range of patient selection, which may contribute to center volume expansion. The new ECLS program's data collection for research and evaluation purposes should be prioritized. A detailed and complete database should be integral to the development of a program.

The ELSO Center of Excellence (Awards of Excellence) provides the Path to Excellence, which guides and supports new centers with tools to develop structures rooted in continuous process improvement. The aim is to offer early guidance, which will position programs to achieve the level of quality that will deserve obtaining the Gold level Award of Excellence and, ultimately, the Platinum level of Excellence (Chapter 55).[5] Adherence to the award's requirements will improve the quality

of programs, which cannot be achieved without continuous improvement and development.

It is essential to follow the five phases to launch a new ECLS program successfully. The Path to Excellence award may contribute to program progression for two years. Within two to three years, the PDCA cycle can be used for each task of improvement or expansion of the program to get the Gold Award of Excellence. Finally, the same cycle might be repeated to keep improving for an extra two years with the goal of achieving the Platinum Award of Excellence. (Figure 52-2).

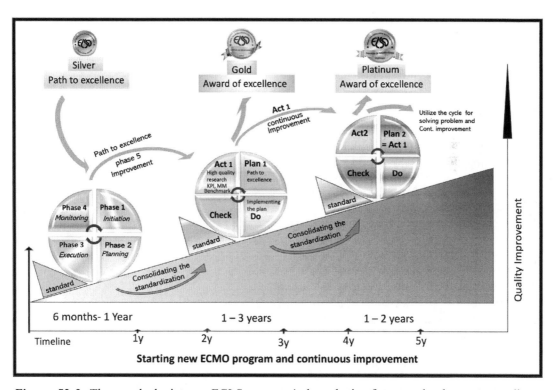

**Figure 52-2.** The graph depicts an ECLS program's launch timeframe and subsequent quality improvement. Using the five phases of development is essential in the first six to twelve months of building the program. Ongoing PDCA cycles and the path to excellence may then help the program's growth and progression for two to three years, with the goal of achieving the gold award of excellence. Finally, within one to two years, the program expands and reinforces itself through repeated PDCA cycles, with the aim of obtaining the Platinum award of excellence.

## New ECLS Centers in Special Situations

### *COVID-19 pandemic*

Previous guidelines recommended against starting new programs during a pandemic.[18] However, updated ELSO Coronavirus Disease 2019 (COVID-19) guidelines suggest that centers may accomplish ECLS support in select cases.[19] The general guidance in starting a new ECLS program during a pandemic is not to jeopardize the preparedness of primary healthcare requirements and infrastructure by diverting critical resources from other patients. Therefore, hospitals may develop a new ECLS program in regions with appropriate healthcare infrastructure and resource capabilities. Supervision by ECLS experts, affiliation with a local ECLS center, education and training assistance, and conservative patient selection are the main requirements for favorable outcomes.[20] The planning mentioned above could be expedited to start a new ECLS program during the pandemic. While ECLS training is crucial before beginning the service, relying on expert centers, experienced clinicians, or ELSO for guidance during a surge is practical. The newly formed ECLS team should manage the first few cases under expert supervision.

### Conclusion

The key to success in starting a new ECLS program is a multidisciplinary team led by a clinical champion who serves as a director, obtains institutional commitment, focuses on continuous education and training, and ensures ECLS program development by continuous improvement. In addition, ELSO plays an essential role in launching and maintaining ECLS programs by providing the required policies, guidelines, education, training, certification, and quality benchmarks to guide and monitor the program's progression.

# References

1. Extracorporeal Life Support Organization/ registered ELSO center worldwide https://www.elso.org/Membership/CenterDirectory.aspx. Accessed January 2022.

2. Combes A, Peek GJ, Hajage D, et al. ECMO for severe ARDS: systematic review and individual patient data meta-analysis. Intensive Care Med. 2020 Nov;46(11):2048-2057.

3. Pleşoianu AF, Pleşoianu CE, Bararu Bojan I, et al. Extracorporeal membrane oxygenation in the management of critically ill patients with coronavirus disease 2019: A narrative review. Exp Ther Med 22: 1296, 2021.

4. Guerguerian AM, Ogino MT, Dalton HJ, et al. Setup and Maintenance of Extracorporeal Life Support Programs: Pediatr Crit Care Med. 2013;14: S84-S93.

5. ELSO Award of Excellence in Extracorporeal Life Support. Extracorporeal Life Support Organization website. https://www.elso.org/AwardofExcellence.aspx. Accessed November 24, 2021.

6. Larson E, Gray C, eds. Project Management: The Managerial Process. 5th ed. New York, NY: McGraw-Hill/Irwin; 2011. Page 101 – 125.

7. https://www.smartsheet.com/blog/demystifying-5-phases-project-management Accessed January 2022.

8. Tague, Nancy R. (2005) [1995]. "Plan–Do–Study–Act cycle". The quality toolbox (2nd ed.). Milwaukee: ASQ Quality Press. pp. 390–392. https://books.google.com.sa/books?id=G3c6S0mzLQgC&sitesec=buy&hl=ar&source=gbs_atb. Accessed January 2022.

9. Tsangaris A, Alexy T, Kalra R, et. al. Overview of Veno-Arterial Extracorporeal Membrane Oxygenation (VA-ECMO) Support for the Management of Cardiogenic Shock. Front Cardiovasc Med 2021; 8: 705.

10. Moll V, Teo EY, Grenda DS, et al. Rapid Development and Implementation of an ECMO Program. ASAIO J. 2016;62(3):354-358.

11. McCallister D, Pilon L, Forrester J, et al. Clinical and Administrative Steps to the ECMO Program Development. In: S. Firstenberg M, ed. Advances in Extracorporeal Membrane Oxygenation - Volume 3. IntechOpen; 2019.

12. Gantt, H.L. (1910). "Work, Wages and Profit". Engineering Magazine. New York.; republished as Work, Wages and Profits. Easton, Pennsylvania: Hive Publishing Company. 1974. ISBN 0-87960-048-9.

13. Connor N, Smith JR. An Innovative ECMO Staffing Model to Reduce Harm. Journal of Perinatal & Neonatal Nursing. 2018;32(3):204-205.

14. ELSO Guideline for ECMO Centers. 1st ed. Extracorporeal Life Support Organization; 2014:17. https://www.elso.org/Portals/0/IGD/Archive/FileManager/faf3f6a3c7cusersshyerdocumentselso guidelinesecmocentersv1.8.pdf. Accessed January 2022.

15. Combes A, Brodie D, Bartlett R, et al. Position paper for the organization of extracorporeal membrane oxygenation programs for acute respiratory failure in adult patients. Am J Resp Crit Care Med. 2014; 190(5): 488-496.

16. Pavlushkov E, Berman M, Valchanov K. Cannulation techniques for extracorporeal life support. Ann Transl Med. 2017;5(4):70. doi:10.21037/atm.2016.11.47.

17. Ogino MT, Chuo J, Short BL. ECMO administrative and training issues, and sustaining quality. In: Annich GM, Lynch WR, MacLaren G, et al., eds. ECMO: Extracorporeal Cardiopulmonary Support in Critical Care. Ann Arbor, MI: Extracorporeal Support 2012: 479-497.

18. ELSO Guidelines for Training and Continuing of ECMO Specialists. Retrieved January 2022, from https://www.elso.org/Resources/Guidelines.aspx. Accessed January 2022.

19. Badulak J, Antonini V, Stead C, et al. ECMO for COVID-19: Updated 2021 guidelines from the Extracorporeal Life Support Organization (ELSO). ASAIO J 2021; 67(5):485-495.

20. Rabie AA, Azzam MH, Al-Fares AA, et al. Implementation of new ECMO centers during the COVID-19 pandemic: experience and results from the Middle East and India. Intensive Care Medicine. 2021;47(8):887-895.

# 53

# Centralization and Regionalization

*Rodrigo Diaz, Marta Velia Antonini, Justyna Swol, Ibrahim Fawzy Hassan, John Beca,*
*Christian A. Bermudez*

## Introduction

Regionalization, or the establishment of healthcare networks at a regional level, can be a huge step towards better care delivery, particularly in medical emergencies such as those requiring ECLS. However, regionalization also comes with challenges, including definitions, difficulties in sharing mental models, stakeholder alignment, and value in health care.

A major barrier to regional network development in some countries is the concern for a decrease in revenue. A value-based care model may be a better approach to regional network development, which emphasizes quality of care, patient experience, and appropriateness of care. In the future, high-quality care at reduced cost (value) will be defined by the ability of the whole system to deliver prompt, coordinated, and patient-centered care.[1]

Healthcare systems that can align resources to assist referring hospitals through regionalization will be better positioned to accomplish this because efficiency can be improved by sharing resources and capabilities across facilities.[2-6] Although difficult to attain when networks cross regional or national boundaries, or those of multiple healthcare systems, shared mental models among stakeholders are essential to pursue this goal.[7]

## Case Volume and Outcome

Over the past 2 decades, there has been considerable growth in both the number of ECLS runs and the number of centers reporting to the ELSO Registry (Figures 53-1 and 53-2).[8] This expansion of case volume is particularly relevant in the adult patient population, although the median number of cases per center is <18 patients/year.

Accumulating evidence demonstrates improved clinical outcomes when patients are managed in higher volume centers by specialized care teams. This has been demonstrated for various surgical procedures and medical conditions, including sepsis, stroke, ARDS, STEMI, and cardiac arrest.[9-25] Lower mortality is reported by high-volume centers for both adult and pediatric patients requiring ECLS,[26-28] although the degree varies among specific patient populations.[26] Previous experience with various configurations of extracorporeal support could contribute to outcome improvement. This favorable impact has been observed in both postcardiotomy VA ECMO[29] and for VV ECMO patients with COVID-19.[30,31]

Nevertheless, data also exist showing that lower ECLS center volume do not necessarily decrease the rate of favorable outcomes.[32,33] It is likely that additional factors influence outcome, including training, protocols, and team leadership, among others. Case volume might be a valid starting point along the pathway to excellence, but a high-quality program is not the same as a high-volume program.

The difference between high-performing teams and poor performers is not necessarily determined by case volume, but more so how they practice. Barbaro et al. state a multidisciplinary team is required to provide care to ECLS patients and the whole team needs to grow together to improve performance.[26] Shutting down low volume programs is not the

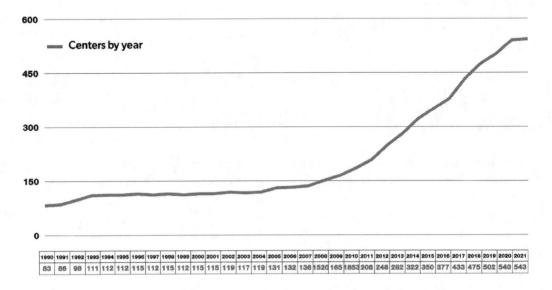

**Figure 53-1.** Centers reporting to ELSO (ELSO ECLS Registry Report International Summary, April 2022).

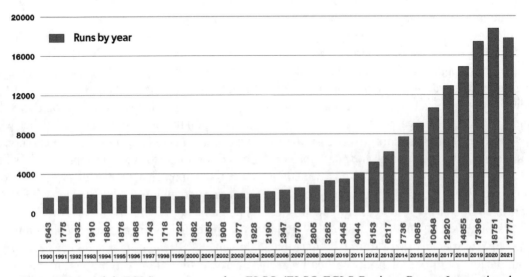

**Figure 53-2.** Adult ECLS runs reported to ELSO (ELSO ECLS Registry Report International Summary, April 2022).

answer.[34-36] Minimum volume requirements may induce a perverse incentive, exposing patients to unnecessary ECLS in order to maintain annual center volume. Similarly, a well-designed ECLS simulation program can mitigate the lack of exposure to ECLS among staff at low-volume centers and help maintain high standards of care for these patients (Figure 53-3)

## Regionalization

Collaboration is essential in regionalization of medical care. Regionalization is particularly appropriate for conditions which are time-sensitive and require specialized resources characterized by a volume-outcome relationship, with the potential benefit of improving the quality of care at a population level. Regionalization is differentiated from 'rationing' and 'centralization'. Rationing is the redistribution of scarce resources to better meet the needs of a given population (ie, relocation of ECMO hardware during a pandemic).

Centralization is the reorganization of highly specialized services into a smaller number of units with more advanced material resources and experienced teams, while regionalization focuses on delivery of specialized care capable of treating more patients more effectively and efficiently.[38,39] Regionalization of care is dynamic and may involve centralization or decentralization.[40]

Importantly, any effort toward regionalization will be ineffective unless the underlying governance and accountability structures are addressed transparently.[37-39] Outcomes will be determined by the right care, at the right place, at the right time.[41] In practice, professionals collaborate in a variety of different dynamic networks, often overcoming limitations imposed by location, with telemedicine and other tools, including messaging applications.[30] Telemedicine can help support parts of a network[42] and expands operational efficiency, including by potentially crossing geographic boundaries.[2]

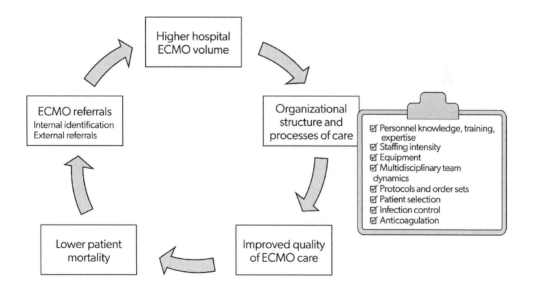

**Figure 53-3.** Conceptual model linking annual age group–specific hospital ECLS volume and outcome; modified from Barbaro et al.[26]

## Practical Experience with Regionalization

The Michigan regional collaborative improvement program (funded by a for-profit insurance company) enhanced healthcare quality related to different clinical conditions and reduced costs in several clinical areas. For vascular surgery, a 2.6% decrease in surgical complications was observed among participating hospitals, with 2,500 fewer patients per year experiencing surgical complications. Estimated savings from this collaborative project approached $20 million annually.[43] In a conference abstract of an observational study including 520 consecutive patients with cardiogenic shock (CS) treated in a regionalized network across 34 spoke hospitals in Maryland which implemented dedicated protocols and expedited transfer algorithms, similar 30-day mortality and associated short-term outcomes were reported for patients initially presenting to either hub or spoke centers.[44]

Welke et al. simulated a model of regionalization for congenital heart surgery in the U.S. to higher volume centers to assess the impact of this type of system. If all congenital heart surgery in the U.S. was done in hospitals that performed more than 300 cases per year, 116 lives could be saved each year.[45] Sweden halved the number of congenital cardiac centers in the 1990s and there was an associated reduction in surgical mortality from 9.5% to 1.9%.[46] Tung and Chang, analyzing acute ischemic stroke admissions through Taiwan's National Health Insurance Research Database, observed that regionalization might improve stroke care, including timely access to thrombolytic therapy, potentially enhancing outcomes.[47] Ely et al. found decreased overall mortality for patients undergoing major pulmonary resection for cancer within their integrated health care system before and after thoracic surgery regionalization.[9] Among patients with STEMI in California from 2006 to 2015 (n=139 494), Shen et al. observed that

regionalization was associated with increased access to a PCI-capable hospital, greater use of PCI, lower 7-day mortality, and lower 30-day readmission rates.[48] These examples provide evidence of the potential benefits of regionalization if thoughtfully constructed.

## Barriers

The main barrier to regionalization may be the need for a cultural shift. Regionalization within the United States, for example, has been historically limited due to the competitive, fee-for-service market-based system. Regionalization demands standardization through cooperation rather than competition and might favorably impact resource utilization and global expenditure. This could promote efforts toward regionalization, together with growing evidence supporting its implementation, as certain conditions are met.[38] Moreover, when debating about regionalization models, the lack of a standardized nomenclature could be an additional limitation.[49]

## Challenges in Regionalization

The following list is comprised of challenges common in regionalization:

1. Sharing mental models (requires collaboration in financial, medical, and political domains);
2. Formal versus informal coordination (this mandates a change in culture, with collaboration as the main tool rather than competition);
3. ECLS is not 'one size fits all' (different patients, pathophysiology, and types of support);
4. Political oversight (local or national political involvement is critical);
5. Financial (eg, fee per service);
6. Hospital status;

7. Data systems (especially important in allocating patients, benchmarking, and accountability); and

8. Nomenclature.

## Integrated Model

The integrated web format has emerged as the ideal model, as both the funnel and hub-and-spoke model demonstrate primarily unidirectional patient flow and a resource hierarchy that is more related to centralization (Figure 53-4). Crafting an integrated web system from healthcare facilities that formed through market forces and largely operate by competitive economic motivation has proven to be an ongoing challenge.[38] Yet, improving

patient outcomes benefits both providers and insurance companies.[50] Martinez and Carr argue for a network of interconnected institutions and providers, sharing quality and performance targets, to replace a system mainly relying on transfer and referral of patients to specialized centers.[1,51] In their vision, this strategy might improve outcomes of emergency care across time and conditions.[1]

In their position paper for the organization of ECLS programs for cardiac failure in adults,[52] Abrams et al. recommend that local and referral centers without the ability to initiate extracorporeal support build networks around regional referral or comprehensive care centers capable of deploying mobile teams to initiate ECLS and transfer patients. The

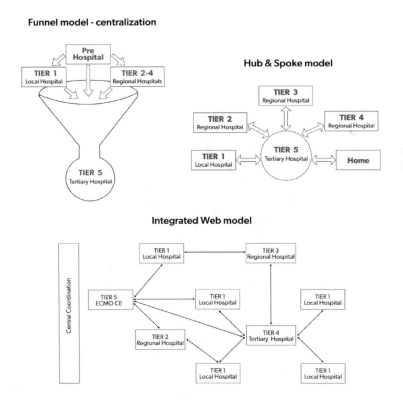

**Figure 53-4.** Integration and organization within regionalized networks of care according to 3 models, with arrows indicating patient flow. The integrated web model has emerged as the desired conception of a regionalized and integrated system of care (modified from Walton et al.[38]).

authors also recommend a formal partnership between local referral centers and regional comprehensive care centers, agreeing on indications, contraindications, criteria for initiation, and cannulation technique. Support should include planning, training, and consultation from experienced personnel, as required, for institutions starting new ECLS programs. Previously, Combes et al. in their position paper for the organization of ECLS programs for respiratory failure in adults,[36] advocated for the creation of networks of hospitals at a local, regional, or inter-regional level around each referral ECLS center. They suggested to introduce among these networks standardized, shared protocols for patient management before ECLS initiation, and for ECLS implementation, and to promote meetings to discuss network activities. In both consensus

papers, the establishment and coordination of mobile experienced ECLS teams available for retrieval 24/7 was deemed advisable for high-volume referring centers. The tiered network designed by Bonadonna et al. (Duke ECLS Transport Program) is shown in Figure 53-5.[53]

**Central Coordination**

In their initial interim guidelines for COVID-19, ELSO recommended employing central coordination of ECLS services to serve the increasing demand for ECLS and ensure equitable care across regions. The updated ELSO guidelines for implementing ECLS during the pandemic[4] stressed that centers should consider pooling available experienced human and material resources to optimize ECLS capacity within regional networks. Over the

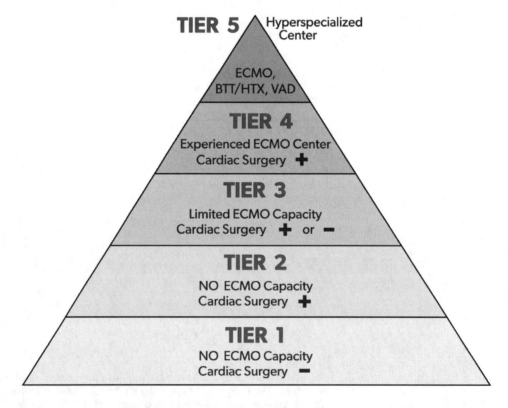

**Figure 53-5.** Levels of ECLS competences per center.

past 2 years of the COVID-19 pandemic, many different experiences of regionalization and central coordination have been implemented to increase ECLS availability safely and effectively. Successful expansion of ECLS availability according to ELSO indications has been reported from the U.S.[54-57] and across the globe.[3,30,58,59] Lebreton and colleagues reported on organization in Greater Paris, where central regulation of ECLS indications and pooling of resources were implemented, with six mobile ECLS teams available for the region. Galvagno et al. described a critical care coordination center in the state of Maryland staffed 24/7 by a critical care physician and emergency medical service clinicians.[56] During a 6-month period, 1,006 critical care consultations were made and directed 578 patient transfers to 58 hospitals within the region. ECLS referrals were requested for 58 patients, 50 of whom were cannulated. Four-hundred twenty-eight patients (42.5%) were not transferred and were managed with consultation only. Rabie et al. reported favorable outcomes for selected ECLS patients managed in newly established centers, thanks to the supervision and training by experienced regional experts.[3] These experiences provide examples of successful integrated regionalization with central coordination.

According to MacLaren et al. "centers should collaborate to identify and disseminate best practices, reduce variation, and improve outcomes".[35] Leung et al. state "transforming the current state of regionalization into a coordinated, accountable system requires a critical assessment of administrative and clinical challenges and barriers.".[2] The ECLS Collaborative Project involved 4 ECLS programs within a single healthcare system serving patients in 47 counties and 52 hospitals in Texas. Standardized guidelines, order sets, data collection, and performance feedback were implemented. The coordination and standardization across the 4 programs led to

improved survival to discharge and transfer in the post-collaborative compared to the pre-collaborative period (107/185, 57.8% vs. 113/243, 46.5%, p=.03), predominantly due to improved outcomes among patients receiving VA ECMO (hazard ratio, 0.61; 95% CI, 0.41-0.91). The proportion of patients successfully weaned from ECLS increased from 58.9% (109/185) to 70% (170/243) (p=0.02). Complication rates decreased by 40% (incidence rate ratio, 0.60; 95% CI, 0.49-0.72). Payment-per-case and contribution-margin-per-case both decreased significantly.[60]

In 2013, The Duke University Medical Center began formalizing their ECLS transport program, promoting relationships between centers through communication; standardized ECLS referral and consultation processes; education; and training, all tailored based on ECLS capability or lack thereof, in a regional network of referring centers. Urgency and geographical location of ECLS cannulation were determined based on patient status, transfer logistics, and local capabilities (no extracorporeal support; post cardiotomy ECLS failure to wean from bypass and no ECLS; limited ECLS capabilities; and established ECLS centers but with no VAD or transplant capability).[53]

Aubin et al. described the implementation of a network for a rapid-response mobile service to apply VA ECMO within a defined regional setting in Germany. In this selected, high-risk cohort of patients with refractory circulatory failure, often with ongoing cardiac arrest, they reported an overall survival of 33% at long term followup, 97% of whom had good neurological outcomes. This favorable outcome supports the feasibility and the effectiveness of such a model in expanding the provision of ECLS support, even in an emergency setting.[61]

The Academic Leaders in Critical Care Medicine Task Force of the Society of Critical Care Medicine stated that systems thinking (a holistic view of the organization in relation to its environment), business planning and control, and essential infrastructure development are critical for assisting critical care organization in regionalization efforts. The authors identified four conditions required for successful regionalization of critical care medicine services: heterogeneity in quality, scarce resources, identifiable centers of excellence (according to ELSO), and identifiable patients. They detailed this for trauma, stroke and ECLS (Figure 53-6).[2]

Regionalization models continue to evolve. There is evidence that support a regionalized model for the provision of ECLS, which can improve access and outcomes, both worthy goals.

## Conclusions

Regionalization and centralization are important concepts to consider when planning effective ECLS services in specific jurisdictions. Concentrating highly complex medical interventions such as ECLS in dedicated centers may lead to better outcomes.[26,36,52] Several countries now have such systems in place with government oversight to ensure equitable access to ECLS services for patients.[62]

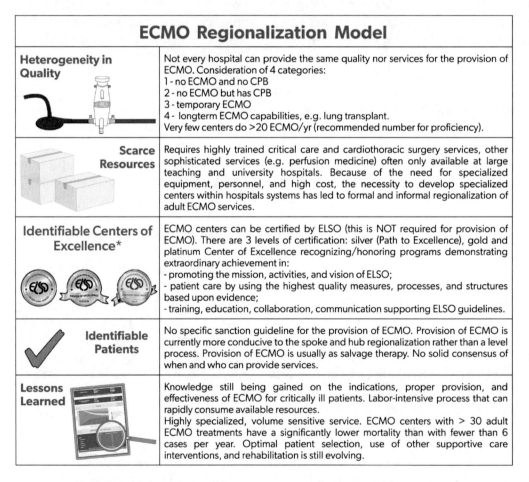

| ECMO Regionalization Model | |
| --- | --- |
| **Heterogeneity in Quality** | Not every hospital can provide the same quality nor services for the provision of ECMO. Consideration of 4 categories:<br>1 - no ECMO and no CPB<br>2 - no ECMO but has CPB<br>3 - temporary ECMO<br>4 - longterm ECMO capabilities, e.g. lung transplant.<br>Very few centers do >20 ECMO/yr (recommended number for proficiency). |
| **Scarce Resources** | Requires highly trained critical care and cardiothoracic surgery services, other sophisticated services (e.g. perfusion medicine) often only available at large teaching and university hospitals. Because of the need for specialized equipment, personnel, and high cost, the necessity to develop specialized centers within hospitals systems has led to formal and informal regionalization of adult ECMO services. |
| **Identifiable Centers of Excellence\*** | ECMO centers can be certified by ELSO (this is NOT required for provision of ECMO). There are 3 levels of certification: silver (Path to Excellence), gold and platinum Center of Excellence recognizing/honoring programs demonstrating extraordinary achievement in:<br>- promoting the mission, activities, and vision of ELSO;<br>- patient care by using the highest quality measures, processes, and structures based upon evidence;<br>- training, education, collaboration, communication supporting ELSO guidelines. |
| **Identifiable Patients** | No specific sanction guideline for the provision of ECMO. Provision of ECMO is currently more conducive to the spoke and hub regionalization rather than a level process. Provision of ECMO is usually as salvage therapy. No solid consensus of when and who can provide services. |
| **Lessons Learned** | Knowledge still being gained on the indications, proper provision, and effectiveness of ECMO for critically ill patients. Labor-intensive process that can rapidly consume available resources.<br>Highly specialized, volume sensitive service. ECMO centers with > 30 adult ECMO treatments have a significantly lower mortality than with fewer than 6 cases per year. Optimal patient selection, use of other supportive care interventions, and rehabilitation is still evolving. |

**Figure 53-6.** Regionalization model for ECLS services: 4 conditions required for success and lessons learned (modified from Leung et al.,[2] *according to ELSO Award for Excellence in Extracorporeal Life Support).

# References

1. Martinez R, Carr B. Creating integrated networks of emergency care: from vision to value. Health Aff (Millwood). 2013;32(12):2082-90.
2. Leung S, Pastores SM, Oropello JM, et al. Regionalization of Critical Care in the United States: Current State and Proposed Framework From the Academic Leaders in Critical Care Medicine Task Force of the Society of Critical Care Medicine. Crit Care Med. 2022;50(1):37-49.
3. Rabie AA, Azzam MH, Al-Fares AA, et al. Implementation of new ECMO centers during the COVID-19 pandemic: experience and results from the Middle East and India. Intensive Care Med. 2021;47(8):887-95.
4. Badulak J, Antonini MV, Stead CM, et al. Extracorporeal Membrane Oxygenation for COVID-19: Updated 2021 Guidelines from the Extracorporeal Life Support Organization. Asaio j. 2021;67(5):485-95.
5. Shekar K, Badulak J, Peek G, et al. Extracorporeal Life Support Organization Coronavirus Disease 2019 Interim Guidelines: A Consensus Document from an International Group of Interdisciplinary Extracorporeal Membrane Oxygenation Providers. Asaio j. 2020;66(7):707-21.
6. Porter ME. What Is Value in Health Care? New England Journal of Medicine. 2010;363(26):2477-81.
7. Wu AW. Reaching common ground: The role of shared mental models in patient safety. Journal of Patient Safety and Risk Management. 2018;23(5):183-4.
8. ECLS Registry Report, International Summary. April 2022 (Reporting data though 2021). [Available from: https://www.elso.org/Registry/InternationalSummaryandReports/InternationalSummary.aspx. Last accessed June 21, 2022.
9. Ely S, Alabaster A, Ashiku SK, et al. Regionalization of thoracic surgery improves short-term cancer esophagectomy outcomes. J Thorac Dis. 2019;11(5):1867-78.
10. Luft S. Regionalization of medical care. American Journal of Public Health. 1985;75(2).
11. Magruder JT, Shah AS, Crawford TC, et al. Simulated Regionalization of Heart and Lung Transplantation in the United States. American Journal of Transplantation. 2017;17(2):485-95.
12. Backer CL, Karamlou T, Welke KF. More Evidence for Regionalization*. Journal of the American College of Cardiology. 2019;74(23):2919-20.
13. Backer CL, Pasquali SK, Dearani JA. Improving National Outcomes in Congenital Heart Surgery: The Time Has Come for Regionalization of Care. Circulation. 2020;141(12):943-5.
14. Goldstone AB, Chiu P, Baiocchi M, et al. Interfacility Transfer of Medicare Beneficiaries With Acute Type A Aortic Dissection and Regionalization of Care in the United States. Circulation. 2019;140(15):1239-50.
15. Subramanian MP, Yang Z, Chang S-H, et al. Regionalization for thoracic surgery: Economic implications of regionalization in the United States. The Journal of Thoracic and Cardiovascular Surgery. 2021;161(5):1705-9.
16. Ike JD, Kempker JA, Kramer MR, et al. The Association Between Acute Respiratory Distress Syndrome Hospital Case Volume and Mortality in a U.S. Cohort, 2002-2011. Crit Care Med. 2018;46(5):764-73.
17. Elmer J, Rittenberger JC, Coppler PJ, et al. Long-term survival benefit from treatment at a specialty center after cardiac arrest. Resuscitation. 2016;108:48-53.
18. Shahian DM, Normand SL. The volume-outcome relationship: from Luft to Leapfrog. Ann Thorac Surg. 2003;75(3):1048-58.
19. Nathens AB, Jurkovich GJ, Maier RV, et al. Relationship between trauma center volume and outcomes. Jama. 2001;285(9):1164-71.
20. Pacella SJ, Butz DA, Comstock MC, et al. Hospital volume outcome and discharge disposition of burn patients. Plast Reconstr Surg. 2006;117(4):1296-305; discussion 306-7.
21. Gorelick PB. Primary and comprehensive stroke centers: history, value and certification criteria. J Stroke. 2013;15(2):78-89.
22. Fanaroff AC, Zakroysky P, Dai D, et al. Outcomes of PCI in Relation to Procedural Characteristics and Operator Volumes in the United States. J Am Coll Cardiol. 2017;69(24):2913-24.
23. Phibbs CS, Baker LC, Caughey AB, et al. Level and volume of neonatal intensive care and mortality in very-low-birth-weight infants. N Engl J Med. 2007;356(21):2165-75.
24. Phibbs CS, Bronstein JM, Buxton E, et al. The effects of patient volume and level of care at the hospital of birth on neonatal mortality. Jama. 1996;276(13):1054-9.
25. Ofoma UR, Dahdah J, Kethireddy S, et al. Case Volume-Outcomes Associations Among Patients With Severe Sepsis Who Underwent Interhospital Transfer. Crit Care Med. 2017;45(4):615-22.
26. Barbaro RP, Odetola FO, Kidwell KM, et al. Association of hospital-level volume of extracorporeal membrane oxygenation cases and mortality. Analysis of the extracorporeal life support organization registry. Am J Respir Crit Care Med. 2015;191(8):894-901.
27. Freeman CL, Bennett TD, Casper TC, et al. Pediatric and neonatal extracorporeal membrane oxygenation: does center volume impact mortality?*. Crit Care Med. 2014;42(3):512-9.

28. Karamlou T, Vafaeezadeh M, Parrish AM, et al. Increased extracorporeal membrane oxygenation center case volume is associated with improved extracorporeal membrane oxygenation survival among pediatric patients. The Journal of Thoracic and Cardiovascular Surgery. 2013;145(2):470-5.

29. Biancari F, Dalén M, Fiore A, et al. Multicenter study on postcardiotomy venoarterial extracorporeal membrane oxygenation. The Journal of Thoracic and Cardiovascular Surgery. 2020;159(5):1844-54.e6.

30. Lebreton G, Schmidt M, Ponnaiah M, et al. Extracorporeal membrane oxygenation network organisation and clinical outcomes during the COVID-19 pandemic in Greater Paris, France: a multicentre cohort study. Lancet Respir Med. 2021;9(8):851-62.

31. Riera J, Alcántara S, Bonilla C, et al. Risk factors for mortality in patients with COVID-19 needing extracorporeal respiratory support. Eur Respir J. 2022;59(2).

32. Ingvarsdottir IL, Vidarsdottir H, Valsson F, et al. Venovenous extracorporeal membrane oxygenation treatment in a low-volume and geographically isolated cardiothoracic centre. Acta Anaesthesiologica Scandinavica. 2019;63(7):879-84.

33. McCarthy FH, McDermott KM, Spragan D, et al. Unconventional Volume-Outcome Associations in Adult Extracorporeal Membrane Oxygenation in the United States. Ann Thorac Surg. 2016;102(2):489-95.

34. Fan E, Brodie D. Higher Volumes, Better Outcomes: The End or Just the Beginning of the Story for Extracorporeal Membrane Oxygenation? American Journal of Respiratory and Critical Care Medicine. 2015;191(8):864-6.

35. Maclaren G, Pasquali SK, Dalton HJ. Volume-outcome relationships in extracorporeal membrane oxygenation: is bigger really better?*. Crit Care Med. 2014;42(3):726-7.

36. Combes A, Brodie D, Bartlett R, et al. Position paper for the organization of extracorporeal membrane oxygenation programs for acute respiratory failure in adult patients. Am J Respir Crit Care Med. 2014;190(5):488-96.

37. Schuurmans JJ, van Pijkeren N, Bal R, et.al. Regionalization in elderly care: what makes up a healthcare region? J Health Organ Manag. 2020;ahead-of-print(ahead-of-print):229-43.

38. Walton NT, Mohr NM. Concept review of regionalized systems of acute care: Is regionalization the next frontier in sepsis care? J Am Coll Emerg Physicians Open. 2022;3(1):e12631.

39. Fallon JM, Axelrod DA. LVAD Volume-Outcome Relationship: Surgeon, Center, or Both? Journal of Cardiac Failure. 2016;22(3):238-9.

40. Bywood PT, Erny-Albrecht KM, editors. Regionalisation of health services: Benefits and impact2016.

41. Hogan AN, Rosenberger R, Fowler RL. Emergency care regionalization. Emergency Medical Services2021. p. 32-42.

42. Bashshur RL, Bashshur MJ, Krupinski EA. Telemedicine, Precision Medicine, and Regionalization. Telemedicine and e-Health. 2021.

43. Share DA, Campbell DA, Birkmeyer N, et al. How a regional collaborative of hospitals and physicians in Michigan cut costs and improved the quality of care. Health Aff (Millwood). 2011;30(4):636-45.

44. Tehrani BN, Sherwood MW, Rosner C, et al. Abstract 12839: A Standardized and Regionalized System of Care Network for Cardiogenic Shock: Insights From the Inova-Shock Registry. Circulation. 2021;144(Suppl_1):A12839-A.

45. Welke KF, Pasquali SK, Lin P, et al. Regionalization of Congenital Heart Surgery in the United States. Semin Thorac Cardiovasc Surg. 2020;32(1):128-37.

46. Lundström NR, Berggren H, Björkhem G, et al. Centralization of pediatric heart surgery in Sweden. Pediatr Cardiol. 2000;21(4):353-7.

47. Tung YC, Chang GM. The Relationships Among Regionalization, Processes, and Outcomes for Stroke Care: A Nationwide Population-based Study. Medicine (Baltimore). 2016;95(15):e3327.

48. Shen YC, Krumholz H, Hsia RY. Association of Cardiac Care Regionalization With Access, Treatment, and Mortality Among Patients With ST-Segment Elevation Myocardial Infarction. Circ Cardiovasc Qual Outcomes. 2021;14(3):e007195.

49. Ghandour HZ, Vervoort D, Welke KF, et al. Regionalization of congenital cardiac surgical care: what it will take. Curr Opin Cardiol. 2022;37(1):137-43.

50. Darling GE. Regionalization in thoracic surgery: The importance of the team. J Thorac Cardiovasc Surg. 2020.

51. Carr BG, Matthew Edwards J, Martinez R. Regionalized care for time-critical conditions: lessons learned from existing networks. Acad Emerg Med. 2010;17(12):1354-8.

52. Abrams D, Garan AR, Abdelbary A, et al. Position paper for the organization of ECMO programs for cardiac failure in adults. Intensive Care Med. 2018;44(6):717-29.

53. Bonadonna D, Barac YD, Ranney DN, et al. Interhospital ECMO Transport: Regional Focus. Semin Thorac Cardiovasc Surg. 2019;31(3):327-34.

54. Gerall C, Cheung EW, Klein-Cloud R, et al. Allocation of resources and development of guidelines for extracorporeal membrane oxygenation (ECMO): Experience from a pediatric center in the epicenter

of the COVID-19 pandemic. J Pediatr Surg. 2020;55(12):2548-54.

55. Bergman ZR, Wothe JK, Alwan FS, et al. The Use of Venovenous Extracorporeal Membrane Oxygenation in COVID-19 Infection: One Region's Comprehensive Experience. Asaio j. 2021;67(5):503-10.

56. Galvagno SM, Jr., Naumann A, Delbridge TR, et al. The Role of a Statewide Critical Care Coordination Center in the Coronavirus Disease 2019 Pandemic- and Beyond. Crit Care Explor. 2021;3(11):e0568.

57. Shih E, DiMaio JM, Squiers JJ, et al. Venovenous extracorporeal membrane oxygenation for patients with refractory coronavirus disease 2019 (COVID-19): Multicenter experience of referral hospitals in a large health care system. J Thorac Cardiovasc Surg. 2022;163(3):1071-9.e3.

58. Diaz RA, Graf J, Zambrano JM, et al. Extracorporeal Membrane Oxygenation for COVID-19-associated Severe Acute Respiratory Distress Syndrome in Chile: A Nationwide Incidence and Cohort Study. Am J Respir Crit Care Med. 2021;204(1):34-43.

59. Japan EfC. Japan ECMOnet for COVID-19: telephone consultations for cases with severe respiratory failure caused by COVID-19. Journal of Intensive Care. 2020;8(1):24.

60. Schwartz G, Huff EA, van Zyl JS, et al. A system-wide extracorporeal membrane oxygenation quality collaborative improves patient outcomes. J Thorac Cardiovasc Surg. 2022; 163:>1366-1374.e9.

61. Aubin H, Petrov G, Dalyanoglu H, et al. A Suprainstitutional Network for Remote Extracorporeal Life Support: A Retrospective Cohort Study. JACC Heart Fail. 2016;4(9):698-708.

62. MacLaren G, Fisher D, Brodie D. Preparing for the most critically ill patients with COVID-19: The potential role of extracorporeal membrane oxygenation. JAMA 2020; 323:1245-1246.

# 54

## Education and Training

*Elizabeth A. Moore, Kollengode Ramanathan, Simon W.C. Sin, Marta Velia Antonini,*
*Bishoy Zakhary, Dana Mullin, Timothy J. Jones, Mark T. Ogino*

## Introduction

The rapid growth of ECLS has pushed practitioners and administrators to reimagine this technology's role within their healthcare systems. The most recent two global pandemics (Influenza A[H1N1] and COVID-19) accelerated the creation of new centers worldwide. While the total global impact is challenging to quantify, in 2009 and the beginning of the influenza A(H1N1) pandemic, the ELSO Registry included 165 member centers internationally. As of the 2021 report, that number has grown to 543 registered member centers. Safe, economical, and effective use of ECLS requires specific institutional resources and effective strategies to maintain optimal quality in care delivery. The foundation of achieving quality clinical care is the presence of an established and institutionally supported ECLS education and training program.

To assist centers by outlining institutional requirements for effective use of ECLS, ELSO developed 'ELSO Guidelines for ECMO Centers' that details the ideal structure and organization of ECMO resources.[1] The 'ELSO Guidelines for Training and Continuing Education of ECMO Specialists' is a guide to design training and educational programs for ECMO specialists.[2] ELSO recognizes that differences in regional and institutional regulations impact each ECMO center, and these variations may result in deviation from these guidelines. Nevertheless, these guidelines establish standards for assessing current and future ECMO centers.

In recent years, further critical work has been completed in the realm of ECMO education. In 2019, a position paper by Zakhary et al. presented a twofold approach to the review of ECMO education. This review described the state of education worldwide, noting limitations and challenges. In addition, it also aimed to create an educational road map that would illustrate a model for a global, standardized, and multidisciplinary approach to ECMO training.[3] Some of the preliminary work of this collaborative will be highlighted in this chapter.

## Educational Process

ECLS education is challenging because of the different skill sets that a member of the patient care team must achieve before being considered knowledgeable and competent to deliver ECLS care. Furthermore, the composition of an institution's ECLS patient care team continues to evolve as different models of care are developed, incorporating advances in technology. The ECLS team is multidisciplinary and includes clinicians with responsibilities to the patient and/or the ECLS circuit. The responsibilities can be divided or provided by a single individual with the appropriate training.

For this chapter, an ECLS physician is defined as a critical care physician or surgeon who has had specific ECLS training outlined by their institutional credentialing guidelines. An ECLS specialist is defined as a technical specialist with a different professional background, trained and experienced in managing the ECLS system and patient's clinical needs on extracorporeal support under the direction and supervision of an ECLS licensed independent practitioner.[1] We have used the term 'ECLS practitioner' to identify all medical professionals who participate in direct ECLS patient care.

With the diversity in ECLS program structures and staffing compositions, each center should develop a training program based on the patient populations served, equipment, and assigned responsibilities of team members. Since the educational backgrounds of ECLS team members differ, each center must tailor its training program to its staff providing direct patient care to the ECLS patient and ECLS system. For example, respiratory care therapists may require more time to learn about transfusion procedures, intravenous pumps, and medications. In contrast, nurses may need more gas physics and circuit component physiology education. Perfusionists may need to know more about the effects of long-term extracorporeal life support and patient care assessment. The interprofessional composition of an ECLS team utilizes the strengths of each discipline to address the multisystem challenges in the care of these complex patients.

ECLS centers must create a training program curriculum based upon guidelines, policies, procedures, and evidence-based practice paradigms. Since educational theories support using an active learning environment, most ECLS centers supplement their traditional didactic courses with practical training to optimize skill acquisitions and maintenance, and the technical and behavioral skills (team interaction, communication, leadership skills) essential to excellent care.[4] Equally important to creating an effective ECLS educational activity is the understanding that the typical learner's attention span wanes after 15 to 20 minutes. After the 20-minute threshold, lectures become less effective.[5] Effective learning can be further enhanced by applying new information to a learner's professional background and previous clinical experience.[6]

The framework for clinical education and assessment was eloquently described by Miller. The essay figuratively describes the ascent to attaining knowledge using a four-tiered triangle as the assessment model; hence the learning process is known as "Miller's Triangle."[7] ELSO recommends that each center develop training programs that accomplish the first three steps of Miller's Triangle framework, to allow the successful implementation of the "does" phase for each learner that should ideally occur in a mentored environment. Adaption of Miller's Triangle to ECLS clinical practice is illustrated in Figure 54-1.

**Establishing ECLS Competency**

The ECLS medical director and coordinator/ manager are responsible for assuring the ongoing competency of the ECLS Team. The Joint Commission International defines competency assessment as the process by which the organization validates, via a defined process, that an individual can perform the task consistent with the education and training provided.[8] Training and education provide the foundation for competency; however, competency assesses three attributes: knowledge, technical skills, and ability. These essential elements are required to provide safe patient care. The roles of the ECLS coordinator/ manager and medical director in competency assessment are to evaluate individual ECLS team member qualifications and job responsibilities, determine competencies required for each role, identify staff development needs, implement a system competency verification, and develop an individual remediation plan for employees who do not meet the defined standards.

Bedside nursing staff (not responsible for ECLS equipment) require specialized training in the care of these patients. Therefore, ECLS coordinator/manager and unit-based nursing educators should develop and implement a competency class for the care of patients on ECLS. The primary objectives should include ECLS physiology, equipment safety, patient safety, cannula care, resource management, and emergency patient management.

Representatives from other patient care services involved with the ECLS program should participate in basic ECLS training.

Multidisciplinary exposure to ECLS improves communication among hospital services, allowing other caregivers to understand and anticipate the needs of the ECLS patient. Good team communication is an essential skill to maintain, and the ECLS training process should include team-building activities across all disciplines. Optimal care of ECLS patients requires specialized knowledge from multiple disciplines to be integrated. Integration is best accomplished through frequent, respectful interaction and competent communication. These skills can be taught and practiced in the training environment. It is recommended that Crisis Resource Management (CRM) proficiencies are embedded in the training program to help understand and develop human factors and behavioral skills required

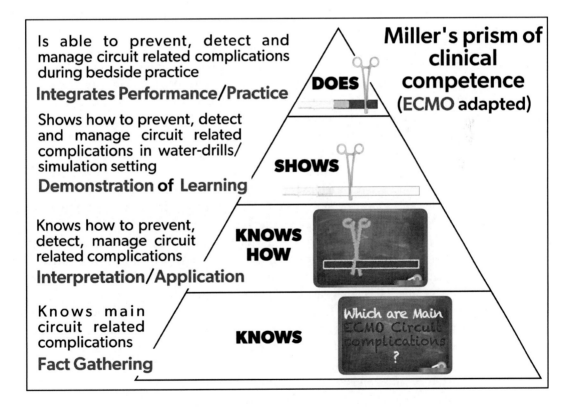

**Figure 54-1:** Miller's Triangle - adapted to ECLS clinical practice.

for effective team working and communication across multiple disciplines.[9]

The training guidelines for experienced centers are very similar; didactic instruction and simulation lab exposure content remain a vital component of ECLS training in experienced centers and bedside orientation with an ECLS preceptor. In addition, ongoing training for the team members provides professional development and, through simulation, the experienced team can improve team communication and focus on human factors.

## Development of Core ECLS Curriculum

The primary goal is to utilize an education program that provides standardized, effective multidisciplinary content where all providers are exposed to a single curriculum for initial ECLS training. This approach alleviates strict dependence on an individual discipline or practitioner to troubleshoot complex ECLS complications.

With the increased global uptake of ECLS over the past decade, there has also been a concurrent upsurge in ECLS educational activity. However, while ongoing education and training are desirable to ensure familiarity and comfort for caring in the ECLS patient and providing high quality patient care, no universal consensus on the structure and delivery of these programs was available.

ELSO guidelines recommend that a new program offer a didactic (lecture) course, followed by water drills using closed-loop priming circuits and/or animal sessions. Although high fidelity simulation is not listed in the guidelines, simulation training in ECLS has gained popularity by providing a standardized and controlled environment to cover challenging clinical scenarios, focusing on the behavioral skills, as opposed to the technical and cognitive skills acquired in other pedagogical forms.[10] A recent study demonstrated that more than 70% of ELSO sites report that ECLS simulation

is active or in development at their center,[11] thus illustrating the increasing popularity and value that simulation adds to ECLS training programs. Most programs require additional time with an instructor or a bedside preceptor until the specialist-in-training has gained a solid understanding of ECLS management principles and is deemed fully competent in managing acute emergencies. In addition, the use of checklists may be beneficial in identifying specific tasks and tracking the volume of the trainee's cases.

### *Didactic Course – Lecture Curriculum*

There are many topics to include in a didactic course. ELSO has developed both educational and clinical practice guidelines for ECLS provision and provides quality assurance for clinical use of ECLS via the ELSO Registry. ELSO continues to be the largest registry of centers across the globe. As such, ELSO was ideally situated to play a key role in setting minimum standards for ECLS education and to developing processes that facilitated course and workshop development as well as the endorsement of training programs. An endorsement process will ensure that a given course or workshop achieves an educational quality as set by ELSO while ensuring standardization and consistency across courses. Using Kern's six-step approach to curriculum development for education and use of the Delphi technique, in the winter of 2021, a standardized core ECLS curriculum was introduced to the ECLS community in the form of an online course called ELSO Foundations.[12,13] A comprehensive list of ELSO's core adult ECLS curriculum can be seen in Figure 54-2. This list can also be found on the ELSO website (www.elso.org) under the Endorsement Course Process section (titled Appendix I).

Centers can now use the Adult ELSO Foundations course curriculum as the basis for their training program, or centers can buy site licenses for their specialists to register for access to the self-paced online course to complete the didactic portion of ECLS training. In addition, work is underway to create a core curriculum for the neonatal and pediatric population utilizing the same educational methodology.

Most centers begin their course with an 'Introduction to ECLS,' which includes a discussion of the history of ECLS (Chapter 1). Understanding of past successes and failures provide a better understanding of the basis for current practice. Other introductory discussions may include different forms of ECLS support, general indications for ECLS, the risks and benefits for specific populations, as well as recent clinical research trials that outline the current status of ECLS therapy and its outcomes.

Other topics recommended for ECLS team member education include the pathophysiology of diseases and current medical therapies in patients with severe respiratory failure. Institutions using ECLS for cardiac support may also have education on the anatomy, circulation, myocardial preservation and recovery, surgical procedures and common operations, cardiopulmonary bypass, postoperative management, the pathophysiology of cardiomyopathy and myocarditis, and principles of transplantation medicine.

Review of the pre-ECLS setting and management are also recommended, including pre-ECLS orders, informed consent for ECLS and blood transfusions, pre-ECLS laboratory sampling tests, neuroimaging studies, and echocardiography. Room setup, circuit priming, ECLS initiation, and necessary documentation tools are also important topics to be reviewed. These topics may also be incorporated into training labs discussed in the next section.

Each ECLS team member must gain a comprehensive understanding of blood gas

| Didactic (Classroom) Course | | |
|---|---|---|
| **Introduction to ECMO** | **Pre-ECMO Procedures, Cannulation, and Initiation** | **Circuit & Circuit Management** |
| History and current status | Notification of the ECMO Team | Circuit design/coatings |
| Pathophysiology of respiratory and cardiac failure | Pre-ECMO evaluation and configuratin selection | Circuit components |
| Patient selection criteria: indications & contraindications | Cannulae and cannulation site selection | Circuit priming |
| Physiology of V-A, V-V ECMO; alternative ECLS configurations | Cannulation procedure (percutaneous, semi-open, open) | ECLS settings |
| Oxygen Content, $DO_2$ and $VO_2$ | POCUS to select configuration and support cannulation | Circuit monitoring and checks |
| Physiology of gas exchange on ECMO | Role and responsibilities of team members | Emergency ECMO cart |
| Literature review and short/long-term outcome | Preparing the patient | Additional organ support (HF, RRT, plasmaphersis) & setup |
| ELSO Registry | Consent process and documentation | circuit |
| Ongoing research and areas for future development | Initiation of ECLS | Orders |
| **Daily Patient Management & Weaning** | | |
| Native lung and cardiac function | Pain control, sedation/awakening | Weaning techniques, trial off, and complications |
| Respiratory management (MV, extubation, tracheostomy, etc) | Neurological exam | Decannulation strategy (percutaneous/surgical/approach) |
| Coagulation management and monitoring (POCT/laboratory) | Infection control | Post-ECMO complications |
| Fluids, electrolytes, and nutrition | PK/PD on ECMO | Short-term follow-up |
| Blood products | Management of complext cases (surgery on ECMO) | Institutional follow-up protocol |
| Bedside care | ECMO transport (inter/intrahospital) | Bridge to transplant and to durable MCS |
| Physical therapy | Assessment of native lung and cardiac function/recovery | ECLS withdrawal |
| Parental and family support | Ethics & economics | |
| **Medical & Mechanical Complications** | | |
| Neurological complications | Pneumothorax | Membrane lung failure |
| Bleeding and thrombosis, consumption coagulopathy & DIC | Recirculation on V-V ECMO | Gas supply interruption |
| Hemolysis | Differential oxygenation and non-ejecting LV on V-A ECMO | Air in the circuit |
| SIRS | Limb ischemia | Circuit disruption |
| Renal failure | Access insufficiency | Inadvertent decannulation |
| Hemodynamic derangements | Return obstruction | Circuit or circuit component exchange |
| Arrhythmias and cardiac arrest | Pump failure | Coming off ECMO emergently |

**Figure 54-2:** Didactic course components.

interpretation and gas exchange. This includes knowledge of the principles involved with oxygen content, delivery, and consumption, and carbon dioxide production and elimination in normal physiologic and extracorporeal support conditions (Chapter 5). In addition, all team members must understand the impact of ECLS pump flow and sweep gas flow changes upon gas exchange. To reinforce the lung protective aspects of ECLS, ventilator and airway management while on ECLS is a vital management discussion to include in the curriculum. A thorough demonstration of ECLS physiology and oxygen physics by the ECLS team members is highly recommended at the conclusion of ECLS training.

Each center may focus training on site-specific ECLS techniques; however, a discussion regarding variations in support in use at other centers may assist interhospital communication and exchange of ideas. Blood product administration, coagulation management, medications commonly used during ECLS, weaning, and decannulation procedures must also be reviewed. In addition, a basic understanding of intrahospital and interhospital ECLS transport requirements is recommended (Chapter 46).

All ECLS team members must obtain a thorough understanding of ECLS equipment and circuit design used in their institution and potential mechanical complications and preventative measures (Chapters 3,6,7). Institutional guidelines need to define the essential equipment and emergency skills each ECLS team member must maintain.

Patient and circuit management lecture topics cover a broad range of subjects, including the fundamentals of the daily management of an ECLS patient and recognition of medical emergencies that may occur during support. ECLS team members in training will also benefit from lectures on ethical and social issues.

### Training Labs – Psychomotor Skills Training

ELSO reported over 17,000 cases of ECLS worldwide in 2021.[14] Despite the increased volume in recent years, ECLS is still considered a high-risk, low-volume therapy in most programs. This creates a challenge for practitioners to the clinical opportunities to practice and maintain necessary skills.

Technical and behavioral skills necessary for effective ECLS team training can be accomplished using different hands-on training methods. These training methods offer a unique opportunity to create, test, refine, and streamline ECLS processes without disrupting patient care or endangering patients. Water drills have been utilized to demonstrate the function of ECLS components and to practice technical skills. Animal labs historically allowed ECLS physiology to be shown in an in vivo model. However, the introduction of high-fidelity simulation into ECLS training sessions has enabled the learner to experience a realtime situation with realistic sensory cues that mimic the acute care setting with an ECLS patient. For this discussion, these hands-on training sessions will be categorized as 'training labs'.

Training lab sessions are recommended to allow additional discussion and demonstration of ECLS equipment, the management of mechanical and medical emergencies, and observation of ECLS team members' bedside care performance. To optimize hands-on experience by each participant, a limited number of participants is recommended to maximize exposure to the circuit and skill. The recommended list of technical skills for training lab sessions is shown in Figure 54-3. Institutional variations will exist based upon equipment and circuit configurations.

The recommended introductory course training lab topics include a discussion and demonstration of all equipment, including an explanation of the circuit configuration and function, alarm functions, and a routine circuit assessment: a 'circuit check'. Basic and emergency procedure drills can also be developed based upon a center's equipment selection and practiced in the training labs. Standard emergency drills include managing power failures, emergency circuit clamping, hand cranking the pump (if applicable), deairing a circuit, and managing accidental decannulation. Individual programs will define each team member's role, thus determining if advanced skills such as priming, replacing a circuit, oxygenator, and/or individual components will be practiced. The goals of these training labs are to prepare each ECLS team member to identify any mechanical circuit problems and promptly initiate the appropriate problem-solving response. The clinician responsible for correcting the problem will depend on the defined responsibilities of a center's ECLS team members.

### Water Drills

Water drill sessions can include ECLS circuits assembled, filled with fluid, and conducted in nonclinical settings. This allows for opportunities to mimic many of the situations that occur during an actual ECLS run. In addition, water drills can assist with mastering technical skills necessary for safe

ECLS management (eg, changing broken segments of an ECLS circuit).

### Animal Labs

Animal labs are performed in accordance with institutional animal care guidelines. The advantage of animal laboratory training is realtime coagulation management and blood gas management, which are difficult to simulate in either water drills or ECLS simulation laboratory settings. During these sessions, participants can practice tasks such as blood product administration, intravenous solution and medication administration, and blood sampling. The physiologic impact of the pump sweep gas regulation and heparin infusion adjustments can be demonstrated in an in vivo model. While animals have played a vital role in learning historically, many centers have difficulty accessing a vivarium for training, causing a decrease in the use of animals for ECLS training. Animal labs have become increasingly difficult to perform due to cost, availability of approved facilities, and rigorous institutional animal care guidelines, prompting the development and adoption of hands-on simulation-based training methods.

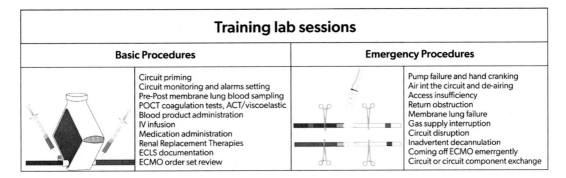

### Training lab sessions

| Basic Procedures | | Emergency Procedures |
|---|---|---|
| Circuit priming<br>Circuit monitoring and alarms setting<br>Pre-Post membrane lung blood sampling<br>POCT coagulation tests, ACT/viscoelastic<br>Blood product administration<br>IV infusion<br>Medication administration<br>Renal Replacement Therapies<br>ECLS documentation<br>ECMO order set review | | Pump failure and hand cranking<br>Air int the circuit and de-airing<br>Access insufficiency<br>Return obstruction<br>Membrane lung failure<br>Gas supply interruption<br>Circuit disruption<br>Inadvertent decannulation<br>Coming off ECMO emerrgently<br>Circuit or circuit component exchange |

**Figure 54-3:** Technical skills for training lab sessions.

## High Fidelity Simulation

High fidelity simulation has become a widely accepted educational tool for anesthesiology, surgery, obstetrics, neonatology, and critical care training programs.[15] High fidelity simulation enhances learning through multiple factors, including repetitive practice, increasing difficulty with attaining skills, addressing various forms of learner strategies, permitting clinical variation in learner responses, and providing immediate feedback.[16] Simulation also addresses the traditional educational method deficiencies of technical and behavioral skill development by immersing the trainee in realistic environments populated with working equipment, a patient simulator capable of generating authentic physiologic cues, and living human beings who respond realistically to the events of the scenario. Creating a highly realistic environment where trainees must respond to problems with both the circuit and the patient creates a more realistic and valuable learning opportunity. To further illustrate the benefits of simulation-based training in ECLS care, a randomized controlled study designed to evaluate simulation based ECLS training vs. training methods in novice critical care fellows demonstrated superior performance in the simulation-based group (SBG). In addition, the SBG had improved long-term scores on written knowledge exams and reductions in the time to critical actions for emergency circuit management.[17]

Simulation training can bridge the educational gap, providing the opportunity for providers to master and demonstrate competency in skills. This training lab environment offers an advantage over water drills and animal labs due to the added ability to adjust the "patient's" physiologic parameters following the participant's ECLS management decisions. This educational tool has been introduced in many ECLS centers as an alternative training tool for both new and experienced specialists and physicians.[18]

High fidelity ECLS simulation and in situ ECLS training provide the opportunity for multidisciplinary team training. Using scripted scenarios, the newly developed and established team can problem solve and practice routine or emergency situations in a realtime setting, such as initiation of ECLS, or equipment failure. These types of simulations can improve patient care and allow the team to develop nontechnical skills such as situational awareness, communication, decisionmaking, teamwork, and leadership. It is widely recognized such human factors independently influence patient outcomes, with good team behaviors being associated with better patient outcomes.

Perhaps the most important aspect of simulation-based learning is the role of debriefing in enhancing the educational experience.[19] As discussed earlier, active participation of the adult learner increases the learning effectiveness. An essential element of successful debriefing is a trained facilitator (the debriefer) who can direct the discussion and extract maximum dialogue from the learners to achieve the defined learning objectives. Formal training for simulation-based healthcare education is recommended for a new facilitator to acquire the basic skill sets to develop into a capable, confident, conversant debriefer.[20] The pairing of a novice debriefer with an expert role model and exposure to a variety of simulation settings are required to develop the skills and comfort level of the debriefer.[21]

## Delivering ECLS Education

As per the ELSO ECLS education taskforce recommendations, delivery of educational content can be achieved through comprehensive courses, workshops, and online education. A Comprehensive Simulation-Based ECLS course meets all ELSO ECLS Practitioner Curricular requirements and maintains an immersive simulation experience with a structured debriefing. Of note, the debriefing is a key feature of this high-level course. The course typically runs over 3-4 days, with simulation making up approximately 50% of course content. ECLS courses are designed to meet the requirements of ECLS curricular knowledge and psychomotor skill learning objectives. In general, they target all healthcare professionals involved in providing direct bedside ECLS care and involve robust learner assessments and course evaluations.

ECLS workshops refer to more focused educational activities that may either be confined to, or expand, beyond the core curriculum. Such settings are ideal for catering to advanced topics or subspecialties not fully addressed in ECLS courses. Thus, they are limited in scope and duration and are often done in collaboration with societal meetings or as standalone workshops that focus on skill sets such as ECLS cannulation or extracorporeal cardiopulmonary resuscitation.

Online ECLS education has garnered more popularity with the advent of travel restrictions following the COVID-19 pandemic. Such platforms enable the global dispersion of standardized learning materials with an opportunity for learners to provide realtime feedback. This tool can also prepare learners ahead of hands-on courses, focusing on flipped classroom strategies during the onsite sessions. ECLS educators are actively exploring the optimal way of delivering telesimulation and its effects on learning when travel restrictions still affect the traditional way of simulation teaching in many countries.[22]

The concept of free open access to medical education (FOAMed), referring to the open sharing of educational resources primarily through social media, emerged in the past decade as a potent tool for developing and/or disseminating valuable educational content. The critical care world, specifically the ECLS community, quickly understood the great potential of social media to support ECLS related education and training, and partially moved to the online space.

In Figure 54-4, some valuable ELSO and non-ELSO online ECLS educational resources and FOAM resources, are highlighted.

## Maintaining Competency Standards- Assessing Competency of ECLS Practitioners

ECLS competency can be assessed by observing actual clinical settings or simulated settings. When assessing competency, the three skills to consider include cognitive (critical thinking), technical, and behavioral. Skill assessment is the objective process of assuring that a staff member can perform competencies based on specific performance criteria used to ensure accurate and safe practice. Performance criteria must be outlined in a policy, procedure, standard, guideline, or reference. Institutional certification of ECLS team members is achieved when performance criteria for clinical competency are fulfilled. The ELSO guidelines recommend that all ECLS specialists take an annual oral and/or written exam.

In 2022, ELSO launched its validated knowledge assessment tool, the ELSO-Adult ECLS Certification Exam (E-AEC). This exam was created in concert with the curriculum development process outlined above, which identified over eighty learning objectives as key elements that programs should include in ECLS Training Program curricula. Exam questions were created that directly tie back to each identified learning objective. This has defined a minimum knowledge and skills standard for those providing ECLS services, allowing for standardization of ECLS practice across sites and healthcare disciplines and recognizing of the unique skill set required for the competent practice of ECLS. The ultimate goal of establishing ECLS certification is to improve the quality of care and patient outcomes.

Technical skills include psychomotor activities within the role's primary responsibilities. Training labs provide a simulated environment to observe the competence of a team member in performing the technical skills necessary for the care of an ECLS patient in routine and emergent situations. Simulation provides the closest assessment of "shows how" competency. True competency, the apex of Miller's Triangle, "does," can only be verified by observing actual patient situations, under real-life, stressful situations.[23] Experience from Advanced Cardiac Life Support training has shown that retention of skills begins to decay after six months.[24] Therefore it is recommended that ECLS team members must practice infrequently used skills regularly.

Behavioral skills reflect the ability to communicate effectively with individuals and groups. Professional communication skills include written, spoken, and nonverbal skills. ECLS team members may identify others who lack the appropriate interpersonal skills. The difficulty lies in objectively identifying those skills. Some behavioral communication indicators include demonstrating courtesy, being respectful, and practicing good listening and feedback skills. The behavioral skills measured by the Stanford CAPE group in their original study measuring the effectiveness of high-fidelity simulation in ECLS training are as follows[25]:

- Familiar with ECLS equipment and bedside environment
- Anticipates and plans for crisis
- Assumes a leadership role
- Communicates effectively

| Virtual ECMO Education Resources | |
|---|---|
| **ELSO and Collaborative Virtual Courses** | **ELSO FOAM Resources** |
| **ELSO Foundations Adult ECMO training course**: self-paced course consisting of 53 modules, covering over 80 learning objectives foundational to adult ECMO patient care (patient selection, configurations including ECMO initiation, cannulation, ECLS physiology, patient monitoring and management, circuit, medical and mechanical complications, weaning) for a total learning time of 7-8 hours, and multiple knowledge checks. Meets "didactic course" definition among criteria to apply for E-AEC. | The **ELSO guidelines** for respiratory circulatory/cardiac support in adult, pediatric, and neonatal patient populations, for ELSO centers organization and ECMO education and training. The guidelines are intended for educational use, to build knowledge of HCPs in assessing and managing ECLS patients, and to support informed decision-making. Regularly updated, guidelines describe what are believed to be useful and safe practices; these are published on ASAIO Journal and are owned and freely available at www.elso.org/resources/guidelines. |
| **ELSO ECMO management course**: 2-day live virtual course designed to train multidisciplinary team on all elements of VV/VA ECMO, and on basics of caring for adults with severe respiratory or cardiac failure requiring ECLS (indications/contraindications, configurations, cannulation techniques, patient physiology, and management on ECMO, decision-making, programmatic design). Meets "didactic course" definition among criteria to apply for E-AEC. | ELSO & its Chapters have channels on **Youtube**, a popular platform for free video sharing, where recording of webinars, selected talks and sessions from annual conferences, presidential addresses and other useful resources are uploaded. **ELSO** channel (also hosting live events) available at bit.ly/ELSOyoutube; **EuroELSO** channel: available at bit.ly/EuroELSOyoutube; **LATAM ELSO** channel: bit.ly/ELSOLATAMyoutube |
| **ECMO Masterclass**: joint courses with other medical societies such as ELSO/SCCM, ELSO/STS, or EuroELSO/ESICM that focus on specific areas of ECLS based on the joint needs established between the organizations. | **ECMO 101**: a web-based course addressing basic elements in ECMO delivery (consisting of 6 modules: introduction and history of ECMO, indications and evidence, circuit, physiology of ECLS, general patient management, common scenarios and complications). The course is an introduction to ECMO for basic orientation; requires ~ 6 hours to complete. |
| **Non-ELSO FOAM Resources\*** | |
| **corECMO**: an e-learning program developed by researchers of University of Washington, as part of a multimodaility ECMO curriculum, along with high-fidelity simulation and bedside clinical training, aimed to facilitate interactive asynchronous education, and composed of core content and simulated interactive cases for both VV and VA ECLS. See www.corECMO.com. | **ED ECMO Project** is aimed to bring extracorporeal life support to Eds and ICUs around the world. This site aims to be a comprehensive resource to learn about the background, logistics, and evidence for resuscitative ECMO, and to raise awareness of ECLS in the Emergency Department. This blog posts interviews with experts in the field. See www.edecmo.org. |
| **ECMOMODEL**: a mathematical model of gas exchange during veno-venous ECMO support, developed by researcher at the University of Milan, suitable simulations of pediatric and adult patients. This software can be a useful teaching tool and might support decision-making for the management of refractory hypoxemia in patients supported by VV ECMO. See www.ecmomodel.unimi.it. | **INTENSIVE blog**: educational website for HCPs training in or practicing intensive care medicine hosted by LITFL and provided by the Alfred ICU in Melbourne, Australia. Blog includes an "Everything ECMO", a developing series of peer-reviewed case-based Q&A posts covering all aspects of ECLS management in critically ill patients. See intensiveblog.com. |
| *\*Note: These are examples and are not an endorsement of these resources from ELSO, nor their sustainability.* | |

**Figure 54-4:** Examples of virtual ECMO courses.

- Distributes workload optimally
- Allocates attention wisely
- Utilizes all available resources
- Calls for help early
- Maintains professional behavior

### *Maintaining ECLS Competency*

Since ECLS is a high-risk, low-volume therapy, centers must establish a process to ensure that all team members obtain the appropriate education and experience to retain their skills. Each center must determine a timeline for competency evaluation based on their specific needs, program patient volumes, and defined responsibilities of the clinician members of the ECLS team. ELSO guidelines recommend that training lab sessions be held at a minimum of every six months and an annual examination be used to verify the knowledge and skills of the ECLS Team. Each program should determine the minimum number of pump hours for ECLS specialists, or the annual volume of patients independently managed by licensed independent practitioners (LIP) within an established time period to maintain institutional certification. If the number of hours is not met, a policy outlining a retraining program is recommended.

Most ECLS centers schedule team meetings on a regularly to discuss clinical and operational issues, quality assurance review findings, and other topics pertinent to the team. Team meetings also provide an opportunity to offer continuing education sessions with case reviews and multidisciplinary morbidity and mortality conferences. The frequency of these meetings is determined based on the size of the team and the volume of ECLS patients treated. Attendance of team members at these meetings is monitored, and criteria for minimal attendance are defined to ensure maintenance of institutional certification. Information on patient followup could be included here, allowing team members to become familiar with patient

outcomes and appreciate the risks and benefits of ECLS.

### *Institutional Certification of ECLS Team Members*

Each institution is responsible for evaluating and certifying its team members and maintaining a written evaluation of the training history of those members. Most centers include documentation of course attendance; successful performance at water drills, animal sessions or training labs; and completion of all required skills lists and competencies in the evaluations. In addition, each specialist must obtain a passing score on written and/or oral exams. After completing the training course requirements and passing the exam, institutional certification can be granted. Sample institutional certification requirements for ECLS specialists are:

- Minimum of 1-year critical care experience prior to training
- Attendance at all didactic sessions
- Attendance at all training lab sessions
- Participation in ECLS emergency drills
- Completion of pump time with a preceptor
- Completion of technical skills list and/or competencies
- Successful completion of written/oral exam with passing score

A periodic review of the ECLS team member's knowledge and skill level is essential. The frequency and skills to be assessed depending on center-specific recertification requirements. All training expectations and criteria indicating success (eg, a passing score on a test and a minimum number of pump hours) must be established. In addition, yearly requirements for attendance and participation in team meetings will need to be fulfilled.

## Feedback

All educational activities should include providing the learner with timely feedback on their knowledge and understanding, including identifying development and further learning areas. The learner must also provide structured feedback on the education and process they have received. All training courses must include formal feedback to ensure the course has met and delivered its educational aims and objectives, including whether the participants have found it helpful, accessible, and effective in gaining new knowledge. All courses should be reviewed and developed based on such feedback.

## Summary

Although providing ECLS to critically ill patients is complex, using many healthcare resources can be very rewarding to the institution, staff, and, especially, the infants, children, adolescents, adults, and families served. The foundation of an exceptional ECLS program relies upon the multidisciplinary ECLS team's education, training, and certification. To assist with the developing these comprehensive programs, the ELSO guidelines exist to provide educational requirements for clinicians responsible for monitoring and maintaining ECLS support. The educational process should follow adult based learning principles and be based upon Miller's Triangle for clinical assessment. Training and education must also address training for new providers and existing providers from all disciplines, including specialists and physicians. This should be enhanced by continuing educational research on the various methods of effective teaching and course and workshop content assessment. Continuing education and assessment of clinical competency should be an integral part of the program, including the competencies of ECLS specialists, physicians, and surgeons. A program can only achieve clinical excellence in life support with robust ECLS education and training.

# References

1. ELSO Guidelines for ECMO Centers. Retrieved May 2022, from https://www.elso.org/ecmo-resources/elso-ecmo-guidelines.aspx.
2. ELSO Guidelines for Training and Continuing Education of ECMO Specialists, https://www.elso.org/ecmo-resources/elso-ecmo-guidelines.aspx.
3. Zakhary B, Shekar K, Diaz R, et al. Position Paper on Global Extracorporeal Membrane Oxygenation Education and Educational Agenda for the Future: A Statement From the Extracorporeal Life Support Organization ECMOed Taskforce. Crit Care Med. 2020;48(3):406-414.
4. Puslecki M, Dabrowski M, Ligowski M, et al. (2021) Comprehensive assessment of a nationwide simulation-based course for artificial life support. PLOS ONE 16(10): e0257162.
5. Jeffries WB. Teaching large groups. In: Jeffries WB, Huggett KN, eds. An Introduction to Medical Teaching. Dordrecht, Netherlands: Springer Netherlands: 2014: 11-26.
6. Knowles MS, Holton E, Swanson R. The Adult Learner. Houston: Gulf Publishing Company, 1998.
7. Miller GE. The Assessment of Clinical Skills, Competence, Performance. Acad Med 1990; 65:S63-7.
8. The Joint Commission. The Joint Commission Edition: Accreditation. Last Reviewed by Standards Interpretation: April 18, 2022. Retrieved on May 2022 from: https://www.jointcommission.org/standards/standard-faqs/ambulatory/human-resources-hr/000002254/.
9. Fanning RM, Goldhaber-Fiebert SA, Udani AD, et al. Crisis Resource Management. In: Levine AI, DeMaria Jr S, Schwartz AD, Sim AJ editors. The Comprehensive Textbook of Healthcare Simulation. New York: Springer;2013. p. 95-109.
10. Sin SWC, Ng PY, Ngai WCW, et al. Simulation training for crises during venoarterial extracorporeal membrane oxygenation. J Thorac Dis. 2019;11(5):2144-2152.
11. Weems MF, Friedlich PS, Nelson LP, et al. The Role of Extracorporeal Membrane Oxygenation Simulation Training at Extracorporeal Life Support Organization Centers in the United States. Simul Healthc. 2017;12(4):233-239.
12. Kern DE, Thomas PA, Hughes MT. Curriculum Development for Medical Education: A Six-Step Approach, 2nd ed. Baltimore, MD: The Johns Hopkins University Press; 2009.
13. McPherson S, Reese C, Wendler MC. Methodology Update: Delphi Studies. Nurs Res. 2018;67(5):404-410.
14. Extracorporeal Life Support Organization (ELSO) ECLS Registry Report, International Summary. Available at: https://www.elso.org/Registry/InternationalSummaryandReports/InternationalSummary.aspx. Accessed April 15, 2022.
15. Helmreich RL, Merritt AC, Wilhelm JA. The evolution of Crew Resource Management training in commercial aviation. Int J Aviat Psychol 1999; 9:19–32.
16. Issenberg S B, McGaghie C, Petrusa E R, et al. What are the features and uses of high-fidelity medical simulations that lead to most effective learning? BEME Guide No 4. Medical Teacher 2005; 27:10-28.
17. Zakhary BM, Kam LM, Kaufman BS, et al. The Utility of High-Fidelity Simulation for Training Critical Care Fellows in the Management of Extracorporeal Membrane Oxygenation Emergencies: A Randomized Controlled Trial. Crit Care Med. 2017;45(8):1367-1373.
18. Johnston L, Oldenburg G. Simulation for neonatal extracorporeal membrane oxygenation teams. InSeminars in Perinatology 2016 Nov 30 (Vol. 40, No. 7, pp. 421-429). WB Saunders.
19. Fanning RM, Gaba DM. The role of debrief- ing in simulation-based learning. Simula- tion in healthcare. 2007 Jul 1;2(2):115-25.
20. McLean M: What can we learn from facili- tator and student perceptions of facilitation skills and roles in the first year of a prob- lem based learning curriculum. Med Educ 2003;3:1–10.
21. Chamberlain D, Smith A, Woollard M, et al. Trials of teaching methods in basic life support (3): Comparison of simulated CPR performance after first training and at 6 months, with a note on the value of re- training. Resuscitation 2002; 53:179–187.
22. Wong AS, Marwali EM, Maclaren G, et al. ECMO simulation training during a worldwide pandemic: The role of ECMO telesimulation [published online ahead of print, 2022 May 11]. Perfusion. 2022;2676591221093868.
23. Miller GE. The Assessment of Clinical Skills, Competence, Performance. Acad Med 1990; 65:S63-7.
24. Chamberlain D, Smith A, Woollard M, et al. Trials of teaching methods in basic life support (3): Comparison of simulated CPR performance after first training and at 6 months, with a note on the value of re- training. Resuscitation 2002; 53:179–187.
25. Anderson J, Boyle K, Murphy A, et al. Simulating Extracorporeal Membrane Oxy- genation emergencies to improve human performance. Part II: Assessment of techni- cal and behavioral skills. Simul Healthcare. 2006; 1(4):228-232.
26. Cadogan M, Thoma B, Chan TM, Lin M. Free Open Access Meducation (FOAM): the rise of emergency medicine and critical care blogs and podcasts (2002-2013). Emerg Med J. 2014 Oct;31(e1):e76-7.
27. Wong A, Ho S, Olusanya O, Antonini MV, et al. The use of social media and online communications in times of pandemic COVID-19. J Intensive Care Soc. 2021 Aug;22(3):255-260.

# 55

## Quality

*Melania M. Bembea, Steven M. Schwartz, Christine Stead, Toshiyuki Aokage, Tracy Morrison, Peter C. Laussen*

### Introduction

ECLS is an invasive, high-risk, low-volume, and expensive tool that is essential to achieving excellent outcomes in most critical care units. Therefore, a robust approach to constantly assess quality and safety of care provided via this technology is an essential aspect of any ECLS program.[1] As will be discussed in detail in this chapter, ECLS quality and safety programs look to continually assess outcomes, complications, team and equipment performance, and resource utilization. In addition to examination of internal program data, participation in registries is helpful to provide benchmarking to understand if a specific center's ECLS program is achieving their goals.

The approach to quality assessment for an ECLS program is built on the standard concepts of quality and safety in medicine popularized by Avedis Donabedian. These include the Model for Improvement and the Define-Measure-Analyze-Improve-Control (DMAIC) approach from Lean/Six Sigma methodology.[2,3] The use of registries dedicated to ECLS, most notably the ELSO Registry, or registries primarily designed for broader populations of critical care patients capture clinical patient data, such as the Pediatric Cardiac Critical Care Consortium (PC[4]), the Virtual Pediatric Systems (VPS), or the American Heart Association Get-With-The-Guidelines – Resuscitation® registries, all of which have been used to study practices and outcomes of ECLS in infants and children.[4-8] Participation in registries can provide both new and established ECLS programs with benchmarking data and communities of like-minded professionals who can support quality efforts.

While collecting data regarding use and outcomes of ECLS is an essential base for any assessment of quality, the way in which data are used to inform organization of the ECLS program and to sustain high-performing ECLS teams ultimately determines the value of the ECLS quality program at a given institution. Resources and references are available including numerous guidelines on the ELSO website (www.elso.org), articles detailing organization of ECLS programs,[1] and models for education and team training, including detailed approaches to simulation to improve performance.[9,10]

This chapter will discuss these concepts and resources, with a focus on

- Commitment to quality and safety,
- Data collection and performance measurement,
- Quality improvement processes for ECLS programs,

- Variability in quality processes among ECLS programs,
- Innovation and new technologies.

## Commitment to Quality and Safety

ECLS is utilized when other therapies are insufficient to sustain life; therefore, its failure could be fatal. Quality and safety are at the forefront of ECLS management and should include evidence-based guidelines, or, when evidence is lacking, expert consensus statements. Quality improvement should be implemented by the ECLS team and supported by the hospital for all disciplines involved in ECLS care (ie, critical care, emergency, and surgical care teams, ECMO specialists, perfusionists, blood bank, pharmacists, and others).

Individual programs typically use published guidelines to educate staff and create detailed, institution-specific policies and protocols that are adapted to their facility's and their country's healthcare system and relevant regulations. ECLS program managers or coordinators are responsible for periodically assessing compliance with institutional policies and protocols, identifying barriers, and developing action plans to overcome barriers to utilization and compliance with institutional policies and protocols; the series of which is called a 'quality improvement program'.

Barrier identification and mitigation procedures should be available at each facility, with a process typically following 5 steps: 1) Assemble the Interdisciplinary Team; 2) Identify Barriers; 3) Summarize Barrier Data; 4) Prioritize the Barriers; and 5) Develop an Action Plan for Each Targeted Barrier.[11]

Similar to other areas in medicine, QI projects related to ECLS may be met with skepticism on the part of physicians or the multidisciplinary team.[12] Concerns may include the lack of high-quality evidence to inform clinical practice guidelines, perception of QI as misplaced priority and focusing on what is measurable rather than what is important for optimal patient outcomes, or fear that quality measurement might be used as a reason for blame. Thoughtful planning, long-term commitment and adequate time and administrative resources are all needed for physicians and other staff to treat ECLS QI initiatives as high priority activities.

## Data Collection and Measuring Quality

Donabedian's quality methodology of measuring structure, process, outcomes create the data elements that inform quality for ECLS programs. Data are available for each of these aspects and should be part of any ECMO program's consistent commitment to improving quality for the patients they serve.

ELSO provides several tools for programs: 1) the ELSO Registry is a global database of data elements that capture important data for each patient run; 2) data definitions provided by ELSO help to achieve a common set of definitions and therefore better data; 3) live registry filtering available for easy access to major data items, available in real time without a data request for quick benchmarking; 4) a quality dashboard that every program has access to; and 5) clinical practice guidelines.[13]

## Performance Measurement

Patient outcomes and complications data relate to performance. Donabedian's approach to measuring quality answers the question 'what goes on here?'.[14] Performance can be assessed through data, observation, and a team commitment to improving performance.

Benchmarking a program's performance relative to others is now available through the ELSO Registry and quality dashboard, which provides a center the ability to review their own data relative to the ELSO Registry in similar patient populations. Risk adjustments were built separately for each age group and support type, enabling benchmarking to understand a center's performance in an appropriate context.

Establishing a system for reviewing performance is essential to providing a high-quality program, which is especially important for new programs. Every case - and the performance data, processes, and outcomes - should be reviewed early on such that the entire ECLS team can learn how their work collectively impacts performance and outcomes (Figure 55-1). ECLS programs are eligible for the ELSO Path to Excellence or the Award of Excellence in Life Support; applications allow self-evaluation as well as external evaluation in seven categories: systems, environment, workforce, knowledge management, quality focus, process optimization, and patient and family (Table 55-1). A Comprehensive

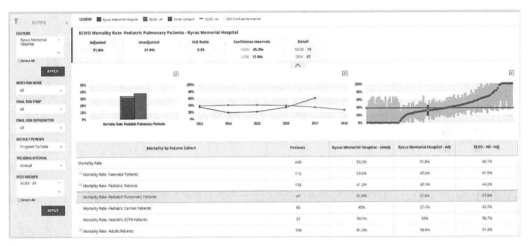

**Figure 55-1.** Sample ELSO Quality Dashboard Output.

| DOMAIN | COMPONENTS (selected) |
|---|---|
| Systems | • Availability of specialty medical services, laboratory, blood bank, operating rooms, occupational and physical therapy, nutrition, pastoral care, etc.<br>• ECLS transport capabilities<br>• Roles and responsibilities of the ECLS medical director and ECLS coordinator |
| Environment | • Single- vs multiple-ICU ECLS program<br>• Back-up equipment and circuit components<br>• Contingency plan for increased census |
| Workforce | • Pre-requisites to become an ECLS Specialist (ES)[a]<br>• Patient to staff (ES, nurse) ratio, primer availability in-hospital or on call<br>• Debriefing and management of staff moral distress |
| Training and competencies | • Initial and continuous credentialing for ECLS for physicians, advanced practice nurses, physician assistants, nurses, ES<br>• Water drills and simulation sessions for basic circuit and emergency management<br>• Annual pump time requirements, bedside training, and exam |
| Quality | • Best practices related to workforce management<br>• Improved value of care delivered<br>• Maintaining knowledge and incorporating current ECLS practice into each center's clinical practice |
| Process optimization | • Process for case reviews (e.g., Morbidity and Mortality Conference)<br>• Review and integration of ELSO benchmarking data<br>• Monitoring process for anticoagulation during ECLS |
| Patient and family | • Educational materials provided to families<br>• Integration of family members into the daily care of ECLS patients<br>• Long-term followup process |
| ECLS=extracorporeal life support; ICU=intensive care unit; ES=ECLS specialist<br>[a]ECLS Specialist: individual designated to care for the ECLS circuit | |

**Table 55-1.** Domains of the ELSO Award for Excellence in Life Support Application.

ELSO Award of Excellence Evaluation and Improvement Tool as well as a Readiness Tool are available on the ELSO website to assist new or growing ECLS centers with the implementation and maintenance of quality improvement programs.[15]

## Quality Improvement Processes for ECLS Using the Model for Improvement

The Model for Improvement is a simple yet powerful tool that has been used successfully by hundreds of health care organizations to improve many different health care processes and outcomes. Developed by Associates in Process Improvement as the framework for the improvement process, the model has three fundamental principles:

- Set clear aims,
- Establish measures that will tell if changes are leading to improvement,
- Identify changes that are likely to lead to improvement.

There are 6 steps to follow using the Model for Improvement.

**Step 1:** Form the QI team. Finding the right people to work on a quality project is critical to the project's success. People who do the work should improve the work, so select team members who are doing or who are affected by the work you are trying to improve. Consider the system that relates to your QI project. Ensure that the team includes members familiar with all the different parts of the process. Bedside staff are the experts at how care processes are delivered to our patients. Ad hoc members from pharmacy, the supply chain, respiratory therapy, or other disciplines should be added to QI teams as needed and might be essential to improving specific ECLS-related processes.

**Step 2:** Define the QI project and establish aims. Choose a topic that is meaningful to ECLS, patients, and/or staff. A meaningful improvement project is much more likely to create buy-in from staff at the bedside.[16]

Ideas for Projects include: improving satisfaction of staff, patients, and/or families; reducing waste and cost of supplies and improving utilization of storage space; reducing loss of instruments, equipment or supplies; reducing the unit's impact on the environment; improving inventory processes (eg, reducing inventory, improving storage, standardizing supplies, and/or reducing costs and expired supplies); improving patient outcomes by reducing central line-associated bloodstream infections (CLABSI), catheter-associated urinary tract infections (CAUTI), or other unit-specific ECLS outcomes.

Improvement work requires a specific SMART aim to help get the work done. SMART aims are specific, measurable, achievable, realistic, and timely. The SMART aim should define the population of patients that will be affected by the improvement project.[17]

Examples of Effective Aim Statements include: increasing the number of days without bloodstream infections in ECLS patients by 50% by [date]; reducing the number of ECLS supplies that expire by 20% by [date]; increasing the number of ECLS patients that are cannulated within [X] hours of the decision to cannulate by 25% by [date]; achieving 100% compliance with anticoagulation protocol in ECLS patients in the ICU by [date]; or improving ECLS staff satisfaction by 20% within 60 days by providing snacks to staff on days they are understaffed.

**Step 3:** Identify quality improvement measures. Measurement is an essential component of the improvement process and can tell you if the change that you made has improved process and/or outcome. Measurement for improvement involves small tests of change that are sequential and build upon each other to accelerate the rate of improvement. Using improvement methods such as the 5 Why's help to identify why changes need to be made.[17]

Outcome measure examples include: ECLS survival; patient satisfaction; adverse drug events/1000 doses.

Process measures include: % ECLS patients rounded on every [X] hours; % access sites on ECLS with alcohol caps; % sepsis patients with lactic acid measured per protocol.

Balancing measures include: number of ECLS with 2nd run; number of reintubations; number of circuit changes.

**Step 4:** Evaluate evidence of improvement. Decisions about patient care should be based on available scientific evidence, of which the highest form of evidence is a well-performed randomized clinical trial. Using evidence-based practices (EBP) should enable the caregiver to provide high quality care, improve processes, and reduce variations in care. A model to using EBP includes the following:

- Recognize that the gap between one's knowledge and the knowledge needed

to answer the relevant clinical question requires review of scientific evidence.

- Formulate a specific question about improving patient care to be answered.
- Search for the relevant evidence to answer the question, which might include print or electronic sources.
- After a review of the evidence, a specific answer to the question is formed.

**Step 5:** Test whether changes result in improvement. While all changes do not all lead to improvement, all improvement does require some type of change. The ability to develop, test, and implement changes is an essential skill to acquire for an organization that wants to continuously improve itself. There are many kinds of changes that will lead to improvement. To support small-scale tests of change in real work settings, one option is using Plan-Do-Study-Act (PDSA) cycles (Figure 55-2). Teams plan a test, try it, observe the results, and act on what is learned. It is critical for tests to be

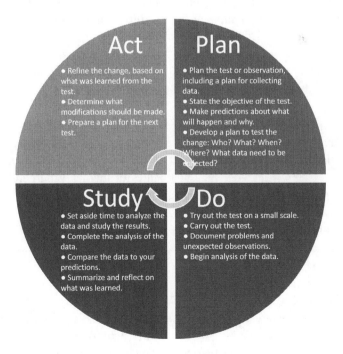

**Figure 55-2.** The Plan-Do-Study-Act Cycle applied to ECLS.

small and rapid (eg, a test with two ICU patients tomorrow). This is the scientific method applied to action-oriented learning.[18] The following are ideas for change: eliminating waste; improving work flow; optimizing inventory; changing the work environment; improving patient/customer satisfaction; managing time; focusing on variation to reduce errors; or error proofing. The last of these, error proofing, can be accomplished by finding ways to redesign the system or processes to make it less likely for people to make errors. One way to error proof a system or process is to make the information necessary to perform a task available by writing it down as a policy, creating a checklist, or by making it inherent in the product or process.

**Step 6:** Implement and evaluate the project. So far you have formed your team, defined your problem and set your aims, measured and collected pre-project data, selected changes based on evidence, and performed small tests of change using PDSA cycles. Now is the time to implement selected changes to a larger population and evaluate how those changes have improved care, flow, etc., and demonstrated success of the project. Implementation is a permanent change to the way work is done and involves building the change into the organization. It may affect documentation, written policies, hiring, training, compensation, and aspects of the organization's infrastructure that are not engaged in the testing phase. Implementation also requires the use of the PDSA cycle.

**Steps for Implementing a Project:** 1) Create a two-way communication plan. 2) Educate staff and other stakeholders. 3) Provide needed documentation (policies, procedures, checklists, doc flow sheets). 4) Create process for monthly data collection to measure how the change is going. 5) Use PDSA cycles when implementing change so you can see if the plan is successful.

**Steps for Spreading Changes:** 1) Creating awareness of the need for change. 2) Tell stories, share data. 3) Create staff desire for supporting the change. 4) Tell patient or staff stories, share data. 5) Educate staff so they have the knowledge to change. 6) Foster ability by providing opportunities for staff to learn new skills or behaviors. 7) Celebrate successes and continuously reinforce new changes with feedback and audits. 8) Continue to use PDSA cycles as needed to continuously improve project.

## Simulation as Quality Improvement Tool for ECMO

Simulation equips learners with the ability to identify and solve problems they might encounter while caring for patients.[19] High-fidelity simulation exercises can build confidence in ECLS teams to emergency situations in a nonpatient setting. This can build confidence, competence, and improve patient outcomes.

Engaging learners in simulated activities fosters deep learning and opportunity to improve the quality of the activity or process being simulated. ECMO processes that can be improved easily using simulation include responses to emergencies, the development of policies, and improving the effectiveness of standardized procedures. Simulation can be thought of as a field experiment to understand the physical patient space, while improving the quality and safety of the procedures created to care for them.[20] Emergencies lend themselves well to simulation with the ability to assess both the individual practitioner's response and the accuracy of available work tools/checklists used by the ECMO specialist to respond to the emergency. Debriefing during simulations will generate ideas, solve problem issues, and improve the way the processes work at the bedside. Costly errors can be prevented when staff provide input as they can readily see "The Why" improvement was needed during debriefing.

Starting a simulation QI project is as simple as asking staff what is not working well.[21] Plan for the upcoming simulation by finding a space that best recreates the environment where ECMO is provided.

- Define your anticipated outcome with a Smart Aim.
- Determine how you will measure improvement.
- Provide background information to staff that will help them analyze current practices and brainstorm during the event. Examples include: literature review, current policy/procedure, reviewing policy from a different organization
- Manage the simulation, providing direction and clarity of intention: attend the event as an observer, facilitating learning and providing feedback.
- Debrief the simulation: evaluate the effectiveness of the event as quality improvement; record ideas for improvement; rewrite policy/procedure/education and complete further testing.
- Document in a PDSA format or hospital preferred format.[19]

It is important to choose the right metrics when using simulation for QI. Sometimes the outcome desired is easy to measure, such as reducing the number of steps to prime a circuit or reducing the time to prime. If you are looking to standardize a process, create a simulation to review process reliability following a guideline or checklist and count the number of vital steps that were completed in the correct order. If you narrow a process down to a few vital steps, compliance in performing these steps could be collected over time. Individual times can be collected on a graph to show overall team improvement.[22] Helping staff to See-Feel-Change using simulation for QI improves buy-in and helps to reinforce changed behavior.[23]

## Variability in Quality Processes

Several studies note variability in outcomes, including a COVID-19 update that demonstrated newer ECLS programs had slightly worse outcomes during the first year of the pandemic.[24] Outcomes represent an indicator of the quality of a program. Reviewing variation in outcomes or other performance indicators can lead to improvements.

ELSO provides variability measures in the international summary reports that are released twice a year. In addition, the Quality Dashboard can provide a real-time view of variability for each program relative to the ELSO Registry.

Peer groups can be created within the quality dashboard[13] to further advance understanding of where variability could be reduced to improve outcomes. Peer groups require agreement among peers, at least 10 centers (Figure 55-3).

Following evidence-based best practices can help with improving quality and reducing variation. ELSO provides guidelines related to clinical practice management for different ECLS patient populations and related ECLS settings. Adherence to guidelines can help reduce variation and generally improve performance.

## Innovation and New Technologies

Data collected through the ELSO Registry provide clinical performance information to ECLS manufacturers. Industry can ask for data on their equipment, which ELSO provides in a manner that maintains the confidentiality of other industry competitors, as well as that of participating centers and patients therein. This information can be important for industry to play a role in improving patient outcomes.

Advances in technology since 2020 include integrated ECMO systems; single-site access, dual-lumen catheters with improvements in patient mobility and catheter placement efficiencies; and oxygenator designs that reduce corners and decrease blood side pressure drop.[25-28] The first was released in 2020 and was also the first device cleared by the FDA for ECMO.[25]

Technology innovations will continue to improve usability, reduce complications, and ultimately improve patient outcomes. These improvements rely on data in nonclinical settings before clinical settings. The ELSO Registry data has increasingly been a source for data on clinical setting equipment performance.

In summary, many play a role in improving quality: ECLS teams; the institutional, national, and global ECLS community; technology partners; health systems; and regulatory agencies. Quality measures connect these different stakeholders together, as does a collective commitment to improving quality and outcomes.

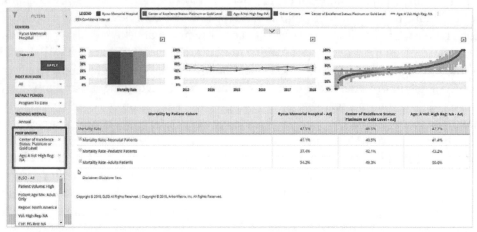

- Benchmark against all ELSO or specific peer groups
- Multiple peer groups can be selected and will be broken out in the legend for all chart types
- You will only be able to select a peer comparison if you are a member of that group and if the group has 10 or more centers.

**Figure 55-3.** Sample Peer Group Data in the ELSO Quality Dashboard.

# References

1. Guerguerian AM, Ogino MT, Dalton HJ, et al. Setup and maintenance of extracorporeal life support programs. Pediatr Crit Care Med. Jun 2013;14(5 Suppl 1):S84-93.

2. Scoville R, Little K. Comparing Lean and Quality Improvement. Cambridge, MA: IHI White Paper; 2014. p. 1-30.

3. Bates KE, Connor J, Chanani NK, et al. Quality Improvement Basics: A Crash Course for Pediatric Cardiac Care. World J Pediatr Congenit Heart Surg. Nov 2019;10(6):733-741.

4. Lorusso R, Alexander P, Rycus P, et al. The Extracorporeal Life Support Organization Registry: update and perspectives. Ann Cardiothorac Surg. 2019:93-98. vol. 1.

5. Beltramo F, DiCarlo J, Gruber JB, et al. Renal Replacement Therapy Modalities in Critically Ill Children. Pediatr Crit Care Med. Jan 2019;20(1):e1-e9.

6. Brunetti MA, Gaynor JW, Retzloff LB, et al. Characteristics, Risk Factors, and Outcomes of Extracorporeal Membrane Oxygenation Use in Pediatric Cardiac ICUs: A Report From the Pediatric Cardiac Critical Care Consortium Registry. Pediatr Crit Care Med. Jun 2018;19(6):544-552.

7. Lasa JJ, Rogers RS, Localio R, et al. Extracorporeal Cardiopulmonary Resuscitation (E-CPR) During Pediatric In-Hospital Cardiopulmonary Arrest Is Associated With Improved Survival to Discharge: A Report from the American Heart Association's Get With The Guidelines-Resuscitation (GWTG-R) Registry. Circulation. Jan 12 2016;133(2):165-76.

8. Bembea MM, Ng DK, Rizkalla N, et al. Outcomes After Extracorporeal Cardiopulmonary Resuscitation of Pediatric In-Hospital Cardiac Arrest: A Report From the Get With the Guidelines-Resuscitation and the Extracorporeal Life Support Organization Registries. Crit Care Med. Apr 2019;47(4):e278-e285.

9. Allan CK, Thiagarajan RR, Beke D, et al. Simulation-based training delivered directly to the pediatric cardiac intensive care unit engenders preparedness, comfort, and decreased anxiety among multidisciplinary resuscitation teams. J Thorac Cardiovasc Surg. Sep 2010;140(3):646-52.

10. Weems MF, Friedlich PS, Nelson LP, et al. The Role of Extracorporeal Membrane Oxygenation Simulation Training at Extracorporeal Life Support Organization Centers in the United States. Simul Healthc. Aug 2017;12(4):233-239.

11. Agency for Healthcare Research and Quality. Barrier Identification and Mitigation Tool. Updated Content last reviewed December 2017. Accessed January 30, 2022. https://www.ahrq.gov/hai/tools/surgery/tools/surgical-complication-prevention/bim.html.

12. Shekelle PG. Why don't physicians enthusiastically support quality improvement programmes? Qual Saf Health Care. Mar 2002;11(1):6.

13. Organization ELS. ELSO Registry Quality Reporting Platform. Accessed January 30, 2022. https://www.elso.org/Registry/QualityReportingPlatform.aspx

14. Donabedian A. Evaluating the quality of medical care. 1966. Milbank Q. 2005;83(4):691-729.

15. ELSO Award of Excellence in Extracorporeal Life Support - Award Evaluation and Improvement Tool. ELSO. Accessed January 30, 2022. https://www.elso.org/awardofexcellence/beforeyouapply.aspx.

16. Langley GJ MR, Nolan KM, Nolan TW, et al. The Improvement Guide. 2nd Edition ed. Jossey-Bass; 2009.

17. Ogrinc GS HL, Barton AJ, Dolansky MA, et al. Fundamentals of Health Care Improvement: A Guide to Improving Your Patients' Care. 3rd Edition ed. Joint Commission Resources; 2018.

18. Evans JR LW. Managing for Quality and Performance Excellence. 11th Edition ed. Cengage Learning; 2019.

19. Riley RH. Manual of Simulation in Healthcare. 2nd Edition ed. Oxford University Press; 2015.

20. Gneezy U List J. The Why Axis: Hidden Motives and the Undiscovered Economics of Everyday Life. PublicAffairs; 2013.

21. Godin S. Poke the Box. The Domino Project; Portfolio, 2011.

22. Brown MG. Keeping Score: Using the Right Metrics to Drive World Class Performance. Taylor and Francis Group; 1996.

23. Cohen DS. The Heart of Change Field Guide: Tools and Tactics for Leading Change in Your Organization. Harvard Business School Publishing; 2005.

24. Barbaro RP, MacLaren G, Boonstra PS, et al. Extracorporeal membrane oxygenation for COVID-19: evolving outcomes from the international Extracorporeal Life Support Organization Registry. Lancet. Oct 2 2021;398(10307):1230-1238.

25. Fresenius. FDA clears Fresenius Medical Care's Novalung for treatment of acute respiratory and cardiopulmonary failure. Accessed January 30, 2022. https://www.fresenius.com/8116.

26. Medtronic. Crescent Jugular Dual Lumen Catheter. Accessed January 30, 2022. medtronic.com/crescent

27. Vijayakumar N, Badheka A, Chegondi M, et al. Successful use of Protek Duo cannula to provide veno-venous extra-corporeal membrane oxygenation and right ventricular support for acute respiratory distress syndrome in an adolescent with complex congenital heart disease. Perfusion. Mar 2021;36(2):200-203.

28. Medtronic. NautilusTM ECMO Oxygenator. Accessed January 30, 2022. https://www.medtronic.com/content/dam/medtronic-com/products/cardiovascular/extracorporeal-life-support-ecls/nautilus-ecmo/documents/nautilus-ecmo-oxygenator-quick-reference-brochure.pdf.

# 56

## Economics

*Kali Barrett, Gordon Morewood, Pranya Sakiyalak, Riyan S. Shetty, Lara Shekerdemian*

## Introduction

Recent years have seen a rapid expansion in the use of ECLS around the globe.[1] Advances in equipment, technology, training, and a more sophisticated understanding of pathophysiology have allowed more patients with cardiopulmonary compromise to benefit from this therapy. Clinical evidence supporting the use of ECLS must be accompanied by an equally rigorous understanding of the economics underlying the deployment of this therapy. Politicians, unelected administrators, and healthcare professionals are all expected to contribute to the value judgements that will shape the services offered within a region.

An exhaustive discussion of the economics of ECLS deployment in every existing healthcare system is beyond the scope of this chapter. Instead, a framework will be presented which can be applied to the general question of how to assess the value of ECLS. Specific attempts to answer this question under focused conditions will be reviewed. The intent is to provide readers with an understanding of how to approach this issue in the context of their own healthcare system, and to participate meaningfully as decisions regarding resource allocation are made.

## Fundamental Considerations

The costs of ECLS include those materials and professional services required to institute, maintain, and wean a patient from extracorporeal support. They can be categorized as fixed or variable, although there is some overlap.

Fixed costs are those that are invoked once an ECLS service is established and do not vary significantly with the volume of services rendered. Fixed costs may include durable equipment (pumps, monitors, lab equipment) and personnel (dedicated technicians, nurses, and physicians). These costs are not fixed in an absolute sense and will vary as the capacity of the planned service is increased or decreased and would be aligned with the market in terms of salaries and/or equipment and related costs. Conceptually, these fixed costs are divided equally amongst all the cases performed. Efficiency is then maximized by supporting the greatest number of ECLS cases possible with the resources allocated.

Variable costs are only incurred when an individual patient undergoes ECLS therapy. Most variable costs are related to consumable goods such as single-use circuit components, pharmaceuticals, and blood products. These costs relate directly to the number of patients supported with ECLS and will rise or fall in direct proportion to service volume, patient complexity, and duration of support.

Despite wide variation in the mechanisms for financing healthcare around the world, there are fundamentally three sources of such revenue—individual patients, health insurers, or governments. Individual patients may be asked to bear the total cost of medical therapies such as ECLS in regions where the medical infrastructure is heterogenous and access is determined largely by free market principles, with little governmental regulation or support. Under such conditions, the total fixed and variable costs per patient for ECLS will typically exceed the financial means of all but the wealthiest. Both private companies and governmental entities may provide insurance that will reimburse healthcare systems for patient care. The reimbursement rates for a broad range of services including ECLS will usually be negotiated between the insurance company and the healthcare entity in advance. Such payment agreements often include stipulations for the appropriate use of particularly expensive or resource intense services. Healthcare professionals should ideally be involved in the creation of such agreements to ensure that the appropriate use criteria are medically reasonable. In some regions, healthcare is centrally funded by government as a public service, either in part or as a comprehensive offering. When government is the sole source of revenue for healthcare providers, the specific services that can be accessed by patients become a matter of public policy. Under such models, the exchange of information between regulators and healthcare professionals is critical to prioritizing resources.

## Costs

It is difficult to accurately estimate the true costs of an episode of healthcare due to many challenges associated with the reporting of costs. Within some healthcare systems, such as the United States, the most readily accessible financial data may be reported as charges. Unfortunately, charges are often closely linked to the structure of payment contracts and may have little or no relationship to actual costs. The internal accounting systems of hospitals may also make tracking the costs allocated to individual patients and services impossible. Even when granular healthcare cost data are available, they still may not accurately account for the total costs incurred by a specific type of care. Direct costs (consumable supplies) may have their acquisition cost linked to an episode of patient care, but indirect costs (equipment, support personnel, facility maintenance) may be simply and grossly divided between all patients cared for, or "rolled up" to specific departmental operating budgets.

With these limitations in mind, a recent systematic review identified 14 studies that reported hospital costs for ECLS for adults after cardiac arrest, post cardiotomy, cardiogenic shock, lung transplantation, and respiratory failure from Europe, the United States, Taiwan, Japan, and Australia.[2] The total reported hospital costs ranged from $22,305 to $334,608 (all costs converted to 2019 US dollars).[2] Reported costs were lower among those studies reporting costs for ECPR and were higher in studies reporting costs for patients with respiratory failure and lung transplantation.

These findings reveal several fundamental principles that can be applied broadly. First, the costs associated with ECLS equipment are high, representing between 11%-20% of the total costs for each hospitalization.[2] Next, labor costs associated with ECLS are also significant drivers of total costs (11%-52%).[2] Additionally, patient factors associated with increased costs include the need for mechanical ventilation, hospital length of stay, and in-hospital mortality.[2] The higher costs among those who die likely reflect the increased resources required to care for the sickest patients, both on and off ECLS, and they may also reflect the "sunk cost effect", when clinicians are hesitant to limit care after significant resources, time, and effort has been invested in a patient.[3]

While hospital costs for those who receive ECLS are high, economic evaluations must also consider the healthcare costs incurred by ECLS survivors after discharge over the remainder of their life. There are no published studies describing the lifetime healthcare costs for ECLS survivors. Previous research has demonstrated that ARDS survivors continue to have high healthcare costs up to 5 years after their critical illness.[4] We might infer the same for ECLS survivors, but the lack of long-term data for ECLS survivors is a critical knowledge gap.

## Outcomes

Expensive technologies can be justified if they result in significant improvements for both survival and quality of life. Unfortunately, there is limited data informing on long-term outcomes for ECLS survivors. The followup time for primary outcomes in the CESAR and EOLIA trials were both less than one year (6 month and 60 days respectively).[5,6] A systematic review of long-term outcomes for patients with respiratory failure who had received ECLS (prior to EOLIA) found that there was a paucity of published data describing these patients' long-term health related quality of life.[7] In analyses pooling data from 3 studies and 245 patients (116 who had received ECLS), and with follow up times ranging from 6-16 months, all survivors had poor long-term quality of life.[7] ECLS recipients had lower overall quality of life as measured by the SF-36 compared to non-ECLS survivors (MWD 5.40; 95% CI, 4.11-6.68).[7] Though a concerning finding, the pooled studies had significant qualitative heterogeneity, were observational, and reported outcomes for a small number of survivors. While there is limited evidence reporting long term data for ECLS survivors, there is a robust and growing body of evidence that clearly demonstrates significant reduction in quality of life and sustained functional disability among many survivors of critical care.[4,8-12] These outcomes data are likely applicable to those who receive ECLS, and they highlight the importance of considering long-term quality of life beyond merely survival when considering outcomes.

## The Quality Adjusted Life Year (QALY)

International best practice guidelines for the conduct of cost-effectiveness analyses recommend that health outcomes be measured using a standardized metric called the 'quality adjusted life year' or 'QALY'.[13] The QALY is a 'quality adjusted survival' score that incorporates both the length of time alive after an intervention, as well as the health-related quality of life (HRQoL) over that time. Health related quality of life is defined as "the value assigned to duration of life as modified by the impairments, functional states, perceptions, and social opportunities that are influenced by disease, injury, treatment, or policy."[14] To calculate QALYs, perfect health is assigned a value of 1 and death is assigned a value of 0. Preference-based weighted scores, or utility weights, are assigned to a range of potential states of health between 0 and 1.[15]

Preference-based utility weights can be derived through time tradeoff or standard gamble exercises with a random sample of individuals chosen from the public.[13] More commonly, they are elicited via indirect, generic, multi-attribute scales such as the EuroQol EQ-5D, the Health Utilities Index, or the SF-6D.[16-18] The EQ-5D, for example, asks respondents to score 5 dimensions of their quality of life (mobility, self-care, usual activities, pain/discomfort, anxiety) with 3 or 5 levels within each attribute.[16] Each potential response to the questionnaire describes a specific 'health state'.[16] Preference-based weightings or utility weights are available for each of the potential health states.

To calculate a QALY, the utility weight for a given health state is multiplied by the amount of time spent in that health state. For example, an individual alive for 1 year in a health state with a utility weight of 0.5, and 2 years in a health state with a utility weight of 0.3, will accumulate 1.1 QALYs over a three-year period.[13,16]

QALYs describe HRQoL in a way that allows decision makers to compare the health gains achieved between different health programs, eg, the number of QALYs gained by funding a new cancer therapy versus funding a new population-based immunization program. When health budgets are constrained, this information can help decision makers identify programs that have the potential to provide the greatest societal benefit.

QALYs are not perfect tools. They are criticized as being biased against the elderly and the disabled.[19] Some have criticized that community-based preference weights derived from the public may undervalue health states compared to the weights that would be elicited from those with lived experience in the health state.[13] Despite these criticisms, the QALY remains the preferred method for reporting health outcomes in economic evaluations because it provides decision-makers with a transparent, empirical, and robust framework within which to assess health outcomes and inform decisionmaking.[13,20]

**Assessing the Value of ECLS**

In scenarios where a technology has the potential to save a life, as with ECLS, international best practice guidelines recommend that value analyses consider the costs and health gains accumulated over a patient's lifetime.[13,20] The relative value is often quantified and reported as the incremental cost-effectiveness ratio (ICER), which reflects the relative costs and health gains between two therapies.[13,20] An

ICER reporting the cost utility of ECLS, for example, would be calculated according to the following formula:

(Total Costs ECMO–Total Costs Standard Therapy) / (Total QALYs ECMO–Total QALYs Standard Therapy)
 = Incremental Cost/QALY with ECMO

The ICER can be plotted on the cost-effectiveness plane (Figure 56-1) to assess its value. When new therapies are more effective and more costly than standard care, the ICER will fall in the upper right quadrant. In these cases, its cost effectiveness is judged against a willingness to pay (WTP) threshold, which is the amount of money a decisionmaker or society is willing to pay for a unit of health outcome.[21] If the cost per unit of a health gain is less than the WTP threshold, the technology could be considered cost effective.

Determining an appropriate "willingness to pay threshold" is challenging. Some jurisdictions use explicit thresholds. The UK National Institute for Health and Care Excellence uses a threshold of £30,000 (GBP) per QALY.[22] In North America, a value of approximately $50,000-$100,000 (USD) per QALY is often cited.[23] The World Health Organization's 2001 Commission on Macroeconomics in Health had suggested thresholds based on multiples of per capita gross domestic product; however, this suggestion has received criticism and was inappropriately interpreted by some as a blunt decision-tool.[24-26]

Some argue that the economics of these thresholds are flawed. Health economists in the UK aimed to identify the ideal WTP threshold considering the opportunity cost, ie, the marginal reductions in funds to extant health and social services resulting from investment in new technologies.[27] Their analysis suggested that a WTP threshold for the UK of £12,936/QALY would best balance the gains in health associated from new investments against the health losses from disinvestment in other areas.[27]

In addition to the uncertainty of the economics of explicit thresholds, analyses of societal value assessments for end-of-life care are mixed. A recent review identified 23 studies reporting societal value assessments for end-of-life care.[28] A premium for end-of-life care was reported in 8 studies, 4 had mixed results, and 11 demonstrated no increased value for end-of-life care.[28] A subsequent study demonstrated that societal value for end-of-life care varies by patient age, severity-of-illness, and the potential magnitude of QALY gain.[29]

The above data demonstrates the challenges associated with determining the appropriate WTP threshold for expensive, potentially life-saving therapies such as ECLS. Given its cost and use in patients who are critically ill and who might otherwise die, a WTP for ECLS must be determined regionally, considering local economic data, opportunity costs, and societal preferences.

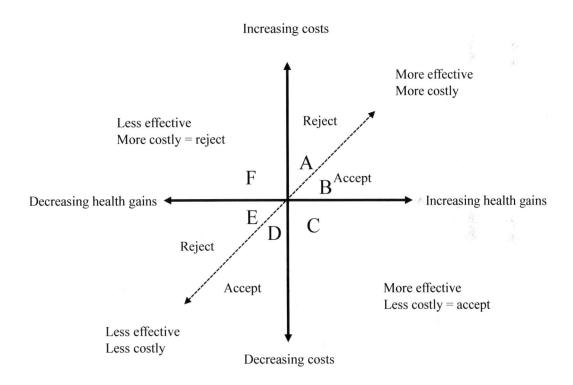

**Figure 56-1.** Incremental cost-effectiveness plane. Each of the quadrants on the cost-effectiveness plane represent potential combinations of incremental costs and incremental health gains associated with a new therapy compared to existing standard therapy. The dashed line represent a given willingness to pay threshold. The incremental cost-effectiveness ratio (ICER) can be plotted on this plane to determine its value. If the ICER falls in either plane C or F, it would be accepted or rejected, respectively. If the ICER is more costly and more effective and falls below the WTP threshold (B), its costs are acceptable, and it would be accepted. If the ICER falls above the WTP threshold (A), its relative costs for health gains are too high, and it would be rejected.

## Assessing the Cost Effectiveness of ECLS

There are a small number of published economic evaluations that report on the cost effectiveness of ECLS, which is dependent on local variables including local health system costs; labor costs; population health; societal preferences and values; and health system infrastructure, capacity, and quality. These studies cannot be taken at face value as transferable to other jurisdictions.

Evidence on the cost effectiveness of ECLS for newborns with hypoxemic respiratory failure was published in 2006. While now over 15 years old, this landmark trial randomized 185 newborns to either ECLS at one of the nation's four ECLS centers (n = 93), or conventional management (n = 92), and then followed the survivors up to 7 years of age.[30] The overall cost effectiveness of neonatal ECLS was expressed in terms of incremental cost per additional life year gained and incremental cost per additional disability-free life year gained. Mean health service costs during the first 7 years of life were £30,270 in the ECLS group and £10,229 in the conventional management group, generating a mean cost difference of £20,041 per patient that was statistically significant.[30] The incremental cost per life year gained was estimated at £13,385.[30] The incremental cost per disability-free life year gained was estimated at £23,566.[30]

The authors of the CESAR trial conducted a parallel economic evaluation alongside their clinical trial.[6,31] In their base-case analysis limited to clinical trial data with a 6-month time-horizon, the ICER for ECLS was £250,162/QALY.[6] The ICER for the life-time time-horizon, calculated using Markov modelling, was £19,252 (95% confidence interval £7622 to £59,200).[6] These results demonstrate that the ICER was sensitive to the time-horizon, and that the QALYs gained over the survivors' lifetime after ECLS were needed to make it cost effective.

A model-based economic evaluation identified similar results. ECLS was not cost effective in their analysis using a 5-year time horizon (ICER of $198,601(CAD)/QALY).[32] It was cost effective using a lifetime time-horizon (ICER $36,001(CAD)/QALY).[32] The authors of this evaluation concluded that ECLS is likely cost effective for adults with respiratory failure, but that it should only be considered in patients with a high likelihood of a good long-term functional outcome.

The use of ECLS in the setting of cardiopulmonary resuscitation (ECPR) is becoming more common and has been endorsed by the AHA.[33] It is not surprising that there have been several economic evaluations published relating to ECPR in the past several years. A Dutch study used Markov modelling to calculate incremental costs and QALYs up to 20 years after ECPR for in-hospital cardiac arrest (IHCA).[34] Their model parameters were informed by published data and they reported an ICER of €10,818/QALY.[34] Bharmal and colleagues used data from their US institution and reported an ICER of $56,156/QALY.[35] However, they only reported costs and outcomes up to hospital discharge and assumed 100% mortality in the comparator group.[35] A Japanese study used clinical trial data from the SAVE-J study, which evaluated outcomes for ECPR with out of hospital cardiac arrest (OHCA) and then modelled lifetime costs and QALYs.[36,37] They reported an ICER of ¥2,619,692/QALY with ECPR.[37] The Health Technology Assessment body in Ontario, Canada, conducted a health technology assessment of ECPR in 2020, and they reported an ICER of $18,722(CAD)/life year gained for IHCA, and $28,792(CAD)/life year gained for OHCA.[38] While these studies indicate that ECPR may be cost effective, successful ECPR programs require significant organization, training, and coordination of the ECPR teams.[39] The budget impact and additional costs required to support these programs have not been included in the above mentioned evaluations. More comprehensive evaluations that consider these system costs are needed to fully evaluate its cost effectiveness. Finally, inequitable access to ECPR as a result of differing geographical proximity to ECLS centers may influence assessments of the cost effectiveness of ECPR. It may have a lower relative societal value if access is not equitable across a region.

**Funding ECLS in Emerging Economies**

Emerging economies face the reality of having only limited or inadequate resources to bear the cost of ECLS, primarily due to low government spending as a percentage of GDP on healthcare. There is, however, significant economic heterogeneity between and within these emerging economies. Most patients rely on self-funding, external charitable organizations, or private healthcare models with limited insurance options.

In India, for example, medical tourism and public-private partnerships are becoming more popular and have contributed to the availability of bringing sophisticated healthcare including ECLS within the reach of many middle and lower income groups. In Thailand, the results of recent health technology assessments and increasing volumes have led to ECLS being reimbursed by the Universal Coverage Scheme. In Indonesia and the Philippines, ECLS is mainly limited to private hospitals, with some access to ECLS in government hospitals funded through hospital budgets with supplementation by universal health schemes.

Many patients in emerging economies have no health insurance, or only minimal coverage, and must therefore pay for health services out of pocket. To improve access, health systems in emerging economies must continually strive to reduce the cost wherever possible, without compromising the quality of care. Countries with large populations can take advantage of economies of scale. India's ECLS programs

are growing rapidly and the total number of ECLS centers has recently increased from 130 to 250. The COVID-19 pandemic has seen significant increases in volumes, including the transport of patients from remote locations for ECLS support, conversions of existing units to ECLS units, and even the use of ECLS to bridge to lung transplant.[40] The expansion of ECLS services in India and other emerging economies has required a careful and strategic approach to the cost of consumables for it to be both accessible and sustainable in the long term. For example, an Indian hospital with a large cardiac surgery program and a high volume ECLS program successfully negotiated lower prices for their consumables given their volume of ECLS cases. This center further reduced costs by adapting ECLS circuits to use locally available products while still adhering to international standards. They have now performed over one thousand ECLS runs over the last 15 years at a substantially reduced cost.

Highly trained personnel are also crucial to the success of ECLS programs in emerging economies. Many of these ECLS centers are led by clinicians who received their ECLS training abroad and who subsequently return and train local staff. Some centers have also adapted staffing models based on local labor markets. Flórez et al. recently reported a successful cost-effective model of care in Columbia, with nurses trained as ECLS specialists supported by a multidisciplinary team.[41] This 'lean' staffing model was combined with reduced (and simpler) circuitry and laboratory monitoring to further reduce costs.

Through reducing the costs of consumables, employing economies of scale, and utilizing alternative reimbursement schemes, ECLS is becoming increasingly available for those living in emerging economies.

## Conclusions

There is a growing body of evidence demonstrating that ECLS is a high-value therapy, with the potential to save lives. Even in emerging economies with a lower per capita GDP, efforts to reduce costs are helping to increase access to this technology. The relative value of ECLS must be determined locally because its value will be highly dependent on the local economy, health system characteristics, societal values and preferences, and the opportunity costs associated with funding ECLS. Patient selection is a key driver of value: the costs associated with the therapy are likely justified when there is the potential for a significant number of QALYs and life years gained. The lack of data on long-term HRQoL and costs for ECLS survivors is a crucial knowledge gap and an important area for future research.

# References

1. Thiagarajan RR, Barbaro RP, Rycus PT, et al. Extracorporeal Life Support Organization Registry International Report 2016. Asaio J. 2017;63(1):60-67.

2. Lansink-Hartgring AO, Minnen O van, Vermeulen KM, et al. Hospital Costs of Extracorporeal Membrane Oxygenation in Adults: A Systematic Review. Pharmacoeconomics - Open. 2021;5(4):613-623.

3. Arkes HR, Blumer C. The psychology of sunk cost. Organ Behav Hum Dec. 1985;35(1):124-140.

4. Herridge MS, Tansey CM, Matte A, et al. Functional disability 5 years after acute respiratory distress syndrome. N Engl J Med. 2011;364(14):1293-1304.

5. Combes A, Hajage D, Capellier G, et al. Extracorporeal Membrane Oxygenation for Severe Acute Respiratory Distress Syndrome: Supplementary Appendix. NEJM. 2018;378(21):1965-1975.

6. Peek GJ, Mugford M, Tiruvoipati R, et al. Efficacy and economic assessment of conventional ventilatory support versus extracorporeal membrane oxygenation for severe adult respiratory failure (CESAR): a multicentre randomised controlled trial. The Lancet. 2009;374(9698):1351-1363.

7. Wilcox ME, Jaramillo-Rocha V, Hodgson C, et al. Long-Term Quality of Life After Extracorporeal Membrane Oxygenation in ARDS Survivors: Systematic Review and Meta-Analysis. Journal of Intensive Care Medicine. 2017;369(6):088506661773703-088506661773711.

8. Hofhuis JGM, Schrijvers AJP, Schermer T, et al. Health-related quality of life in ICU survivors—10 years later. Sci Rep-uk. 2021;11(1):15189.

9. Herridge MS, Chu LM, Matte A, et al. The RECOVER Program: Disability Risk Groups and 1-Year Outcome after 7 or More Days of Mechanical Ventilation. Am J Resp Crit Care. 2016;194(7):831-844.

10. Shankar-Hari M, Rubenfeld GD. Understanding Long-Term Outcomes Following Sepsis: Implications and Challenges. Curr Infect Dis Rep. 2016;18(11):37.

11. Herridge MS, Batt J, Santos CD. ICU-acquired weakness, morbidity, and death. Am J Resp Crit Care. 2014;190(4):360-362.

12. Hodgson CL, Hayes K, Everard T, et al. Long-term quality of life in patients with acute respiratory distress syndrome requiring extracorporeal membrane oxygenation for refractory hypoxaemia. Critical Care. 2012;16(5):R202.

13. Neumann PJ, Sanders GD, Russell LB, Siegel JE, Ganiats TG. Cost-Effectiveness in Health and Medicine Second Edition. Oxford University Press; 2016.

14. Patrick DL, Erickson P. Health Status and Health Policy: Quality of Life in Health Care Evaluation and Resource Allocation. Oxford University Press; 1993.

15. Sinnott P, Joyce V, Barnett P. Preference Measurement in Economics Analysis. Guidebook. Menlo Park VA. VA Palo Alto, Health Economics Resource Center; 2007.

16. Rabin R, Charro F de. EQ-5D: a measure of health status from the EuroQol Group. Ann Med. 2009;33(5):337-343. doi:10.3109/07853890109002087

17. Horsman J, Furlong W, Feeny D, et al. The Health Utilities Index (HUI®): concepts, measurement properties and applications. Health Qual Life Out. 2003;1(1):54.

18. Brazier J, Roberts J, Deverill M. The estimation of a preference-based measure of health from the SF-36. Journal of Health Economics. 2002;21(2):271-292. http://pubmed.gov/11939242.

19. Neumann PJ, Cohen JT. QALYs in 2018—Advantages and Concerns. JAMA. Published online May 24, 2018:1-2.

20. Sanders GD, Neumann PJ, Basu A, et al. Recommendations for Conduct, Methodological Practices, and Reporting of Cost-effectiveness Analyses: Second Panel on Cost-Effectiveness in Health and Medicine. JAMA. 2016;316(10):1093-1103.

21. Consortium YHE. Cost-Effectiveness Threshold [online]. https://yhec.co.uk/glossary/cost-effectiveness-threshold/.

22. Excellence NI for H and C. Guide to the Methods of Technology Appraisal 2013. Published April 4, 2013. nice.org.uk/process/pmg9.

23. Neumann PJ, Cohen JT, Weinstein MC. Updating Cost-Effectiveness — The Curious Resilience of the $50,000-per-QALY Threshold. NEJM. 2014;371(9):796-797.

24. Marseille E, Larson B, Kazi DS, et al. Thresholds for the cost–effectiveness of interventions: alternative approaches. Bull World Health Organ. 2014;93(2):118-124.

25. Bertram MY, Lauer JA, Stenberg K, et al. Methods for the Economic Evaluation of Health Care Interventions for Priority Setting in the Health System: An Update From WHO CHOICE. Int J Heal Policy Management. 2021;10(11):673-677.

26. Macroeconomics and Health: Investing in Health for Economic Development. Report of the Commission on Macroeconomics and Health. World Health Organization; 2001:552. http://apps.who.int/iris/bitstream/10665/42435/1/924154550X.pdf.

27. Claxton K, Martin S, Soares M, et al. Methods for the estimation of the National Institute for Health and Care Excellence cost-effectiveness threshold. Health Technol Assess. 2015;19(14):1-503-v-vi.

28. Shah KK, Tsuchiya A, Wailoo AJ. Valuing health at the end of life: A review of stated preference studies in the social sciences literature. Soc Sci Med. 2018;204:39-50.

29. Reckers-Droog V, Exel J van, et al. Willingness to Pay for Health-Related Quality of Life Gains in Relation to Disease Severity and the Age of Patients. Value Heal J Int Soc Pharmacoeconomics Outcomes Res. 2021;24(8):1182-1192.

30. Petrou S, Bischof M, Bennett C, et al. Cost-Effectiveness of Neonatal Extracorporeal Membrane Oxygenation Based on 7-Year Results From the United Kingdom Collaborative ECMO Trial. Pediatrics. 2006;117(5):1640-1649.

31. Peek G, Elbourne D, Mugford M, et al. Randomised controlled trial and parallel economic evaluation of conventional ventilatory support versus extracorporeal membrane oxygenation for severe adult respiratory failure (CESAR). Health Technol Asses. 2010;14(35):1-46.

32. Barrett KA, Hawkins N, Fan E. Economic Evaluation of Venovenous Extracorporeal Membrane Oxygenation for Severe Acute Respiratory Distress Syndrome. Crit Care Med. 2019;47(2):186-193.

33. Panchal AR, Bartos JA, Cabañas JG, et al. Part 3: Adult Basic and Advanced Life Support: 2020 American Heart Association Guidelines for Cardiopulmonary Resuscitation and Emergency Cardiovascular Care. Circulation. 2020;142(16_suppl_2):S366-S468.

34. Gravesteijn BY, Schluep M, Voormolen DC, et al. Cost-effectiveness of extracorporeal cardiopulmonary resuscitation after in-hospital cardiac arrest: A Markov decision model. Resuscitation. 2019;143:150-157.

35. Bharmal MI, Venturini JM, Chua RFM, et al. Cost-utility of extracorporeal cardiopulmonary resuscitation in patients with cardiac arrest. Resuscitation. 2019;136:126-130.

36. Sakamoto T, Morimura N, Nagao K, et al. Extracorporeal cardiopulmonary resuscitation versus conventional cardiopulmonary resuscitation in adults with out-of-hospital cardiac arrest: a prospective observational study. Resuscitation. 2014;85(6):762-768.

37. Matsuoka Y, Goto R, Atsumi T, et al. Cost-effectiveness of extracorporeal cardiopulmonary resuscitation for out-of-hospital cardiac arrest: A multi-centre prospective cohort study. Resuscitation. 2020;157:32-38.

38. Extracorporeal membrane oxygenation for cardiac indications in adults: a health technology assessment. Ontario Health Technology Assessment Series. 2020;8(20).

39. Hutin A, Loosli F, Lamhaut L, et al. How Physicians Perform PreHospital ECMO on the Streets of Paris. Journal of Emergency Medical Services. Published online 2017. https://www.jems.com/patient-care/how-physicians-perform-prehospital-ecmo-on-the-streets-of-paris/

40. Bharat A, Machuca TN, Querrey M, et al. Early outcomes after lung transplantation for severe COVID-19: a series of the first consecutive cases from four countries. Lancet Respir Medicine. 2021;9(5):487-497.

41. Flórez CX, Bermon A, Castillo VR, Salazar L. Setting Up an ECMO Program in a South American Country: Outcomes of the First 104 Pediatric Patients. World J Pediatric Congenit Hear Surg. 2015;6(3):374-381.

# 57

## Ethics

*Alexander Supady, Darryl Abrams, Katie Moynihan, Wynne Morrison, Xiaotong Hou, Thomas Bein, Daniel Brodie*

### Introduction

In addition to the various clinical and technical aspects of providing ECLS support described throughout this book, those using ECLS in their patients will also be faced with challenging ethical questions. These ethical dilemmas may pertain to the indication and selection of patients eligible for ECLS using a limited evidence base; the need to make decisions of great consequence to patients under time constraints and with varying degrees of uncertainty about history or prognosis; the definition of treatment goals; or the provision of ECLS in situations of resource limitations, as many centers have experienced during the COVID-19 pandemic, among others. These issues apply across all forms of ECLS, while some are more specific. For instance, unique and difficult questions and challenging situations arise specifically from the use of ECLS in children. In this chapter, we will review some of the key ethical questions that practitioners may encounter. By its very nature, this exercise cannot cover all potential scenarios that clinicians will confront during the use of ECLS across adult, pediatric, and neonatal populations and in the setting of the use of VV ECMO, VA ECMO or ECPR, nor can we give definitive answers to most questions. The main goal is to build awareness around the existence of the issues and to inform an ethical approach to these patients.

### Challenges with Patient Selection

A strong evidence base defining the criteria for or against the use of ECLS in individual patients is lacking for VA ECMO and particularly for ECPR, and to a lesser extent for VV ECMO, although the evidence base is growing.[1-10] This is even more true for pediatric patients.[11-15] Therefore, current guidelines still cannot provide absolute certainty surrounding the indications and contraindications for ECMO use.[16-19]

ECLS is offered as part of routine clinical care in some clinical scenarios and settings. Nevertheless, considering the resources that are required to provide ECLS and the uneven distribution of those resources throughout the world, it cannot be available for the treatment of all cases of severe respiratory or cardiac failure in which it is technically indicated. Consequently, in addition to medical criteria, ethical issues, as well as issues of equity, will arise at times in the decision for or against ECLS.

Patients may be able to survive with ongoing ECLS support for weeks or even months. ECLS is not a therapy in the strictest sense, but merely a temporary support option to replace the gas exchange function of the lungs or to attempt to establish and maintain adequate blood circulation, normally provided by the heart. At present, ECLS requires ongoing care be provided in an ICU, therefore, it is most commonly initiated as a bridging measure under one of four conditions; bridge to recovery when organ failure is potentially reversible; bridge to transplant when the patient is eligible for transplantation; bridge to bridge or bridge to device when the patient is eligible for temporary or durable left ventricular assist device (LVAD); or bridge to decision in cases of uncertain prognosis or to facilitate decision-making when the best interests or patient's preferences are uncertain. If ECLS is considered an appropriate support option by the clinical treatment team, it is equally important to involve the patients and surrogate decision-makers in the decision-making process as early as possible.[20,21]

In situations where there is no hope of achieving any of the desired outcomes, ECLS support is not indicated and should therefore not be initiated. In any individual case, the potential benefits and known risks of ECLS must be weighed against each other and the likelihood of any expected short- and long-term outcomes should be determined, to whatever degree that is possible, with guidance from prognostic scores or models, where they exist.[22-26]

### Indications for ECLS in Individual Patients

Medical activities provided by physicians to patients should be guided by two major principles: indication and an individual patient's values and preferences.[27] Indication refers to a rational clinical justification for treatment decisions. Each diagnostic or therapeutic procedure should be based on the careful assessment of the chance for recovery with or without the specific measure, such as ECLS. This assessment should consider the prospects for a certain quality of life and the degree to which therapeutic goals are in accordance with the values and preferences of the individual patient.

In contrast to this, some suggest the use of ECLS as a salvage therapy or *ultima ratio* (or "last resort") support option, even without careful consideration of the prospects for recovery.[28] *Ultima ratio* use of ECLS might leapfrog a careful and ethically valued decision, thus contributing to injudicious use of ECLS in critically ill patients.

The indication for ECLS for the individual patient should be based on a careful assessment of all relevant demographic, medical, and prognostic parameters to avoid nonbeneficial treatments and high ECLS-associated mortality rates.[29] However, even when taking all relevant information into account, individual prognostication is extremely challenging, leaving treating physicians with a high degree of uncertainty surrounding indications.

### Center Characteristics and Patient Logistics

According to several retrospective analyses, survival of patients supported with ECLS may depend on the experience of the centers and the number of ECLS runs performed at these centers.[30-32] The randomized controlled trial Efficacy and Economic Assessment of Conventional Ventilatory Support Versus Extracorporeal Membrane Oxygenation for Severe Adult Respiratory Failure (CESAR) concluded that referral of a patient to an ECLS center improved survival over conventional management at centers not providing ECLS support as part of a comprehensive support algorithm for acute respiratory failure.[5] Therefore, to provide equitable access to the best possible therapy for the maximum possible number of patients, hospitals should consider organizing themselves formally or informally into a so-called hub-and-spoke system, in which patients can be transferred to an ECLS center, if indicated.[31,33]

### Challenges Specific to ECPR

The prognosis of patients undergoing cardiopulmonary resuscitation (CPR) is uncertain and this is equally true for ECPR.[34] ECPR is particularly resource-intensive, and any ECPR program implies significant training needs in addition to high staffing and sophisticated technical requirements.[35] This effort may also touch on important issues of distributive justice, as resources needed for ECPR may be lacking in some areas.[36]

Decisions for or against ECPR often must be made in a high-pressure environment, with considerable time constraints and a high degree of uncertainty about history or prognosis. Moreover, it can be very difficult – and in many cases even impossible – to elicit with reasonable certainty the patients' presumed preferences in such a situation.[37] Consequently, when ECPR is initially able to establish circulation, the ongoing support with VA ECMO in these patients is often intended as a bridge to decision. Yet, like in other contexts of ECMO use, this can lead to a "bridge to nowhere" situation, when a patient may be stabilized with ongoing ECMO support, but recovery, durable device support, or organ transplantation are not options. Therefore, in patients who have undergone ECPR, provisions should be made for these scenarios, including early communication surrounding goals of the therapy, anticipated milestones, frequent updates on progress towards the goals and discussions with the patients' surrogate decision-makers that include discussion of discontinuation of support devices that are no longer clinically beneficial.[38-41]

Many patients supported with ECPR will eventually die in hospital. Survival of patients receiving ECPR is approximately 30% after in-hospital cardiac arrest (IHCA) and only 10% after out-of-hospital cardiac arrest, although selected reports suggest more favorable outcomes may be possible for selected patients with the investment of considerable resources.[8,42] Therefore, treatment and care for patients after ECPR is not only resource intense but it also creates moral distress among the staff that may be further aggravated if the treatment is not felt to be ultimately beneficial to the patient. Families are also often in crisis in the emergent situations where ECLS is required, leading to a need for even greater staff support. These pressures can lead to overwork and burnout among healthcare workers, ultimately resulting in the loss and further depletion of this important, but scarce resource.[43] For these reasons, it may be reasonable for a society to recognize a special responsibility or ethical obligation for the wellbeing of healthcare workers.[44]

### Challenges for Performing ECLS During a Crisis

The need for ECLS as a support option may increase considerably during a crisis, as experienced during the COVID-19 pandemic, and the demand for ECLS may exceed available resources and ultimately rationing may be required.[45,46] On the other hand, there are severe structural inequalities, both within countries and between countries. Globally, there is large variation in access to advanced medical emergency and critical care resources.[47-50]

In the first instance, governments, legislatures, and health administrators are responsible for ensuring that sufficient health care resources are available to meet the needs of the population.[10] Responsible planning must also consider that localized and temporary emergencies can occur, and the need for resources may exceed everyday needs. During the COVID-19 pandemic, large numbers of patients suffering from severe respiratory failure have been treated in ICUs, many of whom were supported with ECLS.[31,51-55] At times, conventional standards of care could not be maintained, and contingency or even crisis standards of care had to be invoked.[56-58]

ECLS was of particular importance because it was increasingly needed for the most severe forms of the disease. However, due to the special resource requirements, increasing use of ECLS may well have an impact on the ability to care for other, less seriously ill patients with potentially better prognoses.[10]

Prior to developing practical approaches to balancing resources between ECLS, mechanical ventilation and other resource-intensive support options, community consensus should be reached with respect to prioritization of ethical principles, including outcome-oriented utilitarian principles and rights-oriented egalitarian principles as the basis for rationing decisions.[36,45,59] Any indicated treatment or support option that would be routinely available under conventional standards of care should not be withheld or reduced under crisis standards of care merely because of its resource demand. Instead, the provision or limitation of any treatment must be balanced against the background of the ethical principles agreed upon.[45] These considerations should also apply when allocating limited resources between VV and VA ECMO support and the provision of ECPR during crisis.[60]

Rationing decisions for the individual patient that may lead to the initiation of ECLS or to the decision to postpone or even withhold ECLS must be made by the treating clinicians at the bedside. However, they should be able to rely on a set of guiding principles and standards, mutually agreed upon in a process of fair and transparent deliberation considering the roles and perspectives of all relevant stakeholders.[10,61]

In addition to focusing on the care of current patients, it is important to also keep an eye on future patients. Therefore, it is absolutely necessary to collect and evaluate clinical data and survival data from past treatments as well as to scrutinize pressing research questions, eg, on indication and selection of suitable patients, within well-designed prospective studies.

As already discussed above in the context of ECPR, the psychological and moral distress of physicians and other healthcare workers caused by rationing decisions must be taken into consideration.[44,62]

Finally, structural poverty and global inequities pose challenges with respect to equitable access to required resources. In many low- and middle-income countries, large parts of the population are without access to even basic emergency and critical care resources due to limited availability.[47-50,63-65] Where available, the quality of services is often inadequate and far below the level that is expected as standard of care in high-income countries and access may be limited to those able to afford to pay for the services out of pocket.[66] Consequently, many that would benefit from ECLS do not have access to such a therapy.[67]

## Challenges with Withdrawal of ECLS Support

The decision to initiate ECLS must sometimes be made under emergency conditions characterized by time constraints and uncertainty. In these situations, relevant data is not always available for a thorough assessment of prognosis, and it is only after initiation of ECLS that it becomes apparent that the prognosis may be poorer than initially expected and continuation of therapy may no longer be considered reasonable. To facilitate a "good death" it may be necessary to align treatment goals with end-of-life planning, establish escalation limits, and ultimately agree on ECLS decannulation and withdrawal of other life-sustaining therapies in regions where this is considered legally and ethically acceptable.[41,68,69]

Similar challenges may arise when patients receive ECLS as a bridge to recovery or bridge to transplant and the expected prognosis has changed since ECLS was started and recovery is no longer deemed possible, or transplantation is no longer an option.[70] In such a situation, often described as a "bridge to nowhere," discontinuation of ECLS should be discussed with the patient or surrogate decision-maker. Although there is general agreement that withholding and withdrawing life-sustaining therapy are ethically equivalent, these decisions will occasionally be very difficult in clinical practice.[38-40]

It is conceivable that a conscious patient may not agree with the discontinuation of ECLS and termination of therapy despite detailed explanations of the prognosis by the treating physicians. In such a case, ECLS should not be discontinued against the patient's declared wish. However, patients and their surrogates are often overwhelmed by the situation and could therefore overlook important issues. It is therefore crucial that patients are not simply faced with the choice of whether or not to continue ECLS support. Instead, it is critical to support a patient through the decision-making process and collaboratively develop a comprehensive treatment plan that can be revised over time in light of the patient's individual wishes, values, goals and preferences, and clinical condition.[21,38] It is legitimate for the treating physicians to recommend discontinuation of treatment that can no longer be considered beneficial.[15,41,68,69,71] It may help a patient to understand that the choice may be between a controlled and comfortable removal of technology with family present vs. awaiting a more emergent and chaotic clinical deterioration or mechanical malfunction where the circumstances are harder to control.[69]

However, decision-making may be different for a patient who is unable to express his or her wishes, and therefore a surrogate decision-maker, representing the patient and acting in the patient's best interest, helps to define the goals and values of the patient as they pertain to the ongoing level of care. If recovery or any other therapeutic goal outside the ICU cannot reasonably be expected, and the continuation of ECLS may merely prolong suffering, treating physicians have reasonable arguments not to delay the patient's death and recommend discontinuation of ECLS, once again, as is appropriate to local customs.[38] In such cases, where the surrogate decision-maker does not agree with discontinuation of therapy, local laws and customs will dictate whether discontinuation of ECLS may proceed.

According to classical thinking for treating competent adults, the treating physicians are primarily obligated to their patients and not to the patients' surrogates. This perspective, however, is challenged by the concept of relational autonomy, arguing that individuals, their preferences and choices, and their decisions are interconnected with and influenced by their cultural environment and their relationships with close relatives and peers.[72,73] The concept of relational autonomy thus acknowledges the importance and the interests of individuals other than the affected patient alone in making decisions about life and death.

In practice, sometimes it may be difficult to reach consensus between the surrogate decision-makers and the treating physicians. Standard patient advance directives frequently cannot give specific enough guidance for decision-making in these situations. Instead, before initiation of ECLS, when obtaining informed consent, the likelihood of such situations in which it may be medically and ethically appropriate to withdraw ECLS support may be described and patients or their surrogates could, at the very least, have a discussion about the discontinuation of ECLS support framed in a way that facilitates later discussions.[41,74] Nonetheless, the resolution of conflicts in these cases will depend heavily on local laws and customs. In these challenging cases, consultation by specialists in ethics and palliative care may be very valuable for all parties involved.

## *Role of Palliative Care Teams and Ethics Consultations*

Discontinuation of ECLS support in patients with no prospect of recovery can be emotionally charged and stressful for the patient, their family members, and the healthcare workers involved. This is particularly true when patients have been treated for a long period of time and personal bonds have developed between caregivers and the patient and surrogates. In such situations, palliative care consultations may be a valuable resource to help support the parties involved and reduce moral distress.[75] When there are perceived challenges with shared decision-making, the goals of care, or specific ethical questions, additional layers of support may be required, eg, in "bridge to nowhere" situations when patients or relatives struggle to accept the hopelessness of the situation.[20,21,76]

### Challenges Specific to ECLS in Children

ECLS support in children brings additional challenges with important clinical implications and nuances for ethical decision-making.[15] With medical and technological advances, pediatric ECLS use has expanded to include high-risk diagnoses and medically complex patients previously considered unsuitable, with formally accepted absolute contraindications now loosely applied or outdated.[12,14] Marked variability exists between providers in their willingness to offer ECLS despite similar severity of illness, creating considerable heterogeneity in indications for support across pediatric populations and variable outcomes for different etiologies limiting capacity for evidence-based prognostication.[11,13,77-80] Pediatric healthcare providers also vary in their desire for medical decisional authority regarding ECLS.[11,13] These clinical issues contribute to ethical dilemmas surrounding ECLS candidacy and discontinuation in children, and underpin why no data-driven decision-support framework currently informs pediatric ECLS decision-making.[15]

It is imperative that ethical considerations specific to children be integrated into ECLS decision-making. First, as most children lack decisional capacity or predefined wishes, the ethical framework most used is the best interest standard. Parents are typically the default decision-makers and collaborate with the medical team in a shared decision-making process to determine those best interests.[21] Substituted judgment is a more common standard for adult patients, where surrogates attempt to judge what the previously autonomous adult would have chosen for themselves.[71] The burdens of decision-making for surrogates may feel different when a substituted judgment framework cannot apply. Second, childhood is also dynamic. The ethical obligation to include children in informed consent, or assent, and decision-making processes varies with developmental status and local custom.[81] An older or more mature child's opinions are important, even when not legally binding, especially when less emergent cases allow for deliberation. Third, pediatric life and death situations are particularly distressing as childhood death violates the natural cycle of one generation preceding the next into death.[71] With pediatric intensive care mortality rates in high-income countries below 3%, survival is expected even in the setting of critical illness.[82]

Furthermore, overlying the clinical complexity is the legal authority and substantial deference afforded to parents or other caregivers in decision-making.[83,84] Although the child's interests are primary, family interests are entwined. This requires thoughtful consideration of the child and family as an interdependent unit. Integration of the parent or other caregiver into decision-making requires effective partnerships between the interdisciplinary critical care team, caregivers, and the patient.[81] This introduces potential for conflict over differential perceptions of benefits and burdens, and acceptability of different outcomes.[15] Growing societal awareness of ECLS as a therapeutic option and high-profile media cases increasing public scrutiny on medical decisions add to the challenges in pediatric (as well as adult) ECLS support.[85-87]

## Challenges with Determining and Declaring Death

As the use of ECLS becomes more widespread, complex questions are emerging about the definitions of life and death, along with the role of extracorporeal interval support for organ retrieval (EISOR) from the deceased. With ongoing ECLS support, it is possible to stabilize patients who would not otherwise survive. Consequently, beyond the dilemmas regarding the "bridge to nowhere" discussed above, concerns may arise as to when to declare death, as ECLS may confound the traditional declaration of cardiocirculatory death.

There is broad consensus that all life support therapies have to be stopped when a patient fulfills criteria for brain death.[88] Yet it may be difficult to decide about continuation or discontinuation of treatment in more ambiguous settings, when criteria for brain death are not met, but prognosis is considered very poor and the likelihood of regaining consciousness, interacting with others, and once again participating in meaningful activities is deemed to be prohibitively low.

It is similarly difficult to decide when vital organs may be procured and donated to another patient. The widely accepted "Dead Donor Rule" (DDR) defines that the procurement of vital organs is only possible after the donor's death has been confirmed, ie, the recovery of organs must not precede or promote the onset of death.[89] This condition is fulfilled when brain death criteria are met (donation after brain death, DBD).[88]

Beyond this, organ donation after circulatory determination of death (DCDD) has been proposed. For declaration of death, DCDD requires a predefined duration of apnea and cessation of circulation to comply with the DDR.[90] However, it remains controversial whether it is possible to determine the irreversibility of death with reasonable certainty after 2-5 minutes of cessation of circulation, as may be used across programs for "controlled DCDD" (organ donation after a patient's or a surrogate's decision to withdraw life sustaining therapy).[90] Similar concerns relate to the conditions for "uncontrolled DCDD" (organ donation after unsuccessful cardiopulmonary resuscitation). A recent analysis revealed overlap between protocols for uncontrolled DCDD and ECPR, raising the possibility of a small but important risk of declaring patients eligible for organ donation even though their lives might yet be saved by ECPR, at least in theory.[91] Extreme care is therefore essential to distinguish efforts that might still save the patient from clinical interventions undertaken purely for organ support.

After circulatory determination of death, ECLS may be used for ongoing perfusion of organs in situ in order to preserve the quality of vital organs before transplantation (Chapter 45).[92] In order to best satisfy the will of the donor, one may argue that the highest possible organ quality should be ensured, and this may well be achieved through ECLS-facilitated organ perfusion.[92] Yet, the evidence supporting the effectiveness of ECLS in this context is still lacking.[93]

## Conclusions

Despite the high resource requirements and considerable demands on the treatment teams, the use of ECLS has been increasing globally for years.[94] ECLS entails complex decision-making for selection of patients, and a careful appreciation for indications, prognostication, and discontinuation of therapy when recovery of a patient no longer can be expected. Throughout this process, ethical issues and dilemmas occur and need to be addressed by the responsible providers at the bedside. Although many questions cannot be definitively answered at this time, open discussion of salient ethical issues within treatment teams and with patients, family members, and surrogate decision-makers can help reduce emotional burdens and moral distress.

# References

1. Combes A, Hajage D, Capellier G, et al. Extracorporeal Membrane Oxygenation for Severe Acute Respiratory Distress Syndrome. N Engl J Med. May 24 2018;378(21):1965-1975.
2. Combes A, Peek GJ, Hajage D, et al. ECMO for severe ARDS: systematic review and individual patient data meta-analysis. Intensive Care Med. Nov 2020;46(11):2048-2057.
3. Goligher EC, Tomlinson G, Hajage D, et al. Extracorporeal Membrane Oxygenation for Severe Acute Respiratory Distress Syndrome and Posterior Probability of Mortality Benefit in a Post Hoc Bayesian Analysis of a Randomized Clinical Trial. JAMA. Dec 4 2018;320(21):2251-2259.
4. Munshi L, Walkey A, Goligher E, et al. Venovenous extracorporeal membrane oxygenation for acute respiratory distress syndrome: a systematic review and meta-analysis. Lancet Respir Med. Feb 2019;7(2):163-172.
5. Peek GJ, Mugford M, Tiruvoipati R, et al. Efficacy and economic assessment of conventional ventilatory support versus extracorporeal membrane oxygenation for severe adult respiratory failure (CESAR): a multicentre randomised controlled trial. Lancet. Oct 17 2009;374(9698):1351-63.
6. Lunz D, Calabro L, Belliato M, et al. Extracorporeal membrane oxygenation for refractory cardiac arrest: a retrospective multicenter study. Intensive Care Med. May 2020;46(5):973-982.
7. Bougouin W, Dumas F, Lamhaut L, et al. Extracorporeal cardiopulmonary resuscitation in out-of-hospital cardiac arrest: a registry study. Eur Heart J. Jun 1 2020;41(21):1961-1971.
8. Yannopoulos D, Bartos J, Raveendran G, et al. Advanced reperfusion strategies for patients with out-of-hospital cardiac arrest and refractory ventricular fibrillation (ARREST): a phase 2, single centre, open-label, randomised controlled trial. Lancet. Dec 5 2020;396(10265):1807-1816.
9. Guglin M, Zucker MJ, Bazan VM, et al. Venoarterial ECMO for Adults: JACC Scientific Expert Panel. J Am Coll Cardiol. Feb 19 2019;73(6):698-716.
10. Supady A, Curtis JR, Abrams D, et al. Allocating scarce intensive care resources during the COVID-19 pandemic: practical challenges to theoretical frameworks. Lancet Respir Med. Apr 2021;9(4):430-434.
11. Chapman RL, Peterec SM, Bizzarro MJ, et al. Patient selection for neonatal extracorporeal membrane oxygenation: beyond severity of illness. J Perinatol. Sep 2009;29(9):606-11.
12. Coleman RD, Goldman J, Moffett B, et al. Extracorporeal Membrane Oxygenation Mortality in High-Risk Populations: An Analysis of the Pediatric Health Information System Database. Asaio j. Mar 2020;66(3):327-331.
13. Kuo KW, Barbaro RP, Gadepalli SK, et al. Should Extracorporeal Membrane Oxygenation Be Offered? An International Survey. J Pediatr. Mar 2017;182:107-113.
14. Steppan DA, Coleman RD, Viamonte HK, et al. Outcomes of pediatric patients with oncologic disease or following hematopoietic stem cell transplant supported on extracorporeal membrane oxygenation: The PEDECOR experience. Pediatr Blood Cancer. Oct 2020;67(10):e28403.
15. Moynihan KM, Dorste A, Siegel BD, et al. Decision-Making, Ethics, and End-of-Life Care in Pediatric Extracorporeal Membrane Oxygenation: A Comprehensive Narrative Review. Pediatr Crit Care Med. Sep 1 2021;22(9):806-812.
16. Tonna JE, Abrams D, Brodie D, et al. Management of Adult Patients Supported with Venovenous Extracorporeal Membrane Oxygenation (VV ECMO): Guideline from the Extracorporeal Life Support Organization (ELSO). ASAIO J. Jun 1 2021;67(6):601-610.
17. Lorusso R, Shekar K, MacLaren G, et al. ELSO Interim Guidelines for Venoarterial Extracorporeal Membrane Oxygenation in Adult Cardiac Patients. Asaio j. Aug 1 2021;67(8):827-844.
18. Maratta C, Potera RM, van Leeuwen G, et al. Extracorporeal Life Support Organization (ELSO): 2020 Pediatric Respiratory ELSO Guideline. Asaio j. Sep/Oct 2020;66(9):975-979.
19. Wild KT, Rintoul N, Kattan J, Gray B. Extracorporeal Life Support Organization (ELSO): Guidelines for Neonatal Respiratory Failure. Asaio j. May 2020;66(5):463-470.
20. Bein T, Brodie D. Understanding ethical decisions for patients on extracorporeal life support. Intensive Care Med. Oct 2017;43(10):1510-1511.
21. Kon AA, Davidson JE, Morrison W, et al. Shared Decision Making in ICUs: An American College of Critical Care Medicine and American Thoracic Society Policy Statement. Crit Care Med. Jan 2016;44(1):188-201.
22. Schmidt M, Bailey M, Sheldrake J, et al. Predicting survival after extracorporeal membrane oxygenation for severe acute respiratory failure. The Respiratory Extracorporeal Membrane Oxygenation Survival Prediction (RESP) score. Am J Respir Crit Care Med. Jun 1 2014;189(11):1374-82.
23. Schmidt M, Burrell A, Roberts L, et al. Predicting survival after ECMO for refractory cardiogenic shock: the survival after veno-arterial-ECMO (SAVE)-score. Eur Heart J. Sep 1 2015;36(33):2246-56.

24. Schmidt M, Zogheib E, Roze H, et al. The PRESERVE mortality risk score and analysis of long-term outcomes after extracorporeal membrane oxygenation for severe acute respiratory distress syndrome. Intensive Care Med. Oct 2013;39(10):1704-13.

25. Rilinger J, Krötzsch K, Bemtgen X, et al. Long-term survival and health-related quality of life in patients with severe acute respiratory distress syndrome and veno-venous extracorporeal membrane oxygenation support. Crit Care. Nov 29 2021;25(1):410.

26. Wengenmayer T, Duerschmied D, Graf E, et al. Development and validation of a prognostic model for survival in patients treated with venoarterial extracorporeal membrane oxygenation: the PREDICT VA-ECMO score. Eur Heart J Acute Cardiovasc Care. Jun 2019;8(4):350-359.

27. Beauchamp TL, Childress JF. Principles of Biomedical Ethics. 8th ed. Oxford University Press; 2019.

28. Abrams D, Ferguson ND, Brochard L, et al. ECMO for ARDS: from salvage to standard of care? Lancet Respir Med. Feb 2019;7(2):108-110.

29. Supady A, Biever PM, Staudacher DL, et al. Choosing the right reference cohort for assessing outcome of venovenous ECMO. Crit Care. Jan 10 2022;26(1):17.

30. Barbaro RP, Odetola FO, Kidwell KM, et al. Association of hospital-level volume of extracorporeal membrane oxygenation cases and mortality. Analysis of the extracorporeal life support organization registry. Am J Respir Crit Care Med. Apr 15 2015;191(8):894-901.

31. Lebreton G, Schmidt M, Ponnaiah M, et al. Extracorporeal membrane oxygenation network organisation and clinical outcomes during the COVID-19 pandemic in Greater Paris, France: a multicentre cohort study. Lancet Respir Med. Apr 19 2021.

32. Kirkland BW, Wilkes J, Bailly DK, et al. Extracorporeal Membrane Oxygenation for Pediatric Respiratory Failure: Risk Factors Associated With Center Volume and Mortality. Pediatr Crit Care Med. Aug 2016;17(8):779-88.

33. Broman LM, Dirnberger DR, Malfertheiner MV, et al. International Survey on Extracorporeal Membrane Oxygenation Transport. ASAIO J. Feb 2020;66(2):214-225.

34. Abrams D, MacLaren G, Lorusso R, et al. Extracorporeal cardiopulmonary resuscitation in adults: evidence and implications. Intensive Care Med. Sep 10 2021:1-15.

35. Henry B, Verbeek PR, Cheskes S. Extracorporeal cardiopulmonary resuscitation in out-of-hospital cardiac arrest: Ethical considerations. Resuscitation. Apr 2019;137:1-6.

36. Persad G, Wertheimer A, Emanuel EJ. Principles for allocation of scarce medical interventions. Lancet. Jan 31 2009;373(9661):423-31.

37. Riggs KR, Becker LB, Sugarman J. Ethics in the use of extracorporeal cardiopulmonary resuscitation in adults. Resuscitation. Jun 2015;91:73-5.

38. Curtis JR, Rubenfeld GD. "No escalation of treatment" as a routine strategy for decision-making in the ICU: con. Intensive Care Med. Sep 2014;40(9):1374-6.

39. Mulaikal TA, Nakagawa S, Prager KM. Extracorporeal Membrane Oxygenation Bridge to No Recovery. Circulation. Jan 22 2019;139(4):428-430.

40. Thompson DR. "No escalation of treatment" as a routine strategy for decision-making in the ICU: pro. Intensive Care Med. Sep 2014;40(9):1372-3.

41. Moynihan KM, Purol N, Alexander PMA, et al. A Communication Guide for Pediatric Extracorporeal Membrane Oxygenation. Pediatr Crit Care Med. Sep 1 2021;22(9):832-841.

42. MacLaren G, Masoumi A, Brodie D. ECPR for out-of-hospital cardiac arrest: more evidence is needed. Crit Care. Jan 7 2020;24(1):7.

43. Costa DK, Moss M. The Cost of Caring: Emotion, Burnout, and Psychological Distress in Critical Care Clinicians. Ann Am Thorac Soc. Jul 2018;15(7):787-790.

44. Supady A, Curtis JR, Brown CE, et al. Ethical obligations for supporting healthcare workers during the COVID-19 pandemic. Eur Respir J. Feb 2021;57(2).

45. Supady A, Badulak J, Evans L, et al. Should we ration extracorporeal membrane oxygenation during the COVID-19 pandemic? Lancet Respir Med. Apr 2021;9(4):326-328.

46. Vincent JL, Creteur J. Ethical aspects of the COVID-19 crisis: How to deal with an overwhelming shortage of acute beds. Eur Heart J Acute Cardiovasc Care. Apr 2020;9(3):248-252.

47. Fowler RA, Adhikari NK, Bhagwanjee S. Clinical review: critical care in the global context--disparities in burden of illness, access, and economics. Crit Care. 2008;12(5):225.

48. Papali A, Schultz MJ, Dünser MW. Recommendations on infrastructure and organization of adult ICUs in resource-limited settings. Intensive Care Med. Jul 2018;44(7):1133-1137.

49. Ouma PO, Maina J, Thuranira PN, et al. Access to emergency hospital care provided by the public sector in sub-Saharan Africa in 2015: a geocoded inventory and spatial analysis. Lancet Glob Health. Mar 2018;6(3):e342-e350.

50. Lee JS, Roberts SWP, Götsch K, et al. Caring for Critically Ill Patients in Humanitarian Settings. Am J Respir Crit Care Med. Mar 1 2019;199(5):572-580.

51. Barbaro RP, MacLaren G, Boonstra PS, et al. Extracorporeal membrane oxygenation for COVID-19: evolving outcomes from the international Extracorporeal Life Support Organization Registry. Lancet. Oct 2 2021;398(10307):1230-1238.

52. Barbaro RP, MacLaren G, Boonstra PS, et al. Extracorporeal membrane oxygenation support in COVID-19: an international cohort study of the Extracorporeal Life Support Organization registry. Lancet. Oct 10 2020;396(10257):1071-1078.

53. Diaz RA, Graf J, Zambrano JM, et al. Extracorporeal Membrane Oxygenation for COVID-19-associated Severe Acute Respiratory Distress Syndrome in Chile: A Nationwide Incidence and Cohort Study. Am J Respir Crit Care Med. Jul 1 2021;204(1):34-43.

54. Schmidt M, Hajage D, Lebreton G, et al. Extracorporeal membrane oxygenation for severe acute respiratory distress syndrome associated with COVID-19: a retrospective cohort study. Lancet Respir Med. Nov 2020;8(11):1121-1131.

55. Schmidt M, Langouet E, Hajage D, et al. Evolving outcomes of extracorporeal membrane oxygenation support for severe COVID-19 ARDS in Sorbonne hospitals, Paris. Crit Care. Oct 9 2021;25(1):355.

56. Cummings MJ, Baldwin MR, Abrams D, et al. Epidemiology, clinical course, and outcomes of critically ill adults with COVID-19 in New York City: a prospective cohort study. Lancet. Jun 6 2020;395(10239):1763-1770.

57. Herreros B, Gella P, Real de Asua D. Triage during the COVID-19 epidemic in Spain: better and worse ethical arguments. J Med Ethics. Jul 2020;46(7):455-458.

58. Rosenbaum L. Facing Covid-19 in Italy - Ethics, Logistics, and Therapeutics on the Epidemic's Front Line. N Engl J Med. May 14 2020;382(20):1873-1875.

59. Emanuel EJ, Persad G, Upshur R, et al. Fair Allocation of Scarce Medical Resources in the Time of Covid-19. N Engl J Med. May 21 2020;382(21):2049-2055.

60. Worku E, Gill D, Brodie D, Lorusso R, et al. Provision of ECPR during COVID-19: evidence, equity, and ethical dilemmas. Crit Care. Jul 27 2020;24(1):462.

61. Supady A, Brodie D, Curtis JR. Ten things to consider when implementing rationing guidelines during a pandemic. Intensive Care Med. May 2021;47(5):605-608.

62. Greenberg N, Docherty M, Gnanapragasam S, et al. Managing mental health challenges faced by healthcare workers during covid-19 pandemic. Bmj. Mar 26 2020;368:m1211.

63. Touray S, Sanyang B, Zandrow G, et al. An assessment of critical care capacity in the Gambia. J Crit Care. Oct 2018;47:245-253.

64. Touray S, Sanyang B. Critical Care in Sub-Saharan Africa: Is It Ready for Prime Time? Ann Am Thorac Soc. Jan 2019;16(1):156-157.

65. Lalani HS, Waweru-Siika W, Kussin PS. Reply: Critical Care in Sub-Saharan Africa: Is It Ready for Prime Time? Ann Am Thorac Soc. Jan 2019;16(1):157-158.

66. Past, present, and future of global health financing: a review of development assistance, government, out-of-pocket, and other private spending on health for 195 countries, 1995-2050. Lancet. Jun 1 2019;393(10187):2233-2260.

67. Lalani HS, Waweru-Siika W, Mwogi T, et al. Intensive Care Outcomes and Mortality Prediction at a National Referral Hospital in Western Kenya. Ann Am Thorac Soc. Nov 2018;15(11):1336-1343.

68. Machado DS, Garros D, Montuno L, et al. Finishing Well: Compassionate Extracorporeal Membrane Oxygenation Discontinuation. J Pain Symptom Manage. Jan 11 2022.

69. Moynihan KM, Ziniel SI, Johnston E, et al. A "Good Death" for Children with Cardiac Disease. Pediatr Cardiol. Dec 2 2021.

70. Truog RD, Thiagarajan RR, Harrison CH. Ethical dilemmas with the use of ECMO as a bridge to transplantation. Lancet Respir Med. Aug 2015;3(8):597-8.

71. Moynihan KM, Jansen MA, Liaw SN, et al. An Ethical Claim for Providing Medical Recommendations in Pediatric Intensive Care. Pediatr Crit Care Med. Aug 2018;19(8):e433-e437.

72. Gómez-Vírseda C, de Maeseneer Y, Gastmans C. Relational autonomy in end-of-life care ethics: a contextualized approach to real-life complexities. BMC Med Ethics. Jun 30 2020;21(1):50.

73. Hedlin M. The Web We Weave. N Engl J Med. Dec 2 2021;385(23):2119-2121.

74. Abrams DC, Prager K, Blinderman CD, et al. Ethical dilemmas encountered with the use of extracorporeal membrane oxygenation in adults. Chest. Apr 2014;145(4):876-882.

75. Wirpsa MJ, Carabini LM, Neely KJ, et al. Mitigating ethical conflict and moral distress in the care of patients on ECMO: impact of an automatic ethics consultation protocol. J Med Ethics. Jan 13 2021.

76. Godfrey S, Sahoo A, Sanchez J, et al. The Role of Palliative Care in Withdrawal of Venoarterial Extracorporeal Membrane Oxygenation for Cardiogenic Shock. J Pain Symptom Manage. Jun 2021;61(6):1139-1146.

77. Bailly DK, Furlong-Dillard JM, Winder M, et al. External validation of the Pediatric Extracorporeal Membrane Oxygenation Prediction model for risk adjusting mortality. Perfusion. May 2021;36(4):407-414.

78. Bailly DK, Reeder RW, Winder M, et al. Development of the Pediatric Extracorporeal Membrane Oxygenation Prediction Model for Risk-Adjusting Mortality. Pediatr Crit Care Med. May 2019;20(5):426-434.

79. Barbaro RP, Bartlett RH, Chapman RL, et al. Development and Validation of the Neonatal Risk Estimate Score for Children Using Extracorporeal Respiratory Support. J Pediatr. Jun 2016;173:56-61.e3.

80. Barbaro RP, Boonstra PS, Paden ML, et al. Development and validation of the pediatric risk estimate score for children using extracorporeal respiratory support (Ped-RESCUERS). Intensive Care Med. May 2016;42(5):879-888.

81. Moynihan KM, Taylor L, Crowe L, et al. Ethical climate in contemporary paediatric intensive care. J Med Ethics. Jan 11 2021;doi:10.1136/medethics-2020-106818.

82. Moynihan KM, Alexander PMA, Schlapbach LJ, et al. Epidemiology of childhood death in Australian and New Zealand intensive care units. Intensive Care Med. Sep 2019;45(9):1262-1271.

83. Gillam L. The zone of parental discretion: An ethical tool for dealing with disagreement between parents and doctors about medical treatment for a child. Clinical Ethics. March 1, 2016 2016;11(1):1-8.

84. McDougall R, Gillam L, Spriggs M, et al. The zone of parental discretion and the complexity of paediatrics: A response to Alderson. Clin Ethics. Dec 2018;13(4):172-174.

85. Lantos JD. The Tragic Case of Charlie Gard. JAMA Pediatr. Oct 1 2017;171(10):935-936.

86. Truog RD. Defining Death: Lessons From the Case of Jahi McMath. Pediatrics. Aug 2020;146(Suppl 1):S75-s80.

87. Fernando SM, Mathew R, Slutsky AS, et al. Media Portrayals of Outcomes After Extracorporeal Membrane Oxygenation. JAMA Intern Med. Mar 1 2021;181(3):391-394.

88. Guidelines for the determination of death. Report of the medical consultants on the diagnosis of death to the President's Commission for the Study of Ethical Problems in Medicine and Biomedical and Behavioral Research. Jama. Nov 13 1981;246(19):2184-6.

89. Robertson JA. The dead donor rule. Hastings Cent Rep. Nov-Dec 1999;29(6):6-14.

90. Bernat JL, Capron AM, Bleck TP, et al. The circulatory-respiratory determination of death in organ donation. Crit Care Med. Mar 2010;38(3):963-70.

91. Dalle Ave AL, Shaw DM, Gardiner D. Extracorporeal membrane oxygenation (ECMO) assisted cardiopulmonary resuscitation or uncontrolled donation after the circulatory determination of death following out-of-hospital refractory cardiac arrest-An ethical analysis of an unresolved clinical dilemma. Resuscitation. Nov 2016;108:87-94.

92. Perez-Villares JM, Rubio JJ, Del Río F, et al. Validation of a new proposal to avoid donor resuscitation in controlled donation after circulatory death with normothermic regional perfusion. Resuscitation. Aug 2017;117:46-49.

93. Dalle Ave AL, Shaw DM, Bernat JL. Ethical Issues in the Use of Extracorporeal Membrane Oxygenation in Controlled Donation After Circulatory Determination of Death. Am J Transplant. Aug 2016;16(8):2293-9.

94. Extracorporeal Life Support Organization. ECLS Registry Report. 2022. Accessed January 26, 2022. https://www.elso.org/Registry/InternationalSummaryandReports/InternationalSummary.aspx.

# 58

## Research

*Eddy Fan, Ryan P. Barbaro, Peta M. A. Alexander, Alain Combes, Carol L. Hodgson, John F. Fraser, Heidi Dalton, Daniel Brodie*

Novel approaches are needed to further reduce morbidity and mortality in patients with heart and/or lung failure. ECLS has emerged as an important tool in the management of select patients with cardiopulmonary failure.[1,2] Given the resource intensity of ECLS, this represents an important challenge for most health systems. Importantly, we lack rigorous data to support such rapid, widespread adoption in some patient populations in which ECLS is already commonly used. Moreover, we lack rigorous data to support many interventions and management strategies (eg, anticoagulation, early rehabilitation) applied in patients supported by ECLS. Therefore, high-quality evidence is needed for stakeholders to make informed decisions on the use of ECLS for many clinical indications and to optimize patient care in those supported with ECLS.

One of the main challenges to obtaining rigorous data on the potential efficacy of ECLS in patients with cardiopulmonary failure is logistical: the likely small number of eligible patients for enrolment into trials at individual centers, the time and resources needed to complete such trials, and the number of centers with expertise in research, critical care, and ECLS. In addition, other substantial, but not insurmountable, considerations are the need to answer simple questions before proceeding to large clinical (efficacy) trials, such as the need

to define many aspects of the standard of care during ECLS support and the correct patient-centered outcomes to measure in these studies.[3,4] A successful program of research focused on answering these questions will necessarily require a collaborative of high-volume ECLS centers, experienced in clinical research. In this chapter, we will provide an overview of some of the key principles that have evolved over time for the conduct of clinical research in extracorporeal support.

### The Need for Collaboration

Given that extracorporeal support is typically applied in relatively small numbers of critically ill patients in any given center, it is often not feasible to conduct rigorous, high-quality clinical trials without collaboration among centers. For example, the CESAR trial[5] took nearly 9 years to complete enrollment of 180 patients (0.03 patients/center/month), while the EOLIA trial[6] took nearly 6 years to complete enrollment of 249 patients (0.06 patients/center/month). Large, international professional societies or research consortia can help to facilitate regional, national, and international collaborative research. ELSO is the largest international society focused exclusively on extracorporeal support with over 500 actively contributing ECLS member centers worldwide. ELSO members represent a large, diverse, and captive collection of ECLS centers that could participate in the research, development, and subsequent implementation of novel management strategies or interventions associated with extracorporeal support. This support for multicenter research is further strengthened by links to the International ECMO Network (ECMONet) and PediECMO. ELSO's infrastructure also includes data management, quality assurance, and statistical support for analyses. Finally, ELSO is actively engaged with a broad group of relevant stakeholders (eg, funding, regulatory, industry representatives), strengthened by regional groups working together, that would be critical to the success of future research in the field of extracorporeal support. A number of successful examples of clinical research in ECLS supported or endorsed

| AUTHOR (Year) | STUDY TITLE | JOURNAL |
|---|---|---|
| O'Rourke (1993) | Extracorporeal membrane oxygenation: support for overwhelming pulmonary failure in the pediatric population. Collective experience from the Extracorporeal Life Support Organization | Journal of Pediatric Surgery |
| Bartlett (2000) | Extracorporeal life support: the University of Michigan experience | JAMA |
| Brogan (2009) | Extracorporeal membrane oxygenation in adults with severe respiratory failure: a multi-center database | Intensive Care Medicine |
| Zabrocki (2011) | Extracorporeal membrane oxygenation for pediatric respiratory failure: Survival and predictors of mortality. | Critical Care Medicine |
| Almond (2011) | Extracorporeal membrane oxygenation for bridge to heart transplantation among children in the United States: analysis of data from the Organ Procurement and Transplant Network and Extracorporeal Life Support Organization Registry | Circulation |
| Fraser (2012) | Prospective trial of a pediatric ventricular assist device. | New England Journal of Medicine |
| Schmidt (2014) | Predicting survival after extracorporeal membrane oxygenation for severe acute respiratory failure. The Respiratory Extracorporeal Membrane Oxygenation Survival Prediction (RESP) score | American Journal of Respiratory and Critical Care Medicine |
| Combes (2014) | Position paper for the organization of extracorporeal membrane oxygenation programs for acute respiratory failure in adult patients | American Journal of Respiratory and Critical Care Medicine |
| Barbaro (2015) | Association of hospital-level volume of extracorporeal membrane oxygenation cases and mortality. Analysis of the Extracorporeal Life Support Organization registry | American Journal of Respiratory and Critical Care Medicine |
| Schmidt (2015) | Predicting survival after ECMO for refractory cardiogenic shock: the survival after veno-arterial-ECMO (SAVE) score | European Heart Journal |
| Barbaro (2015) | Development and validation of the pediatric risk estimate score for children using extracorporeal respiratory support (Ped-RESCUERS) | Intensive Care Medicine |

**Table 58-1.** An overview of influential publications from ELSO, ECMONet, PediECMO. (Table continued on next page.)

by these organizations are summarized in Table 58-1.

**The Importance of Infrastructure–Device-Specific Registries**

ELSO maintains a registry of ECLS cases which included over 175,000 patients at the start of 2022. ELSO and the ELSO Registry provide important infrastructure to efficiently collect data on a variety of practices from member centers, as well the potential ability to embed future clinical trials and evaluations of novel strategies (eg, registry-randomized clinical trial).[7,8] These real-world data are being used for research, quality improvement, and regulatory submissions to the Food and Drug Administration (FDA).[9,10] Any member center

| AUTHOR | STUDY TITLE | JOURNAL |
|---|---|---|
| Abrams (2018) | Position paper for the organization of ECMO programs for cardiac failure in adults | Intensive Care Medicine |
| Conrad (2018) | The Extracorporeal Life Support Organization Maastricht Treaty for nomenclature in extracorporeal life support. A position paper of the Extracorporeal Life Support Organization | American Journal of Respiratory and Critical Care Medicine |
| Combes (2018) | Extracorporeal membrane oxygenation for severe acute respiratory distress syndrome (EOLIA) | New England Journal of Medicine |
| Bembea (2019) | Outcomes after extracorporeal cardiopulmonary resuscitation of pediatric in-hospital cardiac arrest: a report from the Get with the Guidelines-Resuscitation and Extracorporeal Life Support Registries | Critical Care Medicine |
| Zakhary (2020) | Position paper on global extracorporeal membrane oxygenation education and educational agenda for the future: a statement from the Extracorporeal Life Support Organization ECMOed taskforce | Critical Care Medicine |
| DellaVolpe (2020) | Joint Society of Critical Care Medicine-Extracorporeal Life Support Organization task force position paper on the role of the intensivist in the initiation and management of extracorporeal membrane oxygenation | Critical Care Medicine |
| Barbaro (2020) | Extracorporeal membrane oxygenation support in COVID-19: an international cohort study of the Extracorporeal Life Support Organization registry | Lancet |
| Hodgson (2021) | A core outcome set for research in patients on extracorporeal membrane oxygenation | Critical Care Medicine |
| Barbaro (2021) | Extracorporeal membrane oxygenation for COVID-19: evolving outcomes from the international Extracorporeal Life Support Organization Registry | Lancet |

**Table 58-1 (Cont).** An overview of influential publications from ELSO, ECMONet, PediECMO.

can request data from the Registry to conduct research or quality improvement projects. Indeed, in situations where randomized controlled trials are not feasible, the availability of real-world data coupled with modern causal inference techniques (eg, target trial emulation[11]) may provide the best effect estimates for interventions, such as the impact of ECLS support for patients with severe COVID-19.[12] For example, a current ELSO-embedded, National Institutes of Health (NIH)-funded, prospective observational study has harmonized data collection with an ongoing clinical trial to study the long-term outcomes of ECLS-supported children with acute respiratory distress syndrome (ARDS) and will apply causal inference statistical approaches to better understand if and when ECLS should be initiated in clinical trials (ARDS in Children and ECMO initiation strategies impact on Neuro-Development [ASCEND] study).

Research efforts are often hampered by resource limitations needed for data collection, including personnel. Much effort could be minimized by establishing coding between electronic health records (EHR) and research databases, and efforts to improve this capability are underway in many centers. The ability to link data across centers who use similar EHRs by sharing coding schemes may reduce resources needed to obtain data. Existing data sources do not, however, include all the necessary data elements (eg, granular, longitudinal data) or use the standardized definitions needed for research. The International Research Database for Extracorporeal Support (INDEX) and the Australia/New Zealand national ECMO registry (EXCEL) will provide ongoing evaluation of epidemiology, real-world effectiveness, safety, quality, and economic impact across ECLS centers globally. To complement these efforts, a formal consensus process to define core definitions and outcomes for ECLS has been completed and will be progressively implemented in future clinical trials endorsed

by ECMONet.[3,4] Finally, integrating ancillary infrastructure, such as biobanking or long-term followup, in registry sites with the requisite expertise and resources can further enhance the value of these registries. Such efforts will be enhanced by collaboration with other groups such as the COVID Critical Care Consortium, National Heart, Lung and Blood Institute (NHLBI) Hemostasis Consensus group, the Pediatric Critical Care Blood Research Network (BLOODnet), Transfusion and Anemia Expertise Initiative – Continuous Assessment of Blood (TAXICab), and others to maintain similar definitions and goal targets across studies.

## Innovative Clinical Trial Designs

As the pediatric ECLS community is preparing to undertake an RCT of red blood cell transfusion practices in ECLS patients (Trial of Indication-based Transfusion of Red blood cells in ECMO [TITRE]), it is clear that traditional RCTs are challenging in ECLS due to the limited population available for study, as well as the resources and time required for completion. Innovative clinical trial designs would allow more efficient and cost-effective evaluation of ECLS and related interventions. Two examples that could be employed in the field of extracorporeal support include:

1. **Registry RCT (R-RCT).** Using and expanding existing infrastructure such as the ELSO Registry (eg, ASCEND study), EXCEL (eg, the Blend to Limit oxygen in ECMO: a ranDomised controlled Registry Trial [BLENDER]), or INDEX (eg, the Ultra-Low Tidal Volume Mechanical Ventilation in ARDS Through ECMO [ULTIMATE] study) for trial enrollment, randomization, data, and outcomes would enhance the feasibility of ECLS clinical trials.[7,13] Less selective populations will be studied resulting in greater generalizability,

maximizing use of existing data, and increasing relevance of findings to stakeholders.

2. **Adaptive Platform Trial.** A flexible, adaptive algorithm for assigning treatments, evaluating effects, and drawing conclusions would allow simultaneous evaluation of a number of treatments, making it more productive than a traditional RCT.[14] The use of such international Bayesian adaptive platform trials during the COVID-19 pandemic (eg, RECOVERY, REMAP-CAP) has provided real-world examples of the potential timeliness and efficiencies gained through this approach.[15]

For instance, developing an adaptive platform R-RCT across several centers, with a subset used to pilot candidate strategies or interventions (eg, anticoagulation, transfusion thresholds, and best ventilatory strategy, etc.) in ECLS patients, clinicians and researchers could move on quickly from candidate therapies or interventions that are not feasible or successful. A successful pilot could subsequently move forward into an international, multicenter, adaptive R-RCT, using the same design and infrastructure for ECLS and associated interventions.

## The Future

ELSO—along with other major medical organizations, funding bodies, regulatory agencies, device developers, and societies—could organize and lead 'think tank' meetings of relevant stakeholders to establish research priorities and continue to review and update them over time. In this model, given the experience and resources available, as well as the international collaborations available in the ELSO chapters, ELSO could subsequently function as the central hub to coordinate future research efforts prioritized by its members and the community, acting as the clinical coordinating center for such activities to reduce overlap, harmonize, and enhance collaboration between projects, and provide an efficient and effective means to collect data and conduct clinical trials.

There are many important research questions that remain to be answered in the field of extracorporeal support.[16] Coordination by international societies (eg, ELSO, ECMONet, PediECMO, PALISI), exploiting and expanding existing infrastructure (eg, ELSO Registry or INDEX/EXCEL), and utilizing innovative clinical trial designs (eg, step-wedge, R-RCT or Bayesian adaptive platform trials) will help clinicians and researchers achieve these results in a timely, resource-efficient, and rigorous manner.

# References

1. Brodie D, Slutsky AS, Combes A. Extracorporeal Life Support for Adults With Respiratory Failure and Related Indications. Jama. 2019;322(6):557-568.
2. Combes A, Price S, Slutsky AS, et al. Temporary circulatory support for cardiogenic shock. Lancet. 2020;396(10245):199-212.
3. Hodgson CL, Fulcher B, Mariajoseph FP, et al. A Core Outcome Set for Research in Patients on Extracorporeal Membrane Oxygenation. Crit Care Med. 2021;49(12):e1252-e1254.
4. Hodgson CL, Burrell AJC, Engeler DM, et al. Core Outcome Measures for Research in Critically Ill Patients Receiving Extracorporeal Membrane Oxygenation for Acute Respiratory or Cardiac Failure: An International, Multidisciplinary, Modified Delphi Consensus Study. Crit Care Med. Published online August 5, 2019.
5. Peek GJ, Mugford M, Tiruvoipati R, et al. Efficacy and economic assessment of conventional ventilatory support versus extracorporeal membrane oxygenation for severe adult respiratory failure (CESAR): a multicentre randomised controlled trial. Lancet Lond Engl. 2009;374(9698):1351-1363.
6. Combes A, Hajage D, Capellier G, et al. Extracorporeal Membrane Oxygenation for Severe Acute Respiratory Distress Syndrome. New Engl J Med. 2018;378(21):1965-1975.
7. Lauer MS, Gordon D, Wei G, et al. Efficient design of clinical trials and epidemiological research: is it possible? Nat Rev Cardiol. 2017;14(8):493-501.
8. Li G, Sajobi TT, Menon BK, et al. Registry-based randomized controlled trials: advantages, challenges and areas for future research. J Clin Epidemiol. 2016;80:16-24.
9. Kesselheim AS, Avorn J. New "21st Century Cures" Legislation: Speed and Ease vs Science. Jama. 2017;317(6):581-582.
10. Freemantle N, Marston L, Walters K, et al. Making inferences on treatment effects from real world data: propensity scores, confounding by indication, and other perils for the unwary in observational research. Bmj Br Medical J. 2013;347(nov11 3):f6409-f6409.
11. Hernán MA. Methods of Public Health Research — Strengthening Causal Inference from Observational Data. New Engl J Med. 2021;385(15):1345-1348.
12. Shaefi S, Brenner SK, Gupta S, et al. Extracorporeal membrane oxygenation in patients with severe respiratory failure from COVID-19. Intens Care Med. 2021;47(2):208-221.
13. Fröbert O, Lagerqvist B, Olivecrona GK, et al. Thrombus aspiration during ST-segment elevation myocardial infarction. New Engl J Medicine. 2013;369(17):1587-1597.
14. Angus DC, Alexander BM, Berry S, et al. Adaptive platform trials: definition, design, conduct and reporting considerations. Nat Rev Drug Discov. 2019;18(10):797-807.
15. Normand SLT. The RECOVERY Platform. Effect of Hydroxychloroquine in Hospitalized Patients with Covid-19. N Engl J Med. 2020 Nov 19;383(21):2030-2040.
16. Combes A, Brodie D, Chen YS, et al. The ICM research agenda on extracorporeal life support. Intens Care Med. 2017;43(9):1306-1318.

# 59

## Emerging Infectious Diseases

*Graeme MacLaren, Matthieu Schmidt, Rodrigo Diaz, Janet Diaz, Dale Fisher*

## Introduction

Emerging infectious diseases (EIDs) are defined as those which have newly appeared in a population, are rapidly increasing in incidence or geographic range, or which pose the highest threat to national security and public health.[1,2] Historically, EIDs have often facilitated deeper understanding of the utility of ECLS. For example, the influenza A(H1N1) pandemic in 2009 catalyzed interest in ECLS among the adult ICU community,[3] leading to a surge in ECLS use for ARDS which continues to this day. The COVID-19 pandemic demonstrated that clinical outcomes can change rapidly over time, sometimes for the worse, even in the same centers.[4,5] EIDs can also expose weaknesses in regional or national ECLS service provision, such as a lack of inclusion in pandemic preparedness plans, inadequate centralization or coordination of services, or an inability to rapidly conduct relevant clinical trials. However, it is important to emphasize that not all EIDs have pandemic potential. Some EIDs have high fatality rates but low-to-negligible human-to-human transmission, such as many zoonoses. This chapter will summarize major considerations in the use of ECLS for EIDs.

## Preparedness

Enabling ECLS services for a possible EID outbreak with high transmissibility must consider factors relating to personnel, equipment, facilities, and systems.[6] Regional or national coordination of ECLS services should facilitate the creation of a roster of all ECLS-trained clinicians and their respective roles, and comprehensive inventories of all available equipment.[6-9] These should be regularly updated and maintained. Subsequent referral pathways should be widely disseminated to local hospitals. Refresher courses on infection prevention and control (IPC) protocols and ECLS simulation training, while wearing personal protective equipment (PPE) or powered air-purifying respirators (PAPR), should be undertaken among nursing, perfusion, respiratory therapy, and medical staff. ECLS centers within specific regions are advised to agree on common indications and contraindications to provide consistent and equitable care.[7] These may require adaptation or modification over time, especially during crisis standards of care or surge. Standardized data collection ideally should be mandated, while facilitating patient enrollment into clinical trials. Communication networks between healthcare systems must be established to track ECLS utilization rates.[8]

These efforts should be undertaken as part of a preparedness phase rather than trying to implement them in the height of a major outbreak when demand for all clinical services is experiencing surge.[4] The readiness phase is the period in a pandemic where an infectious disease threat is imminent but not yet impacting a region. For example, this would refer to countries other than China from January to March 2020 during the COVID-19 pandemic. In this period, it is important to review all preparedness efforts; research readiness; and standard operating procedures, and organize various strategies aimed at responding to surge by considering different scenarios at a national, state, and institutional level.

## Assessment

Any potential role for ECLS in the management of EIDs will depend upon key characteristics of the pathogen, including the transmissibility, case fatality rate, and mechanisms of death.[10] An early assessment of the potential suitability of ECLS can be made by examining the clinical manifestations of the disease and likely modes of transmission. ECLS only provides support to the heart and lung, so if the mechanisms of death do not include acute respiratory failure, arrhythmias, or cardiogenic shock, and is predominantly due to hypovolemic shock from high-volume gastrointestinal losses for example, then ECLS is unlikely to be helpful. The effects of the illness on other organ systems are important to establish.

As clinical experience grows, the apparent efficacy of ECLS should be assessed, monitored, and rapidly communicated to the scientific community. Preliminary experience with the use of ECLS for Middle East Respiratory Syndrome (MERS), for example, was discouraging but outcomes slowly improved with time and greater experience.[11-13] Similarly, initial reports from China on the use of ECLS for COVID-19 appeared to show very poor outcomes with

ECLS,[14] but this was not borne out by more comprehensive assessment in larger centers in Europe and elsewhere,[15-17] highlighting the dangers of overreliance on observational data. If clinical outcomes remain poor despite substantial case volume in experienced centers, it should be considered whether ECLS can function as a bridge to successful transplantation.[18]

Other outcome measures beyond survival to hospital discharge should also be examined, including long-term mortality, functional and neurological outcomes, and quality of life. Specific strategies which may affect these outcomes should be studied, whether those relate to pre-ECLS care, management during ECLS, or rehabilitation after ICU discharge.[20] EIDs may affect the complication rates typically seen during ECLS, such as the increase in pulmonary emboli observed in some studies of severe COVID-19.[15] Treatment of the EID may also alter the risks of ECLS, such as the use of immunosuppressant therapy for COVID-19 and the subsequent increase in nosocomial infections.[4,5] These may skew the usual risk/benefit assessment against the use of ECLS in some circumstances, especially during crisis standards of care (Chapter 57).

Adherence to strict IPC processes is obviously essential in the management of EIDs, which can pose a substantial danger to staff members and affect ECLS service provision. For example, many centers did not offer ECPR to COVID-19 patients on the grounds that it posed too great a danger to clinicians.[19] Novel pathogens with high case fatality rates and very high transmissibility (eg, those requiring Biosafety level 4 [BSL-4] containment) may render ECLS use impractical.

## Coordination

The emergence of novel pathogens necessitates a coordinated effective response. If ECLS is established as a valid management strategy for a given EID, then organization of

ECLS services at a city, state, or national level is imperative.[6-9] A suitable model of care should be put in place to handle case volumes safely and effectively, such as a regional hub and spoke model (Chapter 53).[7,21] While the establishment of new ECLS centers should ideally not occur during major outbreaks, there are successful examples of this to fulfill otherwise unmet regional needs.[22]

Research coordination is another important issue. If an EID has multiple epicenters with established local transmission and is demonstrating pandemic potential, then ECLS networks should rapidly coordinate multiple clinical trials as to the efficacy, complications, resource consumption, and cost effectiveness of ECLS for that disease.[8] These studies are likely to take a number of different but valid approaches, including prospective observational studies; cluster randomized controlled trials; and adaptive trial designs, such as randomized, embedded, multifactorial, adaptive platform (REMAP) trials.[23] Nonetheless, the difficulty in coordinating and conducting randomized trials of highly complex, supportive interventions such as ECLS under the stress of a rapidly emerging infectious disease outbreak is considerable, and would only likely be successful if the mechanisms and infrastructure were already in place (Chapter 58). ECLS registries, such as that of ELSO, may be helpful in rapidly collecting multicenter data about the disease, with scope to combine with other registries gathering more disease-specific information (Chapter 60).

## Conclusions

Many EIDs will not be amenable to intervention with ECLS, which remains a resource-intensive and costly therapy. Nonetheless, ECLS may have a specific role (ideally, one tested in well-designed clinical trials) in the most critically ill patients suffering from refractory cardiac or pulmonary disease, as part of a broad strategy to mitigate the severe health consequences of emerging pathogens with outbreak potential.[6,8,23]

## References

1.  Emerging infectious diseases. Available at: https://www.niaid.nih.gov/research/emerging-infectious-diseases-pathogens https://www.niaid.nih.gov/ Accessed March 9, 2022.
2.  Prioritizing disease for research and development in emergency contexts. Available at: https://www.who.int/activities/prioritizing-diseases-for-research-and-development-in-emergency-contexts Accessed March 9, 2022.
3.  Noah MA, Peek GJ, Finney SJ, et al. Referral to an extracorporeal membrane oxygenation center and mortality among patients with severe 2009 influenza A(H1N1). JAMA 2011; 306:1659-1668.
4.  Barbaro RP, MacLaren G, Boonstra PS, et al. Extracorporeal membrane oxygenation for COVID-19: Evolving outcomes from the international Extracorporeal Life Support Organization Registry. Lancet 2021; 398:1230-1238.
5.  Schmidt M, Langouet E, Hajage D, et al. Evolving outcomes of extracorporeal membrane oxygenation support for severe COVID-19 ARDS in Sorbonne hospitals, Paris. Crit Care 2021; 25:355.
6.  Ramanathan KR, Antognini D, Combes A, et al. Planning and provision of ECMO services for severe ARDS during the COVID-19 pandemic and other outbreaks of emerging infectious diseases. Lancet Respir Med 2020; 8:518-526.
7.  Lebreton G, Schmidt M, Ponnaiah M, et al; Paris ECMO-COVID-19 investigators. Extracorporeal membrane oxygenation network organization and clinical outcomes during the COVID-19 pandemic in Greater Paris, France: a multicentre cohort study. Lancet Resp Med 2021; 9:851-862.
8.  MacLaren G, Fisher D, Brodie D. Treating the most critically ill patients with COVID-19: The evolving role of extracorporeal membrane oxygenation. JAMA 2022; 327:31-32.
9.  Diaz R, Graf J, Zambrano JM, et al. Extracorporeal membrane oxygenation for COVID-19-associated severe acute respiratory distress syndrome in Chile: a nationwide incidence and cohort study. Am J Respir Crit Care Med 2021; 204:34-43.
10. MacLaren G, Fisher D, Brodie D. Preparing for the most critically ill patients with COVID-19: the potential role of extracorporeal membrane oxygenation. JAMA 2020; 323:1245-1246.
11. Arabi YM, Al-Omari A, Mandourah Y, et al. Critically ill patients with the Middle East Respiratory Syndrome: a multicenter retrospective cohort study. Crit Care Med 2017; 45:1683-1695.
12. Alshahrani M, Sindi A, Alshamsi F, et al. Extracorporeal membrane oxygenation for severe Middle East respiratory syndrome coronavirus. Ann Intensive Care 2018; 8:3.
13. Choi WS, Kang CI, Kim Y, et al. Clinical presentation and outcomes of Middle East Respiratory Syndrome in the Republic of Korea. Infect Chemother 2016; 48:118-26.
14. Henry BM, Lippi G, Poor survival with extracorporeal membrane oxygenation in acute respiratory distress syndrome (ARDS) due to coronavirus disease 2019 (COVID-19): pooled analysis of early reports. J Crit Care 2020; 58:27-28.
15. Schmidt M, Hajage D, Lebreton G, et al. Extracorporeal membrane oxygenation for severe acute respiratory distress syndrome associated with COVID-19: a retrospective cohort study. Lancet Respir Med 2020; 8:1121-1131.
16. Barbaro RP, MacLaren G, Boonstra PS, et al. Extracorporeal membrane oxygenation support in COVID-19: an international cohort study of the Extracorporeal Life Support Organization registry. Lancet 2020; 396:1071-1078.
17. Whebell S, Zhang J, Lewis R, et al. Survival benefit of extracorporeal membrane oxygenation in severe COVID-19: a multi-centre-matched cohort study. Intensive Care Med 2022; 48:467-478.
18. Kurihara C, Manerikar A, Querrey M, et al. Clinical characteristics and outcomes of patients with COVID-19 associated acute respiratory distress syndrome who underwent lung transplant. JAMA 2022; 327:652-661.
19. Worku E, Gill D, Brodie D, et al. Provision of ECPR during COVID-19: evidence, equity, and ethical dilemmas. Crit Care 2020; 24:462.
20. MacLaren G, Combes A, Brodie D. What's new in ECMO for COVID-19? Intensive Care Med 2021; 47:107-109.
21. Combes A, Brodie D, Bartlett R, et al. Position paper for the organization of extracorporeal membrane oxygenation programs for acute respiratory failure in adult patients. Am J Respir Crit Care Med 2014; 190:488-96.
22. Rabie AA, Azzam MH, Al-Fares AA, et al. Implementation of new ECMO centers during the COVID-19 pandemic: experience and results from the Middle East and India. Intensive Care Med 2021; 47:887-895.
23. Brodie D, Abrams D, MacLaren G, et al. ECMO during respiratory pandemics: past, present, and future. Am J Respir Crit Care Med 2022; 205:1382-1390.

# 60

## The ELSO Registry

*Ryan P. Barbaro, Joseph E. Tonna, Peta M. A. Alexander, Rob Hyslop, Jeffrey J. Fanning, Micheal Heard, Matthew L. Paden, Ravi R. Thiagarajan, Matteo Di Nardo, Peter Rycus*

The charter members of the Extracorporeal Life Support Organization (ELSO) believed shared ECLS experience could generate knowledge that benefited future patients.[1,2] That mission remains central to the ELSO Registry, which aims to improve ECLS by: 1) attaining knowledge through scientific research, 2) enhancing centers' quality improvement efforts, 3) supporting advancement and evaluation of ECLS devices, and 4) advancing the quality and usability of ELSO data.

### Knowledge Attainment

The diverse community of member center investigators bring unique experiences to scientific questions. Their scientific research realizes the vision of attaining knowledge through the ELSO Registry. In 2021, more than 200 ELSO Registry data requests were made to address scientific questions.

The ELSO Registry Scientific Oversight Committee (SOC) was established as a subcommittee of the ELSO Registry in 2016. The SOC aimed to facilitate and promote the development of scientific research from the ELSO Registry, and its primary task was to evaluate data requests and release data to ELSO investigators for the purposes of publication or patient care. The SOC is made up of a clinically and geographically diverse group of individuals with ECLS expertise. Each member commits to evaluating and discussing data requests. Members include physicians, nurses, ECLS specialists, respiratory therapists, and statisticians from across the globe.

### Data Request Process

The review of ELSO data requests for scientific research was adapted from the National Institutes of (NIH) grant review process. Submitted requests are administratively processed, assigned for SOC member review, and the reviewers present the data requests to the SOC. Subsequently, the SOC Chair moderates the SOC discussion and data request scoring.

The SOC considers several different factors when rating proposals for approval. These include overlap, significance, innovation, and approach. 'Overlap' with previous data requests is considered because data is released to investigators for a period of 12 months of exclusive access. This approach seeks to mitigate duplicative analyses that hurriedly or competitively race to publish, while also enabling new investigators to ask similar questions. 'Significance' considers what the impact of the work would be if the aims of the research were successfully completed. 'Innovation' considers if the application introduces novel concepts or scientific techniques, or challenges current paradigms. 'Approach' evaluates if the methods and planed analyses are feasible, well-reasoned and rigorous. SOC seeks to encourage new investigators and centers and so it does not evaluate investigators or environment, but it does sometimes suggest new ELSO investigators partner with experienced investigators if questions reflect a lack of familiarity with the strengths and limitations of the ELSO data.

### Large Datasets

Proposals that request entire population categories of ECLS support such as all adult respiratory cases are subject to an additional level of requirements and review. Large dataset requests present a risk of enabling unspecified hypotheses to be addressed and their breadth increases the likelihood the request will overlap with future data requests. Additionally, the potential impact of the research obviates a rigorous analysis. For these reasons, large dataset requests require the collaborative participation of investigators from a minimum of three ELSO member centers and a named biostatistician. Investigators can also only have one large dataset request at a time. After meeting these requirements, the review, if approved by

the SOC, then goes before the Large Dataset Committee for a second review. The Largest Dataset Committee is comprised of, at a minimum, a current or past Registry Chair, the SOC Chair(s), and the ELSO Executive Director. The committee also includes biostatisticians. Finally, proposals approved by the Large Dataset Committee are required to first remit their manuscript prior to journal submission to the SOC to ensure the research remained within the scope of the prespecified hypothesis and aims.

### Transparency

The SOC discloses members, policies, data requests and ELSO publications on the ELSO website.

### Enhancing Center-based Efforts to Improve Quality

Since its inception, the ELSO Registry has reported outcomes, enabling centers to benchmark their performance to the average. The present evolution of that reporting is the result of a collaboration between the ELSO Registry Quality Subcommittee and ArborMetrix in 2016 to create the ELSO Quality Reporting Platform. ArborMetrix is a Michigan-based provider of

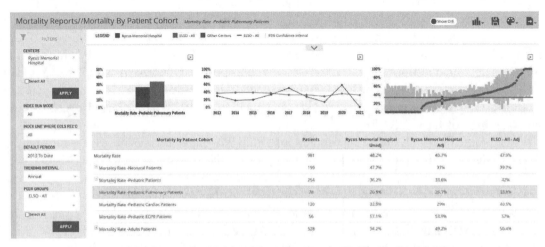

**Figure 60-1.** Example graphic of the ArborMetrix ELSO Quality Platform.

clinically rich, realtime analytics that partners with numerous Registries to provide outcome and process reporting dashboards. ELSO Quality Reporting Platform displays adjusted center-specific ECLS outcomes through tools that benchmark ELSO Member Center performance to center selected peer institutions (Figure 60-1). This application can be used to track and display center-based performance across time and compare performance to peer centers using metrics such as survival, major complications, minor complications, and length of stay. Only the member-center is identified in the ELSO Quality Reporting Platform reports and graphics, and no fewer than 10 centers are presented as comparators.

### Adjustment Models

Risk adjustment for mortality prior to hospital discharge was built into the reporting platform. The platform applied a combination of ELSO-derived published ECLS mortality risk adjustment models,[3-8] and ArborMetrix built pragmatic risk adjustment models. The ArborMetrix models were built with plausible meaningful candidate variables that were missing <10% of time.[9] The methodology was publicized during international conferences, ELSO-hosted webinars, and reported in the

medical literature.[9] The resulting risk adjusted center performance is reported with confidence intervals (Figure 60-1). The risk adjustment models use generalized estimating equations to account for the clustering within hospitals and the models are reliability-adjusted as previously described.[10] This means that if a given center has fewer patients, then the model shrinks the estimate back towards the group average outcome.

### Outcome Reports

The ELSO Quality Reporting Platform includes mortality outcome reports that can be presented according to patient age cohort (neonate, pediatric, or adult), unit where the patient received care (medical, surgical, cardiac, pediatric, or neonatal ICUs), duration of run, as well as per patient or per ECLS run, because some patients have multiple ECLS runs during a hospital admission (Figure 60-2). Complication reports are presented with the same options and can either cluster related complications (eg, Any mechanical complication, Any hemorrhagic complication, etc.), or each individual complication (eg, Oxygenator failure, Pump malfunction, Air in circuit, Surgical site bleeding, Hemolysis). Time to complications,

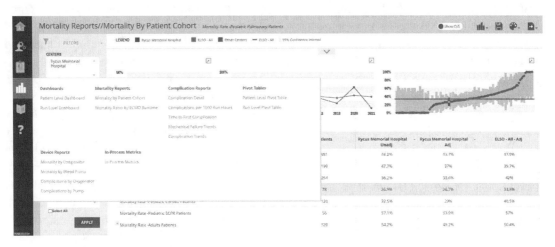

**Figure 60-2.** Example reports included in the ArborMetrix ELSO Quality Platform.

and complications per 1000 ECLS hours are also available as standard outcome reports.

### *Process Metric Reports*

The ELSO Registry Quality Subcommittee has applied process metric reports specific to different populations of patients supported with ECLS. For those patients supported for respiratory indications, PIP $\leq 25$ cmH$_2$O was identified as a potential implementable strategy for 'lung protection' during this support in accordance with established practice.[11-13] No randomized clinical trials have demonstrated that one mechanical ventilation strategy is superior, but the protocol for the ECLS group in the UK neonatal trial used a PIP $<25$ cmH$_2$O, in the CESAR trial a PIP 20-25 cmH$_2$O, and EOLIA a P$_{plat}$ $\leq 24$ cmH$_2$O.[11-13] Thus, a report was added to the Quality Reporting Platform in 2020, reflecting the proportion of patients who were managed with mechanical ventilation PIP $\leq 25$ cmH$_2$O at 24 hours of the ECLS run.

The population of patients cannulated during ECPR represent the most critically ill of the cardiac patients supported with ECLS. As a center level process metric, the proportion of cardiac ECLS patients who were cannulated during ECPR was added to the Quality Reporting Platform as a metric in 2020. There are no established rates of ECPR associated with outcome, so it was chosen to represent the trend of proportion of ECPR in cardiac patients over time, anticipating that centers could chose to use this information to prove uptake of an emerging service in a new ECPR center, to demonstrate the impact of cardiopulmonary arrest prevention strategies in established centers, or to simply visualize utilization of this time-critical, resource-intensive intervention.[14,15] Further process metrics for inclusion in the Quality Platform will be identified by consensus among clinical experts.

### *Peer Groups*

The ELSO Quality Platform presents unadjusted as well as adjusted center-based performance compared to peer centers for each of the included outcomes and process metrics. Preprogrammed peer groups include low/medium/high volume centers, age-mix of patients managed in centers (mixed, neonates, pediatrics, adults), ELSO Center of Excellence status, and ELSO Chapters. In addition, centers can identify and customize peer groups which may be of relevance to their practice. Peer group centers remain blinded in the reports, with only the individual member-center identified. At least 10 centers are included as comparators in each of the reports to ensure member center confidentiality.

### Supporting Development of Devices used in ECLS

In the USA, the 2016 21$^{st}$ Century Cures Act directed regulatory bodies to use real world evidence to support regulatory decision-making. The US Congress characterized real world evidence as data regarding the use, benefits, and risks of a drug using sources other than clinical trials. The United States Food & Drug Administration (FDA) clarified sources of real world data to be electronic health records, product and disease registries, claims and billing activities, patient-generated data, and data gathered from mobile devices. The ELSO Registry receives detailed information on patients, devices, health outcomes, and associated health complications data from over 500 active centers submitting over 20,000 patient cases annually (at the time of writing). This data is valuable for device evaluation by device developers or worldwide regulatory bodies. ELSO believes the extracorporeal community of patients, health care providers, and hospitals are served by sharing ELSO data with partners who strive to bring new devices and services to future patients relying on extracorporeal care.

### *Process*

Consequently, ELSO developed a Device Developer Data Policy that described the process of creating reports for device developers. Reports are composed through a partnership with the device developer, ELSO Registry and Technology committee members, clinician and device experts, ELSO Executive Director, and biostatisticians. ELSO does not release patient level data. Instead, ELSO analyzes the data at the direction of device developers and releases the analysis or aggregate data. Additionally, ELSO does not allow the use of registry data for identification of competitors or for marketing. To date, data from ELSO Reports have been submitted to North American, European, and Asian regulatory bodies.

## Advancing the Reliability and Utility of Registry Data

The ELSO Registry maintains registry development as one of its primary commitments to individual members, member centers, and the international community. This commitment has resulted in the development of multiple key objectives and is supported by the dedicated efforts of the Database Development Committee,[16] a subcommittee of the ELSO Registry Committee.

The first key objective of registry development is to ensure the reliability of entered data. To this end, significant attention is paid to two ongoing projects. First (established in 2017), is the maintenance of registry data definitions, a publicly available resource ensuring continuity of data entry among all member centers. The ELSO Registry Definitions Document identifies mandatory data elements, defines individual data points, sets out data entry rules, and illustrates examples designed to clarify nuance between clinical scenarios. As fields are added, removed, or revised, this document reflects these changes and serves as a baseline for the reliable entry of data. Second (established in 2018), all individuals involved with management, oversight, or collection of registry data are required to complete a data entry certification exam. The exam presents multiple choice questions in patient vignette style designed to educate and ensure data definitions are clear and consistently applied.

Another equally important objective is to maintain the validity of registry data through a two-tiered strategy. First, data elements are internally validated at the time of data entry via programmed hard and soft limits. These minimize inadvertent entry of errors or outliers by flagging elements outside prescribed limits for review. If the user fails to enter reasonable or realistic data, the user is prompted to review the record and address these issues prior to submission. Second, ELSO has launched a pilot program with a small number of member centers affirming a pathway to external data validation through partnership with a vendor. The goal is to validate 10% of each center's patients from the previous year (minimum of 5 and maximum of 25) using 64 data elements selected for audit. Upon completion, centers will receive preliminary results and will be allowed to adjudicate any discrepancies. All processes for internal and external validation as well as the aforementioned processes for ensuring reliability, including those currently under development, are intended to educate the user and improve data integrity in a nonpunitive manner, thus ensuring the highest quality of reported data.

In recent years, the registry has formalized the processes by which registry additions or revisions are evaluated. The first is through revision of primary registry content reviewed by the Registry Development Advisory Group.[16] This group (comprised of the Registry Chair, Database Development chairs, leaders within ELSO, and key ECLS community members) reviews suggested concerns regularly to determine need, process, function, and priority for potential inclusion or revision. Second, potential additions or revisions may be accomplished through optional registry addenda. Currently available addenda include Cardiac, ECPR, SARS CoV-2, and Trauma. Published guidelines for registry changes ask for a demonstration that the addition or revision fulfills a need within the ECLS community, ensures a requisite number of centers agree to participate (10% of active centers), and that funding is considered.[17] Updates following additional registry or addenda development are implemented and communicated to the ECLS community biannually. When circumstances demand greater urgency (eg, the COVID-19 pandemic), the procedural structure may be modified.

While the mainstay of registry reporting has been dissemination of historical outcomes and quality metrics, realtime case reporting has become a necessary and final key objective in registry development. This paradigm shift allows for flexibility in data presentation to meet evolving ECLS community needs. The seminal example of this was demonstrated during the COVID-19 pandemic as international case reporting was rapidly mobilized in response to demand for experiential data to inform clinical care in an evolving and unique patient population.[18] ELSO database development teams in collaboration with ELSO leadership and information technology quickly operationalized dashboard reporting made available to the entire ECLS community. Initial SARS-CoV-2 case reporting included increasingly granular case characteristics including incidence of SARS-CoV-2 ECLS support and survival, patient demographic and ECLS support characteristics, median length of run, patient comorbidities, and complication rates. Need for live reporting is anticipated and expected to remain a key objective in registry development.

## International Engagement of Diverse Membership

The ELSO Registry strives to reflect worldwide use of ECLS. Thus, several initiatives have been developed to foster the engagement of ELSO centers and centers of diverse membership. During the COVID-19 pandemic, ELSO offered free membership to all new centers applying for the ELSO Registry data entry. The main goal of this action was both to recruit new centers in the ELSO community and to have a wider understanding of ECLS use related to COVID-19. With the same purpose, the European chapter of ELSO (EuroELSO), launched several initiatives to monitor the use of ECLS in adult and pediatric COVID-19 patients in Europe.[19-21] The ELSO Registry committees have aimed to have membership that broadly represent different areas of the world. In 2021, the Scientific Oversight Committee established three co-chairs each representing a different chapter of ELSO. The hope is that international leadership will improve ELSO and further engage members from around the world.

## Future Steps

Over the last four decades, the ECLS Registry of ELSO has played a pivotal role in the advancement of ECLS scientific knowledge, improvement in the care of ECLS patients, and ECLS device development. One of the strengths of the registry has been its flexibility and rapidity of data reporting. The registry nimbly adapted to serve as an important repository for outcome information related to ECLS use during the SARS-CoV-2 pandemic and displayed the resultant data to centers in real time, making it an early source of emerging data.[18] The ELSO Registry is the broadest collection of ECLS data in the world and, as it looks to the future, will strive to improve upon its reliability, utility, and flexibility so that it can lead the advancement of knowledge and care in the decades to come.

# References

1. Toomasian JM, Snedecor SM, Cornell RG, et al. National experience with extracorporeal membrane oxygenation for newborn respiratory failure. Data from 715 cases. ASAIO J. 1988;34(2):140-7.
2. Kanto WP, Shapiro MB. The development of prolonged extracorporeal circulation. In: Zwischenberger JB, Bartlett RH, eds. ECMO Extracorporeal Cardiopulmoanry Support in Critical Care. 1 ed. Extracorporeal Life Support Organization; 1995.
3. Maul TM, Kuch BA, Wearden PD. Development of Risk Indices for Neonatal Respiratory Extracorporeal Membrane Oxygenation. ASAIO J. Sep-Oct 2016;62(5):584-90.
4. Barbaro RP, Bartlett RH, Chapman RL, et al. Development and Validation of the Neonatal Risk Estimate Score for Children Using Extracorporeal Respiratory Support. J Pediatr. 2016;173:56-61.e3.
5. Bailly DK, Reeder RW, Zabrocki LA, et al. Development and Validation of a Score to Predict Mortality in Children Undergoing Extracorporeal Membrane Oxygenation for Respiratory Failure: Pediatric Pulmonary Rescue With Extracorporeal Membrane Oxygenation Prediction Score. Crit Care Med. 2017;45(1):e58-e66.
6. Barbaro RP, Boonstra PS, Paden ML, et al. Development and validation of the pediatric risk estimate score for children using extracorporeal respiratory support (Ped-RESCUERS). Intensive Care Med. 2016;42(5):879-888.
7. Schmidt M, Bailey M, Sheldrake J, et al. Predicting survival after extracorporeal membrane oxygenation for severe acute respiratory failure. The Respiratory Extracorporeal Membrane Oxygenation Survival Prediction (RESP) score. Am J Respir Crit Care Med. 2014;189(11):1374-82.
8. Schmidt M, Burrell A, Roberts L, et al. Predicting survival after ECMO for refractory cardiogenic shock: the survival after veno-arterial-ECMO (SAVE)-score. Eur Heart J. Sep 1 2015;36(33):2246-56.
9. Lorusso R, Alexander P, Rycus P, et al. The Extracorporeal Life Support Organization Registry: update and perspectives. Ann Cardiothorac Surg. 2019;8(1):93-98.
10. Dimick JB, Staiger DO, Birkmeyer JD. Ranking hospitals on surgical mortality: the importance of reliability adjustment. Health Serv Res. 2010;45(6 Pt 1):1614-1629.
11. UK collaborative randomised trial of neonatal extracorporeal membrane oxygenation. UK Collaborative ECMO Trail Group. Lancet. Jul 13 1996;348(9020):75-82.
12. Peek GJ, Mugford M, Tiruvoipati R, et al. Efficacy and economic assessment of conventional ventilatory support versus extracorporeal membrane oxygenation for severe adult respiratory failure (CESAR): a multicentre randomised controlled trial. Lancet. 2009;374(9698):1351-63.
13. Combes A, Hajage D, Capellier G, et al. Extracorporeal Membrane Oxygenation for Severe Acute Respiratory Distress Syndrome. N Engl J Med. 24 2018;378(21):1965-1975.
14. Lasa JJ, Banerjee M, Zhang W, et al. Critical Care Unit Organizational and Personnel Factors Impact Cardiac Arrest Prevention and Rescue in the Pediatric Cardiac Population. Pediatr Crit Care Med. 2022.
15. Atkins DL, Sasson C, Hsu A, et al. 2022 Interim Guidance to Healthcare Providers for Basic and Advanced Cardiac Life Support in Adults, Children, and Neonates with Suspected or Confirmed COVID-19: From the Emergency Cardiovascular Care Committee and Get With the Guidelines®-Resuscitation Adult and Pediatric Task Forces of the American Heart Association in Collaboration with the American Academy of Pediatrics, American Association for Respiratory Care, The Society of Critical Care Anesthesiologists, and American Society of Anesthesiologists. Circ Cardiovasc Qual Outcomes. 2022.
16. Extracorporeal Life Support Organization. ELSO Registry Development Committee. Accessed February 9, 2022. https://www.elso.org/Registry/ELSORegistryDatabaseDevelopment.asp.x
17. Extracorporeal Life Support Organization. Policies. Accessed February 9, 2022. https://www.elso.org/AboutUs/Policies.aspx.
18. Barbaro RP, MacLaren G, Boonstra PS, et al. Extracorporeal membrane oxygenation support in COVID-19: an international cohort study of the Extracorporeal Life Support Organization registry. Lancet. Oct 10 2020;396(10257):1071-1078.
19. Lorusso R, Combes A, Lo Coco V, et al. ECMO for COVID-19 patients in Europe and Israel. Intensive Care Med. Mar 2021;47(3):344-348.
20. Di Nardo M, Hoskote A, Thiruchelvam T, et al. Extracorporeal Membrane Oxygenation in Children with Coronavirus Disease 2019: Preliminary Report from the Collaborative European Chapter of the Extracorporeal Life Support Organization Prospective Survey. ASAIO J. Feb 1 2021;67(2):121-124.
21. Broman LM, Eksborg S, Lo Coco V, et al. Extracorporeal membrane oxygenation for COVID-19 during first and second waves. Lancet Respir Med. Aug 2021;9(8):e80-e81.

# Glossary

| | |
|---|---|
| **ACT**: | Activated clotting time |
| **AKI**: | Acute kidney injury |
| **AMI**: | Acute myocardial infarction |
| **APTT**: | Activated partial thromboplastin time |
| **ARDS**: | Acute respiratory distress syndrome |
| **AVCO₂R**: | Arteriovenous carbon dioxide removal |
| **BCPC**: | Bidirectional cavopulmonary connection (Glenn) |
| **BTT shunt**: | Blalock-Thomas-Taussig shunt |
| **CI**: | Cardiac index |
| **CO**: | Cardiac output |
| **CPR**: | Cardiopulmonary resuscitation |
| **CPB**: | Cardiopulmonary bypass |
| **CRRT**: | Continuous renal replacement therapy (also known as CKRT, continuous kidney replacement therapy) |
| **CVP**: | Central venous pressure |
| **CT**: | Computed tomography |
| **CVC**: | Central venous catheter |
| **DIC**: | Disseminated intravascular coagulation |
| **DTI**: | Direct thrombin inhibitor |
| **DO₂**: | Oxygen delivery |
| **ECCO₂R**: | Extracorporeal carbon dioxide removal |
| **ECLS**: | Extracorporeal life support |
| **ECG**: | Electrocardiography |
| **ECMO**: | Extracorporeal membrane oxygenation |
| | **VA**:   Venoarterial |
| | **VV**:   Venovenous |
| | **VVA**:  Venovenoarterial |
| **ECPR**: | Extracorporeal cardiopulmonary resuscitation |
| **EEG**: | Electroencephalography |
| **EF**: | Ejection fraction |
| **ELSO**: | Extracorporeal Life Support Organization |
| **FiO₂**: | Fraction of inspired oxygen concentration |
| **FsO₂**: | Sweep gas inlet oxygen fraction |
| **HFOV**: | High frequency oscillatory ventilation |
| **HIT**: | Heparin-induced thrombocytopenia |
| **IABP**: | Intra-aortic balloon pump |
| **ICU**: | Intensive care unit |
| **IHCA**: | In-hospital cardiac arrest |
| **INR**: | International normalized ratio |
| **IPPV**: | Intermittent positive pressure ventilation |

| | |
|---|---|
| **IVC:** | Inferior vena cava |
| **LA:** | Left atrium |
| **LAP:** | Left atrial pressure |
| **LV:** | Left ventricle |
| **LVEDP:** | Left ventricular end diastolic pressure |
| **MAP:** | Mean arterial pressure (alternatively, mean airway pressure) |
| **MCS:** | Mechanical circulatory support |
| **MRI:** | Magnetic resonance imaging |
| **MOF:** | Multiorgan failure |
| **NICU:** | Neonatal intensive care unit |
| **NIRS:** | Near infrared spectroscopy |
| **NIV:** | Non-invasive ventilation |
| **OHCA:** | Out-of-hospital cardiac arrest |
| **$PCO_2$:** | Partial pressure of carbon dioxide |
| **PA:** | Pulmonary artery |
| **PAP:** | Pulmonary arterial pressure |
| **PCP:** | Pulmonary capillary pressure |
| **$PO_2$:** | Partial pressure of oxygen |
| **PEEP:** | Positive end-expiratory pressure |
| **PICU:** | Pediatric intensive care unit |
| **PIP:** | Peak inspiratory pressure |
| **Pplat:** | Plateau airway pressure |
| **PT:** | Prothrombin time |
| **PVR:** | Pulmonary vascular resistance |
| **RA:** | Right atrium |
| **RAP:** | Right atrial pressure |
| **RPM:** | Revolutions per minute |
| **RV:** | Right ventricle |
| **$ScvO_2$:** | Central venous oxygen saturation |
| **$SvO_2$:** | Mixed venous oxygen saturation |
| **SVC:** | Superior vena cava |
| **SVR:** | Systemic vascular resistance |
| **TCPC:** | Total cavopulmonary connection (Fontan) |
| **TEE:** | Transesophageal echocardiography |
| **TTE:** | Transthoracic echocardiography |
| **VAD:** | Ventricular assist device |
| | **LVAD:** Left ventricular assist device |
| | **RVAD:** Right ventricular assist device |
| | **BiVAD:** Biventricular assist device |
| **VILI:** | Ventilator-induced lung injury |
| **$VO_2$:** | Oxygen consumption |

# Appendix

| Pre ECLS risk factors | On ECLS risk factors | Neuroprotective strategies on ECLS | Post ECLS pre-discharge |
|---|---|---|---|
| Significant duration of hypotension, hypoxemia, acidosis<br><br>Significant hypoxic event<br><br>Any history of cardiac arrest<br><br>Seizures (clinical, aEEG, EEG)<br><br>Perinatal asphyxia, history of cooling<br><br>Associated co-morbidities – prematurity/genetic conditions/syndromes | Seizures (clinical, aEEG, EEG)<br><br>Abnormal neurological examination<br><br>Abnormal EEG / neuro-imaging on USS/CT<br><br>Major mechanical complication<br><br>Cardiac arrest | Protocolized neuromonitoring<br><br>Regular clinical examination<br><br>Cranial ultrasound, EEG, NIRS<br><br>Neuroprotection - cooling (asphyxia), ensure effective ECMO flows, mitigate complications | Neurological examination<br><br>Neuro-imaging<br>• MRI Brain<br><br>Hearing tests<br>• Audiometry<br><br>Community care and family support |

## A schema for multidisciplinary structured longitudinal post discharge follow-up

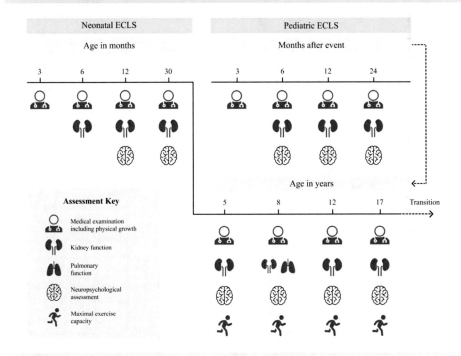

This figure depicts the risk factors during ICU management and a suggested follow-up schedule for neonatal and pediatric ECLS survivors at regular intervals from 0 to 17 years of life. ELSO recommends all children treated with ECLS have a structured follow-up with a multidisciplinary clinic to promote recovery, follow known organ dysfunction/recovery, and detect unanticipated problems such as learning impairment, long-term kidney disease, and long-term pulmonary function. Assessments include medical examination, neuropsychological assessment (all domains), pulmonary function, kidney function (blood pressure, urinary protein/creatinine ratio) and exercise tolerance, wherever possible. For children with congenital heart disease, the screening and surveillance algorithm recommended by the AHA Scientific Statement provides additional guidance. Since ECLS for acute respiratory failure can occur at any age, the initial timing of follow-up is related to hospital discharge while the later follow-up is related to the child's age. After the age of 17 years, transition to adult health care providers is recommended.

*CT – computed tomography, EEG - electroencephalogram and aEEG – amplitude-integrated EEG, ECMO – extracorporeal membrane oxygenation, MRI – magnetic resonance imaging, NIRS – near-infra red spectroscopy, USS – ultrasound*

| | DOMAINS OF INTEREST | ASSESSMENTS | RELEVANCE/ INTERVENTION |
|---|---|---|---|
| **INFANCY**<br><br>0-2 years | Growth | Length, weight, head circumference | Referral to dietician |
| | Kidney function | Blood pressure, urinary protein/creatinine ratio | Early referral to (pediatric) nephrologist |
| | Hearing assessment | Age-appropriate auditory tests | Early referral to audiology |
| | Neurological assessment including imaging | MRI brain (pre-discharge) | Early recognition, referral for neurorehabilitation<br><br>Early referral neurorehabilitation |
| | Mental development | Age-appropriate locally available formal test | Referral to psychiatric professional |
| | Motor development | Age appropriate locally available formal test | Referral to physical therapist |
| **PRESCHOOL AGE**<br><br>2-5 years | Growth (mainly CDH) | Length, weight | Referral to dietician |
| | Kidney function | Blood pressure, urinary protein to creatinine ratio | Early referral to (pediatric) nephrologist |
| | Cognitive development | Age-appropriate locally available formal test | Referral to child development center |
| | Language development | Age-appropriate locally available formal test | Hearing assessment, referral to speech-language pathologist |
| | Motor development | Age-appropriate locally available formal test | Referral to physical therapist |
| **SCHOOL AGE**<br><br>≥6 years | Growth (mainly CDH) | Length, weight | Referral to dietician |
| | Kidney function | Blood pressure, urinary protein-to-creatinine ratio | Early referral to (pediatric) nephrologist |
| | Lung function assessment | Spirometry | Evaluate reversibility of airflow obstruction |
| | Motor development | Age-appropriate locally available formal test | Referral to physical therapist |
| | Exercise capacity | Age-appropriate locally available formal test | Sports participation and/or exercise training |
| | Neuropsychological assessment | Age-appropriate locally available formal test for: | Referral to early school support |
| | Behavior | *Intelligence (only once in follow up) | Referral to cognitive rehabilitation for acquired brain injury |
| | | *Memory | |
| | | *Attention/concentration/information processing | |
| | | Age appropriate locally available formal test for: | |
| | | *Hyperactivity | Referral to psychologist for support/ guidance |
| | | *Somatic problems | |
| **ADOLESCENCE**<br><br>>12 years | Growth (mainly CDH) | Length (pubertal growth spurt), weight | Referral to dietician |
| | Kidney function | Blood pressure, urinary protein-to-creatinin ratio | Referral to (pediatric) nephrologist |
| | Motor function | Age appropriate locally available formal test | Referral physical therapist/sports participation |
| | Exercise capacity | Age appropriate locally available formal test | Sports participation/exercise training<br><br>Referral to school support |
| | Neuropsychological assessment | Age appropriate locally available formal test for: | Career support/choice of profession |
| | | *Memory | Referral to cognitive rehabilitation |
| | | *Attention/concentration/information processing | |
| | Behavior | Age appropriate locally available formal test for:<br>*Hyperactivity | Referral to psychologist for support/guidance |
| | | *Depressed feelings/social problems | |
| | | *Somatic problems | |

Adapted from *Semin Perinatol* 38:114–121, 2014

**Appendix Table-1.** Proposal for, and relevance of, long-term followup after ECMO in neonates and children. Longitudinal multidisciplinary team followup from infancy to adolescence with referral to early intervention services and/or special education services.

# Index